D1247107

Prenatal Diagnosis

NOTICE

Medicine is an ever-changing science. As new research and clinical experience broaden our knowledge, changes in treatment and drug therapy are required. The authors and the publisher of this work have checked with sources believed to be reliable in their efforts to provide information that is complete and generally in accord with the standards accepted at the time of publication. However, in view of the possibility of human error or changes in medical sciences, neither the authors nor the publisher nor any other party who has been involved in the preparation or publication of this work warrants that the information contained herein is in every respect accurate or complete, and they disclaim all responsibility for any errors or omissions or for the results obtained from use of the information contained in this work. Readers are encouraged to confirm the information contained herein with other sources. For example and in particular, readers are advised to check the product information sheet included in the package of each drug they plan to administer to be certain that the information contained in this work is accurate and that changes have not been made in the recommended dose or in the contra-indications for administration. This recommendation is of particular importance in connection with new or infrequently used drugs.

Prenatal Diagnosis

Mark I. Evans, MD

President, Fetal Medicine Foundation of America
Director, Comprehensive Genetics
Professor of Obstetrics and Gynecology
Mt. Sinai School of Medicine
New York, New York

Mark Paul Johnson, MD

Associate Professor of Obstetrics and Gynecology and Pediatric Surgery
Children's Hospital of Philadelphia
University of Pennsylvania
Philadelphia, Pennsylvania

Yuval Yaron, MD

Director, Prenatal Genetic Diagnosis Unit
Genetic Institute
Tel Aviv Sourasky Medical Center
Tel Aviv, Israel

Arie Drugan, MD

Director, Genetics
Department of Obstetrics and Gynecology
Ram Bam Medical Center
Haifa, Israel

McGraw-Hill
Medical Publishing Division

New York   Chicago   San Francisco   Lisbon   London   Madrid   Mexico City
Milan   New Delhi   San Juan   Seoul   Singapore   Sydney   Toronto

Prenatal Diagnosis

1 2 3 4 5 6 7 8 9 0   KGP/KGP   0 9 8 7 6

ISBN: 0-8385-7682-6

This book was set in Times Roman by TechBooks.
The editors were Andrea Seils, Dan Pepper, Michelle Watt, and Karen E. Edmonson.
The production supervisor was Catherine Saggese.
Project management was provided by Stephanie Lentz at TechBooks.
The cover designer was Cathleen Elliott.
The indexer was Bernice Eisen.
Quebecor–Kingsport was printer and binder.

This book is printed on acid-free paper.

Library of Congress Cataloging-in-Publication Data

Prenatal diagnosis / [edited by] Mark I. Evans.
      p. ; cm.
   Includes bibliographical references and index.
   ISBN 0-8385-7682-6
   1. Prenatal diagnosis.   2. Genetic screening.   3. Abnormalities,
Human–Genetic aspects.
   [DNLM: 1. Prenatal Diagnosis–methods.   2. Abnormalities–genetics.
3. Fetal Diseases–diagnosis.   4. Genetic Screening. WQ 209 P92651 2005]
I. Evans, Mark I.
   RG628.P728 2005
   618.3′2075—dc22   2004057883

To the memory of John C. Fletcher, PhD a great friend, educator, mentor, and iconoclast. For more than 30 years, John was truly the "conscience of our field" helping to shape the ethical backbone for care of the dying patient, then moving on to genetic testing, prenatal diagnosis, multiple pregnancy management, and fetal therapy. His steadfast support for developing new approaches involving carefully thought out fetal research helped make possible many of the advances reported in this volume. John was never afraid to do battle with those in power to protect the weak and to challenge existing dogmas even to his own personal and professional detriment. He will be sorely missed.

FOREWORD

This is a *really* big book. Its size and scope are all the more impressive considering the fact that just 40 years ago it would have been a very *small* book, perhaps even non-existent. Human cytogenetics was just developing, amniocentesis for prenatal genetic diagnosis did not appear until 1967, ultrasound use was limited to little more than detecting a midline shift, and talk of the fetus as patient was yet to be heard. Yet just 40 years later a comprehensive book on prenatal diagnosis and associated issues requires 68 chapters to cover the relevant topics. Even as a component of the genetics revolution, this is remarkable growth, matched in only a few other areas of medicine.

Taking on the task of covering this field had to be daunting. We are fortunate that Mark Evans, M.D., expanding on his 1992 book, *Reproductive Risks and Prenatal Diagnosis*, joined with three of his former trainees as co-editors and took on this task. The result provides a great service to the field by documenting how far science has allowed us to progress in providing pregnancy care. It is a remarkable compilation authored by authorities in each topic area, and provides the reader a status report on the whole field of prenatal diagnosis.

John Fletcher, to whom this volume is appropriately dedicated, would have especially loved this book. Coming from a background in theology, conditioned by incomparable experience as the bioethicist (the first one) for the clinical research center at the National Institutes of Health, and channeled by choice into a focus on bioethical issues in reproductive health and maternal-fetal medicine, he played a major role in fostering progress and shaping procedures in this field. John Fletcher firmly believed not only that good ethics begins with good science, but also that understanding science and medical practice was a prerequisite to making sound ethical decisions. He would have enjoyed poring through the pages of this book, with almost every page providing a source of new ethical questions to ponder and deliberate. As his focus became more and more on prenatal diagnosis and pregnancy decision-making, he provided two major valuable services. First, he served as the conscience of the field, asking provocative questions of sometimes-too-cavalier perinatologists about what they were doing and how they were doing it, keeping the focus on the mother/pregnant woman as the person who was the ultimate decision maker. The role he played here was particularly important for its assistance to practitioners and researchers in avoiding many of the pitfalls lurking in the field that could have given well-intentioned efforts a bad name if they were done in an insensitive way. Second, he became also the advocate for the field and the need for research to provide the knowledge base for decision and action. He loved to debate the ethical issues with scientists, physicians, advocates, and politicians, but always wanted to be sure he understood the science before he began.

The reader would do well to approach reading this book emulating John Fletcher, exerting every effort to learn and understand the science, and use that understanding to work through with patients the ethical decision-making process in striving to provide the best care for fetus, child, and mother in the most ethically appropriate manner.

Duane Alexander, M.D.
Director of National Institute of Child Health and Human Development
National Institutes of Health
Bethesda, Maryland

CONTENTS

CONTRIBUTORS   XV

PREFACE   XXI

SECTION ONE

GENETICS & REPRODUCTIVE RISKS / 1

CHAPTER 1   PRINCIPLES OF "CLASSIC" GENETICS   3
             Arie Drugan

CHAPTER 2   EPIDEMIOLOGY OF ANEUPLOIDY   19
             Howard S. Cuckle / Svetlana Arbuzova

CHAPTER 3   NEW GENETIC CONCEPTS   33
             Mark I. Evans / Yuval Yaron / Mark Paul Johnson / Ralph L. Kramer

CHAPTER 4   CHROMOSOMAL ABERRATIONS   41
             Shay Ben Shahar / Avi Orr-Urtreger / Yuval Yaron

CHAPTER 5   MENDELIAN GENETICS IN PRENATAL DIAGNOSIS   51
             Bruce R. Korf

CHAPTER 6   SYNDROME: AN APPROACH TO FETAL DYSMORPHOLOGY   57
             The-Hung Bui

CHAPTER 7   GENES AND DEVELOPMENT   63
             D. Randall Armant

CHAPTER 8   PRENATAL GENETIC COUNSELING   71
             Heather Shane Michaels / Shivani B. Nazareth / Lorien Tambini

CHAPTER 9 | **PRINCIPLES OF TERATOLOGY**   **79**
Robert L. Brent / Lynda Fawcett / David A. Beckman

CHAPTER 10 | **DRUGS**   **113**
Pamela Lewis-Matia / Mitchell Dombrowski

CHAPTER 11 | **THE EFFECTS OF MATERNAL DRINKING DURING PREGNANCY**   **123**
Ernest L. Abel / Robert J. Sokol / John H. Hannigan / Beth A. Nordstrom

CHAPTER 12 | **CHARACTERIZING THE EFFECT OF ENVIRONMENTAL AND OCCUPATIONAL EXPOSURES ON REPRODUCTION AND DEVELOPMENT**   **131**
Donald R. Mattison

CHAPTER 13 | **BACTERIAL INFECTIONS AND PREGNANCY**   **149**
Charles Weber / Christine Kovac

CHAPTER 14 | **VIRAL AGENTS AND REPRODUCTIVE RISKS**   **155**
Jan E. Dickinson / Bernard Gonik

CHAPTER 15 | **EXPOSURE TO IONIZING RADIATION DURING PREGNANCY**   **169**
Daniela Koch / Arie Drugan

CHAPTER 16 | **CHEMOTHERAPY IN PREGNANCY**   **177**
Ralph L. Kramer / Baruch Feldman / Yuval Yaron / Mark I. Evans

SECTION TWO

ULTRASOUND DIAGNOSIS & SCREENING / 185

CHAPTER 17 | **OVERVIEW OF THE COMPREHENSIVE ULTRASOUND EXAMINATION: AN APPROACH TO DIAGNOSIS AND MANAGEMENT OF FETAL ANOMALIES**   **187**
Edith D. Gurewitsch / Frank A. Chervenak

CHAPTER 18 | **IMAGING THE FETAL BRAIN**   **199**
Ana Monteagudo / Ilan E. Timor-Tritsch

CHAPTER 19 | **HEART AND VASCULAR MALFORMATIONS**   **227**
Joshua A. Copel / Charles S. Kleinman

CHAPTER 20   **NORMAL AND ABNORMAL FINDINGS OF THE FETAL ABDOMEN AND ANTERIOR WALL**   **239**
Wayne H. Persutte / John C. Hobbins

CHAPTER 21   **GENITO-URINARY TRACT ABNORMALITIES**   **257**
Marjorie C. Treadwell / Mark Paul Johnson

CHAPTER 22   **SKELETAL DYSPLASIA**   **263**
Jana K. Silva / Lawrence D. Platt / Deborah Krakow

CHAPTER 23   **BIOCHEMICAL SCREENING**   **277**
Mark I. Evans / Robert S. Galen / Arie Drugan

CHAPTER 24   **FIRST TRIMESTER ULTRASOUND SCREENING WITH NUCHAL TRANSLUCENCY**   **289**
Jon Hyett / Kypros Nicolaides

CHAPTER 25   **SECOND TRIMESTER SONOGRAPHIC MARKERS FOR ANEUPLOIDY**   **309**
Bryan Bromley / Beryl R. Benacerraf

CHAPTER 26   **COLOR DOPPLER IN CONGENITAL DEFECTS**   **331**
Asim Kurjak / Sanja Kupesic

CHAPTER 27   **DOPPLER AND FETAL ABNORMALITIES IN THE SECOND TRIMESTER**   **343**
Brian Trudinger / Jill Ablett

CHAPTER 28   **ULTRASOUND IN MULTIPLE GESTATION**   **349**
Yaron Zalel / Zvi Leibovitz

CHAPTER 29   **THREE-DIMENSIONAL ULTRASOUND IN PRENATAL DIAGNOSIS**   **357**
Donna D. Johnson / Dolores H. Pretorius

CHAPTER 30   **THREE-DIMENSIONAL FETAL NEUROSCAN**   **365**
Ilan E. Timor-Tritsch / Ana Monteagudo

CHAPTER 31   **COMPUTER AND ULTRASOUND**   **383**
Sean C. Blackwell / Ivan Zador / Ryan Blackwell

CHAPTER 32 | **FETAL AGE DETERMINATION AND GROWTH ASSESSMENT: THEIR ROLES IN PRENATAL DIAGNOSIS** | **387**
Russell L. Deter

CHAPTER 33 | **ULTRASOUND EVALUATION OF THE PLACENTA** | **407**
Byron Calhoun

SECTION THREE
PROCEDURES / 413

CHAPTER 34 | **AMNIOCENTESIS** | **415**
Arie Drugan / Mark I. Evans

CHAPTER 35 | **EARLY AMNIOCENTESIS: RISK ASSESSMENT** | **423**
R. Douglas Wilson

CHAPTER 36 | **CHORIONIC VILLUS SAMPLING** | **433**
Mark I. Evans / Guy Rosner / Yuval Yaron / Ronald J. Wapner

CHAPTER 37 | **CORDOCENTESIS** | **443**
Carl P. Weiner

CHAPTER 38 | **TISSUE BIOPSIES** | **449**
Mark I. Evans / Wolfgang Holzgreve / Eric L. Krivchenia / Eric P. Hoffman

CHAPTER 39 | **FETAL SKIN SAMPLING AND PRENATAL DIAGNOSIS OF GENODERMATOSES** | **455**
Anthony R. Gregg / Sherman Elias

CHAPTER 40 | **OPERATIVE FETOSCOPY** | **459**
Jan Deprest / Dominique van Schoubroeck / Gerard Barki / Eduardo Gratacos

SECTION FOUR
LABORATORY DIAGNOSTICS / 473

CHAPTER 41 | **CYTOGENETICS AND MOLECULAR CYTOGENETICS** | **475**
Alan E. Donnenfeld / Allen N. Lamb

CHAPTER 42 | **BIOCHEMICAL GENETICS** 485
Yoav Ben-Yoseph

CHAPTER 43 | **MOLECULAR DIAGNOSTICS FOR PRENATAL DIAGNOSIS** 493
Laura S. Martin / Mark I. Evans

CHAPTER 44 | **MOLECULAR SCREENING** 501
Roderick F. Hume, Jr.

CHAPTER 45 | **PRENATAL DIAGNOSIS USING FETAL CELLS FROM MATERNAL BLOOD** 505
Sinhue Hahn / Wolfgang Holzgreve

CHAPTER 46 | **CLINICAL PROTEOMICS** 513
Chris Shimizu / Kevin P. Rosenblatt / Peter K. Bryant-Greenwood

SECTION FIVE

MANAGEMENT OF PROBLEMS / 521

CHAPTER 47 | **PSYCHOLOGICAL REACTION TO PRENATAL DIAGNOSIS AND LOSS** 523
Natalie Gellman

CHAPTER 48 | **COUNSELING FOR ABNORMALITIES** 529
Anne Greb / Jane Wegner

CHAPTER 49 | **TERMINATION OF PREGNANCY** 537
Rony Diukman / James D. Goldberg

CHAPTER 50 | **THE FETAL AUTOPSY** 549
Faisal Qureshi / Suzanne M. Jacques

CHAPTER 51 | **REDUCTION IN MULTIPLE PREGNANCIES** 561
Mark I. Evans / Doina Ciorica / David W. Britt / John C. Fletcher

CHAPTER 52 | **SELECTIVE TERMINATION** 571
Mark I. Evans / Charles H. Rodeck / Mark Paul Johnson / Richard L. Berkowitz

CHAPTER 53 | **THE OBSTETRICAL MANAGEMENT OF FETAL ANOMALIES** | **579**
Peter G. Pryde

CHAPTER 54 | **ASSESSMENT AND MANAGEMENT OF NEONATES WITH CONGENITAL ANOMALIES** | **595**
Mary P. Bedard

SECTION SIX

FETAL THERAPY / 603

CHAPTER 55 | **FETAL SHUNT PROCEDURES** | **605**
Mark Paul Johnson

CHAPTER 56 | **THE EVOLUTION OF FETAL SURGERY FOR TREATMENT OF CONGENITAL DIAPHRAGMATIC HERNIA** | **617**
George B. Mychaliska / Michael R. Harrison

CHAPTER 57 | **FETAL SURGERY—OPEN: CONGENITAL CYSTIC ADENOMATOID MALFORMATION** | **627**
Darrell L. Cass / N. Scott Adzick

CHAPTER 58 | **FETAL PHARMACOLOGIC THERAPY FOR MENDELIAN DISORDERS** | **633**
Roderick F. Hume, Jr.

CHAPTER 59 | **FOLIC ACID AND PREVENTION OF NEURAL TUBE DEFECTS** | **641**
Elisa Llurba / Ellen J. Lansberger / Mark I. Evans

CHAPTER 60 | **EVALUATION OF THE FETAL CARDIOVASCULAR SYSTEM** | **653**
Jack Rychik

CHAPTER 61 | **PRENATAL CARDIAC THERAPY** | **671**
Charles S. Kleinman

CHAPTER 62 | **FETAL GENETIC THERAPY—SOMATIC** | **683**
Yuval Yaron / Avi Orr-Urtreger

CHAPTER 63 | **FETAL GENETIC THERAPY—STEM CELLS** | **691**
Heung Bae Kim / Aimen F. Shaaban / Alan W. Flake

SECTION SEVEN

ETHICAL, LEGAL, AND SOCIAL ISSUES / 699

CHAPTER 64

PSYCHOSOCIAL ISSUES IN PRENATAL DIAGNOSIS   701
David W. Britt

CHAPTER 65

**ETHICS AND PRENATAL DIAGNOSIS:
CROSS-CULTURAL CONSIDERATIONS**   707
John C. Fletcher

CHAPTER 66

AN ETHICAL FRAMEWORK FOR FETAL THERAPY   721
Frank A. Chervenak / Laurence B. McCullough

CHAPTER 67

LEGAL ISSUES IN GENETIC DIAGNOSIS AND COUNSELING   727
Charles W. Fisher / Carol Tarnowsky / Pamela A. Boland

CHAPTER 68

POLITICS AND GENETIC REPRODUCTIVE RISKS   741
Ruth S. Hanft

INDEX   747

CONTRIBUTORS

Ernest L. Abel, MD

Professor
Departments of Obstetrics/Gynecology
   and Psychology
C.S. Mott Center for Human Growth
   and Development
Wayne State University
Detroit, Michigan

Jill Ablett, MD

Westmead Hospital
Westmead New South Wales
Australia

N. Scott Adzick, MD

Professor and Chairman
Department of Surgery
Children's Hospital of Philadelphia
Philadelphia, Pennsylvania

Svetlana Arbuzova, MD

Interregional Medico-Genetic Center
Central Hospital
Donetsk, Ukraine

D. Randall Armant, PhD

C.S. Mott Center for Human Growth
   and Development
Professor, Department of Obstetrics/Gynecology and
   Anatomy and Cell Biology
Wayne State University School of Medicine
Detroit, Michigan

Gerard Barki

Adviser
Karl Storz GmBH and Co.
Tuttlingen, Germany

David A. Beckman

Jefferson Medical College
Philadelphia, Pennsylvania

Mary P. Bedard, MD

Children's Hospital of Michigan
Detroit, Michigan

Beryl R. Benacerraf, MD

Diagnostic Ultrasound Associates
Boston, Massachusetts

Richard L. Berkowitz, MD

Professor of Obstetrics and Gynecology
Columbia University College of Physicians
   and Surgeons
New York, New York

Ryan Blackwell

University Women's Care
Detroit, Michigan

Sean C. Blackwell, MD

Assistant Professor and Medical Director
   of Informatics
Hutzel Hospital
Wayne State University
Detroit, Michigan

Pamela A. Boland, JD

Kitch Drutchas Wagner Valitutti and Sherbrook
Detroit, Michigan

Robert L. Brent, MD, PhD

Distinguished Professor of Pediatrics, Radiology,
   and Pathology
Jefferson Medical College
Philadelphia, Pennsylvania
Head of Clinical Environmental and Teratology
   Laboratory
Alfred I. DuPont Hospital for Children
Wilmington, Delaware

David W. Britt, PhD

Fetal Medicine Foundation of America
New York, New York

Bryan Bromley, MD

Associate Clinical Professor of Obstetrics, Gynecology,
   and Reproductive Biology
Vincent Memorial Obstetrical Ultrasound Division
Massachusetts General Hospital
Boston, Massachusetts

Peter K. Bryant-Greenwood, MD, MBA

Clinical Proteomics Program
Department of Pathology and
   Obstetrics/Gynecology
John A. Burns School of Medicine
Honolulu, Hawaii

The-Hung Bui, MD

Department of Molecular Medicine
Karolinska Hospital
Stockholm, Sweden

Bryon Calhoun, MD, FACOG, FACS, MBA

Professor of Obstetrics and Gynecology
Vice Chair Obstetrics and Gynecology
West Virginia University
Charleston, West Virginia

Darrell L. Cass, MD

Department of Pediatric Surgery
Baylor Medical School
Houston, Texas

Frank A. Chervenak, MD

Given Foundation Professor and Chairman
Obstetrician and Gynecologist In-Chief
Department of Obstetrics and Gynecology
Weill Medical College of Cornell University
New York, New York

Doina Ciorica, RDMS, MD

Maternal Fetal Medicine Associates
New York, New York

Joshua A. Copel, MD

Professor
Department of Obstetrics and
    Gynecology and Reproductive Sciences
Section of Maternal-Fetal Medicine
Yale University School of Medicine
New Haven, Connecticut

Howard S. Cuckle, MD

University of Leeds
Institute of Epidemiology and Health Services
    Research
Research School of Medicine
Leeds, England
United Kingdom

Jan Deprest, MD, PhD

Unit of Fetal Diagnosis and Therapy and Gynecological
    Ultrasound
Department of Obstetrics and Gynecology
University Hospital Gasthuisberg
Leuven, Belgium

Russell L. Deter, MD

Professor, Obstetrics and Gynecology
Baylor College of Medicine
Houston, Texas

Jan E. Dickinson, MBBS, MD

Associate Professor, Maternal Fetal Medicine
School of Women's and Infants Health
University of Western Australia
Maternal Fetal Medicine Specialist
King Edward Memorial Hospital for Women
Perth, Western Australia

Rony Diukman, MD

Tel Aviv, Israel

Mitchell Dombrowski, MD

Chair, Obstetrics and Gynecology
St. John's Hospital
Detroit, Michigan

Alan E. Donnenfeld, MD

Women's Health Care Group of Pennsylvania Main
    Line Perinatal Associates Division
Lankenau Hospital
Wynnewood, Pennsylvania

Arie Drugan, MD

Director, Genetics
Department of Obstetrics and Gynecology
Ram Bam Medical Center
Haifa, Israel

Sherman Elias, MD

Professor and Chairman
Department of Obstetrics and Gynecology
Northwestern University
Chicago, Illinois

Mark I. Evans, MD

President, Fetal Medicine
    Foundation of America
Director, Comprehensive Genetics
Professor of Obstetrics and Gynecology
Mt. Sinai School of Medicine
New York, New York

Lynda Fawcett, PhD

Assistant Professor of Pediatrics
Department of Pediatrics
Alfred I. DuPont Hospital for Children
Wilmington, Delaware

Baruch Feldman, MD

Kfar Saba Medical Center
Kfar Saba, Israel

Charles W. Fisher, JD

Kitch Drutchas Wagner Valitutti and Sherbrook
Detroit, Michigan

Alan W. Flake, MD

Department of Pediatric Surgery
Children's Hospital of Philadelphia
Philadelphia, Pennsylvania

John C. Fletcher, MD

(Deceased)

Robert S. Galen, MD

Professor and Interim Head
Department of Health Administration, Biostatistics,
    and Epidemiology
The University of Georgia College of Medicine
Athens, Georgia

Natalie Gellman, PhD

Psychologist/Director
Humanistic Resources
Warren, Maine

James D. Goldberg, MD

San Francisco Perinatal Associates
San Francisco, California

Bernard Gonik, MD

Department of Obstetrics and Gynecology
Sinai Grace Hospital
Detroit, Michigan

Eduardo Gratacos, MD

Professor
Fetal Medicine and Therapy Programme
Department of Obstetrics
Hospital Clinic Barcelone
Universitat de Barcelona
Barcelona, Spain

Anne Greb, MS

Genetic Counselor
Assistant Professor
Director, Genetic Counseling Graduate Program
Wayne State University School of Medicine
Center for Molecular Medicine and Genetics
Detroit, Michigan

Anthony R. Gregg, MD

Department of Obstetrics and Gynecology
Medical College of South Carolina
Columbia, South Carolina

Edith D. Gurewitsch, MD

Assistant Professor of Gynecology and
    Obstetrics
Division of Maternal Fetal Medicine
Johns Hopkins University School of Medicine
Baltimore, Maryland

Sinhue Hahn, MD

University of Basel
Department of Obstetrics and Gynecology
University Women's University
Basel, Switzerland

Ruth S. Hanft, PhD

Adjunct Associate
Center for Biomedical Ethics
University of Virginia
Charlottesville, Virginia

John H. Hannigan, PhD

C.S. Mott Center for Human Growth
    and Development
Wayne State University

Department of Obstetrics and Gynecology
Detroit, Michigan

Michael R. Harrison, MD

Professor of Surgery, Pediatrics, and Obstetrics,
    Gynecology and Reproductive Sciences
Director, Fetal Treatment Center
Division of Pediatric Surgery
Department of Surgery
Fetal Treatment Center
University of California, San Francisco
San Francisco, California

John C. Hobbins, MD

Professor of Obstetrics and Gynecology
University of Colorado Health Sciences
    Center
Denver, Colorado

Eric P. Hoffman, MD

Children's National Medical Center
Washington, DC

Wolfgang Holzgreve, MD

Professor and Chair
University of Basel
Department of Obstetrics and Gynecology
University Women's Hospital
Basel, Switzerland

Roderick F. Hume, Jr., MD

Hutzel Women's Hospital
Wayne State University
Detroit, Michigan

Jon Hyett, MD

King's College
Denmark Hill
London, England
United Kingdom

Suzanne M. Jacques, MD

Department of Pathology
Hutzel Hospital
Detroit, Michigan

Donna D. Johnson, MD

Assistant Professor
Department of Obstetrics and Gynecology
Medical University of South Carolina
Charleston, South Carolina

Mark Paul Johnson, MD

Associate Professor of Obstetrics and
    Gynecology and Pediatric Surgery
Children's Hospital of Philadelphia
University of Pennsylvania
Philadelphia, Pennsylvania

Heung Bae Kim, MD

Department of Pediatric Surgery
Children's Hospital of Philadelphia
Philadelphia, Pennsylvania

Charles S. Kleinman, MD

Professor of Pediatric Cardiology
Columbia University
New York, New York

Daniela Koch, MD

Rambam Medical Center
Haifa, Israel

Bruce R. Korf, MD, PhD

Professor and Chairman, Department of
    Genetics
University of Alabama at Birminham
Birmingham, Alabama

Christine Kovac, MD

Department of Obstetrics and Gynecology
Madigan Army Medical Center
Tacoma, Washington

Deborah Krakow, MD

Cedars Sinai Hospital
Los Angeles, California

Ralph L. Kramer, MD

Stuart Ob Gyn
Stuart, Virginia

Eric L. Krivchenia, MS

Genetic Counselor
Cherry Hill, New Jersey

Sanja Kupesic, MD

Ultrasonic Institute
University of Zagreb
Zagreb, Croatia

Asim Kurjak, MD

Ultrasonic Institute
University of Zagreb
Zagreb, Croatia

Allen N. Lamb, PhD

Laboratory Director
Molecular Cytogenetics
Genzyme Genetics
Santa Fe, New Mexico

Ellen J. Landsberger, MD

Department of Obstetrics and Gynecology
Albert Einstein College of Medicine
Bronx, New York

Zvi Leibovitz

Genetics Institute
Tel Aviv Sourasky Medical Center
Tel Aviv, Israel

Pamela Lewis-Matia, MD

Greater Washington Maternal Fetal Medicine and Genetics
Rockville, Maryland

Elisa Llurba, MD

Fetal_Maternal Unit
Obstetrics and Gynecology Department
Vall d'Hebron Hospital
Barcelona, Spain

James N. Macri, PhD

Laboratory Director
NTD Laboratories, Inc.
Huntington Station, New York

Laura S. Martin, MD, FAAP, FACMG

Director, Medical Genetics
Rockford Health System
Department of Medical Genetics
Rockford, Illinois

Donald R. Mattison, MD

Senior Advisor
National Institute of Health
Bethesda, Maryland

Laurence B. McCullough, PhD

Professor of Medicine and Medical Ethics
Center for Medical Ethics and Health Policy
Baylor College of Medicine
Houston, Texas

Heather Shane Michaels, MS, MHS, CGC

Genetic Counselor
Genzyme Genetics
New York, New York

Ana Monteagudo, MD

Associate Professor
Department of Obstetrics and Gynecology
New York University Medical Center
New York, New York

George B. Mychaliska, MD

Assistant Professor of Surgery and Obstetrics and Gynecology
Division of Pediatric Surgery
University of Michigan
Ann Arbor, Michigan

Shivani B. Nazareth, MS, CGC

Department of Obstetrics and Gynecology
St. Luke's—Roosevelt Hospital
New York, New York

Kypros Nicolaides, MD

Harris Birthright Research Centre for Fetal Medicine
King's College, London University
London, England
United Kingdom

Beth A. Nordstrom, PhD

Department of Family Medicine
James H. Quillen College of Medicine
Eastern Tennessee State University
Johnson City, Tennessee

Avi Orr-Urtreger

Prenatal Genetic Diagnosis Unit
Genetic Institute
Tel Aviv Sourasky Medical Center
Tel Aviv, Israel

Wayne H. Persutte, MD, RDMS, FAIUM, FSDMS

Director of Sonography
Platte River Perinatal Center
Department of Obstetrics and Gynecology
University of Colorado Health Science Center
Denver, Colorado

Lawrence D. Platt, MD

Professor of Obstetrics and Gynecology
David Geffen School of Medicine at UCLA
Department of Obstetrics and Gynecology
Los Angeles, California

Dolores H. Pretorius, MD

Professor
Department of Radiology
University of California, San Diego
La Jolla, California

Peter G. Pryde, MD

University of Wisconsin
Madison, Wisconsin

Faisal Qureshi, MD

Department of Pathology
Hutzel Hospital
Detroit, Michigan

Charles H. Rodeck, MD

Head, Department of Obstetrics and Gynecology
University College and Middlesex
School of Medicine
University College, London
London, England
United Kingdom

Kevin P. Rosenblatt, MD, PhD

Department of Pathology
Division of Translational Pathology
University of Texas Southwestern Medical Center
Dallas, Texas

Guy Rosner, MD

Prenatal Diagnosis Unit
Genetic Institute
Tel Aviv Sourasky Medical Center
Tel Aviv, Israel

Jack Rychik, MD

Director, Pediatric Cardiology
Children's Hospital of Philadelphia
Philadelphia, Pennsylvania

Aimen F. Shaaban

Genetic Institute
Tel Aviv Sourasky Medical Center
Tel Aviv, Israel

Shay Ben Shahar

Prenatal Genetics Diagnosis Unit
Genetic Institute
Tel Aviv Sourasky Medical Center
Tel Aviv, Israel

Seetha Shankaran, MD

Children's Hospital of Michigan
Detroit, Michigan

Chris Shimizu, MD

Hawaii Pathologists Laboratory
The Queens Medical Center
Honolulu, Hawaii

Jana K. Silva, MD

Assistant Professor
Department of Native Hawaiian Health
Native Hawaiian Center of Excellence
Honolulu, Hawaii

Robert J. Sokol, MD

Distinguished Professor
C.S. Mott Center for Human Growth and Development
Department of Obstetrics and Gynecology
Wayne State University School of Medicine
Detroit, Michigan

Lorien Tambini, MS, CGC

Genetic Counselor
Department of Obstetrics and Gynecology
Division of Genetics
St. Luke's—Roosevelt Hospital
New York, New York

Carol Tarnowsky

Assistant General Counsel
St. Joseph Mercy Oakland
Pontiac, Michigan

Marjorie C. Treadwell, MD

Professor, Obstetrics and Gynecology
Division of Maternal-Fetal Medicine
Director, Obstetric Ultrasound
Center for Fetal Diagnosis and Therapy
Hutzel Women's Hospital
Wayne State University
Detroit, Michigan

Ilan E. Timor-Tritsch, MD

Professor of Obstetrics and Gynecology
Department of Obstetrics and Gynecology
New York University Medical Center
New York, New York

Brian Trudinger, MD

Westmead Hospital
Westmead New South Wales
Australia

Dominique van Schoubroeck, MD
Unit of Fetal Diagnosis and Therapy and Gynecological
    Ultrasound
Department of Obstetrics and Gynecology
University Hospital Gasthuisberg
Leuven, Belgium

Ronald J. Wapner, MD
Professor of Obstetrics and Gynecology
Columbia University College of
    Physicians and Surgeons
New York, New York

Charles Weber, MD
Madigan Army Medical Center
Tacoma, Washington

Carl P. Weiner, MD
Professor and Chairman of Obstetrics and Gynecology
University fo Kansas Medical Center
Kansas City, Kansas

Jane Wegner, MD
Waukesha, Wisconsin

R. Douglas Wilson, MD
Department of Pediatrics General and Thoracic Surgery
The Children's Hospital of Philadelphia
Philadelphia, Pennsylvania

Yuval Yaron, MD
Director, Prenatal Genetic Diagnosis Unit
Genetic Institute
Tel Aviv Sourasky Medical Center
Tel Aviv, Israel

Yoav Ben-Yoseph, PhD
Retired
Wayne State University School of
    Medicine
Detroit, Michigan

Ivan Zador, PhD
Fetal Medicine Foundation of America
Los Angeles, California

Yaron Zalel, MD
Genetic Institute
Tel Aviv Sourasky Medical Center
Tel Aviv, Israel

PREFACE

It has been 15 years since I wrote the preface to *Reproductive Risks and Prenatal Diagnosis* (shown below). The principles have withstood the test of time. I remarked in 1992 how much reproductive genetics had changed in the previous decade. That pattern has not only continued, but it has hastened to WARP speed. The emphasis of advances has shifted from new clinical procedures in the 70s and 80s, to visualization in the 90s, to currently a pre-eminence of changes in the laboratory. These new tools have provided the clinician with a new armamentarium for the earlier, more reliable, and sophisticated ability to diagnose and thereby the option to treat genetic and congenital abnormalities.

The more "bang for the buck" from new biotechnologies has coincided with tremendous challenges to traditional academic institutions that have limited the number that can afford (or have the vision) to invest in the infrastructure necessary to mount extensive research efforts in our field. Thus, more of it has moved "off shore" and outside of the traditional centers. This trend is likely to continue over the next decade.

PREFACE TO REPRODUCTIVE RISKS AND PRENATAL DIAGNOSIS (1992)

I remember my first day of medical school. The Dean gave a fairly standard speech, namely that half of what we were about to learn in the next four years would be wrong, but he didn't know which half. There is perhaps no area of medicine in which that uncertainty and changeability has held truer than in reproductive genetics. Many of the fundamental tenets of genetics have simply been shown in the past decade to be wrong. For the practicing clinician who may not have had genetics since medical school (or even worse since college), the earth-shaking changes are very unsettling, and the field can appear quite alien. The object of this book is to present the radically new approaches to diagnoses of fetal anomalies in such a way as to be understandable, reproducible, and useful in everyday practice. This book is organized such that one starts out getting a foundation in basic principles, gradually moving into their application for clinical tests, the utilization of laboratory techniques, and finally the management of the fetus with a problem. Although each chapter has been written to stand independently of the others, the preceding chapters do, in fact, form a foundation that will make subsequent chapters more understandable.

SECTION
I

Genetics & Reproductive Risks

CHAPTER 1

PRINCIPLES OF "CLASSIC" GENETICS

Arie Drugan

INTRODUCTION

Congenital anomalies affect approximately 2% of liveborns but have a major impact on pregnancy loss as well as on perinatal mortality and morbidity.[1] Although scientists have been intrigued with congenital malformations since early history, glimpses of a true understanding of the origin of genetic defects started with the pioneer work of Mendel in 1865. Mendel's experiments with garden peas defined "inheritance units" (later called genes) that pass separately and randomly into the egg or sperm, allowing parental traits to appear unchanged in subsequent generations. In the following century, only 2 major milestones have been recorded: Garrod's definition of enzymatic defects as "inborn errors of metabolism" and the identification of the 46 human chromosomes in 1956.[2] Chromosomal DNA is the vehicle that carries the "inheritance units" described by Mendel in his early experiments. During cell division, condensation of the DNA allows the chromosomes to be stained and analyzed. Evaluation of the number and gross structure of the chromosomes enabled the correlation of specific chromosome aberrations with severe syndromes of congenital anomalies described many years before.[3,4]

Laboratory techniques to cut and analyze DNA sequences were developed in the early 1970s.[5–7] Restriction enzymes were used to recognize specific base pair sequences and to cut the DNA molecule whenever that sequence appears, thus resulting in DNA strands of differing lengths and velocity on gel electrophoresis. These were called "restriction fragment length polymorphisms" (RFLPs). The DNA strands were then sorted by coupling with molecular probes on the gel. When the actual molecular structure of the gene in investigation is unknown, known RFLPs in close vicinity to the gene can be used as gene markers, enabling us to follow the segregation of the gene within a given family. Direct gene analysis with complementary DNA probes can be used when the sequence of base pairs within the gene is already known. In some families, these techniques enable identification of carrier or affected individuals before they are clinically symptomatic or even before they are born (prenatal diagnosis). Thus, within a relatively short period, the science of genetics evolved from anatomic descriptions of malformation patterns (without an identifiable cause), through the correlation of phenotypic abnormalities with pathology at the microscopic cellular level (i.e., abnormal number or gross structure of the chromosomes) to the current molecular level—an abnormal gene structure causing an abnormal gene product resulting in phenotypic changes.

Genetic disease can be caused by chromosome anomalies, single gene disorders, or multifactorial disorders. In chromosome disorders, the number or the gross structure of the chromosomes is aberrant, resulting in added or missing genetic material. As a group, they are quite common, affecting about 0.7% of live births.[8] The abnormal dose of thousands of genes causes severe malformations in most organ systems, severe growth and mental retardation, and, in some cases, fetal or neonatal death. Some errors in embryogenesis may result in inviability prior to implantation, causing the low fecundity rate (25%) per cycle observed in fertile couples trying to conceive.[1] Others cause loss of pregnancy after it was clinically recognized.

Single gene disorders are caused by "mutations," changes in the structure of an active gene, causing abnormal transmission of genetic information and resulting in an altered or absent gene product. Single gene disorders are inherited following strict Mendelian rules. Knowing the family pedigree and the mode of inheritance of a specific disorder, one can calculate with relative accuracy the risk to other family members.

Multifactorial disorders are the relatively common result of the interaction between genetic predisposition and exogenous factors (e.g., teratogens) to produce a birth defect. Although the risk of multifactorial disorders is higher in families previously affected, the risk of recurrence is significantly lower than in single gene disorders and pedigrees are not characteristic. Overall, multifactorial disorders affect approximately 1% of live births.

THE CHROMOSOMES AND CELL DIVISION

The chromosomes are rod-shaped condensations of DNA formed during cell division. The number and function of the chromosomes is species specific—there are 44 autosomes and 2 sex chromosomes in the human genome (23 pairs of homologous chromosomes). Homologous chromosomes carry the same genes in the same order but are inherited from different parents—1 from the mother, the other from the father. Thus, the human genome is diploid in most of its cells; the only cells in the human body that are haploid (contain only 1 from each chromosome pair, or 23 chromosomes overall) are the gametes—the egg and sperm. At fertilization, the chromosomes in the oocyte and in the sperm combine to form again a diploid zygote from which all cells of the new organism are formed by cell division.

There are 2 types of cell division (Table 1-1). During body growth and repair processes, somatic cells divide by mitosis. In the mitotic process the chromosomes double for each cell division, resulting in end products that are identical to the original parent cell (Fig. 1-1). There are 4 active stages in mitosis (prophase, metaphase, anaphase, and telophase) and a long interphase stage, during which most of the metabolic activities of the cell take place. The duplication of genetic material also takes place in interphase. The chromosomes are best observed at metaphase, when they are maximally condensed.

Meiosis is the reduction division by which gametes are formed. It consists of 2 successive cell divisions with only 1 replication of genetic material, resulting in egg or sperm containing only half the chromosomes (1 from each homologous pair) of the parental cell. Since there are 2 meiotic divisions, 4 haploid cells can be formed from each diploid cell. This

TABLE
1-1 | **DIFFERENCES BETWEEN MITOSIS AND MEIOSIS**

	Mitosis	*Meiosis*
Cell type	Somatic	Gametes
Time span	Hours to days	
	Females—from embryo to ovulation (~45 years)	Males—60 to 72 days
DNA	Duplicated every cell division	Duplicated once every 2 cell divisions
Crossing over[a]	Rare	Very common
End product	46 chromosomes (haploid)	23 chromosomes (diploid)

[a]Crossing over—exchange of genetic material between homologous chromosomes.

is usually the case with spermatogenesis—4 spermatids are formed from every primary spermatocyte in a relatively short and simple process that takes 60–70 days. In contrast, prophase of Meiosis I in the oocyte starts during fetal life, around the fourth month of gestation. The meiotic process is arrested before birth in a stage specific to female meiosis called dictyotene and remains in that stage until that oocyte is ovulated 12–50 years later. The luteinizing hormone (LH) surge stimulates meiosis I to resume, which is now completed in a matter of minutes—1 daughter cell receives most of the ooplasm and 23 chromosomes and becomes a secondary oocyte. The other 23 chromosomes are extruded as the first polar body. The second meiotic division proceeds almost immediately and stops again in metaphase II. Meiosis II is resumed after fertilization in the fallopian tube and is completed with extrusion of the second polar body. Thus, meiotic division in the female is a long and intricate process in which, over many years, only 1 mature haploid oocyte is formed. The complexity of the female meiotic process is the most likely explanation for the strong association between advanced maternal age and increased risk of chromosomal abnormal conceptions.[9] In about 80% of conceptions affected by trisomy 21, nondisjunction (the failure of homologous chromosomes to separate and segregate into different daughter cells during cell division) is of maternal origin, in most cases occurring during maternal meiosis I.[10,11] Molecular studies proved a maternal origin for other autosomal trisomies as well.[12,13] An association between abnormal ovulation patterns and increased risk of chromosomal abnormal conceptions has also been documented.[10] Increased paternal age, however, does not increase the risk of chromosomal abnormal offspring.[14]

A genetic process of major importance occurring during meiosis is chiasma formation and crossing over between homologous chromosomes. This enables infinite variance in genetic material transmitted from generation to generation, which is of utmost importance from the evolutionary point of view. Chiasma formation may be obligatory for normal disjunction, since at least 1 chiasma per chromosome arm is observed. Each crossover event involves only 1 of the 2 sister chromatids of a homologue. In male meiosis about 50 chiasmata are observed—an average of 2.36 chiasmata per chromosome pair. The number of chiasmata is determined by the length of the chromosome. The number of recombination sites is higher

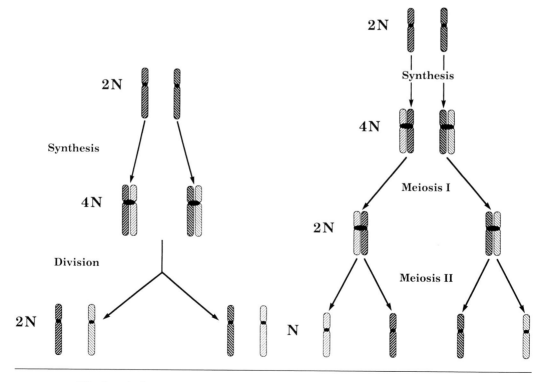

FIGURE 1-1 Mitosis meiosis.

in the female than in the male and nearer to the telomeres (chromosome ends) than to the centromere.

The 44 autosomes and the 2 sex chromosomes of the human genome are unique in function. At first, chromosomes were classified into 7 groups (A through G), according to their size. The X chromosome was placed within the C group and the Y chromosome within the G group. Today, chromosomes are classified according to: their size, the length of the short (p) and long (q) arms, as determined by the location of the centromere, and the banding pattern.

Tissues for chromosome analysis must provide dividing cells—peripheral blood (lymphocytes), bone marrow, skin fibroblasts, amniocytes, or chorionic villi. Common metaphase banding reveal approximately 400 bands per haploid genome. This level of banding is practical for detection of major anomalies in chromosome structure and is most commonly used for karyotype analyses. However, in the late eighties a group of disorders were described in which microdeletions or duplications of a chromosomal region may cause a distinct complex phenotype. These disorders collectively are called contiguous gene syndromes[15] and are thought to result from co-deletion of separate unrelated genes that happen to be contiguous on the deleted chromosomal segment. This type of chromosome anomaly is detected only by high-resolution banding. This technique, performed in only a few laboratories, requires evaluation of the chromosomes in late prophase or early metaphase, when they are less condensed and provides approximately 1000 bands per haploid genome.

CLINICAL ASPECTS OF CHROMOSOMAL ANOMALIES

Chromosome aberrations are a frequent cause of congenital malformations, affecting about 1 of 165 live births.[8] The frequency of chromosome anomalies is much higher in patients with severe mental retardation and in pregnancies affected by congenital anomalies or fetal loss (Table 1-2). About half of all spontaneous abortions in the first trimester are caused by chromosomal problems.[16] Chromosome aberrations have been found in 30–35% of amniocenteses performed following the diagnosis of fetal malformations on ultrasound.[17,18]

Chromosome abnormalities can be classified as numerical or structural. Numerical chromosome anomalies, either additional sets of chromosomes (polyploidy) or additional or missing single chromosomes (aneuploidy), are far more common than structural anomalies, representing more than 95% of recognized chromosomal aberrations.[16] Two different mechanisms are active in the etiology of these disorders. Polyploidy may be caused by failure of cleavage of the fertilized egg at the first mitotic division or, more commonly, by fertilization of the normal oocyte with more than 1 normal sperm (polyspermy). This is a relatively frequent problem, affecting 1–3% of recognized conceptions and approximately 5% of oocytes fertilized in vitro.[19] In contrast, aneuploidy is mainly the result of meiotic nondisjunction and shows a definite association with advanced maternal age.

The vast majority of triploid conceptions are caused by fertilization of a haploid egg by 2 haploid sperm. Thus, triploid conceptions may have the karyotype 69,XXX; 69,XXY; or 69,XYY. Most triploid conceptions will be aborted in the first or early second trimester. About 7% of clinically recognized spontaneous abortions are caused by triploidy.[20] In those cases surviving into the second or third trimester, the placenta undergoes cystic degeneration typical of partial hydatidiform mole. When the fetus survives into the second or third trimester, generally by virtue of fetal mosaicism, it is severely growth retarded and has omphalocele or other associated congenital anomalies. Maternal serum alpha-fetoprotein (MSAFP) is frequently elevated in pregnancies affected by triploidy.[20]

The abnormal development of the fetus and placenta in triploid conceptions demonstrates a new and revolutionary concept in medical genetics, termed genomic imprinting. Gregor Mendel's theory states that hereditary factors, or genes, have equal effects when transmitted from either parent. However, human triploids, which have twice the normal genetic contribution from 1 parent, show differential development dependent on the origin of the double genetic dose (paternal or maternal). Most cases result from dispermy (2 paternal and 1 maternal chromosomal complements) and the abnormalities observed are a large placenta with cystic molar changes and a growth retarded malformed fetus. However, when 2 maternal complements and 1 paternal complement are present, only a small underdeveloped placenta is seen. If a fetus exists, it is markedly underdeveloped, probably related to placental failure. Thus, it appears that paternal genetic information is critical to the development of the placenta and fetal membranes while maternal genetic information is essential for early embryonic development. This has also been substantiated by experiments in pronuclear transplantation and parthenogenetic activation in mice. With only paternally derived chromosomes (androgenetic), only placenta and membranes develop, as seen also in hydatidiform moles. Conversely, with 2 sets of only maternally derived chromosomes there is relatively good embryonic development but poor development of the placenta and membranes.[21]

Tetraploidy (92,XXXX or 92,XXYY) arises almost always from failure of the first mitotic division of a normal diploid zygote, so that 4 copies of each chromosome exist in the multiplying cell. Most of these pregnancies will be miscarried in the first trimester; tetraploidy is observed in about 2% of spontaneous abortions, commonly diagnosed on ultrasonography

TABLE 1-2	FREQUENCY OF CHROMOSOME ANOMALIES	
Live births		0.6 %
Mentally retarded, institutionalized		12 %
Mentally retarded with congenital anomalies		23 %
I-st trimester pregnancy losses		50 %
II-nd trimester pregnancy losses		15–20 %
III-rd trimester losses (stillbirths)		6 %
Major fetal malformations (ultrasound)		35 %
Prenatal diagnosis for maternal age >35y		1–3 %

as an empty sac ("blighted ovum") without embryonic remnants. Isolated cases of liveborn tetraploid fetuses with multiple congenital anomalies have also been reported.[22,23] Mosaic tetraploidy is, however, a relatively common laboratory artifact of amniotic cell cultures and is almost always associated with good outcome.[24] The type of cell and the culture medium (i.e., Chang medium) may affect the percentage of tetraploid cells growing in culture.[25] True tetraploidy should be suspected only if a significant percentage of tetraploid cells is discovered in multiple culture flasks. In these cases, confirmation of cytogenetic results by repeat amniocentesis or percutaneous umbilical blood sampling (PUBS) should be sought before operative decisions are taken.[26]

Aneuploidy refers to the addition or absence of single chromosomes (either autosomes or sex chromosomes), causing trisomy or monosomy, respectively. Most autosomal trisomies and some of the X-chromosome trisomies are caused by maternal nondisjunction and increase in frequency with advanced maternal age.[9–12] For 47,XXY (Kleinfelter syndrome) the frequency of maternal and paternal nondisjunction events is almost equal, with a slight excess (57%) of paternal nondisjunction. The age effect appears to be limited to cases of maternal nondisjunction. Unlike the autosomal trisomies, the diagnosis of monosomy X is observed more frequently in young women.[27] In most cases, the origin of monosomy X is mitotic loss of a paternal sex chromosome post fertilization and during cell division, an event influenced neither by paternal nor by maternal age.[28]

Aneuploidy is the most common type of chromosome anomaly in live births as well as in abortion material.[16] The most commonly observed karyotypes in aneuploid liveborn infants are trisomy of the autosomes 13, 18, or 21 or of the sex chromosomes and monosomy X. Trisomy 21 is the most common chromosome anomaly in liveborns, being diagnosed in about half of all chromosomal abnormal neonates. Rare cases of trisomy 8, 9, 22, or partial trisomies for other chromosomes have also been reported. It is hypothesized that fetuses with full autosomal trisomies surviving to term have a component of mosaicism with a normal cell line in their placenta, facilitating their intrauterine survival.[29] That is true in particular for unusual trisomies such as trisomy 8 or trisomy 9, which are usually diagnosed in neonates only in mosaic form.

Autosomal trisomies occur in about 3% of recognized conceptions and cause about 25% of all pregnancy losses. The most common autosomal trisomy in first trimester miscarriages is trisomy 16, which has never been reported at term. Monosomy X is the most common single chromosome anomaly found in abortion material, occurring in about 18% of all spontaneous miscarriages. It is estimated that 95–99% of all conceptions with monosomy X are miscarried, most commonly in the first trimester.[16]

All autosomal trisomies (except for chromosome 1) have been observed in abortion material, but monosomy is much rarer—only monosomy X have been described. Since trisomy and monosomy are reciprocal events, the results of meiotic nondisjunction, these data imply that autosomal monosomy and trisomy (of chromosome 1) have a stronger negative impact on affected conceptions, causing their loss even before pregnancy is clinically recognized. Thus, whether the aneuploid fetus is destined to be miscarried before or after pregnancy is recognized or is allowed to be delivered, malformed, at term, is determined by the chromosome involved in aneuploidy, meaning the amount and type of added or missing genetic material. Chromosome 21 is the smallest chromosome (only 56,000 kilobases of DNA) and most conceptions affected by trisomy 21 will be delivered as liveborns. Chromosomes 13 and 18 are larger than chromosome 21. About 70% of pregnancies affected by trisomy 13 or 18 are miscarried—the rest are born alive with malformations and severe growth and mental retardation and die soon after birth.[30] Chromosome 1 is the largest human chromosome and pregnancies affected by trisomy 1 are miscarried very early, probably before implantation. Most autosomal monosomies are also miscarried very early, probably because of the effect of uniparental transmission of some genetic information on the developing pregnancy. Likewise, there are definite differences between potentially viable autosomal and sex chromosome trisomy:

1. Mental retardation in sex chromosome aneuploidy is generally mild and some affected individuals may have normal or above normal intelligence. Profound mental retardation is the rule with autosomal trisomies.
2. The phenotypic expression of sex chromosome aneuploidy affects mainly the development and function of sex organs and sex hormones; reproductive failure is common in these cases and may be the presenting symptom. With autosomal trisomies, somatic expression is common and multiple organ systems are frequently affected.

Mosaic aneuploidy (the appearance in culture of 2 cell lines, with different karyotypes) may result from a nondisjunction event during mitosis of a normal zygote. In these cases, the normal and the hypermodal (trisomic) cell lines will continue to develop, but the hypomodal (monosomic) cell line will be lost early after the event. More commonly, however, mosaic aneuploidy is the result of an originally trisomic conception with loss of the extra chromosome in part of the cells. In some of these cases, the diploid cells may have both chromosomes from a uniparental origin, indicating that the only chromosome from the other parent was lost. Uniparental disomy may have important developmental effects due to abnormal genetic imprinting.

Mosaicism with a normal cell line is found in 1–2% of Down syndrome conceptions and up to 20% of liveborns affected by trisomy 13. In general, the phenotype of mosaics should be milder than those of individuals with full aneuploidy. The more severe the effect of aneuploidy, the more likely it is to be mosaic if discovered in a liveborn. It is difficult, however, to predict the outcome in the individual case, since the proportion of normal to abnormal cells in different fetal tissues may vary. An extreme example of such tissue variation is trisomy 20 mosaicism. This abnormality is found at varying rates in different fetal tissues but has never been diagnosed in fetal blood; therefore, cordocentesis does not have a place in the investigation of these cases. Clinical problems associated with trisomy 20 mosaicism are rare, but it is unpredictable which of the involved cases will be affected.[31]

After excluding pseudomosaicism (a single hypermodal cell in culture) chromosomal mosaicism affect 0.2–0.7% of amniotic cell cultures.[32] The chance that pseudomosaicism reflects fetal abnormality is virtually nil. True chromosomal mosaicism in amniotic cell cultures is more ominous, although it should be kept in mind that the culture reflects true fetal mosaicism in only part of these cases. Gosden et al.[26] used cordocentesis to investigate fetal karyotype in cases of mosaicism diagnosed in cultures of amniotic cells. In their study, a normal fetal blood karyotype was obtained in 8 of 10 cases of multiple hypermodal cells confined to 1 culture flask and in 4 of 10 cases in which the abnormality appeared in multiple colonies or in multiple culture flasks. In 16 cases in which autosomal or sex chromosome trisomic mosaicism was the indication for fetal blood karyotyping, trisomic cells were not present in fetal or newborn blood. Fetal blood sampling confirmed the abnormal karyotype in more than 50% of cases involving mosaic translocations, rearrangements or supernumerary markers. These results suggest that all cases of mosaic aneuploidy diagnosed at amniocentesis should be reevaluated by fetal blood sampling, since the chromosome anomaly is probably extraembryonal in most of these cases.

The incidence of mosaicism in chorionic villi specimens is 1–2%.[33] Experience with chorioic villus sampling (CVS) and abortion specimens suggests that it is difficult to predict fetal karyotypes from such results. A recent study suggests that in 90% of cases chromosomal mosaicism is confined to the placenta (CPM), with a normal fetal karyotype.[34] Moreover, it appears that the ratio of normal to abnormal cells may change with time, in favor of the normal cell line (1 clinical example of such changes is the Pallister Killian syndrome—mosaic tetrasomy 12p). Thus, the prognosis in pregnancies diagnosed on CVS to be affected by chromosome mosaicism is commonly favorable. However, unexplained intrauterine fetal death or intrauterine growth retardation may occur in some of these cases.[35,36]

Structural chromosome anomalies affect approximately 0.2% of newborns and are most commonly caused by breakage with abnormal repair of the chromosomes.[37] Chromosome damage can occur spontaneously but is more common after exposure to radiation or to mutagenic agents or in specific genetic disorders such as Bloom syndrome, ataxia telangiectasia or Fanconi anemia. Breaks involving only 1 chromosome may lead to loss of the broken part (deletion) or to inversion of the repaired chromosomal segment. If the breaks involve 2 chromosomes, exchange of the broken segments between the two may lead to a translocation. The translocation may be balanced (when genetic material was not added or lost in the process) or unbalanced (when added or missing chromosomal segments result in partial trisomy or monosomy, respectively). The phenotypic abnormalities depend on the chromosomes involved in the process and whether the rearrangement is bal-

anced. Deletions and duplications are always unbalanced and are always associated with abnormal phenotype and mental retardation. Since deletions or duplications in the offspring may be the product of a balanced structural anomaly in the parents, parental blood karyotypes should be pursued in these cases.

Inversions are the result of 2 breaks in the chromosome with repair of the broken segment in reversed direction. Since genetic material should not be lost in the process, the phenotype is most commonly normal. The population frequency of pericentric inversions is 0.01%[38] and those involving chromosomes 9, 10, or 11 are so common that they are considered normal population variants. The pericentric inversion of chromosome 9 (p11q13) is particularly common in blacks.

When one of the parents carries a balanced inversion the risk of unbalanced offspring at the time of amniocentesis is about 6%.[39] This risk seems to differ with the sex of the carrier. The rate of unbalanced offspring is 4% when the inversion is carried by the father and 7.5% when the mother is the carrier of the balanced inversion. Thus, inversion carriers should receive genetic counseling and should be offered prenatal diagnosis by amniocentesis or CVS, regardless of maternal age. Conversely, when an inversion is diagnosed in an amniocentesis or CVS specimen performed for other indications, parental karyotypes should be obtained. If the inversion is also carried by one of the parents (inherited), a normal phenotype should be expected. However, if the inversion appears de novo in the conceptus and parental karyotypes are normal, mental retardation or abnormal phenotype may occur, due to positional effects on gene activity (moving the coding part of 1 gene next to regulatory sequences of another gene), breaks within a gene or minute deletions at the break lines.

The incidence of balanced inversion or translocation carriers among couples affected by 2 or more pregnancy losses is 2–4%, 10 times higher than the prevalence of translocation carriers in the general population.[38] Among individuals with unbalanced translocations, about one third to one half are inherited from a carrier (balanced) parent—most of the rest arise de novo, commonly in the father's sperm. The pattern of segregation in familial cases exhibits multiple affected siblings and/or multiple miscarriages concentrated on one side of the family. In inherited cases, blood karyotypes of other family members are often necessary to identify additional individuals at risk for unbalanced offspring.

Two main types of translocations are identified—reciprocal and Robertsonian. A reciprocal translocation means that breaks were formed on 2 nonhomologous chromosomes and the segments between the breaks were exchanged between the two. In the balanced carrier, the nomenclature of such a karyotype will be 46, XX or XY, t(a:b), where "a" and "b" represent the numbers of the chromosomes involved in the translocation. Unless minute deletions occurred at the breaking points, the phenotype of reciprocal translocation carriers is normal. Considering the segregation possibilities into gametes of such a carrier, the calculated risk of unbalanced offspring in these cases is 50%; the actual risk of unbalanced offspring when one of the parents is the carrier of a balanced reciprocal translocation is 12–14%.[40]

Robertsonian translocations can take place only between acrocentric chromosomes—numbers 13, 14, 15, 21, and 22. In this translocation, the "p" arms of the translocated chromosomes are lost and the "q" arms unite at the centromere. Thus, a Robertsonian translocation carrier has only 45 chromosomes, but the genetic material is balanced (and the phenotype normal), since the "p" arm of acrocentric chromosomes does not contain euchromatin. The nomenclature of this type of karyotype will be 45, XX or XY, t(a;b). Theoretically, one third of the offspring of a Robertsonian translocation carrier will have an unbalanced karyotype and will be phenotypically abnormal; one third will carry the balanced translocation like the parent and will have a normal phenotype, and one third will have normal chromosomes.[38] The actual risk of unbalanced viable offspring is, however, negligible, unless the translocation involves chromosomes 13 or 21. A significant sex difference in the segregation of Robertsonian translocations is also observed. For a female carrier of a Robertsonian translocation involving chromosome 21, the risk of having a viable trisomic 21 offspring is 10–20%. The exceptions are carriers of 21;21 translocations, in which all conceptions will be abnormal—either monosomic (and therefore nonviable and aborted) or trisomic and potentially viable with Down syndrome. The risk for a liveborn unbalanced offspring for female carriers of other Robertsonian translocations or for male carriers is low (1–2%). Since all conceptions involving trisomy 14, 15, or 22 and most trisomy 13 pregnancies will be miscarried, the rate of spontaneous abortions is increased in carriers of Robertsonian translocations.[38,39]

Structural chromosome rearrangements are often diagnosed incidentally when prenatal diagnosis is performed for unrelated indications (e.g., advanced maternal age). If the rearrangement is unbalanced, the partial monosomy or trisomy implies a serious risk of mental retardation or abnormal phenotype. Available evidence suggests that chromosomal deletions or duplications large enough to be observed by regular cytogenetic techniques usually have serious phenotypic consequences.[41] When the structural rearrangement is seemingly balanced, it is important to determine whether the same rearrangement is carried by one of the parents. The diagnosis of the same chromosome rearrangement in parental karyotype reassures that a normal phenotype is expected in the tested fetus, but may prompt chromosome studies of other family membranes and, obviously, in subsequent pregnancies.

When a balanced chromosome rearrangement is not inherited but appears de novo in the index pregnancy, fetal prognosis is guarded. At amniocentesis, the incidence of de novo balanced translocations or inversions is 0.06%, higher than the 0.04% incidence of these abnormalities reported at term.[41,42] Thus, it appears that about one third of these pregnancies are miscarried between amniocentesis and term. The incidence of dysmorphic features in newborns with de novo rearrangements is 7.6%, 2 to 3 times higher than the incidence of congenital anomalies reported in newborns.[41] Moreover, cases of mental retardation or developmental delay that are not associated with dysmorphism may not be reported at birth. In surveys of the mentally retarded, apparently balanced, de novo chromosome rearrangements were 7 times more frequent than among newborns surveyed at random. Thus, patients that are diagnosed to carry a fetus with de novo chromosome rearrangement should be counseled that the risk of congenital anomalies for that pregnancy is probably in the range of 10–15%. The risk is probably higher with reciprocal translocations or with inversions; the risk for congenital anomalies associated with de novo Robertsonian translocations is probably small.

THE GENES AND MENDELIAN INHERITANCE

The Human Gene—Structure and Function

Human chromosomes are made of DNA, double-helix polynucleotide chains formed of 2 purine and 2 pirimidine bases. In the double helix, Adenine always pairs with Thymine and Guanine with Cytosine (Fig. 1-2). Along the polynucleotide chain, each 3-base sequence (codon) can code for a specific amino acid. Since there are 64 possible arrangements of nucleotide base triplets but only 20 amino acids, the genetic code is said to be redundant, with each amino acid being coded by 1 to 6 codons. Overall, the diploid set of chromosomes contains about 7 billion base pairs.[43] However, not all of it is translated into protein. It is estimated that about half of the DNA is formed by "informative" sequences, that being interspaced with DNA stretches that are not translated and whose function is not exactly defined.

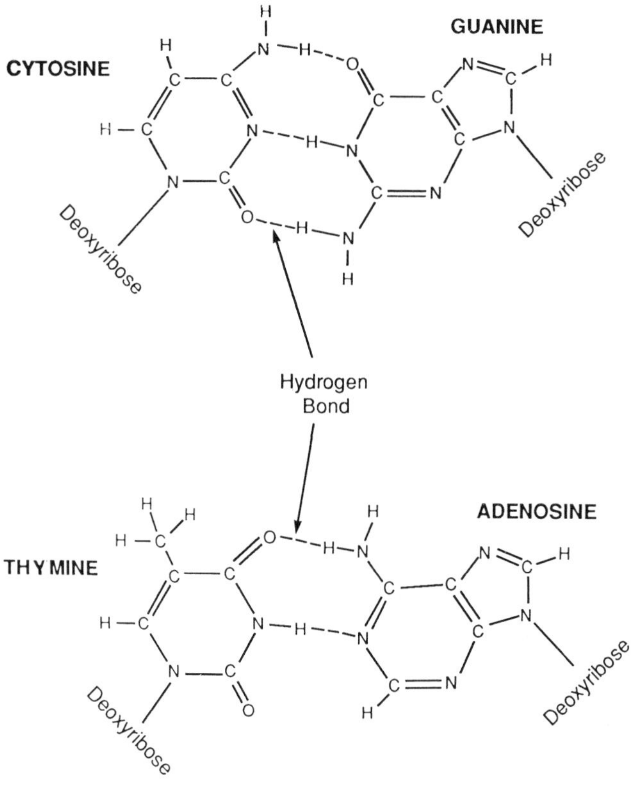

FIGURE 1-2 Nucleotide base pairing.

Three chief classes of DNA are recognized.[44]

1. Unique sequences: Approximately 50–60% of human DNA is formed of single copy stretches about 2000 bases long. The number of protein coding, unique, sequences is probably around 100,000 per haploid genome. They are interspaced with repetitive DNA sequences about 0.3 kb long. The repetitive noncoding DNA sequences probably serve structural or regulatory function.

2. Highly repetitive sequences are found in specific areas such as the heterochromatic region of chromosomes 1, 9, 16, and the Y-chromosome and are usually located near the centromere. These millionfold repetitions of oligonucleotides form about 10% of the human genome. They are highly polymorphic in quantity but without any effect on the phenotype. Since highly repetitive sequences are transmitted from generation to generation in an extremely conserved form, they can be used as markers in population studies.

3. Moderately repetitive sequences (about 30% of the human genome) contain some gene families that are necessary in all cells and in each phase of individual development. Genes for ribosomal RNA, generally located in the nucleolus organizing region (NOR) of human acrocentric chromosomes, immunoglobulins, histones, and transfer RNA are included in this group.

Protein coding genes are formed from exons, the actually translated sequences of nucleotide bases, interspersed with nontranslated sequences called introns (Fig. 1-3). Upstream to the exon-intron complex (toward the 5′ end of the molecule) there are regulatory sequences that control gene expression and initiate transcription. These are called promoter regions and appear to be similar in all genes. They include signals for initiation of transcription (the TATA box, about 30 bases upstream of the gene) and the recognition site for RNA transcriptase (CAT box), about 80 base pair upstream of the transcribed sequence. The signal to stop transcription is given by a regulatory sequence flanking the transcribed complex downstream (toward the 3′ end of the molecule).

Transcription, the transfer of the genetic code from DNA to messenger RNA (mRNA) is always in the same direction, from the 5′ to the 3′ end of the DNA molecule. The mRNA molecule created is complementary to the DNA sequence copied, meaning that it is the exact copy of the DNA strand that was not transcribed (with the exception that Uracyl is substituted for Thymine). After transcription, a poly Adenyl tail is added to the mRNA molecule and the introns are excised (spliced) to form a "mature" form of mRNA that exits the nucleus. In the cytoplasm, the "mature" mRNA serves as a skeleton along which transfer RNA (tRNA) builds the specific protein by sequentially adding amino acids as encoded by mRNA.

Promoter elements modify gene activity by controlling the rate of transcription.[44] Specific mediator proteins (e.g., steroid hormones) may interact with promoter elements to increase their activity. Gene inactivation is effected by DNA methylation of the promoter region.[45] It should be emphasized that DNA methylation is a reversible phenomenon; a decrease in DNA methylation is associated with an increase in gene expression or with reactivation of expression of suppressed genes. Different patterns of DNA methylation are responsible for varying expression of genes in different cells as well as for the decrease in number of genes expressed in mature cells.[45] DNA methylation may also be one of the mechanisms (although not the sole and probably not the primary one) to explain parental genomic imprinting.[21]

MUTATIONS—THE PATHOGENESIS OF SINGLE GENE DISORDERS

Mutation is a change in the normal DNA sequence of nucleotides, caused by absence, addition, or substitution of 1 or more base pairs. If the mutated DNA strand is part of the sequence of base pairs forming a gene, the mutation will result in a different pattern of codons which may cause the formation of an abnormal mRNA template and an abnormal gene product. A single base substitution—"point" mutation—may or may not alter the amino acid sequence coded by the gene since, as previously mentioned, some amino acids are coded by more than 1 codon. For example, the amino acid Leucine is coded by 6 different codons. Sometimes, however, a single base substitution can cause severe disorders. A common example is sickle cell disease. In this disorder a single base substitution in codon 6 of the β globin chain causes the replacement of

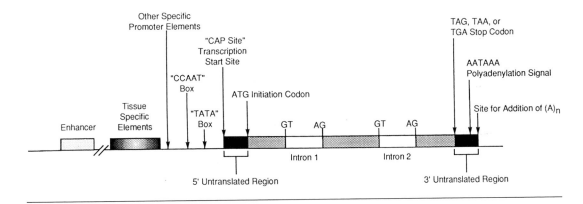

FIGURE 1-3 Exon → intron → protein.

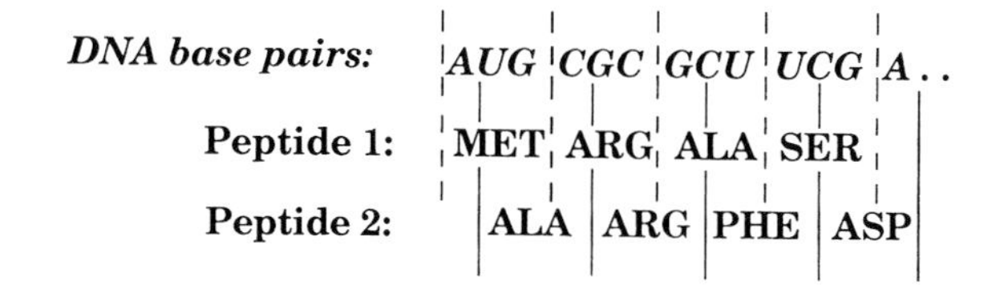

DNA base pairs:	AUG	CGC	GCU	UCG	A . .
Peptide 1:	MET	ARG	ALA	SER	
Peptide 2:	ALA	ARG	PHE	ASP	

FIGURE 1-4 Frameshift mutation.

glutamic acid by valine. Glutamic acid has 2 COOH groups and 1 NH2 group whereas valine has only 1 COOH group. The charge difference between hemoglobin A and hemoglobin S explains the instability of the latter under specific conditions, causing the sickling phenomenon.

"Frameshift" mutations (Fig. 1-4) are caused by insertions or deletions of 1 or more nucleotide bases in the gene sequence altering the whole coding system of the gene caudad to the mutation locus. Since the amino acid sequence coded downstream to the mutation will be entirely different from that coded by the original gene, the gene product in these cases will be grossly abnormal, with obvious phenotypic consequences. Such mutations are observed in part of the β thalassemia genotypes or in the Duchenne Muscular Dystrophy (DMD) locus. Mutations can affect gene activity also by changing the code for termination of transcription (chain termination mutations) or by changing the recognition code for splicing sites. The latter will result in acceptance of part or the whole intron as exon, thus changing significantly the mRNA template. In addition, mutations in regulatory sequences can lead to reduced, abnormal, or absent transcription, by changing the recognition site of RNA polymerase.

Thus, the pathogenesis of genetic disease can be summarized as an alteration of DNA structure causing abnormal gene function and resulting in an abnormal gene product. The abnormal rate of production or the production of abnormal protein may interfere with enzymatic or metabolic pathways or cause structural anomalies or cell membrane dysfunction. Mutations in regulatory genes can be even more detrimental, since cell differentiation and morphologic development may be altered. The existence of regulatory genes has not been substantiated yet in humans, but has been demonstrated in lower life forms.[46]

Genetic disorders that are caused by malfunction of a single gene are inherited following strict Mendelian rules. Based on the diagnosis, the pedigree and knowledge of the pattern of inheritance of a specific disorder, we can calculate the accurate risk for other family members to be affected. Single gene disorders are logged in a useful referral catalog that is updated periodically by Victor McKusick at Johns Hopkins University; the ninth edition contains more than 4400 entries.[47] With a personal computer and modem, the catalog can be available and updated online.

PATTERNS OF SINGLE GENE INHERITANCE

Genes at the same locus on homologous chromosomes are called alleles. According to Mendel, alleles always segregate

during meiosis, each mature sex cell (spermatocyte or oocyte) containing only 1 of each homologous chromosomes (and 1 of each alleles). Since the allocation of chromosomes during meiosis is totally random and independent of segregation of other chromosomes, each fertilized oocyte contains a random assortment of alleles contributed by both parents. Thus, each genetic locus can be either concordant or discordant with regard to the function of a specific allele pair, this being termed homozygous and heterozygous, respectively. Moreover, there is a "gene dosage" effect, each allele contributing half the normal gene product. A trait that is expressed in the heterozygous state is considered dominant. In dominant disorders, 50% reduction of the activity or the quantity of the normal protein coded by the specific gene will cause phenotypic abnormalities. Dominant disorders will be caused mainly by malfunction of genes coding for structural proteins (i.e., collagen) or for proteins regulating complex metabolic pathways, such as membrane receptors. A trait that is expressed clinically only in the homozygous state is called recessive. In recessive conditions, a normal phenotype is maintained with 50% and less of the normal gene function. Disorders associated with enzyme deficiencies ("inborn errors of metabolism") are the main group of diseases in this class.

The pattern of inheritance of a disorder is determined by the location of the abnormal allele (on an autosome or the sex chromosome) and by the dominance of the trait. Building a pedigree helps to identify how a specific disease runs in the family and thus to determine the inheritance pattern and risk of recurrence in other family members. It should be emphasized that dominance and recessiveness are attributes of the phenotype, not the abnormal gene. Since a gene dosage effect always exists (though it may not be fully expressed in the phenotype), we can state that dominance and recessiveness are determined by the sensitivity of the methods used to assay one's phenotype.

AUTOSOMAL DOMINANT INHERITANCE

Autosomal dominant disorders are inherited from 1 parent carrying and, in most cases, showing phenotypic expression of the abnormal gene. For practical purposes, most individuals with a dominant disorder are heterozygotes. Only when both parents have the same autosomal dominant disorder, 25% of their offspring could be affected with the homozygous form of the disease, which will always be more severe than that of the parents due to double dosage of the deleterious gene. In many cases, homozygous autosomal dominant disorders will be lethal in utero or in early infancy. Thus, offspring of achondroplastic individuals, a disease in which marriage between affected individuals is not uncommon, will be either affected (as the parents) or normal; the homozygous form of achondroplasia is always lethal during pregnancy.

Characteristic criteria of autosomal dominant inheritance include:

1. Vertical pattern in a pedigree—the trait appears in every generation without skipping (Fig. 1-5).

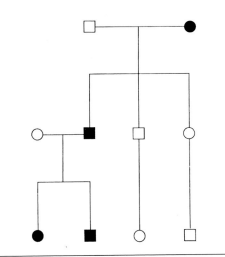

FIGURE 1-5 Autosomal dominant pedigree.

2. Inheritance from only 1 heterozygote parent, with 1:2 risk for offspring of either sex to be affected. Father to son transmission is observed almost exclusively in transmission of autosomal dominant traits.

3. Male and female offspring are affected with equal frequency and equal severity. With some exceptions, the sex of affected individuals does not modify the expression of a dominant trait.

4. The frequency of sporadic cases is in negative correlation with the reproductive fitness of affected individuals. In other words, the proportion of cases caused by new mutations (the first case in the family, not inherited from an affected parent) is highest in disorders that are lethal in utero or in early infancy (e.g., thanatophoric dwarfism). Advanced paternal age has also been associated with a higher risk of autosomal dominant disorders (e.g., achondroplasia or neurofibromatosis) caused by new mutations in offspring. When an autosomal dominant disorder is caused by a new mutation, the risk for other affected offspring (siblings of the affected individual) is very low and probably similar to the frequency of the disorder in the general population.

5. Unaffected family members do not transmit the disorder to their offspring; identification of heterozygotes may be confounded, however, by late or variable age of onset of clinical symptoms and by lack of penetrance or variability in expression of the trait.

Late age of onset is characteristic of Huntington chorea. The mean age of onset of this severe degenerative disorder of the nervous system is 38 years, with some heterozygote carriers not being clinically affected until 70 years of age. Thus, most of the patients are asymptomatic in the reproductive years and do not know whether they carry the deleterious gene, a fact that may have significant implications on the health of both parent and offspring. Although the gene for Huntington disease has been mapped to human chromosome 4p16.3 and, using molecular techniques, prenatal diagnosis of heterozygote fetuses is feasible,[48] ethical and psychological implications obviate the common use of gene probes for Huntington's chorea in clinical practice.

Lack of penetrance is defined as absence of the dominant phenotype in a heterozygote individual known to carry the abnormal gene by means of an affected parent and an affected child. Some autosomal dominant disorders with reduced penetrance are otosclerosis (40%), retinoblastoma (80%), hereditary pancreatitis (80%), and Gardner's syndrome (84%). In some disorders, penetrance may be influenced by age (see Huntington chorea). In disorders with reduced penetrance, the risk for offspring of an apparently normal individual almost never exceeds 10%.

Expression of autosomal dominant traits may vary between heterozygotes. Even within the same family some affected individuals may express severe phenotypic changes while others may manifest only minimal, difficult to detect, symptoms. Variability of expression is evident in neurofibromatosis, tuberous sclerosis, and myotonic dystrophy. In such disorders, detailed clinical examination and, sometimes, special tests may be needed before pronouncing an individual as nonaffected (and therefore not carrying the gene for the disease). That may have obvious implications in terms of genetic risk for affected sibs or offspring. It is important to bare in mind that expression of some disorders may vary between transmitting generations. Thus, the severity of the disorder in the parent does not indicate what will be the expression in the affected offspring. Examples include disorders of late onset, such as Huntington chorea and Myotonic Dystrophy. Approximately 10% of cases of Huntington disease (HD) and 10–20% of cases of myotonic dystrophy are characterized by juvenile onset and a very severe course. In more than 90% of juvenile cases, the gene for the disease is transmitted from a specific parent—in juvenile HD by the father, in congenital myotonic dystrophy by the mother. It appears that parental genomic imprinting plays a major role in determining the appearance of juvenile, severe forms of these disorders.[21]

In summary, autosomal dominant phenotypes are commonly associated with malformations, are clinically variable and, in most cases, are less severe than recessive phenotypes. Variability of expression and incomplete penetrance may confound the vertical pattern of autosomal dominant inheritance. As a rule, individuals affected by autosomal dominant disorders are heterozygous for the disease gene; in the homozygous form, these disorders are almost always lethal in early life. Some genetic disorders with autosomal dominant inheritance are listed in Table 1-3.

AUTOSOMAL RECESSIVE INHERITANCE

Disorders inherited in an autosomal recessive pattern are expressed only in the homozygote who has inherited the diseased gene from 2 heterozygote, phenotypically healthy, parents. Thus, the inheritance pattern is horizontal, with only 1 generation in the pedigree showing clinical manifestations of the disease. Commonly, these disorders are caused by rare

TABLE 1-3	GENETIC DISORDERS WITH AUTOSOMAL DOMINANT INHERITANCE

Achondroplasia
Huntington disease
Hypercholesterolemia
Marfan
Myotonic Dystrophy
Phakomatoses (Neurofibromatosis, Tuberous Sclerosis)
Polycystic Kidney Disease (Adult type)
Polydactyly

enzymatic defects and are termed "inborn errors of metabolism." Since the genotype is homozygous, the phenotype of these disorders is less variable and more severe than in dominant conditions.

Consanguinity or inbreeding in an isolated (ethnic) group have a significant impact on the frequency of recessive disorders in a specific population. A common example is Tay Sachs. This lysosomal storage disease is characterized by accumulation of Ganglioside GM2 in the nervous system, causing mental retardation, blindness, a cherry red spot in the retina, and muscular weakness leading to death in early childhood. The enzymatic defect is absence of Hexoseaminidase A and carrier detection is available by determination of Hex A serum levels.[49] The gene for Tay Sachs, mapped to human chromosome 15q22, is carried with a frequency of 1 in 27 among Ashkenazi Jews and 1 in 300 among the rest of North American population. The chance of random mating between 2 Jewish Tay Sachs carriers can be calculated as 1 in 729, as compared to 1 in 90,000 among non-Jews. Thus, among Ashkenazi Jews, parents of affected children are usually nonrelated, whereas in other populations the consanguinity rate among parents of affected cases is high. Tay Sachs carrier determination should be offered routinely to Jewish couples and should be considered even when only 1 of the parents is Jewish. Other examples of autosomal recessive disorders with obvious ethnic predilection are listed in Tables 1-4 and 1-5. When available, determination of the carrier status for diseases specific to ethnic groups should be offered as a standard of care in pregnancy.

TABLE 1-4	ETHNIC PREDILECTION OF SOME AUTOSOMAL RECESSIVE DISORDERS		
Disease	Ethnic Group	Carrier Frequency	Disease Frequency
Sickle cell	Blacks	1 in 12	1 in 600
Cystic Fibrosis	N. Europeans	1 in 22	1 in 1936
α Thalassemia	Asians, Chinese	1 in 25	1 in 2500
Tay Sachs	Ashkenazi Jews[a]	1 in 27	1 in 2916
β Thalassemia	Mediterranean	1 in 30	1 in 3600
Canavan	Ashkenazi Jews	1 in 37	1 in 5476
Phenylketonuria	E. Europeans	1 in 60	1 in 14400

[a]Niemann-Pick and Gaucher (adult type) are related metabolic disorders more common in this ethnic group.

TABLE 1-5	SINGLE GENE DISORDERS WITH OBVIOUS ETHNIC PREDILECTION	
Ethnic Group	Disorder
Africans	Sickle cell anemia other hemoglobinopathies (Hb C, persistent Hb F, thalassemias)
Ashkenazi Jews	Abetalipoproteinemia
	Bloom's syndrome
	Familial Dysautonomia
	Factor XI deficiency
	Iminoglycinuria
	Sphyngolipidoses (table 3)
Chinese	Alpha thalassemia
Eskimos	Pseudocholinesterase deficiency
Finns	Congenital nephrosis
	Aspartylglucoseaminuria
Japanese	Acatalasia
	Oguchi disease
Mediterranean (Italians, Greeks, Arabs)	Betha thalassemia
	Familial Mediterranean Fever
	G6PD deficiency

The most common autosomal recessive disorder in the white Caucasian population is Cystic Fibrosis, with a carrier frequency of 1 in 22. The gene for cystic fibrosis has been mapped to human chromosome 7p, mutations specific to different ethnic groups have been identified and molecular screening to identify carriers of cystic fibrosis or prenatal diagnosis of affected fetuses is increasingly used in clinical setup.[50–54] Other autosomal recessive disorders in which screening of carriers is used in clinical practice include Canavan, Gaucher (type A), and α1-antitrypsin deficiency.

The following criteria are characteristic of autosomal recessive inheritance:

1. The disorder usually appears only in siblings of an affected case (horizontal pattern of the pedigree). Both parents and offspring (if any) are obligatory carriers, but clinically unaffected (Fig. 1-6).
2. With mating of 2 carriers, each male or female offspring has a 1 in 4 chance of being affected. Half the siblings of an affected individual will be carriers, like the parents, and one fourth will not carry the trait. Thus, two thirds of healthy siblings of an affected person are phenotypically normal but carry the trait.
3. Transmission in consecutive generations is rare and is confined to matings between affected and carrier or affected individuals. In the latter situation, all offspring will be affected.
4. Consanguinity and inbreeding increase the frequency of rare autosomal recessive traits.
5. All humans are heterozygous for 3 to 5 lethal equivalents—disorders that would have been lethal if appearing in the homozygous state. This may account for the increase in perinatal mortality and morbidity associated with

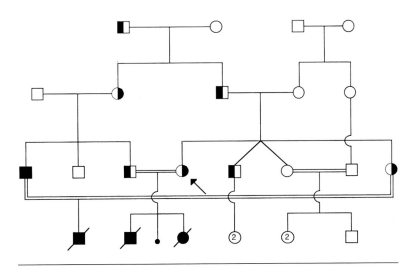

FIGURE 1-6 Autosomal recessive pedigree.

consanguineous marriages or mating within inbred populations or genetic isolates.

DISORDERS INHERITED IN LINKAGE TO THE SEX CHROMOSOMES

For practical purposes, sex-linked inheritance refers mainly to genetic disorders carried on the X chromosome, since the Y chromosome contains only a scarce amount of genetic information (mainly regarding the size of teeth and testes differentiation). For Y-linked inheritance only male-to-male transmission is observed and only males are affected.

X-linked inheritance patterns are influenced by 2 major factors:

1. Women have 2 X chromosomes and can be homozygous or heterozygous to genes on the X. In contrast, males have only 1 X chromosome. Thus, males are said to be hemizygous in respect to X-linked genes.

2. Women have only 1 active X chromosome, the other being inactivated in the early female embryo (the Barr body). Thus, a woman heterozygous for an X-linked gene is an actual mosaic, with the abnormal allele active in about half of her cells.[55,56] The inherited allele on the X chromosome will always be active in the hemizygous male.

The characteristic pattern of X-linked inheritance is oblique (Fig. 1-7), the disease frequently affecting a boy and his maternal uncle. The following model is suggestive of X-linked inheritance:

1. Male-to-male transmission is never observed, since a father does not transmit the X chromosome to his sons.

2. Unaffected males do not transmit the affected phenotype to offspring of either sex.

3. Males are usually affected more severely than females. In X-linked dominant disorders, females tend to be affected twice as frequently (but less severely) than males.

4. All the daughters of an affected male will carry the abnormal gene (and will express it, if dominant).

5. A carrier mother will transmit the mutated gene to half of her offspring, of either sex.

6. The proportion of carrier mothers is positively associated with the severity of the condition. Thus, for disorders that are always lethal in early childhood (e.g., Duchenne Muscular Dystrophy) about a one third of cases are caused by new mutations.

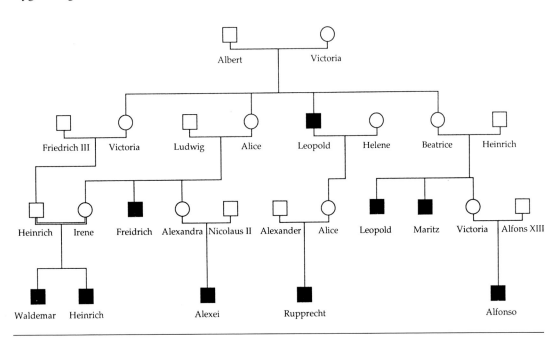

FIGURE 1-7 X-linked pedigree.

TABLE 1-6	GENETIC DISORDERS WITH OBVIOUS X-LINKED INHERITANCE

Color blindness

Duchene Muscular Dystrophy (DMD)

Ectodermal dysplasia

Fragile X syndrome

Hemophylia

Lesch Nyhan syndrome (HGPRT deficiency)

Lowe Oculo-Cerebro-Renal syndrome

Testicular feminization

7. On average, the age of the father of the first heterozygous woman in the pedigree will be advanced.

It appears that the expression of the X-linked phenotype is dependent on a "gene dosage effect." Affected males have only the mutant gene and express its full dosage. Carrier females are mosaic for the abnormal gene and the phenotypic expression will depend on the amount of abnormal gene that was inactivated in early embryonic life. In situations that do not allow inactivation of the specific X chromosome carrying the abnormal gene (e.g., translocation of that X on an autosome), women exhibit the phenotype with the same severity as males. As with autosomal disorders, whether the phenotype is called "recessive" or "dominant" depends on the sensitivity of the assay. Table 1-6 lists some classic examples of genetic disorders transmitted in linkage with the X chromosome.

The most interesting and unusual example of X-linked inheritance in the Fragile X syndrome, delineates another mechanism effective in the transmission of genetic disease to offspring. This most common form of mental retardation heritable in linkage to the X chromosome, affects approximately 1 in 1250 males and 1 in 2000 females; the carrier frequency in the population has been calculated as 1 in 866.[57] The clinical phenotype, which includes an IQ of 20–50, dysmorphic facies, and macroorchidism, is associated with a cytogenetic marker (fragile site) on Xq27, observed in about 35–50% of cells from affected males. A normal sibling of an affected patient may potentially carry the abnormal gene without expressing it and even without exhibiting the fragile site in culture, and yet may transmit it to offspring who subsequently express the disease.[58] Inheritance data suggest that about 20% of hemizygous males may be totally normal. Daughters of such "transmitting males" are almost never retarded yet have a 40% risk of a mentally retarded son and 16% risk of an affected daughter. Moreover, mothers of "transmitting males" have only 9% risk of a mentally retarded son and are never themselves mentally retarded. In contrast, mentally retarded females have a 50% risk for an affected son and 28% risk for an affected daughter. The more severe the mental retardation in the affected woman, the more frequently it is associated with facial dysmorphism. When the pedigree is analyzed, there appears to be a clustering of affected individuals in more recent generations, a phenomenon known as anticipation.

The unusual and puzzling characteristics of inheritance of the fragile X syndrome arise from a "dynamic" mutation: the amplification of a repetitive sequence of 3 nucleotides (cytosine-guanine-guanine). In normal individuals, the DNA segment in Xq27.3 contains between 2–60 copies of CGG. An increase in the number of CGG repeats to 60–200 copies is known as a premutation characteristic of normal transmitting males and some normal carrier females. A premutation is significant because, when passed to offspring, it may develop into a full mutation (many hundreds to thousands of CGG repeats). Expansion to a full mutation is more common when the premutation is maternal rather than paternal and when a male offspring is conceived by a female carrier. The length of the full mutation is unstable during cell division, resulting in marked mosaicism for the number of CGG repeats in the cells of a single individual. Persons carrying the full mutation exhibit the whole range of the FraX/MR phenotype. Molecular testing for clinical diagnosis of patients with mental retardation, carrier detection, and prenatal diagnosis has been accomplished successfully and is more reliable than cytogenetic methods. Prediction of phenotype is relatively straightforward in the normal range ($\leq$50 CGG repeats) or in the premutation range (70–200 CGG repeats). All males and 50% of women carrying far more than 200 CGG copies will be affected. Predicting the phenotype in patients carrying $\approx$200 CGG repeats remains problematic.

Thus, the phenomenon of anticipation and dynamic mutation may explain differences in expression and in penetrance observed in some X-linked dominant disorders as well as the variability in clinical phenotype noted for certain genetic diseases with autosomal dominant inheritance. In specific autosomal dominant disorders, such as Huntington disease, the effect of transmission by either maternal or paternal chromosome on age of onset and severity of symptoms in offspring may be explained by such a dynamic mutation.[59]

MULTIFACTORIAL INHERITANCE

Multifactorial disorders appear to result from the combined effect of genetic and environmental, nongenetic factors. The additive effect of the different components, if above a specific, though ill-defined, threshold, may interfere with developmental processes to cause congenital malformations or to unveil a previously hidden disease. Diabetes, congenital heart defects, neural tube defects, pyloric stenosis, cleft lip and palate, and epilepsy are all examples of disorders with multifactorial inheritance.

In Mendelian (single gene) inheritance, the risk of recurrence in sibs was calculated based on the odds that a specific allele will segregate into the fertilized oocyte. Genetic contribution was equal from both parents and risk for proband was not modified by the number of affected individuals in the pedigree or by environmental influences. With multifactorial disorders, the risk of recurrence is based on empirical data obtained from clinical observations and population studies. Moreover, the population frequency of the disorder, the sex of the proband, and the affected individual and the relationship of the proband

TABLE 1-7	**RISK OF RECURRENCE FOR SOME MULTIFACTORIAL DISORDERS**	
	Population Incidence (%)	*Risk to First-Degree Relatives (%)*
Congenital heart defects	1	2–3
VSD	0.5	2–4
ASD	0.1	3.0
Tetralogy of Fallot	0.07	3.0
Pulmonary stenosis	0.08	2.0
Pyloric stenosis[a] (M:F—5:1)	0.5	3–5
Duodenal ulcer	1.7	10.5
Neural tube defects	0.2	3–4
Cleft lip and/or palate	0.2	2–4
CDH*(F:M—3:1)	0.5	5.0

VSD—ventricular septal defect; ASD—atrial septal defect; CDH—congenital dislocation of hip.

[a]Sex predilection—the risk for relatives is higher if disorder is expressed in member of the less commonly affected sex.

to the latter may all influence recurrence risk. The population frequency of many of these disorders is 1%, with a risk of recurrence of 3–4% in first-degree relatives. Although specific recurrence risks are available for different disorders (Table 1-7), some common rules may apply in many such situations:

1. The risk is highest among closest relatives and decreases rapidly with distance of relationship. The correlation between relatives is proportional to the genes in common. The risk is seldom increased above the risk of the general population in third degree or more distant relatives. In contrast, the risk to subsequent sibs is higher when parents are consanguineous.
2. The risk for affected siblings equals the risk of affected offspring. Dominance and recessiveness do not generally apply in multifactorial inheritance.
3. Recurrence risk depends on the population frequency of the disorder; for first-degree relatives, this risk is approximately the square root of the incidence of the disorder in the population studied. The lower the population risk, the higher the relative risk of recurrence in sibs.
4. When there is unequal sex distribution of a disorder, recurrence risk is higher when a member of the more rarely affected case has the disease. A common example is pyloric stenosis, which is 5 times more frequent in males than in females. The risk of recurrence is 3.8% for brothers of a male index case but 9.2% for brothers of an affected female.
5. Recurrence risk is higher when more than 1 family member is affected.
6. Recurrence risk is higher when the disease in the index case is more severe.

The common denominator of these rules is a higher genetic liability that is associated with increased risk of recurrence in other family members, probably because of genes shared by the affected individuals. A higher genetic liability (lower thresh-

old) may be reflected by many affected members in a family, more severe expression of the disease or members of the more rarely affected sex being affected.[60] The concept of genetic liability is also substantiated by the association of some disorders with specific HLA haplotypes—individuals with the commonly associated HLA haplotype have a significantly higher risk of inheriting the disorder than individuals with other genetic makeups.[61]

Environmental factors (e.g., geographic location or diet) are also essential determinants in the occurrence of multifactorial disorders. A common example is neural tube defects (NTD), a spectrum of disorders of closure of the neural crest that include anencephaly and spina bifida. The overall incidence is approximately 1 in 500 to 1 in 1000 in the United States. Throughout the world, the prevalence of NTD is highest in Northern Ireland (about 8 per 1000 births) and lowest in Japan. For couples of Irish descent that emigrated to the United States the risk for NTD is halved. However, the risk for NTD is doubled for Japanese couples living in Hawaii. Overall in the United States, the highest rate of NTD is observed among the white Appalachian population. For any given place there are marked differences between African and Caucasian population.[62]

Following the birth of 1 child with NTD, the risk of recurrent NTD in another offspring is 3% (in the United States) to 5% (in the United Kingdom). The birth of another affected child increases the risk of recurrent NTD in that family to 10–15%. However, recent evidence suggests that the risk of recurrence can be lowered significantly by preconceptual administration of folic acid, continued until the closure of the neural tube is completed (about 6–8 weeks gestation). In high-risk families, diet complementation with folic acid is advocated to reduce the risk of recurrent NTD to less than 1%.[63] On the other hand, some medications (like valproic acid), maternal diabetes, or operations performed to the mother in the first trimester[64] are reported to be associated with an increased risk for NTD in offspring. Thus, ethnic/genetic and environmental differences may act in common in the production of NTD.

SUMMARY

Genetic diseases are a heterogenous group of disorders whose pathophysiology can be viewed as gene malfunction resulting in abnormal quality or quantity of the gene product. When single genes are involved, these disorders follow strict, mathematical rules of inheritance. Multifactorial disorders are the result of the interaction between genetic predisposition and external (environmental) factors and their inheritance is based on empirical observations. Chromosome anomalies can be viewed as a generalized effect of multiple gene dosage abnormalities, resulting in a pattern of mental and growth retardation and developmental defects of some organ systems specific to the chromosome involved. In many cases these defects will be lethal in the perinatal period.

References

1. Delhanty JDA, Handyside AH. The origin of genetic defects in the human and their detection in the preimplantation embryo. *Human Reproduction Update.* 1995;1:201–215.

2. Tjio HJ, Levan A. The chromosome number of man. *Hereditas.* 1956;42:1.

3. Down JLH. Observations of an ethnic classification of idiots. Clinical Lecture Reports, London Hospital 1866;3:259.

4. Lejeune J, Gauthier M, Turpin R. Etude des chromosomes somatiques de neuf enfants mongoliens. *Cr Acad Sci Paris.* 1959;248:1721.

5. Smith HO, Wilcox KW. A restriction enzyme from Hemophilus Influenza; I. Purification and general properties. *J Mol Biol.* 1970;51:393.

6. Kelly TJ Jr, Smith HO. A restriction enzyme from Hemophilus Influenza; II. Base sequence of the recognition site. *J Mol Biol.* 1970;51:396.

7. Southern EM. Detection of specific sequences among DNA fragments separated by gel electrophoresis. *J Mol Biol.* 1975;98:503.

8. Hsu LYF. Prenatal diagnosis of chromosome anomalies. In: *Genetic Disorders and the Fetus.* 2nd ed. New York and London: Plenum; 1986: 115–183.

9. Hook EB. Rates of chromosomal abnormalities at different maternal ages. *Obstet Gynecol.* 1981;58:292.

10. Juberg RC. Origin of chromosomal abnormalities. Evidence for delayed fertilization in meiotic nondisjunction. *Hum Genet.* 1983;64:122.

11. Jongbloet PH, Mulder AM, Hamers AJ. Seasonality of preovulatory nondisjunction and the etiology of Down syndrome. *Hum Genet.* 1982;62:134.

12. Eggerman T, Nothen MM, Eiben B, et al. Trisomy of human chromosome 18. Molecular studies on parental origin and cell stage of nondisjunction. *Human Genet.* 1996;97:218–223.

13. Fisher JM, Harvey JF, Morton NE, et al. Trisomy 18. Studies of the parent and cell division of origin and the effect of aberrant recombination on nondisjunction. *Am J Hum Genet.* 1995;56:669–675.

14. Martin RH, Rademaker AW. The effect of age on the frequency of sperm chromosomal abnormalities in normal men. *Am J Hum Genet.* 1987;41:484.

15. Emanuel BS. Molecular cytogenetics toward dissection of the contiguous gene syndromes. *Am J Hum Genet.* 1988;43:575.

16. Warburton D. Chromosomal causes of fetal death. *Clin Obstet Gynecol.* 1987;30:268.

17. Williamson RA, Weiner CP, Patil S, et al. Abnormal pregnancy sonogram. Selective indication for fetal karyotype. *Obstet Gynecol.* 1987;69:15.

18. Platt LD, DeVore GR, Lopez E, et al. Role of amniocentesis in ultrasound detected fetal malformations. *Obstet Gynecol.* 1986;68:153.

19. Boyers SP, Diamond MP, Lavy G, et al. The effect of polyploidy on embryo cleavage after in vitro fertilization in humans. *Fertil Steril.* 1987;48:624.

20. O'Brien WF, Knuppel RA, Kousseff B, et al. Elevated maternal serum alpha-fetoprotein in triploidy. *Obstet Gynecol.* 1988;71:994.

21. Hall JG. Genomic imprinting. Review and relevance to human diseases. *Am J Hum Genet.* 1990;46:857.

22. Golbus MS, Bachman R, Wiltse S, et al. Tetraploidy in a liveborn infant. *J Med Genet* 1976;13:329.

23. Scarbrough PR, Hersh J, Kukolich MK, et al. Tetraploidy. A report of three liveborn infants. *Am J Med Genet.* 1984;19:29.

24. Walker S, Lee CY, Gregson NW. Polyploidy in cells cultured from amniotic fluid. *Lancet.* 1970;2:1137.

25. Tegenkamp PR, Hux CH. Incidence of tetraploidy as related to amniotic fluid cell types. *Am J Obstet Gynecol.* 1974;120:1066.

26. Godsen C, Rodeck CH, Nicolaides KH. Fetal blood sampling in the investigation of chromosome mosaicism in amniotic fluid cell culture. *Lancet.* 1988;1:613.

27. Warburton D, Kline J, Stein Z, et al. Monosomy X. A chromosomal anomaly associated with young maternal age. *Lancet.* 1980;1:167.

28. Hassold T, Benham F, Leppert M. Cytogenetics and molecular analysis of sex chromosome monosomy. *Am J Hum Genet.* 1988;42:534.

29. Kalousek DK, Barrett IJ, McGillivray BC. Placental mosaicism and intrauterine survival of trisomies 13 and 18. *Am J Hum Genet.* 1989;44:338.

30. Snijders RJM, Schire NJ, Nicolaides KH. Maternal age and gestational age specific risk for chromosomal defects. *Fetal Diagn Ther.* 1995;10:356–367.

31. Hsu LYF, Kaffe S, Perlis TE. Trisomy 20 mosaicism in prenatal diagnosis. A review and update. *Prenat Diagn.* 1987;7:581.

32. Bell JA, Pearn JH, Smith A. Prenatal cytogenetic diagnosis, amniotic cell culture Vs chorionic villus sampling. *Med J Aust.* 1987;146:27.

33. Wright DJ, Brindley BA, Koppitch FC, et al. Interpretation of chorionic villus sampling laboratory results is just as reliable as amniocentesis. *Obstet Gynecol.* 1989;74:739.

34. Phillips OP, Tharapel AT, Lerner JL, et al. Risk of fetal mosaicism when placental mosaicism is diagnosed by chorionic villus sampling. *Am J Obstet Gynecol.* 1996;174:850–855.

35. Kalousek D. The role of confined chromosomal mosaicism in placental function and human development. *Growth, Genetic & Hormones.* 1988;4:1.

36. Stioui S, Silvestris M, Molinari A, et al. Trisomic 22 placenta in a case of severe intra uterine growth retardation. *Prenat Diagn.* 1989;9:673.

37. Jacobs PA. The epidemiology of chromosome abnormalities in man. *Am J Epidemiol.* 1977;105:180.

38. DeWald GW, Michels VV. Recurrent miscarriages. Cytogenetic causes and genetic counseling of affected families. *Clin Obstet Gynecol.* 1986;29:865.

39. Boue A, Gallano P. A collaborative study of the segregation of inherited chromosome structural rearrangements in 1356 prenatal diagnoses. *Prenat Diagn.* 1984;4:45.

40. Petrosky DL, Borgaonkar DS. Segregation analysis in reciprocal translocation carriers. *Am J Med Genet.* 1984;19:137.

41. Warburton D. Outcome of cases of de novo structural rearrangements diagnosed at amniocentesis. *Prenat Diagn.* 1984;4:69.

42. Hook EB, Schreinmachers DM, Willey AM, et al. Rates of mutant structural chromosome rearrangements in human fetuses. Data from prenatal cytogenetic studies and associations with maternal age and mutagen exposures. *Am J Hum Genet.* 1983;35:96.

43. King CR. Prenatal diagnosis of genetic disease with molecular genetic technology. *Obstet Gynecol. Survey.* 1988;43:493.

44. Thompson JS, Thompson MW. The molecular structure and function of chromosomes and genes. In: Thompson JS, Thompson MW, eds. *Genetics in Medicine,* 4th ed. Philadelphia: WB Saunders; 1986: 27–43.

45. Razin A, Cedar H. DNA methylation in eukaryotic cells. *Int Rev Cytol.* 1984;92:159.

46. Gehring WJ. Homeotic genes, the homeobox and genetic control of development. *Cold Spring Harbor Symp Quant Biol.* 1985;50:243.

47. McKusick VA, ed. *Mendelian inheritance in man,* 8th ed. Baltimore: Johns Hopkins University Press; 1989.

48. Hayden MR, Kastelein JJP, Wilson RD, et al. First trimester prenatal diagnosis for Huntington's disease with DNA probes. *Lancet.* 1987;1:1284.

49. Ben Yoseph Y, Pack BA, Thomas PM, et al. Maternal serum Hexoseaminidase A in pregnancy. Effects of gestational age and fetal genotype. *Am J Med Genet.* 1988;29:891.

50. Gilbert F, Tsao KL, Mendoza A, et al. Prenatal diagnostic options in cystic fibrosis. *Am J Obstet Gynecol.* 1988;158:947.

51. Nugent CE, Gravius T, Green P, et al. Prenatal diagnosis of cystic fibrosis by chorionic villus sampling using 12 polymorphic DNA markers. *Obstet Gynecol.* 1988;71:213.

52. Witt DR, Schaefer C, Hallam P, et al. Cystic fibrosis heterozygote screening in 5161 pregnant women. *Am J Hum Genet.* 1996;58:823–835.

53. Tambor ES, Bernhardt BA, Chase GA, et al. Offering cystic fibrosis carrier screening to an HMO population factors associated with utilization. *Am J Hum Genet.* 1994;55:626–637.

54. Bekker H, Denniss G, Modell M, et al. The impact of population based screening for carriers of cystic fibrosis. *J Med Genet.* 1994;31:364–368.

55. Lyon MF. X-chromosome inactivation and the location and expression of X-linked genes. *Am J Hum Genet.* 1988;29:891.

56. Lyon MF. Gene action in the X-chromosome of the mouse. *Nature* 1961;190:372.

57. Nussbaum RL, Ledbetter DL. The Fragile X Syndrome. In: Scriver CR, Beaudette AL, Sly WS, Valle D, eds. *The metabolic and molecular bases of inherited disease*, 7th edition. New York: McGraw-Hill; 1995:795–810.

58. Weaver DD, Sherman SL. A counseling guide to the Martin Bell syndrome. *Am J Med Genet.* 1987;26:39.

59. Hayden MR, Kremer B. Huntington disease. In: Scriver CR, Beaudette AL, Sly WS, Valle D, eds. *The metabolic and molecular bases of inherited disease*, 7th edition. New York: McGraw-Hill; 1995:4483–4510.

60. Harper PS. Genetic counseling in non Mendelian disorders. In: *Practical genetic counseling*, 2nd ed. Wright, Bristol;1984.

61. Bodmer WF. The HLA system and disease. *JR Coll Physicians.* 1980;14:43.

62. Holmes LB. The health problem: Neural tube defects. In: Maternal serum alpha-fetoprotein. *Issues in the prenatal screening and diagnosis of neural tube defects.* Washington, DC: US Government Printing Office; 1981: 1–4.

63. Milunsky A, Jick H, Bruell Cl, et al. Multivitamin/ Folic acid supplementation in early pregnancy reduces the prevalence of neural tube defects. *JAMA* 1989;262:2847.

64. Kallen B, Mazze RI. Neural tube defects and first trimester operations. *Teratology.* 1990;41:717.

EPIDEMIOLOGY OF ANEUPLOIDY

Howard S. Cuckle / Svetlana Arbuzova

Aneuploidy is a common event in pregnancy with a wide spectrum of medical consequences ranging from the lethal to the benign. Most of the affected zygotes abort spontaneously early in the first trimester, while many abort before there are clinical signs of pregnancy. Those that survive into the second trimester also experience high late-intrauterine mortality and an increased risk of infant death. Viability and clinical outcome vary according to the genotype and this chapter concentrates on the more common forms of aneuploidy which are sufficiently viable and survive to term in relatively large numbers.

The most frequent of these aneuploidies is Down syndrome, which has a birth prevalence, in the absence of prenatal diagnosis and therapeutic abortion, of 1–2 per 1,000 in developed countries. Consequently, it is considered first and more extensive than both Edwards and Patau syndromes, which have, respectively, about one tenth and one twentieth the birth prevalence, and sex-chromosome aneuploidies, which are common but relatively benign.

With the purpose of this book in mind, aspects of the epidemiology that relate to prenatal diagnosis and screening are emphasized. We also show how molecular biology provides a better understanding of the genetic abnormality in Down syndrome. This should eventually help explain the salient epidemiological findings and ultimately lead to the cause of the disorder. The principal etiological hypotheses are outlined.

NATURAL HISTORY OF DOWN SYNDROME

The life-expectancy of those born with Down syndrome today is considerably greater than in the past. Precise estimates are difficult to derive without making assumptions about the long-term consequences of the recent improvements in mortality rates among the young. A Danish study estimated an expectancy of 46 years based on an actuarial analysis of data from 2,466 individuals entering a national register prior to 1980.[1] A similar study, using the records of the Californian State Department of Developmental Services in 1986–1991 found expectancy to relate to the degree of mental disability;[2] 55 years for mild or moderate, 48 for severe and 42 for profound disability. An actuarial analysis was performed using data on the 1,610 births registered up to 1981 in the British Columbia Health Surveillance Register.[3] There was a plateau in the survival curve lasting into the mid 1940s when mortality began to increase markedly. Morbidity has also been improved in recent decades through more effective treatment of associated cardiac, digestive and respiratory symptoms.

Increased survival has placed an even greater burden on those responsible for the educational and social services for individuals with mental disability. Down syndrome remains the most common known cause of severe mental handicap. For example, during the late 1970s, a survey among handicapped young adults in 3 London boroughs found that 20% had Down syndrome.[4] The second largest group with a known cause were the 4% who had cerebral palsy. In addition to the mental handicap, many affected adults may experience cognitive deficits due to pathological changes in the brain normally associated with Alzheimer disease. However, although Alzheimer-like changes are common in the brains of young people with Down syndrome, it is not inevitable that they will develop the clinical disease, and when dementia does occur it is not until middle age. The prevalence of the disorder in Down syndrome is difficult to determine as there are no standardized criteria for dementia in individuals with mental disability. A study from New York State has used operational definitions in an attempt to overcome this lack of standardization.[5] State-wide information systems were used to investigate 2,534 affected individuals and over 16,000 controls with other forms of mental disability. Dementia was defined in terms of declining adaptive behavior. No excess in dementia was seen until age 50. Thereafter, depending on the criteria used, the relative risk compared with controls was 1.7–3.2 at ages 51–60 and 2.7–8.3 at 61–70. In the oldest group the prevalence of dementia was 50% using the most lenient criteria and 15% for the most severe.

GENETICS

In the absence of prenatal diagnosis and selective termination of affected pregnancies Down syndrome occurs in about 1.5 per 1,000 births. In 95% of cases there is non-disjunction of chromosome 21, in 4% a Robertsonian translocation, mostly t(14;21) or t(21;21), and 1% are mosaic.[6] Recent technical advances in molecular biology provide tools for a better understanding of the genetic abnormality. This development helps to explain some of the salient epidemiological findings and in the future may aid in elucidating the etiology.

In cases of apparently non-mosaic free trisomy 21, pericentrometric DNA polymorphisms have been used to determine which parent was the source of the additional chromosome. In the largest series, 724 affected individuals and their parents were tested: 89% of errors were in the mother, 9% the father and 2% had post-zygotic mitotic nondisjunction.[7] These methods also reveal whether the error occurred in the first stage of meiosis (MI) or the second (MII); heterozygous chromosomes implying MI and homozygous MII nondisjunction. In about three quarters of the maternal and half the paternal cases the error was in MI.

Similar methods have shown that trisomy 21 nondisjunction is associated with altered recombination. The initial report of this phenomenon indicated that recombination was reduced,[8] but further studies have shown that the association is complex.[9,10] In the MI cases the generated genetic linkage map is markedly shorter-than-the normal female map, thus indicating a reduction in recombination. There is also an altered distribution of exchanges, so that the reduction is primarily confined to the proximal region of 21q. In contrast, MII cases have a longer-than-normal map with recombination increased near the centromere. One conclusion drawn by the authors of these studies is that 3 configurations render the chromosome susceptible to nondisjunction: absence of chiasmata, distal recombination in MI and proximal recombination in MII. This leads to the suggestion that all maternal nondisjunction could be the result of events occurring in MI, whereas the apparent MII error is a consequence of increased proximal recombination in MI.

Molecular studies have now been performed on large numbers of oocytes and sperm as part of assisted reproduction. Aneuploidy occurs more often in oocytes than sperm, although there are methodological problems in the interpretation of such data.[11] In aneuploid oocytes, extra whole chromosomes are found rarely in comparison to additional free chromatids.[12] A mechanism has been proposed that would account for this observation and explain the recombination data without recourse to MII nondisjunction.[13] The idea is that, if during a long ovarian sojourn time bivalent coherence is lost, then at completion of MI the chromosomes will become 4 single chromatids held together only by chiasmata. At metaphase, stable orientation along the spindle is achieved by tension between the kinetochores and univalent pairs will be rotated until there is a stable reorientation. It can be predicted that distal chiasmata will require 90-degree rotation leading to heterozygous free chromatids, whereas univalent pairs with proximal chiasmata will orientate normally and produce homozygous chromatids without MII nondisjunction.

MATERNAL AGE

The most important risk factor for Down syndrome is maternal age: birth prevalence increases rapidly with age, particularly after age 30. Consequently, the mean maternal age in Down syndrome births is about 5 years greater than unaffected births. The incidence of Down syndrome among pregnancies ending in miscarriage also increases with maternal age. The combined results of 2 large studies, in New York and Hawaii, include 3,395 karyotyped miscarriages.[14] The mean age in 92 cases with trisomy 21 was 30.7 years of age compared with 27.0 in chromosomal normal miscarriages.

The mean maternal age is greater in maternally derived cases of Down syndrome than those in which there is a paternal error: for example, 31.5 compared with 28.2 years in Hasold and Sherman.[7] But the mean maternal age does not differ according to the meiotic stage of the maternal error (MI 31.3 and MII 32.1 years, in the same study) or the paternal error (MI 27.4 and MII 27.5 years).

BIRTH PREVALENCE

The best available estimate for the risk of an affected term pregnancy is obtained from combining data from published series of birth prevalence for individual years of age that were carried out before prenatal diagnosis became common. Four such meta-analyses have been published based on 11 different maternal age-specific birth prevalence series. The difference between the studies was in the number of series included, method of pooling series, type of regression equation and extent to which the maternal age ranges was restricted.

In the first meta-analysis, all 8 series published at that time were included with a total of 4,000–5,000 cases of Down syndrome and more than 5 million unaffected births.[15] For each year of age data were pooled by taking the average birth prevalence rate across the series weighted by the number of births. A 3-parameter additive-exponential regression equation was used of the form $y = a + exp(b + cx)$ where y is prevalence and x is age. A single regression was performed over the entire age range and Figure 2-1 shows that it fitted the data well. In the second study the same 8 series were included but a separate analysis was carried out for the 2 series which the authors regarded to be most complete.[16] Pooling was by summation of the birth prevalence numerators and denominators. Two different additive-exponential regression equations were used: the linear equation above and a 5 parameter version with a cubic exponential component. The maternal age range was restricted in 4 ways (ages 15–49, 20–49, 15–45, 20–45). The third study included 4 series comprising the 2 "most complete" series above, extended by more recent data and 2 newer series.[17] A separate analysis was carried out after excluding one of the new series; pooling was by summation. Three, 5, and 6 parameter additive-exponential regression equations were used, the last having a quartic exponential component; there was no age restriction. The last study included 9 series, 6 of the original 8, including the updated data, the 2 additional series used in the third study and another new series.[18] A separate analysis was carried out after excluding 1 of the original series. Pooling is by the use of a weighting factor which estimates the proportional underascertainment in each series. The regression analysis simultaneously estimates the curve parameters and this proportion. A 3-parameter logistic regression equation is used of the form $y = a + (1 - a)/(1 + exp(-b - cx))$ where a is between 0 and 1; there was no age restriction.

There is little practical difference between the 19 regression curves published in the different meta-analyses over the 15–45 age group range. The real differences emerge at older ages; eg, at age 50 the risks range from 1 in 5 to 1 in 18. There is no simple way of deciding which of the curves is the most accurate since the age-specific rates differ between the component series of the meta-analyses. This is partly due to underascertainment and possibly due to real underlying differences between the populations.

Recently another curve has been published based on a series of 11,000 cases from the National Down Syndrome Cytogenetic Register for England and Wales (NDSCR).[19] It differs significantly in the meta-analyses for older women: birth prevalence was higher at ages 36–41 and considerably lower after age 45. However, the results are subject to potentially strong bias.[20] In the previous series, cases were collected before antenatal screening and prenatal diagnosis became widespread, whereas 45% of the NDSCR cases were diagnosed prenatally and 82% of these ended in termination of pregnancy. Birth prevalence was estimated by assuming an intrauterine survival rate following prenatal diagnosis derived from studies of older women. This rate may not be applicable to women who have undergone prenatal diagnosis because of biochemical and ultrasound screenings. Not only are the women younger, but extreme levels of all screening markers are associated with nonviability and the average marker levels of screen-detected cases vary with age.

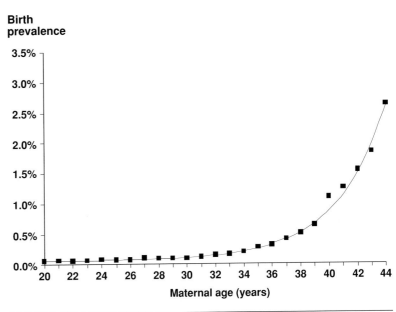

FIGURE 2-1 Down syndrome risk at birth according to maternal age (20–44). Observed birth prevalence and fitted curve.[15]

YOUNG WOMEN

The meta-analyses all applied regression curves that increase monotonically with maternal age. This would not be valid if, as has been claimed, the prevalence of Down syndrome is relatively high at young ages.[21] Examination of the observed single year prevalence in the combined meta-analysis series does not support this claim. The prevalence was 0.00%, 0.06%, 0.07%, 0.06%, and 0.06%, respectively, at ages 15–19 compared with 0.06%, 0.07%, 0.06%, 0.07%, and 0.08% at ages 20–24.[15] Error in recording maternal age is the most likely explanation for the apparent increased prevalence among very young ages in some studies. Down syndrome cases in which maternal age has been under-recorded will tend to make the curve J-shaped.

PATERNAL AGE

Maternal and paternal ages are highly correlated with relatively little variability in the age difference between the 2 parents. As a consequence, an extremely large number of affected couples would have to be investigated in order to discern any independent paternal age effect. Some studies of couples have reported evidence for an effect in births[22] and miscarriages,[23] but many others found no association with age. In a study of French donor insemination centers, where there is a large paternal age difference between donors and recipients, a statistically significant effect of donor age was reported.[24]

If a paternal effect does exist, it is more likely to be present in paternally derived cases. Paternal age has been examined in a series of 67 such cases.[25] The mean age was 29.5 years in 57 meiotic cases and 31.8 in 10 mitotic cases compared with 30.3 in controls. The mean age did not differ according to meiotic stage: MI 29.2 and MII 28.2 years.

Taking the epidemiological and molecular studies together, it can be concluded that when an effect exists it must be much smaller than the maternal age effect.

FETAL LOSS

Although Down syndrome is not associated with extremely high intrauterine lethality, a large proportion of recognized pregnancies with the disorder are not viable.

OVERALL RATES

Studies of prenatal diagnosis are used to estimate fetal loss rates, either by comparing the observed number of cases with that expected from birth prevalence, given the maternal age distribution, or by follow-up of individuals declining termination of pregnancy, using direct or actuarial survival analysis. Published prevalence studies include a total of 341 Down syndrome cases diagnosed at chorionic villus sampling (CVS) and 1,159 at amniocentesis.[26] There are 3 published follow-up series including 110 cases diagnosed at amniocentesis[27] and a series of 126 cases from the NDSCR which has been analyzed according to the gestational age at prenatal diagnosis.[28] However, the NDSCR study is biased, as some miscarriages may have occurred in women who did intend to have a termination; thus, inflating the rates. An actuarial survival analysis of the NDSCR data has now been carried out[29] which overcomes the bias and is more data efficient, since all cases contribute to the estimate and not just those where termination was refused.

Actual and potential heterogeneity between the various studies precludes a grand meta-analysis to estimate the fetal loss rates (Fig. 2-2). But an informal synthesis has been carried out and has reached the conclusion that about one half of Down syndrome pregnancies are lost after first trimester CVS and one quarter after mid-trimester amniocentesis.[30]

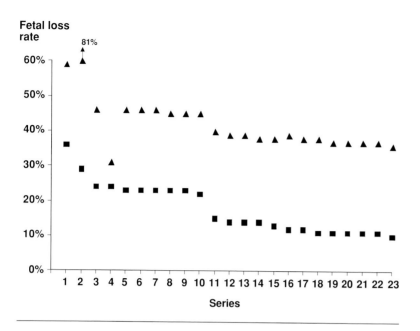

Fetal loss rate

FIGURE 2-2 Estimates of fetal loss rate in 23 series. From the time of CVS (▲) and amniocentesis (■), by comparing observed and expected prevalence directly or from a model (series 16), by follow-up of observed cases that were not terminated (series 1 and 2) or by actuarial survival analysis (series 4).[30]

MATERNAL-AGE SPECIFIC RATES

It is general practice to calculate the maternal age specific risk of Down syndrome at the time of prenatal diagnosis by applying the overall fetal loss rate to the term risk. A formula has also been published, from one of the larger prenatal diagnosis studies, which permits the calculation to be done for individual weeks of gestation.[31]

These calculations assume that fetal loss rates do not vary with maternal age. Since the studies used to calculate the overall rates are largely based on women over age 35 this assumption can only be examined in older women. In the combined results of the prevalence studies the estimated loss rate after CVS, using the birth prevalence curve,[15] was 45% for women ages 35–39 and 47% in those ages 40 and older. For amniocentesis the rates were 28% and 21%, respectively. In the combined results of 3 follow-up studies, the mean maternal age for 29 pregnancies ending in fetal loss was 38.7; for 70 live births it was 39.0; and in 11 cases age was not available.[27] The fourth follow-up study, based on NDSCR data, includes younger women, since many prenatal diagnoses were carried out due to biochemical and ultrasound screening. The gestation standardized mean age for cases diagnosed at 14–21 weeks was 37.5 for 44 fetal deaths and 36.3 for 54 live births (from reference 28).

Thus, the available data do not contradict the assumed lack of correlation between age and Down syndrome viability. Nevertheless, in view of the strong correlation between age and miscarriage in the population,[32] the working assumption should be regarded as tentative and needs to be kept under review.

GENETIC RISK FACTORS

PREVIOUS DOWN SYNDROME

In a small proportion of couples the index case will be shown to have arisen from a parental structural chromosome rearrangement. The recurrence risk in these couples can be quite high, depending on the specific parental genotype. The most frequent is a heterozygous Robertsonian balanced translocation and, for female carriers, the risk is great enough to dwarf the age-specific risk at most ages. For example, among 185 amniocenteses in such women 15% of fetuses had a translocation.[33] In contrast, male carriers of a balanced translocation do not appear to have a high risk; all 70 amniotic fluid samples in the same study had a normal karyotype.

If a woman has had a previous pregnancy with Down syndrome and the additional chromosome 21 was noninherited there is still an increased risk of recurrence. The increase has been estimated at 3 points in pregnancy. In an unpublished study of more than 2,500 women who had first trimester invasive prenatal diagnosis because of a previous affected pregnancy, the Down syndrome incidence was 0.75% higher than that expected from the maternal-age distribution (Kypros Nicolaides, personal communication). Similarly, a meta-analysis of 4 second trimester amniocentesis series totaling 4,953 pregnancies found an excess of 0.54%.[34] A meta-analysis of 433 live births had 5 recurrences, an excess risk of 0.52%.[35] The weighted average of these rates, allowing for fetal losses is 0.77% in the first trimester, 0.54% in the second and 0.42% at term. Examination of the data suggests that the excess is similar at different ages, so the excess can be added to the age-specific risk expressed as a probability. The recurrence risk is relatively large for young women, but by the age of 40 it is not materially different from the risk in women without a family history (see Fig. 2-3). Those with a previous Down syndrome pregnancy also have an increased risk of other types of aneuploidy[35] and neural tube defects.[36]

MULTIPLE RECURRENCE

The recurrence of Down syndrome in older women may be due to chance alone but in young women it is more likely to have a genetic cause. Apart from a parental structural chromosome rearrangement, mosaicism may be involved. In a study of 13 families with recurrent free trisomy 21, for example, 5 were shown to involve parental mosaicism.[37] Even when there is no obvious mosaicism the possibility remains of low level mosaicism confined to the gonads which may be revealed by the use of molecular techniques. In 1 study this approach was used to demonstrate low level maternal mosaicism in 2 couples under 35 years of age, whereas no genetic cause was found for the recurrence in 2 older couples.[38] A serious criticism of all published mosaicism studies is the studies did not include controls from unaffected families. Studies of pre-implantation embryos show that mosaicism is not a rare event.[39]

There are 14 case reports of families with either 2 Down syndrome cases or 1 Down and another aneuploidy in which there were different reproductive partners in the parental or grand-parental generation.[34] In every case recurrence was on the maternal side, except for 1 from a highly inbred population. This suggests the inheritance of a cytoplasmic factor.

POLYMORPHISMS

The $\varepsilon4$ allele of the apolipoprotein (apo) E gene is associated with Alzheimer's disease, both sporadic and familial. Allele frequency in parents of Down syndrome children has been investigated because of the excess risk of this disease in affected families. In a series of 188 Danish cases there was no overall difference in the allele distribution compared to a control population.[40] However, a significantly increased frequency of the $\varepsilon4$ apoE allele was found in young mothers with MII errors.

Abnormal folate and methyl metabolism can lead to DNA hypomethylation and abnormal segregation, which has prompted the investigation of maternal polymorphisms in genes involved in folate metabolism. The common 677C→T polymorphism in the 5,10-methylene-tetrahydrofolate reductase (MTHFR) gene has been reported to occur more frequently than usual in the mothers of children with Down syndrome,[41,42] but this is not a consistent finding.[43–46] An increased frequency of the 66A→G polymorphism in the methionine synthase reductase (MTRR) gene was found in 2 studies.[42,45] Both studies also tested MTHFR alleles in the same women and found that a combination of the 2 mutations conferred a higher risk than either mutation alone.

REPRODUCTIVE RISK FACTORS

PARITY

A number of studies have reported that women of higher parity are at increased Down syndrome risk, while others have failed to confirm such an effect. Most studies either took no account of maternal age or allowed for this co-variable by stratifying the data into broad age groups. However, given the exponential increase in risk after age 30, if stratification is too broad, then residual confounding will remain. Only 3 studies controlled for single-year of maternal age: 2 reported a significant association between Down syndrome risk and parity;[47,48] the third did not.[49]

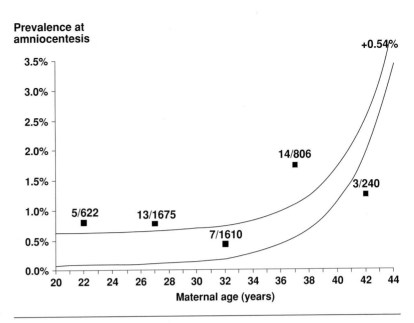

FIGURE 2-3 Recurrence risk according to maternal age. Rate of recurrence observed at amniocentesis compared with curves for incidence at amniocentesis with and without an additive 0.54% risk.[34]

An additional problem of interpretation in this area is that the acceptability of prenatal diagnosis and termination of pregnancies affected by Down syndrome declines with parity. Therefore, analyses which are restricted to births, excluding terminations, are biased towards a positive effect. It is noteworthy that of the 3 fully age-controlled studies only the negative study included terminations.[49] In an attempt to overcome this bias 1 of the positive studies performed a secondary analysis after excluding pregnancies where the birth certificate reported that amniocentesis had been carried out.[48] This resulted in a reduction of the original effect so that it was no longer statistically significant. Moreover, it is known that on US birth certificates the procedure of amniocentesis is only mentioned on roughly half of the pregnancies where the procedure is actually performed. Had complete information been available, it is likely that the effect would have been further reduced. Thus, there is no unbiased information confirming an association with parity.

ASSISTED REPRODUCTION

The risk of Down syndrome does not appear to be greater in pregnancies achieved by assisted reproduction technology than in naturally conceived pregnancies. The prevalence in the combined data from 4 age-matched or age-standardized studies of in vitro fertilization (IVF) was 0.23% (i.e., 32 cases). This result was similar to the weighted average rate of 0.21% in the controls.[50–53] Less data are available on intracytoplasmic sperm injection. In 2 studies the combined prevalence was 0.32% (7 cases) compared with, 0.24%, the rate expected from the average maternal age and gestation of diagnosis.[54,55] Two studies were able to compare the prevalence with a standard IVF series and no difference was found.[56,57]

When calculating the age-specific risk of Down syndrome in pregnancies achieved by IVF, whether conventional or using ICSI, care is needed concerning the maternal age. If a donor egg was used, then the maternal age at term must be calculated from the age of the donor at the time of sampling plus 266 days—the time from conception to term. A similar calculation is done if the woman's own egg was used and it was frozen after sampling. These calculations assume that risk relates to the age of the donor rather than the recipient and that storage has no effect on risk.

FURTHER REPRODUCTIVE FACTORS

Several studies have claimed an association between reduced frequency of coitus and Down syndrome risk: for a review of this subject see Martin-DeLeon et al.[58] Some of the evidence is direct—based on interviews of parents, but much of it is simply by inference. Thus, infrequent coitus has been suggested to underlie occasional reports of the increased Down syndrome frequency in illegitimate births, long marriage, long interval between births and among Catholics, who are assumed to be using the ovulatory method of contraception. More recently, a study in Jerusalem found a higher Down syndrome prevalence in orthodox Jewish couples compared with the nonreligious population.[59] Again infrequent coitus was evoked to explain this result, since orthodox Jews delay coitus until 7 days after the end of the menses at which time there is a religious obligation to resume sexual activity.

Women who have pregnancies affected by Down syndrome experience an early menopause. The evidence for this is presented below (see "Premature ovarian ageing hypothesis" section). In 1 study, use of oral contraceptive was reported to confer increased Down syndrome risk, but this was not confirmed in 3 further studies.[60] Similarly, although an early menarche, a previous miscarriage and consanguinity have been reported to increase risk, yet this has not been found consistent and until further studies are conducted, these variables cannot be regarded as risk factors.

GENERAL RISK FACTORS

TWINS

On theoretical grounds the prior risk of Down syndrome per twin pregnancy should be greater than the risk in singleton pregnancies. Since there are 2 fetuses, the probability of the second being affected is independent of the first and the risk that at least 1 twin is affected would be double that of singletons. In fact the risk will be somewhat less than double because monozygous twins will be concordant for Down syndrome so reducing the overall risk. Theoretical age-specific risks have been published for US Caucasians and African-Americans ages 25–49, based on the observed total twinning rates that increase with age and a monozygous twinning rate assumed to be independent of age.[61] Applying twin risks to US Caucasians for a single year maternal age distribution in

England and Wales in 2000[62] yielded an overall risk for twins 1.88 times greater than the risk for singletons.

However, the observed prevalence of Down syndrome in twin pregnancies is much less than the theoretic calculations predict. A meta-analysis of 5 cohort studies (4 are cited in Wald et al.[63] and a more recent report in Doyle et al.[64]) includes a total of 106 twins with Down syndrome. The overall prevalence was only 3% greater than in singletons. None of the studies was stratified for maternal age and, therefore, this small increase in the crude Down syndrome prevalence rate among twins implies a reduction in the age-specific prevalence rate. Until there is a more precise estimate of age-specific prevalence rates it is probably best to assume that the prior term risk for twins does not differ from that of singletons. The prior risk during pregnancy is even more problematic. The discrepancy between the observed crude rate and that expected from theoretical calculations may be accounted for by a particularly high intrauterine lethality for affected twins. Consequently, the prior risk of Down syndrome in twins at the time of prenatal diagnosis may be much higher than for singletons. There is insufficient published data to clearly judge this at present.

ETHNIC ORIGIN

Those studies with single year of age prevalence rates used to estimate maternal age-specific risk of Down syndrome are based almost entirely on women of European origin. However, there are many individual reports of relatively high or low birth prevalence in other ethnic groups. Some are from countries without reliable systems for collecting information on the maternal date of birth, but 36 studies covering 49 populations provided sufficient detail and reliable age information to be entered into a meta-analyis.[65] An age-standardized index was computed, dividing the observed number of Down syndrome cases by the expected number obtained by applying the age-specific risk curve to the distribution of maternities. Figure 2-4 shows the results. There are two groups with some evidence for rates greater than Europeans. These are women of Mexican and Central American descent living in California (standardized indices 1.19 and 1.30 in 2 studies) and Israeli Jews of Asian or African origin (1.27). The standardized indices were markedly reduced in some populations, including 3 studies in African women, but the authors conclude that this is likely to be due to incomplete ascertainment.

SMOKING

Several early studies reported that smoking was less common in the mothers of infants with Down syndrome, but the latest meta-analysis of 17 published studies failed to find a significant association.[66] Smoking habits are subject to strong birth cohort effects, so it is important to take full account of maternal age. Some of the early studies either did not take account of age or stratified the data using broad age bands, which may not be adequate. This was demonstrated in 1 study which found a relative risk of 0.87 with broad age grouping, 0.89 adjusting for additional variables and 1.00 when age adjustment, with additional variables, was in single years.[67]

One of the studies also categorized subjects according to the parental origin of the additional chromosome 21 and the timing of the error.[68] The overall estimate of the relative risk among all 285 Down syndrome pregnancies combined was 0.96. But when only maternally derived cases were considered the reduction in risk was greater (0.84) and in those cases where the error occurred at MI it was reduced further (0.72).

VAGINAL BLEEDING

There are 5 published studies giving the rate of vaginal bleeding in pregnancies with Down syndrome compared with an unaffected control group of comparable maternal age and in which information on vaginal bleeding had been collected before the outcome of pregnancy was known.[69] In the combined data, including over 300 affected pregnancies, the rate of vaginal bleeding was 1.7-fold higher in pregnancies with Down syndrome than unaffected pregnancies. Since vaginal bleeding is associated with miscarriage, it is possible that the excess relates to nonviable pregnancies. However, in 3 studies restricted to term pregnancies the effect was still present, and in a large study of pregnancies ending in second trimester spontaneous abortion the rate of first trimester bleeding was no higher in chromosomally abnormal fetuses than in those with a normal karyotype.[70]

MEDICAL, PERSONAL, AND ENVIRONMENTAL FACTORS

Several studies have shown that the mothers of children with Down syndrome have either frank thyroid disease or elevated thyroid antibody titers.[71] It is unclear whether the disease process is present before delivery of the affected pregnancy.

Increased risk of Down syndrome has also been related to environmental agents such as fluoride, ionizing radiation, and solar activity as well as personal factors including medical X-rays, premature ageing, grandparental age, dermatoglyphics, and occupation. However, these effects are either small, confounded by maternal age, potentially biased, or they have not been observed consistently. Similarly, reports of variations in prevalence over time, according to the season of conception and geographical clustering, have not been confirmed.

RISK SCREENING

Multi-marker antenatal screening for Down syndrome is now widespread and beginning to have an impact on birth prevalence. Screening uses epidemiological findings for the interpretation of test results and allowance for covariables when calculating marker levels.

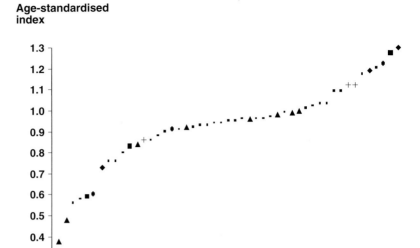

Age-standardised index

Study population

FIGURE 2-4 Relative risk according to ethnic origin. Maternal age-standardized index in 49 study populations: European (∎), African (▲), Latin-American (♦), Asian (●), Jewish (■) and mixed (+).[65]

TEST INTERPRETATION

It can be shown statistically that the optimal way of interpreting the multi-marker profile is to estimate the risk of Down syndrome from the marker levels.[72] This is done by modifying the prior risk that attained before testing, by a factor known as the "likelihood ratio" derived from the marker profile, and then comparing the posterior risk with a fixed cut-off risk. If the posterior is greater than the cut-off risk, then the result is regarded as "screen positive," otherwise it is "screen negative." This approach will yield a higher detection rate for a given false-positive rate than any other method of test interpretation. It also provides a way of encapsulating the result for the purposes of counseling. The method is optimal even if a single marker is used and whether the marker is physical or biochemical.

The prior risk of Down syndrome can be expressed as a probability, say p, or a rate of 1 in 1/p and needs to be converted into an odds of $p:(1-p)$. The posterior risk is calculated by multiplying the left hand side of the odds by the likelihood ratio from the marker profile (x) and the result re-expressed as the rate of 1 in $1 + (1-p)/px$ or the probability $px/(1 + p[x-1])$. The prior risk can relate to the chance of having an affected term pregnancy or the chance of the fetus being affected at the time of testing. In so far as the aim of screening is to reduce birth prevalence the former is more appropriate. However, screening is also about providing women with information on which to base an informed decision about prenatal diagnosis and, therefore, it can be argued that the latter is more relevant.

This calculation assumes that the marker levels and age are independent determinants of risk. When risk is given at the time of the test there is the additional assumption that the marker levels are unrelated to the probability of intra-uterine survival. There is no strong evidence against this, as we have pointed above out in relation to estimating prevalence from screening studies, extreme values of some markers are associated with reduced viability.

ALLOWING FOR COVARIABLES

The levels of all markers currently being used in biochemical or ultrasound screening vary with gestational age. In twin pregnancies the median level of every maternal serum marker is about double that in singletons. All the serum markers investigated so far have shown a tendency to decrease with increasing maternal weight: presumably due to a fixed mass of fetal product diluted in a variable blood volume related to maternal body mass. Some of the biochemical markers are also influenced by maternal smoking, gravidity, ethnic origin, assisted reproduction, and vaginal bleeding.

Of the known covariables gestational age and the presence of twins have a major impact on the discriminatory power of the test. However, all variables can markedly change the risk for an individual woman. Thus, while allowance for gestation and twins is mandatory, most centers also adjust serum marker levels for maternal weight and some take account of the other covariables.

When allowance is made for a co-variable, care is needed to avoid any possible confounding. If the variable is related to the risk of Down syndrome, and when markers are adjusted, then the appropriate prior risk should be used in the risk calculation. From the above, calculating the risk for variables of twins and vaginal bleeding would require this modification, while other variables do not. Furthermore, the standard prior risk may be used in conjunction with maternal weight adjustment. In the only study of maternal weight and Down syndrome the median weight in 51 cases did not differ from that in over 3,000 unaffected controls.[63]

GESTATIONAL AGE

Gestation can be allowed for either by the use of multiples of the gestation specific median (MoMs), deviations from the median, or by taking the ratio between more than one gestation dependent marker. However, none of these methods of adjustment avoid the effect of errors in gestational assessment. Small errors can have a disproportionate effect on the estimated risk of Down syndrome. In practice there are several strategies to minimize error in estimating risk with the intention of increasing detection rate, reducing the false-positive rate or both. One strategy is to organize services so that all women have an ultrasound dating scan prior to screening. However, some centers can only ensure that this is done for those with uncertain dates, pill withdrawal periods and irregular or long cycles. Some centers use only dates to calculate marker levels, but reinterpret the result when a scan is eventually done. However, in practice, those with positive screening results are more likely to have a reinterpretation than negative screenings. Due to "regression to the mean" this leads to a large reduction in the false-positive

rate, and also means a reduction in detection. One way of avoiding this bias is to ensure that borderline negative results are also reinterpreted. Another approach, adopted by many centers, is to reclassify a positive result as negative only if the gestational correction is large (say 2–3 weeks or more).

All of these strategies assume that the ultrasound result is unbiased. This would not be the case if, in pregnancies with Down syndrome, the average gestational age based on the scan differed from the menstrual gestation. A bias could be beneficial or detrimental depending on the direction of bias and the markers used. With the current most used marker combinations a negative bias will reduce detection.

The short stature associated in children with Down syndrome is reflected in utero by short femur lengths measured by ultrasound. Thus, if these biometric measurements were to be used to estimate gestation there would be negative bias. Infants with Down syndrome are growth retarded at term;[73] therefore it is possible that biometric measures in early pregnancy may be reduced. An international multi-center collaborative study has investigated possible bias in 2 main biometric measures of gestation—crown-rump length and biparietal diameter.[74] In 55 case-control sets using the former and 146 the latter the median difference in measurements was 0 for both biometric measures. Therefore, provided the measurement of femur length is avoided, ultrasound should not seriously bias screening results.

ETIOLOGICAL HYPOTHESES

The risk factors highlighted by epidemiological study, particularly the maternal age effect, have given rise to a number of etiological hypotheses. In this section we briefly outline those that are either most plausible or have been considered in most detail.

PRODUCTION LINE HYPOTHESIS

Oocytes formed in late fetal life have fewer chiasmata and more univalents, which render them susceptible to nondisjunction. Therefore, it was proposed that the order in which oocytes ovulate within a woman's reproductive life is determined by the order in which they were produced in utero.[75] The hypothesis has been tested using different experimental methods.

No direct cytological evidence has been produced to show that changes in chromosome pairing at MI prophase can lead to nondisjunction at MI metaphase. The analysis of mice heterozygous for 2 types of inversion showed that the proportion of oocytes with a loop at the MI zygotene and pachytene stages decreases with increasing gestational age, but this effect can be explained by synaptic adjustment.[76] A similar study of mice heterozygous for a translocation compared the proportion of cells with translocation quadrivalent, trivalent and univalent in the MI pachytene stage and MI metaphase but found no correlation between the 2.[77] Moreover, it has been shown that univalents can be produced artificially depending on the chromosomal technique used. In an experiment with rats, chemically marked DNA was used to determine the time that meiosis began. A slight correlation was found with the time primordial follicles were subsequently activated in the mature animals.[78] In contrast, 1 experiment did yield results compatible with a production line affect.[79] Radioactively labeled DNA was used to compare the proportion of oocytes in the pachytene or diplotene stages of MI prophase with the proportion in MI or MII metaphase; a correlation was established between the two. Thus, although different experimental approaches have produced some contradictory results, the majority of investigations do not support the hypothesis.

AGEING OOCYTE HYPOTHESES

Given that errors of female meiosis are more often associated with Down syndrome than errors in male meiosis, irrespective of paternal age, the cause of the disorder has been sought in disturbances during stages of oogenesis, including the period of meiotic arrest of the oocyte.[11]

It has been suggested that the frequency of persistent nucleoli in MI prophase is increased in older women due to the long dictyate stage. Nucleolar fusion, which holds together the short arms of acrocentric chromosomes, predisposes them to errors in meiotic segregation and increases the possibility of nondisjunction.[80] This nucleolus hypothesis and its variants that involve nonhomologous recombination and induction of Robertsonian translocations[81] do not explain the relatively high frequency of trisomy among the nonacrocentric chromosomes.

Several hypotheses are devoted to the damage of spindle components whether by intrinsic factors or by the accumulation of environmental insults over the long meiotic prophase. There are many agents such as irradiation (x-rays, gamma-rays, and ultra-violet) and heavy metal ions that could affect oocytes through intracellular free radical production or oxidative effects. Experimental studies provide unambiguous evidence that the radio-sensitivity of oocytes in the dictyate stage increases with advancing maternal age.[82] Not all chromosomes have equal sensitivity to the effects of radiation and in vitro examinations of radiation-induced mitotic nondisjunction of human lymphocytes have shown a significantly elevated susceptibility of chromosomes 21 and X to abnormal segregation.[83]

RELAXED SELECTION HYPOTHESIS

It has been proposed that the propensity for in utero selection against trisomy, whereby affected fetuses tend to be miscarried, decreases in older mothers.[84] If this were true the mean maternal age would be lower in trisomic miscarriages than trisomic births, provided the chance of miscarriage does not increase rapidly with age.

In the New York and Hawaii studies cited above (see "Maternal age") the mean maternal age in trisomy 21 miscarriages was 30.7 years.[14] Using age-specific prevalence curves the estimated maternal age of Down syndrome births in New York at the time was 30.4–31.0 years, depending on the curve, and for Hawaii it was 29.8 years.[85] So this data appears to contradict the relaxed selection hypothesis. However, the chance of miscarriage is much greater in older women than in the young: in 1 study, for example, 9% at ages 20–24 and 75% at 45 and

older.[32] This increase is so rapid that the mean maternal age in Down syndrome miscarriages is not necessarily less than in Down syndrome births under the relaxed selection hypothesis.

One way of testing the hypothesis in these circumstances is to compare the maternal age difference between miscarriages and births for Down syndrome with that for normal pregnancies. Relaxed selection would imply that the difference is smaller in Down syndrome. In the New York and Hawaii studies the difference for normal pregnancies was 1.0 years[14] compared with 1.2–1.8 years in New York and 0.3 years in Hawaii.[85] The 4 studies above (see "Fetal loss") in which women who declined termination of a Down syndrome pregnancy also provide information on the age difference. In 3 studies combined the difference was −0.3 years[27] and in the fourth it was 1.2 years.[28]

Thus the available data on Down syndrome miscarriages do not provide consistent evidence for the relaxed selection hypothesis. Nor do the results of assisted reproduction using donor oocytes from young women in older recipients.[11] These procedures indicate that it is the quality of the donated oocyte rather than the recipients' ability to select against abnormal embryos that determines a successful outcome. Furthermore, if there is relaxed selection against Down syndrome, the mean maternal age would be increased in *de novo* Robertsonian translocation cases as well as nondisjunction cases, yet it is not.[6]

Even if relaxed selection did contribute to the maternal age effect it could not account for all of it because the incidence of trisomy 21 in miscarriages also increases with maternal age.[14] Moreover, trisomy 21 is only present in about 3% of recognized miscarriages; much less than would be found if selection were efficient at young ages. It remains theoretically possible that the relaxed selection could be taking place before pregnancy is recognized, but this would be difficult to investigate.

PREMATURE REPRODUCTIVE AGEING HYPOTHESIS

This hypothesis contends that physiological ageing of the female reproductive system may be more important than chronological age per se. In particular, a plausible model has been described whereby depletion of the oocyte pool by accelerated atresia would lead to increased risk of trisomy.[86]

Support for the hypothesis comes from experimental work with inbred CBA mice which have a small number of oocytes that are completely depleted by the time ovulation ceases. A large series of mice were given a unilateral oophorectomy which caused increased ovulation in the contra-lateral ovary and an early menopause.[87] The oophorectomized mice had an increased rate of aneuploid embryos at all ages compared with untreated control animals. The treated mice also had earlier onset of irregular cycles indicating premature reproductive ageing.

There is also human evidence in support of the hypothesis. It is of itself suggestive that the rate of decline in the number of available follicles increases exponentially after age 30,[88] just as the exponential rise in Down syndrome risk begins. It is believed that depletion of the oocyte pool below a certain threshold leads to the rapid onset of reproductive ageing, ultimately resulting in menopause. Two studies have reported reduced menopausal age in association with trisomy. In 1 study, menopause occurred on average 10.2 years after a Down syndrome birth compared with 12.8 years for age-matched controls.[89] In the second the mean age of menopause among women with trisomic miscarriages was 1.0 years earlier than those with chromosomally normal losses or births, after adjusting for age at birth.[90] Unilateral oophorectomy in humans is likely to bring forward the age of menopause, although the affect is not great, and in a case-control study surgical removal or congenital absence of 1 ovary was associated with a 9-fold increase in Down syndrome risk.[91] One group who experience an extremely premature menopause are the subset of women with Turner syndrome who do ovulate. Some 221 pregnancies in such women have been reported in the literature (from a systematic review by Tarani et al.[92] and more recent series by Birkebaek et al.[93]) including 4 Down syndrome births, a rate of 1.8%, which represents a very large excess.

Given the long peri-menopausal period the reported age of menopause is subject to considerable subjectivity and is not a reliable measure of ovarian failure. Serum follicle stimulating hormone (FSH) is a more reliable indicator. Elevated FSH levels have also been reported in women who had previously given birth to a child with Down syndrome[94] and in women who were undergoing early abortions for social reasons where karyotyping revealed fetal aneuploidy.[95]

COMPROMISED MICROCIRCULATION HYPOTHESIS

This hypothesis proposes that nondisjunction arises from a series of cascading events, initiated by hormonal imbalance.[96] This causes a less-than-optimal micro-vasculature to develop around the ovarian follicle resulting in reduced blood flow through the area. The oxygen deficit leads to an increase in the concentration of carbon dioxide and lactic acid inside the follicle. This in turn causes a decrease in the intracellular pH of the oocyte which reduces the size of the mitotic spindle with the subsequent displacement and nondisjunction of a chromosome.

Although animal experiments do support the possibility that abnormal pH would lead to nondisjunction,[97] 2 premises of the argument are controversial. First, the proponents of the hypothesis cite studies of the maternal age affect which appear to be J-shaped as evidence for hormonal imbalance. They argue that this would account for both the relatively high prevalence at the time of menarche and the extremely high rates approaching the menopause. However, as we have shown above the curve is not in fact J-shaped. Second, the purported connection between compromised micro-circulation and reduced pH, is that the ovarian follicle has no internal circulation. But both oocytes and spermatocytes are isolated from direct contact with blood and it is known that the ovary is the most highly vascularized organ.[98]

DELAYED FERTILIZATION AND SPERM AGEING HYPOTHESES

The secondary oocyte remains in MII metaphase in the Fallopian tube until it is fertilized. It has been proposed that ageing or over-ripeness of these cells could lead to a higher incidence of spindle defects and so increase the chance of nondisjunction. This hypothesis might explain the maternal age effect, since there is presumed to be a decreased frequency of coitus in older women.[99] Such behavior would reduce the chance of fertilization before the ovum became over-ripe.

There is epidemiological evidence, cited above (see "Further reproduction factors"), which indicates that infrequent coitus may be a risk factor for Down syndrome. Some experiments show that chromosomal errors increase with delayed fertilization in mice, although it is difficult to distinguish this effect from the maternal age *per se*.[100] But there are animal experiments that do not support the hypothesis; for a review see Martin-DeLeon et al.[58]

It has also been proposed that sperm aging, eg as a result of infrequent coitus, could have an etiological role. There is some supportive evidence for this from animal experiments and a possible mechanism has been suggested.[58] This hypothesis claims that chromosomally abnormal sperm are immature and so have a competitive disadvantage over normal sperm, but a delay in utilization would allow them to mature.

In any case, the delayed fertilization hypothesis could only account for a small proportion of cases, since in three quarters of the cases the extra chromosome is derived from a maternal MI error. Moreover, recent studies suggest that all maternal errors are initiated during MI and resolved at MI or MII.[9] Similarly, the ageing sperm hypothesis could account for at most one tenth of cases.

MITOCHONDRIAL (MT) DNA MUTATION HYPOTHESIS

It has been proposed that mtDNA mutations may have a role in the etiology of Down syndrome.[101] Such mutations lead to a decline in ATP level and increased production of free-radicals. This could affect division spindle and chromosome segregation, accelerate telomere shortening, alter recombination and cause nondisjunction of chromosomes.

There are many features of mtDNA which are remarkably consistent with the epidemiology and molecular genetics of the disorder. Thus, unlike nuclear DNA, which is almost entirely of maternal origin, mtDNA mutations in oocytes increase with age[102] and the mutations can be inherited. It may also be relevant that mtDNA mutations are involved in Alzheimer disease, diabetes, and hypothyroidism, disorders which frequently occur in affected families.

There is animal evidence in support of the mtDNA mutation hypothesis. It has been shown, in a mouse model, that mtDNA mutations can modulate the expression of an inheritable MI error in oocytes.[103] In humans, the excess of maternal over paternal remarriages in families with aneuploidy recurrence to different partners is consistent with inheritance of a cytoplasmic factor such at an mtDNA mutation.[34] There is also more direct evidence from humans. The complete mtDNA was sequenced in a peripheral blood sample from the mother of a child with Down syndrome who was the originator of the additional chromosome 21.[101] Four point mutations not previously described were found (1 subsequent to the publication), each of which is likely to disrupt mitochondrial function. Moreover biochemical studies have shown increased free-radical activity in mothers; this could be either a cause or result of mtDNA mutations.[104] Using a chemiluminescent technique there was a statistically significant increase in activity compared with controls, after age-stratification. Recently the entire mtDNA of 3 Down syndrome patients was also sequenced and a high incidence of mtDNA base changes were found, many capable of disrupting mitochondrial function, including several mutations not previously described.[105] While the studies are exciting, they do not themselves constitute proof that mtDNA mutations are involved in Down syndrome etiology. Some of the observed base changes may occur as common polymorphisms in the local population; mtDNA in maternal blood may differ from that in the oocyte and the observed mutations in Down syndrome individuals may reflect premature ageing.

OTHER ANEUPLOIDIES

EDWARDS SYNDROME

This is a lethal condition with about one third dying in the neonatal period, one half surviving 2 months after birth and only a few percent surviving the first year as severely mentally retarded individuals.[106]

The maternal age-specific risk of Edwards syndrome can be taken to be a fixed fraction of the corresponding risk for Down syndrome. The relative frequency of the disorders are one tenth, one fourth, and one third at term, mid-trimester and late in first trimester, respectively. These relative frequencies are derived from the ratio of Edwards and Down syndrome cases in neonates, at amniocentesis and at chorionic villus sampling. When 6 series of routinely karyotyped neonates were combined,[107] there were a total of 7 cases of Edwards' syndrome and 71 of Down syndrome were found (a relative frequency of one tenth). In 5 large amniocentesis series combined[108] together with the multi-center European study[28] there were a total of 241 cases of Edwards syndrome and 1,086 of Down syndrome in women age 35 or more (a relative frequency of one fourth). In 5 large chorionic villus sampling series combined[30] the totals were 67 and 211 respectively (relative frequency one third). These results are consistent with a one tenth relative frequency at term. For example, the late fetal loss rate for Edwards syndrome is higher than for Down syndrome, about two thirds compared with one quarter,[27] so the expected relative frequency at birth for the amniocentesis series would have been (one third of 241) (three quarters of 1,086) or 80/814. In the prenatal diagnosis studies relative frequency of Edwards and Down syndrome appears to be independent of

maternal age. Although they comprised older women it is reasonable to assume that the same relative frequency applies to all ages. Many centers engaged in Down syndrome screening also interpret the result in relation to Edwards syndrome. Again the optimal method of interpretation is to calculate the risk of an affected pregnancy given the marker profile and age.[109,110]

PATAU SYNDROME

The disorder is generally lethal but about 10% will survive for more than a year albeit with profound developmental delay. It is associated with pre-eclampsia and in one study the condition was present in 6 out of 25 cases with a further 4 having other forms of pregnancy induced hypertension.[111] As with Edwards syndrome the prevalence can be derived from that of Down syndrome. The available data on newborns, at amniocentesis and at chorionic villus sampling suggest that the maternal age effect is similar in magnitude to that of both Down and Edwards syndromes.[112] The age-specific prevalence appears to be about one half that of Edwards syndrome or one twentieth, one ninth, and one sixth of Down syndrome at the 3 stages, respectively.

SEX CHROMOSOME ANEUPLOIDY

Turner syndrome is a common, but relatively benign condition in females. Those affected have short stature and are generally infertile, yet there is no intellectual impairment and despite a number of associated medical conditions, life-expectancy is normal. The 45,X genotype, complete or mosaic, is found in 1 per 2,500 female births with a downward trend in frequency with increasing maternal age. However, Turner syndrome is a clinical diagnosis and as such it is not clear what proportion of fetuses with a 45,X karyotype, particularly those with mosaicism, would present clinically.[113]

The other common forms of sex chromosome aneuploidy are 47,XXY and 47,XYY in males, and 47,XXX in females. Much is known about the frequency of these genotypes but there is a biased association with phenotype. Thus, 47,XXY is present in about 1 per 1,000 males, the prevalence increasing with maternal age, although not as steeply as the common autosomal aneuploidies. The clinical phenotype is Klinefelter syndrome which presents with hypogonadism and gynecomastia, associated with a small reduction in intellectual capacity. However, a population based study in North London found that of an estimated 106 males with a 47,XXY genotype only 28 (26%) presented clinically.[114] The implication for prenatal diagnosis is that patients need to be informed that the medical consequences are likely to be less severe than indicated by clinical series. A similar conclusion may be drawn for males with 47,XYY and females with 47,XXX neither of which have marked clinical signs but are associated with a moderate intellectual impairment. The birth prevalence of 47,XYY is also 1 per 1,000 males but this is unrelated to maternal age. High prevalence rates have been found among those in penal institutions. In the North London population based study, of the estimated 89 cases, only 11 (12%) were referred for cytogenetic testing, for reasons of developmental delay, infertility and trans-sexuality.[114] An extra X chromosome is present in about 1 per 1,000 females and the maternal age-specific prevalence of 47,XXX is similar to 47,XXY. There is no comparable information on the relationship between genotype and phenotype and it is likely that, as with the other genotypes, the presenting series are biased.

References

1. Dupont A, Vaeth M, Videbech P. Mortality and life expectancy of Down syndrome in Denmark. *J Ment Defic Res.* 1986;30: 111–120.
2. Strauss D, Eyman RK. Mortality of people with mental retardation in California with and without Down syndrome, 1986–1991. *Am J Ment Retard.* 1996;100:643–653.
3. Baird P, Sadovnick AD. Life expectancy in Down Syndrome adults. *Lancet.* 1988;ii:1354–1356.
4. Mitchell SJ, Woodthorpe J. Young mentally handicapped adults in three London boroughs: prevalence and degree of disability. *J Epid Comm Health.* 1981;35:59–64.
5. Zigman WB, Schuf N, Sersen E, et al. Prevalence of dementia in adults with and without Down syndrome. *Am J Ment Retard.* 1995;100:403–412.
6. Mutton D, Alberman E, Hook EB. Cytogenetic and epidemiological findings in Down syndrome, England and Wales 1989 to 1993. *J Med Genet.* 1996;33:387–384.
7. Hassold T, Sherman S. Down syndrome: genetic recombination and the origin of the extra chromosome 21. *Clin Genet.* 2000;57: 95–100.
8. Warren AC, Chakravarti A, Wong C, et al. Evidence for reduced recombination on the nondisjoined chromosomes 21 in Down syndrome. *Science.* 1987;237:652–654.
9. Lamb NE, Freeman SB, Savage-Austin A, et al. Susceptible chiasma configurations of chromosome 21 predispose to non-disjunction in both maternal meiosis I and meiosis II. *Nat Genet.* 1996;14:400–405.
10. Lamb NE, Feingold E, Savage A, et al. Characterization of susceptible chiasma configurations that increase the risk for maternal nondisjunction of chromosome 21. *Hum Mol Genet.* 1997;6:1391–1399.
11. Eichenlaub-Ritter U. Genetics of oocyte ageing. *Maturitas.* 1998; 30:143–169.
12. Angell RR. First meiotic division disjunction in human oocytes. *Am J Hum Genet.* 1997;61:23–32.
13. Wolstenholme J, Angell RR. Maternal age and trisomy—a unifying mechanism of formation. *Chromosoma.* 2000;109:435–38. Erratum in: *Chromosoma.* 2001;110:130.
14. Hassold T, Warburton D, Kline J, et al. The relationship of maternal age and trisomy among trisomic spontaneous abortions. *Am J Hum Genet.* 1984;36:1349–1356.
15. Cuckle HS, Wald NJ, Thompson SC. Estimating a women's risk of having a pregnancy associated with Down syndrome using her age and serum alpha-fetoprotein level. *Br J Obstet Gynaecol.* 1987;94:387–402.
16. Hecht CA, Hook EB. The imprecision in rates of Down syndrome by 1-year maternal age intervals: a critical analysis of rates used in biochemical screening. *Prenat Diag.* 1994;14:729–738.
17. Hecht CA, Hook EB. Rates of Down syndrome at live birth by one-year maternal age intervals in studies with apparent close to complete ascertainment in populations of European origin: a proposed

rate schedule for use in biochemical screening. *Am J Med Genet.* 1996;62:376–385.
18. Bray I, Wright DE, Davies CJ, et al. Joint estimation of Down syndrome risk and ascertainment rates: a meta-analysis of nine published data sets. *Prenat Diagn.* 1998;18:9–20.
19. Morris JK, Mutton D, Alberman E. Revised estimates of the maternal age specific live birth prevalence of Down syndrome. *J Med Screen.* 2002;9:2–6.
20. Cuckle H. Potential biases in Down syndrome birth prevalence estimation. *J Med Screen.* 2002;9:192.
21. Erickson JD. Down syndrome, paternal age, maternal age and birth order. *Ann Hum Genet.* 1978;41:289–298.
22. Stene E, Stene J, Stengel-Rutkowski S. A reanalysis of the New York State prenatal diagnosis data on Down syndrome and paternal age effects. *Hum Genet.* 1987;77:299–302.
23. Hatch M, Kline J, Levin B, et al. Paternal age and trisomy among spontaneous abortions. *Hum Genet.* 1990;85:355–361.
24. Lansac J, Thepot F, Mayaux MJ, et al. Pregnancy outcome after artificial insemination or IVF with frozen semen donor: a collaborative study of the French CECOS Federation on 21,597 pregnancies. *Eur J Obstet Gynecol Reprod Biol.* 1997;74:223–228.
25. Savage AR, Petersen MB, Pettay D, et al. Elucidating the mechanisms of paternal non-disjunction of chromosome 21 in humans. *Hum Mol Genet.* 1998;7:1221–1227.
26. Bray IC, Wright DE. Estimating the spontaneous loss of Down syndrome fetuses between the time of chorionic villus sampling and livebirth. *Prenat Diag.* 1998;18:1045–1054.
27. Hook EB, Topol BB, Cross PK. The natural history of cytogenetically abnormal fetuses detected at midtrimester amniocentesis which are not terminated electively: new data and estimates of the excess and relative risk of late fetal death associated with 47, +21 and some other abnormal karyotypes. *Am J Hum Genet.* 1989;45: 855–861.
28. Hook EB, Mutton DE, Ide R, et al. The natural history of Down Syndrome conceptions diagnosed prenatally that are not electively terminated. *Am J Hum Genet.* 1995;57: 875–881.
29. Morris JK, Wald NJ, Watt HC. Fetal loss in Down syndrome pregnancies. *Prenat Diag.* 1999;19:142–145.
30. Cuckle H. Down syndrome fetal loss rate in early pregnancy. *Prenat Diag.* 1999;19:1177–1179.
31. Snijders RJ, Sundberg K, Holzgreve W, et al. Maternal age- and gestation-specific risk for trisomy 21. *Ultrasound Obstet Gynecol.* 1999;13:167–170.
32. Nybo Anderson MA, Wohlfahrt J, Christens P, et al. Maternal age and fetal loss: population based register linkage study. *BMJ.* 2000;320:1708–1712.
33. Boué A, Gallano P. A collaborative study of the segregation of inherited chromosome arrangements in 1356 prenatal diagnoses. *Prenat Diagn.* 1984;4:45–67.
34. Arbuzova S, Cuckle H, Mueller R, et al. Familial Down syndrome: evidence supporting cytoplasmic inheritance. *Clin Genet.* 2001;60:456–462.
35. Hook EBH. Chromosome abnormalities: prevalence, risks, and recurrence. In: Brock DJ, Rodeck CH, Ferguson-Smith MA, eds. *Prenatal Diagnosis and Screening.* Edinburgh, England: Churchill Livingstone; 1992:351–392.
36. Barkai G, Arbuzova S, Berkenstadt M, et al. Frequency of Down syndrome and neural-tube defects in the same family. *Lancet.* 2003;361:1331–1335.
37. Pangalos CG, Talbot CC Jr, Lewis JG, et al. DNA polymorphism analysis in families with recurrence of free trisomy 21. *Am J Hum Genet.* 1992;51:1015–1027.
38. James RS, Ellis K, Pettay D, et al. Cytogenetic and molecular study of four couples with multiple trisomy 21 pregnancies. *Eur J Hum Genet.* 1998;6:207–212.

39. Munne S, Cohen J. Chromosome abnormalities in human embryos. *Hum Reprod.* 1998;4:842–855.

40. Avramopoulos D, Mikkelsen M, Vassilopoulos D, et al. Apolipoprotein E allele distribution in parents of Down syndrome children. *Lancet.* 1996;347:862–865.

41. James SJ, Pogribna M, Pogribny IP, et al. Abnormal folate metabolism and mutation in the methylenetetrahydrofolate reductase gene may be maternal risk factors for Down syndrome. *Am J Clin Nutr.* 1999;70:495–501.

42. Hobbs CA, Sherman SL, Ping Y, et al. Polymorphisms in genes involved in folate metabolism as maternal risk factors for Down syndrome. *Am J Hum Genet.* 2000;67:623–630.

43. Petersen MB, Grigoriadou M, Mikkelsen M. A common mutation in the methylenetetrahydrofolate reductase gene is not a risk factor for Down syndrome in a population-based study. *Am J Hum Genet.* 2001;69 suppl:323.

44. Chadefaux-Vekemans B, Coude M, Muller F, et al. Methylenetetrahydrofolate reductase polymorphism in the etiology of Down syndrome. *Pediatr Res.* 2002;51:766–767.

45. O'Leary VB, Parle-McDermott A, Molloy AM, et al. MTRR and MTHFR polymorphism: link to Down syndrome? *Am J Med Genet.* 2002;107:151–155.

46. Stuppia L, Gatta V, Gaspari AR, et al. C677T mutation in the 5,10-MTHFR gene and risk of Down syndrome in Italy. *Eur J Hum Genet.* 2002;10:388–390.

47. Kallen K. Parity and Down syndrome. *Am J Med Genet.* 1997;70:196–201.

48. Doria-Rose VP, Kim HS, Augustine ET, et al. Parity and the risk of Down syndrome. *Am J Epidemiol.* 2003;158:503–508.

49. Chan A, McCaul KA, Keane RJ, et al. Effect of parity, gravidity, previous miscarriage, and age on risk of Down syndrome: population based study. *BMJ.* 1998;317:923–924.

50. Bergh T, Ericson A, Hillensjo T, et al. Deliveries and children born after in-vitro fertilization in Sweden 1982–95: a retrospective cohort study. *Lancet.* 1999;354:1579–1585.

51. Ericson A, Kallen B. Congenital malformations in infants born after IVF: a population-based study. *Hum Reprod.* 2001;16:504–509.

52. Westergaard HB, Johansen AM, Erb K, et al. Danish National In-Vitro Fertilization Registry 1994 and 1995: a controlled study of births, malformations and cytogenetic findings. *Hum Reprod.* 1999;14:1896–1902.

53. Koivurova S, Hartikainen AL, Gissler M, et al. Neonatal outcome and congenital malformations in children born after in-vitro fertilization. *Hum Reprod.* 2002;17:1391–1398.

54. Bonduelle M, Aytoz A, Van Assche E, et al. Incidence of chromosomal aberrations in children born after assisted reproduction through intracytoplasmic sperm injection. *Hum Reprod.* 1998;13:781–782.

55. Loft A, Petersen K, Erb K, et al. A Danish national cohort of 730 infants born after intracytoplasmic sperm injection (ICSI) 1994–1997. *Hum Reprod.* 1999;14:2143–2148.

56. Wennerholm UB, Bergh C, Hamberger L, et al. Obstetric outcome of pregnancies following ICSI, classified according to sperm origin and quality. *Hum Reprod.* 2000;15:1189–1194.

57. Causio F, Fischetto R, Sarcina E, et al. Chromosome analysis of spontaneous abortions after in vitro fertilization (IVF) and intracytoplasmic sperm injection (ICSI). *Eur J Obstet Gynecol Reprod Biol.* 2002;105:44–48.

58. Martin-DeLeon PA, Williams MB. Sexual behavior and Down syndrome: the biological mechanism. *Am J Med Genet.* 1987;27:693–700.

59. Sharav T. Aging gametes in relation to incidence, gender and twinning in Down syndrome. *Am J Med Genet.* 1991;39:116–118.

60. Kullen B. Maternal use of oral contraceptives and Down syndrome. *Contraception.* 1989;39:503–506.

61. Meyers C, Adam R, Dungan J, et al. Aneuploidy in twin gestations: when is maternal age advanced? *Obstet Gynecol.* 1997;89:248–251.

62. Office of National Statistics. Birth Statistics. *Series FM1.* 2002;30:10.

63. Wald NJ, Cuckle HS. Recent advances in screening for neural tube defects and Down syndrome. In: Rodeck CH, ed. *Fetal Diagnosis of Genetic Defects, Baillière's Clinical Obstetrics and Gynaecology.* Vol 1. London, England: Baillière Tindall; 1987:649–676.

64. Doyle PE, Beral V, Botting B, et al. Congenital malformations in twins in England and Wales. *J Epid Comm Health.* 1990;45:43–48.

65. Carothers AD, Hecht CA, Hook EB. International variation in reported live birth prevalence rates of Down syndrome, adjusted for maternal age. *J Med Genet.* 1999;36:386–393.

66. Rudnicka AR, Wald NJ, Huttly W, et al. Influence of maternal smoking on the birth prevalence of Down syndrome and on second trimester screening performance. *Prenat Diagn.* 2002;22:893–897.

67. Chen CL, Gilbert TJ, Daling JR. Maternal smoking and Down syndrome: the confounding effect of maternal age. *Am J Epidemiol.* 1999;149:442–446.

68. Yang Q, Sherman SL, Hassold TJ, et al. Risk factors for trisomy 21: maternal cigarette smoking and oral contraceptive use in a population-based case-control study. *Genet Med.* 1999;1:80–88.

69. Cuckle H, van Oudgaarden ED, Mason G, et al. Taking account of vaginal bleeding in screening for Down syndrome. *Br J Obstet Gynaecol.* 1994;101:948–953.

70. Strobino BA, Pantel-Silverman J. First-trimester vaginal bleeding and the loss of chromosomally normal and abnormal conceptions. *Am J Obstet Gynecol.* 1987;157:1150–1154.

71. Cuckle HS, Wald N, Stone R, et al. Maternal serum thyroid antibodies in early pregnancy and fetal Down syndrome. *Prenat Diagn.* 1998;8:439–445.

72. Royston P, Thompson SG. Model-based screening by risk with application to Down syndrome. *Stat Med.* 1992;11:257–268.

73. Khoury MJ, Erickson JD, Cordero JF, et al. Congenital malformations and intrauterine growth retardation: a population study. *Pediatrics.* 1988;82:83–90.

74. Wald NJ, Smith D, Kennard A, et al. Biparietal diameter and crown-rump length in fetuses with Down syndrome: implications for antenatal serum screening for Down syndrome. *Br J Obstet Gynaecol.* 1993;100:430–435.

75. Henderson SA, Edwards RG. Chiasma frequency and maternal age in mammals. *Nature.* 1968;218:22–28.

76. Tease C, Fisher G. Further examination of the production-line hypothesis in mouse fetal oocytes. II. T(14;15)6Ca heterozygotes. *Chromosoma.* 1986;93:447–452.

77. Tease C, Fisher G. Further examination of the production-line hypothesis in mouse fetal oocytes: inversion heterozygotes (part I). *Chromosoma.* 1989;97:315–320.

78. Meredith S, Doolin D. Timing of activation of primordial follicles in mature rats is only slightly affected by fetal stage at meiotic arrest. *Biol Reprod.* 1997;57:63–67.

79. Polani PE, Crolla JA. A test of the production line hypothesis of mammalian oogenesis. *Hum Genet.* 1991;88:64–70.

80. Polani PE, Briggs JH, Ford CE, et al. A Mongol girl with 46 chromosomes. *Lancet.* 1960;i:721–724.

81. Choo KH. Role of acrocentric cen-pter satellite DNA in Robertsonian translocation and chromosomal non-disjunction. *Mol Biol Med.* 1990;7:437–449.

82. Tease C, Fisher G. The influence of maternal age on radiation-induced chromosome aberrations in mouse oocytes. *Mutat Res.* 1991;262:57–62.

83. Uchida IA, Lee CPV, Byrnes EM. Chromosome aberrations induced in vitro by low doses of radiation: nondisjunction in lymphocytes of young adults. *Am J Hum Genet.* 1975;27:419–429.

84. Ayme S, Lippman-Hand A. Maternal-age effect in aneuploidy: does altered embryonic selection play role? *Am J Hum Genet.* 1982;34:558–565.

85. Hook EB. Down syndrome rates and relaxed selection at older maternal ages. *Am J Hum Genet.* 1983;35:1307–1313.

86. Kline J, Levin B. Trisomy and age at menopause: predicted associations given a link with rate of oocyte atresia. *Paediatr Perinat Epidemiol.* 1992;6:225–239.

87. Brook JD, Gosden RG, Chandley AC. Maternal ageing and aneuploid embryos—evidence from the mouse that biological and not chronological age is the important influence. *Hum Genet.* 1984;66:41–45.

88. Faddy MJ, Gosden RG, Gougeon A, et al. Accelerated disappearance of ovarian follicles in mid-life: implications for forecasting menopause. *Hum Reprod.* 1992;7:1342–1346.

89. Freeman SB, Yang Q, Allran K, et al. Women with a reduced ovarian complement may have an increased risk for a child with Down syndrome. *Am J Hum Genet.* 2000;66:1680–1683.

90. Kline J, Kinney A, Levin B, et al. Trisomic pregnancy and earlier age at menopause. *Am J Hum Genet.* 2000;67:395–404.

91. Phillips OP, Cromwell S, Rivas M, et al. Trisomy 21 and maternal age of menopause: does reproductive age rather than chronological age influence risk of nondisjunction? *Hum Genet.* 1995;95:117–118.

92. Tarani L, Lampariello S, Raguso G, et al. Pregnancy in patients with Turner syndrome: six new cases and review of literature. *Gynecol Endocrinol.* 1998;12:83–87.

93. Birkebaek NH, Cruger D, Hansen J, et al. Fertility and pregnancy outcome in Danish women with Turner syndrome. *Clin Genet.* 2002;61:35–39.

94. van Montfrans JM, Dorland M, Oosterhuis GJ, et al. Increased concentrations of follicle-stimulating hormone in mothers of children with Down syndrome. *Lancet.* 1999;353:1853–1854.

95. Nasseri A, Mukherjee T, Grifo JA, et al. Elevated day 3 serum follicle stimulating hormone and/or estradiol may predict fetal aneuploidy. *Fertil Steril.* 1999;71:715–718.

96. Gaulden ME. Maternal age effect: the enigma of Down syndrome and other trisomic conditions. *Mutat Res.* 1992;296:69–88.

97. Shimada TG, Watanabe G, Ingalls TN. Trisomies and triploidies in hamster embryos: induction by low-pressure hypoxia and pH imbalances. *Arch Environ Health.* 1980;35:101–105.

98. Ellinwood WE, Nett TM, Niswender GD. Ovarian vasculature: structure and function. In Jones RE, ed. *The Vertebrate Ovary, Comparative Biology and Evolution.* New York, NY: Plenum; 1978:583–614.

99. German J. Mongolism, delayed fertilization and human sexual behavior. *Nature.* 1968;217:516–518.

100. Ishikawa H, Endo A. Combined effects of maternal age and delayed fertilization on the frequency of chromosome anomalies in mice. *Hum Reprod.* 1995;10:883–886.

101. Arbuzova S. Why it is necessary to study the role of mitochondrial genome in trisomy 21 pathogenesis? *Down Syndr Res Pract.* 1998;5:126–130.

102. Keefe DL, Niven-Fairchild T, Powell S, et al. Mitochondrial deoxyribonucleic acid deletions in oocytes and reproductive ageing in women. *Fertil Steril.* 1995;64:577–583.

103. Beerman F, Hummler E, Franke U, et al. Maternal modulation of the inheritable meiosis I error Dipl I in mouse oocytes is associated with the type of mitochondrial DNA. *Hum Genet.* 1988;79:338–340.

104. Arbuzova SB. Free radicals in origin and clinical manifestation of Down syndrome. *Cytology & Genetics* 1996;30:25–34.

105. Arbuzova S, Hutchin T, Cuckle H. Mitochondrial DNA mutations in Down syndrome. *Downs Screen News.* 2000;7:31.

106. Goldstein H, Nielsen KG. Rates and survival of individuals with trisomy 13 and 18: data from a 10-year period in Denmark. *Clin Genet.* 1988;34:366–372.

107. Hook EB, Hammerton JL. The frequency of chromosome abnormalities detected in consecutive newborn studies; differences between studies; results by sex and severity of phenotypic involvement. In: Hook EB, Porter IH, eds. *Population Cytogenetics: Studies in Humans.* New York, NY: Academic Press; 1977:63–79.

108. Hook EB, Cross PK, Regal RR. The frequency of 47, +21, 47, +18, and 47 + 13 at the uppermost extremes of maternal ages: results on 56,094 fetuses studied prenatally and comparisons with data on live births. *Hum Genet.* 1984;68:211–220.

109. Barkai G, Goldman B, Ries L, et al. Expanding multiple marker screening for Down syndrome to include Edward syndrome. *Prenat Diag.* 1993;13:843–850.

110. Palomaki GE, Haddow JE, Knight GJ, et al. Risk-based prenatal screening for trisomy 218 using alpha-fetoprotein, unconjugated estriol and human chorionic gonadotropin. *Prenat Diag.* 1995;13:843–850.

111. Toughy JF, James DK. Pre-eclampsia and trisomy 21. *Brit J Obstet Gynaecol.* 1992;99:891–894.

112. Hook EB. Chromosomal abnormalities: prevalence, risks and recurrence. In: Brock DJ, Rodeck CH, Ferguson-Smith MA, eds. *Prenatal Diagnosis and Screening.* Edinburgh, England: Churchill Livingstone; 1992:351–392.

113. Gravholt CH, Juul S, Naeraa RW, et al. Prenatal and postnatal prevalence of Turner syndrome: a registry study. *BMJ.* 1996;312:16–21.

114. Abramsky L, Chapple J. 47,XXY (Klinefelter syndrome) and 47,XYY: estimated rates of and indication for postnatal diagnosis with implications for prenatal counseling. *Prenat Diag.* 1997;17:363–368.

NEW GENETIC CONCEPTS

Mark I. Evans / Yuval Yaron / Mark Paul Johnson / Ralph L. Kramer

Although Mendelian inheritance constitutes the foundation of the science of genetics, recent studies have demonstrated that not all heritable traits follow Mendel's laws. Exceptions to Mendelian inheritance include mitochondrial inheritance, genomic imprinting, uniparental disomy, mosaicism (somatic and germline), and trinucleotide repeat expansion. Understanding of the roles of these modes of inheritance elucidates previously unexplainable patterns of inheritance as well as risks of recurrence. This chapter provides the basic principles of these nontraditional modes of inheritance and is intended for all those who provide genetic counseling.

MITOCHONDRIAL INHERITANCE

Each human cell contains thousands of mitochondria that are the major sites of ATP production. The mitochondrial genome is a circular DNA molecule with 16,569 nucleotides encoding 37 genes (Fig. 3-1). There are 2 to 10 copies of mitochondrial DNA per mitochondrion, amounting to thousands of copies in every nucleated cell. It has highly conserved sequences in divergent species. It encodes for 2 rRNAs, 22 tRNAs, and 13 polypeptide chains (Complexes I–V) which are part of the oxidative phosphorylation system and the respiratory pathway. Complex II is completely encoded by mitochondrial DNA (mtDNA) while Complexes I, III, IV, and V require the products of nuclear genes as well. The mitochondrial genome replicates asynchronously with the cell cycle, and the mitochondria are then randomly distributed to the daughter cells during cytokinesis.

There are several features that differentiate the mitochondrial genome from the nuclear genome. Nearly every nucleotide appears to be part of a coding sequence, either for a protein or for one of the RNAs. Hence, there are very few introns in the mitochondrial genome. Total noncoding DNA is just a little over 1 kb and is thought to be a control region containing both origins of replication for the H (heavy) strand of mtDNA and promoters for H strand and L (light) strand transcription. Both the H and the L strands contain coding sequences.

Comparison of mitochondrial gene sequences and the amino acid sequences of the corresponding proteins indicates that the genetic code in mtDNA is different from that used in the nuclear genome. Four of the 64 codons code for different amino acids in the mitochondrial genome. While greater than 30 tRNAs specify amino acids in the cytoplasm, mitochondrial protein synthesis requires only 22. Many of the tRNA molecules recognize any 1 of the 4 nucleotides in the third position that allows 1 tRNA to pair with any 1 of 4 codons, allowing protein synthesis with fewer tRNAs. In other words, the rules for codon-anticodon pairing appear to be relaxed in the mitocondrial genome.

The rate of nucleotide substitution is much higher in mitochondrial DNA than in nuclear DNA. Comparisons of DNA sequences in different organisms reveal that the rate of nucleotide substitutions during evolution is about 10 times greater in mitochondrial genomes than in nuclear genomes, presumably secondary to the reduced fidelity of mitochondrial DNA replication, a paucity of DNA repair mechanisms, or both. Deletions also occur more frequently.

Variability of phenotypic expression, which is characteristic of mitochondrial disease, is determined by the relative proportion of mutant and normal mtDNA in the affected tissue. Unlike nuclear DNA which is evenly divided between daughter cells, the cytoplasm, and therefore, mtDNA, is randomly distributed to daughter cells. The term heteroplasmy is used to refer to the presence of both normal and abnormal mitochondria, as opposed to homoplasmy, where all the mitochondria are either normal or abnormal. The proportion of normal genomes determines the phenotype of the cell. Once the proportion of either normal or abnormal mitochondria exceeds a certain tissue-specific threshold, the biological behavior of the cell will change. This threshold may be influenced by such factors as energy demands of the cell and age.

The ovum is the source of all mitochondria in the embryo as sperm contain only few mitochondria that are located in the tail region. Since only the nucleus of the sperm fuses with the ovum, the mitochondria from the sperm do not persist in the offspring. Except for a few cases, there is no known disease thought to be inherited through the paternal mitochondrial genome and mitochondrial inheritance is exclusively maternal.

SOMATIC mtDNA MUTATIONS AND AGING

Mitochondria carry out the majority of cellular oxidation and produce most of the cell's ATP. Free radicals are produced in the mitochondria during oxidative phosphorylation and other reactions. Free radical production is increased by inhibition of the electron transport pathways, and is thus a self-perpetuating process. Oxidative damage to mtDNA either directly or indirectly by oxidative products such as lipids and proteins can cause mtDNA mutations which further impair oxidative phosphorylation efficiency. mtDNA is more susceptible to damage by free radicals because of the close proximity of mtDNA to the site of free radical generation, the lack of protective histones, and the relatively poor repair mechanisms of the mitochondrial genome.

With aging there is a decrease in mitochondrial respiratory function. Accumulation of mtDNA mutations in a tissue is inversely proportional to its replicative potential and directly related to its metabolic state, specifically its energy requirements which are met through oxidative phosphorylation. Hence, such mutations are found to a greater extent in the brain and muscle (skeletal and cardiac) than in other tissues. Certain areas within the brain are at greater risk than others. The basal ganglia are at particularly high risk as they are rich in

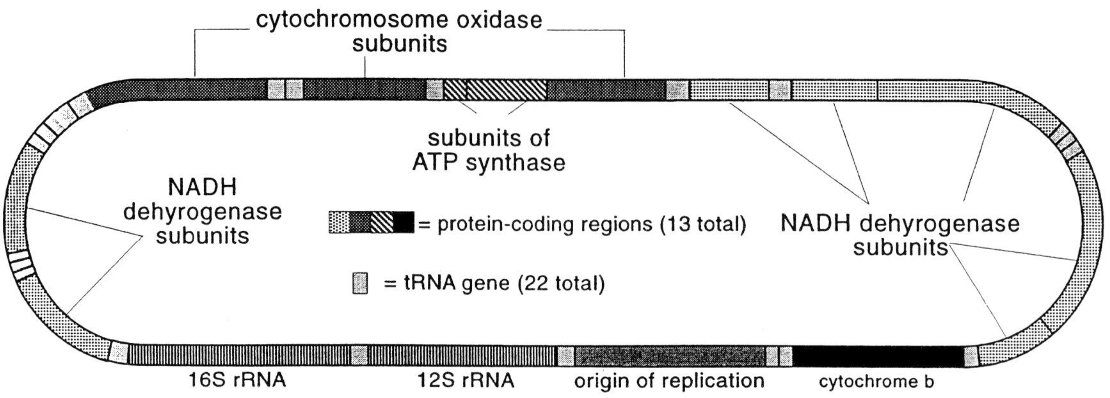

FIGURE 3-1 The mitochondrial genome.

dopaminergic neurons which generate hydrogen peroxide by deamination of dopamine which is catalyzed by monoamine oxidase B(MAO-B). MAO-B levels increase with age concomitantly with the accumulation of mtDNA mutations. By contrast, the cerebellum and myelinated axons, which are not dopaminergic and have a low rate of glucose utilization have the lowest rate of mtDNA mutations.

MITOCHONDRIAL DISEASE

Leber Hereditary Optic Neuropathy (LHON)

LHON is characterized by rapid loss of central vision during early adult life. Eyes may be affected simultaneously or sequentially. LHON patients and their maternal relatives have also been reported to manifest a variety of additional symptoms. Cardiac conduction defects have been noted in some families.[1] Various minor neurological problems including altered reflexes, ataxia, and sensory neuropathy have been described as well as skeletal abnormalities. The penetrance in males who inherit the mutation at basepair (bp) 11778 is about 50% but only 20% in females. This difference cannot be explained by heteroplasmy and is thought to suggest involvement of an X linked gene that may be affected by a variety of mutations.[2]

Myoclonus Epilepsy and Ragged-Red Fibers (MERRF Syndrome)

The term "ragged red fibers" is derived from histologic characteristics observed with the modified Gomori trichome staining of fresh frozen muscle in which accumulated mitochondria appear red, resulting from rearrangements of mtDNA or point mutations affecting tRNA genes. The syndrome consists of myopathy, myoclonus, generalized seizures, hearing loss, intellectual deterioration, and ataxia.

An A-to-G mutation at nucleotide 8344 accounts for 80–90% of cases of MERRF syndrome. The mutation is a missense mutation in the gene for a transfer RNA for lysine, producing multiple deficiencies in the enzyme complexes of the respiratory chain.[3] The clinical phenotype varies greatly within a pedigree, consistent with a heteroplasmic population of mtDNA.

Mitochondrial Myopathy, Encephalopathy, Lactic Acidosis, and Stroke-Like Episodes (MELAS)

Mitochondrial myopathy, encephalopathy, lactic acidosis, and stroke-like episodes (MELAS) is first manifest in childhood as stunted growth, recurrent stroke-like episodes manifest as hemiparesis, hemianopsia, and cortical blindness. Focal or generalized seizures, myoclonic epilepsy, and hearing loss may also be seen. Episodic vomiting may also be present. Death often occurs before the age of 20. MELAS is associated with a point mutation in the tRNA for leucine.[4]

Kearns-Sayre and Chronic Progressive External Ophthalmoplegia (KSS/CPEO)

Kearns-Sayre and chronic progressive external ophthalmoplegia (KSS/CPEO) is characterized by ophthalmoplegia, atypical retinitis pigmentosa, and mitochondrial myopathy. Cardiac conduction defects may be present. The age of onset is usually before age 20. Other features may include ataxia, hearing loss, dementia, short stature, delayed secondary sexual characteristics, hypoparathyroidism, and hypothyroidism. The mtDNA mutations, most commonly deletions, usually occur spontaneously, and hence this disease is not inherited. Heteroplasmy is usually demonstrable in muscle mtDNA.

Neuropathy, Ataxia, and Retinitis Pigmentosa (NARP)

As the name implies, neuropathy, ataxia, and retinitis pigmentosa (NARP) is characterized by a variable combination of retinitis pigmentosa, ataxia, and sensory neuropathy. Other features include developmental delay, dementia, seizures, and proximal limb weakness. NARP was first described in 1990 by Holt et al.[5] and is associated with a mtDNA point mutation in the gene for subunit 6 of mitochondrial H+ -ATPase. This same mutation has also been seen in families with Leigh disease (see below).

Cytochrome C Oxidase Deficiency (Complex IV Deficiency)

There are three established clinical syndromes of cytochrome c oxidase (COX) deficiency, two of which represent variant forms of infantile myopathy. One is benign, characterized by spontaneous recovery by age 2 to 3. The other form presents in the neonatal period and results in respiratory failure. The fatal form is also associated with a renal tubular defect. The fatal form is inherited as a recessive trait and is thought to represent a defect in a nuclear-encoded polypeptide in the respiratory chain. The third form of COX deficiency affects the central nervous system and is known as Leigh syndrome. The typical presentation in the neonatal period is one of hypotonia, recurrent vomiting, and retinitis pigmentosa leading to visual loss. Lactic acid levels are increased in blood and cerebrospinal fluid. Several heteroplasmic mtDNA mutations have been demonstrated in Leigh syndrome.

Maternally Inherited Diabetes Mellitus

Several retrospective studies showed that patients with non-insulin-dependent diabetes mellitus (NIDDM) were much more likely to have a mother who was diagnosed with NIDDM than a father.[6] This was also noted to be true for women with gestational diabetes.[7] These studies may be subject to certain biases, however, as all of them used patient recollection to ascertain affected first-degree relatives.

Glucose intolerance or NIDDM has been reported in some subjects with mitochondrial myopathy. Up to 20% of patients with MELAS have been shown to be diabetic. Diabetes in this group of patients has been associated with nerve deafness and a point mutation in a mitochondrial gene for leucine tRNA.[8] It therefore seems probable that mitochondrial mutations may be involved in the pathogenesis of a small, but clinically significant proportion of cases of NIDDM.

GENOMIC IMPRINTING

Genomic imprinting refers to the process whereby specific genes are differentially marked (imprinted) during parental gametogenesis. The result is differential expression of these genes depending on whether they are inherited either maternally or paternally. The existence of genomic imprinting was first suspected after experiments with pronuclear transplantation. If 1 of the pronuclei is removed and replaced with a pronucleus of the opposite parental origin, the result is lethal. However, depending on whether the pronuclei are of maternal or paternal origin, the consequences are very different. If both are of maternal origin (a gynogenetic embryo), the embryo initially develops normally but development of the placenta and fetal membranes is deficient. If the pronuclei are both male (an androgenetic embryo), the membranes and placenta develop normally while the embryo develops poorly. This latter situation is seen in the case of the triploid conceptus with a partial molar pregnancy. These experiments and observations imply that both maternal and paternal genomes are necessary for normal growth and development. Therefore, their contributions cannot be equivalent.

Several theories have been proposed to explain the existence of genomic imprinting including avoidance of genetic conflict, prevention of parthenogenesis, optimizing placental function while avoiding the development of gestational trophoblastic disease, dominance modification, and gene regulation. Genomic imprinting is also thought to be operative in X inactivation which results in dosage compensation so that structural genes on the X chromosome are expressed at the same levels in males and females.

Genes that are transcriptionally inactive contain 5-methyl-cytosine residues. Transcriptionally active genes generally do not contain 5-methyl-cytosine residues. Methylation of DNA in mammalian cells occurs in CpG dinucleotides, regions of the genome with an unusually high concentration of the dinucleotide 5í-CG-3í. When methylation occurs in the promoter region, the gene becomes transcriptionally inactive. DNA methylation seems to play a major role in the control of transcription, and it appears that selective methylation plays a critical role in genomic imprinting.

GENOMIC IMPRINTING IN HUMAN DISEASE

Prader-Willi and Angelman syndromes have the same deletion but from different parents. Prader-Willi syndrome (PWS) is characterized by short stature, obesity, polyphagia, hypogonadism, and mental retardation. High-resolution chromosome banding studies revealed small interstitial deletions of the 15q11–q13 region in a large proportion of these patients.

An identical deletion was reported in 1987 by Magenis et al. in patients with the much more uncommon Angelman (or "happy puppet") syndrome (AS), characterized by microcephaly, jerky movements, seizures, mental retardation, inappropriate laughter, a large mouth, and protruding tongue.[9] In a rare subset of patients with PWS who did not have detectable cytogenetic deletion, Nicholls et al. reported both copies of chromosome 15 were maternal in origin.[10] It was subsequently discovered in PWS that the deletion always involved the paternally derived chromosome 15, while the deletion was present on the maternal copy in AS.[11] These findings strongly suggest a parent-of-origin effect or genomic imprinting where PWS and AS are caused by 2 closely linked genes which are oppositely imprinted. Both PWS and AS have been documented to result from uniparental disomy where both copies of chromosome 15 are inherited from 1 parent (see below). In the case of PWS, both copies are maternal whereas in AS, both copies are paternal in origin.

BECKWITH-WIEDEMANN SYNDROME (BWS)

This syndrome is characterized by general and regional overgrowth characterized by macrosomia, macroglossia, large kidneys with renal medullary dysplasia, pancreatic hyperplasia, as well as cytomegaly within the fetal adrenal cortex. Omphalocele may also be present. Birthweight averages

4 kilograms, and excessive growth is noted in early childhood. There is a significant predisposition toward the development of certain malignancies, most commonly Wilms's tumor, but also adrenocortical carcinoma, hepatoblastoma, and rhabdomyosarcoma. The gene for BWS has been mapped to 11p15. An increased frequency of several 11p15.5 markers in sporadic cases, paternal duplication in trisomic BWS patients, retention of paternal alleles in Wilms's tumor and adrenocortical carcinoma, as well as higher penetrance in individuals who are born to female carriers all suggest that maternal genomic imprinting is operative. The proposed mechanism is failure of methylation to suppress the maternally derived gene, IGF2 (insulin like growth factor 2).[12]

IMPRINTING AND EPIGENETIC PHENOMENA

Epigenetic refers to post conceptual changes to the genetic material. Imprinting is implemented as an epigenetic event by the process of selective methylation and demethylation of DNA as a function of the parental source. The literature on these two related concepts is expanding geometrically—far beyond the scope possible here.[13–17]

It is becoming increasingly recognized that several diseases follow patterns of imprinting inheritance. For example, there are three genes on maternal chromosome 10 that influence Alzheimer's, male sexual orientation and obesity, a paternal gene on chromosome 9 that influences autism, and paternal genes on chromosomes 2 and 22 influencing schizophrenia.[15] Genes inherited from the "other" parent would be silent and unimportant. However, if there is a disruption of the imprinting pattern either by toxic chemicals, which has been shown experimentally in animal models, or suggested as a by product of assisted reproduction techniques, then there is the potential for significant abnormalities to ensue. The "un-silencing" of the genetic code will be a source of serious investigation over the next decade.

DNA methylation is now appreciated as essentially a second genetic code involving the interaction with chromatin structure and gene expression. Methylation is further implicated in X-Chromosome inactivation and its effects on genomic imprinting and diseases including tumor development. It is likely that the appreciated small, but real increase in congenital abnormalities in babies born following assisted reproductive technologies is likely mediated through this mechanism. Unfortunately, no good method currently exists to predict which embryos are more susceptible than others to such teratogenic effect.[18–20]

In an era in which "cloning" of tissues has been proposed for therapeutic purposes, it is still very unclear how the cloned tissues will behave. Will they retain their imprinted parent of origin or will there be random methylation of different cells? Whatever problems are envisioned for therapeutic cell preparations, they would seem to be several orders of magnitude higher if one were to take it to the next level of reproductive cloning of individuals.

UNIPARENTAL DISOMY (UPD)

Uniparental disomy (UPD) was first suggested by Engel in 1980.[21] UPD refers to the inheritance of 2 copies of a chromosome (or part of a chromosome) from the same parent. When a chromosome or gene is present in duplicate, it is called isodisomy. If both nonidentical homologs are present, it is designated as heterodisomy. UPD can involve both autosomes and the sex chromosomes. Eight years after Engel advanced his hypothesis, cystic fibrosis and growth deficiency were diagnosed in a patient who had inherited 2 copies of the same mutation in the CF gene, but had only 1 carrier parent with that mutation.[22] The patient with CF had evidence of intrauterine growth restriction which was thought to be secondary to the affects of UPD, rather than CF.

As noted above, UPD has been discerned as a cause of both PWS and AS. UPD has since been described for chromosomes 5, 6, 7, 9, 11, 13, 14, 15, 16, 21, 22, and the XY pair.[23] Vidaud et al. described a phenotypically normal boy with sex chromosome UPD which was detected because both the boy, and his father had hemophilia.[24] Maternal isodisomy for chromosome 16 is associated with pregnancy loss, severe IUGR, but can be compatible with a viable pregnancy.[25] The consequences of UPD will depend on the existence of genomic imprinting for a given gene, the presence of recessive mutations in the case of isodisomy, and the extent of mosaicism which may be present in these individuals.

The most common cause of UPD is thought to be "trisomy rescue" which occurs when a trisomic zygote loses the extra chromosome. If the loss happens randomly, two thirds of the cases will not exhibit uniparental disomy, and one third will. Isodisomy results when nondisjunction occurs during meiosis I while heterodisomy results from nondisjunction in meiosis II. The existence of confined placental mosaicism as evidenced on chorionic villus sampling (CVS), is thought to support the theory of trisomy rescue as the most common cause of UPD. Nondisjunction occurs far more commonly in female gametes than in male gametes, and hence, the significantly higher frequency of PWS compared with AS. The role of nondisjunction in the genesis of UPD is supported by the observation of increased risk for PWS or AS with advanced parental age. There are, however, several other proposed mechanisms that are reviewed by Engel.[26]

GERMLINE MOSAICISM

Germline mosaicism is defined as the presence of 2 or more genetically different populations of germline cells. These result from a somatic mutation in a germline precursor that subsequently persists in all the clonal descendants of that cell. Since only the germline cells are affected, the carrier of this mutation is phenotypically normal. Germline mutations are usually suspected when phenotypically normal parents have more than 1 child with a disorder that is known to be inherited as an autosomal dominant or an X-linked trait.

SOMATIC MOSAICISM

If a mutation within the primordial inner cell mass occurs before differentiation of somatic and germline cells, it will be present in both somatic and germline cells. If this mutation were present in progenitor cells from which the germline cells were derived, then all subsequent germline cells would contain this mutation which would be transmissible to all of the offspring, although the transmitting parent will be mosaic. If the mutation occurs only in the somatic cell line after separation of the somatic and germline cells, it will not be transmissible. The carrier of such a somatic mutation will exhibit a segmental or patchy pattern of expression, depending on the proportion and distribution of cells carrying the mutation.

Chromosomal mosaicism may result from postzygotic nondisjunction. The significance of mosaicism is frequently difficult to determine. The effects of mosaicism will depend on the chromosome involved, the proportion of cells containing the abnormal chromosome complement, and the tissues containing this abnormality. The proportion of cells with the abnormal chromosome complement in 1 tissue may not reflect the proportions in another tissue. For example, mosaicism detected in cultured amniocytes may not be detected in fetal or neonatal blood.

One must consider the inherent ascertainment bias in attempting to predict the phenotypic effect of mosaicism, especially when diagnosed prenatally. People who are phenotypically normal are rarely karyotyped. Hence, people who are phenotypically normal but chromosomally mosaic would be unlikely to be ascertained. As a general rule, however, individuals who are mosaic for a given trisomy, are likely to be less severely affected than individuals who are not mosaic for the same trisomy. The ultimate determination of the phenotype depends on many factors.

TRINUCLEOTIDE REPEAT EXPANSION

About three fourths of the linear length of the genome consists of single-copy or unique DNA with the remainder consisting of several classes of repetitive DNA. Tandem (head-to-tail) repeat sequences may be transcriptionally active or inactive. Tandem repeats in coding DNA can vary from short to very large repeat sequences that can include whole genes. Sequence exchange between the repeats can result in either a reduction or an increase (expansion) in the number of tandem repeats.

Expansion of trinucleotide or triplet repeat sequences is now a recognized cause of human disease and provides an explanation of the phenomenon known as genetic anticipation.

Genetic anticipation is defined as the trend toward progressively earlier onset and increased severity of a disease with each subsequent generation. Anticipation was originally thought to reflect ascertainment bias, that is, the family was only studied when a severely affected individual was found. It is now known in at least 10 disorders that anticipation occurs as the result of instability of trinucleotide repeats.[27] In certain disorders such as the fragile-X syndrome, the GC-rich triplet repeats can exist in a "premutation" state where the number of repeats is greater than that found in alleles of the normal population, but insufficient to cause expression of the disease. When the number of repeats exceeds a threshold, which varies with the given disorder, the replication machinery cannot faithfully replicate the sequence with resultant variation in repeat numbers. This can result in amplification of these triplet sequences and is usually thought to occur during meiosis. However, amplification may also occur postconceptionally, during mitosis. The process of amplification may differ in maternal and paternal meiosis.

Fragile-X Syndrome

Fragile-X syndrome was the first disorder recognized to result from trinucleotide repeat expansion. It was originally diagnosed cytogenetically and identified by a fragile site, that is a folate dependent area where the chromatin fails to condense during mitosis, and consequently does not stain when cells are grown in folate-deficient media. On examination the chromosome appears broken or distorted in this region. Fragile-X syndrome is now recognized to be the most common inherited form of moderate mental retardation and the second most common chromosomal cause of mental retardation. Current prevalence estimates suggest that 1 in 1200 males and 1 in 2500 females are affected with fragile-X syndrome. Approximately 1 in 700 females will carry a mutation in the gene for fragile-X syndrome (FMR-1). Males affected with this disorder usually have mental retardation, coarse facial features, and macroorchidism. Affected females are less dysmorphic, but as many as one third will exhibit mild mental retardation.

The expression of the fragile-X mutation depends on the number of CGG repeats within the CpG island in the promoter region of the FMR-1 gene.[28] Amplification of the CGG repeat is associated with subsequent methylation of the CpG island, effectively silencing expression of the gene so that it resembles the FMR-1 locus on the inactive X chromosome. The FMR-1 gene has one of the highest mutation rates of any gene in the human genome. The DNA diagnosis for the fragile-X syndrome is based on the size of the CGG expansion as well as the degree of methylation of the FMR-1 gene.

In fragile-X syndrome, alleles of normal individuals have fewer than 50 copies of the CGG repeat. Small expansions known as premutations involve up to 200 repeats. Males and females carrying the premutation are said to be carriers and are phenotypically normal. The disorder becomes clinically apparent when the triplet is expanded preferentially during maternal meiosis to greater than 200 repeats and the gene is inactivated through methylation with loss of the as yet unknown FMR-1 gene product. However, there is no sharp delineation between the upper limit of normal and the lower limit of the premutation. Forty to 60 copies of the CGG is considered a gray area. Expansion of the repeat from generation to generation varies considerably among families but occurs only when the X chromosome is inherited through a female. Expression also requires inheritance of the X chromosome from a female. Expansion occurs during early embryogenesis so there may be considerable variation between cells in the length of the repeat. It has been observed that the greater the size of the premutation, the greater the risk of expansion to a full mutation (the Sherman Paradox).

Unaffected males who carry the premutation (normal transmitting males) may pass the mutation on to their daughters who will also be unaffected. However, their daughters may pass on the expanded allele to their offspring who are then at risk for expansion to a full mutation and expression of the fragile-X syndrome.

Sutherland and Baker identified a second site of fragility in patients with the cytogenetic changes typical of some patients with fragile-X syndrome but lacking the molecular changes.[29] This site has been designated FRAXE and is 150 to 600 kb distal to FMR-1. FRAXE has since been cloned and patients expressing this site have evidence of amplification of a GCC repeat adjacent to a CpG island in Xq28. Normal individuals have 6 to 25 copies of the repeat whereas patients with mental retardation have more than 200 copies.[30] As with FMR-1, there is also evidence of methylation of the CpG island in affected individuals. Expansion of the GCC repeat at the FRAXE site generally results in a milder degree of mental retardation than that which is seen in patients with the FMR-1 mutation.

Huntington Disease (HD)

Huntington disease (HD) is a progressive neurologic disorder characterized by chorea, dementia, rigidity, seizures, and frequently, psychiatric symptoms. It has been observed that the offspring of affected males have significantly younger age of onset than the offspring of affected females and is thought to result from paternal genomic imprinting involving DNA methylation.[31] Late-onset cases are much more likely to be inherited from an affected mother.

HD is inherited as an autosomal dominant trait. The gene is on the short arm of chromosome 4 and is now known as huntingtin. It contains an expanded, unstable CAG triplet repeat in HD patients. The risk of expansion is greater during spermatogenesis than in oogenesis. The normal range of CAG repeats is 11–34 copies, 30–37 copies define the premutation, and the disease is expressed when 38–86 copies are present.

Myotonic Dystrophy (MD)

Myotonic dystrophy is characterized by myotonia, muscular dystrophy as well as cataracts, hypogonadism, cardiac arrhyth-

mias, and frontal balding. Symptoms usually appear in midlife but age of onset may be considerably earlier. Distal muscles of the extremities are initially affected with later involvement of proximal muscles of the extremities, the extraocular and facial muscles.

The gene is located on chromosome 19 and codes for a protein kinase. The defect is an amplification of a CTG triplet repeat. Less than 30 copies of the repeat is considered normal, 30–50 copies is consistent with the premutation, while overt expression is seen with greater than 50 copies. The severity of the disease is directly correlated with the number of copies. Mildly affected patients will have from 50–80 copies while the most severely affected patients may have over 2000 copies. The expanded repeats affect DNA methylation and chromatin structure and inhibiting expression of adjacent genes. There is no apparent affect on transcription or on the structure of the gene product. Amplification is observed but only when transmission is maternal. The most severe congenital form is seen in offspring of affected women. Thus, MD is both a trinucleotide and imprinting disorder.

Spinocerebellar Ataxia Type I (SCA1)

Spinocerebellar ataxia Type I (SCA1) is a neurodegenerative disease characterized by ataxia, progressive dementia, and spasticity. Symptoms usually begin in the third or fourth decade of life.

The gene for SCA1 has been mapped to chromosome 6. The mutation consists of a CAG repeat expansion. Early-onset disease is associated with a larger number of repeats and paternal transmission. In this disease, 25–36 repeats is considered normal, 35–43 constitutes the premutation, while 42–81 coincides with expression of the disease.

Spinal and Bulbar Muscular Atrophy (Kennedy Disease)

Spinal and bulbar muscular atrophy was first described by Kennedy in 9 males in 2 unrelated kindreds in 1968. Fasciculations followed by muscle weakness and wasting occurred at approximately 40 years of age. Pyramidal, sensory, and cerebellar signs were absent. The disorder is compatible with long life. The main feature of Kennedy disease distinguishing it from autosomal recessive and autosomal dominant forms of SMA, is the presence of sensory abnormalities. Gynecomastia is frequently the first clinical sign suggesting androgen deficiency and estrogen excess.

The gene for spinal and bulbar muscular atrophy has been mapped to Xq11-q12 and is inherited as an X-linked autosomal disorder. La Spada et al. discovered enlargement of a tandem CAG repeat within the first exon of the androgen receptor (AR) gene, in each of 35 unrelated SBMA patients.[34] The AR CAG repeat is normally polymorphic, with an average repeat number of 22 ± 3. In SBMA patients, these investigators found 11 different (CAG)n alleles, with repeat numbers ranging from 40–52. The AR gene abnormality was found to segregate with the disease in 15 SBMA families. The CAG repeat correlates with disease severity such that the mildest clinical manifestations are associated with the smallest CAG repeat. However, other factors seem to contribute to phenotypic variability. As with other diseases resulting from triplet repeat expansion, expansion tends to vary with gender. In the case of Kennedy disease, there is a greater rate of instability and subsequent expansion in male meiosis than in female meiosis.

SUMMARY

Nontraditional inheritance is recognized with increasing frequency, as the explanation for the inheritance of a diverse and increasing number of single gene disorders. Such nonclassical modes of inheritance include mitochondrial inheritance, genomic imprinting, uniparental disomy, mosaicism, and trinucleotide repeat expansion. Examples of disorders associated with each of the above mechanisms will undoubtedly grow as the molecular basis of medical disorders continues to be elucidated and gene defects linked to medical diseases emerge through the Human Genome Project.

The era of epigenetics is just beginning. These heritable changes in gene function, without the need for changes in primary DNA sequence, will be a source of intense investigation over the next decade. It is undoubtedly through such mechanisms that we see variation between supposedly "identical" twins. While only the "tip of the iceberg" is currently evident, we do know that such changes are labile, reversible, and undergo dynamic reprogramming. Such changes are mediated by differential gene expression or other mechanisms involving DNA methylation, chromatin structure, histone modification, and protein changes. Epigenetic programming regulates the combination of genes expressed in each cell and allows tissue specific genes to be programmed to be expressed in certain cells and repressed in others. A decade from now, we will certainly see epigenetic changes as truly a second genetic code with almost as much importance to normal functioning as the original one.

References

1. Nikoskelainen E, Wanne O, Dahl M. Pre-excitation syndrome and Leber's hereditary optic neuroretinopathy. (Letter) *Lancet.* 1985;1:696.
2. Vikki J, Ott J, Savontaus M, et al. Optic atrophy in Leber Hereditary Optic Neuroretinopathy is determined by an X-chromosomal gene closely linked to DXS7. *Am J Hum Genet.* 1991;45:206–211.
3. Shoffner JM, Lott MT, Lezza AMS, et al. Myoclonic epilepsy and ragged-red fiber disease (MERRF) is associated with a mitochondrial DNA tRNA-lys mutation. *Cell.* 1990;61:931–937.
4. Goto Y, Nonaka I, Horai S. A mutation in the tRNA leu(vir) gene associated with the MELAS subgroup of mitochondrial encephalolmyopathy. *Nature.* 1990;348:651–653.
5. Holt IJ, Harding AE, Petty RK, et al. A new mitochondrial disease associated with mitochondrial DNA heteoplasmy. *Am J Hum Genet.* 1990;46:428–433.
6. Alcolado JC, Thomas AW. Maternally inherited diabetes mellitus: the role of mitochondrial DNA defects. *Diabetic Med.* 1995;12:102–108.
7. Martin AO, Simpson JL, Ober C, et al. Frequency of diabetes mellitus in mothers of probands with gestational diabetes: possible maternal influence on the predisposition to gestational diabetes. *Am J Obstet Gynecol.* 1985;151:471–475.
8. Alcolado JC, Majid A, Brockington M, et al. Mitochondrial gene defects in patients with NIDDM. *Diabetologia* 1994;37: 372–376.
9. Magenis RE, Brown MG, Lacy DA, et al. Is Angelman syndrome an alternate result of lel(15)(q11q13)? *Am J Med Genet.* 1987;28:829–838.
10. Nicholls RD, Knoll JH, Butler MG, et al. Genetic imprinting suggested by maternal heterodisomy in non-deletion Prader-Willi syndrome. *Nature.* 1899;342:281–285.
11. Magenis RE, Fejel-Toth S, Allen LJ, et al. Comparison of the 15q deletions in Prader-Willi and Angelman syndromes: Specific regions, extent of deletions, parental origin, and clinical consequences. *Am J Med Genet.* 1990;35:333–349.
12. Weksberg R, Shen DR, Fei YL, et al. Disruption of insulin like growth factor 2 imprinting in Beckwith-Wiedemann syndrome. *Nature Genet.* 1993;5:143–150.
13. Razin A, Kantor B. DNA methylation in epigenetic control of gene expression. *Prog Mol Subcell Biol* 2005;38:151–167.
14. Latham KE: X chromosome imprinting and inactivation in pre-implantation mammalian embryos. *Trends Genet* 2005;21:120–127.
15. Dong C, Geller F, Gorlova OY, et al. Possible genomic imprinting of three human obesity-related genetic loci. *Am J Human Genet* 2005;76:427–437.
16. Seitz H, Royo H, Youngson N, et al. Imprinted small RNA genes. *Biol Chem.* 2004;385:905–911.
17. Wrzeska M, Rejduch B. Genomic imprinting in mammals. *J Appl Genet* 2004; 45:427–433.
18. Maher ER, Afnan M, Barratt CL. Epigenetic risks related to assisted reproductive technologies: epigenetics, imprinting, ART, and icebergs. *Human Reprod* 2003;18:2508–2511.
19. Merlob P, Sapir O, Sulkes J. Fisch B. The prevalence of congenital malformations during two periods of time, 1986–1994 and 1995–2002 in newborns conceived by assisted reproductive technology. *Eur J Med Genet.* 2005;48:5–11.
20. Lidegaard O, Pinborg A, Andersen AN. Imprinting diseases and IVF: Danish national IVF cohort. *Human Reprod.* 2005;20:950–954.
21. Engel E. A new genetic concept. Uniparental disomy and its potential effect, isodisomy. *Am J Med Genet.* 1980;6:137–143.
22. Spence JE, Perciaccante RG, Greig GM, et al. Uniparental disomy as a mechanism for human genetic disease. *Am J Hum Genet.* 1988;42:217–226.
23. Chatkupt S, Antonowicz M, Johnson WG. Parents do matter: genomic imprinting and prenatal sex effects in neurological disorders. *J Neurological Sci.* 1995;130:1–10.
24. Vidaud D, Vidaud M, Plassa F, et al. Father-to-son transmission of hemophilia A due to uniparental disomy. 1989; *40th Ann Meet Am Soc Hum Genet.* Abstract 889.
25. Wolstenholme J. An audit of trisomy 16 in man. *Prenat Diag.* 1995;15:109–121.
26. Engel E. Uniparental disomy revisited: the first twelve years. *Am J Med Genet.* 1993;46:670–674.
27. Erickson RP, Lewis SE. The new human genetics. *Environmental and Molec Mutagenesis.* 1995;25:Supplement 26:7–12.
28. Migeon BR. Role of DNA methylation in X inactivation and the fragile X syndrome. *Am J Med Genet.* 1993;47:685–686.

29. Sutherland GR, Baker E. Characterisation of a new rare fragile site easily confused with the fragile X. *Hum Molec Genet.* 1992;1:111–113.

30. Knight SJL, Voelckel MA, Hirst MC, et al. Triplet repeat expansion at the FRAXE locus and X-linked mild mental handicap. *Am J Hum Genet.* 1994;55:81–86.

31. Ridley RM, Frith CD, Crow TJ, et al. Anticipation in Huntington's disease is inherited through the male line but may originate in the female. *J Med Genet.* 1988;25:589–595.

32. Orr HT, Chung M, Banfi S, et al. Expansion of an unstable trinucleotide CAG repeat in spinocerebellar ataxia type 1. *Nature Genet.* 1993;4:221–226.

33. Kennedy WR, Alter M, Sung JH. Progressive proximal spinal and bulbar muscular atrophy of late onset: a sex-linked recessive trait. *Neurology* 1968;18:671–680.

34. La Spada AR, Wilson EM, Lubahn DB, et al. Androgen receptor gene mutations in X-linked spinal and bulbar muscular atrophy. *Nature.* 1991;352:77–79.

CHROMOSOMAL ABERRATIONS

Shay Ben Shahar / Avi Orr-Urtreger / Yuval Yaron

INTRODUCTION

Cytogenetic disorders such as Down syndrome are at the forefront of both patient's and physician's consciousness when prenatal diagnosis comes to mind. Although Down syndrome represents no more than half of abnormal findings, the mindset of society, the media, and medical practice is geared toward this particular disorder.

To understand the spectrum of chromosomal abnormalities, this chapter will review a number of the more common disorders that are seen. More extensive descriptions are available in pediatrics and genetics textbooks, and the interested reader will have no trouble finding very detailed descriptions of the pediatric, and in some cases adult, sequelae of these disorders.

No chapter on these disorders would be complete without at least some mention of the laboratory analyses necessary to find the diagnosis. A more complete description of the cytogenetics laboratory approaches is presented in Chapter 41.

GENERAL CYTOGENETIC PRINCIPLES

A chromosome within the cell nucleus consists of a continuous molecule of deoxyribonucleic acid (DNA) and specific associated proteins. The DNA molecule is a polymer composed of 3 different subunits, a deoxyribose sugar, a phosphate group, and one of 4 nitrogen-containing bases: adenine, thymine, guanine, and cytosine (A, T, G, and C). The sequence of these nucleotides encodes the genetic information in the form of $\sim$30,000 genes. It is estimated that DNA within a cell contains some 3×10^9 base pairs, and if stretched would be about 1 meter long. The associated proteins, the basic histones, are responsible for the high degree of DNA compaction. With the exception of germ cells (sperm cells and oocytes), each nucleated human cell contains 46 chromosomes in 23 pairs. Of these, 22 pairs are similar in both males and in females—the autosomes—each pair numbered from 1 through 22, from longest to shortest. The remaining pair comprises the sex chromosomes, consisting of two X chromosomes in females, or one X chromosome and one Y chromosome in males (Fig. 4-1). One chromosome of each pair is inherited from the father through the sperm, and the other from the mother, through the oocyte.

Cytogenetics is the study of the genetic material on the chromosomes at the microscopic level. The name chromosome refers to its staining properties with certain biological dyes (chroma = color, soma = body). The chromosomes may be visualized as discrete entities only during prophase and metaphase. During most of the cell cycle however, the chromosomes are decondensed. Hence, specific techniques must

be used to enrich the proportion of cells at the metaphase stage, and various staining protocols are applied to allow visualization of the chromosomes. Chromosome analyses are commonly performed for prenatal diagnosis, birth defects, multiple malformations, familial disorders, mental retardation, infertility, history of recurrent miscarriages, and acquired malignant disorders.

Cytogenetic testing may be performed on most fresh tissues provided its cells undergo replication. This may include such cells as blood lymphocytes, bone marrow cells, skin fibroblasts, amniocytes, chorionic villi, or solid tumors. In general, the investigation of chromosomal abnormalities in humans involves the examination of dividing cells by blocking the cell cycle at, or before, metaphase using an inhibitor of the mitotic spindle formation (e.g., colchicine). Subsequent processing includes treatment with a hypotonic solution to swell the cells, followed by a series of fixations to preserve the cells and enhance the morphology of the chromosomes. After appropriate pretreatment, the cells undergo staining which allows identification of the individual chromosomes. Finally, the cells are visualized and evaluated using light microscopy.

STANDARD CYTOGENETIC TECHNIQUES

The most useful staining technique is the G-banding in which chromosomes are treated with trypsin to denature the associated proteins, and then stained with Giemsa dye. This produces a characteristic pattern of dark and light bands (Fig. 4-1). Other staining techniques included Q-banding wherein chromosomes are stained with quinacrine mustard and viewed with a fluorescence microscope. C-banding highlights centromeric regions and areas containing heterochromatin. NOR-banding allows visualization of the nucleus organizing regions in the satellite stalks. To properly analyze the chromosomes it is necessary to arrange them in order. This was previously done by actually cutting out the chromosomes from a photomicrograph and arranging them according to standard classification, thereby creating the karyotype—a photographic documentation of a representative mitotic spread analyzed in one typical cell. In the karyotype, the chromosomes are arranged in matching pairs aligned at their centromeres, with the shorter arm (p) up and the long arm (q) down.[1] Today these tasks are carried out virtually on a computer screen using dedicated software.

MOLECULAR CYTOGENETIC TECHNIQUES

In addition to the standard cytogenetic techniques, several promising new methods have originated from the interface between cytogenetics and molecular biology, commonly referred to as molecular cytogenetics. In general, these techniques employ labeled DNA probed that allow visualization of specific chromosomal targets.

Fluorescence in situ hybridization (FISH) is a sensitive and a relatively fast method for direct visualization of specific nucleotide sequences. It is based on the fact that

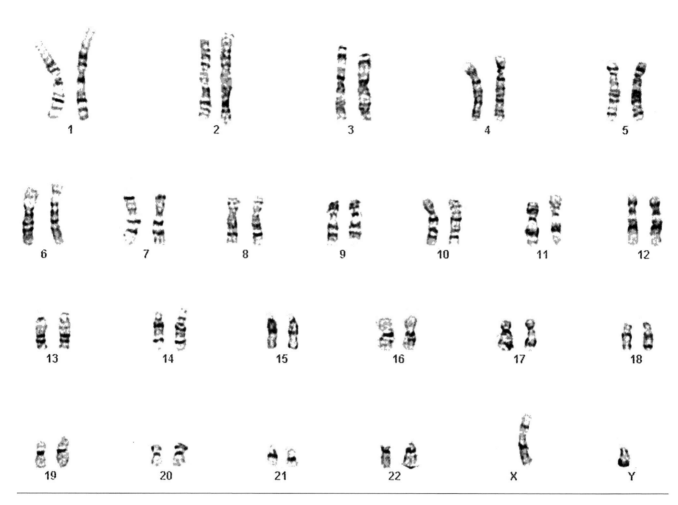

FIGURE 4-1 Normal male karyotype.

single-stranded DNA can anneal to complementary DNA strands to form a double-stranded helix, under proper conditions. The probe is composed of a specific DNA segment that incorporates modified nucleotides that are tagged by fluorescence or other detectable markers. One of the major advantages of FISH over the standard methods is its ability to recognize subtle chromosomal changes such as deletions or duplications. Specific FISH probes are used to recognize specific microdeletions (such DiGeorge/velo-cardio-facial syndrome, or Prader-Willi/Angelman syndrome).[2] In addition, and unlike standard cytogenetic techniques, FISH may be applied to interphase nuclei of nondividing cells, obviating the need for cell culture which usually requires 10–14 days (Fig. 4-2). FISH significantly shortens the procedure time for analysis of numerical aberrations in prenatal diagnosis, and preimplantation genetic diagnosis.[3,4,5] However, structural aberrations cannot usually be detected with this technique. Furthermore, even in cases of known trisomies, not all cells demonstrate three fluorescent signals due to overlapping of the target chromosomes in the interphase nucleus.

FISH is also limited to specific purposes due to the high cost and the need, in most cases to have prior knowledge or suspicion of the specific chromosome aberration. It is currently

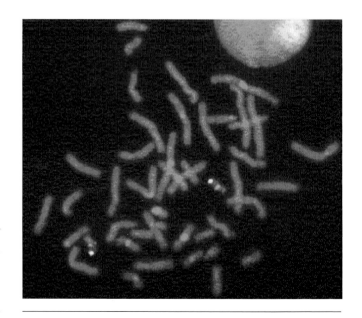

FIGURE 4-2 FISH.

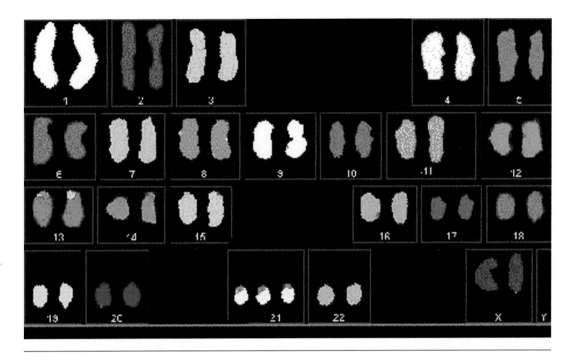

FIGURE 4-3 Multicolored FISH (M-FISH).

advised that this technique does not replace, but rather supplement standard cytogenetic techniques.

Multicolored FISH (M-FISH) is a molecular cytogenetic technique that allows the simultaneous visualization of all 24 chromosomes in a single in situ experiment. With this technique, each chromosome is differentially labeled with a unique combination of fluorescent dyes, which allows the rapid identification of all chromosomes in 24 colors. The analysis may be performed by sequential use of specific filters for each fluorochrome or the use of spectral karyotyping (SKY) which is based on the simultaneous spectral analysis of all fluorescent dyes in the probe mix[6] (Fig. 4-3). SKY may be employed to analyze de novo extra structurally abnormal chromosomes (markers) that cannot be analyzed by standard cytogenetic techniques.[7]

CHROMOSOMAL ABERRATIONS

A precise diploid complement of 46 chromosomes (2n, where n = 23) is required for adequate human development and function. Chromosome abnormalities that can be visualized by standard cytogenetic techniques may potentially involve a concurrent disparity of a large number of genes. Therefore, chromosomal aberrations are commonly incompatible with normal early human development. Indeed, at least 50% of early spontaneous abortions may be due to chromosomal abnormalities. Only a small number of fetuses with chromosomal abnormalities survive, so that the rate of chromosomally abnormal liveborn is only 0.6%. Of these, many succumb within the first weeks or months of postnatal life.

The wide range of chromosome abnormalities may be divided into numerical (aneuploidies) or structural abnormalities (translocations, deletions, and duplications). The frequency of common chromosomal disorders among liveborn infants is presented in Table 4-1.

NUMERICAL ABERRATIONS

Polyploidy (Triploidy and Tetraploidy)

Polyploidy is characterized by the presence of complete extra haploid set(s) of 23 chromosomes in excess of the normal diploid (2n) complement. Examples include triploidy (3n, 69 chromosomes) and tetraploidy (4n, 92 chromosomes). Triploidy may arise as the result of: fertilization by two spermatozoa(dispermy)—the most common cause in humans

TABLE 4-1	FREQUENCY OF COMMON CHROMOSOMAL ABERRATIONS AMONG LIVEBORN INFANTS	
	Disorders	*Frequency*
Autosomal abnormalities	Trisomy 21	1 in 800
	Trisomy 18	1 in 5000
	Trisomy 13	1 in 15,000
Sex chromosome abnormalities	Klinefelter syndrome (47,XXY)	1 in 700 males
	47,XYY syndrome	1 in 800 males
	47,XXX syndrome	1 in 1000 females
	Turner syndrome (45,X or mosaics)	1 in 1500 females

fertilization by a diploid sperm or fertilization of a diploid oocyte, a result of paternal or maternal meiotic error, respectively. Triploidy rarely exists in viable neonates, where it is usually in mosaic form. Triploidy, however, is a common finding in spontaneous abortions accounting for about 16% of cytogenetically abnormal early spontaneous abortions. The phenotypic expression of triploidy depends on the parental origin of the extra haploid set. Triploidy with an extra paternal set is often associated with excessive development of the placenta, resulting in molar pregnancy. Triploidy associated with an extra set of maternal origin most commonly results in spontaneous abortion. Tetraploidy accounts for ~5% of cytogenetically abnormal early spontaneous abortions. Tetraploidies are always 92,XXXX or 92,XXYY suggesting an error in the early division of the zygote.

Aneuploidy

Individuals are referred to as aneuploid if they have fewer or more chromosomes than the exact multiple of the haploid set. These account for slightly over half of the chromosomal anomalies present in liveborn infants. The most prevalent aneuploidies are trisomies (an extra chromosome), monosomies (a missing chromosome), and mosaics (the presence of more than one cell line, each having a different number of chromosomes).

Trisomy

The most frequent numeric abnormality is trisomy, in which three copies of a given chromosome exist in the cell, instead of two, resulting in a total of 47 chromosomes per cell. For example, trisomy 21 implies that all cells of such individuals have 3 copies of chromosome 21. This is described by present nomenclature as 47,XX,+21 or 47,XY,+21 (1). The most frequent cause of trisomy is nondisjunction, whereby the chromosome-pair fails to separate during meiosis I or II. This results in one monosomic daughter cell having 45 chromosomes, a state usually incompatible with cellular viability, and the other daughter cell having an extra chromosome (trisomy). Nondisjunction is more frequent in maternal meiosis than in paternal meiosis. Maternal meiotic nondisjunction occurs with an exponentially increasing frequency with advancing maternal age. Conversely, paternal meiotic nondisjunction is not age-related and thus may be found in offspring of younger parents. The most frequent autosomal trisomies found in liveborn infants (in decreasing order of frequency) are trisomy 21, 18, and 13, respectively. Other autosomal trisomies, such as trisomy 16 and 22, are commonly seen in spontaneous abortions but never in liveborn.

Monosomy

Monosomy is characterized by the presence of only one representative of a given chromosome pair in the cell. Most monosomies are embryologically lethal, the only exception known in humans is monosomy X (45,X; Turner syndrome).

Mosaicism

Nondisjunction can also occur in mitosis, and thus result in mosaicism, a situation where at least two cell lines are present:

the original one, derived from the zygote, and the second, derived after the nondisjunction event. Not uncommonly however, there are more than two cell lines present. The phenotypic expression of the mosaicism depends on the proportion of the different cell lines and their distribution in different tissues and organ systems. The phenotype in these cases is usually an intermediate between the normal and the fully aneuploid. Mosaicism for autosomal trisomy is relatively rare, although some well-described syndromes exist (i.e., mosaic trisomy 8). Mosaicism for sex chromosome aberrations however, is relatively common. These may sometimes be discovered only with the evaluation of infertility in the presence of premature ovarian failure and male infertility.

AUTOSOMAL ANEUPLOIDIES

Trisomy 21 (Down Syndrome)

Down syndrome, is characterized by hypotonicity, brachycepahly with flat facies and mild microcephaly, upslanted palpebral fissures and speckling of the iris (Brushfield spots), small ears, short metacarpals and phalanges, hypoplasia of the midphalanx of the fifth digit with clinodactyly, single palmar crease, wide gap between the first and second toes, joint hypermobility, cardiac anomalies including endocardial cushion defect (A-V canal), ventricular septal defect (VSD), patent ductus arteriosus, increased incidence of leukemia (~1%), gastrointestinal abnormalities including tracheo-esophageal fistulas and duodenal atresia, and mental deficiency. The intelligence quotient (IQ) is usually about 50 although it may approach 65–70 in some individuals. The major cause of early mortality is congenital heart disease. Trisomy 21 occurs in about 1 in 800 births. The incidence of trisomy 21 increases with advanced maternal age (Table 4-2). The likelihood for

TABLE 4-2	MATERNAL AGE-RELATED RISK OF TRISOMY 21 IN LIVEBORNS		
Maternal Age	Risk	Maternal Age	Risk
15–19	1/1560	33	1/545
20	1/1540	34	1/445
21	1/1520	35	1/355
22	1/1490	36	1/280
23	1/1450	37	1/220
24	1/1410	38	1/170
25	1/1350	39	1/130
26	1/1280	40	1/97
27	1/1200	41	1/73
28	1/1110	42	1/55
29	1/1010	43	1/41
30	1/890	44	1/30
31	1/775	45	1/23
32	1/660	46	1/17

Adapted from Hecht CA, Hook EB. The imprecision in rates of Down syndrome by 1-year maternal age intervals: a critical analysis of rates used in biochemical screening. *Prenat Diagn.* 1994;14:729.

recurrence of Down syndrome in a subsequent pregnancy is empirically 1%.

The presence of an extra chromosome 21 is attributed to meiotic nondisjunction in 95% of liveborn with Down syndrome. About 3% are the result of Robertsonian translocations, of which half are inherited and half are de novo, and 2% have trisomy 21 mosaicism. Thus, 98% of all patients with Down syndrome have a noninherited type. Patients having Down syndrome due to a Robertsonian translocation are clinically indistinguishable from those who have an additional free chromosome 21.

Trisomy 18 (Edwards Syndrome)

Trisomy 18 is the second most frequent autosomal chromosome abnormality. The majority of trisomy 18 cases are due to nondisjunction, and empirical recurrence risks for this disorder are less than 1%. More than 130 different structural abnormalities have been reported in patients with trisomy 18, including growth deficiency, hypoplasia of skeletal muscle, subcutaneous and adipose tissue, prominent occiput, narrow forehead, low-set malformed ears, short palpebral fissures and small oral opening, clenched hand with overlapping second finger over third, and fifth finger over forth, short hallux, nail hypoplasia, short sternum, redundant skin with mild hirsutism, and cardiac defects. Less commonly found are cleft lip and palate, hypoplastic to absent thumb, rocker-bottom feet, Meckel's diverticulum, omphalocele, and horse-shoe kidney. The majority of these infants die in the neonatal period despite optimal management due to "failure to thrive," and only 5–10% survive the first year of life. Those that do, have severe mental deficiency though some degree of psychomotor maturation and learning occurs and limited social interaction is possible.

Trisomy 13 (Patau Syndrome)

This is the third most common autosomal trisomy occurring in about 1 in 5000 livebirths. Most cases are due to nondisjunction and advanced maternal age has been implicated. Recurrence risk is presumably low. Trisomy 13 is commonly associated with holoprosencephaly varying in severity from cyclopia or cebocephaly to less severe forms. Other manifestations include microcephaly with sloping forehead, capillary hemangiomata, localized scalp defects, microphthalmia, colobomata, cleft lip and palate, polydactyly, narrow hyperconvex fingernails, cardiac defects, single umbilical artery, structural kidney malformations, and omphalocele. As with trisomy 18, most trisomy 13 conceptions result in miscarriage. Those that survive to term, often succumb within the first days of life, usually of complex heart disease, and only about 5% survive past the first 6 months. Survivors have severe mental deficiency, minor motor seizures with a hypsarrhythmic EEG pattern, and failure to thrive.

Sex Chromosome Aneuploidies

There are four clearly defined syndromes associated with the sex chromosomes (X and Y). These include a monosomy X (Turner syndrome, 45,X), and three trisomies (47,XXY—Klinefelter syndrome, 47,XYY, and 47,XXX). The effects of these chromosomal aberrations on development have been prospectively studied in newborns with sex chromosome aneuploidies.[8]

Monosomy X (Turner Syndrome)

Monosomy X occurs most commonly because of nondisjunction. In the majority the single X chromosome is of maternal origin, suggesting that the nondisjunction event occurred in the father and is therefore unrelated to maternal age. With the advent of ultrasound, these fetuses are increasingly being recognized in utero, presenting with increased nuchal translucency in the first trimester and later with large cystic hygroma of the neck. The cause of the cystic hygroma is usually obstruction at the connection between the lymphatic and venous system at the jugular junction. In some fetuses with monosomy X, it may also be caused by coarctation of the aorta.

Though the incidence of monosomy X in liveborn is rather low (∼1 in 5000 live female births), it is the single most common abnormality found in early spontaneous abortions, accounting for as many as 20% of cytogenetically abnormal gestations. About 99% of such fetuses abort spontaneously and only a minority survive to term. Individuals with Turner syndrome may manifest a characteristic phenotype including swelling of hands and feet at birth, short stature with onset around 6 years of age, gonadal dysgenesis, webbed neck, low hairline, broad chest with widely spaced nipples, congenital heart disease including coarctation of the aorta, and horseshoe kidneys. If untreated, these individuals fail to develop secondary sexual characteristics in puberty and usually present with primary amenorrhea, and later complications of hypoestrogenism. Hormone replacement therapy in the form of combination estrogen and progesterone therapy may alleviate some of the growth deficiency, and induce secondary sexual maturation as well as menses. Growth hormone supplement may assist to gain height if given before bone maturation. While some learning difficulties may be encountered, these individuals are intellectually normal and often lead normal and meaningful lives, although needing in some instances social support. Childbearing for these patients has now become possible using donated oocytes.[9] Most patients with Turner syndrome have 45,X however ∼50% of patients have other karyotypes such as a mosaicism with only a proportion of cells being 45,X, structural abnormalities of the X chromosome, such as deletions of the long or short arm, isochromosomes of the long arm, or translocations.

47,XXY (Klinefelter Syndrome)

Patients with 47,XXY have a normal male phenotype at birth and during childhood. At the onset of puberty however, they appear relatively tall and thin, and in the absence of corrective hormonal therapy, demonstrate signs of hypogonadism, and gynecomastia. Their testes remain small and they are almost invariably infertile. Although no major malformations are associated with this syndrome, patients usually have IQ scores that are 10–15 points lower than their siblings. In addition, there is an increased incidence of learning difficulties, immaturity, and emotional and behavioral problems.

Klinefelter syndrome is one of the most common causes of male infertility with an incidence of about 1 in 1000 liveborn males. It is estimated that about half of the conceptions with a 47,XXY karyotype are spontaneously aborted, despite the fact the phenotype is rather benign. The nondisjunctional error appears to be paternal meiosis I in about 50% of the cases, maternal meiosis I in about 33%, and meiosis II in the remainder. About 15% of Klinefelter syndrome are mosaic, most commonly 47,XXY/46,XY. These are usually the result of mitotic nondisjunction in the early embryonic stages.

47,XYY Syndrome

The estimated incidence is about 1 in 1000, however the physical signs are often so subtle that many cases go undetected. The origin of the XYY karyotype is paternal meiosis II. Abnormal findings may include accelerated growth in mid childhood, reaching a final taller stature than their siblings. Severe nodulocystic acne may develop in adolescence. They are usually fertile, and there have been rare reports of transmission of the abnormal karyotype from father to son. Though initially suspected of mental deficiency and aggressive behavior, this does not appear to be the case in longitudinal studies, albeit a slight decrease in IQ has be observed.[8]

47,XXX (Trisomy X) Syndrome

The incidence of trisomy X is about 1 in 1000 female newborns. There are usually no apparent phenotypic abnormalities although they may be taller than average. Sexual development is usually normal in these women and they are generally fertile with normal offspring. Occasionally, there may be some degree of developmental delay and learning problems in such patients.

RARE SEX-CHROMOSOME ANEUPLOIDIES

Rare sex chromosome aneuploidies are those with more than one extra chromosome including 48,XXXX (tetrasomy X), 49,XXXXX (pentasomy X), 48,XXXY, and 48,XXYY. The presence of a Y chromosome determines the male phenotype, and as a rule of thumb, the more sex chromosomes present, the greater the probability of the dysmorphism and mental deficiency.

STRUCTURAL CHROMOSOMAL ABNORMALITIES

Structural chromosomal rearrangements are caused by initial chromosome breakage, followed by abnormal reconstitution, occurring in about 1 in 500 live births. These abnormalities are generally divided into balanced and unbalanced rearrangements. Balanced rearrangements do not usually have a significant phenotypic presentation in their carriers. This is because all chromosomal material is present, albeit arranged in a different order. The concern in such balanced rearrangements

is for the progeny, since carriers of balanced rearrangements may have chromosomally unbalanced gametes that may lead to chromosomally imbalanced offspring. Rarely however, disruption of genes occurs at the chromosomal breakpoints, resulting in mutation even in "apparently balanced" carriers. Unbalanced rearrangements are characterized by missing or additional chromosomal material, usually manifested by abnormal phenotypes or miscarriages.

BALANCED REARRANGEMENTS

Translocations

There are two basic types of translocations: Robertsonian and reciprocal. Each can be either inherited as a familial trait, or de novo, occurring for the first time in an individual.

Robertsonian Translocations

Robertsonian translocations result in the centric fusion of two acrocentric chromosomes (a chromosome in which the centromere is near the end: 13, 14, 15, 21, or 22). A Robertsonian translocation is said to be balanced, if there are no phenotypic or clinical effects apparent in the carrier. However, carriers of balanced Robertsonian translocations are at risk of having offspring with an unbalanced Robertsonian translocations, with trisomy or monosomy for one of the fused chromosomes, depending on the pattern of segregation at meiosis. A Robertsonian translocation carrier, can theoretically have 6 possible types of gametes leading to 6 theoretically possible zygotes including 1 normal, 1 balanced translocation, and 4 unbalanced forms (trisomy or monosomy). Only the minority of unbalanced Robertsonian monosomic and trisomic conceptions are compatible with life, and most result in a miscarriage. A theoretical risk for spontaneous miscarriages and viable infants having unbalanced translocation can be calculated for each Robertsonian translocation but fortunately the practical risk for unbalanced offspring is much lower. Balanced Robertsonian translocation between chromosome 14 and 21 is the second most common among humans and carry a risk for offspring having trisomy 21 (Down syndrome) with practical incidence of 2.4%.[10] The rare de novo Robertsonian translocation 21;21 inevitably results in trisomy 21 in the offspring.[11]

When a balanced translocation carrier is identified within a family, usually after the birth of a malformed infant with an unbalanced karyotype, it is imperative that other family members be evaluated. This would include chromosomal analysis for all relevant individuals, supportive genetic counseling, and prenatal diagnosis when applicable. On the other hand, recurrence risks for a couple who has had an infant with aneuploidy resulting from a spontaneous, noninherited or de novo Robertsonian translocation are empirically comparable to the recurrence risks for a nondisjunctional event, about 1%. Prenatal diagnosis is indicated in all such situations during a subsequent pregnancy.

Reciprocal Translocations

Balanced reciprocal translocations involve exchange of segments between chromosomes of two different pairs without

TABLE 4-3 | **SOME CHROMOSOME DELETION AND MICRODELETION SYNDROMES**

Syndrome	Deletion	Phenotype
Wolf-Hirschhorn S.	4p–	Hypertelorism, cleft lip/palate, microcephaly, down-turned mouth, MR
Cri du chat S.	5p–	Cat-like cry, microcephaly, downslanting palpebral fissures, MR
Microdeletions		
Prader-Willi S.[a]	15q11.2	Hypotonia, hypogonadism, obesity, small hands and feet, MR
Angelman S.[a]	15q11.2	Severe MR, ataxia, paroxysmal laughter
DiGeorge S.[b]	22q11.2	Absent thymus and parathyroids, heart defects
Velo-cardio-facial S.[b]	22q11.2	Heart defects, cleft palate, developmental delay
Miller-Dieker S.	17p13.3	Lissencephaly, microcephaly, severe MR
Williams S.	7q11.23	Dysmorphic features, cardiac defects, "outgoing" personality, MR

MR—mental retardation.

[a] Although the deletion is similar in both syndromes, the different phenotype is dependent on parent-of-origin, due to genomic imprinting, to be discussed in the chapter on New Genetic Mechanisms.

[b] Both disorders are associated with deletions in similar chromosomal regions and have some overlap.

loss or addition of chromosomal material. Reciprocal translocations occur in about 1 in 500 newborns. As with other balanced chromosomal rearrangements, there is usually no clinical effect on the carrier unless a gene has been disrupted. During meiosis, however, the translocated and normal chromosomes produces different possible gametes according to the different patterns of segregation. The resulting gametes can be both balanced (normal or balanced translocation) or include partial trisomy and partial monosomy of one or the other chromosome. Once a couple has had an infant with an unbalanced karyotype resulting from a parental reciprocal translocation, their risk needs to be assessed on a case by case basis. This is because different translocations carry a different risk for a chromosomally abnormal newborn (between 20% to about 1%.[12] Prenatal diagnosis is strongly indicated in all instances of translocation, and family studies are likewise recommended for all relevant individuals.

INVERSIONS

Inversions occur when two breakpoints are present in a single chromosome and the intervening chromosomal segment is inverted and fused in the opposite direction. There are two types of inversions: pericentric inversions, which include the centromere; and paracentric inversions, not including the centromere. Pericentric inversions may alter the arm ratio in the chromosome and may, in these circumstances, be diagnosed using standard cytogenetic techniques. Some small pericentric inversions (e.g., of chromosome 9) are common and are considered a normal variant. Paracentric inversions, on the other hand, are quite rare. They do not, as a rule, alter the arm ratio of the chromosome and may thus require high-resolution banding for detection. Inversions usually preserve the amount of

chromosomal material, and are therefore considered balanced rearrangements. Occasionally however, the inversion disrupts a gene sequence leading to a mutation (e.g., inversions affecting the factor VIII gene appear to be a common cause of severe hemophilia A.[13] Large pericentric inversions have clinical significance since crossing-over in meiosis may occur within the inversion loop, resulting in an unbalanced chromosomal rearrangement in the gametes (duplication or deletion). Paracentric inversions may result in acentric (having no centromere) or dicentric (having two centromeres) chromosomes, incompatible with embryonic development. Thus the chance that carriers of a paracentric inversion will have abnormal liveborn is very low. When an inversion is discovered for the first time in a prenatal diagnostic setting (CVS or amniocentesis) it is important to obtain the karyotypes of the parents. Inherited balanced translocations, tend to be benign. However, de novo inversions carry an empirical risk of about 6–10% for adverse outcome.

UNBALANCED REARRANGEMENTS

Deletions

Deletions result in a loss of a chromosomal segment leading to partial monosomy. They may arise by one of several mechanisms: (1) chromosome breakage and loss of the distal (acentric) segment, (2) unequal crossing over between misaligned homologous chromosomes or sister chromatids, usually in association with repeated elements, and (3) abnormal segregation from balanced rearrangements (translocations or inversions). Deletions may be terminal involving one breakpoint and loss of the distal, telomeric segment, or interstitial with two breakpoints and fusion of the distal and proximal segments with loss of the intervening segment. A ring chromosome constitutes a special form of deletion, whereby the terminal portions of both arms are lost, with fusion of the 2 proximal ends to form a ring.

The missing chromosomal segment results in partial monosomy and may include numerous genes leading to significant phenotypic abnormalities referred to as contiguous gene syndromes. Some well-described chromosome deletion syndromes are presented in Table 4-3. To detect chromosomal deletions by high-resolution banding to, the size of the deletion has to be at least 2000–3000 Kb in size. Although deletions responsible for clinical syndromes may span large chromosomal regions, the "critical region" that its deletion gives the characteristic appearance of the syndrome may actually be too small to be detected even by such high-resolution techniques.

5p Deletion Syndrome

The partial deletion of the short arm of chromosome 5 is also called "Cri du chat syndrome" because the typical crying of the affected infants resembles a mewing cat. The characteristic facies include microcephaly, hypertelorism, down slanting palpebral fissures and low set ears. Thirty percent of patients have congenital heart disease and mental retardation is invariable. Although most of the cases are sporadic, about 10–15% of the cases are the result of balanced translocation in a parent, with increased risk or recurrence.

4p Deletion Syndrome

The partial deletion of the short arm of chromosome 4 is also called "Wolf-Hirschhorn syndrome." The syndrome includes severe growth and mental retardation, facial anomalies resembling a "Greek mask" including hypertelorism and "fishlike" mouth among other features and hypoplastic dermal ridges. The missing piece may be small in some of the cases and must be investigated thoroughly.

MICRODELETION SYNDROMES

The term microdeletion refers to subtle chromosomal deletions that cannot be seen even with high-resolution standard cytogenetic techniques. Nonetheless, these well-described syndromes are caused by deletions that can be detected with FISH. Some common microdeletions are described in the following sections.

DiGEORGE/VELO CARDIO FACIAL SYNDROME

The clinical spectrum of the deletion of the proximal long arm of chromosome 22 (22q11 deletion syndrome) is variable but can be roughly divided to two syndromes: DiGeorge syndrome and Velocardiofacial (VCF) syndrome with some degree of overlap. The main features of these syndromes include cardiac anomalies, cleft palate, and/or palatal insufficiency particularly velopharyngeal insufficiency, typical faces. Learning disorders with or without mental retardation are commonly observed. Absence of thymus and parathyroid glands with hypocalcaemia are much less common and classically attributed to DiGeorge syndrome and not to VCF. In ~95% of cases, microdeletion of the long arm of chromosome 22 can be detected by FISH. De novo deletions are found in the majority of the cases and only about 5% are inherited from a parent. In the latter, the recurrence arte is 50% in every pregnancy.

PRADER-WILLI AND ANGELMAN SYNDROMES

Prader-Willi and Angelman syndromes are relatively common dysmorphic syndromes characterized by a microdeletion of a specific site in the proximal long arm of chromosome 15, detected in proximally 70% of the cases. Deletion in the paternally derived chromosome results in Prader-Willi syndrome whereas deletion in the maternally derived chromosome results in Angelman syndrome. This is due to imprinting mechanism: a difference in methylation pattern and hence the expression of genes from the paternally and maternally inherited alleles at the same chromosomal locus. These syndromes may also be caused by uniparental disomy or defective methylation.

The clinical phenotype of Prader-Willi syndrome includes mental retardation, hypotonia and hypogonadism. Eating difficulties necessitating gastric-tube feeding are common in early infancy later evolving into eating disorders with obesity.

Angelman syndrome is characterized by severe mental retardation, characteristic facies, paroxysms of laugher and ataxia and arm jerks resemble puppet-like gait (giving the syndrome the inappropriate term "happy puppet").

MILLER-DIEKER SYNDROME

This usually manifests in lissencephaly (incomplete development of the brain cortex) with a smooth surface. The syndrome is caused by a microdeletion of a specific site in the short arm of chromosome 17 that can be detected by FISH. Usually, the deletion is due to unbalanced translocation resulting from balanced translocation of phenotypically normal parents. In addition to lissencephaly, there is often absence of the corpus callosum, microcephaly with bitemporal narrowing, and mental retardation. The forehead is usually high and the nose is small and anteverted.

WILLIAMS SYNDROME

This syndrome results from microdeletion of the long arm of chromosome 7 including the elastin gene. Most cases are sporadic, although familial cases have been described as well. The patients are mentally impaired but have well-preserved language ability and good social skills. There is some degree of facial dysmorphism, and renal anomalies are common as well as cardiac defect. Supravalvular aortic stenosis, a rare cardiac defect is present in 50% of the patients of Williams syndrome. Hypercalcemia can be present in the neonatal period but is uncommon finding later in life.

SUBTELOMERIC REARRANGEMENTS

The subtelomeric chromosomal regions are gene rich and are involved in many instances of rearrangements. Most of the telomeres do not stain with G-banding and therefore small subtelomeric rearrangement are difficult to detect by standard staining techniques. In recent years specific FISH probes were designed to detect subtelomeric rearrangement. Using such probes it was found that 6–9% of patients with idiopathic mental retardation have subtelomeric rearrangements (deletions and duplications).

References

1. An International System for Human Cytogenetic Nomenclature. Report of the Standing Committee on Human Cytogenetic Nomenclature. Mittelman F., ed. Basel: Karger; 1995.

2. Carey AH, Kelly D, Halford S, et al. Molecular genetic study of the frequency of monosomy 22q11 in DiGeorge syndrome. *Am J Hum Genet*. 1992;51:964.

3. Verlinsky Y, Cieslak J, Freidine M, et al. Polar body diagnosis of common aneuploidies by FISH. *J Assist Reprod Genet*. 1996;13:157.

4. Munne S, Weier HU, Stein J, et al. A fast and efficient method for simultaneous X and Y in situ hybridization of human blastomeres. *J Assist Reprod Genet*. 1993;10:82.

5. Munne S, Tang YX, Grifo J, et al. Sex determination of human embryos using the polymerase chain reaction and confirmation by fluorescence in situ hybridization. *Fertil Steril*. 1994;61:111.

6. Schröck E, du Manoir S, Veldman T, et al. Multicolor spectral karyotyping of human chromosomes. *Science* 1996;273:494.

7. Yaron Y, Carmon E, Goldstein M, et al. The clinical application of spectral karyotyping (SKY™) in the analysis of prenatally diagnosed extra structurally abnormal chromosomes (ESACs). *Prenat Diagn*. 2003;23:74–79.

8. Ratcliffe SG, Paul N, eds. Prospective studies on children with sex chromosome aneuploidy. March of Dimes Birth Defects Foundation, Birth Defects Original Article Series 23(3). New York: Alan Liss; 1986.

9. Yaron Y, Ochshorn Y, Amit A, et al. Patients with Turner syndrome may have an inherent endometrial abnormality affecting receptivity in oocyte donation. *Fertil Steril*. 1996;65:1249–1252.

10. Hamerton JL. Robertsonian translocations. In: Jacobs PA, Price WH, Law P, eds. *Human Population Genetics*. Baltimore: Lippincott, Williams & Wilkins; 1970.

11. Steinberg C, Zackai EH, Eunpu DL, et al. Recurrence rate for de novo 21q21q translocation Down syndrome: A study of 112 families. *Am J Med Genet*. 1984;17:523.

12. Gardner RJM, Sutherland GR, eds. *Autosomal Reciprocal Translocations. In: Chromosome Abnormalities and Genetic Counseling*. New York: Oxford University Press; 1996.

13. Lakich D, Kazazian Jr HH, Antonarakis SE, et al. Inversions disrupting the factor VIII gene are a common cause of severe haemophilia A. *Nat Genet*. 1993;5:236.

MENDELIAN GENETICS IN PRENATAL DIAGNOSIS

Bruce R. Korf

The field of medical genetics was launched with the discovery of familial transmission of disorders by the British physician Archibald Garrod. It is therefore fitting that the 20th century ended with the completion of the first draft of the human genome, in which the sequence of the 25,000 or so genes has become known.[1] Molecular genetics has brought new insight into the pathogenesis of disease, as well as new approaches to diagnosis and treatment. Taking a family history, however, remains the cornerstone of the prenatal genetic evaluation, permitting the counselor or physician to identify problems for which a couple may be at risk. In this chapter, we will review the basic principles of single gene inheritance in humans. Although the focus will be on genetic transmission, we will also consider insights from molecular genetics that have elucidated some of the mechanisms that underlie Mendelian inheritance.

BASIC PRINCIPLES

The basis for Mendelian inheritance is the fact that the human is a diploid organism. There are 22 pairs of non-sex chromosomes, and therefore a person inherits a copy of each non-sex-linked gene from each parent. The X and Y chromosomes determine sex: a male is XY, a female XX. Females therefore have 2 copies of every gene, whereas males have 1 copy of each X-linked or Y-linked gene. There is a region of homology at each end of the X and Y chromosome, referred to as the pseudoautosomal regions. Most of the genes on 1 copy of the X chromosome are inactivated early in development in females, achieving dosage compensation between the 2 sexes for X-linked genes. X inactivation occurs at random, so females have mosaic expression, with about 50% of cells expressing 1 X and 50% the other.

The 2 copies of a gene on each homologous chromosome are referred to as alleles. These may be identical in DNA sequence, although molecular genetics studies reveal a high rate of sequence of variation. Most of this variation has no impact on gene function, although some variants are common in the population and are referred to as polymorphisms (technically defined as the occurrence of 2 or more alleles at a gene locus, each having a frequency in the population of at least 1%). Some sequence changes, on the other hand, do affect the function of the gene product. The sequence composition of the 2 alleles is referred to as genotype, whereas the measurable or visible effect on the organism is referred to as phenotype. If, with respect to a particular sequence, the 2 alleles in an individual are identical, the individual is said to be homozygous; if the 2 alleles are different, the individual is described as being heterozygous. As molecular genetic studies have been applied to determining gene sequence, it has become apparent that individuals who are homozygous for mutant alleles often actually have 2 different mutations in the 2 alleles. This is referred to as compound heterozygosity. True homozygosity for the same mutation occurs if a mutation has relatively high frequency in the population, or if the individual has inherited the same mutant allele from each parent via a common ancestor due to consanguinity. Such alleles are described as being identical by descent.

PEDIGREE ANALYSIS

The symbols used for analysis of inheritance in a family are shown in Figure 5-1. Usually a 3-generation family history is obtained as part of a prenatal genetic evaluation. Ideally, both partners are present at the interview and have spoken with their relatives to elicit any important information about medical problems in the family. It is important for the counselor to inquire about a number of issues that may not be volunteered by the couple. These include instances of neonatal or early death, miscarriage, or consanguinity. Inquiry about specific instances of mental retardation, anemia, or congenital anomalies may be revealing, since not all couples realize that these may be hereditary disorders. The counselor should also inquire about racial and ethnic background of both partners, since this may indicate their origin from a group known to have increased risk of carrying specific genetic traits.

PATTERNS OF MENDELIAN TRANSMISSION

The 2 major patterns of Mendelian transmission are recessive and dominant. Traits can also be either autosomal or sex-linked, depending on whether they are carried on a non-sex chromosome, or on the X or the Y. The basic characteristics of Mendelian inheritance will be described in the following section.

AUTOSOMAL RECESSIVE

Autosomal recessive is the pattern first recognized in humans by Garrod. For a recessive trait to be expressed, both alleles must contain a mutation. An affected individual is therefore homozygous, although often he or she is actually a compound heterozygote for 2 distinct mutations. Both parents must carry 1 mutant allele, but for a recessive trait the heterozygous individual does not express a mutant phenotype. Hence the wild-type allele is said to be dominant, the mutant recessive. Autosomal recessive traits are passed from both members of a couple

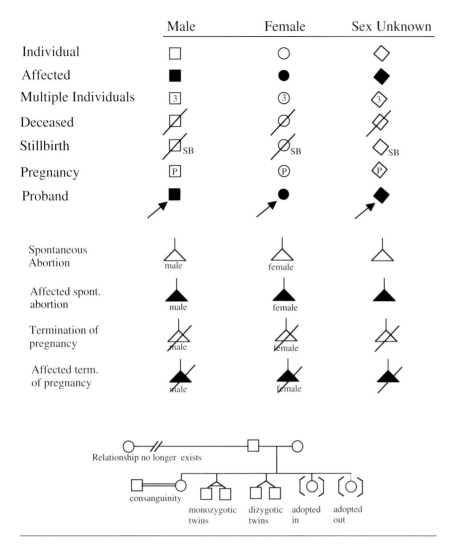

FIGURE 5-1 Symbols used in pedigree analysis. Modified from reference 2.

Autosomal recessive traits may include common or rare disorders. Some mutant alleles are particularly common in specific populations. In some cases, heterozygosity for a mutant allele is preserved in a population because the heterozygote is protected from some environmental risk. This is exemplified by globin mutations, which are particularly common in individuals of African, Mediterranean, or Southeast Asian descent because the mutations exert a protective effect against malaria infection. Some populations will contain an exceptionally high frequency of a particular mutation due to a founder effect, in which the mutation arose in the population in relatively recent times and has been preserved at high frequency due to the population being a closed system with respect to breeding. Often it is a combination of these 2 factors that mold a gene frequency, for example explaining the high frequency of sickle cell globin in Africa, β-thalassemia in the Mediterranean, and α-thalassemia in Asia. Autosomal recessive trades will also appear with increased frequency in individuals whose parents are consanguineous, as noted previously.

AUTOSOMAL DOMINANT

An autosomal dominant trait is expressed in either heterozygotes or homozygotes. Usually, a heterozygous parent transmits the trait to, on average, half of his or her offspring (Fig. 5-3). Males and females are equally likely to be affected, and can transmit to either sex. For rare traits,

to, on average, one quarter of their offspring (Fig. 5-2). About one half of the offspring will be carriers and one quarter inherit the wild-type allele from both parents. The unaffected sibling of a person affected within autosomal recessive trait has a two thirds chance of being a carrier, since of the 4 possible outcomes (1/4 affected, 1/2 carrier, 1/4 wild type), one—being affected—has not occurred, leaving a two thirds chance of being a carrier and one third of being homozygous wild type.

Most autosomal recessive traits are now known to involve mutations in the genes that encode enzymes. Due to the catalytic function of enzymes, heterozygotes have sufficient activity even if there is a 50% reduction in enzyme activity. The affected individuals, in contrast, can be severely deficient, leading both to accumulation of substrate and deficiency of product. Different clinical disorders are the result of either or both of these physiological changes.

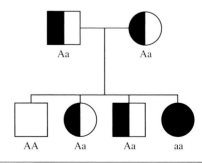

FIGURE 5-2 Pedigree illustrating autosomal recessive inheritance. The "A" allele is dominant, "a" recessive. Both parents are heterozygous carriers, and there is a one quarter chance of any child being homozygous recessive, affected with the disorder.

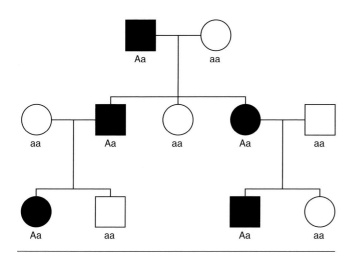

FIGURE 5-3 Pedigree illustrating autosomal dominant inheritance. The "A" allele is dominant to "a." Both males and females are affected, and either sex can transmit to either males or females.

heterozygous affected individuals will far outnumber homozygotes. Often the homozygous phenotype is more severe than the heterozygous, and may be lethal.

Vertical transmission for an autosomal dominant trait may occur for many generations, but sometimes an individual will be the first affected person in the family, due to new mutation. Concluding that a sporadically affected individual represents a new mutation requires careful evaluation of both parents to be sure that one is not subtly affected. Many dominant traits are characterized by variable expressivity, with mild features being easily missed. Some of those who carry a mutation will show no phenotype whatever, and are said to be nonpenetrant. In a disorder with complete penetrance, the unaffected parents of a sporadically affected child can be counseled that their risk of recurrence is low. There remains a possibility, however, of mosaicism, which may be confined to the germline. Recurrence in such cases remains possible and must be remembered when counseling is provided.

A variety of physiological mechanisms has been found to underlie autosomal dominant traits. Product deficiency may result if a mutation substantially reduces the quantity of gene product from the mutant allele. Some structural proteins or transcription factors (proteins that regulate the rate of transcription of specific genes) may be sensitive to gene dosage and result in a phenotype in the haploinsufficient state. In other cases there may be a dominant negative effect, in which the abnormal gene product disrupts the function of a complex structure to which it contributes. Even a small amount of abnormal protein in such a structure may disrupt its stability and yield an abnormal phenotype. Both product deficiency and dominant negative effects occur in Marfan syndrome.[3] Phenotype of the haploinsufficient state tends to be milder than the dominant negative, since a higher proportion of the connective tissue structure is disrupted by the latter. A third mechanism is gain of function, in which the gene product may be constitutively activated or expressed and have aberrantly high levels. This occurs

in achondroplasia, where mutation in gene for the FGF3 receptor is constitutively active, directing the cartilage cells to stop growing in the absence of an external signal, leading to short stature.[4]

One additional molecular mechanism of dominant inheritance deserves mention: the tumor suppressor. Tumor suppressor genes are involved in the formation of neoplasms. It has been found that both copies of a tumor suppressor tend to be inactivated in tumor tissue. Although this implies a recessive mechanism in the tumor cells, tendency to develop tumors is transmitted as a dominant trait. This is explained by the fact of a heterozygous individual has only 1 functional copy of the gene in each cell. The loss of the functional copy will lead to tumor formation in certain tissues. This mechanism accounts for some rare syndromes such as neurofibromatosis or tuberous sclerosis,[5] but also some common forms of cancer such as breast cancer.

SEX LINKAGE

Sex-linked inheritance applies to genes on the X or Y chromosomes, although most medically important sex-linked traits are on the X. X-linked recessive traits are usually expressed in males, who are hemizygous for genes on the X. Carrier females usually are asymptomatic, although nonrandom X inactivation may result in symptoms in some females. Typically, carrier females transmit the trait to half their sons, and carrier status to half their daughters (Fig. 5-4). There is no male-to-male transmission for an X-linked trait.

There are examples of X-linked dominant disorders, in which both males and females are affected. In some cases, males are more severely affected, or the trait may be lethal in

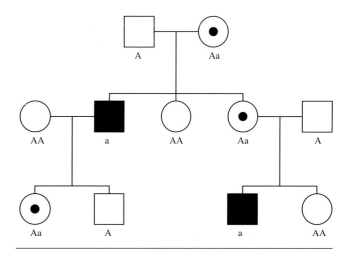

FIGURE 5-4 X-linked recessive pedigree, in which carrier females transmit the disorder to half their sons and carrier status to half their daughters. There is no male-to-male transmission.

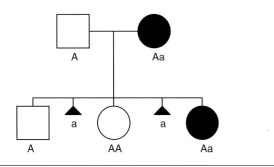

FIGURE 5-5 Pedigree illustrating X-linked dominant inheritance with male lethality in utero.

NON-MENDELIAN INHERITANCE

Some examples of genetic traits have been discovered that do not obey basic Mendelian inheritance.

GENETIC IMPRINTING

Although most genes are expressed from both on the maternal and paternal alleles, there are exceptions in which only 1 allele is expressed.[6] The complete list of imprinted genes is not known, but only a minority of all genes behaves this way. Mutation of an imprinted gene will only result in a phenotype if the mutant allele is inherited from the parent whose allele is expressed. Deletion of the expressed copy of an imprinted gene can also result in a phenotype. Finally, inheritance of both alleles from the same parent—uniparental disomy—can result in over- or underexpression of an imprinted gene. Disorders thought to be due to imprinted genes are listed in Table 5-1.

MITOCHONDRIAL INHERITANCE

Mitochondria are the cellular organelles responsible for oxidative phosphorylation. Each contains multiple copies of a circular, double stranded, 16.5 kb DNA molecule (7). This

TABLE 5-1	DISORDERS ASSOCIATED WITH IMPRINTED GENES
Chromosome Region	**Clinical Effects**
15q12	Prader-Willi or Angelman syndrome
11p	Beckwith-Wiedemann syndrome
7q	Short stature (Possibly Russell-Silver syndrome)
14	Short stature, developmental delay

TABLE 5-2	DISORDERS ASSOCIATED WITH TRIPLET REPEAT EXPANSION
Disorder	**Repeat Unit**
Myotonic Dystrophy	CTG (3' untranslated region)
Friedreich Ataxia	GAA (intron)
Huntington Disease	CAG (polyglutamine)
Spinocerebellar Ataxia (multiple types)	CAG (polyglutamine)
Dentatopallidoluysian Atrophy	CAG (polyglutamne)
Kennedy Disease	CAG (polyglutamine) in androgen receptor
Fragile X Syndrome	CGG (promoter region)

DNA encodes 13 polypeptides involved in mitochondrial energy metabolism, as well as a set of transfer and ribosomal RNAs. Mutations within the coding sequence of some of these genes or tRNAs result in syndromes associated with energy failure, including Leber optic neuropathy or encephalomyopathies. Since mitochondria are maternally inherited, a mutant mitochondrial DNA is transmitted from a mother to all her children. There may be hundreds of mitochondrial DNA molecules in each cell, however, and only a proportion may be mutant, a phenomenon referred to as heteroplasmy. Since mitochondria are segregated passively at each cell division, the proportion of mutant and wild-type mitochondria may vary from cell to cell. This accounts for a wide range of variable expression in mitochondrially inherited traits in a family. It is important to remember that the majority of mitochondrial proteins are encoded in the nucleus, so most mitochondrial dysfunction, even if inherited, is not the maternally transmitted.

TRIPLET REPEATS

A distinct subset of dominant traits result from expansion of repeats of specific triplets of DNA sequence normally found in certain genes.[8] Expansion of the triplet beyond a threshold leads to aberrant expression, producing a phenotype. As indicated in Table 5-2, most triplet repeats expansion syndromes affect the nervous system. Most are autosomal dominant, except for Friedreich ataxia, which is autosomal recessive, and fragile X syndrome, which is X linked. The dominant triplet repeat disorders display the phenomenon of genetic anticipation, in which age of onset decreases and severity increases with each generation. This is because large repeats are unstable at meiosis, and are prone to further expansion with each generation. In fragile X syndrome, carriers have an intermediate expansion of 50–200 CGG repeats, referred to as premutation, whereas affected males or females have more than 200 repeats. Premutation males transmit their alleles to their daughters, but expansion to full mutation only occurs in females. Hence there may be non-manifesting transmitting

males. If the lethality is expressed in utero, only females will be affected and males may miscarry (Fig. 5-5).

males for fragile X syndrome, which is unusual for an X-linked trait.

CONCLUSION

As the twenty-first century opens, the attention of geneticists is turning toward the assessment of complex genetic traits, involving multiple genes and/or environmental effects. Simultaneously, techniques of molecular diagnosis are being developed and refined that will allow screening of multiple genes for pathogenic mutations. The power of genetic testing may some day obviate much of the need to collect detailed family history information, as a couple may be quickly tested for multiple traits that they may be at risk of passing on. The increasing power and scope of genetic analysis will result in a rapidly increasing need for education of the public and health providers, and implementation of novel means of providing counseling, including the use of computer-based systems.

References

1. Collins FS, Green ED, Guttmacher AE, et al. A vision for the future of genomics research. *Nature* 2003;422:835–847.
2. Bennett RL, Steinhaus KA, Uhrich SB, et al. Recommendations for standardized human pedigree nomenclature. *Am J Hum Genet.* 1995; 56:745–752.
3. Robinson PN, Booms P, Katzke S, et al. Mutations of FBN1 and genotype-phenotype correlations in Marfan syndrome and related fibrillinopathies. *Hum Mutat.* 2002;20:153–161.
4. Shiang R, Thompson LM, Zhu Y-Z, et al. Mutations in the transmembrane domain of FGFR3 cause the most common genetic form of dwarfism, achondroplasia. *Cell* 1994;78:335–342.
5. Tucker. National Cancer Institute Workshop Report: the Phakomatoses Revisited. *J Natl Cancer Inst.* 2000;92:530–533.
6. Walter J, Paulsen M. Imprinting and disease. *Semin Cell Dev Biol.* 2003;14:101–110.
7. DiMauro S, Schon EA. Mitochondrial Respiratory-Chain Diseases. *N Engl J Med.* 2003;348:2656–2668.
8. Rosenberg RN. DNA-triplet repeats and neurologic disease. *N Engl J Med.* 1996;335:1222–1224.

SYNDROME: AN APPROACH TO FETAL DYSMORPHOLOGY

The-Hung Bui

In many developed countries, congenital malformations represent the most frequent cause of mortality during the first year of life; for example, they account for more than 20% of all infant deaths in the United States.[1] At birth, about 2–3% of infants are found to have major structural defects and this frequency increases to 3–4% by the age of 1 year. Additionally, birth defects contribute substantially to childhood morbidity and long-term disability.

Today, ultrasound is the main diagnostic tool in the prenatal detection of congenital abnormalities.[2] It allows a detailed examination of fetal anatomy and the detection of not only major defects but also subtle markers of genetic syndromes and chromosomal abnormalities. Due to their family history, medical illness, or to exposure to teratogens such as infection and various drugs, some women are at high risk of fetal abnormalities. However, most congenital defects occur in the low-risk population. For this reason, and despite controversy over its benefits, ultrasound screening is offered routinely to all pregnant women in many countries.[3] The ultrasound scan, which is usually performed at 18–23 weeks of pregnancy, should include systematic examination of the fetus for the detection of both major and minor defects.

Birth defect syndromes number in the thousands, and each condition has its own implications for prognosis, treatment, and recurrence risk. Discriminating among a number of overlapping and, often, ill-defined entities is the most challenging task for the fetal ultrasonographer. A thorough knowledge about human development and its aberrations is required, along with a systematic approach, very detailed examination, and a thorough appreciation of normal variations. The fetal diagnostic process is best achieved within the multidisciplinary team that includes specialists in fetal medicine, pediatrics, and clinical genetics among others.

There are several textbooks and databases that catalogue and describe the thousands of birth defect syndromes reported to date, therefore no attempt has been made to duplicate these sources.[4–9] Instead, this chapter provides a brief review of classification systems for fetal anomalies and birth defects, and outlines a general approach to syndrome diagnosis that has proven to be clinically useful.

CLASSIFICATION OF FETAL AND BIRTH DEFECTS

Congenital defects can be classified in different ways. The most common classification is based on organ systems or body regions. In 1997, the Royal College of Obstetricians and Gynaecologists in the United Kingdom proposed that fetal defects detected during the course of pregnancy could be grouped according to their likely clinical consequences into 4 pragmatic subgroups:

1. Lethal anomalies
2. Anomalies associated with possible survival and long-term morbidity
3. Anomalies that may be amenable to intrauterine therapy
4. Anomalies associated with possible immediate or short-term morbidity[10]

Although this classification has not yet been widely adopted, it has obvious merits for the practicing obstetrician, as information about the clinical effectiveness of routine ultrasound screening in pregnancy can be placed in the context of clinical practice.[3] However, the emphasis of this classification is on potential intervention and not on the diagnostic process of fetal defects. Thus, for diagnostic purposes, more clinically useful systems of classification separate (1) major (medically or surgically significant defects) from minor anomalies, (2) single defect from multiple congenital anomaly syndrome and make use of (3) categorization by pathogenic process and (4) an etiological classification (Tables 6-1 and 6-2).[11–12]

The following 5 major causes of malformations are generally recognized.

1. Chromosome abnormalities including microdeletion/microduplication syndromes
2. Single gene defects
3. Multifactorial disorders (involving both genetic and environmental factors)
4. Teratogenic exposition (environmental factors)
5. Unknown

Table 6-1 lists the main causes of congenital defects in a large investigation conducted in Boston, Massachusetts, USA.[12] Of the 69,277 infants studied, birth defects were found in 1,549 for an incidence of 2.24%. It can be seen that the etiology of two thirds of congenital abnormalities is unknown or multifactorial, that environmental causes of birth defects appear to be infrequent and lastly, that genetic conditions account for about 30% of cases.

The increasing knowledge of the pathogenesis of human congenital defects has led to a better understanding of the developmental relationship of the defects in malformation syndromes. Birth defects can be categorized into the 4 main types of pathogenic processes.[4–6]

MALFORMATION

This term is reserved for intrinsic abnormalities caused by an abnormal completion of 1 or more of the embryonic processes. Thus, such anomalies may be limited to a single anatomic region, involve an entire organ, or produce a malformation syndrome affecting a number of different body systems. The early development of a particular tissue or organ system may be arrested, delayed, or misdirected, resulting in persistent structural abnormalities.[13] Although defining an anomaly as a malformation does not imply any specific etiology, it

TABLE
6-1

CLASSIFICATION AND BIRTH FREQUENCY OF CONGENITAL MALFORMATIONS AND DEFORMATIONS

Classification	Frequency	
	Single	Multiple
Minor malformations	140 per 1000	5 per 1000
Major malformations	30 per 1000	7 per 1000
Deformations	14 per 1000	6 per 1000

Modified from reference 11.

strongly suggests that the developmental error occurred early in gestation, either during tissue differentiation or during organogenesis. During the fetal period, the main events taking place are the growth and maturation of already differentiated systems, and true malformations arising during this time are quite rare.

DEFORMATION

Deformations are secondary events that may be extrinsic or intrinsic to the fetus (Table 6-3).[4] Mechanical forces that alter the shape or position of normally formed body structures can produce them. Although deformations can result in severe changes in the configuration of various body parts, they occur usually in the fetal period and not during embryogenesis. Most deformational abnormalities induced by mechanical forces involve cartilage, bone, and joints, probably because these tissues yield to intrauterine pressure; however, they often tend to resolve spontaneously toward their original forms once the abnormal mechanical stresses are removed.

Abnormal fetal presentation, severe and long-standing oligohydramnios of any cause, or even a pre-existing malformation or disruption that limits fetal mobility can produce a deformation. Other causes include maternal factors such as intrauterine constraint due to primigravidity, a small pelvic outlet, or structural abnormalities of the uterus. Crowding can be produced by multifetal pregnancies. Examples of congenital deformations comprise talipes equinovarus (clubfoot), congenital hip dislocation, congenital postural scoliosis, positional plagiocephaly (flat head), torticollis, and mandibular asymmetry.[13]

TABLE
6-2

CAUSES OF BIRTH DEFECTS IN 1,549 AFFECTED INFANTS

Causes	Percent
Chromosome defects	10.1
Single mutant genes	3.1
Familial disorders	14.5
Multifactorial inheritance	23.0
Teratogens	3.2
Uterine factors	2.5
Twinning	0.4
Unknown	43.2

Modified from reference 12.

TABLE
6-3

CAUSES OF DEFORMATIONS

	Causes of Deformations
Extrinsic	**Mechanical forces**
	Small maternal stature
	Premature rupture of membrane
	Unusual implantation site
	Large uterine leiomyomas
	Uterine malformations
	Multifetal pregnancy
	Breech presentation
Intrinsic	**Malformations**
	Spina bifida
	CNS malformations
	Bilateral renal agenesis
	Severe hypoplastic kidneys
	Severe polycystic kidneys
	Urethral atresia
Dysfunctions	
	Neuromuscular disorders
	Connective tissue defects

Modified from reference 13.

Deformations can be intrinsic and secondary to malformations or neuromuscular disorders (Table 6-3). In such cases the deformity can be progressive after birth.

DISRUPTION

Structural defect of an organ, part of an organ, or a larger region of the body may be caused also by an interference with, or an actual destruction of a previously normal organ or tissue. In contrast to deformities, disruptions may result from mechanical forces as well as by events such as ischemia, hemorrhage, or adhesion of denuded tissues. These secondary abnormalities do not conform to the boundaries normally imposed by the embryonic development, and they commonly affect several different tissue types in a delimited anatomic region. For example, in the amnion band sequence an amniotic band may result in amputation of a limb, or damage the fetal face, penetrating skin, muscle, bone, and soft tissue without regard to their embryonic relationships.[13–14]

Disruptions usually affect structures that had previously developed normally and their presence does not imply intrinsic abnormality of the tissue involved. There is seldom a need for concern about mental deficit or other hidden problems. The recurrence risk is low unless uterine malformation is found in the mother.

DYSPLASIA

The last major category of pathogenic processes that leads to birth defects is dysplasia. The structural changes are caused by a primary defect involving abnormal cellular organization or function within a specific tissue type throughout the body. For an increasing number of these disorders, a specific biochemical deficiency has been defined, often involving abnormalities of enzyme production or synthesis of structural protein.[9] Major mutant genes that may be diagnosed by DNA analysis cause almost all dysplasias.[9] There are, however, some notable exceptions such as the harmatomas. These abnormal admixtures of tissue types often produce discrete tumors such as hemangiomas and nevi. An important feature of most dysplastic conditions is their progressive course. Since the tissue itself is intrinsically abnormal, clinical effects tend to persist or worsen as long as the tissue continues to grow or function.

DIAGNOSTIC APPROACH TO THE DYSMORPHIC FETUS

Pregnancy history is important because a specific nongenetic cause for the structural defect may be revealed such as a teratogenic exposure (infection, drug) or a uterine factor resulting in a deformity or disruption. Other features such as oligohydramnios and lack of fetal movements may provide a clue to the cause of the defect. Information on the family history and a full pedigree is often needed as in any situation where genetic counseling will be provided. Examination of both parents is sometimes needed to arrive at a correct diagnosis.

The vast majority of congenital abnormalities must be dealt with based on incomplete knowledge, and the skills of the fetal sonographer remain among the most useful tools in our diagnostic armamentarium. The fetal scan should be conducted to a high standard using a systematic approach and can be helped by a checklist.[15-16] When examining the fetus, careful measurement is essential especially when a skeletal dysplasia is suspected. Precise measurements allow serial evaluations to be made and compared.

Chromosome analysis should be undertaken in all fetuses with multiple defects and, often also, when the defect appears to be isolated given the limitations of fetal evaluation by ultrasound for minor signs and the possibility of hidden problems.[17] Biochemical studies are currently helpful in only a limited number of dysmorphic fetuses, for example peroxisomal disorders such as Zellweger syndrome and some lysosomal storage diseases.[9] However, consideration should be given to obtaining fetal cells for banking and future analysis if necessary. Molecular analysis is becoming increasingly important in the diagnosis of malformation syndromes and its application will be essential in the future.[9]

Almost all birth defect syndromes are exceedingly rare and general obstetricians would be expected to see only a handful of such cases during their professional lifetime. Yet, there are so many different syndromes that even a specialist in the field will never gain experience with all of them. Therefore the approach set forth here depends not on memorization of the features of rare syndromes but on recognition and analysis of their component anomalies (Fig. 6-1).

The first question to ask when evaluating a fetus with a structural defect is whether the abnormality represents a single, isolated anomaly or is instead part of a broader, organized pattern of malformation, that is, a syndrome. Obviously, an anomaly occurring alone may have considerably different meaning than the same anomaly occurring in conjunction with others.

SINGLE-SYSTEM DEFECT

Malformations that involve only a single organ system of the body make up the largest proportion of birth defects (Table 6-1).[1] Such abnormalities include the most common birth defects: cleft lip and palate, clubfoot, pyloric stenosis,

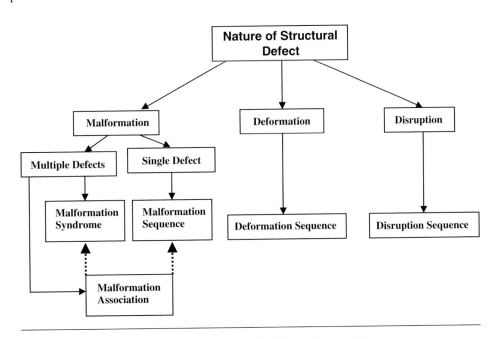

FIGURE 6-1 Categories of structural defects (modified from reference 6.)

congenital hip dislocation, and congenital heart disease. These anomalies occur with increased frequency in some families and ethnic groups but do not follow the classic Mendelian patterns of inheritance expected for disorders caused by major mutant genes. The concordance rate in identical twins for these defects is low, providing strong evidence for the influence of environmental factors in their causation. Most of the disorders in this group are therefore thought to be of multifactorial etiology, implying the additive effects of multiple genes, each contributing a small effect, and presumably an environmental "trigger" of unknown nature. Because these isolated defects appear clinically to be identical with those occurring as part of a syndrome, the pathogenesis may be similar or identical with, presumably, a common pathway that leads to the same defect despite different initial causes.

SYNDROME

When a particular set of primary anomalies thought to originate from a single etiology (e.g., trisomy 18 syndrome) repeatedly occurs in a consistent pattern, it is called a syndrome (from the Greek "running together"). When the underlying cause of a syndrome is discovered, the shorthand designation should be abandoned in favor of a more definitive name; thus, Edwards syndrome should be called trisomy 18 syndrome, Hunter syndrome becomes mucopolysaccharidosis type II. Often the original description of a syndrome is further refined and the limits of variability of its manifestations are explored as more cases are described. Sometimes elucidation of its pathogenesis or etiology is reached. However, prenatal syndrome diagnosis still relies heavily on the ability of the ultrasonographer to detect and correctly interpret morphological and developmental findings, and to recognize a pattern in them. Discussion with a clinical geneticist is therefore often rewarding. In many cases a final syndrome diagnosis can only be reached or confirmed after birth, when additional evaluation can be performed, or following termination of pregnancy after the post-mortem examination.

Diagnoses based on clinical observation show a wide range of latitude, and thus there may be no gold standard. No single congenital malformation is pathognomonic for a specific syndrome. Furthermore, there is inherent variability in the manifestations of most dysmorphic disorders, both in type and in severity of the various structural abnormalities. Table 6-4 indicates the most common multiple congenital anomaly syndromes.[18]

SEQUENCE

Some patterns of multiple malformations appear to be the result of a cascade of related consequences, proceeding often from one primary single-system malformation or event. During intrauterine life, this primary abnormality interferes with normal embryologic and fetal developmental processes resulting at birth in seemingly separate and distinct abnormalities that may involve different body areas and organ systems. The etiology of most sequences is unknown, but some have features compatible with multifactorial inheritance, as might be expected

TABLE 6-4	THE MOST COMMON MULTIPLE CONGENITAL ANOMALY OR DYSPLASIA SYNDROMES
Syndrome	*Cause*
Achondroplasia	Single gene, autosomal dominant
Amnion disruption sequence	Unknown
Cornelia de Lange syndrome	Unknown
Down syndrome (trisomy 21)	Chromosomal
Fetal alcohol syndrome	Teratogenic, excessive alcohol
Klippel-Trenaunay-Weber syndrome	Unknown
Marfan syndrome	Single gene, autosomal dominant
Neurofibromatosis 1, NF1	Single gene, autosomal dominant
Noonan syndrome	Single gene, autosomal dominant
Oligohydramnios sequence	Heterogeneous
Osteogenesis imperfecta	Single gene, heterogeneous inheritance
Prader-Willi syndrome	Microdeletion or maternal uniparental disomy of chromosome 15q11.2–q12
Rubinstein-Taybi syndrome	Single gene, autosomal dominant
Trisomy 13 syndrome	Chromosomal
Trisomy 18 syndrome	Chromosomal
Turner syndrome	Chromosomal (45,X and variants)
VATER/VACTERL association	Unknown
Williams-Beuren syndrome	Microdeletion of chromosome 7q11.2; single gene, autosomal dominant

Modified from reference 18.

by their derivation from often a single underlying malformation. The clinical value of recognizing malformation sequences lies in the differentiation from other multiple defect conditions that may have different implications in terms of prognosis and recurrence risk. The oligohydramnios sequence[19] is the most illustrative example (Fig. 6-2).

Another example is the fetal akinesia deformation sequence (FADS).[19–21] This is a heterogeneous group of neurological, muscular, and skeletal or connective tissue disorders all resulting in the same phenotype with multiple joint contractures, including bilateral talipes and fixed flexion or extension deformities of the hips, knees, elbows, and wrists. This sequence probably covers a number of separate entities comprising several congenital myopathies, congenital lethal arthrogryposis, multiple pterygium, and Pena–Shokeir syndromes.[20,21] The deformities are usually symmetric and, in most cases, all 4 limbs are involved. The severity of the deformities increases

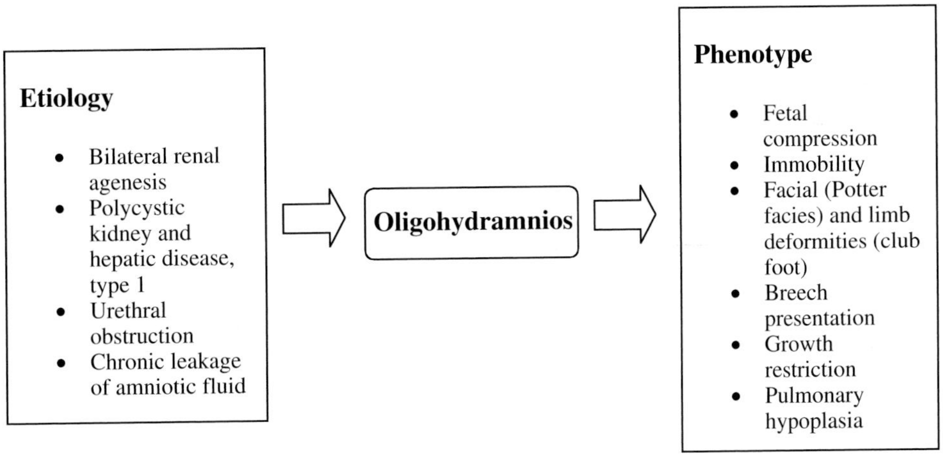

FIGURE 6-2 The oligohydramnios sequence.

distally in the involved limb, with the hands and feet typically being the most severely affected. Polyhydramnios is commonly present after 25 weeks. Other features found are pulmonary hypoplasia, micrognathia and nuchal edema (or increased nuchal translucency at 10–14 weeks).

ASSOCIATION

Several clinical entities have now been described with a nonrandom clustering of embryologically unrelated congenital malformations of unknown origin. These conditions are not consistent enough to justify definition as a syndrome and are referred to as associations to emphasize the lack of uniformity in the clinical presentation from case to case.[6] No genetic basis has yet been found except for the CHARGE association, nor have any teratogenic agents been identified. Most cases are sporadic and the empiric recurrence risk in these conditions is extremely low. The prognosis depends almost entirely on the degree of severity and potential correctability of the individual structural lesions. Mental development often is normal, but statural growth can be affected in children in this category. Thus, the clinical value of an association designation is to prompt the search for hidden abnormalities that might fit the larger pattern.

For example, the well-known acronym, VATER, is used to describe the association of vertebral defects, anal atresia or stenosis, tracheo-esophageal fistula, radial defects, and renal anomalies.[22] Some authors have expanded the acronym to VACTERL to include Cardiac defects and non-radial Limb defects.[23] Most children with this diagnosis, however, do not have all these anomalies but rather varying combination from this list.[23–24] This variability clearly presents a problem for the diagnostician.

Another notable association is CHARGE which is an acronym for Coloboma of iris or retina, Heart defects (of any kind), Atresia of the choanae, Retardation of growth and development, Genital anomalies (mostly in the male where the penis might be small and the testes undescended), and Ear abnormalities.[25–27] These abnormalities consist mostly of simple protruding ears but can include over-folded helices, absent crus of the antihelixes, and deafness, sensorineural, conductive, or both. Obviously, the diagnosis can only be suggested prenatally, as several of the abnormalities included in the CHARGE association cannot be imaged by ultrasonography. However, it appears that temporal bone anomalies, consisting of partial or complete semicircular canal agenesis or hypoplasia, are a major feature of this association and potentially amenable to detection by MRI in utero.[28–29] Recently, a gene (CHD7) has been identified to cause CHARGE "syndrome" in several cases,[30] thus allowing molecular diagnosis pre- or postnatally.

Several thousands of malformation syndromes have been described, and more are added each year.[7–8] For this reason, there is little value in attempting to memorize the features of each disorder. Instead, the approach recommended emphasizes recognition of individual clinical features that, combined with historical information and selected laboratory studies, can help determine the pattern of defects that may define a syndrome. Early in the diagnostic process an analysis of the underlying nature of the abnormalities has to be made (Fig. 6-1). Sometimes, a few pivotal features will immediately suggest a particular syndrome already familiar to the clinician. More often, extensive consultation with other specialists and search of the medical literature are needed. The availability of computerized databases of known and unknown syndromes and other conditions has become an essential tool of the clinical geneticist and is now benefiting the fetal dysmorphologist as well.

Three systems are widely used: Online Mendelian Inheritance in Man (OMIM) for monogenic disorders is available through the web and the London Dysmorphology Database and POSSUM are commercially available on CD-ROM.[7–9] It must be emphasized that these are not expert systems that make the diagnosis for the clinician, rather they are systems for experts and both knowledge and practice are required for their optimal use.

Much effort should be put to reaching a specific diagnosis, as it allows a much more detail and accurate counseling for prognosis and recurrence risk, and provides direction for possible therapeutic intervention. Inevitably, the prenatal diagnostic process sometimes is unsuccessful and no specific syndrome is recognized. It must then be remembered that achieving a fetal diagnosis, important as it is, is only 1 necessary step in the process of providing care and counseling for the pregnant woman and the affected fetus.

ACKNOWLEDGMENTS

Supported in part by the European Commission Biomed 2 Programme (Eurofoetus project) and by funds from the Karolinska Institute.

References

1. Petrini J, Damus K, Johnston RB Jr. An overview of infant mortality and birth defects in the United States. *Teratology.* 1997;56:8–10.
2. Jaffe R, Bui T-H (Ed). *Textbook of Fetal Ultrasound.* New York and London: Parthenon Publishing; 1999.
3. Bricker L, Garcia J, Henderson J, et al. Ultrasound screening in pregnancy: a systematic review of the clinical effectiveness, cost-effectiveness and women's views. *Health Technol Assess.* 2000;4(16).
4. Graham JM Jr. *Smith's Recognizable Patterns of Human Deformation,* 2nd ed. Philadelphia: WB Saunders; 1988.
5. Stevenson RE, Hall JG, Goodman RM. *Human Malformations and Related Anomalies.* New York and Oxford: Oxford University Press; 1993.
6. Jones KL. *Smith's Recognizable Patterns of Human Malformation,* 5th ed. Philadelphia: WB Saunders; 1997.
7. Winter R, Baraitser M. *Winter-Baraitser Dysmorphology Database,* Version 1.0.4. London: London Medical Databases Ltd, 2003. Available from http://www.imdatabases.com
8. Pictures of Standard Syndromes and Undiagnosed Malformations, POSSUM Version 5.6, 2004. Murdoch Children's Research Institute, Royal Children's Hospital, Flemington Road, Parkville, Victoria, Australia, 3052. Available from: http://www.possum.net.au/.
9. Online Mendelian Inheritance in Man, OMIM (TM). McKusick-Nathans Institute for Genetic Medicine, Johns Hopkins University (Baltimore, MD) and National Center for Biotechnology Information, National Library of Medicine (Bethesda, MD), 2005. Available from: http://www.ncbi.nlm.nih.gov
10. Royal College of Obstetricians and Gynaecologists. *Ultrasound screening for fetal abnormalities: report of the RCOG Working Party.* London: RCOG; 1997.
11. Connor JM, Ferguson-Smith MA. *Essential Medical Genetics,* 4th ed. Oxford: Blackwell Scientific Publications; 1993: 193.
12. Nelson K, Holmes LB. Malformations due to spontaneous mutations in newborn infants. *N Engl J Med.* 1989;320:19–23.
13. Cohen MM Jr. *The Child with Multiple Birth Defects.* New York: Raven Press, 1982:10.
14. Evans MI. Amniotic bands. *Ultrasound Obstet Gynecol.* 1997; 10:307–308.
15. American Institute for Ultrasound in Medicine. Guidelines for performance of the antepartum obstetrical ultrasound examination. *J Ultrasound Med.* 2003;22:1116–1125.
16. American College of Obstetricians and Gynecologists. *Ultrasound in Pregnancy.* Washington, DC: ACOG Technical Bulletin Number 187, 1993.
17. Bui T-H, Hume RF Jr, Nicolaides KH, et al. Ultrasonographic screening for fetal chromosomal abnormalities in the first and second trimester of pregnancy. In: Jaffe R, Bui T-H, ed. *Textbook of Fetal Ultrasound.* New York and London: Parthenon Publishing, 1999:287–303.
18. Hall BD. *Genetic Issues in Pediatrics and Obstetrics Practice.* Chicago: Year Book, 1981.
19. Rodriguez JI, Palacios J. Pathogenetic mechanisms of fetal akinesia deformation sequence and oligohydramnios sequence. *Am J Med Genet.* 1991;40:284–289.
20. Beemer FA. The fetal akinesia sequence: pitfalls and difficulties in genetic counseling. *Genetic Counseling.* 1990;1:41–46.
21. Grubben C, Gyselaers W, Moerman P, et al. The echographic diagnosis of fetal akinesia. A challenge towards etiological diagnosis and management. *Genetic Counseling.* 1990;1:35–40.
22. Quan L, Smith DW. The VATER association: vertebral defects, anal atresia, tracheoesophageal fistula with esophageal atresia, radial dysplasia. *BDOAS* 1972;8:75–78.
23. Corsello G, Maresi E, Corrao AM, et al. VATER/VACTERL association: clinical variability and expanding phenotype including laryngeal stenosis. *Am J Med Genet.* 1992;44:813–815.
24. Botto LD, Khoury MJ, Mastroiacovo P, et al. The spectrum of congenital anomalies of the VATER association: an international study. *Am J Med Genet.* 1997;71:8–16.
25. Hall BD. Choanal atresia and associated multiple anomalies. *J Pediatr.* 1979;95:395–398.
26. Pagon RA, Graham JM Jr, Zonana J, et al. Coloboma, congenital heart disease, and choanal atresia with multiple anomalies: CHARGE association. *J Pediatr.* 1981;99:223–227.
27. Tellier A-L, Cormier-Daire V, Abadie V, et al. CHARGE syndrome: Report of 47 cases and review. *Am J Med Genet.* 1998;76:402–409.
28. Graham JM Jr. A recognizable syndrome within CHARGE association: Hall-Hittner syndrome. *Am J Med Genet.* 2001;99:120–123.
29. Amiel J, Attié-Bitach T, Marianowski R, et al. Temporal bone anomaly proposed as a major criteria for diagnosis of CHARGE syndrome. *Am J Med Genet.* 2001;99:124–127.
30. Vissers LE, van Ravens Waaij CM, Admiral R, et al. Mutations in a new member of the chromodomain gene family cause CHARGE syndrome. *Nat Genet* 2004;36:955–957.

CHAPTER 7

GENES AND DEVELOPMENT

D. Randall Armant

OBJECTIVES

It is important to understand the principals that permit genes to determine the countless events that precisely regulate a process as complex as human embryogenesis. Development proceeds through genetically controlled programs that are activated by environmental factors. In this chapter, we will examine the molecular basis of the interacting roles of developmental control genes and environmental cues during development. We will see how individual mutations that impact specific developmental pathways may influence seemingly disparate biological processes, giving rise to multiple defect syndromes. Finally, we will study a specific syndrome that is derived from an inherited mutation in a developmental control gene.

DYSMORPHOLOGY AND DEVELOPMENTAL GENETICS

The field of dysmorphology is concerned with the identification and delineation of syndromes of congenital abnormalities (Epstein, 1995). We have now begun to think of these birth defects as inborn errors of development. Since they are caused by genes that regulate development, efforts are now underway to identify the mutations that cause them.

Because of the complexity of embryogenesis, mutations affecting development often have wide-ranging effects and lead to spontaneous abortion or live births where the individual is afflicted with a multiple defect syndrome that affects 2 or more seemingly unrelated functions. There are over 1750 inherited disorders of morphogenesis, with over 1000 being multiple defect syndromes.

How can single mutations cause multiple defects? The answer lies in an understanding of the molecular basis of mammalian development. Recent discoveries are making it possible to now group some of these genetic disorders according to the functional or structural similarities of the mutant genes. The eventual goal of dysmorphology is to define categories of mutations according to the affected developmental pathways.

Embryonic development requires three processes:

1. Cell proliferation—cells must grow to create body mass.
2. Cell differentiation—this generates unique, specialized cell phenotypes.
3. Morphogenesis—by directing where differentiation takes place within the embryonic mass, the organization of body regions and tissue patterns emerges.

Keep in mind that all cells of an individual, regardless of phenotype, are genetically identical, and that the number, organization, and pattern of differentiated cells within the developing embryo is genetically determined. The immediate surroundings of each cell influence its developmental program, producing the specific patterns of cell differentiation observed during embryonic development.

CELL DIFFERENTIATION

Human development is quite amazing when one considers that the single-cell zygote grows into a multicellular organism with over 200 different cell types. Embryogenesis is genetically controlled in a highly precise manner. Consider the reproducible biological complexity exemplified by identical twins. Their genetic makeup produces identical individuals down to the patterns of their fingerprints. As genetic relationships diverge, so does form. When genetic divergence is great enough, distinct species will emerge.

The relatively simple period of preimplantation embryogenesis provides a useful example for understanding the basis of cell differentiation during embryonic development. After a short period of proliferation that produces 2, 4, and then 8 identical cells through cleavage of the ovum, distinct cell populations are rapidly and precisely generated. Distinct cell types initially differentiate based on their position at the inside (form embryoblast) or outside (form trophoblast) of the morula (Fig. 7-1). The formation of cavities within the conceptus creates new subpopulations of inside and outside cells, which directs further differentiation. Cells at the surface of the embryoblast that line the blastocyst cavity differentiate into hypoblast, while those inside the cell mass form epiblast. After 2 or more cell populations are established, new differentiation may be generated by interactions between different cell types. Embryoblast cells at the edge of the embryonic disc are induced to migrate where they contact the trophoblast, forming Heuser's membrane from the hypoblast and amnioblasts from the epiblast. Thus, complexity is generated within the early ovum though the interaction of environmental cues with the genetic program of embryonic cells.

Cell differentiation is a change of cell phenotype that is brought about by differential gene expression (Alberts et al., 1994). Differentiation often, but not always (e.g., the preimplantation embryo), occurs in association with decreased cell proliferation. Differentiation may occur along a path that permits additional differentiation, but with limited options (e.g., mesoderm). This is known as determination. When the path leads to a "dead end," this is terminal differentiation. Cells that are terminally differentiated generally do not undergo further differentiation into other cell types (e.g., muscle, bone, erythrocytes). Whether cells exit mitosis before differentiating, gene expression becomes altered and new proteins are produced, generating a unique phenotype.

The decision of a cell to differentiate is based on prior developmental programming (regulatory proteins already active within the cell), coupled with environmental cues (signals

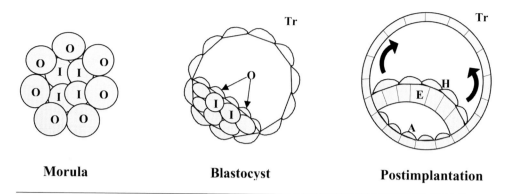

Morula   **Blastocyst**   **Postimplantation**

FIGURE 7-1 Environment influences differentiation during embryogenesis. The location of blastomeres within the morula, either inside (I) or outside (O), determines their fate at the next stage. Inside morula cells form the embryoblast of the blastocyst, based upon cues derived from being completely surrounded by other cells. Outside morula cells that each have a free surface not contacting other cells become the trophoblast (Tr) and pump ions to the embryo interior, which creates an osmotic gradient that forms the blastocyst cavity. Cavities formed within embryonic structures also provide cues for cell differentiation, in this case by creating new environmental cues for subpopulations within the embryoblast. Embryoblast cells adjacent to the blastocyst cavity (O) become hypoblast cells (H) at the postimplantation stage. Cells residing at the interior of the embryoblast (I) form the epiblast (E). Once different fields of cells are created, they can induce further cell differentiation at their interfaces. For example, hypoblast cells at the edge of the embryonic disc are induced to migrate along the inside of the trophoblast cells to form Heuser's membrane (arrows). Epiblast cells at the edge of the disc become amnioblasts (A) after they migrate along trophoblast cells within the newly-formed amnionic cavity that appears within the embryoblast.

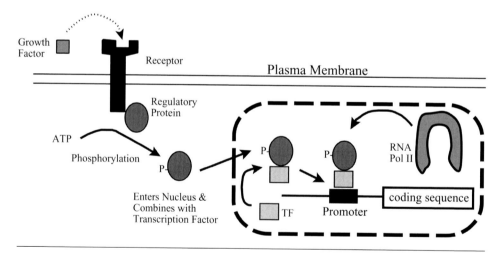

FIGURE 7-2 The interface between environment and gene. In this example, a growth factor encountered by a cell initiates a signaling pathway that alters gene expression. The growth factor binds to the extracellular domain of a specific transmembrane receptor in the plasma membrane. Binding activates enzymatic activity within the cytoplasmic domain of the receptor to phosphorylate a regulatory protein. The phosphorylated form of the regulatory protein can enter the cell nucleus where it combines with a transcription factor (TF). When combined, the protein pair is able to bind to the promoter of the gene, which allows RNA polymerase II to bind and begin transcription of the gene coding sequence. This induction will occur for all genes that contain the specific promoter region that is recognized by the transcription factor complex.

received from the cell's surroundings). Gene transcription is regulated during development on 2 principal levels: (1) expression within a cell of particular transcription factors, which directly regulate gene activity, and (2) the activity of signal transduction pathways, which alter the activity of transcription factors. These pathways are the interface between environmental cues and the nucleus (Fig. 7-2).

Environmental cues are provided in a number of ways. For example the availability of nutrients and trophic factors (growth factors, cytokines, hormones), contact between adjacent fields of cells (inductive processes) and temporal factors (the number of cell divisions that have passed; the time it takes to transcribe, translate, process, and transport gene products). During inductive processes, cells influence each other by (1) cell coupling through gap junctions that pass small signaling molecules and (2) the activation of intracellular signaling pathways through growth factors adhesion molecules on their cell surfaces.

EXAMPLE: MOLECULAR REGULATION OF GENE EXPRESSION DURING OSTEOBLAST DIFFERENTIATION

Osteoprogenitor cells constitute a stem cell population located along the bone surface, in the periosteum, which are maintained as quiescent periosteal cells in normal adult bone. During bone growth or repair, osteoprogenitor cells proliferate and migrate into the bone interior where they differentiate into mature osteoblast cells in response to new environmental cues in the form of steroid hormones, growth factors, new cell contacts, and the extracellular matrix of the bone interior (Stein et al., 1995).

Osteoprogenitor cells manufacture the histone proteins (H3, H4, H2A, and H2B) used by nucleosomes to package newly replicated DNA into condensed chromatin. Upon differentiation, osteoblasts manufacture and secrete fibrous proteins, including osteocalcin, a matrix protein that binds calcium and helps to harden the bone scaffold through mineralization.

Osteoblast differentiation is induced by environmental cues when extracellular signals bind to transmembrane receptors. Examples of such receptors include growth factor receptors and cell adhesion molecules. Alternatively, released steroids can circumvent this step and bind directly to an intracellular receptor. In either case, the ligand-bound receptor alters gene expression through its activation of intracellular signal transduction pathways.

Regulatory molecules associated with these receptors become altered after ligand binding through autophosphorylation or conformational changes, as depicted in Figure 7-2. The ensuing cascade of biochemical reactions culminates with the activation of a transcription factor, which enters the nucleus and binds to a specific region of DNA. The sequence recognized by the transcription factor may be associated with several different genes that are coordinately regulated by its binding. Transcription factors bind either to promoters, which are required for RNA polymerase II binding (like an on/off switch),

or to enhancers which control the level of transcription (like a dimmer switch).

Once all of the requisite transcription factors have bound their respective promoters and enhancers, RNA polymerase II binds to the activated promoter and begins mRNA synthesis. Several transcription factor-promoter interactions may be necessary to bring the DNA into an optimal conformation that can be bound by the RNA polymerase.

H4 HISTONE TRANSCRIPTION

The H4 gene contains 4 promoters, which are each occupied by transcription factors during the S phase of the cell cycle when histone synthesis is maximal. As differentiation of the osteoprogenitor cells into osteoblasts commences, the transcription factors become much less abundant and only one of the promoter sites remains occupied; thus, H4 transcription stops.

OSTEOCALCIN TRANSCRIPTION

The osteocalcin gene contains a TATA box and osteocalcin (OC) box, both promoters that must be bound by the appropriate transcription factors before mRNA synthesis can begin. Several enhancers are also present, including a vitamin D responsive element (VDRE) that binds to the nuclear Vitamin D receptor in the presence of vitamin D.

STRUCTURE-REGULATION PARADIGM

Chromatin-DNA and nuclear matrix-DNA interactions play a critical role in transcriptional regulation. It has been noted that (1) promoters and enhancers are often located far from the transcription initiation site of the gene, yet they regulate polymerase binding; (2) transcription factors are generally produced in low abundance, but they somehow manage to find and combine with their appropriate promoter or enhancer sites within the nucleus; and (3) changes in cell shape are often associated with altered gene expression. Recent studies have demonstrated that DNA folding is regulated to bring promoters and enhancers together and localize them in the region where RNA polymerase must bind. Nucleosomes condense DNA and can thus bring distant promoters into proximity. However, when promoter sites are occupied by nucleosomes, their activity may be blocked. The nuclear matrix influences DNA folding and may concentrate or localize transcription factors to promote their interaction with the promoter or enhancer regions. Transcriptionally active DNA, therefore, tends to be associated with the nuclear matrix. The nuclear matrix binds to DNA or chromatin at specific sites and is continuous with the cytoskeleton. The association between nuclear matrix and cytoskeleton suggests a regulatory coupling.

In the H4 gene of osteoprogenitor cells, the YY1 transcription factor binds to promoter site IV and attaches the H4 DNA to the nuclear matrix. During differentiation to an osteoblast cell, this site becomes incorporated within a nucleosome and cannot become occupied by YY1. This shuts down expression of the H4 gene and stops cell proliferation.

In the osteocalcin gene, nucleosomes are placed in the OC box and VDRE regions during cell proliferation. These regions become free of nucleosomes and can bind transcription factors during osteoblast differentiation. Transcription factors then bind to three other promoter sites and thereby attach the gene to the nuclear matrix. At this point, RNA polymerase II is able to initiate transcription of osteocalcin mRNA.

MORPHOGENESIS

Morphogenesis is driven by cellular processes that determine the final form of the body and individual organs (Table 7-1). Genetic programming controls the spatial arrangement of cells undergoing differentiation, giving rise to patterns of differentiated cells in the developing embryo.

Morphogenesis is controlled by a hierarchy of developmental control genes (Alberts et al., 1994). Polarity genes are responsible for the establishment of the body axes at the onset of morphogenesis. Segmentation genes establish the number and size of subdivisions along the anterior-posterior axis of the embryo. Segments are initially more or less equivalent, although they may vary somewhat according to the anterior-posterior axis.

Pattern Formation is controlled through regional specialization within each body segment that is determined by the homeotic selector genes. Homeotic selector genes specify differences between segments along the body axis and between further subdivisions within the segments. They are targets of the gene products of segmentation genes. Their response to segmentation gene products are tempered by prior exposure of the cells to the polarity gene products. The sequential action of these three groups of genes is responsible for the detailed patterns of cells that constitute the various organ systems and their arrangement.

TABLE 7-1	CELLULAR PROCESSES THAT CONTRIBUTE TO PATTERN FORMATION
Process	*Examples*
Differential cell proliferation	Variable growth rate of various fetal organs
Migration of cells to new sites	Neural crest, primordial germ cells
Mechanical forces generated by altered cell shape	Neural tube formation
Programmed cell death	Syndactyly and triphalangeal thumb
Mechanical and chemical forces generated locally by:	
a. Extracellular matrix	Neural crest migration and integrins
b. Cell adhesion	Cell sorting and cadherin expression
c. Fluid pressure	Blastocyst cavitation via the Na/ATPase pump

Embryonic cells assemble into complex tissues and organs by first establishing gradients of morphogens. A morphogen is a bioactive molecule produced in one region that diffuses toward another region where it may be degraded, thus establishing a concentration gradient of the morphogen across the field of cells (Fig. 7-3). Several morphogen gradients may be produced to define various body polarities (anterior-posterior, dorsal-ventral, proximal-distal). Morphogens are generally gene products that affect the transcription of other genes, causing differential gene expression according to their cellular concentration.

An example of a morphogen is a protein that binds to cell receptors (e.g., growth factors) and induces an intracellular signaling cascade, leading to the activation of a transcription factor. Other examples of morphogens include molecules that can cross the cell membrane and enter the nucleus to activate transcription factors (e.g., vitamin D) or directly serve as a transcription factor. Polarity genes encode morphogens, or proteins that synthesize them, and are expressed very early in development to establish the major body axes.

Target genes may respond to various threshold levels of morphogen in either a positive or a negative manner. Some target genes (e.g., transcription factors) are affected permanently. That is, they and all of their progeny cells will always respond similarly to a variety of cellular signals (confers cell memory). Cell memory can be the result if an activated transcription factor turns on its own gene, permanently keeping it active in a positive feedback loop.

The expression of each set of genes in the hierarchy of polarity, segmentation and homeotic selector genes influences the ability of the next set of genes in the hierarchy to activate each potential gene target. Thus, a positional value (A-I in Fig. 7-3) is assigned to each cell of the embryo according to its history of gene activation, beginning with exposure to the polarity-establishing morphogens. Segmentation genes (there can be very many) are targets of the polarity gene products, and can be morphogens or transcription factors. Multiple morphogens have a combined effect that alternately activates or inhibits the segmentation genes, producing repetitive patterns of expression (see example in Fig. 7-3). As each segment differentiates, additional subdivisions are established by new morphogens, creating finer and finer detail.

Certain products of the polarity and segmentation genes activate the homeotic selector genes according to each cell's positional value. Homeotic selector genes produce transcription factors and contain a DNA-binding homeodomain sequence, called the homeobox. The homeotic selector genes are arranged in 4 complexes on different human chromosomes, named HoxA through HoxD. Each complex contains 9–11 structural genes. These genes apparently arose by gene duplication of homologous genes during evolution. Each Hox complex contains up to 13 structural genes that have homologous counterparts within each complex and are named accordingly as HoxA-1 through HoxA-13, and so on. Not all homologues are represented in each of the 4 human complexes. There are large expanses of noncoding regulatory regions within each

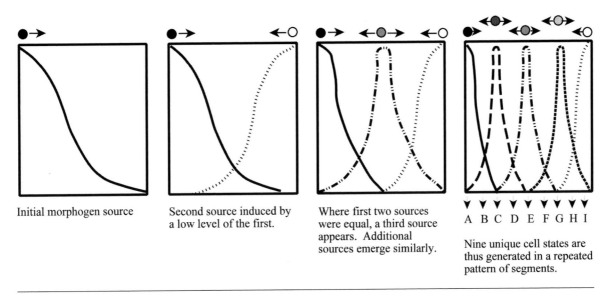

Initial morphogen source

Second source induced by a low level of the first.

Where first two sources were equal, a third source appears. Additional sources emerge similarly.

A B C D E F G H I

Nine unique cell states are thus generated in a repeated pattern of segments.

FIGURE 7-3 Pattern formation through morphogen production. In the first panel, a single point source of a morphogen is produced at one end of a field of cells (polarity gene product), creating the illustrated concentration gradient. A second morphogen is then produced by cells receiving the lowest dose of the first morphogen, creating an opposing concentration gradient. At the point where the two morphogens are of equal concentration, a gene is induced that produces another morphogen with the pattern shown in the third panel. Additional morphogens are produced similarly to generate the complexity shown in the fourth panel. Cells across this field will be exposed to different morphogens and may, therefore, differentiate along unique paths. The repetitious pattern of morphogens locally activates segmentation genes that define body segments (e.g., beginning at morphogen peaks, A,C,E,G,I, and ending at points of equal concentration, B,D,F,H), but the individual segments will be unique (A through I) due to the polarity gene products that have assigned position values to cells along the field. Based on position values, homeotic selector genes will be differentially expressed across the field, assigning different fates to each segment.

complex that contain promoter and enhancer targets for the products of the various developmental control genes.

The homeotic selector genes are physically ordered within each complex according to their temporal and anterio-posterior expression within the embryo. Generally, homeotic selector genes becomes activated beginning at different points along the body axis and continue to be expressed toward the posterior pole, creating an overlapping expression pattern, with the number of Hox genes increasing from the anterior to the posterior segments. An example of this expression pattern, is depicted

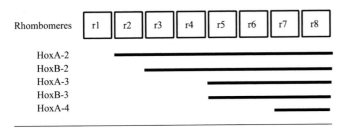

FIGURE 7-4 Expression of homeotic selector genes in the hindbrain. The overlapping pattern of Hox gene expression is exemplified in the hindbrain. Segments of the hindbrain, called rhombomeres, are indicated using a numbering system that begins toward the anterior end of the hindbrain. Below, the expression pattern of several Hox genes is indicated.

in Figure 7-4. The expression of different combinations of these genes within segments along the body axis generates the diversity among individual segments. Consider the vertebral column, which is composed of segments (the vertebrae) that develop from relatively homologous somites. However, each mature vertebra has a unique size, shape and rib association. While segmentation genes are responsible for generating somites of similar proportion, the homeotic selector genes determine the nature of the corresponding vertebrae that eventually form.

Mutation of a "housekeeping gene" may alter an enzymatic activity and inhibit a basic function critical for embryonic survival. Homozygous mutant embryos of this type will die during embryogenesis, giving rise to spontaneous abortion. Mutation of a housekeeping gene that affects a protein critical to a particular differentiated cell type will generate a malfunction limited to a specific organ that may not be an embryonic lethal, but will not affect the body plan. Many such mutations give rise to inborn errors of metabolism (e.g., hemoglobin mutation leads to sickle cell anemia). However, mutations in genes that control positional value will disrupt the body plan by altering the responses of affected cells to environmental queues during development. Cells affected by mutation of developmental control genes may continue to differentiate normally, but in an abnormal pattern. These mutations are the origin of multiple defect syndrome (Epstein, 1995).

Points to remember:

- Control of cell differentiation is built on hierarchies
- Transcription factors control morphogenesis by activating other sets of transcription factors through the induction of morphogens (polarity → segmentation → homeotic selector).
- Morphogenetic transcription factors may also activate genes encoding signal transduction molecules that determine how cells will respond to environmental queues.
- The activated signal transduction pathways may activate sets of structural genes that determine the differentiated state of the cell.

Because of the combinational nature of the interactions among the genes establishing patterns in the embryo, the same gene may be involved in directing the formation of very different body parts in different regions of the embryo.

A single mutation in a developmental control gene will, therefore, cause problems in several areas of the body, perhaps causing problems in several organ systems or disrupting the normal body pattern.

FROM THEORY TO PRACTICE

The following case discusses multiple defect syndrome: a point mutation in the human PAX2 gene (Sanyanusin et al., 1995).

CASE I

At 18 months, a male patient was found to have renal insufficiency, a nonfunctioning right kidney and bilateral grade IV vesicoureteral reflux. At age 7, renal hypoplasia and loss of corticomedullary differentiation was identified. At age 15, he returned with chronic renal failure, as well as severe visual impairment. His renal failure was associated with hypertension and chronic mild proteinuria. Optical examination revealed bilateral optic nerve colobomas. Karyotype, growth, intelligence, and hearing were all normal.

The boy had 2 nonaffected male siblings and 2 brothers with similar problems. One, 10 years old, had bilateral optic nerve colobomas and mild renal dysfunction (grade II vesicoureteral reflux and small hypolastic kidneys with poor corticomedullary differentiation). Otherwise, he had normal growth, intelligence and hearing. The other affected sibling was a 6-year-old with progressive renal failure, having had a renal transplant at age 5. His kidneys had been hypoplastic with poor corticomedullary differentiation, left pyelocaliectasis, grade I vesicoureteral reflux, hypertension and mild proteinuria. This boy was of short stature with mild hypotonia and mild scoliosis; however hearing and intelligence were normal. Optical examination revealed bilateral optic nerve colobomas and megalopapilla.

The father, age 35, also had bilateral optic nerve colobomas, but no recognized renal problems. Closer examination revealed

hypertension, mild proteinuria, elevated serum creatinine, and a mild sensorineural hearing loss. Intelligence was normal. The mother had had 2 early miscarriages, but was otherwise normal except for myopia. No history of similar problems was uncovered in the paternal family.

The reported multiple defect syndrome appeared to be an autosomal dominant mutation inherited from the father and passed on to at least half of the offspring. The 2 miscarriages at 6–10 weeks may have resulted from an embryonic lethal effect of the same gene mutation. Animal experiments have demonstrated that a developmental control gene, PAX2, has a pattern of expression consistent with a phenotype that would include eye malformations, sensorineural hearing loss, and renal hypoplasia. The syndrome described for this family matched this phenotype quite closely.

PAX2 EXPRESSION IN LABORATORY ANIMALS

PAX2 is the human homologue of a class of Drosophila segmentation genes and a member of a homologous human gene family containing nine members (PAX1 through PAX9). It is expressed in mice in the ureteric bud and the ureter during kidney development, as well as in the optic cup, otic vesicle, and other parts of the CNS. The gene product is a transcription factor containing paired box and octapeptide DNA-binding sequences. The PAX gene product binds to enhancers, where gene dose is important; thus, heterozygous loss is detrimental.

In mutant mice lacking the Pax2 gene, epithelial structures of kidney cortex do not differentiate normally, causing reduced renal cortex thickness and glomeruli number. There are also retinal defects within the eye. In mice with a constitutive expression mutation, polycystic kidney abnormalities occur during fetal life. The Pax2 gene is expressed in disparate organ systems where it functions similarly, but impacts unrelated tissues.

PAX2 EXPRESSION IN THE AFFECTED FAMILY

Blood samples were obtained from members of the family described above for molecular analysis of the PAX2 gene. Using a PCR-based technique called single strand conformational polymorphism analysis to broadly search for gene alterations, an abnormal pattern was detected in exon 5 of the PAX2 gene only in affected family members. Detailed sequencing was then conducted within that exon, which revealed a single nucleotide deletion that caused a frameshift mutation. The resulting mutated gene product is a truncated PAX2 protein that contains a normal paired box, but lacks the octapeptide sequence. Therefore, in addition to a reduced level of PAX2 protein, which may be critical, the mutant protein may compete with normal PAX2 protein for DNA binding sites in target genes, further reducing PAX2 activity. That is why the mutation is an autosomal dominant. A pedigree of the PAX2 mutation in three generations of this family demonstrated that the mutation arose spontaneously in the father of the affected boys.

PAX2 illustrates:

1. Multiple birth defect syndromes can arise from a mutation in a single developmental control gene
2. A gene candidate can be identified by comparing patterns of expression during early development in the mouse with clinical syndromes in humans
3. The existence of a phenotypically similar mutant mouse with a known mutation can further support a candidate gene

References

Alberts B, Bray D, Lewis J, et al. *Molecular Biology of The Cell*. New York: Garland; 1994; Chapter 12.

Epstein CJ. The new dysmorphology: application of insights from basic developmental biology to the understanding of human birth defects (REVIEW). *Proc. Natl. Acad. Sci. USA*. 1995;92:8566–8573.

Sanyanusin P, Schimmenti LA, McNoe LA, et al. Mutation of the PAX2 gene in a family with optic nerve colobomas, renal anomalies and vesicoureteral reflux. *Nature Genetics*. 1995;9:358–364.

Stein GS, Stein JL, van Wijnen AJ, et al. The maturation of a cell. *American Scientist*, 1995;84:28–37.

PRENATAL GENETIC COUNSELING

Heather Shane Michaels / Shivani B. Nazareth / Lorien Tambini

GENETIC COUNSELING

Concerning mothers, H. Raban Simeon B. Gamaliel says, "If she produces males and they were circumcised and died, if the first was circumcised and died, the second and he died, the third may be circumcised, but the fourth should not be circumcised."[1]

This Talmudic proscription refers to what is now recognized as hemophilia, indicating that the concept of genetic counseling has existed for centuries.[2] Every culture has recognized and incorporated explanations for familial patterns of disease, birth defects, infertility, and unusual deaths. In many cases, such conditions were ascribed to evil spirits, outside forces of nature, or deserved punishment for a sin. A scientific approach to establishing patterns of inheritance began with Gregor Mendel's observations of garden peas in 1865. Around this same time, Charles Darwin began to describe his theories of evolution, which relied heavily on genetic fitness and survival. Francis Galton, Darwin's cousin, studied twins in an attempt to formulate mathematical models to explain environmental versus hereditary contributions to human traits. A vital step in the application of genetic theory to human disease occurred in 1902, when Sir Archibald Garrod used Mendel's laws of inheritance to describe the familial occurrence of alkaptonuria and other "inborn errors of metabolism."[6]

As the value of genetic knowledge and the inheritance of various disorders became apparent, interest in the field of genetics and preventative medicine exploded. In 1943, Oswald Avery proved that DNA carries genetic information. A decade later, Watson and Crick were credited for delineating the double-helix structure of DNA, and in 1956, Tjio and Levan described the cytogenetic cause of Down syndrome. Concomitant technological advances allowed the field of genetics to advance at an extraordinary pace. Amniocentesis, for example, was used for fetal karyotyping in 1966 with the first identified chromosome anomaly being reported by Jacobson and Barter 1 year later. In recent years, the inception of the Human Genome Project as a collaborative effort to map the nearly 30,000 genes in human DNA has created yet another opportunity to understand familial disease. As genetic research progresses, significant advances will continue to change the way medicine is practiced. The complexity of this new and constantly evolving information has given rise to an organized profession of individuals dedicated to helping patients understand their genetic risks, cope with the implications of these risks, and use the available genetic technology to make important decisions about their future: genetic counselors.

A clear definition of the role of genetic counselors was developed in 1975 by the American Society of Human Genetics as follows:

Genetic counseling is a communication process which deals with the human problems associated with the occurrence or risk of occurrence of a genetic disorder in a family. This process involves an attempt by one or more appropriately trained persons to help the individual or family to: (1) comprehend the medical facts including the diagnosis, probable course of the disorder, and the available management, (2) appreciate the way heredity contributes to the disorder and the risk of recurrence in specified relatives, (3) understand the alternative for dealing with the risk of recurrence, (4) choose a course of action which seems to them appropriate in view of their risk, their family goals, and their ethical and religious standards and act in accordance with that decision, and (5) to make the best possible adjustment to the disorder in an affected family member and/or to the risk of recurrence of that disorder.

This definition was created partly in response to the fears that many people had regarding the use of genetic information for the betterment of the human race. Unfortunately, by the mid-1920s, a eugenics movement had already begun, and laws prohibiting the "mentally defective" from having children were enacted in almost half of the nation's states.[3] Misuse of genetic differences to establish racial inferiority and ethnic cleansing was exemplified by the horrific death of thousands of Jewish people killed in the Holocaust. The repulsiveness of these situations led geneticists to shy away from advising people about their familial risks. In an effort to ameliorate this reaction, the field of genetic counseling moved heavily toward a "non-directive" approach, whereby individuals were encouraged to make their own decisions based on a comprehensive understanding of the benefits, risks, and limitations of all their available options. This approach continues to play a crucial part of the genetic counseling process today, thus allowing genetics professionals to facilitate a discussion around all of the pertinent issues with the goal of helping individuals make decisions that best suit their personal values. To that end, a code of ethics reminding genetic counselors of their professional responsibilities, obligations, and boundaries was established in 1992 by the National Society of Genetic Counselors.[8]

Today, genetic counselors are health professionals with specialized graduate degrees in the areas of medical genetics and counseling. They provide information and support to families who have relatives with birth defects or genetic disorders and to individuals who are at risk of inheriting or passing on genetic disorders. Genetic counselors are responsible for analyzing inheritance patterns, identifying at-risk individuals, providing recurrence risks, and reviewing available options with families who can benefit from such services. Genetic counselors also provide psychosocial counseling to families, serve as patient advocates, and refer individuals and families to social workers and support groups as appropriate to the situation. Since genetic information changes at an alarmingly rapid pace, it is the responsibility of genetics professionals to keep abreast of the advances in molecular genetic testing and to be aware of the clinical availability, utility, and limitations of such testing for accurate risk assessment and counseling.

The field of genetics has grown, and the role of genetic counselors has expanded to include a variety of disciplines, including prenatal, pediatric, adult-onset, and cancer counseling. Specialty clinics, such as hemophilia centers, muscular dystrophy centers, Jewish genetic screening programs, hemoglobinopathy clinics, and cardiogenetic clinics often include genetic counselors as part of their team of healthcare providers. Non-traditional roles for genetic counselors have evolved to include research positions related to the field of medical genetics and genetic counseling, teaching positions, public advocacy, and consulting. Inevitably, the role of genetic counselors will continue to expand with advances in the field of genetics. The focus of this chapter is the role of the prenatal genetic counselor in providing optimal obstetric and gynecologic care.

INDICATIONS FOR PRENATAL GENETIC COUNSELING

During the course of obstetric care, the physician or midwife may encounter issues with which he or she has limited familiarity. Obstetric providers may have a working knowledge of many genetic diseases, but limited experience with the inheritance patterns of these conditions, carrier frequencies, recurrence risks, and available genetic tests. Information presented during the review of family medical history or pregnancy history often requires the expertise of those trained specifically in genetics. A primary role of genetic counselors is to obtain a detailed 3-generation family and medical history in order to assess risk. In the prenatal setting, the following represent the most common medical indication for a referral to a genetic counselor:

- Advanced maternal age (maternal age greater than 34 years)
- Positive maternal serum screen
- Patient or family member with a known mendelian disorder
- Prior pregnancy with a chromosomal disorder
- Family history of mental retardation or birth defect
- Fetal anomalies or markers detected by sonogram
- Recurrent pregnancy loss/stillbirth
- Infertility
- Ethnic-based carrier screening
- Consanguinity
- Maternal disease and/or teratogen exposure
- Parental concern

ADVANCED MATERNAL AGE

The occurrence of meiotic nondisjunction is largely influenced by maternal age. During fetal development, females amass their lifetime supply of oocytes, a significant proportion of which regress over time. Although the mechanisms are not well understood, experts agree that the aging process of the oocytes and/or environmental influences adversely affect the meiotic spindle. Consequently, advanced maternal age is associated with an increased risk for fetal aneuploidy. Although the increase is gradual during the first decades of life, a more pronounced risk is notable by age 35. Traditionally, a woman's risk to have a fetal chromosome anomaly at age 35 has been comparable to the risk of pregnancy loss associated with amniocentesis. That is, the risks are both equivalent to approximately 1/200, or 0.5%. As a result, maternal age greater than 34 years is an indication for offering genetic counseling to review the benefits, risks, and limitations of prenatal diagnostic procedures. As the risk from these procedures is determined to be less than previously reported, the age at which such referrals should be made is likely to decrease.

POSITIVE MATERNAL SERUM SCREEN

Although advanced maternal age has been established as a known risk factor for fetal aneuploidy, any couple can have an affected pregnancy. In fact, most babies with Down syndrome are born to women under the age of 35. Although the individual risk per fetus in younger women is lower than that of older women, young women collectively have more babies and do not typically pursue prenatal diagnostic testing. To help address this issue, second-trimester maternal marker screening using maternal serum was developed as a means to identify pregnancies at increased risk for certain birth defects or chromosomal disorders. Four analytes—alpha-feto protein (AFP), human chorionic gonadotropin (hCG), unconjugated estriol (uE3), and inhibin—have been utilized as components of this screening to assess risk. Maternal age, weight, race, gestational age, diabetic status, and number of fetuses influence the analyte levels, and specific patterns of these analytes have been correlated with risk for certain conditions. For instance, elevated maternal serum alpha-feto protein levels have been correlated with open neural tube defects, abdominal wall defects, renal anomalies, fetal demise, and other adverse pregnancy outcomes. On the other hand, suboptimal levels of maternal serum AFP are associated with certain chromosomal disorders, such as Down syndrome, for which the detection rate associated with traditional second-trimester maternal marker screening is approximately 60%.

First-trimester screening in conjunction with early sonographic findings has shown substantial merit in the detection of chromosomal disorders and is rapidly gaining favor as a more effective method of fetal screening. Screening in the first trimester involves measurement of free beta hCG and pregnancy-associated plasma protein A (PAPP-A) from maternal serum, with adjuvant sonogram measurement of fetal nuchal translucency. Assessment of these 2 values appears to detect approximately 85% of fetuses with Down syndrome, and can allow for early diagnostic testing using chorionic villus sampling (CVS).

Generally, any patient with an abnormal screen should be referred to a genetic counselor to discuss pregnancy management options, such as a repeat screen, high-resolution sonogram, or utilization of prenatal tests, including amniocentesis with acetylcholinesterase testing.

PATIENT OR FAMILY MEMBER WITH A KNOWN MENDELIAN GENETIC DISORDER

Many couples enter a pregnancy with the knowledge that they are at risk of transmitting a genetic disorder to their offspring. Couples in this situation may feel guilt, not only about the risk, but also about choosing to test and possibly terminate a pregnancy affected with the same condition from which a loved one suffers. Such patients often benefit from the psychosocial aspects of a genetic counseling session, where the emotional impact of the decision can be addressed and the genetics professional can help facilitate a discussion around all the pertinent issues. Equally important, a genetic counselor can offer these couples medical information about the chance of passing on the disease gene in question and the availability and accuracy of molecular prenatal testing for the specific disorder. In these cases, the specialized training of the genetic counselor plays a critical role in both education and psychosocial support.

PRIOR PREGNANCY WITH A CHROMOSOMAL DISORDER

Couples who have had a prior anomalous pregnancy are likely to have significant concern about the recurrence risk for future pregnancies. For couples with a previous pregnancy affected with a common chromosome disorder, such as Trisomy 13, 18, or 21, the estimated recurrence risk is approximately 1% or the patient's age-related risk, whichever is higher. Other chromosomal conditions may be inherited and associated with greater recurrence risks. All couples in this situation should be referred to a genetic counselor and offered prenatal diagnosis through CVS or amniocentesis.

FAMILY HISTORY OF MENTAL RETARDATION OR BIRTH DEFECTS

Mental retardation and/or congenital anomalies result from numerous causes, including genetic diseases, chromosomal disorders, and in-utero exposures. The recurrence risk for future pregnancies or other family members typically depends on the type of anomaly, an association with an underlying disorder, and the sex of the affected child. Genetic counselors can discuss the estimated recurrence risk with the couple and offer them appropriate testing.

Many relatively common conditions follow a multifactorial inheritance pattern, meaning that both genetic and environmental factors contribute to their development. While taking a family history, one must attempt to differentiate between isolated conditions and problems that occur as part of a larger constellation of findings. For example, establishment of a genetic etiology would be more pressing for an expecting couple with a family history of a ventricular septal defect and cleft lip and palate, as compared to a family history of a 60-year old with heart disease acquired over time. The latter scenario suggests a multifactorial condition, whereas the former may represent an underlying genetic disorder for which there is a risk for recurrence.

FETAL ANOMALIES OR MARKERS DETECTED BY SONOGRAM

In many cases, ultrasound abnormalities are identified in pregnancies of couples with no particular risk factors. The unexpected finding of an anomaly during routine ultrasound can cause extreme parental concern. Some ultrasound markers detected as early as the first trimester can be associated with increased risks for genetic and chromosomal disorders. In other cases, true anomalies are detected, but it may be unclear if they are associated with an underlying genetic or chromosomal disorder. Family medical history information, maternal serum screening results, and other pertinent information must be gathered to allow for better assessment of genetic risk. Genetic counselors can assist patients by explaining the significance of the finding and the availability of further testing through CVS, amniocentesis, or fetal echocardiogram. They can also interpret genetic test results for the patient and aid in the follow-up decisions based on these tests. Interpretation of findings and test results as well as information about any underlying disorder may be critical determinants in helping couples make decisions about the management of their pregnancy.

RECURRENT PREGNANCY LOSS/STILLBIRTH

Approximately 15% of identified pregnancies end in spontaneous abortion in the first trimester, and more than 50% of these losses are chromosomally abnormal. When possible, fetal losses should be karyotyped to determine recurrence risks for future pregnancies. Couples with a history of recurrent pregnancy loss or stillborn child should be referred to genetics for blood chromosome analysis. In approximately 5% of couples with multiple fetal losses, 1 parent carries a rearrangement of the chromosomes called a translocation. The usual translocation found with recurrent pregnancy loss involves a reciprocal exchange of segments of chromosomal information. The rearrangement is deemed "balanced" in the carrier, as there is no significant amount of functional genetic material lost. However, segregation of chromosomal derivatives to progeny may involve a gain or loss of genetic material and can result in an "unbalanced" arrangement. Aneuploidy of a chromosome segment can affect the viability of a pregnancy and may result in fetal loss or stillbirth. It may also result in the birth of a child with congenital anomalies and/or mental retardation. Referral to a genetic counselor for a discussion and evaluation of risks after adverse pregnancy outcomes should be a component of the work-up.

INFERTILITY

Assessment of infertility is a multidisciplinary approach, often involving evaluation by specialists in urology, obstetrics, endocrinology, genetics, and others. Among healthy individuals with difficulty conceiving, a significant proportion may have a chromosomal rearrangement or numerical chromosome disorder contributing to their fertility problems (Chromosomal Factors of Infertility in ICSI). These may include sex chromosome disorders, translocations, inversions, or deletions. Healthy males with impaired fertility may carry a deletion on the Y chromosome in a region crucial for spermatogenesis in 10–15% of cases. Further, a significant proportion of males with fertility problems are carriers for a mutation in the Cystic Fibrosis Transmembrane Regulator gene. The available assisted reproductive techniques such as IVF and ICSI may put these couples at risk for offspring with associated birth defects and/or mental retardation, or for offspring with similar fertility problems.[4] Couples having difficulty achieving pregnancy should be referred to a genetic specialist for evaluation and appropriate testing.

ETHNIC-BASED CARRIER SCREENING

Since every individual is thought to be a carrier of approximately 5–10 recessive genetic disorders, ethnic-based carrier screening is an important aspect of responsible obstetric care. Different ethnic groups are known to have higher carrier frequencies of specific recessive alleles. For instance, in individuals who are Jewish and from Eastern or Central Europe, also known as Ashkenazi Jews, there are several disease genes that are more frequent than in the general population. To date, there are 11 such diseases for which clinical carrier screening is available: Tay-Sachs disease, Canavan disease, Niemann-Pick disease, Gaucher disease, cystic fibrosis, Fanconi anemia, Bloom syndrome, familial dysautonomia, and mucolipidosis type IV, glycogen storage disease Type 1a, Maple Syrup Urine disease (see Table 8-1). Since these diseases also occur, though with lower frequency, in the non-Jewish population, carrier screening is recommended for all couples in which one or both individuals is of Ashkenazi Jewish descent.

Cystic fibrosis (CF) is not exclusive to the Ashkenazi Jewish population; it is a pan-ethnic disorder with a relatively higher frequency in both Northern European Caucasians and Ashkenazi Jews. In October 2001, The American College of Obstetrics and Gynecology (ACOG) issued a recommendation that all pregnant couples belonging to this ethnic group be offered carrier screening for cystic fibrosis.[10] In addition, ACOG

TABLE 8-1	DISEASE CARRIER FREQUENCIES IN ASHKENAZI JEWISH POPULATION
Disease	*Carrier Frequency in Ashkenazi Jewish Population*
Tay Sachs disease	1 in 25
Cystic fibrosis	1 in 25 – same for all Caucasians
Gaucher disease	1 in 18
Canavan disease	1 in 40
Niemann-Pick disease	1 in 70
Fanconi anemia	1 in 90
Bloom syndrome	1 in 100
Familial dysautonomia	1 in 35
Mucolipidosis type IV	1 in 122
Glycogen storage disease	1 in 71
Maple Syrup Urine disease	1 in 113[14]

recommends that couples in a lower risk category should be made aware of the availability of CF screening. In accordance with these guidelines, many obstetric providers are incorporating CF carrier screening into routine prenatal blood work. A referral to a genetic counselor is warranted when 1 or both members of a couple are determined to be a CF carrier.

Given the wide variety of ethnicity-based screening tests and differing patient opinions about what to do with the information, a referral to a genetic counselor should be made whenever a patient is determined to be a carrier. This is optimally prior to conception or early in the pregnancy. The genetic counselor can help clarify the distinction between being a carrier versus being affected with the disease, not only for educational purposes, but also to reduce the feeling of stigmatization that can accompany such results. The patient's partner must also be offered carrier testing so that risks for affected offspring can be assessed and prenatal testing can be offered if applicable. The genetics professional plays a crucial role in coordinating prenatal DNA and biochemical testing for identified at-risk couples, acting as a liaison between the molecular, cytogenetic, and biochemical laboratories and the patient.

CONSANGUINITY

When partners are related to each other by blood, it increases the likelihood of having children with certain birth defects. There are a number of harmful or lethal genetic mutations that follow autosomal recessive inheritance and since consanguineous couples have a higher proportion of their genes in common, they are more likely to carry the same rare genetic mutation.[13] A genetic counselor can assess family medical histories, ethnicity, and coefficient of relationship for such couples, educate them about their risks, and offer genetic testing when appropriate.

MATERNAL DISEASE/TERATOGEN EXPOSURE

Teratogens refer to exposures, chemical, radiological, or otherwise, that have the potential to interfere with normal fetal development. At least half of the pregnancies in North America are unplanned, and every year, thousands of women expose their fetuses to drugs prior to learning of their pregnancy.[11] In such cases, the specific agents involved, as well as the dosage and timing of the exposure are essential to determining risks. Patients in this situation should be referred to a genetic counselor to discuss the effects of the exposures on the developing fetus and pregnancy management options.

In some cases, the teratogen is the maternal disease itself; for example, thyroid dysfunction, phenylketonuria (PKU), insulin dependent diabetes mellitus (IDDM), seizure disorders, and lupus are among the maternal diseases that can adversely affect a developing fetus. In such cases, it may be unclear whether the maternal pathology itself or the medication used to treat the disorder is implicated in the risk. Patients suffering from such conditions should be referred to a genetic counselor to discuss the potential risks versus benefits of medication use during pregnancy. In this regard, a genetic counselor will work with the physician to determine the best course of action for the patient. Ideally, risk assessment will take place prior to conception, so that the patients can best prepare for the pregnancy.

PARENTAL CONCERN

Some couples are not considered at increased risk based on age or family history, but may request genetic evaluation due to their own anxiety. Frequently, these patients know or have worked with an individual that is mentally or physically challenged, and may feel concern about similar problems in their own pregnancy. These sessions, like all genetic counseling sessions, involve a review of the family medical history, pregnancy, and discussion, and can provide reassurance to couples regarding the likelihood of a normal pregnancy outcome.

PSYCHOSOCIAL GENETIC COUNSELING

The interaction of the genetic counselor and patient is highly influenced by psychosocial factors, including the patient's personal beliefs about the cause of birth defects and genetic disorders, the patient's emotional reaction to unforeseen risk, and the complex process of making a decision to suit one's personal belief system. The patient is often thrust into a position of choosing options based on risks that tread in unfamiliar territory. The genetic counselor has the responsibility of presenting this information in a way that encourages open dialogue, addresses the potential impact on the entire family, and ensures support for the patient's best interests. Establishment of this dynamic is crucial to the success of any genetic counseling session.

An important aspect of psychosocial genetic counseling is an awareness of the nongenetic factors that are "transmitted" within families, such as culture and religion. Such factors inevitably shape patients' capacity to cope, willingness to trust scientific information, and ability to accept a particular diagnosis. While the patient's upbringing does influence his or her decision-making process, the genetic counselor must take great care in treating each person as an individual and avoid making assumptions based on the religious or cultural experience of the patient.[3] Regardless of their background, parents faced with difficult decisions concerning the health of their unborn children often struggle with feelings of denial, fear, guilt, shame, depression, and anger. The astute genetic counselor can assess these emotional responses, assist patients in dealing with these feelings, and ultimately help to redirect the patient's energy toward a solution.

For particularly complex cases, genetic counselors work together with other healthcare professionals to ensure that patients receive extensive psychosocial support. These include, but are not limited to, social workers, grief counselors, and psychologists. Genetic counselors often have access to a network of support groups to help parents deal with a variety of genetic issues, including a new diagnosis, pregnancy loss, or the death of a child. The genetic counselor may also choose to put families in similar circumstances in touch with each other to facilitate healing and decision-making.

FROM THEORY TO PRACTICE

The following cases demonstrate the utility of genetic counseling in providing complete obstetric care:

CASE I

SB was a G3 P1011 39-year-old patient of Indian descent referred for genetic counseling secondary to advanced maternal age at 6 weeks and 6 days gestation. Her partner, JB, was a 42-year-old man of Irish Czechoslovakian descent. The couple had a healthy daughter who was 15 months old. Pregnancy history revealed that the couple's prior pregnancy had Trisomy 21 determined through amniocentesis testing, and the pregnancy was terminated at 18 weeks gestation. Given their anxiety about these events, SB and JB expressed interest in pursuing first-trimester prenatal diagnosis for their current pregnancy. As is standard in a genetic counseling session, a 3-generation family history was obtained to assess heritable risks and determine the need for additional tests. No other risk factors were noted.

The genetic counselor explained the option of CVS and compared the procedure to the amniocentesis in terms of its benefits, risks, and limitations. SB signed an informed consent to pursue CVS testing, and approximately 2 weeks after she underwent the procedure, the genetic counselor obtained the following results: 47,XY, +mar. A follow-up counseling session was scheduled with the couple, and at that time, the genetic counselor explained that a small piece of an extra chromosome, also called a "marker," was detected. The counselor reviewed that the marker chromosome may have been inherited from either parent, or may have occurred spontaneously (de novo) in the fetal cells. In order to determine the origin and significance of the marker chromosome, blood was drawn from both SB and JB for karyotyping.

Approximately 1 week later, it was determined that the marker chromosome was not familial, but rather de novo. Since about 40% of marker chromosomes originate from chromosome 15, further testing was offered to determine if the marker fell into this category. At this point, the genetic counselor reviewed in detail the benefits, risks, and limitations of further testing, while taking into consideration the timing of the pregnancy, cost, and turn around time of the tests. SB and JB decided to pursue further testing, and after several weeks, it was determined that the marker chromosome indeed originated from chromosome number 15.

In a follow-up consultation, the genetic counselor discussed the finding with the couple and explained the significance of a marker chromosome 15. It was reviewed that chromosome number 15 is 1 of the few chromosomes that are "imprinted," in other words, the expression of genes on chromosome 15 was influenced by the parent of origin. Typically, within a pair of chromosomes, 1 is inherited from each parent. If both chromosomes within a pair are inherited from the same parent, however, particularly in the case of an imprinted chromosome, the developing fetus will be adversely affected. The genetic counselor explained that this phenomenon is known as uniparental disomy (UPD).

The genetic counselor went on to explain the four mechanisms by which uniparental disomy could arise. The first and most common is referred to as trisomy rescue, whereby a trisomic cell recognizes the presence of an extra chromosome, and through cell division, "discards" it. In one third of these cases, the 2 remaining chromosomes are derived from the same parent, resulting in UPD. Another mechanism is called monosomy rescue, whereby a cell that is missing a chromosome undergoes mitotic duplication to produce a more viable cell line. Again, the resulting 2 chromosomes arose from the same parent. A third mechanism called gamete complementation is possible, although highly unlikely, whereby a sperm cell, for example, that is missing a chromosome fertilizes an egg that is disomic for that exact same chromosome. Finally, a fourth mechanism called somatic crossing over can occur and results in UPD for a chromosome segment.

In this case, the genetic counselor reviewed the clinical manifestations of UPD for a marker chromosome 15, including the possibility of Prader-Willi syndrome, mental retardation, or autistic-like behaviors. The couple felt that this information would help them decide whether to continue or terminate the pregnancy. Accordingly, the counselor coordinated UPD studies with the genetics laboratory. At 16 weeks gestation, the final report was complete, and the genetic counselor informed the couple that UPD was not present. SB and JB opted to continue the pregnancy and gave birth to a healthy baby boy.

CASE II

RG had a routine 18-week Level II sonogram that revealed the fetus had isolated echogenic bowel. RG, age 27, and her spouse, ML, age 30, were referred for genetic counseling to discuss the potential implication of this finding. The couple was understandably anxious, as this was their first pregnancy and no pregnancy complications had been noted previously. As is standard in any genetic counseling session, a 3-generation family history is obtained. No relatives with mental retardation, birth defects, or genetic disorders were reported on either side of the family. The genetic counselor explained the ultrasound finding and informed the couple that the majority of fetuses with isolated echogenic bowel are born without associated problems. Given the finding, however, several possibilities were reviewed.

The first possibility was that of a maternal infection, such as toxoplasmosis or CMV. Since approximately 3–4% of cases of echogenic bowel are related to such infections, the genetic counselor contacted the obstetrician and confirmed that RG did not have any known infection during her pregnancy.

The couple inquired about other causes of echogenic bowel, and the genetic counselor explained that an underlying chromosomal abnormality, such as Down syndrome, can also cause echogenic bowel. ML expressed confusion because he thought that only women over age 35 could have babies with Down syndrome. The genetic counselor proceeded to review the concepts behind chromosomes and nondisjunction, and informed the couple that while fetal chromosome problems are unlikely for most 27-year-old women, approximately 3% of fetuses with isolated echogenic bowel have aneuploidy.[9] Amniocentesis as a prenatal tool to detect such abnormalities was discussed and offered to the couple.

Finally, the genetic counselor discussed the association of echogenic bowel with obstruction, as seen in pregnancies with CF. RG stated that she already had CF testing and was indeed found to be a carrier. At that time, her husband was tested for CF and found to be negative. The genetic counselor obtained these reports from the obstetrician and confirmed that RG was tested for the standard panel of 31 mutations and was identified as a carrier of the deltaF508 mutation. ML was also tested for this standard panel and was found to be negative. The genetic counselor notes, however, that RG was half Northern European and her husband was entirely Puerto Rican. The couple is informed that many different mutations can lead to CF, and the detection rate for Puerto Rican mutations using the standard CF panel is low. To err on the side of caution, an expanded panel of CF mutations was offered to the patient's husband and his blood was drawn for carrier screening.

The ability of amniocentesis to prenatally detect CF in addition to chromosome abnormalities was reviewed. Since RG was already 18 weeks pregnant, and prenatal diagnosis for CF can take up to four weeks, she opted to pursue the amniocentesis procedure immediately following the counseling session. This would allow time to consider the option of termination if the fetus was determined as affected with either a chromosome abnormality or CF.

Two weeks later, the fetus was found to have normal chromosomes; however, ML was found to be a carrier of a CF mutation that was not part of his original screening panel. The genetic counselor reviewed autosomal recessive inheritance with the couple and they learned that their risk was one quarter, or 25%, to have a child with CF. The genetic counselor coordinated CF testing on the available cultured fetal cells. Approximately, 3 weeks later, it was determined that the fetus inherited 2 CF mutations and was therefore affected with CF.

At 23 weeks of pregnancy, the couple was in the predicament of choosing between continuation or termination of pregnancy prior to the 24-week legal limit for termination in most states. The genetic counselor helped the couple deal with the emotional reaction to this news and answered their questions regarding the clinical manifestations of CF. The supportive treatments available for CF were reviewed and the counselor informed the couple that while research is progressing, no cure existed for the disorder. The counselor facilitated a discussion between the couple about their options for the current pregnancy. Literature was provided to the couple and the genetic counselor remained open to phone calls and follow-up visits to help the couple make a decision that best suited their values. In the end, they elected to terminate the pregnancy, mainly because of the inability of genetic testing to determine the degree of severity of the CF.

The genetic counselor reviewed the information with RG's obstetrician, and it was discussed that while the standard panel of CF mutations picks up the majority of carriers, ethnic-based screening can be used to increase the detection rate and clinical utility of genetic testing. When RG was initially determined to be a CF carrier, a consultation with a genetic counselor would have helped the obstetrician determine which test to proceed with for her husband. If the couple had learned this information earlier in the pregnancy, prenatal testing and diagnosis could have been offered in the first trimester.

CASE III

JS was a 35-year-old G2P1001 Caucasian woman referred for prenatal genetic counseling at 13.5 weeks gestation to discuss her age-related risk for fetal aneuploidy. A 3-generation family history was obtained, and it was noted that her maternal first cousin had mental retardation of unknown etiology. The patient was counseled regarding origins of mental impairment, including genetic, chromosomal, and external causes and informed that the recurrence risk for her pregnancy would depend on the nature of her cousin's condition. It was suggested that she contact her maternal aunt for additional diagnostic information regarding her cousin's condition. JS also revealed that her 3-year-old son was undergoing evaluation by a psychologist for hyperactivity and language delay, and had been preliminarily diagnosed with autism. He was never evaluated by a medical geneticist, although such an examination was suggested by the genetic counselor. During the remainder of the genetic counseling session, the patient's age-associated risk for fetal chromosome disorders was discussed and the benefits, risks, and limitations of amniocentesis were explained. JS scheduled an amniocentesis at 16 weeks gestation.

JS elected to contact her aunt about her cousin's diagnosis and to return later in the week for appropriate testing. She learned that her cousin has been diagnosed with Fragile X syndrome, one of the most common forms of inherited mental impairment. At a follow-up genetic counseling session, the nature and etiology of Fragile X was described. Specifically, JS was counseled about the X-linked inheritance pattern of Fragile X. It was explained that Fragile X results from an expansion of a trinucleotide base pair repeat (CGG) within the Fragile X Mental Retardation (FMR-1) gene on the X chromosome. The genetic counselor reviewed that the normal size allele consists of less than 50 repeats. The range of 50–200 is considered the pre-mutation or carrier state, containing an unstably methylated number of repeats which can expand in 1 generation to a full mutation of greater than 200 repeats. JS was counseled that males who inherit a full mutation are expected to have a Fragile X phenotype, including mental impairment, subtle physical findings, and behavioral problems. Females with the full mutation may have normal intelligence,

although up to 60% may have learning disabilities or mental retardation. Due to limited correlation between the number of CGG repeats and the clinical presentation of the disease, the counselor explained that prediction of the phenotype of an affected female from molecular testing was limited.

JS was informed that the chance of her being a Fragile X carrier based on her cousin's diagnosis was one quarter. However, if her son were likewise affected, she would be considered an obligate carrier. Blood testing was offered to JS to quantify the number of CGG repeats on each of her FMR1 alleles. The results indicated that JS had 1 allele within the normal range, containing 29 CGG repeats. The other allele at the Fragile X locus was determined to contain 100 CGG repeats, consistent with the Fragile X pre-mutation state. JS was counseled that she had a 50% chance of passing on the expanded CGG repeats to each of her pregnancies, which would be anticipated to expand to a full mutation. After a discussion of the ability of amniocentesis to identify fetal chromosome disorders and to determine Fragile X status in the fetus, JS consented to pursue the procedure.

The chromosome analysis revealed a 46, XY karyotype and amniotic fluid AFP levels within expected limits. However, a full Fragile X mutation was identified in the pregnancy. After a follow-up genetic counseling session during which the results were reviewed and the prognosis was discussed, JS elected to terminate the pregnancy. Options for future pregnancies including CVS and pre-implantation genetic diagnosis of Fragile X were explained. Soon after, JS brought her son to see a geneticist, who diagnosed him with Fragile X. JS and her family were put in touch with another couple with a child with Fragile X for support.

JS returned for genetic counseling 6 months later, 10 weeks into her third pregnancy. She was offered CVS testing for chromosome analysis and Fragile X testing and the CVS procedure was explained. She consented to undergo CVS analysis and the pregnancy was determined to have a 46,XX karyotype and a full Fragile X mutation. The potential spectrum of clinical findings in affected females was reviewed, ranging from normal intellectual development to variable mental impairment. JS expressed an inability to care for another child with special needs, given the amount of time and attention her son required. After much deliberation, the patient elected to terminate the pregnancy. JS noted her eagerness to have another child but decided that she could not face the possibility of another affected pregnancy. During genetic counseling, it had been discussed that Fragile X carriers have been noted to have an increased rate of premature ovarian failure.[5] JS began to worry about her future ability to conceive. She was put in contact with a center that provided pre-implantation genetic diagnosis for Fragile X. The procedure involves removal of a single undifferentiated cell from a developing blastocyst after in-vitro fertilization. Molecular testing for Fragile X was performed on the cell and those embryos unaffected with Fragile X were transferred. CVS was utilized to confirm the diagnosis and to determine if fetal aneuploidy associated with maternal age was present. Today, JS has a baby girl unaffected with Fragile X.

SUMMARY

As demonstrated in all of these cases, genetic counseling involves risk assessment, discussion of appropriate genetic testing, psychosocial support, patient education, and follow-up to ensure the provision of both immediate and longer-term care. For information about how to contact a genetic counselor in your area, contact the National Society of Genetic Counselors at *www.nsgc.org*.[8]

References

1. [T. Shab. 15:8A-C].
2. *The Talmud of Babylonia: An American Translation*. Translated by Jacob Neusner. Number 251. Volume XIII.B: Tractate Yebamot, Chapters 4–6. Program in Judaic Studies Brown University. Atlanta: Scholars Press. 1992.
3. Baker DL, Schuette JL, Uhlmann WR. *A Guide to Genetic Counseling*. Mississauga, Ontario, Canada: John Wiley & Sons, Inc.; 1998.
4. Kim ED, Bischoff FZ, Lipshultz LI, et al. Genetic concerns for the subfertile male in the era of ICSI. *Prenatal Diagnosis* 1998;18:1349–1365.
5. Sherman SL. Premature ovarian failure in the fragile X syndrome. *Am J Med Genet*. 200;97:189–194.
6. Jorde LB, Carey JC, White RL. *Medical Genetics*. 2nd ed. St. Louis, MO: Mosby, Inc.; 1999.
7. *http://www.ornl.gov/hgmis/project/about.html*
8. National Society of Genetic Counselors (www.nsgc.org)
9. Bianchi OW, Crombleholme TM, D'Alton MI. *Fetology: Diagnosis & Management of the Fetal Patient*. New York: McGraw-Hill; 2000.
10. American College of Obstetricians and Gynecologists. *Preconception and Prenatal Carrier Screening for Cystic Fibrosis: Clinical and Laboratory Guidelines*. Washington, DC: Author; 2001.
11. Koren G, Pastuszak A, Ito S. Drugs in pregnancy. *N Engl J Med*. 1998; 338:1128–1137.
12. Gardner RJM, Sutherland GR. *Chromosome Abnormalities and Genetic Counseling*, 2nd ed. New York: Oxford University Press; 1996.
13. Bridge P. *The Calculation of Genetic Risks: Worked Examples in DNA Diagnostics*, 2nd ed. Baltimore: Johns Hopkins University Press; 1997.
14. Edelmann L, Wasserstein MP, Kornreich R, et al. Maple Syrup Urine Disease: Identification and carrier-frequency determination of a novel founder mutation in the Ashkenazi Jewish population. *Am J Hum Genlt* 2001;69:863–868.

PRINCIPLES OF TERATOLOGY

Robert L. Brent / Lynda Fawcett / David A. Beckman

INTRODUCTION

There have been dramatic advances in understanding of the causes of human birth defects. In earlier times, superstition, ignorance, and prejudice predominated in these explanations. The stigma associated with birth defects has primitive beginnings and persists today. In the minds of many, even the most sophisticated, a birth defect is felt to be some form of punishment. At the beginning of the last century the predominant cause was believed to be genetic; the rest of the causes consisted of totally unsolvable clinical problems. At this point in the history of birth defect research, the etiology of congenital malformations can be divided into 3 categories: unknown, genetic, and environmental factors (Table 9-1).

The etiology of the majority of human malformations, approximately 65–75%, is still unknown.[1–3] However, a significant proportion of congenital malformations of unknown etiology is likely to be polygenic (i.e., due to 2 or more genetic loci[4,5]) or at least to have an important genetic component. Malformations with an increased recurrent risk, such as cleft lip and palate, anencephaly, spina bifida, certain congenital heart diseases, pyloric stenosis, hypospadias, inguinal hernia, talipes equinovarus, and congenital dislocation of the hip, can fit the category of multifactorial disease, as well as the category of polygenic inherited disease.[4,5] The multifactorial threshold hypothesis involves the modulation of a continuum of genetic characteristics by intrinsic and extrinsic (environmental) factors.[5] Although the modulating factors are not known, they probably include placental blood flow, placental transport, site of implantation, maternal disease states, infections, drugs, chemicals, and spontaneous errors of development.

Spontaneous errors of development may account for some of the malformations that occur without apparent abnormalities of the genome or the imposition of environmental influences. We postulate that there is some probability for error during embryonic development based on the fact that embryonic development is a complicated process, similar to the concept of spontaneous mutations.[2,6] It has been estimated that up to 50% of all fertilized ova in the human are lost within the first 3 weeks of development.[7] The World Health Organization estimated that 15% of all clinically recognizable pregnancies end in a spontaneous abortion, with 50–60% of the spontaneously aborted fetuses having chromosomal abnormalities.[8–10] As a conservative estimate, 1173 clinically recognized pregnancies will result in approximately 173 miscarriages and 30–60 of the infants in the remaining 1000 live births will have congenital anomalies. The true incidence of pregnancy loss is much higher, but undocumented pregnancies are not included in this risk estimate. The 3–6% incidence of malformed offspring represents the background risk for human maldevelopment. Although we know little about the mechanisms that result in the in utero death of defective embryos, it is more important to understand the circumstances that permit abnormal embryos to survive to term.[11]

Understanding the pathogenesis for the large group of malformations with unknown etiology will depend on identifying the genes involved in polygenic or pleurogenic processes, the interacting genetic and environmental determinants of multifactorial traits, and the statistical risks for error during embryonic development.

The known etiologies of teratogenesis include genetic and environmental factors that affect the embryo during development (e.g., drugs, chemicals, radiation, hyperthermia, infections, abnormal maternal metabolic states, or mechanical factors). Environmental and genetic causes of malformations have different pathologic processes that result in abnormal development. Congenital malformations due to genetic etiology have a spectrum of pathologic processes that are the result of a gene deficiency, a gene abnormality, chromosome deletion, or chromosome excess. The pathologic nature of this process is determined before conception, or at least before differentiation, because of inherited or newly acquired genetic abnormalities present in all or most of the cells of the embryo. Although environmental factors may modify the development of the genetically abnormal embryo, the genetic abnormality is usually the predominant contributor to the pathologic process.

The remainder of this review will focus on prescription drugs and therapeutic agents that cause congenital malformations in the human. Although these agents account for less than 1% of all malformations, they are important because these exposures are preventable.

OVERALL TERATOGENIC RISK

To appreciate the difficulty in predicting the effect that an exposure to a drug or therapeutic agent will have on the developing embryo, we shall briefly discuss factors that influence this prediction. The baseline risk of human reproduction is based on epidemiologic studies that have determined the incidence of fetal death and maldevelopment. A substantial proportion of all conceptions are lost before term, and 50% of those are lost within the first 3 weeks.[7,12] Of the liveborn infants, 3% will have major malformations. Reproductive problems encompass a multiplicity of diseases including sterility, infertility, abortion (miscarriage), stillbirth, congenital malformations (due to environmental or hereditary etiologies), fetal growth retardation, prematurity, and others (Table 9-2). These diseases occur commonly in the general population and therefore environmental causes are not always easy to corroborate. Since severe congenital malformations, which have multiple causes (genetic, environmental, and unknown), occur in 3% of births, this means that each year in the United States, 120,000 newborns are born with severe birth defects. Genetic diseases occur

TABLE 9-1	ETIOLOGY OF HUMAN CONGENITAL MALFORMATIONS OBSERVED DURING THE FIRST YEAR OF LIFE

Suspected Cause	Percent of Total
UNKNOWN	65–75
Polygenic	
Multifactorial (gene-environment interactions)	
Spontaneous errors of development	
Synergistic interactions of teratogens	
GENETIC	15–25
Autosomal and sex-linked inherited genetic disease	
Cytogenetic (chromosomal abnormalities)	
New mutations	
ENVIRONMENTAL	10
Maternal conditions: alcoholism; diabetes; endocrinopathies; phenylketonuria; smoking and nicotine; starvation; nutritional deficits	4
Infectious agents: rubella, toxoplasmosis, syphilis, herpes simplex, cytomegalovirus, varicella-zoster, Venezuelan equine encephalitis, parvovirus B19	3
Mechanical problems (deformations): Amniotic band constrictions; umbilical cord constraint; disparity in uterine size and uterine contents	1–2
Chemicals, drugs, high dose ionizing radiation, hyperthermia	<1

Modified from references 2, 507, 508.

TABLE 9-2	FREQUENCY OF REPRODUCTIVE RISKS IN THE HUMAN

Reproductive Risk	Frequency
Immunologically and clinically diagnosed spontaneous abortions per 10^6 or million conceptions	350,000
Clinically recognized spontaneous abortions per 10^6 or million pregnancies	150,000
Genetic diseases per 10^6 or million births	110,000
Multifactorial or polygenic (genetic-environmental interactions)	90,000
Dominantly inherited disease	10,000
Autosomal and sex-linked genetic disease	1,200
Cytogenetic (chromosomal abnormalities)	5,000
New mutations[a]	3,000
Major congenital malformations per 10^6 or million births[b]	30,000
Prematurity per 10^6 or million births	40,000
Fetal growth retardation per 10^6 or million births	30,000
Stillbirths per 10^6 or million pregnancies (>20 wks)	20,900

Modified from reference 2.
[a] The mutation rate for many genetic diseases can be calculated. This can be readily performed with dominantly inherited diseases when offspring are born with a dominant genetic disease and neither parent has the disease.
[b] Congenital malformations have multiple etiologies including a significant proportion that are genetic.

in approximately 11% of births and include the congenital malformations with a genetic etiology. Genetic diseases due to new (uninherited) mutations at individual loci (spontaneous mutations) account for less than 2–3% of genetic disease.[13] Therefore, mutations induced from preconception exposures of environmental mutagens are difficult endpoints to document.[13]

ENVIRONMENTAL RISK PARAMETERS OR MODIFIERS

See Table 9-3.

THE IMPORTANCE OF THE STAGE OF EXPOSURE

The susceptibility of an embryo or fetus to teratogenic influences is related to the stage of development at which the exposure occurs. The explanation for this phenomenon is that the fetus is constantly changing during its development with respect to tissue receptors, metabolism, drug distribution, and

cell proliferation. Thus, tissue response to an exposure and the ability of the fetus to recuperate from the insult vary with the gestational stage. Although detrimental effects can be induced at any time during pregnancy, most major malformations result from exposures during days 18–40 of post conception in the human (Table 9-4). However, the palate, central nervous system, and genital structures can be affected at later stages of development. Our knowledge of the time of resistance or susceptibility of the embryo to various environmental influences has expanded over the past 30 years. This information is vital in evaluating the significance of individual exposures or epidemiologic studies.

THE THRESHOLD CONCEPT AND THE IMPORTANCE OF THE MAGNITUDE OF EXPOSURE (DOSE AND DOSE RATE)

Every teratogenic agent that has been tested in mammals has exhibited a dose-response relationship and a threshold dose response—that is, a dose below which there is no difference between the exposed and nonexposed in the incidence of malformations (Table 9-5). The dose to which the fetus is exposed is determined by maternal pharmacokinetics, placental exchange, fetal, and placental metabolism of the substance (and the teratogenic activity of the metabolites), the fetal distribution of the substance, and the presence of tissue-specific receptors. Factors that influence the response include maternal

TABLE 9-3	FACTORS THAT INFLUENCE SUSCEPTIBILITY TO DEVELOPMENTAL TOXICANTS

Stage of development: The developmental period at which an exposure occurs will determine which structures are most susceptible to the adverse effects of chemicals and drugs and to what extent the embryo can repair the damage.

Magnitude of the exposure: Both the severity and incidence of toxic effects increase with dose.

Threshold phenomena: The threshold dose is the dose below which the incidence of death, malformation, growth retardation, or functional deficit is not statistically greater than that of non-exposed subjects.

Pharmacokinetics and metabolism: The physiologic changes in the pregnant woman and during fetal development and the bioconversion of compounds can significantly influence the developmental toxicity of drugs and chemicals by affecting absorption, body distribution, active metabolites and excretion.

Maternal diseases: A maternal disease may increase the risk of fetal anomalies or abortion with or without exposure to a chemical or drug.

Placental transport: Most drugs and chemicals cross the placenta. The rate and extent to which a drug or chemical crosses the placenta are influenced by molecular weight, lipid solubility, polarity or degree of ionization, plasma protein binding, receptor mediation, placental blood flow, pH gradient between the maternal and fetal serum and tissues, and placental metabolism of the chemical or drug.

Genotype: The maternal and fetal genotypes may result in differences in cell sensitivity, placental transport, absorption, metabolism, receptor binding and distribution of an agent, and account for some variations in toxic effects among individual subjects and species.

---

toxicity and drug-drug interactions. Additionally, more than 30 drug-related disorders are related to genotype.[12] Although genetic variations have not been proved to alter drug teratogenicity in human beings, such proof exists for experimental animals.[14,15]

It is important that the significance of dose is not ignored when characterizing the manifestations of exposures to any reproductive toxicant. One cannot evaluate the biological effects and the risks of environmental agents without knowing the type of drug or chemical, its dose rate and the actual exposure. It has been demonstrated that both the genetic (preconception) and intrauterine effects of teratogens are reduced if the exposure is protracted, due to the reparability of the genome and the embryo. Acute exposures below the threshold for teratogenesis to the developing embryo or fetus represent no risk for deterministic reproductive effects and the embryo can be exposed to higher protracted exposures of a teratogen without sustaining any permanent reproductive effects.

Too often, the principle advocated by Paracelsus in the sixteenth century is ignored: "What is there that is not poison? All things are poison and nothing is without poison. Solely the dose determines that a thing is not a poison."

The most significant mistake by scientists or lay individuals uneducated in the fields of general and radiation toxicology is to ignore the importance of the dose or the exposure of the environmental agent. Environmental chemicals and physical agents (such as radiation) have deleterious effects at high exposures and represent no measurable risk at low exposures. This includes all environmental agents, even water.

MATERNAL DISEASE STATES

Maternal disease states may produce deleterious effects on the fetus that are difficult to separate from a possible teratogenic effect of a therapeutic agent. This is an especially relevant consideration for long-standing conditions such as diabetes or the autoimmune diseases.

BASIC PRINCIPLES OF TERATOLOGY (BIOLOGICAL PLAUSIBILITY)

The suggested reproductive effect should be biologically plausible and not contradict established scientific principles.[16–19] When evaluating studies dealing with the reproductive effects of any environmental agent, important principles should guide the analysis of reproductive human and animal studies. Paramount to this evaluation is the application of the basic science principles of genetics, teratology, and developmental biology. These principles are as follows:

1. Exposure to teratogens follows a toxicological dose response curve. There is a threshold below which no effect will be observed and as the dose of the teratogen is increased both the severity and frequency of reproductive effects will increase (Table 9-5).
2. The period of exposure is critical in determining what effects will be produced and whether any effects can be produced by a known teratogen. Some teratogenic effects have a broad, and others, a very narrow period of sensitivity.
3. Even the most potent teratogenic agent cannot produce every malformation.
4. Most teratogens have a confined group of congenital malformations that result after exposure during a critical period of embryonic development. This confined group of malformations is referred to as the syndrome that describes the agent's teratogenic effect.
5. While a group of malformations may suggest the possibility of certain teratogens, they cannot definitively confirm the causal agent. On the other hand the presence of certain malformations can eliminate the possibility that a particular teratogenic agent was responsible.

This approach is of greatest value when utilized for the evaluation of environmental agents that have been in use for some time or for evaluating new agents that have a similar mechanism of action, function, chemical structure, pharmacology, or physical effects of other agents that have been extensively studied. Of course, it is best to have data that pertains to the agent of interest.

TABLE 9-4	ESTIMATED OUTCOME OF 100 PREGNANCIES VERSUS TIME FROM CONCEPTION	
Time Conception	*From Percent Survival to Term[a]*	*Last Time for Induction of Selected Malformations[b]*
Preimplantation		
0–6 days	25	
Postimplantation		
7–13 days	55	
14–20 days	73	
3–5 wk	79.5	22–23 days; cyclopia; sirenomelia, microtia
		26 days; anencephaly
		28 days; meningomyelocele
		34 days; transposition of great vessels
6–9 wk	90	36 days; cleft lip,
		6 wk; diaphragmatic hernia, rectal atresia, ventricular septal defect, syndactyly
		9 wk; cleft palate
10–13 wk	92	10 wk; omphalocele
14–17 wk	96.26	12 wk; hypospadias
18–21 wk	97.56	
22–25 wk	98.39	
26–29 wk	98.69	
30–33 wk	98.98	
34–37 wk	99.26	
38+ wk	99.32	38+ wk; CNS cell depletion

[a] Data from reference 509.
[b] Modified from reference 47.

When counseling patients, especially in our litigious climate, 3 confounding influences are at work:

1. Because of the anxiety created by unfounded reports and misinformation, reported associations of drugs and their effect on the fetus must be evaluated critically.[20]
2. Pregnancy is not without risk, and congenital malformations occur in the absence of drug or chemical exposures.

3. Teratogenic agents do exist and new ones could be introduced.

MECHANISMS OF TERATOGENESIS

Based on his review of the literature, Wilson provided a format of theoretical teratogenic mechanisms: mutation; chromosomal aberrations; mitotic interference; altered nucleic acid synthesis and function; lack of precursors, substrates, or coenzymes for biosynthesis; altered energy sources; enzyme inhibition; osmolar imbalance, alterations in fluid pressures, viscosities, and osmotic pressures; and altered membrane characteristics.[1] Even though an agent can produce 1 or more of these pathologic processes, exposure to such an agent does not guarantee that maldevelopment will occur. Furthermore, it is likely that a drug, chemical, or other agent can have more than 1 effect on the pregnant women and the developing conceptus, and therefore the nature of the drug or its biochemical or pharmacologic effects will not in themselves predict a human teratogenic effect. Wilson's list of pathologic processes leading to teratogenesis has been modified in Table 9-6 to take into consideration some of the newer concepts pertaining to the mechanisms of teratogenesis, that is, the induction of somatic mutation and chromosomal abnormalities play no role in the teratogenic process except as they are responsible for cell death. Notwithstanding the importance of animal testing, the fact is that the discovery of human teratogens has

TABLE 9-5	STOCHASTIC AND THRESHOLD DOSE-RESPONSE RELATIONSHIPS OF DISEASES PRODUCED BY ENVIRONMENTAL AGENTS				
Relationship	*Pathology*	*Site*	*Diseases*	*Risk*	*Definition*
Stochastic phenomena	Damage to a single cell may result in disease	DNA	Cancer, mutation	Some risk exists at all dosages; at low exposures the risk is below the spontaneous risk	Incidence of disease increases but severity and nature of the disease remain the same
Threshold phenomena	Multicellular injury	High variation in etiology, affecting many cell and organ processes	Malformation, growth retardation, death, chemical toxicity, etc.	No increased risk below the threshold dose	Both severity and incidence of the disease increase with dose

Modified from reference 508.

TABLE 9-6	**MECHANISMS OF TERATOGENESIS**

1. Cell death or mitotic delay beyond the recuperative capacity of the embryo or fetus.
2. Inhibition of cell migration, differentiation and cell communication.
3. Interference with histogenesis by processes such as cell depletion, necrosis, calcification, or scarring.
4. Biologic and pharmacological receptor-mediated developmental effects.
5. Metabolic inhibition or nutritional deficiencies.
6. Physical constraint, vascular disruption, inflammatory lesions, amniotic band syndrome.
7. Interference with nutritional support of the embryo due to abnormalities of yolk sac or chorioplacental transport.

come primarily from observations and studies in human populations. Animal studies and in vitro studies can be very helpful in determining the mechanism of teratogenesis and the pharmacokinetics related to teratogenesis.[21] We have proposed a list of mechanisms (Table 9-6) that we shall use in our discussion of the known teratogenic drugs and therapeutic agents in man. However, even if one understands the pathologic effects of an agent, one cannot predict the teratogenic risk of an exposure without taking into consideration the developmental stage, the magnitude of the exposure, and the reparability of the embryo.

TERATOGENIC THERAPEUTIC AGENTS AND DRUGS

See Table 9-7.

AMINOPTERIN AND METHOTREXATE

Aminopterin and methotrexate (methylaminopterin) are folic acid antagonists that inhibit dihydrofolate reductase, resulting in cell death during the S phase of the cell cycle.[22] Aminopterin-induced therapeutic abortions have resulted in malformations (hydrocephalus, cleft palate, meningomyelocele and growth retardation) in some of the abortuses.[11,23,24] Three case reports of children exposed to aminopterin in utero included observations of growth retardation, abnormal cranial ossification, high-arched palate, and reduction in derivatives of the first branchial arch.[25] The pattern of malformations associated with exposure to either compound has been referred to as the fetal aminopterin/methotrexate syndrome.[26] Key features of this pattern of malformations include prenatal growth deficiency, abnormal cranial ossification, micrognathia, small low-set ears, and limb abnormalities. There have also been 3 case reports to date of severe developmental delay in children with methotrexate syndrome.[27–29] It is unclear if cognitive deficits occur as a direct result of exposure or are because of complicating factors of prematurity.

Methotrexate is used therapeutically as an abortifacient, treatment of rheumatoid arthritis and other autoimmune disorders, and as an antineoplastic agent. Skalko and Gold demonstrated a threshold effect and a dose-dependent increase in malformations in mice exposed to methotrexate in utero.[30] Analysis of human data indicate a critical period of exposure to methotrexate from 6–8 weeks from conception at a dose above 10 mg per week for the development of amniopterin/methotrexate syndrome.[31]

ANDROGENS

Masculinization of the external genitalia of the female has been reported following in utero exposure to large doses of testosterone, methyltestosterone, and testosterone enanthate.[32–34] The masculinization is characterized by clitoromegaly with or without fusion of the labia minora and no indication of nongenital malformations. Affected females experience normal secondary sexual development at puberty.[35]

Many animal models show the masculinizing effects of androgens. Well-known studies were performed by Greene and coworkers in the rat, Raynaud in the mouse, Bruner and Witschi in the hamster, Jost in the rabbit, and Wells and Van Wagenen in the monkey.[36–40] These studies demonstrated the masculinization of the urogenital sinus, its derivatives, and the external genitalia, although there was little effect on the mullerian ducts, and ovarian inversion did not occur. Based on experimental animal studies of altered sexually dimorphic behavior in female guinea pigs, rats, and monkeys,[41–46] behavioral masculinization of the female due to prenatal exposure to androgens in the human will be rare. The available literature indicates that the effects of androgens on the fetus are dependent on the dose and stage of development during which exposure occurred.

ANTICONVULSANTS

Although individual anticonvulsant drugs will be discussed in detail later, important aspects of anticonvulsants as a group should be discussed now.

Chronic administration of anticonvulsant drugs, with the exception of the succinimides (ethosuximide, methsuximide, phensuximide), have been associated with an increased teratogenic risk: barbiturates (phenobarbital, primaclone), hydantoins (phenytoin), oxazolidinediones (trimethadione, paramethadione), and a miscellaneous group (valproic acid, carbamazepine).[47] The increased teratogenic risk estimates for the anticonvulsants are 6% for barbiturate-hydantoin exposure, 80% for oxazolidinedione exposure, and about 1% for valproic acid induced neural tube defects. The mechanism of teratogenic action for the anticonvulsants has been difficult to define for several reasons: many are given in combination therapeutically, dose-response relationships are difficult to demonstrate, and the exposure is chronic. Since the increased teratogenic risk is small relative to the risk in nontreated pregnancies, it is likely that the chronic nature of anticonvulsant therapy is an important contributor to the increased teratogenic risk.

| TABLE 9-7 | EFFECTS AND ESTIMATED RISKS OF SELECTED PRESCRIBED AND SELF-ADMINISTERED DRUGS ON HUMAN PREGNANCY | |

Selected Drugs	*Reported Effects or Associations and Estimated Risks*	*Comments*[a]
Alcohol	Fetal alcohol syndrome: intrauterine growth retardation, maxillary hypoplasia, reduction in width of palpebral fissures, characteristic but not diagnostic facial features, microcephaly, mental retardation. An increase in spontaneous abortion has been reported but since mothers who abuse alcohol during pregnancy have multiple other risk factors, it is difficult to determine whether this is a direct effect on the embryo. Consumption of 6 oz of alcohol or more per day constitutes a high risk but it is likely that detrimental effects can occur at lower exposures.	Quality of available information: good to excellent. Direct cytotoxic effects of ethanol and indirect effects of alcoholism. While a threshold teratogenic dose is likely it will vary in individuals because of a multiplicity of factors.
Aminopterin, methotrexate	Microcephaly, hydrocephaly, cleft palate, meningomyelocele, intrauterine growth retardation, abnormal cranial ossification, reduction in derivatives of first branchial arch, mental retardation, postnatal growth retardation. Aminopterin can induce abortion within its therapeutic range; it is used for this purpose to eliminate ectopic embryos. Risk from therapeutic doses is unknown but appears to be moderate to high.	Quality of available information: good. Anticancer, antimetabolic agents; folic acid antagonists that inhibit dihydrofolate reductase, resulting in cell death.
Androgens	Masculinization of female embryo: clitoromegaly with or without fusion of labia minora. Nongenital malformations are not a reported risk. Androgen exposures which result in masculinization have little potential for inducing abortion. Based on animal studies, behavioral masculinization of the female human will be rare.	Quality of available information: good. Effects are dose and stage dependent; stimulates growth and differentiation of sex steroid receptor-containing tissue.
Angiotensin-converting enzyme (ACE) inhibitors	The therapeutic use of ACE inhibitors has neither a teratogenic effect nor an abortigenic effect in the first trimester. Since this group of drugs does not interfere with organogenesis, they can be used in a woman of reproductive age; if the woman becomes pregnant, therapy can be changed during the first trimester without an increase in the risk of teratogenesis. Later in gestation these drugs can result in fetal and neonatal death, oligohydramnios, pulmonary hypoplasia, neonatal anuria, intrauterine growth retardation, and skull hypoplasia. Risk is dependent on dose and length of exposure.	Quality of available information: good. Antihypertensive agents; adverse fetal effects are related to severe fetal hypotension over a long period during the second or third trimester.
Antibiotics	Streptomycin: Streptomycin and a group of ototoxic drugs can affect the 8th nerve and interfere with hearing; it is a relatively low risk phenomenon. There are not enough data to estimate the abortigenic potential of streptomycin. Because the deleterious effect of streptomycin is limited to the 8th nerve, it is unlikely to affect the incidence of abortion.	Quality of available information: fair to good. Long duration maternal therapy during pregnancy is associated with hearing deficiency in offspring.
	Tetracycline: Bone staining and tooth staining can occur with therapeutic doses. Persistent high doses can cause hypoplastic tooth enamel. No other congenital malformations are at increased risk. The usual therapeutic doses present no increased risk of abortion to the embryo or fetus.	Quality of available information: good. Effects seen only if exposure is late in the first or during second or third trimester, since tetracyclines have to interact with calcified tissue.

(continued)

TABLE
9-7

**EFFECTS AND ESTIMATED RISKS OF SELECTED PRESCRIBED AND
SELF-ADMINISTERED DRUGS ON HUMAN PREGNANCY** (*Continued*)

Selected Drugs	Reported Effects or Associations and Estimated Risks	Comments[a]
	Penicillin G benzathine used for the treatment of syphilis produces no adverse fetal effects in the usual therapeutic regimens:	These antibiotics are used in late pregnancy for the treatment of sexually transmitted diseases.
	Ceftriaxone and doxycycline used for the treatment of gonorrhea produces no adverse fetal effects in the usual therapeutic regimens.	
	Erythromycin base or stearate used for the treatment of Chlamydia involves a possible increased risk of cholestatic hepatitis in the usual therapeutic regimens.	
Antihypertensives (excluding ACE inhibitors)	Clonidine: a direct alpha adrenergic agonist that appears to be relatively safe during pregnancy but there are few available data.	
	Hydralazine: a vasodilator often used in combination with methyldopa and is considered to be safe.	
	Methyldopa: a centrally acting adrenergic antagonist and currently the safest antihypertensive drug available for use during pregnancy with no reported adverse effects on the fetus or on mental and physical development.	
	Nifedipine: a calcium channel blocker whose potential for adverse effects with its long term use in the treatment of hypertension is unknown.	
	Propranolol: a beta-blocker whose prolonged use may increase the risk of intrauterine growth retardation.	
Anti-tuberculosis therapy	Drugs prescribed for the treatment of tuberculosis include aminoglycosides, ethambutol, isoniazid, rifampin, and ethionamide. The ototoxic effects of streptomycin (discussed above) are the only proven adverse effects of these drugs on the fetus. Therapeutic exposures to other tuberculostatic drugs appear to represent a very small risk of teratogenesis and even less risk of abortion.	
Aspirin	No increased risk for malformations or abortion low dose regimen (60–150 mg per day). Aspirin should be discontinued 1 week before anticipated delivery to reduce the risk for maternal or neonatal bleeding.	Used for treatment of preeclampsia, idiopathic placental insufficiency, systemic lupus erythematosus, increased platelet aggregation.
Benzodiazepines	Benzodiazepines appear to have minimal or no increased risk of malformations at therapeutic ranges; higher exposures may increase the risk. The risk for abortion is unknown.	The benzodiazepines are widely used as tranquilizers during pregnancy.
	Chlordiazepoxide (Librium), appears to have a minimal risk for congenital anomalies and no increased risk for abortion at therapeutic doses. Higher exposures are likely to increase the risk of adverse effects on the fetus but the magnitude of the increase is not known.	
	Diazepam (Valium): third trimester exposure can reversibly affect the fetus and neonate there is minimal increased risk of congenital malformations and no demonstrated increased risk of abortions from therapeutic exposures.	

(*continued*)

| TABLE 9-7 | **EFFECTS AND ESTIMATED RISKS OF SELECTED PRESCRIBED AND SELF-ADMINISTERED DRUGS ON HUMAN PREGNANCY** (Continued) |

Selected Drugs	Reported Effects or Associations and Estimated Risks	Comments[a]
	Meprobamate: weakly associated with a variety of congenital malformations but the data are not sufficient to confirm or rule out a small increase risk of malformations due to exposures early in pregnancy.	
Caffeine	Caffeine is teratogenic in rodent species with doses of 150 mg/kg. There is no convincing data that moderate or usual exposures (300 mg per day or less) present a measurable risk in the human for any malformation or group of malformations. On the other hand, excessive caffeine consumption (exceeding 300 mg per day) during pregnancy is associated with growth retardation and embryonic loss.	Quality of available information: fair to good. Behavioral effects have been reported and appear to be transient or temporary; more information is needed concerning the population with higher exposures.
Carbamazepine	Minor craniofacial defects (upslanting palpebral fissures, epicanthal folds, short nose with long philtrum), fingernail hypoplasia, and developmental delay. Teratogenic risk is not known but likely to be significant for minor defects. There are too few data to determine whether carbamazepine presents an increased risk for abortion. Since embryos with multiple malformations are more likely to abort, it would appear that carbamazepine presents little risk because an increase in these types of malformations has not been reported.	Quality of available information: fair to good. Anticonvulsant; little is known concerning mechanism. Epilepsy may itself contribute to an increased risk for fetal anomalies.
Cocaine	Preterm delivery; fetal loss; placental abruption; intrauterine growth retardation; microcephaly; neurobehavioral abnormalities; vascular disruptive phenomena resulting in limb amputation, cerebral infarctions and certain types of visceral and urinary tract malformations. There are few data to indicate that cocaine increases the risk of first trimester abortion. The low but increased risk of vascular disruptive phenomena due to vascular compromise of the pregnant uterus would more likely result in midgestation abortion or stillbirth. It is possible that higher doses could result in early abortion. Risk for deleterious effects on fetal outcome is significant; risk for major disruptive effects is low, but can occur in the latter portion of the first trimester as well as the second and third trimesters.	Quality of available information: fair to good. Cocaine causes a complex pattern of cardiovascular effects due to its local anesthetic and sympathomimetic activities in the mother. Fetopathology is likely to be due to decreased uterine blood flow and fetal vascular effects. Because of the mechanism of cocaine teratogenicity, a well-defined cocaine syndrome is not likely. Poor nutrition accompanies drug abuse and multiple drug abuse is common.
Coumarin derivatives	Nasal hypoplasia; stippling of secondary epiphysis; intrauterine growth retardation; anomalies of eyes, hands, neck; variable central nervous system anatomical defects (absent corpus callosum, hydrocephalus, asymmetrical brain hypoplasia). Risk from exposure 10% to 25% during 8th to 14th week of gestation. There is also an increased risk of pregnancy loss. There is a risk to the mother and fetus from bleeding at the time of labor and delivery.	Quality of available information: good. Anticoagulant; bleeding is an unlikely explanation for effects produced in the first trimester. Central nervous system defects may occur anytime during second and third trimester and may be related to bleeding.
Cyclophosphamide	Growth retardation, ectrodactyly, syndactyly, cardiovascular anomalies, and other minor anomalies. Teratogenic risk appears to be increased but the magnitude of the risk is uncertain. Almost all chemotherapeutic agents have the potential for inducing abortion. This risk is dose-related; at the lowest therapeutic doses the risk is small.	Quality of available information: fair. Anticancer, alkylating agent; requires cytochrome P450 mono-oxydase activation; interacts with DNA, resulting in cell death.

(continued)

TABLE 9-7 | EFFECTS AND ESTIMATED RISKS OF SELECTED PRESCRIBED AND SELF-ADMINISTERED DRUGS ON HUMAN PREGNANCY *(Continued)*

Selected Drugs	Reported Effects or Associations and Estimated Risks	Comments[a]
Diethylstilbestrol (DES)	Clear cell adenocarcinoma of the vagina occurs in about 1:1,000 to 1:10,000 females who were exposed in utero. Vaginal adenosis occurs in about 75% of females exposed in utero before the 9th week of pregnancy. Anomalies of the uterus and cervix may play a role in decreased fertility and an increased incidence of prematurity although the majority of women exposed to DES in utero can conceive and deliver normal babies. In utero exposure to DES increased the incidence of genitourinary lesions and infertility in males. DES can interfere with zygote survival, but it does not interfere with embryonic survival when given in its usual dosage after implantation. Offspring who were exposed to DES in utero have an increased risk for delivering prematurely, but do not appear to be at increased risk for first trimester abortion.	Quality of available information: fair to good. Synthetic estrogen; stimulates estrogen receptor-containing tissue, may cause misplaced genital tissue which has a greater propensity to develop cancer.
Digoxin	No adverse fetal effects reported with usual therapeutic regimens.	Used for treatment of fetal dysrhythmia.
Diphenylhydantoin	Hydantoin syndrome: microcephaly, mental retardation, cleft lip/palate, hypoplastic nails and distal phalanges; characteristic, but not diagnostic facial features. Associations documented only with chronic exposure. Wide variation in reported risk of malformations but appears to be no greater than 10%. The few epidemiological data indicate a small risk of abortion for therapeutic exposures for the treatment of epilepsy. For short term treatment, i.e. prophylactic therapy for a head injury, there is no appreciable risk.	Quality of available information: fair to good. Anticonvulsant; direct effect on cell membranes, folate, and vitamin K metabolism. Metabolic intermediate (epoxide) has been suggested as the teratogenic agent.
Glucocorticoids	Dexamethasone, Betamethasone, Hydrocortisone, Methylprednisone: Glucocorticoids have not been shown to be teratogenic but chronic glucocorticoid therapy may result in prematurity and intrauterine growth retardation.	Glucocorticoids are used late in pregnancy to reduce respiratory distress in premature infants and to treat congenital adrenal hyperplasia. They are also used in the treatment of rheumatic diseases, other acute and chronic inflammatory diseases, and organ transplantation.
Indomethacin	Can prolong labor and may predispose neonate to necrotizing enterocolitis when used as a tocolytic.	Used for the prevention or reduction of intraventricular hemorrhage in premature infant and for treatment of polyhydramnious.
Lithium carbonate	Although animal studies have demonstrated a clear teratogenic risk, the effect in humans is uncertain. Early reports indicated an increased incidence of Ebstein's anomaly, other heart and great vessel defects, but as more studies are reported the strength of this association has diminished. Lithium levels within the therapeutic range (<1.2 mg%) do not increase the risk of abortion.	Quality of available information: fair to good. Antidepressant; mechanism has not been defined.
Methylene blue	Hemolytic anemia and jaundice in neonatal period after exposure late in pregnancy. There may be a small risk for intestinal atresia. No indication of increased risk of abortion.	Quality of available information: poor to fair. Used to mark amniotic cavity during amniocentesis.
Misoprostol	Misoprostol is a synthetic prostaglandin analog that has been used by millions of women for illegal abortion. A low incidence of vascular disruptive phenomenon, such as limb reduction defects and Mobius syndrome, has been reported.	Quality of available information: fair: Classical animal teratology studies would not be helpful in discovering these effects, because vascular disruptive effects occur after the period of early organogenesis.

(continued)

TABLE 9-7	EFFECTS AND ESTIMATED RISKS OF SELECTED PRESCRIBED AND SELF-ADMINISTERED DRUGS ON HUMAN PREGNANCY (Continued)	
Selected Drugs	**Reported Effects or Associations and Estimated Risks**	**Comments**[a]
Oxazolidine-2,4-diones (trimethadione, paramethadione)	Fetal trimethadione syndrome: V-shaped eye brows, low-set ears with anteriorly folded helix, high-arched palate, irregular teeth, CNS anomalies, severe developmental delay. Wide variation in reported risk. Characteristic facial features are documented only with chronic exposure. The abortifacient potential has not been adequately studied, but appears to be minimal.	Quality of available information: good to excellent. Anticonvulsants; affects cell membrane permeability. Actual mechanism of action has not been determined.
D-Penicillamine	Cutis laxa, hyperflexibility of joints. Condition appears to be reversible and the risk is low. There are no human data on the risk of abortion.	Quality of available information: fair to good. Copper chelating agent; produces copper deficiency inhibiting collagen synthesis and maturation.
Phenobarbitol	No adverse fetal effects reported for usual therapeutic regimens.	May be used for the prevention or reduction of intraventricular hemorrhage in premature infant.
Progestins	Masculinization of female embryo exposed to high doses of some testosterone-derived progestins and may interact with progesterone receptors in the liver and brain later in gestation. The dose of progestins present in modern oral contraceptives presents no masculinization or feminization risks. All progestins present no risk for non-genital malformations. Many synthetic progestins and natural progesterone have been used to treat luteal phase deficiency, embryos implanted via IVF, threatened abortion or bleeding in pregnancy with variable results. Conversely, synthetic progestins that interfere with progesterone function may cause early pregnancy loss; RU-486 is presently used specifically for this purpose.	Quality of available information: good. Stimulates or interferes with sex steroid receptor-containing tissue.
Retinoids, systemic (isotretinoin, etrentinate)	Increased risk of central nervous system, cardio-aortic, ear and clefting defects. Microtia, anotia, thymic aplasia and other branchial arch, aortic arch abnormalities and certain congenital heart malformations. Exposed embryos are at greater risk for abortion. This is plausible since many of the malformations, such as neural tube defects, are associated with an increased risk of abortion.	Quality of available information: fair. Used in treatment of chronic dermatoses. Retinoids can cause direct cytotoxicity and alter programmed cell death; affect many cell types but neural crest cells are particularly sensitive.
Retinoids, topical (tretinoin)	Epidemiological studies, animal studies and absorption studies in humans do not suggest a teratogenic risk. Regardless of the risks associated with systemically administered retinoids, topical retinoids present little or no risk for intrauterine growth retardation, teratogenesis or abortion because they are minimally absorbed and only a small percentage of skin is exposed.	Quality of available information: poor. Topical administration of tretinoin in animals in therapeutic doses is not teratogenic, although massive exposures can produce maternal toxicity and reproductive effects. More importantly, topical administration in humans results in nonmeasurable blood levels.
Rh immune globulin	No adverse fetal effects have been associated with Rh-Ig prophylaxis against Rh immunization.	
Smoking and nicotine	Placental lesions; intrauterine growth retardation; increased postnatal morbidity and mortality. While there have been some studies reporting increases in anatomical malformations, most studies do not report an association. There is no syndrome associated with maternal smoking. Maternal or placental complications can result in fetal death. Exposures to nicotine and tobacco smoke are a significant risk for pregnancy loss in the first and second trimester.	Quality of available information: good to excellent. While tobacco smoke contains many components, nicotine can result in vascular spasm vasculitis which has resulted in a higher incidence of placental pathology.

(continued)

TABLE
9-7

**EFFECTS AND ESTIMATED RISKS OF SELECTED PRESCRIBED AND
SELF-ADMINISTERED DRUGS ON HUMAN PREGNANCY** (Continued)

Selected Drugs	*Reported Effects or Associations and Estimated Risks*	*Comments[a]*
Thalidomide	Limb reduction defects (preaxial preferential effects, phocomelia), facial hemangioma, esophageal or duodenal atresia, anomalies of external ears, eyes, kidneys, and heart, increased incidence of neonatal and infant mortality. The thalidomide syndrome, while characteristic and recognizable, can be mimicked by some genetic diseases. Although there are fewer data pertaining to its abortigenic potential, there appears to be an increased risk of abortion.	Quality of available information: good to excellent. Sedative-hypnotic agent. The etiology of thalidomide teratogenesis has not been definitively determined.
Thyroid: iodides, antithyroid drugs (thioamides)	Fetal hypothyroidism or goiter with variable neurologic and aural damage. Maternal hypothyroidism is associated with an increase in infertility and abortion. Maternal intake of 12 mg of iodide per day or more increases the risk of fetal goiter. Thioamides may cause fetal goiter but dose can be adjusted to minimize this effect.	Quality of available information: good. Fetopathic effect of iodides and antithyroid drugs involves metabolic block, decreased thyroid hormone synthesis and gland development.
Tocolytics	There are no reports of adverse fetal outcome resulting from exposure to therapeutic doses of terbutaline, ritodrine, or magnesium sulfate.	
Toluene	Intrauterine growth retardation; craniofacial anomalies; microcephaly. It is likely that high exposures from abuse or intoxication increase the risk of teratogenesis and abortion. Occupational exposures should present no increase in the teratogenic or abortigenic risk. The magnitude of the increased risk for teratogenesis and abortion in abusers is not known because the exposure in abusers is too variable.	Quality of available information: poor to fair. Neurotoxicity is produced in adults who abuse toluene; a similar effect may occur in the fetus.
Valproic acid	Malformations are primarily neural tube defects and facial dysmorphology. The facial characteristics associated with this drug are not diagnostic. Small head size and developmental delay have been reported with high doses. The risk for spina bifida is about 1% but the risk for facial dysmorphology may be greater. Because therapeutic exposures increase the incidence of neural tube defects, one would expect a slight increase in the incidence of abortion.	Quality of available information: good. Anticonvulsant; little is known about the teratogenic action of valproic acid.
Vitamins	Biotin: No adverse fetal effects for the usual therapeutic regimen	Used for treatment of multiple carboxylase deficiency
	Cyanocobalamin: No adverse fetal effects for the usual therapeutic regimen.	Used for treatment of vitamin B12-responsive methylmalonic acidemia
	Folic acid: The efficacy of folic acid supplementation for reducing the risk of neural tube defect recurrence may be limited to a select portion of the population. There are no adverse fetal effects for the usual therapeutic regimen.	Used for reduction in recurrence of neural tube defects
	Vitamin A: The same malformations that have been reported with the retinoids have been reported with very high doses of vitamin A (retinol). Exposures below 10,000 I.U. present no risk to the fetus. Vitamin A in its recommended dose presents no increased risk for abortion.	Quality of available information: good. High concentrations of retinoic acid are cytotoxic; it may interact with DNA to delay differentiation and/or inhibit protein synthesis.
	Vitamin D: Large doses given in vitamin D prophylaxis are possibly involved in the etiology of supravalvular aortic stenosis, elfin faces, and mental retardation. There is no data on the abortigenic effect of vitamin D.	Quality of available information: poor. Mechanism is likely to involve a disruption of cell calcium regulation with excessive doses.

[a]Quality of available information is modified from reference 510.

ANTI-TUBERCULOSIS THERAPY

Drugs prescribed for the treatment of tuberculosis include aminoglycosides, ethambutol, isoniazid, rifampin, and ethionamide. The ototoxic effects of streptomycin are the only proven adverse effects of these drugs on the fetus. Other aminoglycosides have not been associated with fetal effects. Neither ethambutol nor rifampin have been associated with an increase in the incidence of growth retardation, premature birth or malformations.[48–51]

Early reports did not associate therapeutic exposures to isoniazid with an increased risk of malformations[50–51] but there is an unconfirmed association with central nervous system dysfunction.[52,53] There was one attempted suicide involving 50 tablets of isoniazid per day during the twelfth week that resulted in a stillbirth with arthogyryposis multiplex congenita syndrome.[54] Isoniazid may have small increased risk for adverse effects on the central nervous system but there is no apparent increase in risk for congenital malformations or abortions with therapeutic exposures.

Only 1 report associated ethionamide with an increased risk of teratogenic effects.[55] However, this association is tenuous and not supported by other case reports.[56]

As a general observation, the anti-tuberculosis drugs produce adverse effects on the fetus of experimental animals in greater doses than those equivalent to therapeutic exposures and not in all species. Embryotoxicity can be demonstrated for streptomycin in the mouse, kanamycin in the guinea pig, isoniazid in the rat, rifampin in the rat, and ethionamide in the rabbit.[57–59]

The only anti-tuberculosis drug with confirmed developmental toxicity is streptomycin—a small risk of ototoxicity associated with high exposures over a prolonged period. While this does not eliminate the possibility of adverse effects on the fetus following exposure to the other prescribed tuberculostatic medications discussed, therapeutic exposures appear to represent a very small risk of teratogenesis and even less risk of abortion.

BENZODIAZEPINES

The benzodiazepines, such as chlordiazepoxide (Librium), diazepam (Valium), and meprobamate, are widely used as tranquilizers during pregnancy and, therefore, it is not surprising that they have been associated with congenital malformations in some publications.

Chlordiazepoxide was associated with various anomalies after exposure during early pregnancy but no syndrome was identified.[60,61] Other studies were inconclusive[62] or found no association.[63–65] Animal studies reported dose-dependent maternal and developmental toxicity from doses that exceed therapeutic exposures.[63,64] Chlordiazepoxide appears to have a minimal risk for congenital anomalies and no increased risk for abortion at therapeutic doses. Higher exposures are likely to increase the risk of adverse effects on the fetus but the magnitude of the increase is not known.

Some studies reported an association between diazepam and increased incidence of congenital malformations (65, 66). However, a follow-up study found no associations.[67] The majority of studies of fetal outcome following in utero exposure to diazepam are negative.[63,68–70] Behavior alterations have been reported in infants exposed to benzodiazepines, mostly diazepam,[71] but this observation must be confirmed and the long-term developmental outcome evaluated before it can be appropriately interpreted.

Dose-dependent developmental toxicity can be demonstrated in laboratory animals at doses that greatly exceed therapeutic exposures.[72,73] Although third-trimester exposure to diazepam can reversibly affect the fetus and neonate[74] there is minimal increased risk of congenital malformations and no demonstrated increased risk of abortions from therapeutic exposures.

Meprobamate has been weakly associated with a variety of congenital malformations.[75–77] Other studies found no associations.[3,64,78] Malformations and fetal loss can be induced in experimental animals at doses equivalent to many times the therapeutic range.[79–81] Because of inconsistencies, the data are not sufficient to confirm or rule out a small increase risk of malformations due to exposures early in pregnancy.

Benzodiazepines appear to have minimal increased risk of malformations at therapeutic ranges; higher exposures may increase the risk. The risk for abortion is unknown.

CAFFEINE

Caffeine is a methylated xanthine that acts as a central nervous system stimulant. It is contained in many beverages including coffee, tea, and colas, as well as chocolate. Caffeine constitutes 1–2% of roasted coffee beans, 3.5% of fresh tea leaves, and about 2% of mate leaves.[82–84] Caffeine is also present in many over-the-counter medications, such as cold and allergy tablets, analgesics, diuretics, and stimulants; the latter lead to relatively minimal population intakes. Caffeine containing food and beverages are consumed in large quantities by most of the human populations of the world. The per capita consumption of caffeine from all sources is estimated to be about 200 mg/day, or about 3–7 mg/kg per day.[85] Consumption of caffeinated beverages during pregnancy is quite common and is estimated to be approximately 144 mg per day.[86]

Current evidence, does not appear to implicate the usual exposure of caffeine as a human teratogen, however, associations between maternal coffee drinking during pregnancy and miscarriage or poor fetal growth have been reported in epidemiological studies.[87–97] In many instances these associations are largely attributable to confounding effects of maternal cigarette smoking (87) or other factors. Some of these studies[98] have serious methodological limitations. If maternal consumption of caffeine-containing beverages in conventional amounts during pregnancy does have an association with the rate of miscarriage or fetal growth retardation, the effect appears to be relatively small.

In other studies no association has been found between caffeine consumption during pregnancy and congenital defects (3, 99–102). For instance, Rosenberg et al.[103] analyzed 6 selected birth defects in relation to maternal ingestion of more than 8 mg/kg per day of tea, coffee, or cola. The defects were inguinal hernia, cleft lip/cleft palate, cardiac defects, pyloric stenosis, cleft palate (isolated), and neural tube fusion defects. None of the point estimates of relative risk was significantly greater than unity, suggesting that caffeine was not a major teratogen, at least for the defects evaluated.

In animal studies caffeine is teratogenic only at very high doses. Nishimura and Nakai[104] reported that caffeine injected into mice at a dose of 250 mg/kg at selected times during organogenesis resulted in 43% of the offspring with cleft palate and digital defects. Fetal growth retardation and embryolethality were observed at maternally toxic doses.[105]

The teratogenic effect in rats and mice has been confirmed by the oral (gavage) route,[106–108] by dietary feeding[109] by addition to the drinking water,[110,111] by fetal injection,[112] and by the subcutaneous route.[113] The teratogenic response varies with the dose, route, and species, but limb hypoplasia and digital defects (ectrodactyly) were a common finding. The rabbit exhibited 9% digital defects following oral administration during the first half of gestation.[107] Teratogenic effects have not been produced in hamsters.[114] An increased frequency of malformations, especially of the limbs and palate, has been observed among the offspring of rats or mice treated with caffeine during pregnancy in doses equivalent to the human consumption of 40 or more cups of coffee per day.[114,115] Fetal death, growth retardation, and skeletal variations are often seen in these experiments after maternal treatment with very high doses of caffeine during pregnancy. In addition paraxanthine, a metabolite of caffeine, induced increased resorption, cleft palate, and limb defects similar to those of caffeine when given intraperitoneally to rats.[116]

In the majority of animal studies in which lower doses of caffeine were administered (equivalent to 5–20 cups of coffee per day), adverse effects on development were either not observed or were mild.[111,117,118] In one study an increased frequency of cleft palate was observed among the offspring of rats given the human equivalent of 5–19 cups of coffee a day during pregnancy.[111] In another study, an increased rate of cardiac defects was observed among the offspring of rats treated during pregnancy with the equivalent of 15 or more cups of coffee per day.[119] However, most investigations do not show an increased frequency of malformations among the offspring of rodents treated during pregnancy with these high doses of caffeine.[110,114,120,122] An extensive study showed that the no-observable-effect level for frank teratogenesis in the rat was 40 mg/kg per day on days 0–19 post-conception and that both the severity and frequency of the effects increase with dose. The overall result of this large study was that embryotoxicity did not occur unless the exposure was significantly above the usual human exposure.

Several groups of investigators maintain that prenatal caffeine may result in subtle, but lasting, physical and behavioral impairments.[123] Persistent behavioral alterations have been reported to occur among the offspring of rats and mice treated during pregnancy with doses of caffeine equivalent to 10–60 cups of coffee a day.[123–128] The developmental toxicity profile of caffeine in animals was reviewed in detail by Nolen.[122]

In primates, teratogenicity due to caffeine consumption has not been observed. However, stillbirths and miscarriages were observed with increased frequency among the offspring of Macaca fascicularis female monkeys treated during pregnancy with caffeine in a dose equivalent to 5–7 or 12–17 cups of coffee per day.[128] The cause for the stillbirths was not apparent on necropsy. Behavioral alterations have also been recorded among the offspring of monkeys born to mothers treated with an unspecified dose of caffeine during pregnancy.[129] The relevance of these observations to the risks in infants born to women who drink large amounts of caffeinated beverages during pregnancy is unknown, but many of the whole animal pregnancy studies indicate that if exposures are very high and the administration technique can attain high blood levels, reproductive effects may occur.

Interpretation of the available information pertaining to the animal and human studies regarding the teratogenicity of caffeine leads us to conclude that the usual exposure of caffeine does not present a measurable risk in the human for any 1 malformation or group of malformations. There is a clear indication that the consumer must ingest a substantial amount of caffeine in order to have an effect on the developing embryo or fetus; total consumption of 300 mg/day may be a safe upper daily limit. Most reviewers and investigators concluded that there is a threshold, below which caffeine does not exert a detrimental effect, and the usual human consumption falls in this nontoxic range. The quantity of caffeine consumed in an average cup of coffee, about 1.4–2.1 mg/kg,[130] is believed to be below the amount that induces congenital defects in animals. Quantities of caffeine in tea and soft drinks would be even less.

CARBAMAZEPINE

Carbamazepine is a tricyclic compound that is widely used for the treatment of epilepsy and various psychiatric disorders. Although carbamazepine has been considered a relatively safe drug for pregnant women requiring anticonvulsant therapy, epidemiologic and case report studies have not yielded consistent results regarding the teratogenicity of this compound. Initially reports in the literature suggested that carbamazepine presented no increased risk of major malformations.[131] More recently however exposure to carbamazepine has been associated with craniofacial defects, fingernail hypoplasia, developmental delay,[132–134] reduced birth weight, length, and head circumference,[135–137] and neural tube defects.[138,139] Confounding the issue is the possibility that epilepsy itself increases the risk for malformations.[140] However, an attempted suicide involving carbamazepine produced blood levels of 27–28 ug/ml (the therapeutic range is 8–12 ug/ml) during what was estimated to be 3–4 wk postconception.[141] The fetus was later determined to have myeloschisis, with carbamazepine being the only known exogenous risk factor.

Results from animal studies vary considerably[142,143] with some studies reporting no effects[144–146] and others reporting abnormalities at doses well above the human therapeutic range, often associated with maternal toxicity,[147,148] although fetal weight reduction occurred at lower doses.

There remains some question as to whether carbamazepine is the primary teratogen, or whether a metabolite is responsible for the adverse effects reported. Carbamazepine is metabolized to a pharmacologically active, stable epoxide, carbamazepine 10, 11-epoxide. Although the epoxide metabolite has been reported to induce malformations in mice,[149] it did not induce embryonic dysmorphology in either rat or mouse embryo culture in vitro at doses comparable to the parent compound.[150] Although the available data is insufficient for a definitive estimation, carbamazepine does appear to present a risk to the fetus.

CHORIONIC VILLOUS SAMPLING

There are now numerous reports relating chorionic villous sampling (CVS) to transverse limb reduction defects and other malformations with some studies reporting as much as a 6-fold increase in the risk for transverse digital deficiency following exposure to CVS (0.03%).[151–153] However other studies report no associated increased risk.[154,155] A NICHD workshop evaluated reports indicating that there was an increased prevalence of limb reduction defects (LRD) in the offspring of women who had undergone first trimester diagnostic CVS.[156] While there was not unanimous agreement, there appeared to be a low risk of vascular disruption-type malformations following CVS. Not all of the research groups who studied the malformation rates following CVS were able to corroborate these findings, but the report concluded the following:

1. There was an increase in the prevalence of vascular disruption-type malformations (congenital amputations of the nonsymmetrical type, orofacial malformations such as mandibular hypoplasia, cleft palate, and Moebius syndrome).
2. There appeared to be a sensitive period (i.e., 50–70 days of gestation) for the induction of these malformations, probably because the bleeding that accompanies the CVS may result in hypo-perfusion of the limbs, the face, and other structures sensitive to minimal reductions in organ perfusion. This may indicate that a shift of a few weeks in the timing of CVS might eliminate or markedly reduce the risk to the embryo.
3. The occurrence of these types of malformations is biologically plausible based on the experimental induction of LRD using uterine vascular clamping and uterine trauma[16,157–161] and the description of malformations due to vascular disruption reported in clinical reports.[162]

Associations between bleeding in early pregnancy and suboptimal pregnancy outcome and/or increased presence of malformations in offspring have previously been reported, however there has been disagreement about whether pregnancy bleeding was responsible for the malformations or visa versa.[163–176] The conclusions of the NICHD workshop support the hypothesis that sometimes the bleeding may be causal and not just a marker for the presence of the malformation. Previous investigations and reports support this concept.

Research has suggested that increased risk of defects following CVS may be correlated with fetal age[151] and may be particularly prevalent in fetuses under 10 weeks gestational age.[153,177] Since there is an obvious discrepancy in the results obtained by the various research and clinical groups, these differences may be related to the stage of the procedure, the amount of material removed, the experience of the operator, and the technique used. At this time the consensus is that the procedure presents a real but small risk to the fetus. Because CVS offers advantages to certain patients, it will be important to determine whether a totally safe procedure can be designed.

COUMADIN DERIVATIVES

Nasal hypoplasia following exposure to several drugs, including warfarin, during pregnancy was reported by DiSaia.[178] Kerber and colleagues[179] were the first to suggest warfarin as the teratogenic agent. Coumadin anticoagulants have since been associated with nasal hypoplasia, calcific stippling of the secondary epiphysis, and central nervous system (CNS) abnormalities. Warfarin embryopathy has been described and an overview of the difficulties in relating a congenital malformation to an environmental cause has been published.[179–187] There is an estimated 10–25% risk for affected infants following exposure during the period from the eighth through the 14th week of pregnancy, although this risk has been reported to be much lower in some series, and other factors besides dose and gestational stage seem to play a role.[182] Low-dose warfarin (5 mg/day or less) throughout pregnancy did not result in any adverse effects in 20 offspring.[188]

Coumadin has been shown to inhibit the formation of carboxyglutamyl residues from glutamyl residues, decreasing the ability of proteins to bind calcium.[189] The inhibition of calcium binding by proteins during embryonic-fetal development, especially during a critical period of ossification, could explain the nasal hypoplasia, stippled calcification, and skeletal abnormalities of warfarin embryopathy.[182] Microscopic bleeding does not seem to be responsible for these problems early in development.[190]

One case report was unique in that the time of exposure to warfarin was between 8 and 12 weeks of gestation, and the infant presented with Dandy-Walker malformation, eye defects, and agenesis of the corpus callosum.[191] This case report represents the clearest evidence for a direct effect of warfarin on the developing central nervous system rather than an effect mediated by hemorrhage, because the exposure was well defined and occurred before the appearance of vitamin K-dependent clotting factors. Similar embryopathies have been described in infants with vitamin K deficiency secondary to maternal malabsorption.[192] Further supportive evidence for a direct pathogenic role of warfarin is the report of an infant with an inherited deficiency of multiple vitamin K dependent coagulation factors whose congenital anomalies were similar to warfarin syndrome without exposure to warfarin.[193]

The risk of stillbirths and spontaneous abortions is increased in pregnant women treated with warfarin[182,194-196] but the risk may be less if the exposure occurs in the last half of pregnancy. The risk of adverse effects due to hemorrhaging increases later in gestation. Fetal hemorrhage in the second or third trimester has been reported to account for various brain abnormalities and may be present without the presence of the abnormalities associated with first-trimester exposures.[182,183]

No increase in major malformations was reported in mice,[197] rats,[198] or rabbits[199] exposed to warfarin at greater than therapeutic doses. In the rat however, increased fetal hemorrhaging was reported,[198] and maxillonasal hypoplasia occurred after postnatal administration.[200] One difficulty in producing an appropriate animal model to study warfarin teratogenicity is that the period of human skeletal maturation that is susceptible to the detrimental effects of warfarin occurs postnatally in the rat.

CYCLOPHOSPHAMIDE

Cyclophosphamide is an antineoplastic agent widely used for treatment of cancer and autoimmune disease[201] with an apparent risk of malformation in the human of approximately 1:6.[47] Animal studies with several species have demonstrated teratogenicity in the rat,[202,203] mouse,[204] and rabbit[205] with distinct developmental-stage specificity, dose-effect relationships, and a high sensitivity of nervous system and mesenchymal tissues.[206] There have been isolated case reports of congenital anomalies in exposed human infants, however conclusive epidemiologic evidence for cyclophosphamide teratogenesis in the human is lacking. Defects reported in exposed human infants include growth retardation, ectrodactyly, syndactyly, cardiovascular anomalies, and other minor anomalies.[207,208] Ten normal pregnancies have been reported after cyclophosphamide exposure.[209] Recently a possible distinctive phenotype of human congenital malformation following cyclophosphamide exposure has been described.[201] Defects common to all exposures included growth deficiency, developmental delay, craniosynostosis, flat nasal bridge, abnormal ears, and distal limb defects as well as other minor anomalies.[201]

The current knowledge of the mechanism of cyclophosphamide teratogenesis has recently been reviewed: cytochrome P-450 monooxygenases convert cyclophosphamide to 4-hydroxycyclophosphamide, which in turn breaks down to phosphoramide mustard and acrolein.[206] Phosphoramide mustard may produce teratogenic effects by interacting with cellular DNA in an as yet undefined manner whereas acrolein appears to act differently, possibly by affecting sulfhydryl linkages in proteins.[210] Tissue sensitivity to phosphoramide mustard and acrolein is thought to be related to such processes as detoxification and cellular repair.

DIETHYLSTILBESTROL

The first abnormality reported following exposure to diethylstilbestrol (DES) during the first trimester was clitoromegaly in female newborns.[211] Much later, Herbst and coworkers[212,213] and Greenwald and associates[214] reported an association of vaginal adenocarcinoma in adolescent females who were exposed during their pregnancy. Further studies revealed that almost all the cancers occurred after 14 years of age and only in those exposed before the eighteenth week of gestation.[215-217] There is a 75% risk for vaginal adenosis for exposures occurring before the ninth week of pregnancy; however, the risk of developing adenocarcinoma is extremely low (1 in 10,000).[218]

Although there does not appear to be an adverse effect on the rate of conception,[219] the anatomical abnormalities of the uterus and cervix induced by intrauterine exposure to DES including T-shaped uterus, transverse fibrous ridges, and uterine hypoplasia increase the probability of reproductive problems such as ectopic pregnancy, spontaneous abortions and premature delivery in pregnancies of women exposed to DES in utero.[219-226]

There have been reports that males exposed to DES in utero exhibited genital lesions and abnormal spermatozoa.[227-230] Other studies reported no increase in the risk in the male for genitourinary abnormalities or infertility.[231,232] The controversial nature of the effects of DES exposure on the male may be attributable to study design or, more likely, to the facts that dose levels have varied greatly according to different regimens.[223]

Teratogenic and transplacental carcinogenic effects following in utero exposure to DES have been demonstrated in the rat,[233] mouse,[234,235] hamster,[214] and monkey.[236-239] A major difficulty in studies of the mechanism of action of DES is the extensive biotransformation that occurs in the adult and fetus. These transformations recently have been demonstrated in the hamster fetus.[240,241]

DES is a potent nonsteroidal estrogen and, as in the case of steroidal estrogens, must interact with the receptor proteins present only in estrogen-responsive tissues before exerting its effects by stimulating RNA, protein, and DNA synthesis. The carcinogenic effect of DES is most likely indirect: DES exposure results in the presence of columnar epithelium in the vagina, and this "misplaced tissue" may have a greater susceptibility to developing the adenocarcinoma—much as teratomas and other misplaced tissues are more susceptible to malignant degeneration.

DIPHENYLHYDANTOIN

Chronic exposure to diphenylhydantoin has been suggested to present a maximum of 10% risk for the full syndrome and a maximum of 30% risk for some anomalies.[242-245] Although cleft lip and palate, congenital heart disease, and microcephaly have been reported, hypoplasias of the nails and distal phalanges may be more specific malformations in the exposed fetuses although they occur in many other syndromes.[180,246]

Hanson and associates noted that, although the hydantoin syndrome is observed in 11% of the subjects in their study, 3 times that number exhibit mental deficits.[247,248] Prospective studies demonstrate a much lower frequency of effects, and some do not demonstrate any effect; thus, the overall prospective risk may be much lower for the classically reported effects.

Factors associated with epilepsy may contribute to the etiology of these malformations: based on the United States Collaborative Perinatal Project and a large Finnish registry, the incidence of malformations was 10.5% when the mother was epileptic, 8.3% when the father was epileptic, and 6.4% when neither parent was affected.

Cleft lip and palate, skeletal anomalies, and cardiac defects have been produced in rabbits,[248,249] mice,[250–253] and rats,[254,255] and the malformation rate was dosedependent.[251,256]

The teratogenic action of diphenylhydantoin has been postulated to involve the cytochrome P-450 metabolism of phenytoin to produce a reactive epoxide metabolite. The arene oxide would covalently bind to macromolecules and interfere with their function.[105–108] Further studies have not confirmed this or other hypothesis.

LITHIUM CARBONATE

Lithium carbonate, widely used for treatment of manic-depressive disorders, was first associated with human congenital malformations in 1970.[257,258] The malformations described include heart and large-vessel anomalies, Epstein's anomaly, neural tube defects, talipes, microtia, and thyroid abnormalities.[47,259,260] Lithium readily crosses the placenta,[261] and appears to be a human teratogen at therapeutic dosages but it represents a small risk. Early reports suggested a strong association of prenatal lithium exposure with cardiac defects, in particular Epstein's anomaly. More recent evidence from controlled epidemiologic studies suggests that the risk for malformations is much lower than initially thought.[262,263] The results of a retrospective study suggest that lithium may also increase the risk for premature delivery[264] but again the magnitude of the risk is likely to be small. Only 1 follow-up study has been published examining long-term effects of lithium on early development. In this study children exposed prenatally to lithium with no congenital abnormalities at birth did not show any signs of developmental delay at 7.3 years follow up.[265]

Fetal toxicity has been associated with late gestational maternal lithium use with and without obvious maternal toxicity. One reported side effect is nephrogenic diabetes insipidus[266–268] and associated polyhydramnios which may increase the likelihood of premature labor.[264,266] Transient toxic effects have also been reported in neonates exposed late in pregnancy. These include hypothyroidism, lethargy, hypotomia, cardiac murmur, renal toxicity, persistent fetal circulation, and diabetes insipidus.[269–272] To prevent lithium intoxication in the neonate the lithium dosage of the patient should be adjusted to avoid high serum levels in the second and third trimester.[262]

Lithium can induce abnormal development in several laboratory animals, but the mechanisms of the teratogenic action of lithium is not known.[273–275] The neurotropic activity of lithium suggests that central nervous system malformations may result from cell membrane disturbances which affect neural tube closure.[276]

Because of the value of lithium carbonate for treating manic-depressive psychosis, the risk associated with psychiatric relapse on removing the drug may be more important clinically than the teratogenic risk. Moreover, the risk of alternative pharmacologic agents for treatment of bipolar disorder may exceed the risk from lithium carbonate.[277]

METHYLENE BLUE

Methylene blue has been used clinically for a variety of purposes including the identification of anatomic structures, the treatment of methemoglobinemia, and to mark the amniotic cavity during amniocentesis. Use of methylene blue in late gestation to detect rupture of fetal membranes has been associated with adverse fetal effects including hyperbilirubinemia, hemolytic anemia and staining of the skin.[278–281] There is currently not enough data to determine whether respiratory distress in these infants may also result from late gestation methylene blue exposure.[282]

There have been several reports of an increased prevalence of small intestinal atresia in twins with intra-amniotic exposure to methylene blue. Twinning itself results in an increased prevalence of intestinal atresia, increasing from approximately 2–2.5 per 10,000 in singletons to 5–7.3 per 10,000 amongst twins.[283] However, in twins exposed to midgestational amniocentesis in which methylene blue was used to mark the amniotic cavity the prevalence of small intestinal atresia has been reported as high as 9.6%.[284] The strongest evidence indicating that methylene blue is a teratogen is a retrospective study from Amsterdam. In this study methylene blue was injected into 1 amniotic cavity of 86 twin pregnancies undergoing midgestation amniocentesis. Jejunal atresia occurred in 17 infants, each from different pregnancies.[284] In 15 of these cases it was possible to determine which twin was exposed to methylene blue, and in each case the twin exposed to methylene blue had jejunal atresia. Based on this evidence and several other reports there appears to be a significant risk of small intestinal atresia associated with exposure to methylene blue during midgestation amniocentesis.[278,285–289] Intra-amniotic exposure to methylene blue has not been associated with any other malformation.[282] Whether midgestation exposure to methylene blue increases the incidence of fetal death has not been clearly established.[290,291] However in rats, intra-amniotic injection of methylene blue increased fetal loss.[292]

MISOPROSTOL

Misoprostol is a synthetic prostaglandin E1 methyl analogue used for the prevention of gastric ulcers induced by nonsteroidal antiinflammatory drugs. It has known, but not very effective, abortifacient properties.[293] Gonzalez et al.[294] recently reported 7 newborns with vascular disruptive phenomena (limb reduction defects, Moebius syndrome) whose mothers used misoprostol early in pregnancy in an attempt to induce abortion. Although there is evidence that misoprostol is used illegally by thousands of pregnant Brazilian women as an abortifacient[295–297] controlled cohort or case control epidemiological studies of the fetal outcome of failed abortions are not available. Coelho et al.[295] indicate that the World Health Organization estimated that there are 5 million illegal abortions in Brazil each year. Although the data available are not conclusive, the uterine bleeding produced by misoprostol[293] and type of malformations produced suggest a vascular disruption mechanism for misoprostol induced teratogenesis.

Most of the animal studies dealing with the teratogenic potential of prostaglandins were negative, although Marks et al.[298] did report hydrocephaly, anophthalmia, and microphthalmia at maternally toxic doses (2.0 mg/kg prostaglandin E1, alprostadil) in pregnant rats. If one is looking for vascular disruption, it will more likely be produced later in gestation. Therefore, classical animal teratology experiments will not detect the vascular disruptive effect of drugs or chemicals unless they are exposed beyond the period of early organogenesis.[158] Furthermore, it has become clear that if an agent produces vascular disruption, it is a rare event and therefore large populations would need to be studied before the effect can be demonstrated.[156,299]

Previous case reports are also of little assistance. Collins and Mahoney[300] reported an infant with hydrocephalus and attenuated digital phalanges after exposure intravaginally to 15-methyl F2alpha prostaglandin 5 weeks after conception. Schuler et al.[301] reported that 29% of women who used misoprostol in Brazil as an abortifacient failed to abort. Seventeen children who failed to abort were observed to have no malformations. Wood et al.[302] reported an infant exposed to oxytocin and prostaglandin E2 for the purpose of termination to have hydrocephaly and growth retardation. Schonhofer[303] and Fonesca et al.[304] reported 5 Brazilian infants with defects of the skull and overlying scalp who were exposed to misoprostol in utero. These case reports indicate the low risk of misoprostol exposure and the possibility that some of the features reported may or may not be due to misoprostol.[305] It is too early to know the extent of the effects of misoprostol, but it is biologically plausible that they should include all of the features of vascular disruption.

OXAZOLIDINE-2,4-DIONES

Trimethadione and paramethadione are antiepileptic oxazolidine-2,4-diones that distribute uniformly throughout body tissues and exert their effects by means of the action of their metabolism. These drugs affect cell membrane permeability and vitamin K-dependent clotting factors, but their primary mode of action is unknown. The N-demethylated metabolite of trimethadione is believed to be the proximate teratogen.[306]

German and coworkers reported the fetal trimethadione syndrome characterized by development delay, V-shaped eyebrows, low-set ears with anterior folded helix, high-arched palate, and irregular teeth plus cardiac anomalies.[307] Zackai and colleagues described similar findings.[308] Feldman and associates and Goldman and Yaffe have reviewed the clinical findings in the literature and from their own observations.[309,310] There are wide variations in reported risk, with estimates as high as 80% for major or minor defects. Because the number of exposures is small, the actual risk could vary considerably from these figures. It is unlikely that we will ever be able to ascertain the risk accurately, because the drug is no longer used in pregnant women.

Mice exposed to high doses of trimethadione on days 8–10 or 11–13 of gestation had a high incidence of fetal growth retardation and abnormalities of the viscera and skeleton; aortic arch and vertebral defects were especially common.[311]

PENICILLAMINE

Human exposure to D-penicillamine can induce a connective tissue defect, including generalized cutix laxa, hyperflexibility of the joints, varicosities, and impaired wound healing.[312] The exposure must be long enough to induce a copper deficiency sufficient to inhibit collagen synthesis and maturation. However, the condition appears to be reversible, and the risk is low,[313] approximately 4% to 5%.[47]

D-penicillamine is a copper chelator shown to induce cleft palate and skeletal defects in the rat.[314,315] Copper deficiency appears to be the mechanism for teratogenicity.[316]

PROGESTINS (FEMALE SEX HORMONES)

For the purpose of discussion, expediency justifies grouping together many compounds by generically using the term "sex hormones." Similarly, there are common references to "progestogens" or "progestational agents." This expediency is unfortunate when it occurs in epidemiologic studies, which may not list the specific sex hormone exposures.[60,317,318] It also is often overlooked that, although various progestogens act by means of similar receptors, their potential androgenic effects can differ markedly. This point is critical for the appreciation of the virilizing effects of these compounds in the human. It has been shown, for example, that the pharmacokinetic parameters that estimate steroid bioavailability and metabolism show great variability among subjects and between steroids conveniently grouped together, such as "progestins."[319] One must assume that these differences in bioavailability and metabolism reflect differences in the biologic activity of these steroids in humans.

In contrast to progesterone and 17-alpha-hydroxyprogesterone caproate, high doses of some of the synthetic progestins have been reported to cause virilizing effects in humans. Exposure during the first trimester to large doses of 17-alpha-ethinyltestosterone has been associated with masculinization of the external genitalia of female fetuses.[320,321] Similar associations result from exposure to large doses of 17-alpha-ethinyl-19-nortestosterone (norethandrolone)[321] and 17-alpha-ethinyl-17-OH-5(10)estren-3-one (Enovid-R).[322] The synthetic progestins, like progesterone, can influence only those tissues with the appropriate steroid receptor proteins. The preparations with androgenic properties may cause abnormalities in the genital development of females only if present in sufficient amounts during critical periods of development.[320,321,323] In 1959, Grumbach and coworkers pointed out that labioscrotal fusion could be produced with large doses if the fetuses were exposed before the thirteenth week of pregnancy, whereas clitoromegaly could be produced after this period, illustrating that a specific form of maldevelopment can be induced only when the embryonic or fetal tissues are in a susceptible stage of development.[322]

The World Health Organization reported that there is a suspicion that combined oral contraceptives or progestogens may be weakly teratogenic but that the magnitude of the relative risk is small.[324] In a large retrospective study, Heinonen and associates reported a positive association between cardiovascular defects and in utero exposure to female sex hormones.[60] A re-evaluation of some of the base data by Wiseman and Dodds-Smith, however, did not support the reported association.[325] Another retrospective study, conducted by Ferencz and colleagues, did not find a positive association between female sex hormone therapy and congenital heart defects.[326] Although neither study disproved the positive association reported by Heinonen and coworkers, their findings made the association less likely.[60]

Epidemiologic studies have reported an association between exposures to female sex hormones, hormone pregnancy tests, oral contraceptives or progestogens, and congenital neural tube defects[327,328] and limb defects.[317,318] Further studies and reevaluations have not supported either of these associations.[329-332] Several reviews have discussed the evidence against the involvement of female sex hormones in nongenital teratogenesis.[1,333,334]

Further support for the absence of a nongenital effect of progestins comes from a negative correlation between sex hormone usage during pregnancy and malformations[333,335] that showed no increased incidence in malformations following progesterone therapy to maintain pregnancy,[336] and no increased incidence in malformations following first-trimester exposure to progestogens (mostly medroxyprogesterone) administered to pregnant women who had signs of bleeding.[337,338] The Food and Drug Administration has recently recognized that the evidence does not support an increased risk of limb reduction defects, congenital heart disease, or neural tube defects following exposure to oral contraceptives or progestins.[339]

As has been stated, it is generally accepted that the actions of steroid hormones are mediated by specific steroid receptors,[340,341] and therefore only those tissues with the specific receptors can be affected by steroid hormones. It has been shown that medroxyprogesterone (Provera) and 17-alpha-hydroxyprogesterone caproate (Delalutin) do not cause developmental abnormalities in nonreproductive organs of mice.[342-344]

RADIOACTIVE ISOTOPES

All forms of irradiation are not identical. The effects of external irradiation (discussed later) with x-rays or gamma rays differ from those of radioisotopes. Medically administered radioactive isotopes (or the compound containing the isotope) have a predictable distribution in the embryo determined by several factors that include placental exchange, tissue affinity, and nature of the radiation(s) emitted (alpha particle, beta particle, gamma ray).

In addition to the administered isotope, background radiation contributes to the total exposure. Background radiation has been estimated to contribute greater than 100 mrad over the course of pregnancy to the dose absorbed by soft tissue, which presents no increased risk of deleterious effects for the embryo.[18] This is an important concept because many of the exposures from nuclear medicine procedures are within the same order of magnitude as background radiation.

Estimating the absorbed dose and hazard to the fetus is complex because the radioisotope may locate on specific target organs, it may or may not cross the placenta, the distribution of irradiation may not be random, metabolism of the element or compound may be affected by disease or genotype, and the radiation dose rate decreases exponentially with time.

Radioactive iodine in the form of ^{131}I is used primarily for uptake studies and radioactive scanning. It may be in the form of the inorganic ion or it may be bound to protein. ^{125}I is used to label hormones for in vivo and in vitro studies. Radioactive iodine is a potential risk to the fetal thyroid, especially once the fetal thyroid begins to concentrate iodide at 10–12 weeks of gestation. Inorganic iodides readily cross the placenta, and in time, a substantial amount of bound iodide will be released and become available to the fetus.[345] In all likelihood, there is no compound containing radioisotope of iodide that does not expose the fetus to some radioactivity.

Fetal thyroid avidity for iodides is greater than maternal thyroid avidity.[346] Reported fetal effects from therapeutic (ablative) doses of ^{131}I administered to pregnant women include total fetal thyroid destruction. In a retrospective study of fetuses accidentally exposed to ^{131}I during the first or first and second trimesters, 6 neonates out of 178 live births had hypothyroidism, although other anomalies were not statistically increased above the general population.[347] Although there are few case reports in the literature, there is a definite risk of thyroid dysfunction in the offspring.

The use of radioactive iodine should be avoided during pregnancy unless it is essential for the medical care of the mother and there is no substitute.

Inorganic radioactive potassium, sodium, phosphorus, cesium, thallium, selenium, chromium, iron, and strontium readily cross the placenta. Experiments in animals with radioactive phosphorus and strontium indicate that if the dose is large enough, embryonic abnormality and death can result.[348] These isotopes are used in less than 1% of procedures; only radioactive phosphorus or gold may be used therapeutically (e.g., in the treatment of polycythemia or management of malignancies involving peritoneal surfaces). Most new isotopic agents are bound to some complex macromolecule or macroaggregate, cross the placenta in minuscule amounts, and therefore deliver extremely low doses to the embryo.

When radioisotopes are to be used in a woman of child-bearing age, the following procedure is recommended:

1. Record the date of the last menstrual period and determine whether the woman could be pregnant.
2. If pregnancy is a possibility, determine the stage of gestation and the estimated dose to the fetus or fetal target organs.
3. Communicate this information to the patient or a responsible member of the family. Record this information, the time and place of the communication, and an informed consent in the patient's record.

For each procedure, the dose to the embryo must be calculated individually and is dependent on the form of the isotope, the site of administration, and the nature of the disease. Estimates of approximate fetal and maternal exposure for standard doses and procedures have been published.[346] In the vast majority of instances a careful analysis will reveal that the exposure is too low to represent a significant risk to the embryo.

EXTERNAL IONIZING IRRADIATION

The classic effects of radiation are cell death or mitotic delay. These effects are due to direct damage to the cell chromatin and are expressed in the offspring as gross malformations, intrauterine growth retardation, or embryonic death, each having a dose-response relationship and a threshold exposure below which no difference between an exposed and a nonexposed control population can be demonstrated.[349] Offspring born to patients receiving radiation therapy for various conditions exhibited growth retardation, eye malformations, and CNS defects.[350-352] Microcephaly is probably the most common manifestation observed following in utero exposure to high levels of radiation in the human.[353] Fetal exposure to radiation at Hiroshima and Nagasaki resulted in microcephaly, growth retardation, and mental retardation.[354-356] In a recent review of radiation teratogenesis, Brent pointed out that no malformation of the limb, viscera, or other tissue has been observed unless the child also exhibits intrauterine growth retardation, microcephaly, or eye malformations.[349] The risk of major anatomical malformations is not increased by in utero exposure of 5 rads (.05 Sv) or less.[349]

Experimental animal models have shown that radiation-induced effects on the developing organism are the result of the direct action of ionizing radiation on the embryo and are not due to a maternal effect.[349] Prior to implantation, the mammalian embryo is minimally sensitive to the teratogenic and growth-retarding effects of radiation and very sensitive to the lethal effects.[357-359] Organogenesis is a stage sensitive to the teratogenic, growth-retarding, and lethal effects of irradiation, but the embryo has some recuperative capacity.[357,360-362] Sensitivity to the teratogenic effects of radiation decreased during the fetal stage, but the fetus may still sustain permanent cell depletion, since the recuperative capacity is less.[349] Permanent growth retardation is thus more severe following mid-gestation radiation.[363,364] Because of its extended periods of organogenesis and histogenesis, the CNS retains the greatest sensitivity of all organ systems to the detrimental effects of radiation through the later fetal stages. The documented effects of prenatal exposure to ionizing radiation, which leads to histopathologic abnormalities of the brain in experimental animals, are cell death and inhibition of cell migration.[365]

RETINOIDS SYSTEMIC ADMINISTRATION (ISOTRETINOIN, ETRETINATE)

There are few case reports of congenital defects in humans associated with massive vitamin A ingestion during pregnancy: 2 have cited urogenital anomalies,[366,367] and 1 described Goldenhar's syndrome.[368] Historically, vitamin A has played an important role in experimental and clinical teratology. Vitamin A deficiency in swine was the first experimental model of teratogenesis in a mammal.[369-372] Vitamin A congeners, including retinol, retinal, all-trans-retinoic acid (tretinoin) and 13-cis-retinoic acid (isotretinoin), are all teratogenic in numerous species (reviewed by Schardein).[47]

Both isotretinoin (Accutane), marketed for treating severe acne, and etretinate (Tegison), marketed for treating psoriasis, contained warnings by the manufacturers against exposure during pregnancy. Unfortunately, exposures occurred. Analyses of the resulting malformations have been reviewed.[373,374] Human malformations include malformations of the central nervous system, cardioaortic malformations, microtia, and clefting defects. Similar defects may result from vitamin A supplements (as retinol-retinyl esters) at high dosage. "Recommendations for Vitamin A Use During Pregnancy" is a position paper published by the Teratology Society reviewing the literature concerning retinoids and birth defects.[375] Supplementation of 8000 IU vitamin A per day should be the maximum during pregnancy, and high dosages (above 10,000 IU) are not recommended.

Experimental evidence[376] suggests that endogenous retinoic acid may act as a natural morphogen. Cellular binding protein-retinoic acid complexes enter the nucleus to affect gene activity, and the resulting regulation of gene transcription influences digit formation. Exogenous retinoids appear to act either directly, to result in cytotoxicity, or via receptor-mediated pathways, to interact with DNA and alter programmed cell death.[377-381]

We are beginning to understand how retinoid metabolism and placental transfer affect the teratogenic potency of various retinoids. In mice, the metabolites of isotretinoin, 4-oxo-isotretinoin and tretinoin, are more efficiently transferred across the placenta than isotretinoin and are more potent teratogens.[382,383] It is likely that different specificities of retinoid-binding proteins[384] account for the variations in placental transfer. Although retinoids can influence many types of cells, Lammer has recently emphasized that neuroectodermally derived cells of the rhomboencephalon are particularly sensitive and that the resulting neural crest cell abnormality differs from that resulting in oculoauriculo-vertebral dysplasia or Goldenhar syndrome.[381] It has been postulated that the susceptibility of specific cell types to the effects of the retinoids is determined by the intracellular concentration of cellular retinoic binding protein.[381]

RETINOIDS (TOPICAL ADMINISTRATION)

There have been several case reports of congenital malformations occurring in the offspring of mothers who used topical tretinoin during pregnancy.[385–387] However, evidence from epidemiologic and animal studies have not supported an association with topical tretinoin use during pregnancy and increased risk of congenital malformations.[388–394] Jick and colleagues reported a relative risk of 0.7 for birth defects from comparison of 215 pregnancies exposed to topical tretinoin with 430 nonexposed mothers using data from the Group Health Cooperative of Puget Sound.[394] In another study DeWals[393] evaluated the association of holoprosencephaly with topical tretinoin exposure. Among 502,189 births there were 31 infants with holoprosencephaly. Eight patients had an abnormal karyotype and 16 had a normal karyotype. None of the patients with a normal karyotype were exposed to topical tretinoin during pregnancy. More recently Shapiro et al.[392] published the results of a prospective study based on 94 topical tretinoin exposed pregnancies and 133 controls and found no increased risk of congenital malformation associated with exposure.

Animal studies examining topical tretinoin exposure and fetal outcome have been conducted with rats,[389,395] hamsters,[388] and rabbits.[390] None of these studies have reported an increased incidence of congenital malformations associated with topical tretinoin exposure at doses that greatly exceeded human therapeutic doses. Decreases in fetal weight and increases in fetal loss have been reported at doses that produced overt maternal toxicity.[389,390,395] Seegmiller and colleagues reported an increase in the incidence of supernumerary ribs in offspring of rats exposed to 2.5 mg/kg and above.[389] Based on the lack of correlation of these effects with the dose administered, the plasma levels achieved and the absence of malformations consistent with tretinoin exposure these fetal effects were most likely attributable to nonspecific, maternally mediated effects associated with maternal toxicity.

All teratogens that have been appropriately studied have a no-effect dose. Thus in order to have an effect on the developing fetus, topically applied tretinoin would have to result in an internal tretinoin concentration at or above the developmentally toxic threshold established for oral administration. Pharmacokinetic data have shown that absorption of tretinoin from the skin is minimal.[390,396,397] At conventional doses, blood levels from topical administration are far below the teratogenic dose and add negligibly to normal, endogenous levels.[390,396–398] Studies estimate the dose absorbed from daily therapeutic application of topical tretinoin is several orders of magnitude below the minimal teratogenic dose for oral administration.[391,396,398–400] It would appear that prudent use of this topical medication presents no risk to the embryo. The pharmacokinetics, animal studies, and human studies support this conclusion.

STREPTOMYCIN

Based on case reports, there appears to be a small increased risk of sensorineural deafness in offspring of women treated with streptomycin for tuberculosis during pregnancy.[50,51,401] Other congenital anomalies have not been associated with in utero exposure to streptomycin in the human[3] or in mice.[402,403] Since auditory nerve damage is a toxic effect of streptomycin in the adult and animal data show inner ear damage after high exposures in utero,[58] it is likely that there is a small increased risk of deafness but not of malformations after in utero exposure to streptomycin. A related drug, kanamycin, appears to have minimal risk of causing similar adverse effects.[404,405]

TETRACYCLINE

The antimicrobial tetracyclines inhibit bacterial protein synthesis by preventing access of aminoacyl transfer RNA (tRNA) to the messenger RNA (mRNA)-ribosome complex.[406]

Tetracycline crosses the placenta but is not concentrated by the fetus.[407] It has been shown to discolor teeth,[408] and very high doses may depress skeletal bone growth and result in hypoplasia of tooth enamel.[409] No congenital malformations of any other organ system have been associated with antenatal tetracycline exposures. Several case reports of limb reduction defects in human embryos exposed to tetracycline are not supported by epidemiologic studies or animal studies. Tetracyclines complex with calcium and the organic matrix of newly forming bone without altering the crystalline structure of hydroxyapatite.[409]

Although stunting has been produced in rats,[382] other experimental animal studies have found either no teratogenic effect[382] or ambiguous effects.[383]

THALIDOMIDE

Lenz and Knapp were the first to describe the thalidomide-induced limb reduction defects and other features of the thalidomide syndrome.[384,410,411] Limb defects resulted from exposure limited to a 2-week period from the 22nd to the 36th day post-conception. Exposures, early during this period, most often affected only the arm, whereas exposures from the 30th to the 33rd days resulted in abnormalities of both leg and arm.[410–412] Although there was no association of mental retardation, brain malformations, or cleft palate, other abnormalities included facial hemangioma, microtia, esophageal or duodenal atresia, deafness, and anomalies of the kidneys, heart, and external ears; and increased incidence of miscarriages and neonatal mortality.[384,412–416] Approximately 20% of the fetuses exposed during the critical period were affected. The current use of thalidomide in South America for the treatment of leprosy has resulted in more recent cases of embryopathy including at least 29 children born with thalidomide syndrome.[417–419]

McCredie proposed that the segmental pattern of limb reduction defects was determined by the peripheral nerves derived from the neural crest.[420] Stephens and McNulty confirmed that limb development exhibits a segmental pattern.[421] However, recent studies by Strecker and Stephens have refuted the proposed role of peripheral nerve damage in thalidomide-induced embryopathy.[422] A foil barrier was placed lateral to the chick neural tube to block the innervation of the wing field by the brachial plexus. A reduced source of innervation from spinal nerves anterior or posterior to the brachial plexus resulted in muscular atrophy but not in reductions or malformations of the skeleton of the wing.

Lash and Saxen have postulated that thalidomide indirectly exerts its effects on limb chondrogenesis by acting on the kidney primordia.[423] Based on an association between nephric tissue and limb development[423-425] in vitro evidence suggests that thalidomide inhibits an interaction between metanephric tissue and associated mesenchymal tissue necessary for normal limb development.[423] Other postulated mechanisms involve the known properties of thalidomide to inhibit angiogenesis and the production of TNF. Although the mechanism of teratogenic action for thalidomide is not yet defined, the subject has been reviewed.[426,427]

THYROID: IODINE DEFICIENCY, IODIDES, ANTITHYROID DRUGS

Iodine deficiency, reviewed by Warkany,[428] is the primary cause of endemic cretinism. The damage to the embryo is due to iodine deficiency, occurs early in gestation, and results in irreversible neurologic and aural damage with variable severity. Goiter in a female of reproductive age due to endemic iodine deficiency is an indicator for iodine supplementation prior to conception to prevent harmful teratogenic effects.

Several drugs used to treat maternal hyperthyroidism (^{131}I and antithyroid drugs) and non-thyroid conditions (especially iodide-containing compounds for bronchitis and asthma) affect thyroid function. In utero exposure to these drugs may result in congenitally hypothyroid infants who will not reach their potential for physical or mental development unless treated very early after birth with thyroid hormone.

There are several case reports of congenital goiter due to in utero exposures to iodide-containing drugs.[429,430] Maternal intake as low as 12 mg per day may result in fetal goiter.[430] Iodinated diagnostic X-ray contrast agents used for amniofetography have been reported to affect fetal thyroid function adversely.[431]

Propylthiouracil and methimazole, used to treat thyrotoxicosis, readily cross the placenta.[432] Methimazole has been associated with aplasia cutis.[433,434] Propylthiouracil is safer because the incidence of fetal goiter is low,[432,435] and there have been no observed detrimental effects on mental development.[435,436]

VALPROIC ACID

Valproic acid (dipropylacetic acid) is approved for the treatment of various types of epilepsy. Valproic acid had been iden-

tified as a teratogen in animal studies,[437-441] but Dalens and coworkers were the first to report the association of valproic acid and congenital malformations in the human.[442] Although other reports followed, Robert and colleagues described the associated malformations, consisting primarily of neural tube defects, usually spina bifida in the lumbar or sacral region.[443-447] Therapeutic dosages during pregnancy represent a teratogenic risk for spina bifida of about 1%,[47] but the risk for facial dysmorphology may be greater.

Valproic acid crosses the human placenta,[448,449] but the fetal serum concentrations are not known. In the rhesus monkey, the fetus is exposed to approximately one half of the free valproic acid concentration present in the maternal plasma; craniofacial and skeletal anomalies and fetal death are observed.[450,451] Little is known of its mechanism of action or of the effects of various dosages of valproic acid on human development.

VITAMIN D

Because the vitamins as a group are essential for normal metabolism, it seems unlikely that a severe deficiency would be compatible with reproduction and therefore would result in reproductive loss. Excess of vitamin D has been associated with increased incidence of congenital malformations. Huge doses of vitamin D administered for rickets prophylaxis resulted in a markedly increased incidence of a syndrome consisting of supravalvular aortic stenosis, elfin facies, and mental retardation in the human.[452,453]

OTHER HUMAN TERATOGENIC AGENTS: ALCOHOL

Table 9-3 lists other human teratogenic agents. Alcohol will be discussed here because of its relatively large social impact. Jones and associates described the fetal alcohol syndrome (FAS) in children with intrauterine growth retardation, microcephaly, mental retardation, maxillary hypoplasia, flat philtrum, thin upper lip, and reduction in the width of palpebral fissures (cardiac abnormalities also were seen).[133] Many children of alcoholic mothers had FAS, and all the affected children evidenced developmental delay.[404,454,455]

A period of greatest susceptibility and a dose-response relationship have not yet been established. Although we are reluctant to claim that malformations are due to single exposures to alcohol in the human, binge drinking early in pregnancy has been suggested to be associated with neural tube defects.[456] The neural tube defects, if real, are a minor risk when compared to the risk of decreased brain growth and differentiation that results from high alcohol consumption during the second and third trimester. Chronic consumption of 6 ounces of alcohol per day constitutes a high risk, whereas FAS is not likely when the mother drinks fewer than 2 drinks (equivalent to 2 ounces of alcohol) per day.[457] Reduction of alcohol consumption at any time in pregnancy reduces the severity of FAS but may not significantly reduce the risk of some degree of physical or behavioral impairment. The human syndrome is likely to involve the direct effects of ethanol and the indirect effects of genetic susceptibility and poor nutrition. Although alcoholic mothers frequently smoke and consume other drugs, there is little doubt that alcohol ingestion alone can have a disastrous effect on the developing embryo or fetus. It is estimated that at least several hundred children each year are born with the full FAS and probably several thousand children are born with fetal alcohol effects.

COCAINE

Cocaine (benzoylmethylecgonine) is one of the most commonly used illicit drugs by women of reproductive age. Reported estimates for cocaine use during pregnancy range from 3–17%,[458] the highest rates occurring in inner city populations. Because of its widespread use during pregnancy and the growing cost of caring for cocaine exposed neonates,[459] there has been increasing concern over the risks associated with prenatal cocaine use to maternal and fetal health. Despite numerous clinical studies linking prenatal cocaine use with a variety of adverse maternal and fetal effects, methodological limitations in these studies have made it difficult to establish a causal relationship between these effects and maternal cocaine use. Not only are the timing, frequency and dose of cocaine use hard to determine, but adverse effects due to low socioeconomic status, poor nutrition, multiple drug use, infections, and a lack of prenatal care are difficult to dissociate from effects due to cocaine use alone.[458,460] As such the issue of how much risk to the fetus is associated with cocaine use during pregnancy remains unresolved. Nonetheless a growing body of literature supports the concept that cocaine is a developmental toxicant. Adverse effects attributed to prenatal cocaine exposure include a higher incidence of spontaneous abortion, placental abruption, still birth, prematurity, low birth weight, growth retardation, decreased head circumference, intracerebral hemorrhage, congenital defects, neurobehavioral abnormalities,[458,461] and a possible association with increased risk of SIDS.[462] These effects are reduced but not eliminated in mothers receiving appropriate prenatal care.[463] Like other developmental toxins, outcome is dependent on dose and time of use.

The majority of adverse effects associated with cocaine use during pregnancy appear to be due to high levels of cocaine abuse in later stages of gestation.[464] Reports indicate that moderate usage of cocaine only in the first trimester does not appear to result in adverse fetal outcome and may not pose an increased risk to the fetus.[465] However, studies in both humans and animals suggest that first trimester usage can result in neurological and urogenital abnormalities.[460,466]

When taken systemically cocaine blocks presynaptic reuptake of monoamines leading to stimulation of the sympathetic nervous system.[467] Cocaine also directly affects the heart.[468] Physiologic effects include vasoconstriction, tachycardia, cardiac dysrythmias, and hypertension. It is thought that the increased incidence of placental abruption reported in cocaine users results from this latter effect.[464,468] Altered cocaine metabolism during pregnancy may increase the susceptibility of pregnant women and their fetuses to the cardiovas-

cular effects of cocaine.[460,469] Enhanced hypertensive effects due to cocaine have been demonstrated in non-pregnant animals treated with progesterone suggesting these changes are hormonally mediated.[469]

Adverse fetal outcomes associated with maternal cocaine use are thought to primarily result from the vasoconstrictive effects of cocaine on both the maternal and fetal vasculature.[464] Additionally, cocaine may inhibit the maternal-fetal transfer of nutrients such as amino acids[470,471] contributing to growth retardation.[468,469,471] The combination of fetal hypertension combined with increased cerebral blood flow may result in intracerebral hemorrhage or infarction which has been reported to occur in cocaine exposed fetuses in both human and animal studies.[466,472–476]

A significant association between cocaine use and an increased incidence of genitourinary tract malformations has been reported.[458,475,477,478] Other defects reported include limb reduction defects,[475,477] nonduodenal intestinal atresia,[475] cardiac anomalies, renal defects such as hypospadius, prune belly syndrome, hydronephrosis,[468] crossed renal ectopia,[479] and limb-body wall complex.[480] With the exception of genitourinary tract malformations, the sample size in these clinical studies has not been sufficient to determine a statistically significant relationship between cocaine use and these congenital anomalies.[481]

In one study, light to moderate usage with decreased usage after the first trimester did not result in adverse fetal outcome.[(482)] In other studies the incidence of anomalies for cocaine exposed infants was reported to be anywhere from 3 to 6 times the incidence in controls or higher.[461,477,478,480,483]

In rodents cocaine is teratogenic during the late organogenic to post-organogenic period.[484] Defects reported in these studies are similar in nature to those reported in human studies and include genitourinary malformations, limb reduction defects, and cerebral hemorrhages.[474,484,485] These defects share similarities in that they have an etiology suggestive of vascular disruptive phenomena.[464,475,484–486] Decreased uterine/placental blood flow alone or in conjunction with direct effects on fetal vasculature may lead to hemorrhage/edema, followed by necrosis and reabsorption of affected tissues[484,486] and resulting in the destruction of already formed structures.[464,486] Temporary clamping of the uterine arteries in the rat results in similar malformations.[158] Recent evidence indicates that reperfusion of tissues following cocaine induced ischemia may also result in tissue damage due to free radicals generated by the mother,[487] and later in gestation by the fetus.[488]

Various neurobehavioral effects have also been described in infants following in utero cocaine exposure including tremors, seizures, irritability, excessive high pitched crying, poor feeding, sleeping abnormalities, poor state regulation, and abnormal EEG.[461,489] A majority of studies using the Brazelton neonatal assessment scale also indicate that neonates exposed to cocaine in utero have altered behavioral responses, especially in orientation and habituation, when compared to nonexposed controls,[461,490] although there are conflicting reports.

Many of the behavioral patterns observed can be ascribed to the direct toxic/physiologic effects of cocaine on the neonate and disappear as cocaine and its metabolites are eliminated.[491,492] However, impaired organizational ability, orientation and state control have also been observed in neonates exposed to cocaine only during the first trimester indicating a more direct effect of cocaine on CNS development and maturation.[463,466] Sensory deficits and altered auditory brain stem response has also been reported but normalize by 3 months of age in the human.[461] Other studies indicate that deficient performance on developmental tests may persist up to 2 years in some exposed groups.[493] One other study demonstrated no difference in IQ scores between the cocaine exposed and unexposed groups at 3 years of age.[490] Unfortunately these studies have methodological complications due to confounding variables such as alcohol abuse.

Studies in rodents, however, suggest that cocaine may produce permanent neurochemical alterations in the brain and may alter behavior and learning.[494–496] Studies have also demonstrated that in utero exposure to cocaine may lead to lasting changes in cholinergic,[497] dopaminergic,[498] seratonergic,[498,499] and noradrenergic[500] systems. In addition, cocaine reduces DNA synthesis in the brain,[(501)] and inhibits macromolecular synthesis by glial cells in vitro.[502] Alterations in brain ornithine decarboxylase activity have also been reported in both fetal rabbits[492] and rats[503] exposed to cocaine. In utero cocaine exposure also resulted in delayed auditory brainstem response in adult[504] and 22 day rat pups[505] possibly due to delayed myelination. Hypomyelination has been demonstrated in rat pups exposed to cocaine in the fetal period of gestation.[506] These studies and others suggest that cocaine may subtly alter CNS development and maturation leading to the altered behavior and learning patterns that have been observed. Further studies are necessary to determine if permanent subtle alterations in learning and behavior are indeed apparent in human infants and how long these changes persist. Until carefully controlled follow-up studies are performed, it is not possible to determine whether cocaine has direct neuroteratogenic properties in the human.

SUMMARY

Environmental causes of human malformations account for approximately 10% of malformations, and less than 1% of all human malformations are related to prescription drug exposure, environmental chemicals, or ionizing radiation. However, malformations caused by drugs and other therapeutic agents are important because these exposures may be preventable, just as preventing or treating maternal disease states such as diabetes, alcoholism or teratogenic infection have the potential for preventing birth defects. Research has expanded our horizons in epidemiology and animal research to enable the scientific community to monitor human populations and improve the predictability of animal testing with regard to the teratogenic risk of drugs and chemicals. As we better understand the mechanisms of teratogenesis from all etiologies we may learn how best to predict, prevent, and test for teratogenicity.

ACKNOWLEDGMENTS

We thank Mrs. Yvonne G. Edney for her assistance in the preparation of this manuscript. This work was supported in part by funds from The Nemours Foundation, and the Harry Bock Charities.

References

1. Wilson JG, ed. *Environment and Birth Defects.* New York: Academic Press; 1973.
2. Brent RL. Environmental factors: Miscellaneous. In: Brent RL and Harris MI, ed. *Prevention of Embryonic Fetal and Perinatal Disease.* Bethesda, MD: DHEW (NIH); 1976:211–218.
3. Heinonen OP, Slone D, Shapiro S, eds. *Birth Defects and Drugs in Pregnancy.* Littleton, CO: Publishing Sciences Group; 1977.
4. Carter CO. Genetics of common single malformations. *Br Med Bull.* 1976;32:21–26.
5. Fraser FC. The multifactorial/threshold concept-uses and misuses. *Teratology.* 1976;14:762–770.
6. Brent RL. Drug testing in animals for teratogenic effects: Thalidomide in the pregnant rat. *J Pediatr.* 1964;64:762–770.
7. Hertig AT. The overall problem in man. In Benirschke K, ed. *Comparative Aspects of Reproductive Failure.* Berlin: Springer-Verlag; 1967:11–41.
8. Boue J, Boue A, Lazar P. Retrospective and prospective epidemiological studies of 1,500 karyotyped spontaneous abortions. *Teratology.* 1975;12:11–26.
9. World Health Organization. *Spontaneous and Induced Abortion.* Geneva: World Health Organization; 1970.
10. Simpson JL. Genes, chromosomes and reproductive failure. *Fertil Steril.* 1980;33:116–778.
11. Warkany J. Aminopterin and methotrexate: Folic acid deficiency. *Teratology.* 1978;17:353–358.
12. Robert CJ, Lowe CR. Where have all the conceptions gone? *Lancet.* 1975;1:498–499.
13. National Research Council. *Health Effects of Exposure to Low Levels of Ionizing Radiation: BEIRV.* Washington, DC.: National Academy Press; 1990.
14. Biddle FG, Fraser FC. Genetics of cortisone-induced cleft palate in the mouse-embryonic and maternal effects. *Genetics.* 1976;84:743.
15. Biddle FG. Use of dose-response relationships to discriminate between the mechanism of cleft-palate induction by different teratogens: An argument for discussion. *Teratology.* 1978;18:247.
16. Brent RL. Method of evaluating alleged human teratogens (Editorial). *Teratology.* 1978;17:83.
17. Brent RL. The effects of embryonic and fetal exposure to x-ray, microwaves and ultrasound. *Clin Ob/Gyn.* 1983;26:484–512.
18. Brent RL, Beckman DA, Jensh RP. The relationship of animal experiments in predicting the effect of intrauterine effects in the human. In Kriegel H, et al., ed. *Radiation Risks to the Developing Nervous System.* New York: Gustav Fisher; 1986:367–397.
19. Shepard TH, ed. *Catalog of Teratogenic Agents.* 5th ed. Baltimore: Johns Hopkins University Press; 1986.

20. Wilson JG. Misinformation about risks of congenital anomalies. In Maurois M, ed. *Prevention of Physical and Mental Congenital Defects Part C: Basic and Medical Science, Education and Future Strategies.* New York: Alan R. Liss; 1985:165.

21. Brent RL. Predicting teratogenic and reproductive risks in humans from exposure to various environmental agents using in vitro techniques and in vivo animal studies. *Cong Anom.* 1988;28:S41–S55.

22. Skipper HT, Schabel FM Jr. Quantitative and cytokinetic studies in experimental tumor models. In Holland JF and Frei E III, ed. *Cancer Medicine.* Philadelphia: Lea and Febieger; 1973: 629–650.

23. Thiersch JB. Therapeutic abortions with a folic acid (4-amino P.G.A.). *Am J Obstet Gynecol.* 1952;63:1298–1304.

24. Goetsch C. An evaluation of amniopterin as an abortifacient. *Am J Obstet Gynecol.* 1962;83:1474–1477.

25. Warkany J, Beautry PH, Horstein S. Attempted abortion with amniopterin (4-aminopteroylglutamic acid). *Am J Dis Child.* 1959;97:274–281.

26. Jones KL. Fetal amniopterin/methotrexate syndrome. In Jones KL, ed. *Smith's Recognizable Patterns of Human Malformation.* Philadelphia: Saunders; 1997:570–571.

27. Del Campo M, Kosaki K, Bennett FC, et al. Developmental delay in fetal aminopterin/methotrexate syndrome. *Teratology.* 1999;60:10–12.

28. Bawle EV, Conard JV, Weiss L. Adult and two children with fetal methotrexate syndrome. *Teratology.* 1998;57:51–55.

29. Shaw EB, Steinbach HL. Amniopterin-induced fetal malformation: Survival of infant after attempted abortion. *Am J Dis Child.* 1968;115:477–482.

30. Skalko RG, Gold MP. Teratogenicity of methotrexate in mice. *Teratology.* 1974;9:159–164.

31. Feldkamp M, Carey JC. Clinical teratology, counseling and consultation case report: Low dose methotrexate exposure in the early weeks of pregnancy. *Teratology.* 1993;47:533–539.

32. Grumbach MM, Conte FA. Disorders of sex differentiation. In Williams RH, (ed.): *Textbook of Endocrinology.* Philadelphia, WB Saunders, 1981:422–514.

33. Moncrieff A. Nonadrenal female pseudohermaphroditism associated with hormone administration in pregnancy. *Lancet.* 1958;2: 267.

34. Hoffman F, Overzier C, Uhde G. Zur frage der hormonalen erzengung fotaler zwittenbildugen beim menschen. *Geburtshife Frauerheikd* 1955;15:1061–1070.

35. Reschini E, Giustina G, D'Alberton A, et al. Female pseudohermaphroditism due to maternal androgen administration: 25-year follow-up. *Lancet.* 1985;1:1226.

36. Greene RR, Burrill MW, Ivy AC. Experimental intersexuality: the effect of antenatal androgens on sexual development of female rats. *Am J Anat.* 1939;65:415–469.

37. Raynaud A. Observations dur de development normal des ebauches de la glande mammaire des foetus maleset femele de souris. *Ann Endocrinol.* 1947;8:349–359.

38. Brunner JA, Witschi E. Testosterone-induced modifications of sexual development in female hamsters. *Am J Anat.* 1946;79:293–320.

39. Jost A. Problems of fetal endocrinology: the gonadal and hypophyseal hormones. *Rec Prog Horm Res.* 1953;8:379–418.

40. Wells LJ, Van Wagenen G. Androgen induced female pseudohermaphroditism in the monkey (macaca mulatta) anatomy of the reproductive organs. *Carnegie Institute Contrib Embryol.* 1954;35:93–106.

41. Dohler KD, Hancke JL, Srivastava SS, et al. Participation of estrogens in female sexual differentiation of the brain: neuroanatomical, neuroendocrine and behavioral evidence. *Prog Brain Res.* 1984;6:99–117.

42. Goy RW, Bercovitch FB, McBrair MC. Behavioral masculinization is independent of genital masculinization in prenatally androgenized female rhesus macaques. *Horm Behav.* 1988;22:552–571.

43. Goy RW, Bridson WE, Young WC. Period of maximal susceptibility of the prenatal female guinea pig to masculinizing actions of the testosterone propionate. *J Comp Physiol Psychol.* 1964;57:166–174.

44. Hoepfner BA, Ward IL. Prenatal and neonatal androgen exposure interact to affect sexual differentiation in female rats. *Behav Neurosci.* 1988;102:61–65.

45. Huffman L, Hendricks SE. Prenatally injected testosterone propionate and sexual behavior of female rats. *Physiol Behav.* 1981;26:773–778.

46. Phoenix CH, Goy RW, Gerall AA, et al. Organizing action of prenatally administered testosterone propionate on the tissues mediating mating behavior in the female guinea pig. *Endocrinology.* 1959;65:369–382.

47. Schardein JL, ed. *Chemically Induced Birth Defects.* New York: Marcel Dekker; 1993.

48. Bobrowitz ID. Ethambutol in pregnancy. *Chest.* 1974;66:20–24.

49. Lewit T, Nebel L, Terracina S, et al. Ethambutol in pregnancy: Observations on embryogenesis. *Chest.* 1974;66:25–26.

50. Snider DE, Layde PM, Johnson MW, et al. Treatment of turberculosis during pregnancy. *Am Rev Respir Dis.* 1980;122:65–79.

51. Warkany J. Antituberculosis drugs. *Teratology.* 1979;20:133–138.

52. Monnet P, Kalb JC, Pujol M. Harmful effects of isoniazid on the fetus and infants. *Lyon Med.* 1967;218:431–455.

53. Varpela E. On the effect exerted by the first line turberculosis medicines on the fetus. *Acta Tuberc Scand.* 1964;35:53–69.

54. Lenke RR, Turkel SB, Monsen R. Severe fatal deformities associated with ingestion of excessive isoniazid in early pregnancy. *Acta Obstet Gynecol. Scand.* 1985;64:281–282.

55. Potworowska M, Sianoz-Ecka E, Szufladowicz R. Treatment with ethionamide in pregnancy. *Gruzlica.* 1966;34:341–347.

56. Zierski M. Effects of ethionamide on the development of the human fetus. *Gruzlica.* 1966;34:349–352.

57. Dluzniewski A, Gastol-Lewinska L. The search for teratogenic activity of some tuberculostatic drugs. *Diss Pharm Pharmacol.* 1971;23:383–392.

58. Nakamoto Y, Otani H, Tanaka O. Effects of aminoglycosides administered to pregnant mice on postnatal development of inner ear in their offspring. *Teratology.* 1985;2:604–605.

59. Steen JSM, Stainton-Eldis DM. Rifampicin in pregnancy. *Lancet.* 1977;2:604–605.

60. Heinonen OP, Slone D, Monson RR, et al. Cardiovascular birth defects and antenatal exposure to female sex hormones. *N Engl J Med.* 1977;296:67–70.

61. Kullander S, Kallen B. A prospective study of drugs and pregnancy. *Acta Obstet Gynecol. Scand.* 1976;55:25–33.

62. Crombie DL, Pinsent RJ, Fleming DM, et al. Fetal effects of tranquilizers in pregnancy. *N Engl J Med.* 1975;293:198–199.

63. Czeizel A. Lack of evidence of teratogenicity of benzodiazepine drugs in Hungary. *Reprod Toxicol.* 1988;1:183–188.

64. Hartz SC, Heinonen OP, Shapiro S, et al. Antenatal exposure to meprobamate and chloridiazepoxide in relation to malformations, mental development, and childhood mortality. *N Engl J Med.* 1975;292:726–728.

65. Rothman KJ, Fyler DC, Goldblatt A, et al. Exogenous hormones and other drug exposures of children with congenital heart disease. *Am J Epidemiol.* 1979;109:433–439.

66. Bracken MB, Holford TR. Exposure to prescribed drugs in pregnancy and association with congenital malformations. *Obstet Gynecol.* 1981;58:336–344.

67. Zierler S, Rothman KJ. Congenital heart disease in relation to maternal use of Bendectin and other drugs in early pregnancy. *N Engl J Med.* 1985;313:347–352.

68. Aselton P, Jick H, Milunsky A, et al. First-trimester drug use and congenital disorders. *Obstet Gynecol.* 1985;65:451–455.

69. Safra MJ, Oakley GP. Association between cleft lip with or without cleft palate and prenatal exposure to diazepam. *Lancet.* 1975;2:478–479.

70. Tikkanen J, Heinonen OP. Risk factors for conal malformations of the heart. *Eur J Epidemiol.* 1992;8:48–57.

71. Laegried L, Hagberg G, Lundberg A. Neurodevelopment in late infancy after prenatal exposure to benzodiazepines—A prospective study. *Neuropediatrics.* 1992;23:60–67.

72. Gill TS, Guram MS, Geber WF. Comparative study of the teratogenic effects of chlorodiazepoxide and diazepam in the fetal hamster. *Life Sci.* 1981;29:2141–2147.

73. Weber LWD. Benzodiazepines in pregnancy—academic debate or teratogenic risk? *Biol Res Pregnancy.* 1985;6:151–167.

74. Rementeria JL, Bhatt K. Withdrawal symptoms in neonates from intrauterine exposure to diazepam. *J Pediatr.* 1977;90:123–126.

75. Jick H, Holmes LB, Hunter JR, et al. First trimester drug use and congenital disorders. *J Am Med Assoc.* 1981;246:343–346.

76. Milkovich L, van den Berg BJ. Effects of prenatal meprobamate and chlordiazepoxide hydrochloride on human embryonic and fetal development. *N Engl J Med.* 1974;291:1268–1271.

77. Saxen I. Association between oral clefts and drugs taken during pregnancy. *Int J Epidemiol.* 1975;4:37–44.

78. Belafsky HA, Breslow S, Hirsch LM, et al. Meprobamate during pregnancy. *Obstet Gynecol.* 1969;34:378–386.

79. Hoffeld DR, McNew J, Webster RL. Effect of tranquilizing drugs during pregnancy on activity of offspring. *Nature.* 1968;218:357–358.

80. Murai N. Effect of maternal medication during pregnancy upon behavioral development of offspring. *Tohoku J Exp Med.* 1966;89:265–272.

81. Werboff J, Kesner R. Learning deficits of offspring after administration of tranquilizing drugs to the mothers. *Nature.* 1963;197:106–107.

82. Graham HN. Mate. In Spiller GA, ed. *The Methylxanthine Beverages and Foods: Chemistry Consumption and Health Effects.* New York: Alan R. Liss; 1984a:179–183.

83. Graham HN. Tea: The plant and its manufacture, chemistry and consumption of the beverage. In Spiller GA, ed. *The Methylxanthine Beverage and Foods: Chemistry, Consumption and Health Effects.* New York: Alan R. Liss; 1984b:29–74.

84. Spiller GA. The chemical components of coffee. *Prog Clin Biol Res.* 1984;158:47–91.

85. Barone JJ, Roberts H. Human consumption of caffeine. In Dewes PB, ed. *Caffeine.* New York: Springer-Verlag; 1984:59–73.

86. Hill RM, Craig JP, Chaney MD, et al. Utilization of over-the-counter drugs during pregnancy. *Clin Obstet Gynecol.* 1977;20:281–394.

87. Beaulac-Baillargeon L, Desrosiers C. Caffeine-cigarette interaction on fetal growth. *Am J Obstet Gynecol.* 1987;157:1236–1240.

88. Brooke OG, Anderson HR, Bland JM, et al. Effects on birth weight of smoking, alcohol, caffeine, socioeconomic factors and psychosocial stress. *Br Med J.* 1989;298:795–801.

89. Caan BJ, Goldhaber MK. Caffeinated beverages and low birth weight—A case control study. *Am J Public Health.* 1989;79:1299–1300.

90. Fenster L, Eskenazi B, Windham GC, et al. Caffeine consumption during pregnancy and fetal growth. *Am J Public Health.* 1991;81:458–461.

91. Martin TR, Bracken MB. The association between low birth weight and caffeine consumption during pregnancy. *Am J Epidemiol.* 1987;126:813–821.

92. Mau G, Netter P. Kaffee und alkoholkonsum, risikofaktoren in der schwangerschaft. *Geburtsh Frauenheilkd.* 1974;34:1018–1022.

93. Srisuphan W, Bracken MB. Caffeine-consumption during pregnancy and association with late spontaneous abortion. *Am J Obstet Gynecol.* 1986;154:14–20.

94. van der Berg BJ. Epidemiological observations of prematurity: Effects of tobacco, coffee and alcohol. In Reed DM and Stanley FJ ed. *The Epidemiology. of Prematurity.* Baltimore: Urban & Schwarzenberg; 1977:157–177.

95. Watkinson B, Fried PA. Maternal caffeine use before, during and after pregnancy and effects upon offspring. *Neurobehav Toxicol Teratol.* 1985;7:9–17.

96. Weathersbee PS, Olsen LK, Lodge JR. Caffeine and pregnancy: a retrospective survey. *Postgrad Med.* 1977;62:64–69.

97. Wilcox AJ, Weinberg CR, Baird DD. Risk factors for early pregnancy loss. *Epidemiology.* 1990;1:382–385.

98. Berger A. Effects of caffeine consumption on pregnancy outcome — A review. *J Reprod Med.* 1988;33:945–956.

99. Kurppa K, Holmberg PC, Kuosma E, et al. Coffee consumption during pregnancy. *N Engl J Med.* 1982;306:1548.

100. Kurppa K, Holmberg PC, Kuosma E, et al. Coffee consumption during pregnancy and selected congenital malformations: a nationwide case-control study. *Am J Public Health.* 1983;73:1397–1399.

101. Linn S, Lieberman E, Schoenbaum SC, et al. No association between coffee consumption and adverse outcomes of pregnancy. *N Engl J Med.* 1982;306:141–144.

102. van't Hoff W. Caffeine in pregnancy. *Lancet.* 1982;1:1020.

103. Rosenberg L, Mitchell AA, Shapiro S, et al. Selected birth defects in relation to caffeine-containing beverages. *J Am Med Assoc.* 1982;247:1429–1432.

104. Nishimura H, Nakai K. Congenital malformations in offspring of mice treated with caffeine. *Proc Soc Exp Biol Med.* 1960;104:140–142.

105. Gilbert EF, Pistey WR. Effect on the offspring of repeated caffeine administration to pregnant rats. *J Reprod Fertil.* 1973;34:495–499.

106. Bertrand M, Schwam E, Frandon A, et al. Sur un effet teratogene systematique et specifique de la cafeine chez les rongeurs. *C R Soc Biol (Paris).* 1966;159:2199–2202.

107. Betrand M, Girod J, Rigaud MF. Ectrodactylie provoquee par la cafeine chez les rongeurs: role des facteurs specificques et genetiques. *C R Soc Biol (Paris).* 1970;164:1488–1489.

108. Knoche C, Konig J. Zur prantalen toxizitat von diphenylpyralin-8-chlortheophyllinat unterbercksichtgung von erfahrungen mit thalidomid und caffein. *Arzneimittelforschung.* 1964;14:415–424.

109. Fujii T, Nishimura H. Adverse effects of prolonged administration of caffeine on rat fetus. *Toxicol Appl Pharmacol.* 1972;22:449–457.

110. Elmazar MMA, McElhatton PR, Sullivan FM. Studies on the teratogenic effects of different oral preparations of caffeine in mice. *Toxicology.* 1982;23:57–72.

111. Palm PE, Arnold EP, Rachwall PC, et al. Evaluation of the teratogenic potential of fresh-brewed coffee and caffeine in the rat. *Toxicol Appl Pharmacol.* 1978;44:1–16.

112. Pitel M, Lerman S. Further studies on the effects of intrauterine vasoconstrictors on the fetal rat lens. *Am J Ophthalmol.* 1964;58:464–470.

113. Fujii T, Sasaki H, Nishimura H. Teratogenicity of caffeine in mice related to its mode of administration. *Jpn J Pharmacol.* 1969;19:134–138.

114. Collins TFX, Welsch JJ, Black TN, et al. A study of the teratogenic potential of caffeine given by oral intubation to rats. *Regul Toxicol Pharmacol.* 1981;1:355–378.

115. Christian MS, Brent RL. Teratogen Update: Evaluation of the reproductive and developmental risks of caffeine. Teratology 2001;64:51–78.

116. York RG, Randall JL, Scott WJ Jr. Reduction of caffeine teratogenicity in mice by inducing maternal drug metabolism with b-Naphthoflavone. *Teratology.* 1985;31:217–225.

117. Murphy SJ, Benjamin CP. The effects of coffee on mouse development. *Microbios Lett.* 1981;17:91–99.

118. Nolen GA. A reproduction/teratology study of decaffeinated coffees. *Toxicologist* 1981;1:104.

119. Matsuoka R, Uno H, Tanaka H, et al. Caffeine induces cardiac and other malformations in the rat. *Am J Med. Genet Suppl.* 1987;3:433–443.

120. Collins T, Welsh J, Black T, et al. Potential reversibility of skeletal effects in rats exposed in utero to caffeine. *Food Chem Toxicol.* 1987;25:647–666.

121. Kavlock RJ, Chernoff N, Rogers EH. The effect of acute maternal toxicity on fetal development in the mouse. *Teratogen Carcinogen Mutagens.* 1985;5:3–13.

122. Nolen GA. The developmental toxicity of caffeine. In Kalter H, ed. *Issues and Reviews in Teratology.* New York: Plenum Press; 1989: 305–350.

123. Grimm VE, Frieder B. Prenatal caffeine causes long lasting behavioral and neurochemical changes. *Int J Neurosci.* 1988;41:15–28.

124. Groisser DS, Rosso P, Winick M. Coffee consumption during pregnancy: subsequent behavioral abnormalities of the offspring. *J Nutr.* 1982;112:829–832.

125. Hughes RN, Beveridge IJ. Behavioral effects of prenatal exposure to caffeine in rats. *Life Sci.* 1986;38:861–868.

126. Hughes RN, Beveridge IJ. Effects of prenatal exposure to chronic caffeine on locomotor and emotional behavior. *Psychobiology.* 1987;15:179–185.

127. Sobotka TJ, Spaid SL, Brodie RE. Neurobehavioral teratology of caffeine exposure in rats. *Neurotoxicology.* 1979;1:403–416.

128. Gilbert SG, Rice DC, Reuhl KR, et al. Adverse pregnancy outcome in the monkey (macaca fascicularis) after chronic caffeine exposure. *J Pharmacol Exp Ther.* 1988;245:1048–1053.

129. Rice DC, Gilbert SG. Automated behavioral procedures for infant monkeys. *Neurotoxicol Teratol.* 1990;12:429–439.

130. Klebanoff MA, Levine RJ, Dersimonian R, et al. Serum caffeine and paraxanthine as markers for reported caffeine intake in pregnancy. *Ann Epidemiol.* 1998;8:107–111.

131. Nakane Y, Okuma T, Takahashi R, et al. Multi-institutional study on the teratogenicity and fetal toxicity of antiepileptic drugs: a report of a collaborative study group in Japan. *Epilepsia.* 1980;21:663.

132. Nielsen M, Froscher W. Finger and toenail hypoplasia after carbamazepine monotherapy in late pregnancy. *Neuropediatrics.* 1985;16:167–168.

133. Jones KL, Lacro RV, Johnson KA, et al. Pattern of malformations in the children of women treated with carbamazepine during pregnancy. *New Engl J Med.* 1989;320:1661–1666.

134. Ornoy A, Cohen E. Outcome of children born to epileptic mothers treated with carbamazepine during pregnancy. *Arch Dis Child.* 1996;75:517–520.

135. Wide K, Windbladh B, Tomson T, et al. Body dimensions in infants exposed to antiepileptic drugs in utero: observations spanning 25 years. *Epilepsia.* 2000;41:854–861.

136. Hilesmaa VK, Teramo K, Granstrom ML, et al. Fetal head growth retardation associated with maternal antiepileptic drugs. *Lancet.* 1981;2:165–167.

137. Bertollini R, Kallen B, Mastroiacovo P, et al. Anticonvulsant drugs in monotherapy: effect on the fetus. *Eur J Epidemiol.* 1987;3:164–167.

138. Rosa FW. Spina bifida in infants of women treated with carbamazepine during pregnancy. *N Engl J Med.* 1991;10:674–677.

139. Kallen AJ. Maternal carbamazepine and infant spina bifida. *Repro Tox.* 1994;8:203–205.

140. Nulman I, Scolinik D, Chitayat D, et al. Findings in children exposed in utero to phenytoin and carbamazepine monotherapy: independent effects of epilepsy and medications. *Am J Med. Gen.* 1997;68:18–24.

141. Little BB, Santos-Ramos R, Newell JF, et al. Megadose carbamazepine during the period of neural tube closure. *Obstet Gynecol.* 1993;82:705–708.

142. Lindhout D, Hoppener RJE, Meinardi H. Teratogenicity of antiepileptic drug combinations with special emphasis of epoxidation (of carbamazepine). *Epilepsia.* 1984;25:77–83.

143. Paulson RB, Paulson GW, Jreissaty S. Phenytoin and carbamazepine in production of cleft palates in mice. Comparison of the teratogenic effects. *Arch Neurol.* 1979;36:832–836.

144. Fritz H, Muller D, Hess R. Comparative study of the teratogenicity of phenobarbitone, diphenylhydantoin and carbamazapine in mice. *Toxicology.* 1976;6:323–330.

145. Finnell RH, Mohl VK, Bennett GD, et al. Failure of epoxide formation to influence carbamazapine-induced teratogenesis in a mouse model. *Teratogenesis, Carcinogenesis and Mutagenesis.* 1986;6:393–401.

146. Wray SD, Hassell TM, Phillips C, et al. Preliminary study of the effects of carbamazepine on congenital orofacial defects in offspring of A/J mice. *Epilepsia.* 1982;23:101–110.

147. Vorhees CV, Acuff KD, Weisenburger WP, et al. Teratogenicity of carbamazepine in rats. *Teratology.* 1990;41:311–317.

148. Eluma FO, Sucheston ME, Hayes TG, et al. Teratogenic effects of dosage levels and time of administration of carbamazapine, sodium valproate, and diphenylhydantoin on craniofacial development in the CD-1 mouse fetus. *J Craniofacial Genetics and Developmental Biology* 1984;4:191–210.

149. Bennett GD, Amore BM, Finnell RH, et al. Teratogenicity of carbamazepine-10, 11-epoxide and oxycarbazapine in the SWV mouse. *J Pharmacol and Exper Therapeutics.* 1996;279:1237–1242.

150. Hansen DK, Dial SL, Terry KK, et al. In vitro embryotoxicity of carbamazapine and carbamazapine-10, 11-epoxide. *Teratology.* 1996;54:45–51.

151. Olney RS, Khoury MJ, Alo CJ, et al. Increased risk for transverse digital deficiency after chorionic villus sampling: results of the United States Mulktistate Case-Control Study, 1988–1992. *Teratology.* 1995;51:20–29.

152. Firth HV, Boyd PA, Chamberlain PF, et al. Analysis of limb reduction defects in babies exposed to chorionic villus sampling. *Lancet.* 1994;343:1069–1071.

153. Mastrioacovo P, Tozzi AE, Agosti S, et al. Transverse limb reduction defects after chrion villus sampling: a retrospective cohort study. GIDEF-Gruppo Italiano Diagnosi Embrio-Fetali. *Prenatal Diagnosis.* 1993;13:1051–1056.

154. Kuliev A, Jackson L, Froster U, et al. Chorionic villus sampling safety. Report of World Health Organization/EURO meeting in association with the Seventh International Conference on Early Prenatal Diagnosis of Genetic Diseases. Tel Aviv, Israel, May 21, 1994. *Am J Obstet Gynecol.* 1996;174:807–811.

155. Silver RK, MacGregor SN, Muhlbach LH, et al. Congenital malformations subsequent to chorionic villus sampling: outcome analysis of 1048 consecutive procedures. *Prenatal Diagnosis.* 1994;14:417–427.

156. NICHD Workshop. CVS and limb reduction defects. *Teratology.* 1993;48:7–13.

157. Brent RL. The indirect effect of irradiation on embryonic development. II. Irradiation of the placenta. *Am J Dis Child.* 1960;100:103–108.

158. Brent RL. Relationship between uterine vascular clamping, vascular disruption, and cocaine teratogenicity (Editorial). *Teratology.* 1990;41:757–760.

159. Brent RL. What is the relationship between birth defects and pregnancy bleeding? New perspectives provided by the NICHD workshop dealing with the association of chorionic villous sampling and the occurrence of limb reduction defects. *Teratology.* 1993;48:93–95.

160. Brent RL, Franklin JB. Uterine vascular clamping: New procedures for the study of congenital malformations. *Science.* 1960;132:89–91.

161. Webster WS, Lipson AH, Brown-Woodman PDC. Uterine trauma and limb defects. *Teratology.* 1987;35:253–260.

162. Hoyme EH, Jones KL, Van Allen MI, et al. The vascular pathogenesis of transverse limb reduction defects. *J Pediatr.* 1982;101:839–843.

163. Funderburk SJ, Guthrie D, Meldrum D. Outcome of pregnancies complicated by early vaginal bleeding. *Brit J Obstet Gynecol.* 1980;87:100–105.

164. Asanti R, Vesanto T. Effect of threatened abortion on fetal prognosis. *Acta Obstet Gynec Scand.* 1963;42:107.

165. Burge ES. The relationship of threatened abortion to fetal anomalies. *Am J Obstet Gynec.* 1951;61:615–621.

166. Evans JH, Beicher NA. The prognosis of threatened abortion. *Med J Aust.* 1970;2:165–168.

167. King AG. Threatened and repeated abortion. *Status Ther.* 1953;1:104.

168. Matsunaga E, Shiota K. Threatened abortion, hormone therapy and malformed embryos. *Teratology.* 1979;20:69–80.

169. Matsunaga E, Shiota K. Ectopic pregnancy and myoma uteri: teratogenic effects of maternal characteristics. *Teratology.* 1980;20:61–69.

170. Nishimura H, Uwabe C, Semba R. Examination of teratogenicity of progestogens and/or estrogens by observation of the induced abortuses. *Teratology.* 1974;10:93.

171. Ornoy A, Benady S, Kohen-Raz R, et al. Association between maternal bleeding during gestation and congenital anomalies. *Amer J Obstet Gynec.* 1976;124:474–478.

172. Peckham CH. Uterine bleeding during pregnancy: I. When not followed by immediate termination of pregnancy. *Obstet Gynec.* 1970;35:937–941.

173. Smith DW. Teratogenicity of anticonvulsive medications. *Am J Dis Child.* 1977;131:1337–1339.

174. South J. The effect of vaginal bleeding in early pregnancy on the infant born after the 28 week of pregnancy. *J Obstet Gynec.* 1973;80:236–241.

175. Stevenson SS, Worchester V, Rice RG. Congenitally malformed infants and associated gestational characteristics. *Pediatr.* 1950;6:37.

176. Turnbull EPN, Walker J. The outcome of pregnancy complicated by threatened abortion. *J Obstetr Gynecol Br Emp.* 1956;63:553–559.

177. Mastrioacovo P, Botto LD, Cavalcanti DP, et al. Limb anomalies following chorionic villus sampling: a registry based case-control study. *Am J Med. Genet.* 1992;44:856–864.

178. DiSaia PJ. Pregnancy and delivery of a patient with a Starr-Edwards mitral valve prosthesis: Report of a case. *Obstet Gynecol.* 1966;29:469–472.

179. Kerber IJ, Warr OS, Richardson C. Pregnancy in a patient with prosthetic mitral valve. *J Am Med Assoc.* 1968;203:223–225.

180. Barr M, Pozanski AK, Shmickel RD. Digital hypoplasia and anticonvulsants during gestation, a teratogenic syndrome. *J Pediatr.* 1974;4:254–256.

181. Pettiflor JM, Benson R. Congenital malformations associated with the administration of oral anticoagulants during pregnancy. *J Pediatr.* 1975;86:459–462.

182. Hall JG, Pauli RM, Wilson RM. Maternal and fetal sequelae of anticoagulation during pregnancy. *Am J Med.* 1980;68:122–140.

183. Warkany J. A warfarin embryopathy? *Am J Dis Child.* 1975;129:287–288.

184. Warkany J. Warfarin embryopathy. *Teratology.* 1976;14:205–209.

185. Stevenson RE, Burton OM, Furlauto GJ, et al. Hazards of oral anticoagulants during pregnancy. *JAMA.* 1980;243:1549–1551.

186. Khera KS. Maternal toxicity of drugs and metabolic disorders—a possible etiologic factor in the interuterine death and congenital malformation: a critique on human data. *CRC Crit Rev Toxicol.* 1987;17:345–375.

187. Zakzouk MS. The congenital warfarin syndrome. *J Laryngol Otol.* 1986;100:215–219.

188. Cotrufo M, deLuca TSL, Calabro R, et al. Coumarin anticoagulation during pregnancy in patients with mechanical vale prostheses. *Eur J Cardiothorac Surg.* 1991;5:300–305.

189. Stenflo J, Suttie JW. Vitamin K-dependent formation of gamma-carboxyglutamic acid. *Ann Rev Biochem.* 1977;46:157–172.

190. Barr M, Burdi AR. Warfarin-associated embryopathy in a 17-week abortus. *Teratology.* 1976;14:129–134.

191. Kaplan LC. Congenital Dandy Walker malformation associated with first trimester warfarin: a case report and literature review. *Teratology.* 1985;32:333–337.

192. Menger H, Lin AE, Toriello HV, et al. Vitamin K deficiency embryopathy: a phenocopy of the warfarin embryopathy due to a disorder of embryonic vitamin K metabolism. *Am J Med. Genet.* 1997;72:129–134.

193. Pauli RM, Lian JB, Mosher DF. Association of congenital deficiency of multiple vitamin K-dependent coagulation factors and the phenotype of the warfarin embryopathy: clues to the mechanism of coumarin derivatives. *Am J Hum Genet.* 1987;41:566–583.

194. Salazar E, Sajarias A, Gutierrez N, et al. The problem of cardiac valve prostheses, anticoagulants and pregnancy. *Circulation.* 1984;70:1169–1177.

195. Sheikhazadeh A, Ghabusi P, Hamim SH, et al. Congestive heart failure in valvular heart disease in pregnancies with and without valvular prostheses and anticoagulant therapy. *Clin Cardiol.* 1983;6:465–470.

196. Vitali E, Donatelli F, Quaini E, et al. Pregnancy in patients with mechanical prosthetic heart valves. *J Cardiovasc Surg.* 1986;27:221–227.

197. Kronic J, Phelps NE, McCallion DJ, et al. Effects of sodium warfarin administered during pregnancy in mice. *Am J Obstet Gynecol.* 1974;118:819–823.

198. Howe AM, Webster WS. Exposure of the pregnancy rat to warfarin and vitamin K1: an animal model of intraventricular hemorrhage in the fetus. *Teratology.* 1990;42:413–420.

199. Grote VW, Weinmann I. Examination of the active substances coumarin and rutin in a teratogenic trial with rabbits. *Arzneimittelforch.* 1973;23:1319–1320.

200. Howse AM, Webster WS. The warfarin embryopathy: a rat model showing maxillonasal hypoplasia and other skeletal disturbances. *Teratology.* 1992;46:379–390.

201. Enns GM, Roeder E, Chan RT, et al. Apparent cyclophosphamide (cytoxan) embryopathy: a distinct phenotype? *Ann J Med Gen.* 1999;86:237–241.

202. Chaube S, Kury G, Murphy ML. Teratogenic effects of cyclophosphamide (NSC-26271) in the rat. *Cancer Chemother Rep.* 1967;51:363–376.

203. Singh S. The teratogenicity of cyclophosphamide (Endoran-Asta) in rats. *Indian J Med Res.* 1971;59:1128–1135.

204. Gibson JE, Becker BA. The teratogenicity of cyclophosphamide in mice. *Cancer Res.* 1968;28:475–480.

205. Fritz H, Hess R. Effects of cyclophosphamide on embryonic development in the rabbit. *Agents Actions.* 1971;2:83–86.

206. Mirkes PE. Cyclophosphamide teratogenesis: A review. *Teratogen Carcinogen Mutagen.* 1985;5:75–88.

207. Greenberg LH, Tanaka KR. Congenital anomalies probably induced by cyclophosphamide. *J Am Med Assoc.* 1964;188:423–426.

208. Toledo TM, Harper RC, Moser RH. Fetal effects during cyclophosphamide and irradiation therapy. *Ann Intern Med.* 1971;74:87–91.

209. Blatt J, Mulvihill JJ, Ziegler JL, et al. Pregnancy outcome following cancer chemotherapy. *Am J Med.* 1980;69:828–832.

210. Hales BF. Effects of phosphoramide mustard and acrolein, cytotoxic metabolites of cyclophosphamide, on mouse limb development in vitro. *Teratology.* 1989;40:11–20.

211. Bongiovanni AM, DiGeorge AM, Grumbach MM. Masculinization of the female infant associated with estrogenic therapy alone during gestation: Four cases. *J Clin Endocrinol Metab.* 1959;19:1004–1011.

212. Herbst AL, Ulfelder H, Poskanzer DC. Adenocarcinoma of the vagina: Association of maternal stilbestrol therapy with tumor appearance in young women. *N Engl J Med.* 1971;284:878–881.

213. Herbst AL, Kurman RJ, Scully RE, et al. Clear-cell adenocarcinoma of the genital tract in young females. *N Engl J Med.* 1972;287:1259–1264.

214. Greenwald P, Barlow JJ, Nasca PC, et al. Vaginal cancer after maternal treatment with synthetic estrogens. *N Engl J Med.* 1971;285:390–392.

215. Herbst AL, Poskanzer DC, Robboy SJ, et al. Prenatal exposure to stilbestrol: A prospective comparison of exposed female offspring with unexposed controls. *N Engl J Med.* 1975;292:334–339.

216. Herbst AL, Scully RE, Robboy SJ. Effects of maternal DES ingestion on the female genital tract. *Hosp Pract.* 1975;10:51–57.

217. Ulfelder H. DES-transplacental teratogen and possibly also carcinogen. *Teratology.* 1976;13:101–104.

218. O'Brien PC, Noller KL, Robboy SJ, et al. Vaginal epithelial changes in young women enrolled in the National Cooperation Diethylstilbestrol Adenosis (DESAD) project. *Obstet Gynecol.* 1979;53:300–308.

219. Barnes AB, Colton T, Gundersen J, et al. Fertility and outcome of pregnancy in women exposed in utero to diethylstilbestrol. *N Engl J Med.* 1980;302:609–613.

220. Berger MJ, Goldstein DP. Impaired reproductive performance in DES-exposed women. *Obstet Gynecol.* 1980;55:25–27.

221. Veridiano NP, Delk I, Rogers J, et al. Reproductive performance of DES exposed female progeny. *Obstet Gynecol.* 1981;58:58–61.

222. deHass I, Harlow BL, Cramer DW, et al. Spontaneous preterm birth: a case-control study. *Am J Obstet Gynecol.* 1991;165:1290–1296.

223. Herbst AL, Hubby MM, Azizl F, et al. Reproductive and gynecologic surgical experience in diethylstilbestrol exposed daughter. *Am J Obstet Gynecol.* 1981;141:1019.

224. Herbst AL, Hubby MM, Blough RR, et al. A comparison of pregnancy experience in DES-exposed and DES-unexposed daughters. *J Reprod Med.* 1980;24:62–69.

225. Linn S, Liberman E, Schoenbaum SC, et al. Adverse outcome of pregnancy in women exposed to diethylstilbestrol in utero. *J Reprod Med.* 1988;33:3–7.

226. Sanberg EC, Riffle NL, Higdon JV, et al. Pregnancy outcome in women exposed to diethylstilbestrol in utero. *Am J Obstet Gynecol.* 1981;110:194–205.

227. Bibbo M. Transplacental effects of diethylstilbestrol. in Grundman, E (ed.): Perinatal Pathology. New York, Springer-Verlag, 1979: p 191–211.

228. Gill WB, Schumacher GFB, Bibbo M, et al. Association of diethylstilbestrol exposure in utero with cryptorchidism, testicular hypoplasia and semen abnormalities. *J Urol.* 1979;122:36–39.

229. Shy KK, Stenchever MA, Karp LE, et al. Genital tract examinations and zona-free hamster egg penetration tests from men exposed in utero to diethylstilbestrol. *Fert Steril.* 1984;42:772–778.

230. Gill WB, Schumacher GFB, Bibbo M. Structural and functional abnormalities in the sex organs of male offspring of mothers treated with diethylstilbestrol (DES). *J Reprod Med.* 1976;16:147–153.

231. Leary FJ, Resseguie LJ, Kurland LT, et al. Males exposed to diethylstilbestrol. *J Am Med Assoc.* 1984;252:2984–2989.

232. Vessey MP. Epidemiological studies of the effects of diethylstilbestrol. *Int Agency Res Canc Sci Publ.* 1989;96:335–348.

233. Miller RW, Heckman ME, McKenzie RC. Diethylstilbestrol: Placental transfer, metabolism, covalent binding and fetal distribution in the Wistar rat. *J Pharmacol Exp Ther.* 1982;220:358–365.

234. McLaughlin JA. Prenatal exposure to diethylstilbestrol in mice: toxicological studies. *J Toxicol Environ Health.* 1977;2:527–537.

235. Newbold RR, Bullock BC, McLachlan JA. Exposure of diethylstilbestrol during pregnancy permanently alters the ovary and oviduct. *Biol Reprod.* 1983;28:735–744.

236. Hendrickx AG, Benirschke K, Thompson RS, et al. The effects of prenatal diethylstilbestrol (DES) exposure on the genitalia of pubertal Macaca mulatta. I. Female offspring. *J Reprod Med.* 1979;22:233–240.

237. Hendrickx AG, Prahalada S, Binkerd PE. Long-term evaluation of the diethylstilbestrol (DES) syndrome in adult female rhesus monkeys (Macaca mulatta). *Reprod Toxicol.* 1988;1:253–261.

238. Johnson LD, Palmer AE, King NW, et al. Vaginal adenosis in Cebus apella monkeys exposed to DES in utero. *Obstet Gynecol.* 1981;57:629–635.

239. Thompson RS, Hess DL, Binkerd PE, et al. The effects of prenatal diethylstilbestrol exposure on the genitalia of pubertal Macaca mulatta. II. Male offspring. *J Reprod Med.* 1981;26:309–316.

240. Madl R, Metzler M. Oxidative metabolites of diethylstilbestrol in the fetal Syrian golden hamster. *Teratology.* 1984;30:351–357.

241. Metzler M. The metabolism of diethylstilbestrol. *CRC Crit Rev Biochem.* 1981;10:171–212.

242. Speidel BD, Meadow SR. Maternal epilepsy and abnormalities of the fetus and newborn. *Lancet.* 1972;2:839–843.

243. Frederick J. Epilepsy and pregnancy: a report from Oxford record linkage study. *Br Med J.* 1973;2:442–448.

244. Monson RR, Rosenberg L, Hartz SC, et al. Diphenylhydantoin and selected malformations. *N Engl J Med.* 1973;289:1049.

245. Albengres E, Tillement JP. Phenytoin in pregnancy: a review of the reported risks. *Biol Res Pregnancy Perinatol.* 1983;4:71–74.

246. Hill RM, Verland WM, Horning MG, et al. Infants exposed in utero to antiepileptic drugs. *Am J Dis Child.* 1974;127:645–653.

247. Hanson JW, Myrianthopoulos NC, Harvey, MAS, et al. Risks to the offspring of women treated with hydantoin anticonvulsants, with emphasis on the fetal hydantoin syndrome. *J Pediatr.* 1976;89:662–668.

248. Hanson JW. Teratogen Update: Fetal hydantoin effects. *Teratology.* 1986;33:349–353.

249. McClain RM, Langhoff L. Teratogenicity of diphenylhydantoin in the New Zealand White rabbit. *Teratology.* 1980;21:371–379.

250. Collins MD, Fradkin R, Scott WI. Induction of postaxial forelimb ectrodactyly with anticonvulsant agents in A/J mice. *Teratology.* 1990;41:61–70.

251. Finnell RH, Abbott LC, Taylor SM. The fetal hydantoin syndrome: answers from a mouse model. *Reprod Toxicol.* 1989;3:127–133.

252. Elshave J. Cleft palate in the offspring of female mice treated with phenytoin. *Lancet.* 1969;2:1074.

253. Harbinson RD, Becker BA. Relation of dosage and time of administration of diphenylhydantoin to its teratogenic effect in mice. *Teratology.* 1969;2:305–312.

254. Rowland JF, Binkerd PE, Hendrickx AG. Developmental toxicity and pharmacokinetics of oral and intravenous phenytoin in the rat. *Reprod Toxicol.* 1990;4:191–202.

255. Zengel AE, Keith DA, Tassinari MS. Prenatal exposure to phenyltoin and its effect on postnatal growth and craniofacial proportion in the rat. *J Craniofac Genet Dev Biol.* 1989;9:147–160.

256. Finnell RH. Phenytoin-induced teratogenesis: a mouse model. *Science.* 1981;211:483–484.

257. Lewis WH, Suris OR. Treatment with lithium carbonate: results in 35 cases. *Tex Med.* 1970;66:58–63.

258. Vacaflor L, Lehmann HE, Ban TA. Side effects and teratogenicity of lithium carbonate treatment. *J Clin Pharmacol.* 1970;10:387–389.

259. Frankenberg RR, Lipinski JF. Congenital malformations. *N Engl J Med.* 1983;309:311–312.

260. Warkany J. Teratogen Update: lithium. *Teratology.* 1988;38:593–596.

261. Rane A, Tomson G, Bjarke B. Effects of maternal lithium therapy in a newborn infant. *J Pediatr.* 1974;93:296–297.

262. Cohen LS, Friedman JM, Jefferson JW, et al. A reevaluation of risk of in utero exposure to lithium. *J Am Med Assoc.* 1994;271:146–150.

263. Jacobson SJ, Jones K, Johnson K, et al. Prospective multicentre study of pregnancy outcome after lithium exposure during first trimester. *Lancet.* 1992;339:530–533.

264. Troyer WA, Pereira G, Lannon RA, et al. Association of maternal lithium exposure and premature delivery. *J Perinatol.* 1993;13:123–127.

265. Schou M. What happened later to the lithium babies? A follow-up study of children born without malformations. *Acta Psychiatr Scand.* 1976;54:193–197.

266. Krause S, Ebbsen F, Lange AP. Polyhydramnios with maternal lithium treatment. *Obstet & Gynecol.* 1990;75:504–506.

267. Lam SS, Kjellstrand C. Emergency treatment of lithium-induced diabetes insipidus with non-steroidal anti-inflammatory drugs. *Renal Failure.* 1997;19:183–188.

268. Holtzman EJ, Ausiello DA. Nephrogenic diabetes insipidus: causes revealed. *Hospital Practice.* 1994;29:89–93, 97–98, 103–104.

269. Nars PW, Girad J. Lithium carbonate intake during pregnancy leading to a large goiter in a premature infant. *Am J Dis Child.* 1977;131:123–127.

270. Wilson N, Forfar JD, Godman MJ. Atrial flutter in the newborn resulting from lithium ingestion. *Arch Dis Child.* 1983;58:538–539.

271. Morrell P, Sutherland GR, Buamah PK, et al. Lithium toxicity in the neonate. *Arch Dis Child.* 1983;58:539–541.

272. Filtenborg JA. Persistent pulmonary hypertension after lithium intoxication in the newborn. *Eur J Pediatr.* 1982;138:321–323.

273. Klug S, Collins M, Nagao T, et al. Effect of lithium on rat embryos in culture: Growth, development, compartmental distribution and lack of protective effect of inositol. *Arch Toxicol.* 1992;66:719–728.

274. Hansen DK, Walker RC, Grafton TF. Effect of lithium carbonate on mouse and rat embryos in vitro. *Teratology.* 1990;41:155–160.

275. Weinstein MR, Goldfield M. Cardiovascular malformations with lithium use during pregnancy. *Am J Psych.* 1975;132:529–531.

276. Jurand A. Teratogenic activity of lithium carbonate: an experimental update. *Teratology.* 1988;38:101–111.

277. Llewellyn A, Stowe ZN, Strader JR. The use of lithium and management of women with bipolar disorder during pregnancy and lactation. *J Clin Psychiatry.* 1998;59:57–64.

278. Dolk H. Methylene blue and atresia or stenosis of ileum and jejunum. *Lancet.* 1991;338:1021–1022.

279. Cowett RM, Hakanson DO, Kocon RW, et al. Untoward neonatal effect of intra-amniotic administration of methylene blue. *Obstet Gynecol.* 1976;48:745–755.

280. Crooks J. Haemolytic jaundice in a neonate after intra-amniotic injection of methylene blue. *Arch Dis Child.* 1982;57:872–886.

281. Serota FT, Bernbaum JC, Schwartz E. The methylene blue baby. *Lancet.* 1979;2:1142–1143.

282. Cragan JD. Teratogen Update: Methylene blue. *Teratology.* 1999;60:42–48.

283. Cragan JD, Martin ML, Waters GD, et al. Increased risk of small intestinal atresia among twins in the United States. *Arch Pediatr Adolesc Med.* 1994;148:733–739.

284. van der Pol JG, Wolf H, Boer K, et al. Jejunal atresia related to the use of methylene blue in genetic amniocentesis in twins. *Br J Obstet Gynecol.* 1992;99:141–143.

285. Moorman-Voestermans CGM, Heig HA, Vos A. Jejunal atresia in twins. *J Pediatr. Surg.* 1990;25:638–639.

286. Nicolini U, Monni G. Intestinal obstruction in babies exposed in utero to methylene blue. *Lancet.* 1990;336:1258–1259.

287. Cragen JD, Martin L, Khoury MJ, et al. Dye use during amniocentesis and birth defects (letter). *Lancet.* 1993;341:1352–1353.

288. Gluer S. Intestinal atresia following intra-amniotic use of dyes. *Eur J Pediatr. Surg.* 1995;5:240–242.

289. Moorman-Voestermans CGM, Heij HA, Vos A. Letter to the Editor. *J Pediatr. Surg.* 1992;27:133.

290. Kidd SA, Lancaster PA, Anderson JC, et al. Fetal death after exposure to methylene blue dye during mid-trimester amniocentesis. *Prenatal Diagnosis.* 1996;16:39–47.

291. Kidd SA, Lancaster PA, Anderson JC, et al. A cohort study of pregnancy outcome after amniocentesis in twin pregnancy. *Pediatric and Perinatal Epidemiology.* 1997;11:200–213.

292. Piersma AH, Verhoet A, DeLiefde A, et al. Embryotoxicity of methylene blue in the rat. *Teratology.* 1991;43:458–459.

293. Rabe T, Basse H, Thuro H, et al. Wirkung des PGE1-methylanalogens misoprostol auf den schwangeren uterus im erstentrimester. *Geburtsch Frauenheilk.* 1987;47:324–331.

294. Gonzalez CH, Vargas FR, Perez ABA, et al. Limb deficiency with or without Moebius sequence in seven Brazilian children associated with misoprotol use in the first trimester of pregnancy. *Am J Med. Genet.* 1993;46:59–64.

295. Coelho HLL, Misago C, Fonsecam WVC, et al. Selling abortifacients over the counter in pharmacies in Fortaleza, Brazil. *Lancet.* 1991;338:247.

296. Costa SH, Vessey MP. Misoprostol and illegal abortion in Rio de Janeiro, Brazil. *Lancet.* 1993;341:1258–1261.

297. Luna-Coelho HL, Teixeria AC, Santos AP, et al. Misoprostol and illegal abortion in Fortaleza, Brazil. *Lancet.* 1993;341:1261–1263.

298. Marks TA, Morris DF, Weeks JR. Developmental toxicity of alprostadil in rats after subcutaneous administration or intravenous infusion. *Toxicol Appl Pharmacol.* 1987;91:341–357.

299. Firth HV, Boyd PA, Chamberlain P, et al. Severe limb abnormalities after chorionic villus sampling at 56–66 days gestation. *Lancet.* 1991;337:762–763.

300. Collins FS, Mahoney MJ. Hydrocephalus and abnormal digits after failed first trimester prostaglandin abortion attempt. *J Pediatr.* 1983;102:620–621.

301. Schuler LS, Ashto PW, Sanseverino MT. Teratogenicity of misoprostol. *Lancet.* 1992;339:437.

302. Woods JR, Plessinger MA, Clark KE. Effect on cocaine on uterine blood flow and fetal oxygenation. *J Am Med Assoc.* 1987;257:957–961.

303. Schonhofer PS. Brazil: Misuse of misoprostol as a abortifacient may induce malformations. *Lancet.* 1991;337:1534.

304. Fonseca W, Alencar AJC, Mota FSB, et al. Misoprostol and congenital malformations. *Lancet.* 1991;336:56.

305. Brent RL: Congenital malformation case reports: The editor's and reviewer's dilemma. *Am J Med Gen.* 1993;47:872–874.

306. Midha KK, Buttar HS, Rowe M, et al. Metabolism and disposition of trimethadione in pregnant rats. *Epilepsia.* 1979;20:417–423.

307. Zackai EH, Melmen WJ, Neiderer B, et al. The fetal trimethadione syndrome. *J Pediatr.* 1975;87:280–284.

308. German J, Kowal A, Ehlers KH. Trimethadione and human teratogenesis. *Teratology.* 1970;3:349–362.

309. Feldman GL, Weaver DD, Lovrien EW. The fetal trimethadione syndrome. *Am J Dis Child.* 1977;131:1389–1392.

310. Goldman AS, Yaffe SJ. Fetal trimethadione syndrome. *Teratology.* 1978;17:103.

311. Brown NA, Schull G, Fabro S. Assessment of the teratogenic potential of trimethadione in the CD-1 mouse. *Toxicol Appl Pharmacol.* 1979;51:59–71.

312. Mjolnerod OK, Rasmussen K, Dommerud SA, et al. Congenital connective-tissue defect probably due to D-penicillamine treatment in pregnancy. *Lancet.* 1971;1:673–675.

313. Endres W. D-penicillamine in pregnancy—to ban or not to ban. *Klin Worchenschr.* 1981;59:535–538.

314. Steffek AJ, Verrusio AC, Watkins CA. Cleft palate in rodents after maternal treatment with various lathrogenic agents. *Teratology.* 1972;5:33–40.

315. Mark-Savage P, Keen CL, Lonnerdal B, et al. Teratogenicity of D-penicillamine in rats. *Teratology.* 1981;23:50A.

316. Keen CL, Mark-Savage P, Lonnerdal B, et al. Teratogenesis and low copper status resulting from D-penicillamine in rats. *Teratology.* 1982;26:163–165.

317. Janerich DT, Piper JM, Glebatis DM. Oral contraceptives and congenital limb reduction defects. *N Engl J Med.* 1974;291:697–700.

318. Janerich DT, Dugan JM, Standfast SJ, et al. Congenital heart disease and prenatal exposure to exogenus sex hormones. *Br Med J*. 1977;1:1058–1060.

319. Fotherby K. A new look at progestins. *Clin Obstet Gynecol*. 1984;11:701–722.

320. Wilkins L, Jones HW, Holman GH, et al. Masculinization of the female fetus associated with administration of oral and intramuscular progestins during gestation: nonadrenal female pseudo-hermaphrodism. *J Clin Endocrinol Metab*. 1958;18:559–585.

321. Wilkins L. Masculinization due to orally given progestins. *J Am Med Assoc*. 1960;172:1028–1032.

322. Grumbach MM, Ducharine JR, Moloshok RE. On the fetal masculinizing action of certain oral progestins. *J Clin Endocrinol Metab*. 1959;19:1369–1380.

323. Van Wyk J, Grumbach MM. Disorders of sex differentiation. In Williams RH, ed. *Textbook of Endocrinology*. Philadelphia: W. B. Saunders, 1968: 537–612.

324. World Health Organization. *The effect of female sex hormones on fetal development and infant health*. Geneva: Author; 1981.

325. Wiseman RA, Dodds-Smith IC. Cardiovascular birth defects and antenatal exposure to female sex hormones: A reevaluation of some base data. *Teratology*. 1984;30:359–370.

326. Ferencz C, Matanoski GM, Wilson PD, et al. Maternal hormone therapy and congenital heart disease. *Teratology*. 1980;21:225–239.

327. Gal I, Kirman B, Stern J. Hormonal pregnancy tests and congenital malformations. *Nature*. 1967;216:83.

328. Gal I. Risks and benefits of the use of hormonal pregnancy test tablets. *Nature*. 1972;240:241–242.

329. Laurence M, Miller M, Vowles M, et al. Hormonal pregnancy tests and neural tube malformations. *Nature*. 1971;233:495–496.

330. Laurence KM, James N, Miller MH, et al. Double-blind randomized controlled trial of folate treatment before conception to prevent recurrence of neural tube defects. *Br Med J*. 1981;282:1509–1511.

331. Laurence KM. Reply to Gal. *Nature*. 1972;240:242.

332. Sever LE. Hormonal pregnancy tests and spina bifida. *Nature*. 1973;242:410–411.

333. Briggs MH, Briggs M. Sex hormone exposure during pregnancy and malformations. In Briggs MH and Corbin A, ed. *Advances in Steroid Biochemistry and Pharmacology*. London: Academic Press, 1979: 51–89.

334. Wilson JG, Brent RL. Are female sex hormones teratogenic? *Am J Obstet Gynecol*. 1981;114:567–580.

335. Wiseman RA. Negative correlation between sex hormone usage and malformations. In Maurois M, ed. *Prevention of Physical and Mental Congenital Defects Part C Basic and Medical Science, Education and Future Strategies*. New York: Alan R. Liss; 1985: 171–175.

336. Rock JA, Wentz AC, Cole KA, et al. Fetal malformations following progesterone therapy during pregnancy: a preliminary report. *Fertil Steril*. 1985;44:17–19.

337. Katz K, Lancet M, Skornick J, et al. Teratogenicity of progestagens given during the first trimester of pregnancy. *Obstet Gynecol*. 1985;65:775–780.

338. Yovich JL, Turner SR, Draper R. Medroxyprogesterone acetate therapy in early pregnancy has no apparent fetal effects. *Teratology*. 1988;38:135–144.

339. Brent RL. Editorial Comment: Kudos to the Food and Drug Administration: reversal of the package insert warning for birth defects for oral contraceptives. *Teratology*. 1989;39:93.

340. King RJB, Mainwaring WP, eds. *Steroid-Cell Interactions*, Vol. 1. Baltimore: University Park Press; 1974.

341. FDA. 1999. Progestational Drug Products for Human Use; Requirements for Labeling Directed to the Patient. Federal Register, Vol. 64, No. 70, Proposed Rules, Department of Health and Human Services (HHS), Public Health Service (PHS), Food and Drug Administration (FDA), 21 CFR Part 310, [Docket No. 99N-0188], 64 FR 17985, Date: Tuesday, April 13, 1999.

342. Seegmiller RE, Nelson BW, Johnson CK. Evaluation of the teratogenic potential of Delalutin (17 alpha-hydroxyprogesterone caproate) in mice. *Teratology*. 1983;28:201–208.

343. Carbone JP, Figurska K, Buck S, et al. Effect of gestational sex steroid exposure on limb development and endochondral ossification in the pregnant C57B1/6J mouse: I. Medroxyprogesterone acetate. *Teratology*. 1990;42:121–130.

344. Carbone JP, Brent RL. Genital and nongenital teratogenesis of prenatal progestogen therapy: The effects of 17 alpha-hydroxyprogesterone caproate on embryonic and fetal development and endochondral ossification in the C57B1/6J mouse. *Am J Obstet Gynecol*. 1993;169:1292–1298.

345. Speert H, Quimby EH, Werner SC. Radioiodine uptake by the fetal mouse thyroid and resultant effects in later life. *Surg Gynecol Obstet*. 1951;93:230–242.

346. Book S, Goldman M. Thyroidal iodine exposure of the fetus. *Health Phys*. 1975;29:874.

347. Stoffer SS, Hamber JI. Inadvertent 131I therapy for hyperthyroidism in the first trimester of pregnancy. *J Nucl Med*. 1976;17:146–149.

348. Sikov MR, Noonan TR. Anomalous development induced in embryonic rat by the maternal administration of radiophosphorous. *Am J Anat*. 1958;103:137.

349. Brent RL. Radiation teratogenesis. *Teratology*. 1980;21:281–298.

350. Dekaban AS. Abnormalities in children exposed to x-radiation during various stages of gestation: tentative timetable of radiation half-lives of the drug in mother and baby. *J Pediatr*. 1968;94:832–835.

351. Goldstein L, Murphy DP. Microcephalic idiocy following radium therapy for uterine cancer during pregnancy. *Am J Obstet Gynecol*. 1929;18:189–195, 281–283.

352. Murphy DP, Goldstein L. Micromelia in a child irradiated in utero. *Surg Gynecol Obstet*. 1930;50:79–80.

353. Miller RW, Mulvihill JJ. Small head size after atomic irradiation. *Teratology*. 1976;14:355–358.

354. Miller RW. Delayed radiation effects in atomic bomb survivors. *Science*. 1969;166:569–574.

355. Wood JW, Johnson KG, Omori Y, et al. Mental retardation in children exposed in utero to the atomic bombs in Hiroshima and Nagasaki. *Am J Public Health*. 1967;57:1381.

356. Wood JW, Johnson KG, Omori Y. In utero exposure to the Hiroshima atomic bomb. An evaluation of head size and mental retardation: Twenty years later. *Pediatrics*. 1967;39:385–392.

357. Russell LB. X-ray induced developmental abnormalities in the mouse and their use in the analysis of embryological patterns. I. External and gross visceral changes. *J Exp Zool*. 1950;114:545–602.

358. Russell LB, Russell WL. The effects of radiation on the preimplantation stages of the mouse embryo. *Anat Res*. 1950;108:521.

359. Brent RL, Bolden BT. The indirect effect of irradiation on embryonic development. IV. The lethal effects of maternal irradiation on the first day of gestation in the rat. *Proc Soc Exp Biol Med*. 1967;125:709–712.

360. Russell LB. X-ray induced developmental abnormalities in the mouse and their use in the analysis of embryonical patterns. II. Abnormalities of the vertebral column and thorax. *J Exp Zool*. 1956;131:329–395.

361. Russell LB, Russell WL. An analysis of the changing radiation response of the developing mouse embryo. *J Cell Comp Physiol*. 1954;43:103–149.

362. Brent RL, Bolden BT. The indirect effect of irradiation on embryonic development. III. The contribution of ovarian irradiation, uterine irradiation, oviduct irradiation, and zygote irradiation of fetal mortality and growth retardation in the rat. *Radiat Res*. 1967;30:759–773.

363. Jensh RP, Brent RL. Effects of prenatal X-irradiation on postnatal testicular development and function in the Wistar rat: Developmental/*Teratology*./behavioral/radiation. *Teratology*. 1988;39:443–449.

364. Jensh RP, Brent RL. Effects of prenatal x-irradiation on the 14th–18th days of gestation on postnatal growth and development in the rat. *Teratology.* 1988;38:431–441.

365. Ferrer I, Xumetra A, Santamaria J. Cerebral malformation induced by prenatal x-irradiation: An autoradiographic and Golgi study. *J Anat.* 1984;138:81–93.

366. Bernhardt IB, Dorsey DJ. Hypervitaminosis A and congenital renal anomalies in a human infant. *Obstet Gynecol.* 1974;43:750–755.

367. Fantel AG, Shepard TH, Newell-Morris LL, et al. Teratogenic effects of retinoic acid in pigtail monkeys (macaca nemistrinal). *Teratology.* 1977;15:65–72.

368. Mounoud RL, Klein D, Weber F. A propos d'un cas de syndrome de Goldenhar intoxication aigue a la vitamin A chez la mere pendent la grossesse. *J Genet Hum.* 1975;23:135–154.

369. Zilva SS, Golding J, Drummond JC, et al. The relation of the fat-soluble factor to rickets and growth in pigs. *Biochem J.* 1921;15:427–437.

370. Hale F. Pigs born without eyeballs. *J Hered.* 1933;24:105–106.

371. Hale F. Relation of vitamin A to anophthalmos in pigs. *Am J Ophthalmol.* 1935;18:1087–1093.

372. Hale R. Relation of maternal vitamin A deficiency to microphthalmia in pigs. *Tex State J Med.* 1937;33:228–232.

373. Rosa FW. Teratogen Update: Penicillamine. *Teratology.* 1986;33:127–131.

374. Lammer EJ. Developmental toxicity of synthetic retinoids in humans. *Prog Clin Biol Res.* 1988;281:193–202.

375. Teratology Society. Teratology Society position paper: recommendation for vitamin A use during pregnancy. *Teratology.* 1987;35:269–275.

376. Thaller C, Eichele G. Identification and spatial distribution of retinoids in developing chick limb bud. *Nature.* 1987;327:625.

377. Kay ED. Cranofacial dysmorphogenesis following hypervitaminosis A in mice. *Teratology.* 1987;35:105–117.

378. Sulik KK, Johnston MC, Dehart DB. Potlentiation of programmed cell death by 13-cis-retinoic acid: A common mechanism for early craniofacial and limb malformation? *Teratology.* 1987;35:32A.

379. Yasuda Y, Konishi H, Kihara T, et al. Developmental anomalies induced by all-trans-retinoic acid in fetal mice.: II. Induction of abnormal neuroepithelium. *Teratology.* 1987;35:355–366.

380. Sulik KK, Dehart DB. Retinoic-acid-induced limb malformations resulting from apical ectodermal ridge cell death. *Teratology.* 1988;37:527–537.

381. Alles AJ, Sulik KK. Retinoic-acid-induced limb-reduction defects: perturbation of zones of programmed cell death as a pathogenetic mechanism. *Teratology.* 1989;40:163–171.

382. Hurley LS, Tuchmann-Duplessis H. Influence de la tetracycline sur la developpement pre-et post-natal du rat. *C R Acad Sci.* 1963;257:302–304.

383. Fillippi B. Antibiotics and congenital malformations: Evaluation of the teratogenicity of antibiotics. In Woolam DHM, ed. *Advances in Teratology.* New York: Academic Press; 1967:237–256.

384. Lenz W, Knapp K. Thalidomide embryopathy. *Arch Environ Health.* 1962;5:100–105.

385. Camera G, Pregliasco P. Ear malformation in baby born to mother using tretinoin cream. *Lancet.* 1992;339:687.

386. Lipson A, Collins FWW. Multiple congenital defects associated with maternal use of topical tretinoin. *Lancet.* 1993;341:22.

387. Selcen D, Seidman S, Nigro MA. Otocerebral anomalies associated with topical tretinoin use. *Brain and Development.* 2000;22:218–220.

388. Willhite CC, Sharma RP, Allen PV, et al. Percutaneous retinoid absorption and embryotoxicity. *J Inves Dermatol.* 1990;95:523–529.

389. Seegmiller RE, Ford WH, Carter MW, et al. A developmental toxicity study of tretinoin administered topically and orally to pregnant Wistar rats. *Journal of the American Academy Dermatology.* 1997;36:S60–S66.

390. Christian MS, Mitala JJ, Powers WJ Jr, et al. A developmental toxicity study of tretinoin emollient cream (Renova) applied topically to New Zealand white rabbits. *Journal of American Academy of Dermatology.* 1997;36:S67–S76.

391. Johnson EM. A risk assessment of topical tretinoin as a potential human developmental toxin based on animal and comparative human data. *Journal of the American Academy of Dermatology.* 1997;36:S86–S90.

392. Shapiro L, Patzuzak A, Curto G, et al. Safety of first trimester exposure to topical tretinoin: a prospective cohort study. *Lancet.* 1997;350:1143–1144.

393. DeWals P, Bloch D, Calabro A, et al. Association between holoprosencephaly and exposure to topical retinoids: Results of the EUROCAT survey. *Neonatal Perinatal Epidemiol.* 1991;5:445–447.

394. Jick SS, Terris BZ, Jick H. First trimester topical tretinoin and congenital disorders. *Lancet.* 1993;341:1181–1182.

395. Seegmiller RE, Carter MW, Ford WH, et al. Induction of maternal toxicity in the rat by dermal application of retinoic acid and its effect on fetal outcome. *Reprod Toxicol.* 1990;4:277–281.

396. Clewell HJ III, Anderson ME, Wills RJ, et al. A physiologically based pharmacokinetic model for retinoic acid and its metabolites. *Journal of the American Academy of Dermatology.* 1997;36:S77–S85.

397. Latriano L, Tzima G, Wong F, et al. The percutaneous absorption of topically applied tretinoin and its effect on endogenous concentrations of tretinoin and its metabolites after a single dose or long term use. *Journal of the American Academy of Dermatology.* 1997;36:S37–S46.

398. van Hoogdalem EJ. Transdermal absorption of topical anti-acne agents in man; review of clinical pharmacokinetic data. *Journal of the European Academy of Dermatology and Venereology.* 1998;11:S9-S13.

399. Nau H. Embryotoxicity and teratogenicity of topical retinoic acid. *Skin Pharmacology.* 1993;6:35–44.

400. Kochhar DM, Christian MS. Tretinoin: a review of the nonclinical developmental toxicology experience. *Journal of the American Academy of Dermatology.* 1997;36:S47–S59.

401. Donald PR, Sellars SL. Streptomycin ototoxicity in the unborn child. *S Afr Med J.* 1981;60:316–318.

402. Ericson-Strandvik B, Gyllensten L. The central nervous system of foetal mice after administration of streptomycin. *Acta Pathol Microbiol Scand.* 1963;59:292–300.

403. Nomura T, Kimura S, Kanzaki T, et al. Induction of tumors and malformations in mice after prenatal treatment with some antibiotic drugs. *Med J Osaka Univ.* 1984;35:13–17.

404. Jones KL, Smith DW. Recognition of the fetal alcohol syndrome in early infancy. *Lancet.* 1973;2:99.

405. Nishimura H, Tanimura T, eds. *Clinical Aspects of the Teratogenicity of Drugs.* New York: American Elsevier, Excerpta Medica; 1976.

406. Weisblum B, Davies J. Antibiotic inhibitors of the bacterial ribosome. *Bacteriol Rev.* 1968;32:493–528.

407. Bevelander G, Cohlan SW. The effect of the rat fetus of transplacentally acquired tetracycline. *Biol Neonate.* 1962;4:365–370.

408. Baden E. Environmental pathology of the teeth. In Gorlin RJ and Goldman HM, ed. *Thomas' Oral Pathology.* St. Louis: Mosby; 1970:189–191.

409. Cohlan SQ, Bevelander G, Tiamsic T. Growth inhibition of prematures receiving tetracycline: clinical and laboratory investigation. *Am J Dis Child.* 1963;105:453–461.

410. Lenz W. Thalidomide embryopathy in Germany, 1959–1961. In Maurois M, ed. *Prevention of Physical and Mental Congenital Defects, Part C Basic and Medical Science, Education, and Future Strategies.* New York: Alan R. Liss; 1985:77–83.

411. Lenz W. A short history of thalidomide embryopathy. *Teratology.* 1988;38:203–215.

412. Brent RL, Holmes LB. Clinical and basic science lessons from the thalidomide tragedy: what have we learned about the causes of limb defects? *Teratology.* 1988;38:241–251.

413. Kida M. *Thalidomide Embryopathy in Japan.* Tokyo, Japan: Kodnasha; 1987.

414. Ruffing L. Evaluation of thalidomide children. *Birth Defects.* 1977;13:287–300.

415. Smithells RW. Defects and disabilities of thalidomide children. *Br Med J.* 1973;1:269–272.

416. Knapp K, Lenz W, Nowack E. Multiple congenital abnormalities. *Lancet.* 1962;2:725.

417. Cutler J. Thalidomide revisited. *Lancet.* 1994;343:795–796.

418. Gollop TR, Eigier A, Guiduglio-Nto J. Prenatal diagnosis of thalidomide syndrome. *Prenat Diagn.* 1987;7:295–298.

419. Jones GRN. Thalidomide: 35 years on and still deforming. *Lancet.* 1994;343:1041.

420. McCredie J. Sclerotome subtraction: A radiologic interpretation of reduction deformities of the limbs. In Bergsman D and Lowry RB, ed. *Birth Defects: Original Article Series.* New York: Alan R. Liss; 1977: 65–77.

421. Stephens TD, McNulty TR. Evidence for a metameric pattern in the development of the chick humerus. *J Emb Exp Morph.* 1981;61:191–205.

422. Strecker TR, Stephen TD. Peripheral nerves do not play a trophic role in limb skeletal morphogenesis. *Teratology.* 1983;27:159–167.

423. Lash JW, Saxen L. Human teratogenesis: In vitro studies on thalidomide-inhibited chondrogenesis. *Develop Biol.* 1972;28:61–70.

424. Lash JW. Studies on the ability of embryonic mesonephros explants to form cartilage. *Develop Biol.* 1963;6:219–232.

425. Lash JW. Normal embryology and teratogenesis. *Am J Obstet Gynecol.* 1964;90:1193–1207.

426. Stephens TD. Proposed mechanisms of action in thalidomide embryopathy. *Teratology.* 1988;38:229–239.

427. Miller MT, Stromland K. Teratogen Update: thalidomide: a review, with focus on ocular findings and new potential uses. *Teratology.* 1999;60:306–321.

428. Warkany J. Teratogen Update: iodine deficiency. *Teratology.* 1985;31:309–311.

429. Martin MM, Rento RD. Iodide goiter with hypothyroidism in two newborn infants. *J Pediatr.* 1962;61:94–99.

430. Carswell F, Kerr MM, Hutchinson JH. Congenital goiter and hypothyroidism produced by maternal ingestion of iodides. *Lancet.* 1970;1:1241–1243.

431. Rodesch F, Camus M, Ermans AM, et al. Adverse effect of amniofetography on fetal thyroid function. *Am J Obstet Gynecol.* 1976; 126:723–726.

432. Cheron RG, Kaplan MM, Larsen PR, et al. Neonatal thyroid function after propylthiouracil therapy for maternal Graves disease. *N Engl J Med.* 1981;304:525–528.

433. Milham S Jr, Elledge W. Maternal methimazole and congenital defects in children. *Teratology.* 1972;5:125.

434. Mujtaba Q, Burrow GM. Treatment of hyperthyroidism in pregnancy with propylthiouracil and methimazole. *Obstet Gynecol.* 1975; 46:282–286.

435. Burrow GN. Neonatal goiter after maternal propylthiouracil therapy. *J Clin Endocrinol.* 1965;25:403–408.

436. McCarroll AM, McCarroll AM, Hutchinson M, et al. Long-term assessment of children exposed in utero to carbimazole. *Arch Dis Child.* 1976;51:532–536.

437. Whittle BA. Pre-clinical teratological studies on sodium valproate (Epilim) and other anticonvulsants. In Legg NJ, ed. *Clinical and Pharmacological Aspects of Sodium Valproate (Epilim) in the Treatment of Epilepsy.* Turnbridge Wells, UK: MCS Consultants; 1976: 105–110.

438. Kao J, Brown NA, Schmid B, et al. Teratogenicity of valproic acid: In vivo and in vitro investigations. *Teratogen Carcinogen Mutagen.* 1981;1:367–376.

439. Bruckner A, Lee YJ, O'Shea KS, et al. Teratogenic effects of valproic acid and diphenylhydantoin on mouse embryos in culture. *Teratology.* 1983;27:29–42.

440. Nau H, Spielmann H. Embryotoxicity testing of valproic acid. *Lancet.* 1983;1:763–764.

441. Loscher W, Nau H, Marescaux C, et al. Comparative evaluation of anticonvulsant and toxic potencies of valproic acid and 2-en-valproic acid in different animal models of epilepsy. *Eur J Pharmacol.* 1984;99:211–218.

442. Dalens B, Raynaud E-J, Gaulme J. Teratogenicity of valproic acid. *J Pediatr.* 1980;97:332–333.

443. Lindhout D, Omtzigt JGC, Cornel MC. Spectrum of neural tube defects in 34 infants prenatally exposed to antiepileptic drugs. *Neurology.* 1992;42:111–118.

444. Lindhout D, Meinardi H, Meijer JWA, et al. Antiepileptic drugs and teratogenesis in two consecutive cohorts: changes in prescription policy paralleled by changes in pattern of malformations. *Neurology.* 1992;42:94–110.

445. Robert E, Guibaud P. Maternal valproic acid and congenital neural tube defects. *Lancet.* 1982;2:1142.

446. Robert E. Valproic acid and spina bifida: a preliminary report. *France Morb Mortal Wkly Rep.* 1982;31:515–566.

447. Robert E, Rosa F. Valproate and birth defects. *Lancet.* 1983;2: 1142.

448. Dickinson RG, Hapland RC, Lynn RK, et al. Transmission of valproic acid across the placenta: Half-lives of the drug in mother and baby. *J Pediatr.* 1979;94:832–835.

449. Nau H, Zierer R, Spielmann H, et al. A new model for embryotoxicity testing: Teratogenicity and pharmacokinetics of valproic acid following constant-rate administration in the mouse using human therapeutic drug and metabolite concentrations. *Life Sci.* 1981;29: 2803–2814.

450. Hendrickx AG, Nau H, Binkerd P. Valproic acid developmental toxicity and pharmacokinetics in the rhesus monkey: an interspecies comparison. *Teratology.* 1988;38:329–345.

451. Mast TJ, Cukierski MA, Nau H, et al. Predicting the human teratogenic potential of the anticonvulsant, valproic acid from a nonhuman primate model. *Toxicology.* 1986;39:111–119.

452. Garcia RE, Friedman WF, Kaback MM, et al. Idiopathic hypercalcemia and supravalvular stenosis: documentation of a new syndrome. *N Engl J Med.* 1964;271:117–120.

453. Friedman WF. Vitamin D and the supravalvular aortic stenosis syndrome. In Woollam DHM (ed.): *Advances in Teratology.* New York, Academic Press, 1968:p 83–96.

454. Jones KL, Smith DW. The fetal alcohol syndrome. *Teratology.* 1975;12:1.

455. Jones KL, Smith DW, Streissguth AP, et al. Outcome in offspring of chronic alcoholic women. *Lancet.* 1974;1:1076–1078.

456. Graham JM Jr. The effects of alcohol consumption during pregnancy. In Marois M, ed. *Prevention of Physical and Mental Congenital Defect Part C Basic and Medical Science, Education and Future Strategies.* New York: Alan R. Liss; 1985:335–339.

457. Streissguth AP, Landesman-Dwyer C, Martin JC, et al. Teratogenic effect of alcohol in humans and laboratory animals. *Science.* 1980;209:353–361.

458. Slutsker L. Risk associated with cocaine use during pregnancy. *Obstet Gynecol.* 1992;79:778–779.

459. Phibbs CS, Bateman DA, Schwartz RM. The neonatal costs of maternal cocaine use. *J Am Med Assoc.* 1991;266:1521–1526.

460. Gingras JL, Weese-Mayer DE, Hume RF, et al. Cocaine and development: mechanisms of fetal toxicity and neonatal consequences of prenatal cocaine exposure. *Early Hum Dev.* 1992;31:1–24.

461. Young SL, Vosper HJ, Phillips SA. Cocaine: its effects on maternal and child health. *Pharmacotherapy.* 1992;12:2–17.

462. Gingras JL, O'Donnell KJ, Hume RF. Maternal cocaine addiction and fetal behavioral state: a human model for study of sudden infant death syndrome. *Med Hypoth.* 1990;33:227–230.

463. MacGregor SN, Keith LG, Chasnoff IJ, et al. Cocaine use during pregnancy: adverse perionatal outcome. *Am J Obstet Gynecol.* 1987;157:686–690.

464. Jones KL. Developmental pathogenesis of defects associated with prenatal cocaine exposure: fetal vascular disruption. *Clin Perinatol.* 1991;18:139–146.

465. Koren G, Graham K. Cocaine in pregnancy: analysis of fetal risk. *Vet Hum Toxicol.* 1992;34:263–264.

466. Chasnoff IJ, Griffith DR. Cocaine: clinical studies of pregnancy and the newborn. *Ann NY Acad Sci.* 1989;562:260–266.

467. Ritchie JM, Greene NM. Local anesthetics. In Tillman AG, et al., ed. *The Pharmacological Basis of Therapeutics.* New York: MacMillan Publishing; 1985:309.

468. Plessinger MA, Woods JR. Maternal placental, and fetal pathophysiology of cocaine exposure during pregnancy. *Clin Obstet Gynecol.* 1993;36:267–278.

469. Woods JR, Plessinger MA. Maternal-fetal cardiovascular system: a target of cocaine. *NIDA Res Monogr.* 1991;108:7–27.

470. Barnwell SL, Sastry BVR. Depression of amino acid uptake by human placental villus by cocaine, morphine and nicotine. *Trophoblast Res.* 1983;1:101–202.

471. Dicke JM, Verges DK, Polakoski KL. Cocaine inhibits alanine uptake by human placental microvillus membrane visicles. *Am J Obstet Gynecol.* 1993;169:515–521.

472. Dixon SD, Bejar R. Brain lesions in cocaine and methamphetamine exposed neonates. *Pediatr Res.* 1988;23:405A.

473. Dogra VS, Menon PA, Poblete J, et al. Neurosonographic imaging of small for gestational age neonates exposed and not exposed to cocaine and cytomegalovirus. *J Clin Ultrasound.* 1994;22:93–102.

474. El-Bizri H, Guest I, Varma R. Effects of cocaine on rat embryo development in vivo and in cultures. *Pediatr Res.* 1991;29:187–190.

475. Hoyme EH, Jones KL, Dixon SD. Prenatal cocaine exposure and prenatal vascular disruption. *Pediatrics.* 1990;85:743.

476. Webster WS, Brown-Woodman PDC, Lipson AH, et al. Fetal brain damage in the rat following prenatal exposure to cocaine. *Neurotoxicol Teratol.* 1991;13:621–626.

477. Chasnoff IJ, Chisum GM, Kaplan WE. Maternal cocaine use and genitourinary tract malformations. *Teratology.* 1988;37:201–204.

478. Chavez GF, Mulinare J, Cordero JF. Maternal cocaine use during early pregnancy as a risk factor for congenital urogenital anomalies. *J Am Med Assoc.* 1989;262:795–798.

479. Lezcano L, Antia DE, Sahdeve S, et al. Crossed renal ectopia associated with maternal alkaloid cocaine abuse: a case report. *J Perinatol.* 1994;14:230–233.

480. Viscarello RR, Ferguson DD, Nores J, et al. Limb-body wall complex associated with cocaine abuse: further evidence of cocaine's teratogenicity. *Obstet Gynecol.* 1992;80:523–526.

481. Lutiger BK, Graham K, Einarson TR, et al. Relationship between gestational cocaine use and pregnancy outcome: a meta analysis. *Teratology.* 1991;44:405–414.

482. Richardson GA, Day NL. Maternal and neonatal effects of moderate cocaine use during pregnancy. *Neurotoxicol Teratol.* 1991;13:455–460.

483. Bingol J, Fuchs M, Diaz V, et al. Teratogenicity of cocaine in humans. *J Pediatr.* 1987;10:93–97.

484. Webster WS, Brown-Woodman PDC. Cocaine as a cause of congenital malformations of vascular origin: experimental evidence in the rat. *Teratology.* 1990;41:689–697.

485. Finnell RH, Toloyan S, van Waes M, et al. Preliminary evidence for cocaine-induced embryopathy in mice. *Teratol Appl Pharmacol.* 1990;103:228–237.

486. Van Allen MI. Structural anomalies resulting from vascular disruption. *Pediatr Clin N Am.* 1992;39:255–277.

487. Zimmerman EF, Potturi RB, Resnick E, et al. Role of oxygen free radicals in cocaine-induced vascular disruption in mice. *Teratology.* 1994;49:192–201.

488. Fantel AG, Barber CV, Carda MB, et al. Studies on the role of ischemia/reperfusion and superoxide anion radical production in the teratogenicity of cocaine. *Teratology.* 1992;46:293–300.

489. Peters H, Theorell CJ. Fetal and neonatal effects of maternal cocaine use. *J Obstet Gynecol. Neonatal Nursing.* 1990;20:121–126.

490. Singer L, Arendt R, Minnes S. Neurodevelopmental effects of cocaine. *Clin Perinatol.* 1993;20:245–262.

491. Doberczak T, Shanzer S, Senie R, et al. Neonatal, neurologic, and electroencephalographic effects of intrauterine cocaine exposure. *J Pediatr.* 1988;113:354–358.

492. Gingras JL, Weese-Mayer DF, Dalley LB, et al. Prenatal cocaine exposure alters postnatal ornithine decarboxylase activity in rabbit brain. *Biochem Med Metab Biol.* 1993;50:284–291.

493. Singer LT, Yamashita TS, Hawkins C, et al. Increased incidence of intraventricular hemorrhage and development delay in cocaine-exposed, very low birth weight infants. *J Pediatr.* 1994;124:765–771.

494. Heyser CJ, McKinzie DL, Athalie F, et al. Effects of prenatal exposure to cocaine on heart rate and nonassociative learning and retention in infant rats. *Teratology.* 1994;49:470–478.

495. Simonik DK, Robinson SR, Smotherman WP. Cocaine alters behavior in the rat fetus. *Behav Neurosci.* 1993;107:867–875.

496. Spear LP, Kirstein CL, Bell J, et al. Effects of prenatal cocaine exposure on behavior during the early postnatal period. *Neurotoxicol Teratol.* 1989;11:57–63.

497. Tyrala EE, Mathews SV, Rao GS. Effect of intrauterine exposure to cocaine on acetylcholinesterase in primary cultures of fetal mouse brain cells. *Neurotoxicol Teratol.* 1992;14:229–233.

498. Henderson MG, McMillen B. Changes in dopamine, serotonin, and their metabolites in discrete brain areas of rat offspring after in utero exposure to cocaine or related drugs. *Teratology.* 1993;48:421–430.

499. Cabrera TM, Yracheta JM, Li Q, et al. Prenatal cocaine produced deficits in serotonin mediated neuroendocrine responses in adult rat progeny: evidence for long-term functional alterations in brain serotonin pathways. *Synapse.* 1993;15:158–168.

500. Seidler FJ, Slotkin TA. Fetal cocaine exposure causes persistent noradrenergic hyperactivity in rat brain regions: effects on neurotransmitter turnover and receptors. *J Pharmacol Exp Ther.* 1992;263:413–421.

501. Anderson-Brown T, Slotkin TA, Seidler FJ. Cocaine acutely inhibits DNA synthesis in developing rat brain regions: evidence for direct actions. *Brain Res.* 1990;537:197–202.

502. Garg UC, Turndorf H, Bansinath M. Effect of cocaine on macromolecular synthesis and cell proliferation in cultured glial cells. *Neuroscience.* 1993;57:467–472.

503. Seidler FJ, Slotkin TA. Prenatal cocaine and cell development in rat brain regions: effect on ornithine decarboxylase and macromolecules. *Brain Res Bull.* 1993;30:91–99.

504. Church MW, Overbeck GW. Sensorineural hearing loss as evidenced by the auditory brainstem response following prenatal cocaine exposure in the Long-Evans rat. *Teratology.* 1991;43:561–570.

505. Salamy A, Dark K, Salfi M, et al. Perinatal cocaine exposure and functional brain stem development in the rat. *Brain Res.* 1992;598:307–310.

506. Wiggins RC, Ruiz B. Development under the influence of cocaine. II. Comparison of the effects of maternal cocaine and associated undernutrition on brain myelin development in offspring. *Metab Brain Dis.* 1990;5:101–109.

507. Brent RL. The magnitude of the problem of congenital malformations. In: Marois M, ed. *Prevention of Physical and Mental Congenital Defect Part A Basic and Medical Science, Education and Future Strategies*. New York: Alan R. Liss; 1985:55–68.

508. Brent RL. Editorial: definition of a teratogen and the relationship of teratogenicity to carcinogenicity. *Teratology.* 1986;34:359–360.

509. Kline J, Stein Z, Susser M, et al. Environmental influences on early reproductive loss in a current New York City study. In Porter IM and Hook EM, ed. *Human Embryonic and Fetal Death*. New York: Academic Press; 1980:225.

510. TERIS. *Teratogenic Effects of Drugs: A Resource for Clinicians.* Baltimore: The Johns Hopkins University Press; 1994.

DRUGS

Pamela Lewis/Mitchell Dombrowski

The purpose of this chapter is to review the teratogenic risks of therapeutic drugs, a subject too complex for even a comprehensive text to cover in any depth. Because of length constraints, this chapter will be limited to a synopsis of only a few drugs. The Wayne State University Teratogen Rating System, which currently includes over 80 drugs and can be useful for clinical care, is also included.

Over the past several decades the physician's pharmacological armamentarium has increased geometrically. It is perhaps remarkable that there have not been other drug-teratogenic tragedies to rival that of thalidomide. With the possible exception of isotretinoin, no other widely used drug has approached thalidomide's teratogenic potential. Drugs with relatively little teratogenic potential, but which are widely ingested by pregnant women, now probably represent the greatest net risk.

It is virtually impossible to prove that a drug is not teratogenic. Conversely, it is very difficult to prove that a drug is teratogenic unless it is relatively potent. Major malformations are apparent at birth in about 3% of the general population and in about 4.5% by 5 years of age.[1] In a system that monitors 25,000 births per year, it would take up to 20 years to show a significant increase in the number of anomalies over background even with a relative risk of 20–25.[2] Weak teratogens, those with relative risk of 2–5 may never be identified. Detecting drug-induced subtle, minor malformations is even more difficult.

Because of these limitations, much of our knowledge has been based on case reports and retrospective studies. Both of these are biased to associate bad outcomes with specific events such as drug ingestion; this is technically termed ascertainment bias. For example, women who deliver malformed children are more likely to remember and report drugs they took as compared to controls. It is therefore likely that any widely used drug in pregnancy will be found to be "associated" with anomalies unless one is careful to compare the incidence of that specific anomaly to the expected incidence in the general population. This is especially difficult when analyzing the teratogenic potential of drugs which are used to treat patients who may have a baseline risk of anomalies which is greater than the general population, such as anticonvulsants and epileptics.

A number of factors influence the absolute risk a given drug has for inducing anomalies. These include its teratogenic potential, host susceptibility, dosage, synergism with other drugs and/or environmental factors, duration, timing in gestation, and the number of individuals exposed to the drug. The extent of exposure to potentially teratogenic drugs is remarkable. Piper et al. (1988) reported the use of prescribed drugs among 18,886 Michigan Medicaid recipients during pregnancy.[3] Of these, drug use per 1,000 gravid women included: tetracycline = 43.1; sulfonamides = 25.4; phenobarbital = 15.8; phenytoin = 2.6; warfarin = 0.4; valproate = 0.3; lithium = 0.3; diethylstilbestrol = 0.2; anticholinergics = 16.3. The use of nonprescription and illicit drugs would certainly be far more common than those in this partial list.

Because drug use is so common during pregnancy, one of the most frequently asked questions is "will the drug I took cause birth defects?". This is most often a difficult question to answer with the exception of a few drugs, either the known teratogens, or those with a long and broad clinical use with no known effects. However, parents are neither informed nor satisfied by being told that the risks are unknown. It is the health care provider's responsibility to provide an informed estimate of the risk for anomaly secondary to drug exposure during pregnancy.

The United States Food and Drug Administration (FDA) has developed a rating system which balances the potential risks and benefits of a drug during pregnancy (Table 10-1). This system was developed as an aid to guide therapeutic management during pregnancy based on potential risk versus benefits.

For its designed purpose, the FDA rating system is helpful. However, these categories are not necessarily appropriate for counseling a pregnant woman who is concerned about potential teratogenicity based on prior drug exposure. For example, oral contraceptives have a rating of "X," contraindicated in pregnancy, while trimethadione has a rating of "D," positive evidence of risk. However, there is no evidence of increased risk of fetal anomalies from inadvertent exposure early in pregnancy with oral contraceptives.[4] In contrast, trimethadione has been associated with a 60–80% risk of anomaly or spontaneous abortion.[5] The FDA ratings are accurate in that oral contraceptives should never be prescribed during pregnancy while there are indications for trimethadione use. Yet, they do not reflect the representative teratogenic risk for these 2 drugs, or for many others.

At our institution (Hutzel Hospital, Department of Maternal Fetal Medicine), we counsel several thousand parents per year about their risks for birth defects. To facilitate counseling, we have developed a system which rates a drug's probable potential for inducing human teratogenicity at "typical" therapeutic doses during the first trimester (Tables 10-2 and 10-3). The Wayne State University Teratogen Rating System ranks a drug's probable risk in 1 of 5 categories: "0-Nominal," "1-Minimal," "2-Small," "3-Moderate," and "4-Potent." These compiled estimations of teratogenic risks were developed with extensive review of the literature. Frequently consulted references include Drugs in Pregnancy and Lactation: A Reference to Fetal and Neonatal Risk,[5] Birth Defects and Drugs in Pregnancy,[6] and Catalog of Teratogenic Agents.[7] Computer databases are now available as well that provide current reviews of the literature. Some of the more commonly used databases are listed (Table 10-4).

In our ranking system, oral contraceptives are given a probable teratogenic risk rating of "minimal" while trimethadione is rated "potent." Based on reports in the literature, these ratings more accurately convey the probable teratogenic risks than do the respective FDA classifications of "X" and "D." This teratogen rating system is not meant to be a substitution for a careful literature search and individualized counseling. Rather,

TABLE 10-1	THE UNITED STATES FOOD AND DRUG ADMINISTRATION (FDA) USE IN PREGNANCY RATINGS
Category:	*Interpretation*
A	Controlled studies show no risk. Adequate, well-controlled studies in pregnant women have failed to demonstrate risk to the fetus.
B	No evidence of risk in humans. Either animal findings show risk, but human findings do not; or, if no adequate human studies have been done, animal findings are negative.
C	Risk cannot be ruled out. Human studies are lacking, and animal studies are either positive for fetal risk, or lacking as well. However, potential benefits may justify the potential risk.
D	Positive evidence of risk. Investigational or post-marketing data show risk to the fetus. Never-the-less, potential benefits may outweigh the potential risk.
X	Contraindicated in pregnancy. Studies in animals or human, or investigation or post-marketing reports have shown fetal risk which clearly outweighs any possible benefit to the patient.

Modified from reference 50.

we developed this system to apply some standard by which the teratogenic potential of drugs may be compared. These ratings should only be used to compliment and summarize individualized counseling. The ratings for individual drugs are updated as new data and information become available.

SYNOPSES OF COMMONLY USED AND POTENT TERATOGENS

ANTICONVULSANT DRUGS

Epileptic women have a 2- to 3-fold increased incidence of congenital anomalies.[8] However, it is unclear how much of this increased incidence is due to epilepsy per se or to inherent teratogenicity of anticonvulsant drugs. A recent study by Meadow (1991) reported infants born to epileptic mothers not on anticonvulsant therapy did not have an increased frequency of malformations.[9] Moreover, the incidence of congenital malformations in the offspring of epileptic men was also not increased. In contrast to this, Janz (1982) and Shapiro (1976) reported that the incidence of malformations was increased among children of epileptic fathers.[10,11] Gaily et al. (1988) reported that several minor anomalies associated with anticonvulsant therapy appear to be genetically linked to epilepsy.[12] In contrast, Friis (1989) suggested that genetic factors play a minor role in the incidence of facial clefts among children of epileptic parents.[13] A review of 15 epidemiological studies found wide variation in the reported incidence (2.2–26.1%) of birth defects among offspring of treated epileptics.[14]

Recent evidence suggests that the pathophysiology of congenital malformation associated with epilepsy is a combination of exposure to anticonvulsant medication in an individual who may be "genetically" susceptible. Data suggest that an enzyme deficiency may be responsible for certain malformations seen with anticonvulsant use. The enzyme, epoxide hydrolase, is required to metabolize intermediary oxidative metabolites of anticonvulsants that utilize the arene oxide pathway. Buehler et al. conducted a prospective study of 19 pregnant women receiving phenytoin. These authors found 4 fetuses who demonstrated decreased epoxide hydrolase activity and all had characteristic features of the phenytoin embryopathy. The 15 fetuses with normal enzyme activity did not have these features. Epoxide hydrolase is regulated by a single gene which has 2 allelic forms. Thus, it would appear that in fetuses homozygous for the recessive allele would have a lower enzyme activity and therefore be at a greater risk of malformation from anticonvulsant use.[15]

Multiple drug therapy appears to increase the risk of anomalies. A prospective study by Kaneko et al. (1988) found a 6.5% malformation rate among 31 patients treated with a single drug and a 15.6% malformation rate among 141 patients treated with several drugs.[16] Folic acid supplementation has been reported to decrease the incidence of congenital malformations due to single or multiple anticonvulsant drugs.[17] All anticonvulsants interfere with folic acid metabolism and therefore, patients taking anticonvulsants may develop a folic acid deficiency. Thus, it is recommended that patients taking anticonvulsants take a folic acid supplement both pre- and post conceptually. The dose currently recommended is 4mg/d.[18] Neonates of women treated with anticonvulsants, especially barbiturates, should receive vitamin K at birth to reduce the risk of hemorrhage.[19]

The possibility of an increased baseline rate of congenital malformations among epileptics should be remembered when counseling patients about the potential teratogenic risks of phenytoin or other anticonvulsant drugs. The risks of possible drug teratogenicity must also be balanced against increased fetal and maternal morbidity due to generalized convulsions.[8] Anticonvulsant drugs should not routinely be discontinued during pregnancy. Because of increased metabolism, the dosage of anticonvulsant drugs frequently needs to be increased during pregnancy.[20] Consensus guidelines regarding preconceptual counselling, mangagement, and care of the pregnant woman with epilepsy have been published.[21]

PHENYTOIN

Phenytoin (diphenylhydantoin) is probably the most commonly used anticonvulsant in pregnancy. Phenytoin has been reported to cause a pattern of malformations known as the

| TABLE 10-2 | RANKING OF DRUGS BY PROBABLE RISK OF TERATOGENICITY |

Class 0: Nominal Risk of Teratogenicity

Acetaminophen B
Aspirin C
Caffeine B
Cephalosporins B
Erythromycin C
Insulin B
Levothyroxine A
Penicillins B
Ritodrine B
Terbutaline B

Class 1: Minimal Risk of Teratogenicity

Acyclovir C
Aminoglycosides C
Antistamines
Atenolol C
Cimetidine B
Codeine C
Corticosteroids B
Bromocriptine C
Diazepam D
Digoxin C
Diphenhydramine C
Fluoxetine B
Furosemide C
Haloperidal C
Heparin C
Hydralazine C
Ibuprofen B
Imipramine D
Indomethacin B
Isoniazid C
Isoproterenol C
Labetalol C
Magnesium sulfate B
Meperidine B
Metaproterenol C
Metronidazole B
Methyldopa C
Miconazole B
Morphine B
Nitrofurantoin B
Opiates B
Oral contraceptives X

Progesterone D
Propranolol C
Propylthiouracil D
Reserpine D
Sulfasalazine B
Sulfonylureas D
Sulfonamides B
Tetracyclines D
Theophylline C
Thiazide diuretics D
Trimethobenzamide C
Trimethoprin C
Vancomycin C
Verapamil C
Zidovidine C

Class 2: Small Risk of Teratogenicity

Azothioprine D
Captopril C
Cocaine X
Ethosuximide C
Gold compounds C
Meprobamate D
Phenobarbital D
Phenothiazines C
Rifampin C
Nifedipine C
Penicillamine D

Class 3: Moderate Risk of Teratogenicity

Amantadine C
Carbamazepine C
Ethanol X
Fluorouracil D
Lithium D
Mercaptopurine D
Methimazole D
Phenytoin D
Valproic acid D

Class 4: Potent Teratogens

Aminopterin X
Coumarin derivatives D
Cyclophosphamide D
Isotretinoin X
Methotrexate D
Trimethadione D

Modified from reference 50.

fetal hydantoin syndrome (FHS).[22] This syndrome includes intrauterine growth retardation, distal digital and nail hypoplasia, mental retardation, cleft lip/palate, depressed nasal bridge, low-set ears, ocular hypertelorism, cardiac, and other anomalies.[23] This pattern of malformations has recently been linked to individual epoxide hydroxolase levels. Thus, it would appear that certain individuals may be genetically susceptable to FHS.[15]

The incidence of FHS is controversial. Hanson et al. (1976) estimated the risk of FHS to be approximately 11%.[23] In contrast, Gaily et al. (1988) estimated the risk of serious developmental disturbances among phenytoin exposed children to be only 1–2%.[12] Among a cohort of 305 epileptic patients, Shapiro et al. (1976) did not find a significant difference in the malformation rates according to the use of phenytoin.[11] Tumors may be another risk of phenytoin exposure. Briggs (1994) reviewed 11 case reports of tumors, including 5 neuroblastomas, among children exposed to phenytoin in utero.[3]

CARBAMAZEPINE

Carbamazepine (Tegeretol) is a commonly prescribed anticonvulsant that was originally thought to be ideal for use in pregnancy as initial reports showed no teratogenic risks above baseline. Later, Jones et al. (1989) described a pattern of malformations similar to those seen in fetal hydantoin syndrome. Like phenytoin, carbamezepine is metabolized into oxidative intermediates (epoxides). Clearance of these metabolites relies on epoxide hydroxolase activity. Infants with a decreased enzyme activity would likely be at an increased risk for this pattern of malformations if their mother used carbamezapine during pregnancy.[15]

VALPROIC ACID

Valproic acid, an anticonvulsant most efficacious for the treatment of absence seizures, is also used for the treatment of grand mal epilepsy. Valproic acid exposure in the first trimester has been associated with an increased risk of neural tube defects. The relative risk ratio for spina bifida from 2 studies has been reported to be 20.6 and 25.8; the absolute risk for spina bifida has been estimated at 1–2%.[24]

TABLE 10-3	WAYNE STATE UNIVERSITY TERATOGEN RATING SYSTEM	

Probable Agent	*Reported Associations or Effects*	*Risk*
Acetaminophen B	Limb	Nominal
Acyclovir C	Teratogenic in rats; potential for chromosomal breaks	Minimal
Amantadine C	Teratogenic in animals	Moderate
Aminoglycosides C	8 Cranial nerve toxicity	Minimal
Aminopterin X	CNS, facial, limb defects, spontaneous abortions	Potent
Antihistamines		
H1 Antagonists C	Cleft palate, GU, cardiac	Minimal
H2 Antagonists B	No known teratogenic effects	Minimal
Atenolol C	No known teratogenic effects	Minimal
Aspirin C	Clefts, cardiac; IUGR, closure of ductus, facial	Nominal
Azothioprine D	Bone marrow hypoplasia, cardiac	Small
Caffeine B	CNS, limb, GU, other	Nominal (in moderation)
Captopril C	Limb, cranial, stillbirth in animals	Small
Carbamazepine C	Craniofacial, fingernail hypoplasia	Moderate
Cephalosporins B	No known teratogenic associations	Nominal
Cocaine X (illicit use)	GU, cardiac, IUGR, prematurity, death	Small
Codeine C	Respiratory, GU, limb	Minimal
Corticosteroids B	Facial clefts in animals	Minimal
Coumarin	Fetal warfarin syndrome, CNS, cardiac	Potent
Derivatives D	Vertebral, limb	Probable risk = 5–25%
Bromocriptine C	CNS, urinary, talipes, limb, hemangioma	Minimal
Cimetidine B	Antiandrogenic effects in rats	Minimal
Cyclophosphamide D	Facial, limb, IUGR, teratogenic	Potent in animals
Diazepam D	Cleft lip and palate	Minimal
Digoxin C	Variation in rat lumbar ribs	Minimal
Diphenyhydramine C	GU, hernia, eye, ear	Minimal
Disulfiram X	Limb, vertebral	Moderate
Erythromycin C	No known teratogenic associations	Nominal
Ethanol X[a]	Fetal alcohol syndrome in chronic	Moderate[a]; dependency, excessive consumption
Ethosuximide C	Facial clefts, PDA	Small
Fluorouracil D	Skeletal, CNS in rats	Moderate
Flouxetine (B)	Increase minor anomalies	Minimal
Furosemide C	No known teratogenetic effects	Minimal
Gold compounds C	Limb, anomalies in rats	Small
Haloperidal C	Limb	Minimal
Heparin C	Prematurity, fetal death	Minimal
Hydralazine C	Teratogenic in mice	Minimal
Ibuprofen B	Constrict ductus arteriosus	Minimal
Imipramine D	Craniofacial, limb	Minimal
Indomethacin B	Oligohydramnious, constrict ductus, arteriosus	Minimal
Insulin B	CNS, limb, vertebral, cardiac, not cross placenta, control of diabetes may decrease risk of anomalies	Nominal[a]
Isoniazid C	Neural tube defects, talipes	Minimal
Isoproterenol C	Teratogenic in chick embryos	Minimal
Isotretinoin X	CNS, cardiovascular, facial (probable teratogenic risk 15–20%)	Potent
Labetalol C	No known teratogenic effects	Minimal
Levothyroxine A	Cardiovascular, Down's, does not cross placenta	Nominal
Lithium D	Ebstein's, other cardiovascular (probable risk = 2–10%)	Moderate

(continued)

TABLE 10-3 | Wayne State University Teratogen Rating System (*Continued*)

Probable Agent	Reported Associations or Effects	Risk
Magnesium sulfate B	No known teratogenic effects	Minimal
Meperidine B	No consistent teratogenic effects	Minimal
Meprobamate D	Cardiac, eye, CNS	Small
Mercaptopurine D	Abortion, stillbirth, facial	Moderate
Metaproterenol C	Teratogenic in rodents	Minimal
Methimazole D	Aplasia cutis, cardiac, fetal hypothyroidism	Moderate
Methotrexate D	(See aminopterin)	Potent
Methyldopa C	No known teratogenic effects	Minimal
Metronidazole B	CNS, midline facial	Minimal[a]
Miconazole B	No known teratogenic effects	Minimal
Morphine B	No consistent teratogenic effects	Minimal
Nifedipine C	Teratogenic and fetal demise in animals	Small
Nitrofurantoin B	Hemolytic anemia in G6PD	Minimal
Oral contraceptives X	Cardiac, CNS, eye, limb reduction, ear, masculinization	Minimal
Penicillamine D	Cutis laxa, inguinal hernia	Small
Penicillins B	No known teratogenic effects	Nominal
Phenytoin D	Mental retardation, craniofacial, limb, fetal tumors and hemorrhage (probable risk = 2–11%)	Moderate
Phenobarbital D	CNS, heart, limb and face defects	Small
Phenothiazines C	CNS, limb, cardiac, facial clefts, extrapyramidal syndrome	Small
Progesterone D	Hypospadias, cardiac, CNS, eye	Minimal
Propranolol C	IUGR, fetal hypoglycemia, bradycardia	Minimal
Propylthiouracil D	Non-specific anomalies	Minimal
Reserpine D	Microcephaly, hydronephrosis, hydroureter	Minimal
Rifampin C	CNS, limb, renal	Small
Ritodrine B	No known teratogenic effects (use after 20 weeks gestation)	Nominal[a]
Sulfasalazine B	No known teratogenic effects	Minimal
Sulfonylureas D	Teratogenic in animals	Minimal
Sulfonamides B	No consistent malformations	Minimal
Terbutaline B	No known teratogenic effects (use after 20 weeks gestation)	Nominal[a]
Tetracyclines D	Potent for discolored teeth, limb, hypoplasia, inguinal hernia	Minimal[a]
Theophylline C	Teratogenic in animals	Minimal
Thiazide diuretics D	Neonatal thrombocytopenia	Minimal
Thyroxine A	(See levothyroxine)	
Trimethadione D	Craniofacial, cardiac, limb, GU esophageal, IUGR (probable risk = 60–80%)	Potent
Trimethobenzamide C	No known teratogenic effects	Minimal
Trimethoprim C	Teratogenic in rat	Minimal
Valproic acid D	Neural tube defects, craniofacial (probable risk = 1–2%)	Moderate
Vancomycin C	No known teratogenic effects	Minimal
Verapamil C	No known teratogenic effects	Minimal
Zidovudine C	No known teratogenic effects	Minimal[a]

KEY: Probable potential for inducing human teratogenicity at "typical" therapeutic doses during the first trimester; Risk Levels: 0. nominal—no apparent teratogenic effects with extensive clinical experience; 1. minimal—no apparent teratogenic effects with limited clinical experience, or minimal evidence of animal or human teratogenicity with extensive clinical experience; 2. small-limited evidence of teratogenicity in humans, or known animal teratogen with limited human clinical use; 3. moderate—clinical studies with evidence of human teratogenicity or potent animal teratogen with limited clinical experience, probable teratogenic risk < 5%; 4. potent-probable teratogenic risk > 5%.
CNS—central nervous system; IUGR—intrauterine growth retardation; GU—genitourinary; PDA—patent ductus arteriosus.
[a] Drug added since last edition, or category changed.

TABLE 10-4	COMPUTER REPRODUCTIVE RISK INFORMATION DATABASES

Micromedex, Inc.
REPRORISK (REPROTEXT, REPROTOX, Sheperd's Catalog
  of Teratogenic Agents and TERIS)
Englewood, CO
(800) 525-9083

Reproductive Toxicology Center
REPROTOX
Columbia Hospital for Women Medical Center
Washington, DC
(202) 293-5137

National Library of Medicine, MEDLARS Service Desk
GRATEFUL MED (TOXLINE, TOXNET, and MEDLINE)
Bethesda MD
(800) 638-8480

Shepard's Catalog of Teratologic Agents
University of Washington
Seattle, WA
(206) 543-3373

Teratogen Information System
TERIS and Sheperd's Catalog of Teratogenic Agents
Seattle, WA
(206) 543-2465

Modified from reference 1.

Based on the cumulative data from 13 prospectively recorded cohort studies, Lindhout et al. (1986) examined the incidence of neural tube defects and valproate exposure.[25] Of 120 women taking valproate as a single agent, 3 had neonates with spina bifida. There were an additional 3 cases among 273 epileptic mothers who took other anticonvulsants in addition to valproate. These authors estimated the cumulative absolute risk of spina bifida from valproate exposure to be 1.5%. This risk of neural tube defect is comparable to that of a proband with an affected first degree relative.

Valproate has also been associated with increased risks for orofacial clefts and congenital heart defects. From the case-controlled Lyon Birth Defect Registry, Robert and Rosa (1983), reported 11 infants with heart defects among 38 exposed to valproate.[26] There were also 5 cases of facial clefts among the 38 exposures. They reported odds ratio of 4.3 (95% CL 1.8–10.3) for heart defects and 5.4 (95% CL 1.7–16.3) for orofacial clefting and valproate exposure.

Mastroiacovo et al. (1983) analyzed the teratogenic effects of anticonvulsants during the first trimester while taking into account the confounding effects of epilepsy itself.[27] They concluded that the association of valproate and congenital heart defects or clefts can be attributed to maternal epilepsy per se, and not anticonvulsants. However, they did confirm the association of spina bifida with valproate exposure.

Jager-Roman et al. (1986) prospectively studied 14 cases of valproate monotherapy and 12 cases of valproate in combination with other anticonvulsants.[28] Four neonates in the monotherapy group had major malformations. Interestingly, they reported a median number of 4 minor anomalies per infant exposed to valproate monotherapy. This compares to a median of 4.8 minor anomalies after valproate combination therapy among 12 infants, and a median of 1.1 minor anomalies in the control group. These were predominantly anomalies of the face, skull, ears, and digits.

It is advisable to evaluate valproate exposed fetuses for neural tube defects. This should include careful sonographic evaluation and maternal serum alpha fetoprotein with consideration for amniocentesis for acetylcholinesterase and alpha fetoprotein determination.

TRIMETHADIONE

Trimethadione is indicated for the treatment of petit mal seizures which are refractory to other anticonvulsant drugs. Zackai et al. (1975) described the fetal trimethadione syndrome consisting of developmental delay, V-shaped eyebrows, low-set ears with anteriorly folded helix, high-arched palate, and irregular dentition.[29] Other associated anomalies include mental retardation, speech impairment, hernias, cardiac, limb, and genitourinary defects.[30]

The risk of birth defects or spontaneous abortion following first trimester trimethadione exposure has been estimated at 60–80%.[1] Briggs reviewed the histories of 9 families and found a 69% incidence of congenital anomalies from 36 pregnancies. Feldman et al. (1977) summarized the reports of 53 pregnancies.[31] Perinatal losses were 32.5% and only 17% of the exposed children were without any apparent defects.

ANTIDEPRESSANTS

Drugs used to treat depression include the tricyclic derivatives, the monoamine oxidase inhibitors (MAOIs), and the selective serotonin reuptake inhibitors (SSRIs). Use of tricyclic antidepressants in pregnancy has not been associated with congenital malformations. (Indanpaan) MAOIs should be avoided as they have been shown to be teratogenic in animals.[32] Also, there is a risk of severe maternal hypertensive reaction with these medications. The SSRIs are newer to the market and include fluoxetine (Prozac) and sertraline (Zoloft). Currently fluoxetine is the most frequently prescribed antidepressant drug in the United States. Its use in pregnancy is described in the following section.

FLUOXETINE

Fluoxetine is a SSRI and is used to treat major depression, Tourette's syndrome, obsessive-compulsive disorder, and premenstrual syndrome. The manufacturer (Eli Lilly and Company) maintained a patient register that included 544 pregnancies. The fluoxetine exposed pregnancies did not have an increased incidence of major malformations.[33] The manufacturer has also reported no toxologic effects in the rat and rabbit in doses 11 times the maximum human daily dose.[34] Chambers et al. (1996) identified 228 pregnant women taking fluoxetine and matched them to controls.[35] There was no increased incidence of major anomalies in the fluoxetine exposed group. There were, however, more infants with 3 or more minor anomalies identified in the fluoxetine group (15.5% vs. 6.5% p = 0.03). Interestingly, third-trimester exposure to fluoxetine was associated with higher rates of premature delivery (relative risk = 4.8).

Neurobehavioral testing of 55 children with exposure to fluoxetine in utero showed no difference in IQ when compared to either children with exposure to tricyclics or children with no antidepressant exposure.[36]

LITHIUM

Lithium, used for the treatment of manic-depressive disorders, has been associated with Ebstein anomaly and other cardiovascular defects. Ebstein anomaly is characterized by a dysplasia of the tricuspid valve with caudadal displacement of the septal and posterior leaflets. By 1980, 225 infants exposed to lithium during the first trimester, were reported to the International Registry for Lithium. Of these, 25 (11%) had major congenital anomalies, 18 (8%) had cardiovascular defects including 6 (3%) with Ebstein anomaly.[37] The risk for cardiac malformations due to first-trimester exposure has also been reported to occur in approximately 2% of cases.[1] Other cardiovascular defects associated with lithium ingestion include mitral atresia, patent ductus arteriosus, ventricular septal defects, hypoplasia of the left ventricle, dextrocardia, and anomalies of the great vessels.[5]

More recently, of 16 children with Ebstein anomaly, only 1 was exposed to lithium in utero.[38] Kallen reported a joint case-control study from New Zealand, Hungary, Sweden, and Denmark. Of 25 cases of Ebstein's anomaly, none were known to be exposed to lithium. Nor was there any known exposures to lithium among the 15 cases of Ebstein's identified by the French Rhone-Alps-Auvergne monitoring system.[39]

Ebstein anomaly is rare, only 300 cases have been recorded in the literature.[38] Therefore, the occurrence of this anomaly among women treated with lithium is cause for concern. However, these more recent data demonstrate that most cases of Ebstein are not associated with lithium ingestion, and suggest that the association between lithium and Ebstein is weak.[39]

H2 BLOCKERS

Since the introduction of cimetidine into the pharmacuetical market in the 1970s the number of H2 blockers on the market, and their use has increased worldwide. Many H2 blockers are now available over-the-counter. As pregnancy is commonly complicated by gastroesophageal reflux there is a clear need to assess the safety of these antisecretory drugs.

CIMETIDINE

Magee et al. (1996) published a prospective cohort study addressing the safety of first-trimester exposure to histimine H2 blockers.[40] In this study, 178 patients were identified who used an H2 blocker in the first trimester. These patients were matched with controls. Pregnancy outcome did not differ between the 2 groups. There was no increased incidence of major malformations in the H2 blocker exposed group. No significant difference was noted for incidence of jaundice among the infants or attainment of developmental milestones.

Animal studies have been performed addressing development of secondary sex characteristics in male rats after perinatal cimetidine exposure. There are conflicting data on postnatal feminization following exposure to cimetidine in utero. A recent study published by Hoie et al. (1994) shows that with the exception of a shorter distance from the anus to the genitalia in the cimetidine-exposed newborn rats, no statistically significant differences were observed in the measured parameters between the cimetidine exposed and control groups.[41]

ISOTRETINOIN

Isotretinoin is the vitamin A analogue that is singularly effective for the treatment of severe, recalcitrant cystic acne. However, isotretinoin (Accutane) is one of the most potent known human teratogens. Thus is the therapeutic dilemma that women who stand to benefit most from this drug are also the group at greatest risk for unplanned pregnancies and subsequent embryopathy. It is estimated that up to 60,000 premenopausal women per year are being treated with isotretinoin.[42] Remarkably, of women conceiving on isotretinoin, no contraceptive was used in 50% and up to one third were pregnant at initiation of therapy.[42]

Isotretinoin has been associated with an increased rate of spontaneous abortions and up to an 18% incidence of fetal malformations, when exposure occurred between 5 and 70 days of conception.[43] This has been compared to thalidomide in risk of major malformations. In contrast to the remarkable risk of taking isotretinoin during pregnancy, there appears to be no increased risk if this drug is discontinued prior to conception.[44]

The most common abnormalities associated with isotretinoin are craniofacial, followed by cardiac thymus and CNS.[43,45] Craniofacial abnormalities include: microtic ears, agenesis or stenosis of the external ear canal, micrognathia, malformed calvarium, flattened and depressed nasal bridge, and hypertelorism.

Cardiac malformations include: transposition of the great vessels, tetralogy of Fallot, double-outlet right ventricle, truncus arteriosus communis, ventricular septal defects, aortic arch hypoplasia, and retroesophageal right subclavian artery.[43] Thymic ectopia, hypoplasia, and aplasia occurred most commonly in conjunction with cardiac malformations.

Hydrocephalus was the most common central nervous system malformation.[43] Other anomalies included microcephaly, cortical lesions, cerebellar hypoplasia, agenesis, or dysgenesis.

To avoid isotretinoin embryopathy, guidelines have been developed by the FDA and the manufacturer, Hoffman-La Roche, Inc., a summary of which include:

1. Isotretinoin and etretinate should not be used by women who are pregnant or who may become pregnant while taking the drug.
2. Pregnancy should be ruled out before treatment begins. This precaution may be best accomplished by obtaining a negative pregnancy test no more than 2 weeks prior to the beginning of therapy and starting therapy on the second or third day of the patient's next normal menstrual period.
3. An effective form of contraception should be used for at least 1 month before therapy begins, and during therapy.
4. Women who have received isotretinoin should continue using an effective form of contraception for 1 month after discontinuing treatment.
5. The period of time during which pregnancy must be avoided after treatment is discontinued has not been determined for women who have received etretinate.
6. Female patients should be counseled on the risk of major birth defects associated with first-trimester exposure to isotretinoin or etretinate. Should a pregnancy occur during treatment, the woman should consult her physician about the management of her pregnancy.[46]

COUMARIN DERIVATIVES

Coumarin derivatives (warfarin, dicumarol, phenindione) are oral vitamin K antagonists which are widely used anticoagulants. These agents appear to be capable of inducing fetal malformations in all trimesters. Hall et al. (1980) compiled 418 cases of exposure to coumarin derivatives during pregnancy.[47] Of these, there were only 293 liveborns without complications, 57 liveborns with complications (malformations, prematurity, hemorrhage), 32 stillbirths, and 36 spontaneous abortions.

Exposure to these anticoagulants during the first trimester can cause specific anomalies known as fetal warfarin syndrome (FWS). The most consistent features of this syndrome are nasal hypoplasia, depression of the bridge of the nose and stippled epiphyses. All cases of FWS appear to result from exposure between the s6th and 9th weeks of gestation.[47]

Other, non-FWS associated anomalies also occur. Bony deformities include: vertebral malformations, short limbs and fingers, and stipled epiphyses; malformations similar to those seen in chondroplasia punctata. CNS defects include hydrocephalus, mental retardation, microcephaly, cerebellar atrophy, meningocoele, and others. Other abnormalities include, deafness, optic atrophy, blindness, and microphthalmia.[5,47] The CNS and eye abnormalities have been reported in cases where exposure was limited to the second and third trimesters.[47] The pathophysiology of coumarin derivative embryopathy may involve interference with calcium binding by proteins, possibly due to interference of polypeptide post-translational modification by vitamin K, and/or fetal hemorrhage.[5,47]

Briggs compiled a total of 463 reported cases, 255 first-trimester exposures and 208 cases in the second and third trimesters. First-trimester exposures resulted in an 8% incidence of FWS and a 4% incidence of CNS and other defects. Exposure in the second and third trimesters resulted in a 5% incidence of CNS and other defects. However, coumarin derivative use in the first trimester has been associated with up to a 15–25% incidence of abnormalities when used in the first trimester according to ACOG technical bulletin #236.[1]

The use of coumarin derivatives in all trimesters appears to cause significant fetal risk. However, it is not clear that heparin is a better alternative.[48] Since warfarin has not been detected in the milk of lactating women breastfeeding does not appear to be contraindicated.[49]

SUMMARY

A common concern of expectant parents is the potential of birth defects from over-the-counter or prescription drugs. There is limited and often conflicting data in regards to the teratogenicity of most drugs. Fortunately, most drugs appear to have limited human teratogenic potential; reassurance is usually appropriate. Limitation of unnecessary drug exposure during pregnancy and avoidance of the known teratogens will minimize drug induced malformations.

ACKNOWLEDGMENT

The publisher acknowledges that parts of this chapter are based on the contribution of Mitchell P. Dombrowski, MD. The editor would also like to thank Dr. Mitchell P. Dombrowski who was also a main contributor to this particular chapter.

References

1. ACOG Technical Bulletin: *Teratology*. 1997;236.
2. Khoury MJ, Holtzman NA. On the ability of birth defects monitoring to detect new teratogens. *Am J Epidemiology*. 1987;126:136–143.

3. Piper JM, Baum C, Kennedy DL, et al. Maternal use of prescribed drugs associated with recognized fetal adverse drug reactions. *Am J Obstet Gynecol.* 1988;159:1173–1177.

4. ACOG Technical Bulletin: Hormonal Contraception. Number 198, October 1994.

5. Briggs GG, Freeman RK, Yaffe SJ. *Drugs in Pregnancy and Lactation: A Reference Guide to Fetal and Neonatal Risk.* Fourth ed. Baltimore: Willians and Wilkins; 1994.

6. Heinonen OP, Slone D, Shapiro S. *Birth Defects and Drugs in Pregnancy.* Little Publishing Sciences Group, 1982.

7. Shepard TH. *Catalog of Teratogenic Agents.* 8th ed. Baltimore, MD: The Johns Hopkins University Press; 1995.

8. Yerby MS. Problems and management of the pregnant woman with epilepsy. *Epilepsia.* 1987;28:S29–S36.

9. Meadow R. Anticonvulsants in pregnancy. *Arch Child Dis.* 1991; 66:62.

10. Janz D. Antiepileptic drugs and pregnancy: altered utilization patterns and teratogenesis. *Epilepsia.* 1982;23:S53–S63.

11. Shapiro S, Hartz SC, Siskind V, et al. Anticonvulsants and parental epilepsy in the development of birth defects. *Lancet.* 1976;i:272.

12. Gaily E, Granstrom ML. Minor anomalies in offspring of epileptic mothers. *J Pediatr.* 1998;112:520–529.

13. Friis ML. Facial clefts and heart defects in children of parents with epilepsy: genetic and environmental etiologic factors. *Acta Neurologica Scandinavica.* 1989;79:433–459.

14. Hanson JW, Buehler BA. Fetal hydantoin syndrome: current status. *J Pediatr.* 1982;101:816–818.

15. Buehler BA, Delimont D, van Waes M, et al. Prenatal prediction of risk of the fetal hydantoin syndrome. *N Engl J Med.* 1990;322:1567.

16. Kaneko S, Otani K, Fukushima Y, et al. Teratogenicity of antiepileptic drugs: Analysis of possible risk factors. *Epilepsia.* 1988;29:459–467.

17. Biale Y, Lewenthal H. Effect of folic acid supplementation on congenital malformations due to anticonvulsant drugs. *Europ J Obstet Gyned Reprod Biol* 1984;18:211–216.

18. ACOG Siezure Disorders in Pregnancy #231 December 1996.

19. Mountain KR, Hirsh J, Gallus AS. Neonatal coagulation defect due to aniconvulsant drug treatment in pregnancy. *Lancet.* 1970;1:265.

20. Dalessio DJ. Current concepts: seizure disorders in pregnancy. *N Engl J Med.* 1985;312:559.

21. Delgado-Escueta AV, Janz D. Concensus guidelines: preconceptual counselling, management and care of the pregnant women with epilepsy. *Neurology.* 1992;42:149–160.

22. Hanson JW, Smith DW. The fetal hydantoin syndrome. *J Pediatr.* 1975;87:285.

23. Hanson JW, Myrianthopoulos NC, Sedgwick Harvey MA, et al. Risks to the offspring of women treated with hydantoin anticonvulsants, with emphasis on the fetal hydantoin syndrome. *J Pediatr.* 1976;89:662–668.

24. Lammer EJ, Lowell ES, Oakley GP. Teratogen update: valproic acid. *Teratology.* 1987;35:465–473.

25. Lindhout D, Schmidt D. In utero exposure to valproate and neural tube defects. *Lancet.* 1986;i:1392–393.

26. Robert E, Rosa F. Valproate and birth defects. *Lancet.* 1983;ii:1142.

27. Mastroiacovo P, Bertollini R, Morandini S, et al. Maternal epilepsy, valproate exposure and birth defects. *Lancet.* 1983;ii:1499.

28. Jager-Roman E, Deichl A, Jakob S, et al. Fetal growth, major malformations, and minor anomalies in infants born to women receiving valproic acid. *J Pediatr.* 1986;108:997–1004.

29. Zackai EH, Mellman WJ, Neiderer B, et al. The fetal trimethadione syndrome. *J Pediatr.* 1975;87:280–284.

30. Schardein JL. *Chemically Induced Birth Defects.* New York: Marcel Dekker; 1985.

31. Feldman GL, Weaver DD, Lovrien EW. The fetal trimethadione syndrome: report of an additional family and further delineation of this syndrome. *Am J Dis Child.* 1977;131:1389–1392.

32. Indanpaan-Heikkila J, Saxen L. Possible teratogenicity of imipramine-chloropyramine, *Lancet.* 1973;2:282–284.

33. Goldstien DJ, Marvel DE. Psychotropic medications during pregnancy: risk to the fetus. *JAMA.* 1993;270:2177.

34. Byrd RA, Markham JK. Developmental toxicology: studies of fluoxetine hydrochloride administered orally to rats and rabbits. *Fundamental and Applied Toxicology.* 1994;22:511–518.

35. Chambers CD, Johnson KA, Dick LM, et al. Birth outcomes in pregnant women taking fluoxetine. *N Engl J Med* 1996;335:1010–1015.

36. Nulman I, Rovet J, Stewart DE, et al. Neurodevelopment of children exposed in utero to antidepressant drugs. *N Engl J Med.* 1997;336:258–262.

37. Frankenberg RR, Lipinski JF. Congenital malformations. *N Engl J Med.* 1983;309:311–312.

38. Warkany J. Teratogen update: lithium. *Teratol.* 1988;38:593–596.

39. Kallen B. Comments on teratogen update: lithium. *Teratol.* 1988; 38:597.

40. Magee LA, Inocencion G, Kamboj L, et al. Safety of first trimester exposure to histamine H2 blockers. *Digestive Diseases and Sciences.* 1996;41:1145–1149.

41. Hoie EB, Swigart SA, Nelson RM, et al. Development of secondary sex characteristics in male rats after fetal and prenatal cimetidine exposure. *Journal of Pharmaceutical Sciences.* 1994;83:107–109.

42. Strauss JS, Cunningham WJ, Leyden JL, et al. Isotreinoin and teratogenicity. *J Am Acad Deratol.* 1988;19:353–354.

43. Lammer EJ, Chen DT, Hoar RM, et al. Retinoic acid embryopathy. *N Engl J Med.* 1985;313:837–841.

44. Dai WS, Hsu MA, Itri LM. Safety of pregnancy after discontinuation of isotretinoin. *Arch Dermatol* 1989;125:362–365.

45. Rappaport EB, Knapp M. Isotretionin embryopathy: a continuing problem. *J Clin Pharmacol.* 1989;29:463–465.

46. Leads from the MMWR. Birth defects caused by isotretinoin: New Jersey. *JAMA.* 1988;259:2362–2365.

47. Hall JG, Pauli RM, Wilson KM. Maternal and fetal sequelae of anticoagulation during pregnancy. *Am J Med.* 1980;68:122–140.

48. Howie PW. Anticoagulants in pregnancy. *Clin Obstet Gynecol.* 1986;13:349–363.

49. L'E Orme M, Lewis PJ, DeSwiet M, et al. May mothers given warfarin breast-feed their infants? *Br J Med.* 1977;1:564–565.

50. *Physician's Desk Reference.* 44th ed. Oradell, NJ: Medical Economics; 1990.

CHAPTER 11

THE EFFECTS OF MATERNAL DRINKING DURING PREGNANCY

Ernest L. Abel / Robert J. Sokol / John H. Hannigan / Beth A. Nordstrom

Current awareness of the clinical effects of alcohol abuse during pregnancy in children began in the early 1970s.[1,2] Since then, these effects have been widely recognized[3] and include a pattern of cognitive, growth-related, and physical abnormalities called fetal alcohol syndrome (FAS), or more recently "fetal alcohol abuse sydrome"[4] to reflect the fact that this disorder only occurs in connection with maternal alcohol abuse. This chapter examines some of the concerns that we believe are of particular interest to readers of this book. Related topics, such as psychological concomitants of alcohol abuse in pregnancy, associated patterns of family stress, and treatment of alcohol intoxication and withdrawal syndromes, have been examined elsewhere.[5,6]

GENERAL ASPECTS OF MEDICAL CARE IN PREGNANCY

Current recognition of alcohol's teratogenic potential can be traced to the early 1970s,[1,2] when a pattern of cognitive growth and facial anomalies called the fetal alcohol syndrome (FAS) was identified. Several hundred cases of FAS have now been documented.[7] Prior to 1980, however, standardized criteria for FAS were not available. In 1980, such criteria were developed by the Fetal Alcohol Study Group of the Research Society on Alcoholism.[8] These criteria required the presence of at least 1 feature from each of the following three categories for a formal clinical diagnosis of FAS:

1. Prenatal or postnatal growth retardation (weight, length, or height below the 10th percentile when corrected for gestational age).
2. A pattern of abnormal features of the head, such as microcephaly, or the face, such as short palpebral fissures, midfacial hypoplasia, flattened nasal bridge, or decreased prominence of the philtrum (the vertical groove between the nose and mouth).
3. Evidence of central nervous system abnormality, such as hyperactivity or mental retardation.

Other nonspecific abnormalities subsequently described in conjunction with FAS have included ocular retinal tortuosity; cardiac abnormalities, particularly septal defects; genital anomalies, such as hypospadias and undescended testes; hemangiomas; dermatoglyphic abnormalities; and cognitive anomalies, such as hearing and visual impairments, and speech pathology. These latter effects in the absence of FAS have been referred to as fetal alcohol spectrum disorders (FASD) or alcohol-related birth defects (ARBDs).

In 1996, the Institute of Medicine[9] described a new classification which includes five categories of diagnoses. Category 1 contains essentially the same criteria as the FAS Study Group's paradigm except that it now includes a history of maternal alcohol abuse as part of its diagnosis. A Category 2 diagnosis is the same as Category 1, except that it does not require a confirmed diagnosis of maternal alcohol abuse during pregnancy. Category 3 refers to conditions in which some, but not all, of the symptoms associated with Categories 1 and 2 are present. A Category 3 diagnosis, which the IOM designated as "partial FAS," is not intended to refer to conditions less severe than those in Categories 1 or 2. The IOM committee also created 2 additional diagnostic categories. Category 4 refers to physical anomalies or ARBDs, whereas Category 5 refers to cognitive and behavioral anomalies, designated alcohol-related neurodevelopmental disorders (ARNDs). Categories 4 and 5 were created to include clinical conditions for which the link to maternal alcohol abuse during pregnancy is more circumspect than those associated with Categories 1–3, but nevertheless is reasonably certain based on epidemiological or animal research.

The reported incidence of FAS is still variable and no firm national data for the United States are available. Depending on location and population under study, the overall incidence has varied from 0.4 per 1000 in Cleveland to 3.1 per 1000 in Boston. Estimates in Europe have ranged from 1.6 per 1000 in Sweden to 2.9 per 1000 in France. The overall prevalence of FAS in the Western World appears to be about 1 case per 1000 live births.[10] When only women identified as problem drinkers or alcohol abusers are considered, estimates of the frequency of FAS are more consistent and higher, with the overall average about 59 per 1000.[11]

Although relatively few children may be born with enough stigmata to be diagnosed as FAS, maternal alcohol abuse during pregnancy may be responsible for about 5% of all congenital anomalies.[12] Mental retardation is the most serious and damaging of all these anomalies, and maternal alcohol abuse during pregnancy may be the most common teratogenic cause of mental retardation in the industrialized world.[11]

It is now clear from clinical observations, epidemiological studies, and experimental studies in animals, that while alcohol abuse is a necessary element in FASD, it is not a sufficient cause.[13] For instance, a clinical case in which 1 fraternal twin was more severely affected with FAS than the other indicates that genetic factors influence fetal susceptibility to alcohol's damaging effects.[13] This may explain in part why 2 women can consume the same amount of alcohol, yet one may give birth to a child with FAS and the other may not. However, what should not be lost sight of is that alcohol abuse, not simply alcohol consumption, is the necessary condition (see "Alcohol Abuse" section).

Observational studies involving large numbers of patients rather than single cases can be more difficult to interpret. Critical reviews of such studies have identified some of the reasons for this difficulty.[7,14,15] One involves the issue of bias. In many published case reports and studies, the diagnosis of alcohol-related birth defects has been based on foreknowledge of maternal alcohol abuse. This leads to the possibility that some of the observed associations may be artifactual (i.e., found purely because they were being looked for).

Another problem is confounding. Alcohol is 1 of a multitude of possible pregnancy risks (cofactors), which include smoking, poverty, medical diseases, pregnancy complications, exposure to environmental pollutants, and lifestyle factors.[7,13,16] Epidemiologic studies employ complex statistical techniques to control and adjust for as many factors as possible to support inferences linking observed effects to alcohol, but many pregnancy risks remain unknown, and there are limitations in these statistical techniques.[7] Therefore, it is not possible to adjust completely for confounding. Although epidemiological studies can document associations between alcohol and adverse pregnancy outcome, they cannot prove causality.[17] While studies in animals allow greater control and greater certainty in inferring a causal role for alcohol as a teratogen, here too confounding cannot be entirely eliminated.[7,13] Nevertheless, alcohol-related birth effects comparable to those occurring in humans have been observed in many animal models and studies have documented dose-response effects of alcohol on perinatal mortality, infant weight, and cognitive and behavioral anomalies.[7,11]

Additional compelling evidence for a direct effect of alcohol as a teratogen comes from in vitro models. In 1 study, 18 rat embryos exposed to 0.15 or 0.3 g of alcohol per 100 mL of culture medium (0.1 g per 100 mL blood is considered intoxicating) had decreased crown-rump and head lengths, decreased total cell counts, and retarded development compared to controls after 24 hours of exposure. Because rat embryos at this stage cannot metabolize alcohol to their primary metabolite, acetaldehyde, this study strongly supports a causative role of alcohol as an agent directly toxic to the fetus.

ALCOHOL ABUSE

Approximately 60% of American women drink alcoholic beverages, and approximately 3% can be classified as problem drinkers.[7] The proportion of women in their reproductive years (age 18–34) who drink an average of at least 2 drinks per day (i.e., 14 drinks per week) is about 5.5%. During pregnancy, the proportion of women who drink this much decreases to about 2%.[7] Different populations of gravidas, however, have different drinking habits. In a study in California,[19] 0.5% of gravidas reportedly drank 14 or more drinks per week; in Buffalo it was 16%.[20]

These estimates pose some interesting issues: (1) because alcohol crosses the placenta, most people in the United States probably have been exposed to some alcohol prenatally; and (2) a considerable number of fetuses probably have been exposed to a lot of alcohol. Despite such exposures, however, relatively few Americans have suffered adverse consequences. Statements to the effect that "social" or "moderate" drinking (defined as drinking that does not result in intoxication) is inex-

orably damaging to the fetus are therefore untenable. We firmly believe that statements about the dangers of such drinking during pregnancy are groundlessly alarmist. The IOM[9] clearly states that FAS, partial FAS, ARBDs, and ARNDs are associated with "a pattern of excessive intake (of alcohol) characterized by substantial, regular intake or heavy episodic drinking" (p. 77) and Abel[7] has suggested that FAS be renamed "fetal alcohol abuse syndrome" to reflect the more clinically accurate relationship between these alcohol-related birth effects and the kind of maternal drinking that is their etiological factor. Whereas abstinence is still the surest way of avoiding FASD, we should nevertheless be forthright in acknowledging that FASD like FAS are the consequences of alcohol abuse and not an occasional drink.

One reason for misinformation regarding the alleged dangers of "moderate" drinking is that determinations of drinking behavior depend on self-reports and are usually imprecise. A drink, for instance, can vary from 1–8 oz depending on the respondent and the way questions are posed.[21] Using self-report data to estimate relations between numbers of drinks per day and a particular risk to the fetus also is problematic because of denial or inability to recall actual alcohol intake. In many cases, the greater the drinking, the more inaccurate the response, and the lower the estimate compared with actual intake.[22,23] Such underreporting will have the effect of exaggerating the risk to the fetus from relatively low levels of drinking such as 2 drinks per day. For example, Ernhart et al.[24] found that 41% of the women they sampled 4 to 5 years after an index pregnancy, reported higher levels of drinking during pregnancy than those obtained contemporary with that pregnancy. Especially noteworthy was the fact that the retrospective report was a better predictor of ARBDs than the reports given during pregnancy. This improved predictive validity suggests the higher reports were more accurate and, the higher the drinking, the greater the underreporting. The implication is that women most at risk for fetuses with ARBDs are those most likely to grossly underestimate their drinking. The corollary is that the risk to the fetus of what might appear to be 2 drinks a day is likely to be the result of much more than 2 drinks.[7]

A second stumbling block in estimating risk levels of drinking is the multitude of definitions of problem drinking, abusive drinking, heavy drinking, and alcohol dependence. For example, in a Boston study, heavy drinking was defined as consumption of 45 drinks per month and at least five drinks on some occasions;[25] in Loma Linda, California, it was defined as consumption of at least 2 oz of absolute alcohol per day (about 4 drinks per day);[26] in Seattle, where much of the early work in this area was conducted, heavy drinking was defined as daily consumption of 1 oz of absolute alcohol (about 2 drinks per day).[27] In Cleveland, risk was based not on drinking level but on responses to the Michigan Alcoholism Screening Test (MAST), a well-validated, widely used instrument for identifying individuals with drinking-related psychosocial disruption.[28] Such differences in definition and approach make comparisons across studies and estimates of fetal risk from maternal drinking difficult. Uncertainties associated with terms such as "light," "moderate," and "heavy" drinking,[29] further complicate attempts to estimate risk levels of drinking.

Assessing risk levels is further complicated by the well-documented spontaneous decrease in drinking as pregnancy progresses.[11,21,28,30] This is a salubrious occurrence inasmuch as decreases in drinking should improve pregnancy outcome. However, it underscores the problem of trying to summarize an individual's alcohol consumption throughout pregnancy by a single number (e.g., 2 drinks per day) calculated to 2-decimal-place precision. The variability and complexity of human drinking behavior must always be kept in mind when interpreting studies of drinking during pregnancy.

PATERNAL DRINKING

Women who drink heavily tend to consort with men who drink heavily,[31] a phenomenon known as "assortive mating." Conceivably, some ARBEs could be caused by paternal drinking, although this area of research has received relatively little attention. Nevertheless, virtually all of the effects associated with maternal alcohol exposure, including physical malformations, decreased birth weight, and cognitive anomalies, have been observed experimentally in animal offspring sired by alcohol-consuming fathers.[32] Also, some of the effects attributed to in utero alcohol exposure may be caused by mutagenic effects of alcohol on sperm.

EFFECTS OF ALCOHOL

SPONTANEOUS ABORTION AND STILLBIRTHS

Maternal consumption of intoxicating levels of alcohol over prolonged periods is clearly associated with a range of specific adverse fetal outcomes. The risk for spontaneous abortion may be increased 2-fold in pregnancies complicated by maternal alcohol abuse (about 3–5% of women).[33] Pregnant monkeys also tend to abort after high levels of alcohol exposure, but not at lower levels.[34] Reports of an increased risk for spontaneous abortion resulting from "moderate" drinking[35] are more likely the result of statistical artifact or confounding.[34]

Although some studies have reported an increase in stillbirths associated with maternal alcohol consumption, most studies have not found any such association.[7]

LOW BIRTH WEIGHT

Lowered birth weight is the most reliably documented effect of maternal alcohol abuse. In a recent review of more than 550 reported cases of FAS, the average birth weight of such children was 2100 g,[6] compared to the median birth weight for all infants in the United States of more than 3300 g.[36] Decreased birth weight also has been noted in the absence of full FAS.[6] Alcohol-related decreases in birth weight are primarily due to intrauterine growth retardation (IUGR). In a study by Sokol et al.[16] of more than 12,000 pregnancies, birth weight

was decreased by about 190 g in 204 pregnancies complicated by alcohol abuse with no effect on pregnancy duration.[26] Comparable findings have been reported in numerous animal studies.[6,7,11] The IUGR is related to treatment period. In animals, exposure during the third trimester has a more severe effect on birth weight than exposure earlier in gestation.[6,7,11] This observation in animals is consistent with studies in humans that indicate that women who reduce drinking during the third trimester give birth to infants with higher birth weights than women who do not reduce drinking during this period.[37]

Indirect evidence from studies in animals implicates fetal hypoxia in alcohol-related IUGR.[6,11,13] Other possible mechanisms include alcohol-induced fetal hypoglycemia,[38] interference with the passage of amino acids across the placenta,[39] and decreased incorporation of amino acids into protein in fetuses.[40] Although alcohol-related decreased maternal zinc levels also have been suggested to contribute to growth retardation,[41] the evidence on this issue is contradictory.[42]

An indicated above, the lower birth weight of infants prenatally exposed to alcohol does not appear to be attributable to preterm delivery. Although some studies have found a statistically significant increase in preterm births associated with maternal drinking, most epidemiological studies have not found this effect except at high levels of consumption.[43]

NEUROBEHAVIORAL AND NEURAL ABNORMALITY

If the fetus survives, arguably the most severe ARBDs are those involving the central nervous system, effects which the IOM calls alcohol-related neurodevelopmental disorders (ARNDs).

The adverse effects of alcohol on behavioral development can be detected in the neonatal period. Neonates born to heavy drinkers are more restless during sleep and sleep less than other children.[44] Abnormal electroencephalographic (EEG) activity during sleep has been noted for as long as 6 weeks after birth in some of these children. In fact, the EEG during some stages of sleep may be so unusual in these children that trained investigators have been able to identify 20 of 22 children whose mothers were alcoholics on the basis of the EEG records alone.[45]

Slower mental and motor development in 8-month-old infants prenatally exposed to alcohol who did not exhibit full FAS has also been reported.[46,47] One study reported that children born to mothers who had an average of three or more drinks per day during pregnancy, had IQ scores at 4 years of age, about five points below those whose mothers drank less.[48] Although the authors interpreted these results as evidence that maternal consumption of more than an average of three drinks per day in early pregnancy may "triple the risk of subnormal IQ," a decrease of five points in IQ does not constitute subnormal IQ. In fact, IQ scores for these children were not stated except for noting that they were in the "normal range." Furthermore, while the authors attributed this effect to an average of three drinks a day, examination of this study indicates that the effect is attributable to "lumping" children in this category with children born to alcohol-abusing mothers.[7] Alcohol abuse leading to FAS is decidedly linked to considerably lower IQ scores in several studies.[7] About 50% of all individuals with FAS have IQs below 70.[6]

Hyperactivity in children with FAS has been noted in several clinical case studies[7,11] and in children who do not exhibit physical abnormalities consistent with FAS.[49] Although IQ scores for the latter may be within normal limits, in many cases these children may eventually recommended for special education services because of restlessness, short attention spans, and distractibility.

As is the case of physical anomalies, studies in animals have been able to duplicate many of the behavioral abnormalities associated with maternal alcohol abuse in humans. For example, hyperactivity and learning difficulties have been noted in rats prenatally exposed to alcohol; these effects may be related to an underlying problem in response inhibition.[11,50]

NEURAL DEVELOPMENT

Neuroanatomic and biochemical abnormalities undoubtedly underlie the abnormal behavioral development observed in conjunction with fetal alcohol exposure. Microcephaly, a frequent characteristic of FAS, reflects an overall decrease in brain growth. Specific anatomic abnormalities observed in brains of children born to alcoholic women as studied at autopsy, as well as in animals prenatally exposed to alcohol, include absence of the corpus callosum, and abnormal migration of nerve and supportive glial cells.[51]

More subtle changes in brain structure have been noted in animals prenatally exposed to alcohol, such as abnormally distributed nerve fibers in the hippocampus,[52] decreased cell numbers in the hippocampus,[7] and decreased dendritic arborization of hippocampal nerve cells.[53] The latter also has been observed in the hippocampus of a child with FAS.[54] Because the hippocampus is known to be involved in learning and memory inhibitory control of behavior, these anatomic abnormalities may be the structural basis for some of the behavioral abnormalities observed in humans and animal studies.

RESEARCH ISSUES

Differential alcohol-related birth defects depend, in part, on at least three major questions concerning alcohol and pregnancy: How do timing of alcohol exposure, pattern of exposure, and beverage source affect pregnancy outcome? Is there a threshold for alcohol exposure below which there is no danger to the conceptus? Can women who are susceptible to alcohol-related birth defects be identified?

TIMING, PATTERN, AND BEVERAGE SOURCE

There is no "safe" time during pregnancy for drinking. Different alcohol-related birth defects can result from drinking during different critical periods (e.g., early or late in pregnancy). Knowing when exposure occurs is important in anticipating different kinds of alcohol-related abnormalities (e.g.,

facial versus central nervous system). A large brief exposure to alcohol (bingeing) does not necessarily cause significant biologic damage to the human conceptus, but is more likely to do so than exposure to the same amount of alcohol spread out during the day.[7] For reliable damage to occur, drinking must be heavy and sustained.[7,55]

Beverage source is not a major determinant of infant outcome in animal studies.[56,57] Beer has been found to produce a small but significant risk for alcohol-related birth defects in several epidemiologic studies.[7,26] Beer, however, may be a surrogate for low socioeconomic status,[7] a known contributing factor in FAS.[7]

THRESHOLD

One of the most frequently asked questions about alcohol and pregnancy is whether there is a safe level of alcohol intake and, if so, what it is. In July of 1981, the Surgeon General advised "women who are pregnant or considering pregnancy not to drink alcoholic beverages ..."[58] This advice is reasonable, conservative ... and simplistic. Recommending abstinence to an alcoholic has no more chance of eliminating alcohol-related birth defects than it has of preventing alcohol abuse in general. ARBDs are a generic problem within the framework of alcohol abuse and alcohol dependence. Failing abstinence, specifying a safe level of alcohol intake might be useful for some patients.

Recent data from ongoing epidemiologic studies now places the threshold for ARBDs at five drinks per day.[7] One study[59] contributing to this estimate focused on 25 cases of FAS out of 1290 prospectively studied pregnancies. These pregnancies were divided into three exposure groups consisting of zero, more than zero but less than 2 drinks per day, up to 6 or more drinks per day. There were no significant increments in risk up to 6 drinks per day. When projected to the total study population, less than 1% of the women were drinking at or above this amount, but in this group, the risk for FAS was substantial.

Studies in animals similarly indicate that blood alcohol levels below 150 mg/100 mL, have either no or biologically trivial effects in offspring.[7] Reports of low levels of alcohol intake producing lowered birth weight, abnormal neurobehavioral development, and spontaneous abortion are dependent on questionable reported intakes (typically underreported), artifactual methods of data analysis (lumping "heavy" drinkers and alcohol abusers together with "moderate" drinkers), and the particular populations being sampled (overwhelmingly low socioeconomic status).

In the ongoing debate as to whether there is a safe level of alcohol, less is better, but abstinence is not the only alternative. In the United States, about 60% of all women drink to some extent.[7] This means that most Americans were very likely exposed to some alcohol in utero. Either most of us and our children are less than we might be as a result of a drink or 2 during our gestations, or there is a "no effect" zone of exposure that appears to be about 1–2 drinks per day. Although statistically significant effects have occasionally been reported at this level, none of these are biologically significant. Even in pregnancies complicated by very heavy alcohol use, only 5% of the offspring exhibit Category 1 or 2 FAS.[11]

The identification of thresholds for alcohol-related birth effects provides some guidelines for advising women in clinical care. Since there is no benefit from drinking during pregnancy, there is no reason to advise alcohol consumption at levels below any threshold. On the other hand, there is no reason for alarm if drinking does occur occasionally at sub-threshold levels. In terms of public health, however, we will achieve the greatest impact by focusing our efforts on women who are risk-drinkers, that is, those consuming alcohol above the threshold.

SUSCEPTIBILITY

Although differential susceptibility in twins indicates genetic factors contribute to alcohol's impact on the developing fetus (see above), such differences should not be interpreted to mean that relatively small amounts of alcohol are damaging depending on genetic susceptibility. Twins in these studies are born to alcohol-abusing women, not "social" drinkers. Instead, the implication is that if drinking is great enough (i.e., abused enough) to produce damage, genetic factors will contribute to the severity of such damage. Susceptibility also might be affected by the presence or absence of other pregnancy risks, such as poor nutrition, smoking, or medical illnesses. A profile of patients particularly at risk for the adverse effects of in utero alcohol exposure would be useful to clinicians who provide direct patient care. Indeed, in a carefully controlled study, we have reported that above a high threshold of exposure, African American, low socioeconomic status infants, are about 7-fold more likely to develop FAS than white infants.[59] The most important factor contributing to alcohol's potential for producing FAS, however, is low SES not race.[7,11,13]

PREVENTION

The most conservative advice from a prevention standpoint is abstention from alcohol from the time of conception throughout the entire perinatal period.[60] Such advice has been disseminated through public and professional education efforts.[10,60] Broad media coverage has been obtained for public health advisories regarding the use of alcohol during pregnancy. In 1 survey, 90% of the respondents were aware that drinking during pregnancy might be harmful.[61] The assumption that increased awareness will necessarily translate into altered behavior, however, is unrealistic. For example, 1 study found that as many as 20% of those being surveyed drank more during pregnancy than what they themselves considered harmful.[62] This suggests that public education programs may not be as successful as desired in modifying attitudes toward drinking during pregnancy. This is especially evident from the low impact of the alcohol warning label.[63,64] Since it is a limited proportion of the pop-

ulation, probably less than 5%, that incurs the greatest risk for alcohol-related birth effects, these findings suggest that mass media-based public education efforts are unlikely to modify attitudes or behavior sufficiently and therefore are not the way to prevent the kind of abusive drinking during pregnancy that results in ARBDs.

An alternative approach is to focus on prevention in the clinic or physician's office. Considerable evidence exists that this approach is more effective in decreasing alcohol intake or attaining abstinence during pregnancy and in improving pregnancy outcome than public health education.[65] The major problem here is that obstetricians and gynecologists are not yet expert in identifying alcohol abuse in their patients.

DIAGNOSING ALCOHOL ABUSE

The first step in managing alcohol abuse is detecting the problem. We have no valid biologic markers for detecting alcohol abuse. Obtaining an alcohol history as a routine part of an obstetric or gynecologic history and physical examination is a viable alternative, but these histories are subject to denial.[16] Detailed history-taking might reveal alcohol abuse, but the ability of this approach is limited by the time available to the physician to devote to such activity.

We have described a new validated questionnaire that takes little time and is more sensitive than other available questionnaires, such as the Michigan Alcohol Screening Test (MAST) and CAGE, for identifying pregnant alcohol abusers.[23] It is called T-ACE, and it is a variant of the CAGE. It asks 4 questions having to do with tolerance (T), annoyance at being asked about drinking (A), attempts to cut down (C), and drinking early in the morning (E). The questionnaire identified 69% of a group of risk drinkers and is the first validated questionnaire for use in obstetric and gynecologic practice.[23]

CONCLUSION

Alcohol abuse has been clearly established as a teratogen in humans. The effects of in utero exposure to alcohol include a characteristic collection of anomalies called fetal alcohol syndrome (FAS) and subtle behavioral disturbances in children who bear no physical stigmata of prenatal alcohol exposure.

Extensive public education efforts have alerted women to the dangers of drinking during pregnancy, but warning labels on alcoholic beverages have had little effect. Women who are heavy or abusive drinkers may have difficulty in decreasing their drinking, whether they are pregnant or not. But if they are pregnant, these women (about 5–10%) may be subjecting their unborn children to a significant risk for well-documented embryotoxic and teratogenic effects. If women are able to cut their drinking down below five drinks per occasion, and reduce the number of such occasions, the evidence from animal and human studies suggests that their babies will be much healthier.

The greater the decrease, the better the anticipated outcome. The operative advice should be "less is better."

Effective prevention strategies for FAS and alcohol-related birth defects probably relate to prevention of alcohol abuse in general. More information is needed about alcohol abuse and dependence in young women, so that more focused approaches to prevention can be developed. Professional education and involvement of physicians, nurses, and other health care providers may offer a rational and cost-effective approach to prevention of alcohol-related birth defects. If these individuals take an active role in influencing the drinking habits of their patients, it may be possible to decrease the occurrence of alcohol-related birth defects and improve pregnancy outcome.

References

1. Jones KL, Smith DW, Ulleland CN, et al. Pattern of malformation in offspring of chronic alcoholic mothers. *Lancet*. 1973;1:1267.
2. Jones KL, Smith DW. Recognition of the fetal alcohol syndrome in early infancy. *Lancet*. 1973;2:999.
3. Abel EL. *New Literature on Fetal Alcohol Exposure and Effects*. Westport, CT: Greenwood Press; 1990.
4. Abel EL. *Fetal Alcohol Abuse Syndrome*. New York: Plenum. 1998.
5. Bowen OR, Sammons JH. The alcohol-abusing patient: a challenge to the profession. *JAMA*. 1988;260:2267.
6. Jessup M, Green JR. Treatment of the pregnant alcohol-dependent woman. *J Psychoact Drugs*. 1987;19:193.
7. Abel EL. *Fetal Alcohol Syndrome: Historical, Epidemiological, Medical and Economic Aspects*. Oradell, NJ: Medical Economics; 1990.
8. Rosett HL. A clinical perspective of the fetal alcohol syndrome. *Alcohol Clin Exp Res*. 1980;4:119.
9. Institute of Medicine. *Fetal Alcohol Syndrome*. Washington, DC: National Academy Press; 1996.
10. Abel EL. An update on incidence of FAS: FAS is not an equal opportunity birth defect. *Neurotoxicol Teratol*. 1995;17:437.
11. Abel EL. Fetal Alcohol Syndrome and Fetal Alcohol Effects. New York: Plenum; 1984.
12. Sokol RJ. Alcohol and abnormal outcomes of pregnancy. *Can Med Assoc J*. 1981;125:143.
13. Abel EL, Hannigan JH. Maternal risk factor in fetal alcohol syndrome: provocative and permissive influences. *Neurotoxicol Teratol*. 1995;17:445.
14. Abel EL, Sokol RJ. Alcohol consumption during pregnancy: the dangers of moderate drinking. In: Goedde HW, Agarwal DP, eds. *Alcoholism: Biochemical and Genetic Aspects*. New York: Pergamon; 1989: 228.
15. Neugut RH. Epidemiological appraisal of the literature on the fetal alcohol syndrome in humans. *Early Human Develop*. 1981;5:411.
16. Sokol RJ, Miller SI, Reed G. Alcohol abuse during pregnancy: an epidemiologic study. *Alcohol Clin Exp Res*. 1980;4:135.
17. Sokol RJ. Alcohol abuse during pregnancy: clinical research problems. *Neurobehav Toxicol*. 1980;2:157.
18. Brown NA, Goulding EH, Fabro S, et al. Ethanol embryotoxicity: direct effects on mammalian embryos in vitro. *Science*. 1979;206:573.
19. Harlap S, Shiono PH. Alcohol, smoking and incidence of spontaneous abortions in the first and second trimester. *Lancet*. 1980;2:173.
20. Russell M, Bigler LR. Screening for alcohol-related problems in an outpatient obstetric-gynecologic clinic. *Am J Obstet Gynecol*. 1979;34:4.
21. Weiner L, Rosett HL, Edelin KC, et al. Alcohol consumption by pregnant women. *Obstet Gynecol*. 1983;61:6.
22. Morrow-Tlucak M, Ernhart C, Sokol RJ, et al. Underreporting of alcohol use in pregnancy: relationship to alcohol problem history. *Alcohol Clin Exp Res*. 1989;13:399.
23. Sokol RJ, Martier SS, Ager JW. The T-ACE questions: practical prenatal detection of risk-drinking. *Am J Obstet Gynecol*. 1989;160:863.
24. Ernhart CB, Morrow-Tlucak M, Sokol RJ, et al. Underreporting of alcohol use in pregnancy. *Alcohol Clin Exp Res*. 1988;12:506.
25. Rosett HL, Weiner L. Identifying and treating pregnant patients at risk from alcohol. *Can Med Assoc J*. 1981;125:149.
26. Kuzma JW, Sokol RJ. Maternal drinking behavior and decreased intrauterine growth. *Alcohol Clin Exp Res*. 1983;6:396.
27. Hanson JW, Streissguth AP, Smith DW. The effects of moderate alcohol consumption during pregnancy on fetal growth and morphogenesis. *J Pediatr*. 1978;92:457.
28. Sokol RJ, Miller SI, Debanne S, et al. The Cleveland NIAAA prospective alcohol-in-pregnancy study: the first year. *Neurobehav Toxicol Teratol*. 1981;3:203.
29. Abel EL, Kruger ML. Hon v. Stroh Brewing Co: what do we mean by "moderate" and "heavy" drinking? *Alcohol Clin Exp Res*. 1995;19:1024.
30. Little RE, Schultz FA, Mandell W, et al. Drinking during pregnancy. *J Stud Alc*. 1976;37:375.
31. Abel EL. Paternal exposure to alcohol. In: Sonderegger TB, ed. *Perinatal Substance Abuse*. Baltimore, MD: Johns Hopkins Univ Press; 1992:132.
32. Bielawski D, Abel EL. Acute treatment of paternal alcohol exposure produces malformations in offspring. *Alcohol*. In press, 1997.
33. Sokol RJ. Alcohol and spontaneous abortion. *Lancet*. 1980;2:1079.
34. Abel EL. Maternal alcohol consumption and spontaneous abortion. *Alc Alcohol*. 1997;32:211.
35. Kline J, Shrout P, Stein Z, et al. Drinking during pregnancy and spontaneous abortion. *Lancet*. 1980;2:176.
36. National Center for Health Statistics. *Monthly Vital Statistics Report: Annual Summary for the United States, 1979*. Hyattsville, MD: National Center for Health Statistics; 1980.
37. Rosett HL, Ouellette EM, Weiner L, et al. Therapy of heavy drinking during pregnancy. *Am J Obstet Gynecol*. 1978;51:41.
38. Tanaka H, Suzuki N, Arima M, et al. Hypoglycemia in the fetal alcohol syndrome in the rat. *Brain Develop*. 1982;4:97.
39. Henderson GI, Turner D, Patwardhan RV, et al. Inhibition of placental valine uptake after acute and chronic maternal ethanol consumption. *J Pharmacol Exp Ther*. 1981;216:465.
40. Henderson GI, Hoyumpa AM Jr, Rothschild MA, et al. Effect of ethanol and ethanol-induced hypothermia on protein synthesis in pregnant and fetal rats. *Alcohol Clin Exp Res*. 1980;4:165.
41. Flynn A, Miller SI, Martier SS, et al. Zinc status of pregnant alcoholic women: a determinant of fetal outcome. *Lancet*. 1981;1:572.
42. Fisher SE, Alcock NW, Amirian J, et al. Neonatal and maternal hair zinc levels in a nonhuman primate model of the fetal alcohol syndrome. *Alcohol Clin Exp Res*. 1988;12:417.
43. Abel EL, Hannigan JH. "J-shaped" relationship between drinking during pregnancy and birth weight. Reanalysis of prospective epidemiological data. *Alc Alcohol*. 1995;30:345.
44. Rosett HL, Synder P, Sander LW, et al. Effects of maternal drinking on neonatal state regulation. *Develop Med Child Neurol*. 1979;21:464.
45. Havlicek V, Childiaeva R, Chernick V, et al. EEG frequency spectrum characteristics of sleep rates in infants of alcoholic mothers. *Neuropaediat*. 1977;8:360.
46. Golden NL, Sokol RJ, Kuhnert BR, et al. Maternal alcohol use and infant development. *Pediatrics*. 1982;70:931.
47. Streissguth AP, Barr HM, Martin DC, et al. Effects of maternal alcohol, nicotine and caffeine use during pregnancy on infant mental and motor developments at eight months. *Alcohol Clin Exp Res*. 1980;4:152.
48. Streissguth AP, Barr HM, Sampson PD, et al. IQ at age 4 in relation to maternal alcohol use and smoking during pregnancy. *Develop Psychol*. 1989;25:3.

49. Shaywitz SE, Cohen DJ, Shaywitz BA, et al. Behavior and learning deficits in children of normal intelligence born to alcoholic mothers. *J Pediatr*. 1980;96:978.

50. Meyer LS, Riley EP. Behavioral teratology of alcohol. In: Riley EP, Vorhees CL, eds. *Handbook of Behavioral Teratology*. New York: Plenum Press; 1986:101.

51. Mattson SN, Riley E. Brain anomalies in fetal alcohol syndrome. In: Abel EL, ed. *Fetal Alcohol Syndrome: From Mechanism to Prevention*. Boca Raton, FL: CRC Press; 1996:51.

52. West JR, Hodges CA, Black AC, et al. Prenatal exposure to ethanol alters the organization of hippocampal mossy fibers in rats. *Science*. 1981;211:957.

53. Berman RF, Krahl SE. Neurophysiological correlates of fetal alcohol syndrome. In: Abel EL, ed. *Fetal Alcohol Syndrome: From Mechanism to Prevention*. Boca Raton, FL: CRC Press; 1996:69.

54. Ferrer I, Galofre E. Dendritic spine anomalies in fetal alcohol syndrome. *Neuropediatrics*. 1987;18:161.

55. Majewski F. Alcohol embryopathy: some facts and speculations about pathogenesis. *Neurobehav Toxicol Teratol*. 1981;3:129.

56. Abel EL. Prenatal effects of beverage alcohol on fetal growth. In: Messiha FS, Tyner GS, eds. *Endocrinology Aspects of Alcoholism. Progress in Biochemical Pharmacology*. 18th ed. Basel, Switzerland: Karger; 1981:111.

57. Abel EL, Dintcheff BA, Bush R, et al. Behavioral teratology of alcoholic beverages compared to ethanol. *Neurobehav Toxicol Teratol*. 1981;3:339.

58. US Department of Health and Human Services. Surgeon General's Advisory on Alcohol and Pregnancy. *FDA Drug Bull*. 1981;11:9.

59. Sokol RJ, Ager J, Martier S, et al. Significant determinants of susceptibility to alcohol teratogenicity. *Ann New York Acad Sci*. 1986; 477:87.

60. Rosett HL, Weiner L. Prevention of fetal alcohol effects. *Pediatrics*. 1982; 69:813.

61. Little RE, Grathwohl HL, Streissguth AP, et al. Public awareness and knowledge about the risks of drinking during pregnancy in Mulnomah County, Oregon. *Am J Publ Hlth*. 1981;71:312.

62. Minor MJ, Van Dort B. Prevention research in the teratogenic effects of alcohol. *Prevent Med*. 1982;11:346.

63. Hankin J, Sloan J, Firestone I, et al. The Alcohol Beverage Warning Label: when did knowledge increase? *Alcohol Clin Exp Res*. 1993;17:428.

64. Hankin J, Sloan J, Firestone I, et al. A time series analysis of the impact of the alcohol warning label on antenatal drinking. *Alcohol Clin Exp Res*. 1993;17:284.

65. Rosett HL, Weiner L, Edelin KC, et al. Strategies for prevention of fetal alcohol effects. *Obstet Gynecol*. 1981;57:1.

CHARACTERIZING THE EFFECT OF ENVIRONMENTAL AND OCCUPATIONAL EXPOSURES ON REPRODUCTION AND DEVELOPMENT

Donald R. Mattison

INTRODUCTION

Reproduction and development are essential for maintenance of all species, and like other biological processes, are vulnerable to impairment.[1-5] As recognition of this vulnerability has spread, individuals have become increasingly concerned about their working and living environments and exposures to drugs or chemicals that can affect their fertility, reproduction, pregnancy, or offspring.[2,6-9] In addressing these issues it is important to understand how to define exposures that represent potential risks to reproduction or development. Similarly, it is important to correctly identify exposures that do not represent a risk to fertility, pregnancy, the fetus, or the infant. In either situation, accurate and appropriate guidance concerning the extent of reproductive and developmental risk, if any, must be provided.

When clinicians are asked for advice on the relationship between workplace or environmental exposures and adverse outcome, the questions typically represent 1 of 2 different concerns: (1) what is the effect of this exposure on my ability to become pregnant or on my offspring? (2) I have had an adverse outcome (i.e., inability to conceive, spontaneous abortion, premature delivery, fetal or neonatal death, or my baby has a malformation); were any of these adverse outcomes caused by any workplace or environmental exposures before or during my pregnancy?

Although quantification of the actual risk following exposure to a chemical (or group of chemicals), radiation, or biological agent(s) is complex, there is a well-defined process for reaching a reasonable scientific and medically sound determination of risk to reproduction[7] and development.[8] This process is called *risk assessment*, a formal scientific method applicable to both the definition of risk and assessment of causation. The risk assessment process utilized in this chapter was formulated by the National Academy of Sciences[10-13] and is used by U.S. federal regulatory agencies for a range of health hazard evaluations.[14,15]

The goals of this chapter are to (1) define the steps that are used in risk assessment for reproduction and development; (2) review the epidemiology of reproductive and developmental failure; and (3) explore the risks for reproduction and development that may be associated with occupational or environmental exposures.

RISK ASSESSMENT FOR REPRODUCTION AND DEVELOPMENT

The process of risk assessment for human reproduction and development incorporates 4 interrelated exercises.[10,11,14,15] The first is hazard identification—can this agent or mixture of agents produce adverse reproductive or developmental effects in humans or experimental animals? If so, what type of effect is produced and what is the window of susceptibility for the effect(s)? The second step is hazard characterization—at a minimum this requires dose-response data. Note that dose-response relationships in developmental toxicity can be complicated by multiple competing endpoints, such as reduced fetal weight, disruption of fetal development, and fetal death. Because of this, dose-response relationships may not always have the familiar sigmoidal shape.[16] In addition, the use of toxicity data in risk assessment implies extrapolation of animal data to humans; therefore, it is important to obtain as much information as possible on the site of toxicity and mechanism of action. The third step is exposure assessment—what is the likely amount and duration of exposure and how much of the agent was absorbed and distributed to the reproductive system, fetus, or placenta? The final step is risk characterization—how likely is the given exposure to result in an adverse reproductive or developmental outcome and what degree of uncertainty is inherent in that estimation?[11]

HAZARD IDENTIFICATION

The goal of reproductive and developmental toxicology is to identify chemical, physical, or biological agents that alter or impair reproduction or development before humans are exposed and suffer adverse effects. This means that chemical, physical, or biological agents are initially evaluated in experimental animals and data from those experiments are translated into exposure levels, which are thought to protect human populations from reproductive or developmental toxicity. It is not always possible, however, to identify all reproductive or developmental toxicants in animal models. Therefore epidemiological studies are also conducted to define the human effects of the exposure(s) of interest.[17,18] This means that it is necessary to consider both animal and human endpoints of concern for reproductive and developmental toxicity and define methods for relating these endpoints across species.[14,15,19-21]

REPRODUCTIVE AND DEVELOPMENTAL ENDPOINTS IN HUMANS

Human reproductive[7] and developmental[8] toxicity outcomes include alterations of male and female reproductive function (gametogenesis and gamete release), conception, transport, implantation, embryonic and fetal growth, fetal structure,

TABLE 12-1	EXAMPLES OF HUMAN ENDPOINTS OF REPRODUCTIVE AND DEVELOPMENTAL TOXICITY

Reproductive
  Hypothalamic dysfunction
  Pituitary dysfunction
  Gonadal dysfunction
  Anatomic changes in reproductive organs
Developmental
  Embryonic or fetal death
  Infant mortality
  Placental, cord, and fetal membrane abnormalities
  Intrauterine or postnatal growth retardation
  Change in gestation age at delivery (premature, postmature)
  Altered sex ratio
Birth defects
  Major, minor, mild
  Malformations, deformations, disruptions
  Single defects, syndromes, sequences, patterns
  Mutations, chromosomal defects, monogenic disorders
Developmental disabilities
  Abnormal maturation
  Abnormal sexual development or function
  Mental retardation/learning disability
  Specific organ system dysfunction
  Visual impairment
  Hearing impairment
  Cerebral palsy and other motor handicaps
  Other sensory disturbances
  Behavioral disorders
Transplacental carcinogenesis and mutagenesis (genotoxicity)

and function and embryonic or fetal death (Table 12-1). As indicated previously, many of these endpoints may not be independent events. For many developmental toxicants there is a spectrum of adverse developmental outcomes that may vary in frequency, severity, and type.[14–16] For example, at low doses a toxicant may produce growth retardation. At higher doses, a specific malformation may occur. At even higher doses, fetal death may occur. For reproductive toxicants, low doses may be associated with decreased fertility, as reflected in time to achieve pregnancy, while higher doses may be associated with infertility.

It is also possible among a population exposed to a known developmental toxicant to find individuals who do not display all the structural and functional consequences attributable to that exposure. This may reflect variability in the amount of the toxicant reaching the fetus due to genetic or any other factors that affect the absorption, distribution, metabolism, or elimination of the toxicant. The net result is that both outcome and severity of the reproductive or developmental effect may be variable. The sources of this variability include differences in dose, timing of exposure, host susceptibility (male, female, maternal, and fetal), and interactions with other environmental factors such as nutrition.

REPRODUCTIVE AND DEVELOPMENTAL ENDPOINTS IN ANIMALS

Reproductive and developmental toxicity in animals is defined as the adverse effect of a chemical on the male, female, or conceptus associated with exposure prior to or during pregnancy. These effects may be manifest during the embryonic or fetal periods, or postnatally. Reproductive or developmental toxicity can include decreased fertility, growth retardation, death of the conceptus, structural malformation, and functional deficits.

The endpoints of reproductive and developmental toxicity encountered in experimental animals may not mimic those observed in humans exposed to the same toxicant. This is an important concept to grasp so as not to discard the results from animal studies when they have different outcomes from that observed in humans. Similarly, specific toxic endpoints observed in humans are not always reproduced in experimental animals. The absence of absolute uniformity of response across species is not surprising, however, when the differences that exist between the anatomy and physiology of reproduction and development and the conditions of human exposure and experimental animal dosing are considered. For example, differences in dosage, gonadal physiology, reproductive tract control and function, placentation, metabolism, pharmacokinetics, critical periods of development or gonadal function, and duration of gestation can influence the expression or reproductive and developmental toxicity.

In general, reproductive and developmental toxicity experiments should include a dose that is toxic to the male, female, or pregnant female. This may or may not result in toxic effect to reproduction or the conceptus (death, morphological alteration, delayed development, and/or functional impairment). One important component of the identification of a developmental toxicant is to determine the relative toxicity of the substance to the adult mother and the developing conceptus.[22] In humans, there appear to be exposures that produce developmental toxicity in the absence of apparent maternal toxicity (e.g., diethylstilbestrol, ionizing radiation) and exposures that produce developmental toxicity at therapeutic levels or that result in maternal physiological or toxicological changes (e.g., tobacco, steroid hormones, alcohol, methylmercury, 13-cis-retinoic acid, phenytoin, and valproic acid).

TIMING OF EXPOSURE IN REPRODUCTIVE AND DEVELOPMENTAL TOXICITY

Reproduction and development are dependent on the completion of multiple sequential processes. As a result, the timing of exposure in relationship to either reproduction or development is important in defining the consequences of exposure.

Our understanding of the differential impact of exposure at various stages of oocyte development and maturation remains

TABLE 12-2 | CRITICAL PERIODS FOR DEVELOPMENTAL TOXICITY IN THE HUMAN[a]

Days Form LMP	Days From Conception	Biological Event
14	0	Ovulation
15–16	1	Conception
19–21	5–7	Implantation/blastula
38–39	24–25	Anterior neuropore closes
40–41	26–27	Posterior neuropore closes
41–42	27–28	Upper limb bud develops
43–44	29–30	Lower limb bud develops
51	37	Crown-rump (10 mm)
60–61	46–47	Heart septation
70–72	56–58	Palate closed
98	84	Second trimester begins

[a]Based on day 28 of menstrual cycle.

incomplete. Exposure at different stages of spermatogenesis is associated with varying degrees of vulnerability and consequences.

Most developmental toxicants produce their effects during specific critical developmental periods. These periods of developmental vulnerability vary across both agents and species. A fundamental concept of developmental toxicology is that some stages of embryonic and fetal development are more vulnerable than others. The time of exposure to a developmental toxicant influences both the severity of damage and the type of defect (Table 12-2).

For some animal developmental toxicants, detailed studies have been conducted at different doses and times during pregnancy.[2,3] For these chemicals, a critical period, sensitive developmental processes, and potential mechanisms of action can be defined. Such studies indicate that the susceptible period is generally the time of maximal tissue proliferation and differentiation in a particular organ. Time specificity has been found in nearly all cases where developmental toxicity of the human has been proven and studied in detail.

It is generally thought that exposure during the preimplantation or presomite periods (0 to 14 days after fertilization) produces little altered morphogenesis because the embryo either dies or regenerates completely. However, this hypothesis may be incorrect.[23–25] During organogenesis the embryo is highly sensitive to developmental toxicity and exposure can produce major morphologic changes. After this period, the fetus is less sensitive to morphologic alterations, but functional changes can occur in selected organs throughout pregnancy and even during postnatal development (e.g., effects of lead on the central nervous system).

By the third trimester, much of the structure of the fetus has been defined. During this period, many functional characteristics of the fetus are being developed. For example, cellular communication (e.g., neuronal contacts) is developing, and the cell number in many organ systems is increasing. The fetus remains vulnerable to cytotoxic or disruptive processes during the third trimester.

HAZARD IDENTIFICATION WITH INCOMPLETE DATA

If there is no animal or human data available that addresses the reproductive or developmental hazard posed by a chemical, it is difficult to estimate the risk at any exposure. The most that can be said is that the risk to reproduction or development is unknown. The one caveat is if exposure is at a level that produces male, female, or maternal toxicity, then an indirect effect is always possible. If, however, there are any human reports or animal studies that suggest a possible hazard or there are physical or chemical properties of the compound that would make it more or less likely to be a hazard, then, depending on the weight of the evidence, it is important to proceed further in defining the exposure and calculating the effect.

In characterizing the potential for reproductive or developmental toxicity of an untested chemical, it is important to know if the physical structure is similar to a known reproductive or developmental toxicant (e.g., methyl testosterone and testosterone). Does the compound belong to a class of compounds known to be reproductive or developmental toxicants (e.g., antimetabolites or antithyroid compounds)? Does the drug or compound have a mechanism of action similar to that of a known reproductive or developmental toxicant (e.g., bind with an estrogen receptor)? Is the compound a mutagen or cytotoxic agent (e.g., cyclophosphamide)? Any of these characteristics heighten suspicion, suggesting the potential for reproductive or developmental toxicity even when there are no animal or human data available.

If there are human studies that evaluate reproductive or developmental toxicity, it is important to define the outcome pattern for each study and the timing of exposure associated with that outcome. Risk assessment should provide an estimate for each different possible outcome. Some outcomes are less "severe" than others and their risk might be acceptable compared to other possible outcomes.

If there are animal studies that explore reproductive or developmental toxicity of the agent, it is important to characterize the pattern of toxicity in each animal species, as well as the highest no-observed-adverse effect level for each study. Are there any weaknesses of study design that would lower confidence in the study?

Implicit in this first step in risk assessment is the assumption that reproductive or developmental hazards identified in animals are predictive of reproductive or developmental hazards in humans. Note that the converse, failure to demonstrate reproductive or developmental hazards, is also generally assumed to reflect safety following human exposure. It is important to critically review the accuracy of this assumption.

Frankos has reviewed the concordance of animal and human data for 38 drugs reported to be developmental toxicants in humans and 165 reported not to produce developmental toxicity.[26] Of the 38 drugs identified as human teratogens, 37 were positive in at least 1 species of experimental animal and 29 were positive in more than 1 test species. Among 165 compounds identified as nonteratogenic in humans, only 47 were negative in all species tested.

Jelovsek et al. have also conducted an analysis of the predictive power of developmental toxicity testing in experimental animals using statistical techniques.[27] These studies suggest that combining animal data using statistical models is generally useful for predicting human developmental toxicants. Unfortunately, positive or negative animal studies do not always mean hazard or safety for humans. However, that evidence should be evaluated for hazard identification. A more detailed assessment of the rules used by developmental toxicologists to assign hazard for developmental toxicity has been assembled and may assist the process of hazard identification.[21]

HAZARD CHARACTERIZATION

At a minimum, hazard characterization requires demonstration of a dose-response relationship for the reproductive or developmental toxicant. Given differences in development among animal species, it is desirable to have information on the site of toxicity and mechanism of action in the animal species studied. Like hazard identification, hazard characterization also suffers from the lack of published peer-reviewed data.[1–6,28] As a result, even the minimal requirement for dose-response information is often not available for risk assessment.

For any chemical that has been identified as a reproductive or developmental toxicant in either a human or animal study, it is important to know if the offending agent is the parent compound or a metabolite. This is especially true when animal studies are positive because the metabolic pathway may be different in humans. The metabolite that produced the reproductive or developmental toxicity in the animals studied may not be produced in the human. What is the compound's absorption by different likely routes of exposure and what is the likely gonadal or fetal exposure at different doses (extent of placental transport)? In addition, one should extract from the studies different levels of effect such as lowest-observed-adverse effect level (LOAEL), the no-observed-adverse effect level (NOAEL), the toxic effect level, and for drugs, the therapeutic effect level. All of these levels will play a role in assessing the likelihood that a given exposure is above or below the threshold for developmental toxicity.

EXPOSURE ASSESSMENT

The goal of exposure assessment is to determine if there was exposure to a dose that could cause an indirect or direct reproductive or developmental effect. If the exposure was at or near toxic levels, or if the exposed individual manifests toxic side effects, then there is always the possibility of an indirect effect

whether the compound is known or suspected to be a hazard. If the compound is a known or suspected hazard, the toxic side effects are evidence that the chemical(s) did get into the bloodstream and thus reproductive or developmental processes are at greater risk. The route of exposure and absorption via that route bring into play our knowledge of reproductive and developmental physiology and its likely effect on the pharmacokinetics of the compound. All of this information is used to estimate the dose to which the reproductive system, placenta, or fetus was exposed.

Because of unique windows of vulnerability for reproduction and development, exposure assessment requires accurate determination of the dose, duration of exposure, and relationship of exposure to timing of reproductive or developmental processes. If, for example, the exposure occurred prior to conception and clearance of the parent compound and its metabolites also occurred prior to conception, it is unlikely that any excess fetal risk would result. Although the health care professional may have some knowledge of dose, duration of exposure, and relationship of exposure to stages of reproduction or fetal development for prescription drugs, information on environmental or occupational exposures is likely to be scant.

RISK CHARACTERIZATION

Risk characterization, the final step of risk assessment, requires a methodology for translating toxicity data in animals and humans and estimates of time and duration of exposure into a qualitative or quantitative estimate of excess risk. On a population level there are methods for estimating human risk from animal studies. However, there is still disagreement on the validity of these methods because they do not consider species differences in reproduction or development, nor do they consider species differences in site or mechanism of action of the reproductive or developmental toxicants.

If the window of exposure is inconsistent with a known or suspected effect and yet the compound is a known teratogen, how much reassurance will an exposed individual get from our calculation?[6] It is at this point that the risk assessment procedure becomes somewhat subjective and we must admit the lack of hard and fast rules for assigning the final risk. However, some groups have developed explicit approaches for characterizing both the data and risk for developmental toxicity (Teris). Finally, we must clearly communicate the quality and quantity of data from which our estimates of reproductive and developmental risk are derived.[11,12]

SUCCESSFUL REPRODUCTION AND DEVELOPMENT

In the sexually mature couple, successful reproduction assumes conception at the desired time. After conception, the

TABLE 12-3	**INDIVIDUAL AND COUPLE DEPENDENT FACTORS THAT MAY INFLUENCE REPRODUCTION**	
Reproductive Endpoint	*Factor or Exposure*	*Potential Impact on Endpoint*
Male fecundity	Vasectomy	Decrease sperm release
	Mumps	Decrease sperm production
	Fever	Decrease sperm production
	Varicocoele	Decrease sperm production
	Diabetes	Decrease libido
	Hypertension	Decrease libido
	Prescription drugs	Decrease libido, spermatogenesis
	Smoking	Decrease libido, spermatogenesis
	Alcohol	Decrease testicular function
	Recreational drugs	Impair testicular function
Female fecundity	Contraception	Decrease fecundity
	Tubal ligation	Decrease fecundity
	Infection	Decrease fecundity, impair fallopian tube function
	Prescription drugs	Impair ovulation and fecundity
	Smoking	Impair fecundity
	Alcohol	Impair fecundity
	Recreational drugs	Impair fecundity
	Age	Decrease fecundity
Frequency of intercourse	Infection	Decrease fertility
	Prescription drugs	Decrease fertility
	Alcohol	Decrease fertility
	Recreational drugs	Decrease fertility
Spontaneous abortion	Maternal age	Increase abortion
	Smoking	Increase abortion
	Alcohol	Increase abortion
	Recreational drugs	Increase abortion
	Infection	Increase abortion
	History of prior spontaneous abortion	Increase abortion

embryo implants within the uterus and develops normally, both structurally and functionally. Some abnormalities of reproduction, fetal development, or maternal adaptation to the pregnancy will lead to early pregnancy loss (unrecognized or recognized spontaneous abortion). Successful reproduction and development also assumes that the pregnancy progresses to term (38 to 42 weeks) when labor occurs. Correct timing of delivery is essential because prematurity and postmaturity are associated with increased morbidity and mortality. Note that age at birth and weight at birth are critical determinants of postnatal adaptation. Finally, successful reproduction requires that the infant adapt to life outside the uterus and grow and develop normally, including subsequent sexual development.

Successful reproduction is dependent on both individual and couple factors (Fig. 12-1, Table 12-3). Fecundity is the capacity of a male, female, or couple to produce offspring. Fertility is the actual production of offspring by a couple. Factors that impair male or female fecundity will have an adverse impact on fertility. Trivial examples of factors impairing fecundity are surgical sterilization (vasectomy or tubal ligation). Some infections can alter testicular function, either by direct

cell destruction or fever. Diabetes and hypertension both produce vascular damage that can impair libido or sexual responsiveness. Finally, smoking, alcohol consumption, and use of recreational drugs or substances of abuse are also associated with impairment of male and female fecundity.

In the female, contraceptives impair ovulation (oral contraceptives), block sperm-egg interaction or fertilization (barrier methods, condom, diaphragm, cervical cap), or implantation (intrauterine devices). Infections can alter the structure and function of the cervix, uterus, or tubes and as a result impair fecundity. Some prescription drugs have been demonstrated to alter the frequency of ovulation and impair fecundity.

Couple-dependent factors, such as the frequency of intercourse, may also alter fertility. Belsey[29] evaluated the effect of frequency of intercourse on the number of conceptions within 6 months of stopping contraception (Table 12-4). If intercourse occurred at least 4 times per week, more than 80% of the couples were able to conceive within 6 months. If, however, intercourse occurred less than once per week, only 16.7% of the couples were able to conceive within 6 months. Similar studies by Barrett[30,31] provided data that can be used to define the impact of intercourse frequency and the cycle day

TABLE 12-4	EFFECT OF FREQUENCY OF INTERCOURSE ON NUMBER OF CONCEPTIONS WITHIN SIX MONTHS	
Frequency of Intercourse (per Week)	Number of Cases	Conceptions Within 6 Months (%)
<1	24	16.7
1–2	109	32.1
2–3	123	46.3
3–4	100	51
>=4	72	83.3

Data from reference 30.

on which intercourse occurred, on the cycle specific fertility, that is, the proportion of couples that conceive within a given menstrual cycle. These data suggest that frequency of intercourse has an impact on fertility, including the amount of time needed to achieve pregnancy. In addition, it appears that both female fecundity and the likelihood of spontaneous abortion (Table 12-5) are dependent on the timing of intercourse with respect to the time of ovulation.[22,31]

Spontaneous abortion is considered an endpoint of reproductive toxicity because it occurs early in pregnancy and in some cases is incorrectly identified as infertility. A range of factors is associated with increased risk for spontaneous abortion. These include maternal age and poorly defined ovarian and uterine physiological and endocrine factors. It has been recognized for some time that risk of chromosome errors increases with maternal age.[17] Other factors associated with increased risk for spontaneous abortion include cigarette smoking, probably due to altered endocrine milieu or uterine function. Although alcohol and recreational drugs have been associated with increased risk for spontaneous abortion it is not known if this association is a result of these exposures or other associated lifestyle factors. Finally, women with a history of prior spontaneous abortions are at increased risk for a miscarriage.

TABLE 12-5	EFFECT OF CYCLE DAY ON FEMALE FECUNDITY AND RISK OF SPONTANEOUS ABORTION	
Cycle Day	Female Fecundity	Miscarriage Rate
−5	0.26	0.106
−4	0.33	0.118
−3	0.33	0.055
−2	0.41	0.032
−1	0.28	0.070
0-Ovulation	0.28	0.075
+1	0.11	0.055
+2	0.05	0.091
+3	0.03	0.240
+4	0.03	0.90
+5	0.03	0.90

Data from references 32 and 33.

Reproduction involves processes in the male and female leading to the production and release of mature sperm and eggs such that fertilization and subsequent development occurs. Development generally is considered to begin after implantation and formation of the embryo. Note that there are clearly overlapping temporal periods associated with reproductive failure. For example, if ovarian function is impaired early in the pregnancy, miscarriage can occur. This is one possible explanation for the increased risk for spontaneous abortion among smoking women.[32–35]

Reproductive toxicity has many unique differences from toxicity to other systems. Other forms of occupational or environmental toxicity typically involve the development of disease in an exposed individual. Reproduction however, requires interaction between 2 individuals. Therefore, when reproductive toxicity occurs, it will be expressed within a reproductive unit, or couple. This unique, albeit obvious, couple-dependent aspect makes reproductive toxicology distinct since it is possible that exposure to a toxicant by 1 member of a reproductive couple (e.g., male) will be manifest by adverse reproductive outcome in the other member of the couple (e.g., increased frequency of spontaneous abortion or birth defect). Therefore, any attempt to deal with environmental or occupational causes of reproductive (as well as developmental) toxicity must address the couple-specific aspect of reproduction (Table 12-3); more detailed considerations of reproductive toxicity can be found in several reviews.[36,37]

There are other unique aspects of reproductive toxicity. Reproduction, unlike renal, cardiac, or pulmonary function, occurs intermittently. This means that environmental exposures may interfere with reproduction, but go unnoticed during periods when fertility and conception are not desired. This intermittent characteristic of reproduction can make the identification of a reproductive toxicant in humans more difficult. Complete assessment of the functional integrity of the reproductive system requires that the couple attempt pregnancy.

EPIDEMIOLOGY OF REPRODUCTIVE FAILURE

Given the biological and social events needed for successful reproduction and the many "common" factors associated with reproductive failure, it is not surprising that reproductive failure should occur. However, the actual role of environmental and occupational exposures in reproductive failure is less well defined. To appreciate the potential impact of environmental or occupational exposures on reproduction it is necessary to explore the epidemiology of reproductive failure.

Recent data from the National Survey of Family Growth[38] suggest that from 10–20% of married women, depending on age, have impaired fertility (Table 12-6). While impaired

| TABLE 12-6 | DISTRIBUTION OF REPRODUCTIVE STATUS AMONG CURRENTLY MARRIED WOMEN |

Fertility Status	Age of Married Woman		
	15–24	25–34	35–44
Surgically sterile			
Contraceptive	5.6%	26.0%	51.5%
Noncontraceptive	0.3%	1.1%	7.3%
Impaired fertility	10.0%	12.5%	13.9%
Fertile	84.1%	60.4%	27.3%

Data from reference 39.

| TABLE 12-8 | CAUSES OF INFERTILITY IN COUPLES EVALUATED IN INFERTILITY CLINICS |

Etiology	Range Reported
Male factors	20–50%
Azospermia	5–15%
Oligospermia	15–40%
Female factors	25–85%
Tubal function	5–85%
Impaired ovulation	5–50%
Abnormal cervic/uterus	5–50%
Multiple causes	10–25%
Unexplained	0–20%

Modified from reference 32.

fertility is slightly less frequent among younger women (10% among those less than 25 years, 13.9% among those greater than 35) fertility clearly changes with age, but primarily due to surgical sterilization.

One way to explore the potential impact of environmental factors (infection, biological, and chemical) influencing fertility is to look at time dependent trends in infertility (Table 12-7). Between 1965 and 1982 there has been a 3-fold increase in infertility among couples between 15 and 24 years of age. Although there have been smaller increases in infertility over this period among some older age groups, they do not appear to be as strongly affected. The high incidence of surgical sterilization and completion of family size among older women makes it possible, however, that adverse reproductive effects may be missed. Given that fertility is traditionally highest among younger couples,[29,38] this increase in impaired fertility among women between 15 and 24 is of heightened concern. Causes for this 3-fold increase in infertility are not known. While most available evidence suggests that infectious diseases are responsible for a significant component of this increase, this does not rule out an adverse impact of environmental factors on reproduction.

In general, the causes of infertility are thought to be roughly one third male, one third female, and one third couple.[29,38,39,40] The actual breakdown, however, varies from clinic to clinic (Table 12-8). Data from the National Survey of Family Growth[38] suggest that 15.4% of women between the ages 15–44 have received services to either assist conception or prevent miscarriage, drugs for ovulation were used on 3% and surgery for blocked tubes on 1.5%.

Although it is expected that sperm count, sperm motility, sperm morphology, and semen composition all impact on male fecundity,[40-46] only sperm count and motility have been demonstrated to have an effect. Female fecundity has been shown to be influenced by age.[47,48]

As suggested by these data, impaired fecundity is not uncommon. Factors associated with impaired fecundity, or fertility, need to be considered in exploring putative environmental causes of impaired reproduction. Failure to do so may obscure the identification of a reproductive toxicant, or falsely identify a compound as a reproductive toxicant. Both courses have unnecessary economic and human health costs.

EPIDEMIOLOGY OF SPONTANEOUS ABORTION

Spontaneous abortion or miscarriage is often defined as involuntary pregnancy loss prior to fetal viability (Table 12-9). Spontaneous abortion is influenced by maternal age[8,17,30] and prior reproductive history.

| TABLE 12-7 | PERCENTAGE OF MARRIED WOMEN WHO ARE INFERTILE (EXCLUDING SURGICAL STERILIZATION) |

Age	1965	1976	1982
15–19	0.6	2.1	2.1
20–24	3.6	6.7	10.6
25–29	7.2	10.8	8.7
30–34	14.0	16.1	13.6
35–39	18.4	22.8	24.4
40–44	27.7	31.1	27.2

Data from reference 38.

| TABLE 12-9 | DISTRIBUTION OF PREGNANCY LOSS AMONG MARRIED COUPLES |

Pregnancy Amount of Loss	Maternal Age and % Loss		
	15–24	25–34	35–44
All	11.6	19.7	31.1
1	9.8	14.1	19.9
2	1.0	3.7	6.6
3+	0.8	1.9	4.6

Data from "Reproductive Impairments Among Married Couples." United States National Survey of Family Growth. Series 23, Number 11.

TABLE 12-10	**DISTRIBUTION OF EARLY PREGNANCY LOSS BY GESTATIONAL AGE**

Gestational Age (Weeks)	Percentage of Pregnancy Loss
<7	10
>7–11	45
>11–15	30
>15–19	10
>19–23	5
>23–27	2

Data from reference 52.

TABLE 12-11	**LIFE TABLE OF REPRODUCTIVE SUCCESS**

Reproductive Event	Outcome
Couples attempting pregnancy	1000
Conceptions (occurs midcycle, 14 days before menses)	600–1000
Preimplantation loss (About 50% between conception and implantation)	(300–500)[a]
Chemical Pregnancies (+hCG, about 7 days before, missed menses until 7 weeks)	300–500
Urecognized loss (15% to 30% up to 7 weeks)	(100–150)
Clinical pregnancy (clinically recognized)	200–350
Recognized loss (15% between 7 and 28 weeks)	(30–50)
Continuing pregnancies (>28 weeks)	170–300
Stillbirths (<10%)	(20–30)
Premature births (>10%)	(20–30)
Term births	110–240

Data modified from references 17, 18, and 52.
[a]The numbers in parentheses represent reproductive loss.

While early pregnancy loss occurs "early in pregnancy" it is becoming more common to have information concerning the frequency of this adverse outcome in some settings. There are several reasons for our growing knowledge about this previously undefined outcome. One is the increasing availability of sensitive and specific assays for hCG (human chorionic gonadotropin). They have been used in several studies as research tools to define the presence of the very early pregnancy.[50,51] However, early in pregnancy the woman or her physician may assume that a delayed period is simply that and not an early pregnancy lost by miscarriage. In addition, many women, with known or suspected pregnancy, who have an early pregnancy loss do not seek medical care. For these reasons the body of knowledge on early pregnancy loss is incomplete. This is unfortunate as general knowledge of the rate of early pregnancy loss by age, race, and other factors is essential for evaluation of studies (or allegations) exploring the impact of occupational or environmental factors on miscarriage.

The timing of early pregnancy loss (and all pregnancy loss) has been studied in some detail.[17,52] Earlier studies, conducted prior to the availability of sensitive assays for detection of pregnancy relied on the clinical detection of pregnancy (Table 12-10). These studies suggest that among pregnancies that end in miscarriage, most end within the first trimester and are frequently associated with chromosomal abnormalities. More recent studies using sensitive and specific hCG assays suggest that about 15% of pregnancies are lost around the time of expected menses[50,51] and another 15% are lost after 1 diagnosis of pregnancy during the first trimester.

The number of couples attempting pregnancy during a cycle of unprotected intercourse resulting in a living infant born at term is quite small (Table 12-11). Even these term births will not all be normal. In addition, there are other factors—such as maternal and paternal age, smoking habits, lifestyle factors, and so on—which influence the success of *all* these stages of reproduction.

Between 10 and 20% of all recognized pregnancies will end in spontaneous abortion.[50] It is also estimated that an additional 10–20% of pregnancies are lost prior to the recognition of pregnancy.[47] These pregnancies are lost before the pregnancy is confirmed, either by a missed or delayed menstrual period. Some studies have suggested that as many as 75% of all conceptions are lost before delivery—either as preimplantation or postimplantation loss before the recognition of pregnancy or as miscarriage after the recognition of pregnancy. Clearly, miscarriage early in the pregnancy is a common outcome of many pregnancies.

Another characteristic of spontaneous abortion is that it is a heterogeneous reproductive outcome, with many defined (as well as uncharacterized) causes. Some miscarriages are chromosomally normal; others are not. Some miscarriages are structurally normal; others have a malformed embryo or fetus.

One survey examined 2607 early pregnancy losses[49] among women admitted to hospitals in London. In 804 of those pregnancies, no identifiable tissue was found. Malformations were identified in 73 of the pregnancies. Most of the malformations were of the central nervous system.

A substantial proportion of miscarriages—between 30 and 50%—have abnormal chromosomes. In most of the cases, these anomalies are incompatible with survival. This is higher than the proportion of chromosomal anomalies among stillbirths (about 5%) and livebirths (about 0.5%). Approximately 90% of those embryos with abnormal chromosome number will be spontaneously aborted, an additional 1% will be stillborn and the remaining approximately 10% will be born alive.

Knowledge that a miscarriage, stillbirth, or liveborn child has a chromosome anomaly provides information on the timing of the abnormality and relation to putative exposures. Chromosome anomalies occur prior to the time of conception in either sperm or egg, or at the time of conception. In addition, studies of miscarriages, stillbirths, or livebirths suggest that the extra chromosome in trisomies is more often from the mother than the father.[51] It has been estimated that 25% of all early pregnancy loss is produced by errors of maternal gametogenesis, 5% by errors of paternal gametogenesis, 5% by errors of fertilization, and 5% by errors in early division of the zygote.[14]

The risk that a chromosomally normal conception will miscarry is approximately 10%. In these pregnancies however the embryo or fetus may be absent or grossly deformed, suggesting the influence of early disruption of the developmental process. Because miscarriage occurs frequently, it has been possible to define several factors associated with an increased risk including: maternal age, maternal smoking, use of an intrauterine device, and history of prior spontaneous abortion. The impact of age on miscarriage appears to effect both the chromosomally normal and abnormal embryos. With increasing maternal age there is an increase in the incidence of conceptions with abnormal chromosome number, including trisomy 21 (Down syndrome). Smoking also increases the risk of miscarriage. Interestingly the increase appears to be a result of an increased loss of chromosomally normal embryos.[52–54] The presence of an intrauterine device also increases the risk of miscarriage of a chromosomally normal conceptus.[55–57]

There are other suspected causes of early pregnancy loss. Gynecologic pathology or abnormalities of the female reproductive tract have been associated with early pregnancy loss. Immunological factors have been postulated; this remains a hypothesis that requires more detailed exploration.

Early in pregnancy, progesterone production by the ovary (corpus luteum) is needed to maintain the pregnancy. Some have suggested that early pregnancy loss among some women is a result of inadequate progesterone production. Additional effort will be needed to move this suggestion beyond the hypothesis stage.

Infections (viral, bacterial, and mycoplasma), and their associated fevers and/or endotoxins have also been associated with early pregnancy loss. Several studies have suggested that the presence of an intrauterine device increases the risk of early pregnancy loss.[49] As oocytes and sperm age in the reproductive tract (i.e., the time between insemination and ovulation increases) there is an increase in chromosomal abnormalities.[35] This suggests that the incidence of early pregnancy loss will increase when the time between ovulation and insemination increases (see Table 12-5). In these studies the risk of early pregnancy loss increased when insemination and ovulation were separated by more than 3 days.

MATERNAL OCCUPATIONAL OR ENVIRONMENTAL EXPOSURES AND MISCARRIAGE

While this section explores the impact of maternal exposures on pregnancy loss it is important to note that paternal exposures may also have an effect.[59] In general, many studies exploring occupational or environmental influences on early pregnancy loss have used location of resident, job title, or simply reported estimates of exposure by the woman or couple. This is a potentially serious disadvantage of many other reproductive effects studies as well. The disadvantage created by this loose classification of exposure is that errors in the identification of reproductive and developmental toxicants can occur. Another corollary of this misclassification of exposure is inability to group individuals by reproductive characteristics. This also can lead to misidentification of chemicals or exposures as reproductive or developmental toxicants when in fact they are not.

Although several epidemiological studies have explored the relationship between maternal occupation and miscarriage, a small number appear to have a strong association.[50] Among women employed in health care settings, exposure to anesthesia, cytostatic drugs, and ethylene oxide has been suggested to increase the risk for early pregnancy loss. Among women exposed to anesthetic gasses there appears to be an increase in the risk of spontaneous abortion, and recent studies have also suggested a decrease in the cycle specific fertility.

Data from studies exploring the effect of cytostatic (anticancer) drug exposure to nursing personnel have similar findings to those of the anesthetic gas studies.[50] There is a single study exploring the effect of ethylene oxide—used as a gas sterilizing agent in medical facilities—on early pregnancy loss. This Finnish study suggests that exposure to high concentrations of ethylene oxide early in pregnancy was associated with an approximate 2-fold increased risk for spontaneous abortion.[58]

Other occupations have also been explored for an association with spontaneous abortion. By focusing on occupation and not quantitating exposure, these studies do not identify specific chemicals which increase the risk for spontaneous abortion. In addition, many of these studies should be viewed more as hypothesis gathering rather than providing confirmation of a relationship between given exposures and miscarriage or early pregnancy loss.

PREMATURE BIRTHS

The World Health Organization and International Federation of Obstetricians and Gynecologists definition of gestational age at delivery is: preterm, <37 completed weeks (<259 days); term, 37 to <42 week (259–293 days); and postterm, ≥42 weeks (≥294 days).[60] Premature birth, at less than 37 completed weeks of gestation, is a major cause of perinatal morbidity and mortality. Differences in neonatal mortality across countries or regions within countries can frequently be explained by differences in prematurity. While defining a birth as premature requires the length of gestation, some of the older (and even recent) literature confuses birthweight and gestation length. In the past, newborns weighing less than 2500 grams have been considered premature; however only about half of the infants weighing less than 2500 grams at birth are actually less than 37 weeks gestation. Similarly only about half of the infants born with gestational age less than 37 weeks weigh less than 2500 grams. Therefore, defining the actual risk for adverse outcome for a given newborn requires knowledge of both the length of gestation and birthweight.

Part of the reason to substitute low birthweight for prematurity has been a traditional distrust of the woman's recollection of her last menstrual period (LMP). However, with more careful analysis it has become clear that the LMP alone and in combination with early ultrasound is a good predictor of the gestational length.[14] With these developments it became possible to consider that infants born prematurely were either growth retarded (small for gestational age), normally grown (appropriate for gestational age), or larger than normal (large for gestational age). The same 3 weight categories can be applied to infants born at term or beyond. Although the distinction may seem slight, these categories are generally thought to be important in understanding the risks facing the infant at birth. Infants of different ages, but of the same size, have different risks for morbidity and mortality.

In a study of women with regular menstrual cycles who delivered infants weighing 3000 grams or more, the normal length of gestation was 284 ± 15 days.[61] Gestational age assessment is easiest in women with regular menstrual cycles of 28-day durations. Women with regular cycles of longer duration can also have gestational age estimated from the LMP. However, for women with irregular and infrequent menstrual cycles, it will be difficult to predict the estimated date of delivery. The reasons for this derive from the relationship between the first day of the last menstrual period and the time of ovulation. In a normal 28-day cycle the first day of menses is day 1 of the cycle. Ovulation occurs on day 14 and if conception and implantation do not occur, the next menstrual period will begin 14 days later. Detailed analysis of menstrual cycles[33,62] has demonstrated that the most constant part of the cycle is the time from ovulation to the beginning of menses. The most variable time of the cycle however is the time from the beginning of menses to ovulation. This variability is what leads to uncertainty in assigning the length of gestation and the estimated date of delivery.

Factors associated with premature birth include demographic characteristics (age and education), maternal habits (smoking, contraceptive use, planned pregnancy), and previous history of prematurity.[60] Among women less than 20 years of age, approximately 12% of pregnancies end in premature birth. This proposition falls to 5% among women between the ages of 25–34 and then begins to increase in women above 35 years of age (to 9%). Prematurity is also inversely correlated with both maternal and paternal education and paternal occupation: The greater the amount of education (and the educational attainment required for the occupation) the lower the risk for prematurity.

There is a clear relationship between smoking and prematurity.[27,28] Among women who do not smoke the risk for prematurity is about 5%. Among women who stopped before pregnancy the risk is essentially the same as among the nonsmokers. Among smokers the risk is approximately 8%. Also of interest, if the pregnancy was planned, the risk for prematurity was lower (5%) than when the pregnancy was not planned (7%) or when the pregnancy occurred outside of marriage (8%). Two factors that were substantial risk factors

for prematurity included a previous pregnancy which ended before 37 weeks or a previous delivery of an infant weighing <2500 grams.

Other factors associated with prematurity include abnormal anatomy of the reproductive system and pregnancy complications. Alterations in the structure of the cervix are associated with increased risk for premature delivery. For example, women who have had multiple voluntary terminations of pregnancy may have cervical damage that increases the risk for premature delivery in a subsequent pregnancy. In addition women who were exposed to diethystilbestrol in utero generally have a shortened cervix. This shortened cervix is more prone to dilate during pregnancy leading to premature delivery.

Anatomical factors associated with the volume of the uterus also are associated with prematurity. For example, with multiple gestation (e.g., twins, triplets, and so on) the volume of the developing infants is greater than normal; increase intrauterine volume appears to put these pregnancies at increased risk for premature delivery. Indeed any factor that increases intrauterine volume (e.g., polyhydramnios) increases the risk for prematurity. Other factors that alter the shape of the intrauterine cavity increase the risk for prematurity and include leiomyomata (benign smooth muscle tumors of the uterus), congenital uterine defects, and prior uterine surgery. Infections, especially urinary tract infections, during pregnancy increase the risk for premature delivery, presumably by causing uterine contractions or irritability.

DEVELOPMENTAL TOXICITY OR BIRTH DEFECTS

Structural and/or functional developmental defects complicate a significant number of pregnancies.[63] Between 3 and 5% of all infants are born with a congenital malformation, 1–2% with a severe malformation. As the child grows and develops, more congenital defects are identified.[64] The causes of these congenital defects fall into 3 general areas: (1) the action of a mutated gene or chromosome anomaly, for example, achondroplasia or maternal phenylketonuria; (2) the action of an environmental agent, for example congenital rubella, ionizing radiation or the drug aminopterin;[65] (3) a combination of genetic and environmental factors, for example fetal phenytoin syndrome, a collection of malformations associated with the use of the anticonvulsant phenytoin.[66]

Among all congenital defects, 20–25% are associated with a chromosomal or genetic (spontaneous or Mendelian inheritance) anomaly, 7–10% are due to infection or maternal disease, and drugs and environmental chemicals account for approximately 2%. Approximately two thirds of all developmental defects have no identifiable cause. It has been estimated that 7–10% of developmental defects are potentially preventable.[67] However, analysis of a unique data set from Norway suggests that a substantial proportion of those infants born with a structural malformation may have an environmental etiology.[68]

Spranger and other investigators have proposed a practical classification for developmental abnormalities.[69-71] This system separates developmental defects into 3 categories: malformations, disruptions, and deformations.

MALFORMATION

A malformation is a morphologic defect that results from an intrinsically abnormal developmental process. This implies that the developmental potential of the structure was abnormal at conception or very early in embryogenesis. Many malformations are considered defects of a developmental region. The whole developmental region responds as a coordinated unit during embryogenesis. Therefore, abnormal development of the developmental region can result in complex or multiple malformations. For example, defects associated with Down syndrome can include abnormalities of the central nervous system, face, skeleton, cardiovascular system, skin, hair, and reproductive systems. The impact of this intrinsically abnormal developmental process is manifest in multiple developmental regions.

DISRUPTION

A disruption is a developmental defect which results from an extrinsic or intrinsic factor producing the breakdown of, or interference with, an originally normal developmental process. In the absence of the extrinsic or intrinsic factor (a deficiency state or chemical, biological, or physical exposure), development would have been normal. Therefore, developmental alterations following exposure to developmental toxicants should be considered disruptions.

A disruption cannot be inherited. However, the genetic composition of the maternal or fetal organism may predispose to and influence the development of a disruption. For example, in some cases development of fetal phenytoin syndrome has been demonstrated to depend on fetal genotype.[66] Similarly, experiments using genetically defined experimental animals have demonstrated clearly the interaction of extrinsic factors with genotype in the production of developmental defects including orofacial clefts[72] or neural tube defects.[73]

DEFORMATION

A deformation is an abnormal form, shape, or position of a part of the body that is caused by mechanical forces acting on that part of the body during development.[74] For example, in pregnancies complicated by oligohydramnios (i.e., insufficient amniotic fluid to cushion and protect the fetus), intrauterine compression can produce alterations in the shape of the legs and feet. Another example of a deformation is the hypoplastic lung associated with herniation of the gut into the thorax during fetal development.

MULTIPLE DEVELOPMENTAL DEFECTS

Investigation of the child with multiple anomalies requires detailed consideration of developmental processes to determine which represents the earliest malformation and temporal sequence of subsequent malformations. Once the developmentally earliest malformation is identified, consideration of the subsequent developmental processes altered may indicate that all the malformations resulted from the first. For example, if fetal kidneys do not form, a malformation, amniotic fluid volume will be lower than normal or may even be completely absent. In the absence of amniotic fluid, multiple deformations of the fetus will occur. These multiple anomalies are all secondary to the renal malformation and so would form a malformation sequence known as the oligohydramnios sequence or Potter syndrome.

TERATOGENICITY OF DRUGS

Using the approaches outlined in the previous sections a selected list of drugs and chemicals have been reviewed for potential hazards to the developing fetus (Tables 12-12 and 12-13). Most drug-induced teratogenicity shows effects that would be categorized as disruption; occasionally drugs produce effects in the category of multiple developmental defects, although it is likely that those too are from disruptions of a more generalized field or process. The cancer chemotherapeutic drugs listed in Table 12-12 are representative examples. These tend to produce multiple malformations, abortions, and unusual disruptions.

Antibiotics and antipyretic drugs can often have an effect manifesting toxicity in the fetus, just as they might in the adult. Renal and hepatic toxicity as well as ototoxicity are not uncommon in this group. Similarly, drugs which manifest any neurological effects may also demonstrate fetal neurotoxic effects. Many of the antiepileptic drugs, as well as tranquilizers, sedatives, narcotics, and alcohol, are suspect for various disruptions, multiple malformations, and direct toxic effects on the central nervous system.

While it is considered that almost any drug can cause developmental harm at levels of maternal toxicity, the majority of drugs which have been identified as teratogens have an effect at therapeutic rather than at toxic doses. Compounds that have their effects at much higher doses associated with maternal

TABLE
12-12 | **IMPACT OF DRUGS ON THE FETUS**

Class and Compound (FDA Category)	Use During Pregnancy	Known or Suspected Developmental Effect
Analgesics/Antipyretics		
Aspirin (C/D)	Safe	Chronic exposure to large doses may be too toxic to mother and fetus, hemorrhage, prolonged gestation, premature closure of the ductus anteriosis
Acetaminophen (B)	Safe	Fetal renal and maternal and fetal hepatic toxicity may occur following chronic ingestion of large doses
Narcotic Analgesics		
Codeine (C/D)	Caution	Malformations, respiratory depression, withdrawal
Pentazocine (C)	Safe	Withdrawal with chronic use
Meperidine (B/D)	Safe	Withdrawal with chronic use
Antibiotics		
Penicillins (B)	Safe	Routine use for infections during pregnancy without risk
Cephalosporins (Bm)	Caution	Probably safe, few epidemiologic studies
Tetracyclines (D)	Known	Incorporation in fetal teeth and bones, malformations, maternal hepatic toxicity and acute fatty metamorphosis
Streptomycin (D)	Caution	Ototoxicity at high doses, interaction with $MgSO_4$
Gentamicin (C)	Caution	Ototoxicity not reported, interaction with $MgSO_4$
Tobramycin (C/D)	Caution	Ototoxicity not reported, interaction with $MgSO_4$
Amikacin (C/D)	Caution	Ototoxicity not reported, interaction with $MgSO_4$
Chloramphenicol (C)	Caution	Cardiovascular collapse (gray syndrome)
Sulfonamides (B/D)	Safe	Displace bilirubin from albumen
Nitrofurantoin (B)	Safe	Hemolysis, anemia and hyperbilirubinemia in G6PD deficiency
Metronidazole (Bm)	Caution	Avoid during first trimester
Trimethoprim (Cm)/ Sulfamethoxazole (B/D)	Caution	Folic acid antagonist
Antituberculosis		
Isoniazid (C)	Safe	Drug of choice for tuberculosis treatment during pregnancy
Rifampin (C)	Safe	Drug of choice for tuberculosis treatment during pregnancy
Ethambutol (B)	Safe	Drug of choice for tuberculosis treatment during pregnancy
para-Aminosalicylic acid (C)	Caution	Drug of choice for tuberculosis treatment during pregnancy
Antihistamine/Antiemetic		
Cyclizine (B)	Safe	
Buclizine (C)	Safe	Retrolental fibroplasia in premature infants associated with treatment during last 2 weeks of pregnancy
Meclizine (Bm)	Safe	
Antihistamines		
Diphenhydramine (Bm)	Caution	Possible association with malformations
Chlorpheniramine (B)	Safe	
Brompheniramine (Cm)	Safe	Retrolental fibroplasia in premature infants associated with treatment during last 2 weeks of pregnancy
Sedatives		
Barbituates	Caution	Conflicting data on malformations, dependence with prolonged use
Ethanol (D)	Known	Fetal alcohol syndrome, craniofacial, limb abnormalities, and microcephaly

(continued)

| TABLE 12-12 | IMPACT OF DRUGS ON THE FETUS (Continued) |

Class and Compound (FDA Category)	Use During Pregnancy	Known or Suspected Developmental Effect
Tranquilizers/Sedative		
Chlordiazepoxide (D)	Caution	Conflicting data on malformations, dependence with prolonged use
Meprobamate (D)	Caution	Conflicting data on malformations, dependence with prolonged use
Diazepam (D)	Caution	Possible association with oral clefts and other malformations
Antidepressants		
Lithium	Known	Cardiovascular anomalies, neonatal toxicity
Imipramine (D)	Caution	Malformations, neonatal withdrawal
Amitriptyline (D)	Caution	Neonatal withdrawal
Doxepin(C)	Caution	Possible association with malformations
Anesthetics		
Inhalational	Caution	Spontaneous abortion, decreased fertility with occupational exposure
Tranquilizer/Antiemetic		
Prochlorperazine (C)	Safe	
Antiemetic		
Trimethobenzamide (C)	Safe	
Anticonvulsants		
Phenytoin	Caution	Fetal hydantoin syndrome, define benefit : risk ratio
Carbamazepine	Caution	Conflicting data on malformations
Ethosuximide	Caution	Conflicting data on malformations, drug of choice for petit mal in pregnancy
Primidone	Caution	Conflicting data on malformations
Valproic acid	Known	CNS, neural tube defects
Trimethadione	known	Congenital malformations, abortion
Paramethadione	Known	Congenital malformations, abortion
Aminophyllines		
Theophylline	Safe	Bronchodilator of choice in pregnancy
Diuretics	Caution	Initiation of use during pregnancy
Reserpine and Rauwolfia Alkaloids		
Reserpine	Caution	
Methyldopa	Caution	
Vasodilators		
Hydralizine	Caution	Drug of choice in pre-eclampsia, eclampsia
Sodium nitroprusside	Caution	Produces increased cyanide levels in fetus
Digitalis	Safe	
Hypoglycemics		
Tolbutamide	Known	Not indicated during pregnancy
Antithyroid and Iodine		
Propylthiouracil	Known	Mild fetal hypothyroidism and goiter, drug of choice for hyperthyroidism in pregnancy
Potassium iodide	Known	Fetal hypothyroidism and goiter
Providone iodide	Known	Fetal hypothyroidism and goiter

(continued)

TABLE 12-12	**IMPACT OF DRUGS ON THE FETUS** *(Continued)*

Class and Compound (FDA Category)	*Use During Pregnancy*	*Known or Suspected Developmental Effect*
Steroids		
Cortisone	Caution	
Betamethasone	Caution	Prevention of respiratory distress
Diethylstilbestrol	Known	Uterine and vaginal malformations (adenosis), epididymal cysts, hypotrophic testes, infertility
Estradiol	Known	Congenital defects
Medroxyprogesterone	Caution	Possible congenital defects
Methyltestosterone	Known	Masculinization
Anticoagulants		
Heparin	Safe	Anticoagulant of choice, prolonged use associated w/maternal osteopernia
Coumarins	Known	Nasal hypoplasia, shortened extremities, abortion
Antimalarials		
Chloroquine	Caution	Drug of choice for malaria, small increased risk for malformations
Quinine	Caution	Abortion, conflicting data on malformations
Pyimethamine	Caution	Folic acid antagonist
Cancer Chemotherapeutic Drugs		
Aminopterin	Known	Malformations, spontaneous abortion
Busulfan	Known	Multiple visceral malformations, abortion
Chlorambucil	Known	Renal agenesis
Cyclophosphamide	Known	Conflicting data on malformations, ovarian and testicular toxicity
Cytarabine	Known	Malformations and chromosome abnormalities
Fluorouracil	Known	Multiple anomalies
Mechlorethamine	Known	
Methotrexate	Known	Malformations similar to aminopterin folic acid antagonist
Procarbazine	Known	Malformations, decreased spermatogenesis
Antiacne		
Retinoic acid	Known	Spontaneous abortion, hydrocephalus, microcephalus, ear/eye abnormalities, cardiovascular malformations
Miscellaneous		
Penicillamine	Known	Skin lesion (cutis laxa)
Disulfiram	Known	Multiple anomalies

Safe—safe in normal exposure doses; Caution—caution, therapeutic indication should outweigh possible small risk; Known—known, human developmental toxicant, use during pregnancy requires careful risk benefit analysis.

toxicity (e.g., alcohol and cocaine) have been identified only recently as teratogens. This is probably because the pattern of effects are more subtle and represent a generalized set of disruptions resulting in multiple developmental defects.

Lessons we should learn from this are that any medication or compound at maternally toxic levels should be suspected as being a developmental toxicant. Similarly, any drug that is known to interfere with basic metabolic processes such as DNA replication, energy metabolism, and so on, should also be considered as a potential developmental toxicant even at less than maternally toxic doses. The therapeutic doses of these drugs often have a narrow range between beneficial levels and toxic levels.

Finally, any compound that has a mechanism of action similar to a know teratogen (e.g., affect estrogen receptor, antithyroid compound, antimetabolite) would raise a caution flag even though it had not yet been tested for developmental toxicity in humans.

TABLE 12-13 **IMPACT OF CHEMICALS IN INDUSTRY AND THE ENVIRONMENT ON THE FETUS**

Class and Compound	Risk	Known or Suspected Developmental Effect
Methyl mercury	Known	Microcephaly, mental retardation including cerebral palsy
Acetone	Caution	Sacral abnormalities, camptomelic syndrome
Benzene	Caution	Spontaneous abortions, premature births
Boric acid	Caution	Conflicting data on malformation rate
Carbon disulfide	Caution	Spontaneous abortions, sperm abnormalities, abnormal menses
Carbon monoxide	Known	Stillbirth with maternal toxicity
Chloroprene	Caution	Possible mental defects, chromosomal abnormalities
1,2-dibromo-3-chloropropane	Caution	Testicular toxicity, spontaneous abortions
Dichloromethane	Caution	Spontaneous abortions
Dinitro-dipropylsufanilamide	Caution	Miscarriage, heart defects
Ethylene dibromide	Caution	Decreased fertility
Formaldehyde	Caution	Spontaneous abortions
Hexachlorobenzene	Caution	Stillbirth
Lead	Known	Increased abortion rate, stillbirth, central nervous system toxicity
Mercuric chloride	Caution	Spontaneous abortions
Methyl ethyl ketone	Caution	Spontaneous abortions
Methyl parathion	Caution	Malformations
Polychlorinated biphenyls	Known	Brown skin in newborns, growth retardation, exophthalmos
Sodium selenite	Caution	Spontaneous abortions, limb defects
Styrene	Caution	Spontaneous abortions
Toluene	Caution	Growth retardation, malformations
Trichloroethylene	Caution	Malformations, sacral agenesis
Vinyl chloride	Caution	Spontaneous abortions
Xylene	Caution	Sacral agenesis

INDUSTRIAL AND ENVIRONMENTAL EXPOSURES

Among the occupational and environmental exposures listed, only 3 are identified as known human developmental toxicants, methyl mercury, lead, and polychlorinated biphenyls. Caution is indicated for all the others. Does that mean that these chemicals actually pose risks to human reproduction and development? The data for each chemical are quite variable and careful assessment of potential for reproductive or developmental hazard is necessary. Even if the chemical of concern is determined to represent a reproductive or developmental hazard, additional exposure information is needed to define the actual risk to the patient since the exposure is often unmeasured or minimal.

The review by Barlow and Sullivan[1] is a good summarization of environmental chemicals that are hazards. Exposures from industry and the environment, however, are just in their infancy in being defined.[12,13,15,28,60,85] Often patients are exposed to multiple chemicals and it is difficult to determine the contribution to risk of each separate compound. While drugs frequently appear on lists of definite developmental hazards, experts are much less certain about environmental chemicals and as a result these compounds are included on lists of suspected reproductive and developmental toxicants

rather than definite hazards.[1-3] Often the effect associated with these chemicals is suspected to be spontaneous abortion or stillbirth.[60,85] When the pattern of developmental toxicity is as general as that, it can be difficult to determine what part the compound plays in the overall process. The environmental or occupational exposures may be causing disruptions that are so severe as to cause the pregnancies not to continue; they may be causing very early genetic damage that results in abortion; or they may be toxic to the maternal system with a resultant early disturbance in implantation. The metals such as lead, mercury, and cadmium are especially implicated in these types of embryotoxic effects. Volatile organic chemicals also appear on these lists although their effects, if they produce developmental toxicity, are likely to occur at much higher doses where maternal toxicity is manifest.

The entire area of environmental exposures needs much more research along with well-designed epidemiological studies to screen for possible hazards. The recent consumer interest in this area that has resulted in the mandate expressed by California's Proposition 65[2,5] may lead to such new knowledge. For the present time, we have observed that this is a major area of questions to teratogen information services for women who work in various industrial settings and who question whether they are exposed to any substance that may alter their fertility or pregnancy outcomes. Even normal, daily nonemployment activities such as having pets, houses, and yards sprayed for insect infestations, or even being exposed to various cosmetic products may bring these questions to a woman's mind. The list of potential environmental exposures far exceeds the different exposures to drugs, both prescribed and available over the counter. Many compounds for which human environmental or occupational exposure occurs are completely untested for their reproductive and developmental effects, and they are unlikely to be tested in the near future. This further compounds the risk assessment process since little data are likely to be available to someone counseling about present or potential exposures during pregnancy.

CONCLUSION

The need to define the impact of a drug or a chemical exposure on pregnancy is heightened by patient awareness, interest, and concern. The risk-assessment process has been outlined and should be studied by the person giving counsel to pregnant patients concerning such exposures. While it might be easy to say that in many cases the data is too scanty to make an assessment, patients want some sort of advice regarding the potential health of their offspring. They can often be made to understand the uncertainty that one must give this assessment, but any information influencing the patient's decision either toward an increased risk or toward no-increased-risk is helpful for their decision making.

Patients will often err on the side of deciding to terminate a pregnancy when in fact the data does not support any increased incidence of abnormality;[4] they tend to perceive an even greater risk if they are not told anything. Finally, risk assessment often requires an interdisciplinary team, not only to formulate whether the exposure constitutes a hazardous one but also to determine the likely amount of maternal exposure and any metabolic and physiologic changes that would affect exposure to the fetus. Pharmacologist, physiologist, obstetricians, and geneticists often must pool their knowledge about an exposure scenario in order to render the best possible information to a concerned patient.

ACKNOWLEDGMENTS

This chapter is intended as a survey of the previous edition.

References

1. Barlow SM, Sullivan FM. *Reproductive Hazards of Industrial Chemicals. An Evaluation of Animal and Human Data.* New York, Academic Press, 1982.

2. Schardein JL. *Chemically Induced Birth Defects*, 3rd ed. New York, Marcel Dekker, 2000.

3. Shepard TH. *Catalog of Teratologic Agents*, 9th ed. Baltimore, Johns Hopkins University Press, 1998.

4. Briggs GG, Freeman RK, Yaffee SJ. *Drugs in Pregnancy and Lactation*, 5th ed. Baltimore, Williams and Wilkins, 1998.

5. The development of on line databases has, to some extent, eased the access to data on reproductive and developmental toxicity. Databases of particular interest include: www.modimes.org, Reprotox, Teris (others?).

6. Koren G, ed. *Maternal-Fetal Toxicology. A Clinician's Guide*, New York, Marcel Dekker, 1989.

7. Mattison DR, Working PK, Blazak WF, et al. Criteria for identifying and listing substances known to cause reproductive toxicity under California's Proposition 65. *Reproductive Toxicology.* 1990;4:163.

8. Mattison DR, Hanson J, Kochhar DM, et al. Criteria for identifying and listing substances known to cause developmental toxicity under California's Proposition 65. *Reproductive Toxicology.* 1989;3:3.

9. Etzel RA, Balk SJ, eds. *Handbook of Pediatric Environmental Health.* Elk Grove Village, Illinois, American Academy of Pediatrics, 1999.

10. National Research Council. Committee on the Institutional Means for the Assessment of Risks to Public Health. *Risk assessment in the federal government: managing the process.* Commission on Life Sciences, National Research Council. Washington, DC, National Academy Press, 1983.

11. Committee on Risk Assessment of Hazardous Air Pollutants. *Science and Judgement in Risk Assessment*, Washington, DC, National Academy Press, 1994.

12. Stern PC, Feinberg H, eds. Committee on Risk Characterization. *Understanding Risk, Informing Decisions in a Democratic Society*, Washington, DC, National Academy Press, Washington, DC, 1996.

13. Committee on Hormonally Active Agents in the Environment. *Hormonally Active Agents in the Environment.* Washington, DC, National Academy Press, 1999.

14. *Guidelines for Reproductive Toxicity Risk Assessment.* EPA 630R96009, USEPA, Washington, DC.

15. *Guidelines for Developmental Toxicity Risk Assessment.* EPA 600FR91001, USEPA, Washington, DC.

16. Selevan SG, Lemasters GK. The dose-response fallacy in human reproductive studies of toxic exposures. *J Occup Med.* 1987; 29:451.

17. Kline J, Stein Z, Susser M. *Conception to Birth. Epidemiology of Prenatal Development.* New York, Oxford University Press, 1989.

18. Bracken MB. *Perinatal Epidemiology.* New York, Oxford University, 1984.

19. Schardein JL. Teratogenic risk assessment: Past, present, and future. In: Kalter, H. ed. *Issues and Reviews in Teratology.* Vol 1. New York, Plenum, 1983:181–214.

20. Fabro S. On predicting environmentally-inducted human reproductive hazards: an overview and historical perspective. *Fund Appl Toxicol.* 1985;5:609.

21. Jelovsek FR, Mattison DR, Young JF. Eliciting principles of hazard identification from experts. *Teratology.* 1990;45:521.

22. Fabro S, Schull G, Brown NA. The relative teratogenic index and teratogenic potency: Proposed components of developmental toxicity risk assessment. *Teratogen, Carcinog, Mutagen.* 1982;2:61.

23. Rutledge JC, Generoso WM. Fetal pathology produced by ethylene oxide treatment of the murine zygote. *Teratology.* 1989;39:563.

24. Katoh M, Cacheiro NL, Cornett CV, et al. Fetal anomalies produced subsequent to treatment of zygotes with ethylene oxide or ethyl methanesulfonate are not likely due to the usual genetic causes. *Mutat Res.* 1989;210:337.

25. Generoso WM, Katoh M, Cain KT, et al. Chromosome malsegregation and embryonic lethality induced by treatment of normally

ovulated mouse oocytes with nocodazole. *Mutat Res.* 1989;210: 313.

26. Frankos VH. FDA perspectives on the use of teratology data for human risk assessment. *Fund Appl Toxicol.* 1985;5:615.

27. Jelovsek FR, Mattison DR, Chen J. Prediction of risk for human development toxicity: How important are animal studies? *Obstet and Gynecol.* 1989;74:624.

28. National Research Council. Toxicity Testing. Strategies to Determine Needs and Priorities. Steering Committee on Identification of Toxic and Potentially Toxic Chemicals for Consideration by the National Toxicology Program. Board on Toxicology and Environmental Health Hazards. Commission on Life Sciences. Washington, DC, National Academy Press, 1984.

29. Belsey MA. Infertility: prevalence, etiology, and natural history. In: Bracken MB, ed. *Perinatal Epidemiology.* New York, Oxford University Press, 1984:255–282.

30. Barrett JC. Fecundability and coital frequency. *Pop Studies.* 1971;25: 309.

31. Barrett JC, Marshall J. The risk of conception on different days of the menstrual cycle. *Pop Studies.* 1969;23:455.

32. Gurrero VR, Rojas OI. Spontaneous abortion and aging of human ova and spermatozoa. *N Engl J Med.* 1975;293:573.

33. Mattison DR. The effects of smoking on reproduction from gametogenesis to implantation. *Environ Res.* 1982;28:410.

34. Mattison DR, Plowchalk DR, Meadows MJ, et al. The effect of smoking on oogenesis, fertilization and implantation. *Seminars in Reproductive Endocrinology.* 1989;7:291.

35. Baird DD, Wilcox AJ. Cigarette smoking associated with conception delay. *JAMA.* 1985;253:2979.

36. Working PK. *Toxicology of the Male and Female Reproductive Systems,* New York, Hemisphere Publishing Corp, 1989.

37. Scialli AR. *A Clinical Guide to Reproductive and Developmental Toxicology.* Boca Raton, CRC Press.

38. Fertility, Family Planning and Women's Health: New Data From the 1995 National Survey of Family Growth, *National Survey of Family Growth,* Series 23, #19, 1997 (PHS 97–1995)

39. Mosher WD, Pratt WF. Fecundity and infertility in the United States, 1965–1982 *NCHS Advancedata.* 104:1, Feb. 1985 (PHS 85–1250).

40. Milby TH, Whorton D. Epidemiological assessment of occupationally related, chemically induced sperm-count suppression. *J Occup Med.* 1980;22:77.

41. Rosenberg MJ, Wyrobek AJ, Ratcliffe J, et al. Sperm as an indicator of reproductive risk among petroleum.

42. Whorton MD, Krauss RM, Marshall S, et al. Infertility in male pesticide workers. *Lancet.* 1977;ii:1259.

43. Whorton MD, Milby TH, Stubbs HA, et al. Testicular functions among carbaryl-exposed employees. *J Toxicol Environ Health.* 1979;5:929.

44. Wyrobek AJ, Gordon FLA, Burkhart JG, et al. An evaluation of human sperm as indicators of chemically induced alterations of spermatogenic function. *Mutation Research.* 1983;115: 73.

45. Wyrobeck AJ, Brodsky J, Gordon L, et al. Sperm studies in anesthesiologists. *Anesthesiology.* 1981;55:527.

46. Wyrobek AJ, Watchmaker G, Gordon L, et al. Sperm shape abnormalities in carbaryl-exposed employees. *Environ Health Perspect.* 1981;40:255.

47. Menker J, Trussel J, Larsen U. Age and infertility. *Science.* 1987; 233:1389.

48. Schwartz D, Magauz MJ. Female fecundity as a function of age. Results of artificial insemination in 2193 nulliparous women with azospermic husbands. *N Engl J Med.* 1982;306:404.

49. Paul M. Occupational reproductive hazards. *Lancet.* 1997;349: 1385–1388.

50. Wilcox AJ, Weinberg CR, O'Connor JF, et al. Incidence of early loss of pregnancy. *N Engl J Med.* 1988;319:189.

51. Canfield RD, O'Connor JF, Birken S, et al. Development of an assay for a biomarker of pregnancy and early fetal loss. *Environ Health Perspect.* 1987;74:57.

52. Roman E, Stevenson AC. Spontaneous abortion. In: Berin SL, Thomson AM, eds. *Obstetrical Epidemiology.* New York, Academic Press, 1983:61–87.

53. Kline JK. Maternal occupation: effects on spontaneous abortions and malformations. *Occupational Medicine: State of the Art Review.* 1986;1:381.

54. Hassold T, Chiud, Yamaneja. Parental origin of autosomal trisomies. *Ann Hum Genet.* 1984;48:129.

55. Kline J, Stein Z, Susser M, et al. Environmental influences on early reproductive loss in a current New York City study. In: Porter IH, Hook EB. eds. *Human Embryonic and Fetal Death.* New York, Academic Press, 1980.

56. Kline J, Levin B, Stein Z, et al. Epidemiological detection of low dose effects on the developing fetus. *Environ Health Perspect.* 1981;42:119.

57. Stein Z, Kline J, Levin B, et al. Epidemiologic studies of environmental exposures in toxic reproduction. In: Burg GC, Maillie HD. Eds. *Measurement of Risks.* New York, Plenum, 1981.

58. Harlap S, Shiono P, Ramcharan S. Spontaneous fetal losses in women using different contraceptives around the time of conception. *Inter J Epidem.* 1980;9:49.

59. Vessey MP, Dahl R, Johnson B, et al. Outcome of pregnancy in women using an interuterine device. *Lancet.* 1974;1:495.

60. Vessey MP, Meiser L, Flavel R, et al. Outcome of pregnancy in women using different methods of contraception. *Brit J Obstet Gynecol.* 1979;86:548.

61. Hemminki K, Mutanen P, Saloniemi I, et al: Spontaneous abortions in hospital staff engaged in sterilizing instruments with chemical agents. *Brit Med J.* 1982;285:1461.

62. Refer to Journal issue on prematurity.

63. Vandenberg BJ, Oechsli FW. Prematurity. In: Bracken M. ed. *Perinatal Epidemiology.* New York and Oxford, Oxford University Press, 1984:69–85.

64. Andersen F, Johnson TRB, Flora JD, et al. A gestational age assessment. 1. Analysis of individual clinical observations. *Am J Obstet and Gynecol.* 1981;139:173.

65. Andersen F, Johnson TRB, Flora JD, et al. A gestational age assessment. 2. Prediction from combined clinical observations. *Am J Obstet Gynecol.* 1981;140:770.

66. Scott RT Jr, Hodgen GD. The ovarian follicle: life cycle of a pelvic clock. *Clin Obst and Gynecol.* 1990;33:551.

67. MOD data

68. Myrianthopoulos NC. *Malformations in Children from One to Seven Years. A Report from the Perinatal Project.* New York, Alan R. Liss, 1985.

69. Spranger J, Bernischke K, Hall JG, et al. Errors of morphogenesis: Concepts and terms. *J Pediatr.* 1982;100:160.

70. Persaud TVN. Classification and epidemiology of developmental defects. In: Persaud TVN, Chudley AE, Skalko RG, eds. *Basic Concepts in Teratology.* New York, Alan R. Liss, 1985:13–22.

71. Sever JL, Brent RL. *Teratogen Update. Environmentally Induced Birth Defect Risks.* New York, Alan R. Liss, 1986.

72. Hanson JW. Fetal hydantoin effects. In: Sever JL, Brent RL. *Teratogen Update. Environmentally Induced Birth Defect Risks.* New York, Alan R. Liss, 1986:29–34.

73. Brent RL. The complexities of solving the problem of human malformations. In: Sever JL, Brent RL. *Teratogen Update. Environmentally Induced Birth Defect Risks.* New York, Alan R. Liss, 1986:189–197.

74. Wilcox—Norwegian data.

75. Persaud TVN, Chudley AE, Skalko RG. *Basic Concepts in Teratology.* New York, Alan R. Liss, 1985.

76. Pratt RM. Hormones, growth factors, and their receptors in normal and abnormal prenatal development. In: Kalter H. ed. *Issues and Reviews in Teratology.* Vol 2. New York, Plenum, 1983:189–218.

77. NTD—gene/environment interactions.

78. Graham JM Jr. *Smith's Recognizable Patterns of Human Deformation,* 2nd ed. Philadelphia, WB Saunders, 1988.

79. Wang GM, Schwetz BA. An evaluation system of ranking chemicals with teratogenic potential. *Teratogen, Carcinogen, Mutagen.* 1987;7:133.

80. Hart WL, Reynolds RC, Krasavage WJ, et al. Evaluation of developmental toxicity data: a discussion of some pertinent factors and a proposal. *Risk Analysis.* 1988;8:59.

81. Kimmel CA, Wellington DG, Farland W, et al. Overview of a workshop on quantitative models for developmental toxicity risk assessment. *Environ Health Perspect.* 1989;79:209.

82. Jones KL. *Smith's Recognizable Patterns of Human Malformation,* 4th ed. Philadelphia, WB Saunders, 1988.

83. Karonfsky DA. Drugs as teratogens in animals and man. *Ann Rev Pharmacol.* 1965;5:447.

84. Seller MJ. Neural-tube defects: cause and prevention. In: Matteo A, Benson P, Giannelli F, Seller M, eds. *Pediatric Research: A Genetic Approach. Spastics International Medical Publication.* Lavenham, Suffolk, Lavenham Press, 1982.

85. US Congress. Office of Technology Assessment. *Reproductive Health Hazards in the Workplace.* Washington, DC, US Government Printing Office (OTA-BA-266), 1985.

CHAPTER 13

BACTERIAL INFECTIONS AND PREGNANCY

Charles Weber / Christine Kovac

Bacterial infections have become a part of our life, either as a symbiotic portion of our life or when overgrowth occurs, as a pathological process. This cycle does not cease when a woman becomes pregnant. Pregnancy poses another aspect of the infectious process. The mother must downregulate her immune system to prevent rejection of the fetus as well as upregulate to fight off infections. The 2 processes do not necessarily counteract each other, but one must be aware of their co-existence. The bacterial infections most often associated with pregnancy are urinary tract infections, genital tract infections, and pulmonary and some other rarer cases of dermatological and central nervous system involvements.

A simple discussion of the normal immune process in the nonpregnant and pregnant state is in order. The normal immune system consists of the innate and adaptive system. Both systems complement each other, one utilizing the strengths of the other. The innate consists of physical and biochemical barriers, such as our skin, the natural killer cells, macrophages, or other antigen-presenting cells in the various organs. The adaptive system consists of humoral and cellular responses to combat the invasion of microorganisms. Responses from the adaptive utilize the T- and B-cell lines to generate the limitless combination of antigen recognition sites, which will attract and produce the troops known as T- or B-cell proliferation. The T-cells mediate the cellular immunity while the B-cells produce the antibodies producing the humoral responses that are needed for long-term memory of our immune system.

The fetus adds another aspect of the immune system as another potential target that needs the mother's immune system to remain intact in order to stave off the onslaught from the bacteria world. Some of the barriers, which exist for the pregnant female, are different from the nonpregnant state. Under normal physiological conditions the endometrial cavity has no normal flora. Only when the functional tissue undergoes changes in mucosal integrity and the presence of blood and necrotic decidua can it sustain bacterial colonization. The fetus has its own innate immune system: that of amniotic fluid, which surrounds the fetus. It has bacteriostatic properties, which actually inhibit bacterial growth. Amniotic fluid has been shown to be ineffective in suppressing growth of common organisms in premature gestations, yet at term it can suppress growth of bacteria for up to 32 hours. If pregnancy is interrupted prematurely or if there is placental insufficiency, the serum IgG level in the newborn infant is reduced.[1–3]

One of the risks associated with bacterial infections, not specific to any one organism, is preterm labor. The cascade of events that have been hypothesized to cause premature labor consist of bacteria-releasing endotoxins (lipopolysaccharides) or exotoxins that initiate cytokine and interleukin responses. These responses in turn effect the decidua, membranes, or prostaglandin production that leads to uterine contractions. With these contractions come cervical dilation and a potential opening for more microbes into the uterus.

Evidence that preterm birth is associated with infections includes the following observations:

1. Histologic chorioamnionitis is increased in preterm births.
2. Clinical infection is increased after preterm births.
3. Positive cultures from amniotic fluid or membranes from preterm births.
4. Inflammatory process of membranes in association with preterm births.
5. Bacteria or their products induce preterm births in animal models.
6. Some antibiotic trials have shown a decreased incidence of preterm birth.[18,21]

Other risks associated with bacterial infection include maternal or neonatal sepsis, fetal distress, and fetal demise.

The bacteria that we will discuss may enter the amniotic cavity by the following pathways:

1. Ascending from either the cervix or vagina.
2. Hematogenous spread with transplacental passage, usually associated with maternal bacteremia.
3. Entry through the fallopian tubes or peritoneal cavity.
4. Nosocomial through amniocentesis, chorionic villus sampling or funipuncture.

The most common of these pathways is ascending infection.

The most prevalent bacteria associated with maternal or fetal risks during gestation include many exogenous and endogenous organisms. Exogenous pathogens include *Chlamydia trachomatis*, *Bordetella pertussis*, *Calmymmatobacterium granulomatis*, *Hemophilus Ducreyi-Chancroid*, *Hemophilus Influenza*, *Listeria Monocytogenes*, *Neissiera Gonorrhoeae*, *Salmonella Typhi*, and Group A B-hemolytic Streptococci (*Streptococcus pyogenes*). Endogenous pathogens include Bacteroidacea, Clostridia, *Escherichia coli*, *Gardnerella vaginallis* (*Hemophilus vaginallis*), *Proteus*, *Staphylococcus aureus*, *Staphylococcus epidermidis*, and Group B-hemolytic Streptococci.[3] Following is a discussion of these various pathogens, the risks they pose, and management options.

GROUP B BETA-HEMOLYTIC STREPTOCOCCI (GBS)

GBS are Gram-positive cocci that grow in chains. Because it lacks a protein, which exists on the Group A streptococci, it has a much different virulence. GBS is a normal constituent of the vaginal flora and the gastrointestinal tract. Fecal colonization exceeds any other colonization rates. Between 14 and 25% of pregnant women may be continually, intermittently or transiently colonized. GBS is rarely a cause of maternal morbidity. It is, however, the most common cause of neonatal sepsis, meningitis and pneumonia in the United States. Often associated with PPROM, the patient is at risk of developing chorioamnionitis and/or postpartum endometritis. Although studies in Great Britain failed to identify preterm labor associated with GBS positive gravid females, it was noted that GBS positive pregnancies were more common with low birth weight infants.[15,16]

The most recent data suggests that judicial culturing and liberal use of prophylactic antibiotics does not significantly reduce nor limit the incidence or mortality of GBS-related sepsis. Although decreased incidences of chorioamnionitis have been universally recorded.[17] The mother's response to the GBS, or any infection, has been the usual cause of poor fetal outcomes. Although chorioamnionitis has been noted to be present in as high as 68% of all healthy deliveries and 87% in stillborn deliveries, the most common finding was an inflammatory process in the decidua basalis *along with* a predominant bacteria cultured. Risks doubled if both inflammation and bacteria were present.[18]

There is a great amount of controversy in the literature about how best to treat patients to reduce the risk of GBS sepsis in the neonate. Options include treating selective patients (those with risk factors), selective screening with antibiotic treatment for those with positive cultures, or universal screening. The best method often varies with the patient population to which it is being applied. Issues in this controversy include concern for developing drug resistance, efficacy of each protocol in different populations or settings, cost, and impact on other organisms. Universal screening has shown a decrease in early neonatal GBS infections, chorioamnionitis, and endometritis, but this difference may not be significant in populations with a lower incidence of GBS.[19]

GROUP A BETA-HEMOLYTIC STREPTOCOCCUS (*STREPTOCOCCUS PYOGENES*)

Streptococcus pyogenes is a gram-positive cocci. Its capsule contains hyaluronic acid, which lyses endothelium cells, and it has the M protein to interfere with phagocytic cells. Infections are associated with puerperal sepsis, prepubertal vulvovaginitis, endometritis-salpingitis-peritonitis, and necrotizing fascitis.

In gravid women *Streptococcus pyogenes* can be present as part of the normal vaginal flora; however, infections can occur. For an infection to occur, it is theorized that there needs to be a break in the mucosal-epithelial barrier. Clinically, it presents as a high maternal fever and uterine tenderness. Other evidence of infection of the uterus and pelvis can include leukocytosis, tachycardia, edematous soft uterus, and a serosanguinous vaginal discharge. Maternal septicemia will occur before fetal involvement occurs, but with ruptured membranes, it can ascend to infect the fetus, amniotic fluid and chorion. Exten-

sion beyond the pelvis can result in peritonitis. Treatment can include penicillin, ampicillin, or vancomycin.[3,18]

LISTERIA MONOCYTOGENES

Listeria monocytogenes is a Gram-positive, catalase positive bacillus in the corynebacteriaceae family. Infections occur more frequently in pregnant women compared to the general population at a rate of 12 per 100,000. The gastrointestinal tract is the most likely usual reservoir for *Listeria monocytogenes*. The depressed cell-mediated immunity during pregnancy may be responsible for the unusual high incidence in pregnant women.[5–7] Maternal infections can present as a mononucleosis-like syndrome with a short duration. However, fetal death may occur. Contaminated food may be a likely source. If Listeria chorioamnionitis is diagnosed preterm, in utero therapy with high dose penicillin or trimethoprim-sulfamethoxazole should be attempted in order to avoid the high risk of preterm delivery. Preterm labor occurs in 50% of cases.

When fetal or neonatal infections do occur, the mode of transmission is transplacental. It does not colonize the vaginal canal well, although cases of ascending infection have been noted. Like GBS, there is an early and late onset neonatal disease. Risks to the fetus include preterm delivery, fetal distress (35%) and meconium-stained amniotic fluid in (75%).[6,7] Spontaneous abortions or intrauterine fetal demise have been most recently documented as occurring from 4–10.9% depending on the study[7,8] and are associated with areas of necrosis on the placenta.

Treatment may include ampicillin with clavulanic acid, erythromycin, or trimethoprim-sulfamethoxazole (may have better efficacy but is a class C associated with neonatal kernicterus). The most effective strategy to prevent this disease is to eliminate the most likely source: contaminated food. Monitoring of dairy products by the FDA, CDC and of meats by the USDA has decreased the incidence of *Listeria* infections from 17.4 per 100,000 births in 1989 to 8.6 per 100,000 in 1993, a 44% decrease.[9]

HAEMOPHILUS INFLUENZAE

Haemophilus influenzae is a Gram-negative capsulated cocci that form short chains. Its prevalence is low, but it has a high infectious rate. Infections associated with this organism include meningitis, epiglotitis, pneumonia, otitis, and bronchitis. Chorioamnionitis can occur with PROM. There is a higher correlation with postpartum maternal infections than neonatal disease. Treatment includes cefotaxime, ceftriaxone, or trimethoprim-sulfamethoxazole.

CHLAMYDIA TRACHOMATIS

Chlamydia trachomatis is an obligate intracellular Gram-negative organism that utilizes the host cells' ATP production. They have a 2-part life cycle: 1 as an elementary body and the other as a reticulate body. The elementary body is the dormant version, which allows it protection in the extracellular environment. The reticulate body is metabolically active, shedding its coat and living only in the intracellular environment. The cell takes up the elementary body by endocytosis. Antibodies do not necessarily play a major role in the immune response against this organism. Therefore the body must rely on the cell-mediated response, which is suppressed in the gravid female. As with most cell-mediated responses, it appears that our own immune system is responsible for the scar tissue that results in Pelvic Inflammatory Disease (PID), which can complicate subsequent pregnancies.

Chlamydia is the most common sexually transmitted disease in United States. It is the known pathogen for inclusion conjunctivitis in the newborn and lymphogranuloma venerum (LGV). Serious long-term effects include pelvic inflammatory disease, tubal infertility, and ectopic pregnancy. Newborn-associated diseases are fetal wastage, premature ruptured membranes, preterm labor and delivery, and postpartum endometritis.

Diagnostic Tests for Chlamydia Trachomatis

Inclusion bodies can be seen on cytologic smears such as the Papanicolau smear. The sensitivity and specificity are not very high; therefore confirmation is usually by either culture or a specific nonculture test such as the Chlamydia-specific monoclonal antibodies or DNA identification using PCR. Treatment may include azithromycin or erythromycin base. Doxycycline, the drug of choice in the nonpregnant population, is contraindicated in pregnancy.

NEISSERIA GONORRHOEAE

Neisseria gonorrhoeae is a Gram-negative diplococci that infects columnar and transitional epithelium. In the nongravid woman, the cervical mucous acts as a barrier to ascending infections. Menstruation not only negates the effect of the cervical mucous, but also destroys the barrier formed by the endometrium as it is "sloughed" off. Pelvic inflammatory disease is the residual of a post-gonococcal infection. It has a higher incidence of ectopic pregnancy and infertility. Septicemia can progress to lead to endocarditis (rarely) and gonococcal arthritis. Peritonitis can occur and infection can produce paravertebral adhesions known as the Curtis-Fitz-Hughes syndrome (Gonococcal perihepatitis). Ascending infections are very rare in pregnancy because of the role of the cervical mucous and fetal membranes. Infection of the fetus is extremely rare with intact membranes. Infections during pregnancy are associated with preterm delivery, PPROM, and neonatal infections. Neonatal infections are associated with blindness and should be treated with silver nitrate.[10] Maternal treatment is with penicillin.

TREPONEMA PALLIDUM: SYPHILIS

Syphilis is caused by *Treponema pallidum*, a bacteria in the order of Spirochaetaceae, a strict anaerobe. With the exception of transmission from congenital means, it is a sexually transmitted organism. Its cell wall is still very susceptible to penicillin, which is the treatment for both gravid and nongravid females. The primary chancre of syphilis is characteristic of a painless ulcer having a smooth raised border with clean surfaces. Most females will get the primary lesion on the labia, vaginal wall, or cervix. Without identification of the primary chancre, usually presenting 10 days to 12 weeks after initial sexual contact the disease process enters the incubation period leading to secondary syphilis.

The secondary syphilis is usually associated with dermatological findings, lymphadenopathy and a spirochetemia. This will last anywhere from 2–6 weeks. Without treatment about one third of all patients will develop tertiary syphilis. Tertiary syphilis involves the central nervous system, cardiac and musculoskeletal structures. Another sign of tertiary syphilis is that of the Argyll-Robertson pupil (accommodates, but does not react).

Syphilis is known to cross the placenta as early as 8 weeks of gestation.[20] Women in their primary or secondary stage of syphilis are more likely to transmit the disease to the fetus than at the later stage of the disease. Without treatment, infection rates have been as high as 100% of fetuses, with 50% probability of congenital syphilis, of which 50% could result in a fetal demise.[20] Congenital syphilis includes clinical signs of hepatosplenomegaly, characteristic rash, condyloma lata, snuffles, jaundice, pseudoparalysis, anemia, thrombocytopenia, or edema. In children greater than 2 years old other signs might include saddle nose, Hutchinson's teeth, rhagades or Clutton's joints, nerve deafness, anterior bowing of shins, frontal boring, and mulberry molars.

Diagnosis is best achieved from direct fresh specimens from the primary lesion under dark field as quickly as possible. The direct fluorescent antibody test is similar but the slide is treated with 10% methanol and allowed to air dry or heat fixation. Unfortunately, most patients are in the latent portion of the test and need serological tests. There are nonspecific and specific antitreponemal antibody tests, which include the VDRL and the RPR-rapid plasma reagent test. The specific tests for confirmation are the FTA-ABS (Fluorescent treponemal antibody absorption test) and the MHA-TP (microhemagglutination assay). The FTA-ABS test will become positive earlier than the VDRL test.

ESCHERICHIA COLI

Escherichia coli is a motile Gram-negative bacillus, which is part of the normal flora of the intestine and vagina. It is by far, the most common cause of urinary tract infections (UTI) and neonatal sepsis with an incidence is 0.5–1.5 cases per 1000 live births. It is also associated with chorioamnionitis, postpartum endometritis, and septic abortions, often a part of a polymicrobial infection.[12,13]

Pregnancy-related hormonal factors that may increase susceptibility to UTIs include progesterone-mediated ureteral and vesicular smooth muscle relaxation and estrogen facilitated upper urinary tract bacterial infection, particularly with *E. coli* strains.[14] UTIs in pregnancy are associated with pyelonephritis and preterm labor. They have also been known to increase IgM lymphoblastic responses in neonates. Treatment is with cephalosporins, trimethoprim-sulfamethaxazole, ampicillin with clavulanic acid, or gentamicin, depending on the site.

PROTEUS GROUP

Proteus consists of a group of motile Gram-negative bacilli with pleomorphic shape. Urease production is characteristic to this species. Urinary, wound, and neonatal infections are the predominant infections in a gravid female. Neonatal infections are rare, yet if they occur they will present with respiratory findings, rash, and intracerebral hemorrhage. Treatment includes ampicillin or cefazolin.

BACTEROIDACEAE

This family of bacteria consists of Gram-negative anaerobic bacilli, which includes *Bacteriodes fragilis*. It is abscess forming and poses a risk in the gravid woman with an incomplete abortion or retained products of conception. The patient is not only at risk of an abscess, but also of sepsis. It can also be a source for infection at episiotomy sites with rates ranging from 0.2–4%.[11] These infections can progress to necrotizing fasciitis or deeper invasion leading to myonecrosis and perineal abscesses. At times when infection occurs, one should always utilize broad spectrum antibiotics that covers *Bacteriodes fragilis* in addition to the Gram-positive skin pathogens such as *Staphylococcus aureus* and *S. epidermis*. Treatment may include clindamycin, hyperbaric oxygen therapy is still controversial, surgery to remove the abscess, metronidazole, doxycycline, and ampicillin.

GARDNERELLA VAGINALLIS (HEMOPHILUS VAGINALLIS)

Hemophilus vaginallis is an anaerobic, nonmotile, Gram-variable bacilli or coccobacilli associated with bacterial vaginosis. Bacterial vaginosis occurs in 10–30% of pregnant women. The usual complaint is a malodorous vaginal discharge. Symptoms such as irritation, dysuria, and dysparuenia may also be present. It can be diagnosed with the presence of clue cells on a wet mount.

Although *Hemophilus vaginallis* is a normal variant of the vaginal flora, bacterial vaginosis is associated with preterm labor. Septicemia with this organism, if it happens, will happen in the obstetrical patient. Usually it will present itself in 1 of these 3 scenarios: septic abortion, post-cesarean-section, and post-partum endometritis. If isolated from the blood, severe pyrexia will also be present. It will not usually affect the fetus directly, except in the form of maternal chorioamnionitis. Treatment includes intravaginal medications such as metronidazole, oral metronidazole, or ampicillin with clavulanic acid.

HEMOPHILUS DUCREYI

Hemophilus ducreyi is a chancroid forming Gram-negative rod. It is sexually transmitted and needs blood to grow. If a chancroid is found an exam test for syphilis should also be performed. Treatment is with sulfanamide, or chloramphenicol if resistant, but should be used with caution in pregnancy.

ACTINOMYCES ISRAELII

Actinomyces israelii is a Gram-positive anaerobic. It causes a progressive inflammatory disease with local or systemic manifestations. The female genital tract can be involved through direct dissemination from a contiguous area, lymphatic spread, or hematogenous dissemination during a systemic infection. It is possible to be associated with ascending infection, but this is rare. Treatment is with penicillins, ampicillin, tetracycline, chloramphericol, clindamycin, and some aminoglycosides.

CALYMMATOBACTERIUM GRANULOMATIS

Calymmatobacterium granulomatis is a Gram-negative organism, thought to be sexually transmitted. It is associated with a higher rate of malignancy of the vulva, which does not decrease during pregnancy. Treatment usually consists of chloramphenicol, tetracycline, ampicillin, or streptomycin. During pregnancy ampicillin should be used.

CLOSTRIDIA

Clostridia consist of larger Gram-positive rods that produce elaborate endotoxins and can result in gas gangrene from *Clostridium perfringens* and others as well as exotoxic neurotoxins of the tetani and botulism subclass. *C. perfringens* is found in the soil, intestinal tract, and female genital tract and is a major human pathogen. It is associated with postabortion and puerperal uterine infections and low-grade endometritis with or without gas formation. Clinically, these infections present with vaginal discharge, uterine tenderness, and fever. Clostridia can also cause soft-tissue infections. Treatments may consist of metronidazole, clindamycin, or vancomycin.

STAPHYLOCOCCUS AUREUS

Staphylococcus aureus is a coagulase positive, Gram-positive cluster of cocci that can replicate under aerobic or anaerobic conditions. It is usually responsible for wound infections, bacterial gangrene, UTI, septicemia, mastitis, toxic shock syndrome, and endocarditis. Wound infections are usually purulent in nature with local tenderness, edema, and erythema. The usual spread is hematogenous rather than an ascending infection. If there is renal or perinephric abscess involvement then the patient presents with rigors, spiking fevers and flank pain. The biggest risk for obstetrics is septicemia. Culture tubes from two different sites should be drawn and all indwelling catheters should be removed if *Staphylococcus* is suspected. Treatment should be with a penicillinase resistant penicillin, or vancomycin. Methicillin-resistant *Staphylococcus aureus* (MRSA) is a concern and knowing the hospitals prevalence for MRSA would be beneficial for choosing the appropriate therapy.

Staphylococcus Epidermis

Staphylococcus epidermis is a coagulase-negative, Gram-positive cocci. It is the second most common cause of UTIs in young women with no renal abnormality. Cultures from wound infections and neonatal scalp abscesses will frequently grow *S. epidermis*. The treatment of choice is vancomycin.

SALMONELLA TYPHI

Salmonella typhi is a Gram-negative, nonencapsulated, motile bacilli with a predilection for the reticuloendothelial system. The gastrointestinal tract is usually the site of infection, but it can also be involved in gallbladder disease. If there is gallbladder disease then the patient can become a chronic carrier. It disseminates through the lymphatics. It can cross the placenta and cause fetal infection, and is associated with an increased incidence of spontaneous abortion and preterm labor. Treatment is with amoxacillin in pregnancy since chloramphenicol is contraindicated.

References

1. Barton L, Hodgman JE, Pavlova Z. Causes of death in the extremely low birth weight infant. *Pediatrics.* 1999;103:446–451.
2. Goldman AS. Host responses to infection. *Pediatrics in Review.* 2000;21:342–349.
3. Monif G. *Infectious Diseases in Obstetrics and Gynecology* 2nd ed. Philadelphia: Harper & Row; 1982.
4. Andrews W. The preterm prediction study: association of second-trimester genitourinary chlamydia infection with subsequent spontaneous preterm birth. *Amer J Obstet Gynecol.* 2000;183:662–668.
5. Bortolussi R, McGregor D, Kongshavn P, et al. Host defense mechanisms to perinatal and neonatal Listeria monocytogenes infection. *Surv Synth Path Res.* 1984;3:311–312.
6. Lennon D, Lewis B, Mantell C, et al. Epidemic perinatal listeriosis. *Pediatric Infectious Disease.* 1984;3:30–34.
7. Mazor M, Froimovich M, Lazer E, et al. Listeria monocytogenes: the role of transabdominal amniocentesis in febrile patients with preterm labor. *Arch Gynecol Obstet.* 1992;252:109–112.
8. McLauchlin J. Human listerosis in Britain, 1967–1985: a summary of 722 cases. Listeriosis during pregnancy and in the newborn. *Epidermiology Infection.* 1990;104:181–189.
9. Tappero J, Schuchat A, Deaver K, et al. Reduction in the incidence of human listeriosis in the United States. *J Am Med Association.* 1995;273:1118–1122.
10. Stoll BJ, Kanto WP Jr, Glass RI, et al. Treated maternal gonorrhea without adverse effect on outcome of pregnancy. *South Medicine J.* 1982;75:1236–1238.
11. Pastorek JG. *Obstet Gynecol Infectious Disease.* New York: Raven Press; 1994.
12. Larsen B, Galask RP. Host resistance to intra-amniotic infection. *Obstet Gynecol Survey.* 1976;30:675–691.
13. Cherry SH, Filer M, Harvey H. Lysozyme content of amniotic fluid. *American J Obstet Gynecol.* 1973;116:639–642.
14. Andrews W. The preterm prediction study: association of second-trimester genitourinary chlamydia infection with subsequent spontaneous preterm birth. *American J Obstet and Gynecol.* 2000;183:662–668.
15. Lancet RF, Taylor Robinson D, Newman M, et al. Spontaneous early preterm labor associated with abnormal genital bacterial colonization. *British J Obstet Gynecol.* 1986;93:804–810.
16. Smeltzer J, Cruikshank D, Lewis J, et al. Group B streptococcal colonization as an independent risk factor for premature birth. *8th Annual Meeting of the Society of Perinatal Obstetricians.* Las Vegas, NV, 1988.
17. Katz PF. Group B streptococcus: to culture or not to culture? *J Perinatology.* 1999;19:337–342.
18. Sweet R, Gibbs R. *Infectious Diseases of the Female Genital Tract,* 3rd ed. Baltimore, MD: Williams and Wilkins; 1995.
19. Main E, Slagle T. Prevention of early-onset invasive neonatal group B streptococcal disease in a private hospital setting: the superiority of culture based protocols. *Am J Obstet Gynecol.* 2000;182:1344–1354.
20. Harter CA, Benirschke K. Fetal syphilis in the first trimester. *Am J Obstet Gynecol.* 1976;124:705–711.
21. Minkoff H. Prematurity: infection as an etiologic factor. *Obstet Gynecol.* 1983;6:137.
22. Goldman AS. Host responses to infection. *Pediatrics in Review.* 2000;21:446–451.

VIRAL AGENTS AND REPRODUCTIVE RISKS

Jan E. Dickinson / Bernard Gonik

INTRODUCTION

Viruses are ubiquitous in our environment, producing a wide variety of clinical phenomena when infecting the human organism. It is therefore not surprising that viral agents may infect the pregnant human host and that such infections may traverse the maternal-placental barrier to result in a variety of outcomes for the fetus. These outcomes vary depending on the specific viral agent, the period of gestation at which the infection occurs, the maternal immune status and the mechanism of action of the virus on the fetal host. The impact of a maternal viral infection on the fetus range from no discernible effects through to abortion, stillbirth, preterm labor and delivery, physical defects, intrauterine growth disturbances and the postnatal persistence of infection (Table 14-1). A wide variety of viral agents have been reported to affect the developing fetus in utero, transmission occurring by the transplacental passage of the virus during the period of maternal viremia. Ascending infection from the lower genital tract or local extension from adjacent upper genital or gastrointestinal tract infections are also portals of entry for viruses to the fetoplacental unit. Fetal viral transmission does not necessarily produce adverse fetal effects. Serologic changes may be the only evidence of fetal infection. For example, most neonates with congenital cytomegalovirus infection display no signs of congenital disease at birth.

The mechanisms by which viral agents may produce adverse effects on the fetus include placental dysfunction secondary to maternal infection (fever, toxins, altered placental circulation, thrombosis, or placentitis producing hypoxia with altered cell growth and subsequent fetal damage), chromosomal damage, cellular necrosis, and antigen-antibody formation. Both the infecting viral agent and the resultant fetal inflammatory response produce the observed organ damage, the relative contribution of each being uncertain.

DIAGNOSTIC APPROACH TO CONGENITAL VIRAL INFECTIONS

Fetal viral infections are usually not clinically apparent. The mother may provide a history of rubella or varicella infection, but usually either no reported illness or nonspecific symptoms (e.g., malaise, rash, fever, or lymphadenopathy) are elicited on direct questioning. Certain lifestyle factors may provide diagnostic assistance: intravenous drug use (hepatitis B and C, HIV infections), occupational exposure to cytomegalovirus in health care workers, or parvovirus in childcare employees.

When the community prevalence of a teratogenic or otherwise obstetrically detrimental viral agent is high and the background seropositivity low, maternal serologic screening is useful, particularly if a specific therapy is available. Universal maternal serum screening for rubella virus immunity is standard obstetric practice. Ideally, all reproductive age women should have their rubella status assessed preconception and vaccination of those who are nonimmune performed, a practice that could virtually eliminate congenital rubella syndrome. Maternal screening for other viral agents is less clear and is based on the population prevalence of the particular agent, the potential impact of the viral agent on the pregnancy and the availability of an appropriate screening test. Evidence of maternal hepatitis B viral exposure is usually assessed antenatally and vaccination provided after birth to the infant and family members of those at risk. Other viral agents may be selectively screened for in the mother. Cytomegalovirus, a common viral agent in pregnancy with known potential adverse fetal effects, is usually not screened for in the general obstetric population because the background seropositivity rate is high and management protocols uncertain. In selected populations, however, viral screening may be appropriate. A maternal history of exposure to varicella should prompt serologic screening for prior exposure, the information gleaned usually acting to reassure the mother of her existing immune status. In high-risk groups, preconception CMV serologic testing may be indicated to clarify the clinical scenario. HIV serologic screening is being offered routinely, and in all viral screening programs adequate counseling and follow up is mandatory. Similarly, discussions with the testing laboratory are important for correct interpretation of the screening tests. For example, cross-reaction of IgG and IgM antibodies is a recognized phenomenon and can lead to false-positive diagnoses. Serial studies may be required and viral IgM positive results should be interpreted with caution.

Assessment of the fetal environment is required when investigating viral exposures in the second and third trimesters. Sonography of the fetus may provide the first clue that a viral infection has occurred. Conversely, in cases of documented maternal viremia, the fetal sonogram is usually unremarkable. It is not certain what percentage of virally infected fetuses that will display sonographic abnormalities. Sonography may demonstrate the presence of fetal hydrops, classically observed in instances of fetal viral infections with parvovirus but also reported in cases of congenital CMV. Abnormal central nervous system findings in the form of intracranial calcification, hydrocephalus or microcephaly may be demonstrated in congenital CMV and varicella infection. It is important to emphasize that normality of the fetal sonogram does not exclude the later development of viral-induced sequelae.

Invasive prenatal diagnostic testing should be tailored to the individual clinical circumstance and specific viral agent. Careful, accurate pretest counseling is important prior to and following any testing procedures. Demonstration of fetal infection does not necessarily imply an adverse fetal effect from the

TABLE 14-1	FETAL EFFECTS OF INTRAUTERINE VIRAL INFECTIONS
Pregnancy loss	
Abortion	
Stillbirth	
Preterm labor and birth	
Intrauterine growth restriction	
Teratogenic malformations	
Hydrops fetalis	
Central nervous system	Microcephaly, hydrocephaly, intracranial calcification chorioretinitis, cataracts, microphthalmia
Cardiorespiratory system	Pericardial/pleural effusions, cardiac failure, myocarditis
	Congenital cardiac defects
Gastrointestinal system	Hepatosplenomegaly, ascites, intraabdominal calcification
Peripheries	Limb reduction defects, cicatricial scarring
Hematologic system	Pancytopenia, aplastic anemia, thrombocytopenia, leukopenia, leucocytosis
Chronic infection	

viral agent and invasive testing procedures should probably be performed only if the result will directly alter pregnancy management.

Amniocentesis is the principal diagnostic modality in the assessment of fetal CMV infection, due to the renal excretion by the fetus of this virus. Herpes simplex virus and rubella have also been isolated from the amniotic fluid.[1] Amniocentesis is probably the best medium for culturing CMV in the infected fetus, although a positive culture does not predict the final outcome.[2] The techniques of polymerase chain reaction (PCR) are increasingly being used in viral infection investigation, although false-positive amplification is possible.

Fetal blood sampling may be used in the assessment of suspected fetal viral infection. The most useful criterion for assessment of fetal infection is the detection of viral-specific IgM, antigen or culture/polymerase chain reaction techniques from fetal blood. The fetal full blood count (with assessment of fetal platelet count, hemoglobin, and white cell count), hepatic biochemistry and total IgM may be used as indirect indicators of infection. The fetus does not appear to generate a detectable IgM response to infection until after 20 weeks gestation, although IgG will be detectable due to maternal placental transfer.

Other invasive fetal techniques such as chorion villus sampling (CVS) and thin-gauge embryofetoscopy are investigational tools in the assessment of fetal viral infections. There is a potential to employ CVS and viral PCR in the assessment process, particularly in the first trimester of infections such as rubella. As PCR is extremely sensitive, contamination by maternal body fluids and tissue need to be considered prior to specific testing.

Should a fetus be demonstrated antenatally to be infected with a specific viral agent, appropriate information transfer antenatally and assessment post-delivery is required in a multidisciplinary team setting.

SPECIFIC VIRAL AGENTS AND REPRODUCTIVE RISKS

Rubella

The rubella virus produces an acute, contagious exanthem that usually occurs in epidemics. A single-stranded RNA togavirus, the rubella virus is spread by nasopharyngeal droplets from which the virus implants and multiplies in the respiratory epithelium, with an incubation period of 14–21 days. The typical maculopapular rash and generalized lymphadenopathy of rubella infection is preceded by a short period of prodromal symptomatology with malaise, fever, headache, conjunctivitis, and pharyngitis. The duration of the rash is usually 3 days, commencing on the face and migrating caudally.

Infectivity is greatest in the prodromal and rash period. Infection may be asymptomatic, with only 60–70% of those infected developing a rash. Therefore, confirmation of disease should be based on serologic evidence.

It is the potential teratogenic effect of the rubella virus in pregnancy that produces most concern. During periods of epidemics, almost 4% of pregnant women may become infected, compared with only 0.1–0.2% of pregnant women at other times. Intrauterine transmission of the virus occurs after primary infection of the mother. The gestational age of the fetus at the time of maternal infection is the principal factor determining pregnancy outcome. Defects attributable to rubella result from infections occurring before 16 weeks of gestation. Infections beyond 16–20 weeks of gestation do not appear to result in congenital anomalies, probably because of fetal structural development and developing immunologic competence. The frequency of fetal rubella infection after clinical maternal infection is more than 80% during the first 12 weeks of pregnancy, 54% at 13–14 weeks, and 25% at the end of the second trimester.[3] Enders et al.,[4] in a prospective study of periconceptional maternal rubella, reported a negligible fetal risk when rubella occurred before the last menstrual period and a universal, fetal infection when rash occurred 3–6 weeks after the last normal menstruation. Infection of the embryo during the first 8 weeks of gestation often leads to the full congenital rubella syndrome, whereas after this period, fetal damage is less severe and is confined to individual organs. Severe congenital malformations and fetal damage occur in approximately 22% of infants following first trimester rubella and in 10% following second-trimester rubella.[5]

First trimester rubella virus infection has been investigated with CVS to detect placental viral presence by viral culture and antigen identification. In the second trimester, fetal blood sampling may be used to detect rubella-specific IgM. To minimize false negative results due to the immature fetal immune system, such sampling should not be performed prior to 22 weeks gestation.[6,7]

Immunization programs have significantly reduced the incidence of rubella. Although the incidence of rubella in women of childbearing age has declined accordingly, 10–15% still are susceptible to infection. It is thus important that fertile, nonimmune women are identified and actively vaccinated prior to pregnancy. By effective and aggressive immunization programs it should be possible to virtually eliminate congenital rubella.

Maternal viremia may be followed by placental infection and secondary fetal viremia, with subsequent infection of fetal organs. Vascular endothelial cellular necrosis has been noted on histologic examination of rubella-infected abortuses.[3] The placenta may contain virus in the absence of fetal viral infection. Fetal disease is associated with major structural anomalies, destruction of normal tissue, and chronic infection that persists months to years after birth. Congenital rubella infection is characterized by a prolonged period of viral shedding. Virus can be recovered from the throats of 88% of infected babies at 1 month of age, decreasing to 33% at 5–8 months of age.

The clinical manifestations of congenital rubella are diverse (Table 14-2). The classic congenital rubella triad comprises cataracts, sensorineural deafness, and congenital heart disease. Other defects following fetal infection include intrauterine growth restriction, retinopathy, central nervous system disease with meningoencephalitis, and secondary intellectual handicap. Also included in the spectrum of congenital rubella are pneumonitis and bony lesions, immunologic disorders, chromosomal abnormalities, hepatitis, and thrombocytopenic purpura. Not all the defects associated with congenital rubella are recognizable at birth. Deafness is usually not diagnosed until late infancy. Other anomalies, such as the progressive panencephalitis and the endocrinopathies, do not develop for several years.[8] Continued viral replication may contribute to these chronic defects. It is estimated that one third

of neonates with congenital rubella syndrome have expanded syndromes and are asymptomatic at birth, but ultimately manifest evidence of developmental injury.[9]

The mechanisms involved in the growth anomalies of congenital rubella are now more precisely understood. Infection with rubella virus in fibroblasts can induce mitotic arrest without morphologic defect. A soluble factor produced by the infected cells has been shown to inhibit mitosis in uninfected cells.[10] Chronically infected human mesenchymal cells demonstrate slower growth responses to epidermal growth factor (EGF), possibly because of suboptimal utilization of the EGF.[11] Chromosomal abnormalities have been associated with congenital rubella infections, and these may contribute to altered growth. Persistent viral presence and antigenemia may induce autoimmune phenomena. These phenomena may be involved in a variety of chronic sequelae, most notably the endocrine diseases.

The management of women with rubella infection in pregnancy centers around the accurate diagnosis of the viral infection. There is no evidence to support the use of immunoglobulin to reduce the risk of fetal disease, nor the effectiveness of antiviral agents in this setting. Serial ultrasound to assess fetal growth may be used and fetal echocardiography for cardiac structural evaluation, but normally sonography does not imply an absence of viral effect. Pregnancy interruption should be included in discussions of early pregnancy rubella infection.

Cytomegalovirus

Cytomegalovirus (CMV) is a double-stranded DNA herpes virus and is highly species specific. The *herpesvirus* family are characterized by latency and reactivation phenomena. CMV is ubiquitous in human society, its incidence being influenced by several lifestyle factors. In middle-upper class socioeconomic groups in the United States and England, 40–60% of adults are seropositive to CMV compared with 80% of those from lower socioeconomic groups.[12–14] Most infections with CMV are not clinically apparent, although it can manifest as an infectious mononucleosis-like illness. Early childhood, adolescence, and reproductive age groups appear to have an increased risk of viral acquisition.[15,16] An estimated 57% of women of reproductive age are seropositive, and cervical viral secretion occurs in 14%.[17]

CMV is not highly contagious; spread occurs by close contact with infected secretions. CMV may be excreted in the urine and bodily secretions of those infected and viral transmission to an uninfected host occurs by close body contact. Human blood, marrow, or organs may be a source of infection if received from a seropositive donor. The newborn may be congenitally infected by the transplacental passage of virus from mother to fetus in utero or the virus may be perinatally acquired from contact with maternal genital tract secretions or breast milk.

Cytomegalovirus is the most common viral infection to be transmitted to the fetus in utero, with a reported incidence of 1% of all live births.[18,19] Most primary CMV infections in pregnancy are asymptomatic, and occur in some 0.7–4.1% of

TABLE 14-2	CONGENITAL RUBELLA SEQUELAE	
Congenital rubella triad	Cataracts
	Sensorineural deafness
	Congenital cardiac defects
Expanded rubella syndrome	Intrauterine growth restriction
	Meningoencephalitis
	Retinopathy
	Chromosomal abnormalities
	Hepatitis
	Thrombocytopenia
	Pneumonitis
	Immunologic disease

pregnancies. Approximately 10% of neonates with congenital CMV are symptomatic of this viral infection at birth, with some 30% of these dying and the majority of survivors demonstrating severe neurologic sequelae of this disease. Of those asymptomatic neonates, 10–15% will develop disease manifestations such as neurologic abnormalities and deafness.[20] The pathogenesis of prenatal infection appears similar to that of rubella. Maternal infection is followed by maternal viremia and probable transplacental infection. Placental infection does not imply fetal infection, and fetal infection does not always imply fetal effect. An ascending route of infection is possible but less likely.

Unlike most viral infections, the presence of maternal humoral antibody does not preclude subsequent reinfection or reactivation of latent virus and secondary transplacental viral passage. Latent CMV may reside in monocytes, bone marrow, and kidney. The virulence of infection in the fetus and neonate is obtunded in recurrent infections, implying that the maternal immune response has some protective effect. The woman who develops primary CMV infection during pregnancy is at greatest risk of severe fetal pathology.

The severity of congenital infection appears to be related to the gestational age at the time of exposure to the virus. Infection occurs with similar frequency in all trimesters although in the first half of pregnancy the risk of significant fetal anomalies is greater.[12,14] The overall rate of vertical transmission for CMV is in the order of 35–40%.[20–22]

Congenital CMV infection may be associated with a variety of congenital anomalies (Table 14-3), primarily CNS and oculo-auditory lesions, but 90% of infected neonates have no clinical manifestations of disease at birth. Approximately 5% of infected neonates have classic CMV inclusion disease, with hepatosplenomegaly, thrombocytopenia with purpura and petecchiae, mental retardation (microcephaly, encephalitis, intracranial calcification), chorioretinitis, pneumonitis, and intrauterine growth restriction. This group usually develops long-term complications. An additional 5% of congenitally infected infants have atypical disease with varying degrees of neurologic, psychomotor, and behavioral disorders. Not all long-term sequelae are evident at birth. Ninety percent of infected asymptomatic infants appear to have a good long-term outcome. Conboy et al. noted that in a group of asymptomatic

TABLE 14-3	CONGENITAL CMV INFECTION SEQUELAE
Intracranial calcification
Microcephaly
Chorioretinitis
Intrauterine growth restriction
Thrombocytopenia
Hepatosplenomegaly
Sensorineural deafness
Pneumonitis

congenitally infected children without auditory involvement there was no later intelligence deficit.[23]

Cellular injury by CMV may occur by direct or indirect viral cytolysis, with or without an immunologic destructive reaction. The direct cytocidal effects of CMV produce intranuclear inclusions and destruction of cells. Cytomegalovirus may persist in tissue culture for long periods without cytopathic changes,[24] implying that latent or persistent CMV infections may be cytologically occult. CMV also may have rubella-like noncytocidal effects on cellular proliferation, with intrauterine growth restriction resulting from a reduction in the number of cells in the fetal organs.

Indirect mechanisms of cellular injury are those mediated by secondary inflammatory responses and vasculitis. Vasculitis causes ischemia and secondary tissue destruction. The presence of circulating immune complexes in congenitally infected infants provides evidence for immune complex disease-mediated destruction. Destruction of host cells carrying less than the cytocidal dose of virus occurs by a cell-immune reaction mediated by T lymphocytes.[24]

The exact role of immune complex disease in congenital CMV is undetermined. There are several immunologic anomalies in the congenital CMV-infected infant: elevated immunoglobulins M and G, circulating immune complexes, and a specific defect in cell-mediated immunity.[25,26] The cell-mediated immune defect appears to be due to an abnormality in helper T cells. This defect in T lymphocyte function does resolve over several years, and normalization is associated with the cessation of viral secretion. This abnormal immune response of congenital CMV may contribute to persistent viral replication and continued damage.

The diagnosis of congenital CMV may be assisted by serologic testing. Seventy percent of congenitally infected infants have a positive CMV ELISA IgM, while those in whom infection is acquired perinatally will demonstrate increasing IgG titers with an absent IgM. The most sensitive method for the diagnosis of CMV however is isolation of the virus from blood, urine, or amniotic fluid using tissue culture techniques, in situ hybridization or polymerase chain reaction. Antenatal diagnosis of CMV infection is centered around sonographic suspicion (e.g., periventricular calcification, intra-abdominal calcification, hydrocephaly, fetal hydrops, intrauterine growth restriction) and subsequent viral culture from the amniotic fluid. Fetal blood sampling is used in some centers to supplement information (e.g., fetal thrombocytopenia, presence of CMV-specific IgM). Isolation of CMV from the amniotic fluid does not discriminate between fetal infection and long-term outcome. When fetal sonographic abnormalities such as microcephaly, intracranial calcification, ventriculomegaly, abnormal intracavity fluid collections, and intrauterine growth restriction are present, the incidence of CMV on culture of the amniotic fluid is much higher than if the sonogram is normal. A negative amniotic fluid culture for CMV probably excludes the diagnosis, although further studies are needed to solidify this impression. The gestation at which the amniocentesis is performed appears important in terms of diagnostic accuracy. Amniocentesis performed beyond 21 weeks gestation is associated with an 81–100% sensitivity, while those performed prior to this time demonstrate a lower diagnostic sensitivity of 45%, but maintain a 100% specificity.[27]

The use of antiviral agents as part of the therapeutic approach in the treatment of infants with CMV is currently being investigated.[28,29] Ganciclovir treatment has been demonstrated to decrease viral shedding during therapy in infants with congenital CMV.[30,31] This drug has been associated with neutropenia and thrombocytopenia in humans. Ganciclovir does not traverse the placenta, and therefore is of limited use in utero. Certain orally administered agents such as valacyclovir have the theoretical advantage of maintaining high maternal serum levels, and thus may cross the placenta in high enough a concentration to attenuate fetal infection. Valacyclovir and pharmacologically similar drugs have been shown effective against CMV infection when used in high concentrations. The use of immunoglobulin and antiviral agents to ameliorate or prevent fetal effects in the pregnant woman with primary CMV infection has yet to be adequately investigated.

Herpes Simplex Virus

Herpes simplex virus (HSV), a double-stranded DNA virus, produces a range of infections. HSV type 2 is most often associated with genital herpes infection. The herpes virus has the ability to reactivate intermittently after a primary infection, between periods of latency in the body. The sites of latency are the central nervous system sensory ganglia. Most herpes infections in pregnancy represent recurrent disease, with the recurrence rate increasing as gestation advances.[32]

Herpes simplex virus damages the neonate mainly through *intrapartum* infections, but can also cause congenital disease. Congenital HSV is a distinct entity and not related to perinatally acquired HSV occurring around the time of birth.[33] There is an associated increase in spontaneous abortions and stillbirths with primary HSV infections, especially in the first half of pregnancy.[34] The incidence of fetal HSV is unknown, but it is probably uncommon; however, there are reported cases of congenital malformations associated with primary maternal HSV, usually in the first trimester.[35–37] The fetal effects that have been reported include cutaneous defects (scars, calcifications, vesicles), microcephaly, hydranencephaly, cerebral and cerebellar necrosis, intracranial calcification, microphthalmia, hepatosplenomegaly, chorioretinitis, and bone anomalies. Primary HSV infection in early pregnancy has been associated with as high as a 10% incidence of central nervous system and musculoskeletal defects in the fetus. The transplacental transmission of HSV and secondary fetal infection may produce a severe in utero infection leading to fetal death. In the survivors, there is a 40% perinatal morbidity and major chronic neurologic sequelae.[38]

The isolation of HSV virus in tissue culture is the gold standard for diagnosis, requiring 7–10 days of culture to defini-

tively exclude the presence of infection. Using HSV-specific ELISA with tissue culture allows for a more rapid preliminary result to be available in 24–48 hours. Maternal serology is usually not helpful in the diagnosis of maternal HSV infection because of the high background rate of seropositivity. The level of antibody present is not predictive of the presence or absence of infection.

The intrapartum exposure of the fetus to HSV in the genital tract is the usual method of neonatal viral acquisition. Less commonly, the virus may be acquired in the postpartum period. The reported incidence of neonatal HSV varies from 1 in 3000 livebirths to 1 in 7000 live births.[39,40] In asymptomatic women, active viral shedding has been reported in 0.4% at delivery,[41] with 35% of these women experiencing a primary HSV episode on the basis of serology. In those women deemed to have an asymptomatic primary HSV episode at the time of delivery, the neonatal infection rate was 33% compared with 3% in the remaining women deemed to have had a reactivation of HSV. The higher viral load, longer duration of viral shedding and absence of protective maternal IgG in primary HSV is presumed to account for the higher observed neonatal infection rates.

Neonatal HSV infection may present clinically with localized infection of the skin, eyes, and mouth, central nervous system infection (seizures, irritability, hypotonia, lethargy), or as disseminated disease. Outcome following neonatal HSV infection depends on the clinical extent of the disease (virtually zero in localized cases, 15% with central nervous system involvement and 57% with disseminated disease in the presence of appropriate antiviral therapy), gestation, presence or absence of coagulopathy, and presence or absence of coma and seizures.[40] Therapy centers around isolation, antiviral agents, and adjunctive intensive care.

The obstetric management strategies involve identification of women with HSV shedding and reduction of the risk to the neonate of viral transmission. First-episode HSV genital infection during pregnancy is associated with a 30–50% incidence of preterm birth[38,42] and vaginal delivery with an approximate transmission rate of 40%.[39] It is uncertain if the use of acyclovir antenatally during an initial viral infection ameliorates the obstetric sequelae. Delivery by cesarean section is now standard obstetric practice in the setting of active primary genital HSV[39,43,44] although this delivery route does not completely protect the fetus with 20–30% of neonatal HSV cases being delivered by cesarean section.[45–48] Unfortunately, many women are not aware of HSV genital infections and such obstetric strategies therefore cannot be applied in asymptomatic first-episode cases. Recurrent genital HSV with active lesions present at the time of delivery are also best treated with cesarean route of delivery, although the neonatal transmission rate is much lower. In cases of unavoidable vaginal delivery in primary genital HSV infection therapy with acyclovir is commenced, while in recurrent infections treatment may be individualized with therapy for positive cultures or clinical evidence of infection.

Other Herpesviruses

Epstein-Barr Virus

Epstein-Barr virus (EBV) is a common childhood infection, and therefore, most adults are seropositive. The seronegative rate among pregnant women is low, with 95% having serologic evidence of prior EBV exposure. Primary EBV infection in pregnancy is therefore very unusual. A 7% seroconversion rate has been reported in pregnancy in 1 study of 46 seronegative women,[49] however, others have not reported such a high conversion rate.[35,50]

As primary EBV infection in pregnancy is rare, it is difficult to establish if transplacental viral transmission occurs and if the fetus becomes infected. The studies performed have not shown a significant fetal infection rate.[34,51–53] A few studies, however, have reported congenital malformations associated with virologic and serologic evidence of EBV infection.[54–57] The anomalies include congenital heart disease, CNS malformations, cataracts, biliary atresia, microphthalmia, metaphysitis, and low birth weight. Although the impact of primary EBV infection in pregnancy is uncertain, it would seem prudent to perform a detailed assessement of fetal cardiac anatomy in the second trimester following a documented first-trimester EBV infection and consideration be given to serial sonographic evaluation of fetal growth.

Varicella-Zoster Virus

Varicella-zoster virus (VZV), a DNA herpes virus, is an extremely common childhood infection, such that the majority of the adult population in developed countries are seropositive. It clinically manifests as chickenpox (varicella) and shingles (zoster), the latter arising from reactivation of latent VZV.

Varicella is a highly contagious respiratory infection characterized by cutaneous lesions. The incubation period varies from 10–21 days, usually averaging 14–16 days. A transient viremia precedes the development of fever, malaise, and crops of intensely pruritic vesicles. The vesicles subsequently break open and crust over, resulting in a rash that usually lasts 7–10 days. Viral transmission occurs from 2 days prior to the development of cutaneous manifestations until the vesicles crust over. Varicella pneumonia and hepatitis are the most serious complications although encephalitis, pericarditis, glomerulitis, and arthritis may occasionally occur.

The diagnosis is usually based on the clinical manifestations, particularly the characteristic skin lesions. The virus may be cultured from the cutaneous vesicles or identified using antigen-detection tests on samples from skin lesions. More than 95% of women of childbearing age have serologic evidence of prior exposure to varicella, hence the incidence in pregnancy is low, on the order of 1–7 in 10,000 pregnancies.[34,58] It was believed that varicella complicating pregnancy was associated with severe maternal disease, but contemporary studies have not supported this belief.[59] Nonimmune pregnant women exposed to varicella should be offered varicella immune globulin in an attempt to ameliorate the maternal disease. In maternal varicella, therapy with acyclovir may be required if symptoms

are severe. Zoster infection occurs long after primary varicella and presents as a unilateral skin eruption in a dermatomal distribution. Herpes zoster in pregnancy is rare, occurring in 0.5 in 10,000 pregnancies.

In the small number of women who are seronegative, VZV can cause serious intrauterine infection, with the virus presumably reaching the fetus by way of the transplacental route after maternal viremia. Viremia is presumed to occur only during the acute rash evolution phase of a primary chickenpox illness; viremia is rare during zoster illness. Therefore, transplacental infection may occur with maternal chickenpox, but is not a significant risk in maternal zoster. The frequency with which VZV reaches the placenta and fetus during maternal chickenpox is unknown, although it is clear that a fetus is not invariably infected during such maternal infections.

Maternal IgG antibodies cross the placenta, the transplacental passage increasing with advancing gestation. The maternal antibody response protects the neonate and infants lacking protective transplacental varicella antibody may become very ill with perinatal varicella. Approximately 5 days is required to generate an adequate maternal antibody response. Zoster immune globulin is recommended for neonates at risk of perinatal varicella to modify the disease severity.[60]

Serologic tests are available to ascertain the susceptibility of the mother to varicella and previous viral exposure. The diagnosis of in-utero infection may be assisted in the presence of abnormal fetal sonography (ventriculomegaly, microcephaly, intrauterine growth restriction, intra-abdominal calcification). The roles of placental biopsy, amniocentesis, and fetal blood sampling is uncertain and should probably be restricted to only those cases in which the fetus is abnormal on ultrasound.

Varicella in the first half of pregnancy has been associated with congenital anomalies in the fetus. Later infections generally have not been associated with malformations, although in the last 3 weeks of pregnancy the incidence of neonatal varicella is 25%. The manifestations of congenital varicella are primarily cutaneous (cicatricial skin lesions, denuded skin), neurologic (microcephaly, cerebellar and cortical atrophy, focal brain calcification), ocular (chorioretinitis, microphthalmia, optic atrophy), and musculoskeletal (limb hypoplasia, muscular atrophy, rudimentary digits, talipes), and include intrauterine growth restriction and congenital-neonatal zoster. A neuropathy secondary to damage of dorsal ganglia and anterior spinal cord is believed to be responsible for the observed limb abnormalities. The frequency of congenital varicella syndrome developing in offspring of mothers with chickenpox is in the order of 1–2% based on the published prospective studies.[58,59] In a recent series,[59] no cases of congenital varicella syndrome were reported in those women receiving varicella immune globulin.

Maternal zoster infection does not appear to be associated with such a high incidence of congenital anomalies, although a small number of infants with malformations following maternal zoster have been described;[61–63] malformations are predominantly microcephaly, microphthalmia, cataracts, and talipes. A recent study involving 366 women with gestational herpes zoster did not report 1 case of congenital varicella.[59]

Parvovirus

Parvovirus B19 is a human-specific single-stranded DNA virus which most usually manifests clinically as erythema infectiosum, or fifth disease, in children. In adults an immune-mediated arthralgia and exanthematous illness may occur, although infection is frequently asymptomatic. Viral transmission is via contact with respiratory secretions. Parvovirus replicate intracellularly in the nucleus and its presence is characterized by inclusions ("lantern cells") visible with light microscopy. The virus preferentially infects rapidly dividing cells such as bone marrow erythroid precursors.

Acquisition rates for parvovirus B19 are associated to occupation, with the highest attack rates seen in school teachers and childcare workers. The prevalence of parvovirus antibody is less than 5% in preschool-aged children, increasing to 40% by age 20 years and in older age groups the seroprevalence may exceed 75%.

The seroprevalence of parvovirus B19 in women of reproductive age is 35–50%. The incidence of parvovirus infection in pregnancy has recently been reported as 3.7%.[64] Maternal infection with parvovirus B19 is associated with a fetal infection rate of approximately 20% (range 11–33%)[64,65] and a perinatal loss rate of 10% (range 0.5–16%) in women who seroconvert during pregnancy.[64–66] Maternal infection with parvovirus B19 is associated with an immunoglobulin response of IgG and IgM, the former persisting for life and offering protection, the latter usually declining to undetectable levels by 60–90 days.

Parvovirus does not appear to induce fetal structural abnormalities although a viral myocarditis has been reported. In the fetus, destruction of erythrocyte precursors produces anemia with secondary cardiac failure and nonimmune hydrops. Fetal death may result if the viral infection is not recognized and supportive therapy with intravascular fetal blood transfusion not provided.[67,68]

The management of pregnant women in whom acute parvovirus is diagnosed is controversial. A baseline ultrasound is reasonable practice and serial sonography advisable to assess for evidence of fetal hydrops. Fetal parvovirus infection is manifest within 12 weeks of maternal infection. It has been suggested that elevated maternal serum alpha-fetoprotein levels may predict fetal hydrops but the usefulness of this test is yet to be determined on a practical basis.

Hepatitis C Virus

Hepatitis C is an RNA virus, definitively identified in 1989 and a significant cause of non-A, non-B transfusion-related hepatitis. An increasing number of humans appear to be acquiring this virus with an international prevalence of 0.14–6%[69,70] and 1.4% of people in the United States being currently infected with hepatitis C.[71] This virus is readily transmitted via blood exposure and the primary known risk factors for hepatitis C include intravenous drug use, previous blood transfusion, tat-

tooing and organ transplantation. Although in 50% of antibody positive cases there is no revealed risk factor, undisclosed parenteral exposures and illicit drug use are present in more than 80% of circumstances.[72] Chronic hepatitis C occurs in 50–70% of people with hepatitis C, with 50% of all cases of chronic viral hepatitis attributable to this viral agent. Data from hepatitis C blood transfusion acquisition indicates high morbidity rates with approximately 35% of those with acute hepatitis C progressing to cirrhosis at 20 years and 20–25% develop hepatocellular carcinoma.[73,74]

Antibody screening is available using ELISA and recombinant immunoblot assay with a 90–95% sensitivity. Antibody presence indicated prior or current infection with hepatitis C but does not imply protection against the virus. The hepatitis C virus is detectable in blood using polymerase chain reaction techniques and this is the most sensitive test although this assay is subject to greater laboratory error. The earliest serologic test to be positive, hepatitis C RNA is detectable 2 weeks after viral exposure and disease activity may be reflected by the quantitative viral-specific RNA levels.

As with other hematogenously transmitted viruses, there have been reported instances of perinatal hepatitis C transmission, with the risk of transmission being greatest in the third trimester.[75,76] There is a broad range of transmission rates reported, varying from 0–36%.[77,78] Women who are hepatitis C positive, HIV-negative appear to have a 0–18% risk of vertical transmission of hepatitis C. Women who are also HIV-positive have the greatest risk of perinatal hepatitis C transmission, with rates of 6–36% reported.[78] Other factors increasing the vertical transmission rate of hepatitis C are high levels of hepatitis C RNA[77,79,80] and active intravenous drug use.[81] In the absence of hepatitis C RNA maternal-neonatal transmission does not appear to occur.[79] There are limited data on acute hepatitis C viral infection in pregnancy, although reports of vertical transmission following third-trimester infection are published.[82] It would seem prudent to assess the infants of women acutely infected with hepatitis C during pregnancy at 1 year of age. Sexual transmission of hepatitis C appears low, with a reported transmission rate in those without parenteral exposure or HIV of <1%.[83] Similarly, spread of hepatitis C from mother to child in the absence of parenteral exposure is rare.[83]

Screening for hepatitis C should be offered to women at-risk preconception (e.g., intravenous drug use, unscreened blood transfusion recipients). Women known to have hepatitis C infection who are considering pregnancy should undergo hepatitis C RNA quantitation to assess the probable viral vertical transmission risk. Vertical transmission does not appear to occur in the presence of a repeatedly negative hepatitis C RNA, in contrast, if maternal hepatitis C RNA levels exceed 1 million copies/ml the risk is substantial. There is no data to suggest alteration to standard intrapartum protocols in the presence of maternal hepatitis C infection, although avoidance of invasive intrapartum procedures would seem prudent. Hepatitis C transmission from breastmilk does not appear to occur and therefore breastfeeding is not contra-indicated in hepatitis C positive women.[84] At 1 year of age, children of women infected with hepatitis C should undergo testing for hepatitis C RNA, or antibody assessment at 18–24 months of age.

Other RNA Viruses

Enteroviruses

The enteroviruses are single-stranded RNA viruses and include poliomyelitis, coxsackie A, coxsackie B, and echoviruses. The diagnostic technique for enterovirus identification is by tissue culture. Infection with enteroviruses is common, occurring predominantly in children and lower socioeconomic groups, and typically occur in seasonal outbreaks. Viral transmission occurs by respiratory or gastrointestinal routes, followed by generalized viremia. The clinical evidence of infection is variable; it is often asymptomatic or associated with fever, nonspecific rash, and upper respiratory tract infection. More severe disease may be seen, in the form of poliomyelitis, hand-foot-mouth disease, meningoencephalitis, or pleurodynia. The secondary antibody response to enteroviruses is type-specific and appears to provide permanent immunity. Prolonged fecal viral shedding is characteristic, especially in the immunocompromised host.

There is evidence in experimental models that pregnancy alters the immune response to enterovirus, producing a shorter incubation period, more prolonged viremia, and increased susceptibility to infection.[85] Most enterovirus infections in pregnancy are asymptomatic, with the National Institutes of Health Collaborative Perinatal Project reporting a 9% seroconversion rate in 198 pregnant women without significant perinatal disease.[86] Spontaneous abortion rates of 13–24% have been reported in pregnancies complicated by poliomyelitis and coxsackie A16 infections (hand-foot-mouth disease). Echovirus and coxsackie B infections have been associated with stillbirths after late gestational infections.[87,88] These are associated mainly with coxsackie B virus infections, in which a small increase in the incidence of congenital cardiac (coxsackie B3 and B4 in all trimesters) and urologic (first-trimester coxsackie B4) defects was noted. Gastrointestinal tract anomalies have been associated with gestational coxsackie A9 infections throughout all trimesters. All of these malformations are of a wide variety and nonspecific and there is no good evidence to support congenital enterovirus syndromes. The mode of transmission in utero is believed to be transplacental: echovirus 11 is recoverable from cord blood and coxsackie B1 virus in amniotic fluid in infants with evidence of viral infections at birth. Echovirus infections have been associated with severe neonatal disease and death. Coxsackie B virus antigen has been found in 25% of stillbirths and infant deaths in the presence of myocarditis,[89] suggesting that intrauterine infections may lead to cardiac disease as a long-term sequelae.

Influenza Virus

Influenza is a common viral infection and hence is frequently seen in pregnancy, especially during epidemics. Little is known about fetal effects of the influenza virus, and the reported literature is unclear with respect to teratogenic potential. The influenza virus produces an acute respiratory tract infection with postinfective malaise. Several epidemics have occurred during the twentieth century. Symptomatology alone is poor evidence of infection; serology is required to make a definitive diagnosis. Pregnancy does not appear to alter the disease course although the virus is associated with an increased incidence of preterm labor.

The influenza virus appears to cross the placenta: IgG and IgM are found in cord blood, and virus can be cultured from the amniotic fluid. The virus has not been cultured from fetal blood, although a fetal viremia is believed to occur.

Influenza has been associated with congenital anomalies, but there is no defined syndrome or consistent defects. It is known that the virus is subject to antigenic shifts and drifts, and so comparisons of effects between epidemics may not be valid. The diagnostic criteria are often based on symptoms; however, because this basis for diagnosis is unreliable in this viral illness, observed defects may not be real. Influenza virus infection may modify the naturally occurring malformation incidence and not in its own right be a discrete teratogen.[90]

Mumps

Infection with the mumps virus in pregnancy is uncommon; estimates of incidence in pregnancy are of the order of 0.8–10/10,000. The illness symptomatology does not seem to alter in the presence of the gravid state.

An increased incidence of spontaneous abortion has been reported in early pregnancies complicated by mumps.[91] The relationship of the mumps virus to congenital malformations is undetermined. There are scattered case reports of anomalies occurring in association between gestational, but in larger series[91] there is no significant anomaly trend. There was believed to be an association between gestational mumps and endocardial fibroelastosis, however this is now not considered significant.

Human Immunodeficiency Virus

The human immunodeficiency virus (HIV), an RNA retrovirus, has had a significant medical impact, and with this virus now established in the heterosexual population HIV infections complicating pregnancy have become a major obstetric and pediatric issue. It is recognized that maternal-fetal transmission of the virus may occur with a risk of vertical transmission of HIV infection of approximately 25% (range 14–40%)[92] of cases of HIV-seropositive pregnancies.[93] The risk of perinatal HIV is greatest when the maternal disease is advanced, with transmission rates of 65% reported.[94] A decline in the incidence of maternal-fetal transmission in the United States since 1994 has occurred, probably secondary to the use of perinatal zidovudine and avoidance of invasive intrapartum fetal procedures. There is a potential risk of fetal infection during invasive procedures such as amniocentesis, CVS, and fetal blood sampling.[95] Any factor that increases fetal exposure to maternal body fluids may influence vertical transmission rates. The presence

TABLE 14-4 | **PERINATAL HIV TRANSMISSION: RISK FACTORS**

HIV-disease related	Advanced maternal disease status
	High viral RNA load
	Low CD4 count
	Co-existent sexually transmitted diseases
Perinatal factors	Cigarette smoking
	Preterm birth
	Prolonged ruptured membranes
	Chorioamnionitis
	Invasive fetal procedures
	Breastfeeding

of sexually transmitted diseases and chorioamnionitis have been associated with increased transmission rates.

Maternal-fetal transmission of HIV is more likely in the presence of advanced maternal disease, low CD4 counts, and high viral loads.[96-98] (Table 14-4) The maternal viral load appears to be the most reliable correlate of vertical transmission. With improved techniques for HIV RNA measurement now available it appears that discriminants of vertical transmission relate to mean levels of viral RNA.[99,100] However, no absolute viral load threshold has been determinable for maternal-fetal transmission, and vertical transmission is well reported in circumstances of women with no detectable viral RNA and conversely in those with very high viral RNA levels in whom vertical transmission did not occur. Pregnancy does not appear to shorten the temporal progression from HIV seropositivity to acquired immunodeficiency syndrome (AIDS). There is no evidence that primary HIV infection occurring in pregnancy increases the incidence of vertical transmission, although theoretically the higher viral load at this time may increase the fetal infection acquisition risk. Assessment of markers such as p24 antigen at the time of fetal blood sampling may be predictive of fetal acquisition of infection with the presence of p24 antigenemia associated with increased likelihood of neonatal disease if present in cord blood. The fetus and mother are not concordant for p24 antigen status.[101]

The temporal relationship of maternal-fetal HIV-infection is uncertain. Intra-uterine viral infection occurs, probably accounting for 24–50% of cases,[94] supported by the identification of the virus in products of conception,[102,103] presence of HIV in amniotic fluid,[104] and virus present in the blood of neonates.[105,106] The remaining congenital HIV cases appear to occur through intrapartum transmission,[107] with more than 50% of HIV-infected infants having negative viral detection in the first few days and a rapid increase in the detection of virus in the first week after birth. Postnatal acquisition of HIV is predominantly secondary to breast feeding, estimated to account for an additional 14% transmission risk.[108] Formula feeding of infants is recommended for HIV-positive women in developed countries. Bryson et al.[109] have proposed a temporal description of infection based on probable timing acquisition of HIV:

early (intra-uterine) infection in the presence of a positive viral detection within 48 hours of life and late (intrapartum or late gestation) where no virus is detectable in the first week of life but is positive by 3 months of age. Using this definition, an estimated 40–80% of perinatal HIV infection occur in the late period.

The prevention or reduction of perinatal transmission of HIV from mother to infant has received much attention this decade. The use of antiretroviral agents has become an important preventative strategy since the publication of the pediatric AIDS Clinical Trial Group protocol 076 in 1994.[99] A prospective randomized controlled trial, this study demonstrated a significant reduction in perinatal transmission of HIV in those infants whose mothers received zidovudine antepartum and intrapartum compared to those who received placebo (8.3% versus 25.5%, p = 0.006). This study did not assist in determining the optimal time for administration of antiretroviral therapy, nor did it assist in the management of women with disease profiles differing from those in the study (disease enrollment criteria: CD4 counts >200 cells/mm^3 and less than 6 months of previous antiretroviral therapy). Guidelines on the use of antiretroviral agents have been developed and although uptake is variable a consistent reduction in maternal-fetal transmission has been observed with the use of zidovudine. Other antiretroviral agents may also be of use in this scenario and studies are ongoing assessing these plus triple therapy regimens (combination antiretroviral therapy, reverse transcriptase inhibitors and protease inhibitors). The latter may reduce the HIV load to non-detectable levels, thus further reducing vertical transmission rates.

Obstetric practices have been altered as information appears concerning maternal-fetal transmission of HIV. The impact of delivery mode on transmission rates is controversial and conflicting results have been published. All published studies have been observational to date and may be criticized for issues such as failure to control for confounding variables and inadequate sample size. The results have variously reported a reduction in the risk of vertical transmission with cesarean section[110-112] or demonstrated no benefit to cesarean delivery.[113-118] A policy of routine cesarean delivery for HIV-positive women is not supported by the current literature. A randomized controlled trial is currently being performed in Europe to assess the impact of delivery mode on perinatal HIV transmission, and alterations to clinical practice should await the availability of such data.

Minimizing exposure of the fetus to maternal body fluids is central to current intrapartum policies in the management of women infected with HIV. Thus the avoidance of artificial membrane rupture and invasive fetal procedures should be adhered to wherever possible. The presence of intact fetal membranes appears to decrease the risk of vertical viral transmission.[116,119] Antiseptic cleansing of the lower genital tract has been proposed as a method to reduce vertical transmission, but a clinical trial in Malawi of 0.25% chlorhexidine did not demonstrate any alteration in the viral transmission rates.[120] Interruption of the fetal epithelial integrity by procedures such as fetal scalp electrode application and fetal scalp blood sampling may increase the fetal risk of infection, although conflicting results have been reported to date.[110,115,120,121] It would seem prudent to avoid such procedures in women known to be HIV-infected.

Because of the transplacental passage of maternal IgG antibody to the fetus, all neonates exposed to HIV perinatally are HIV antibody positive on testing. HIV antibody testing is reliable for the diagnosis of HIV in perinatally exposed children only after the age of 15–18 months. Prior to this time, the diagnosis rests with clinical suspicion, viral culture, and polymerase chain reaction-based tests. The mean time to the onset of HIV-related disease is shorter in perinatally infected children than adults. Presentations strongly suggestive of HIV-related disease after perinatal exposure include *Pneumocystis carinii* pneumonia, lymphoid interstitial pneumonitis, nonsuppurative parotitis, hyperglobulinemia, and esophageal candidiasis. Failure to thrive, chronic diarrhea, cardiomyopathy, encephalopathy, extensive lymphadenopathy, and developmental delay, in a clinical context of known maternal HIV infection, are indications for infant assessment of HIV status.

In 1986, Marion et al.[122] described a dysmorphic syndrome in 20 children exposed to human T-lymphocyte Virus III (HTLV-III) infection in utero. The embryopathy was further expanded in a subsequent publication in 1987.[123] This HTLV-III embryopathy is characterized by growth failure (75%), microcephaly (70%), and craniofacial abnormalities. The children with the most marked dysmorphic features developed immune dysfunction phenomena earlier than those with less prominent features. The variable expression of HIV-associated embryopathy may relate to timing of exposure to the virus in gestation. Postulated mechanisms for this embryopathy include direct viral infection of the fetus or infection secondary to postnatal disease from HIV infection. The 1991 European Collaborative Study, in evaluating 600 infants, did not detect 1 case of HIV dysmorphic syndrome, and the existence of this disorder as a discrete entity is doubtful given the multiple confounding variables arising from the associated maternal illicit drug use and infections in the mothers.[124]

References

1. Grose C, Itani O, Weiner CP. Prenatal diagnosis of fetal infection: advances from amniocentesis to cordocentesis-congenital toxoplasmosis, rubella, cytomegalovirus, varicella virus, parvovirus, and human immunodeficiency virus. *Pediatr Infect Dis J.* 1989;8:459–468.
2. Weiner CP, Grose CF, Naides SJ. Diagnosis of fetal infection in the patient with an ultrasonographically detected abnormality but a negative clinical history. *Am J Obstet Gynecol.* 1993;168:6–11.
3. Miller E, Cradock-Watson JE, Pollock TM. Consequences of confirmed maternal rubella at successive stages of pregnancy. *Lancet.* 1982;2:781–784.
4. Enders G, Nickerl-Pacher U, Miller E, et al. Outcome of confirmed periconceptional maternal rubella. *Lancet.* 1988;1:1445–1447.
5. Sever JL, Hardy JB, Nelson KB, et al. Rubella in the collaborative perinatal research study: clinical and laboratory findings in children through 3 years of age: Part II. *Am J Dis Child.* 1969;118:123–132.
6. Daffos F, Forestier F, Grangeot-Keros L, et al. Prenatal diagnosis of congenital rubella. *Lancet.* 1984;2:1–3.
7. Morgan-Capner P, Rodeck CH, Nicolaides K, et al. Prenatal diagnosis of rubella (letter). *Lancet.* 1984;2:343.
8. Sever JL, South MA, Shaver KA. Delayed manifestations of congenital rubella. *Rev Infect Dis.* 1985;7:164–169.
9. ACOG. Perinatal viral and parasitic infections. *ACOG Tech Bull.* 1993;177.
10. Plotkin SA, Vaheri A. Human fibroblasts infected with rubella virus produce a growth inhibitor. *Science.* 1967;156:659–661.
11. Yoneda T, Urade M, Sakuda M, et al. Altered growth, differentiation and responsiveness to epidermal growth factor of human embryonic mesenchymal cells of the palate by persistent rubella virus infection. *J Clin Invest.* 1986;77:1613–1621.
12. Griffiths PD, Baboonian C. A prospective study of primary cytomegalovirus infection during pregnancy: final report. *Br J Obstet Gynaecol.* 1984;91:307–315.
13. Stagno S, Pass RF, Dworsky ME, et al. Congenital cytomegalovirus infection: the relative importance of primary and recurrent maternal infection. *N Eng J Med.* 1982;306:945–949.
14. Yow MD, Williamson DW, Leeds LJ, et al. Epidemiologic characteristics of cytomegalovirus infection in mothers and their infants. *Am J Obstet Gynecol.* 1988;158:1189–1195.
15. White NH, Yow MD, Demmler GJ, et al. Prevalence of cytomegalovirus antibody in subjects between the ages of 6 and 22 years. *J Infect Dis.* 1989;159:1013–1017.
16. Yow MD, White NH, Taber LH, et al. Acquisition of cytomegalovirus infection from birth to 10 years: a longitudinal serologic study. *J Pediatr.* 1987;110:37–42.
17. Chandler SH, Alexander ER, Holmes KK. Epidemiology of cytomegaloviral infection in a heterogeneous population of pregnant women. *J Infect Dis.* 1985;152:249–256.
18. Stagno S. Significance of cytomegaloviral infections in pregnancy and early childhood. *Pediatr Infect Dis J.* 1990;9:763–764.
19. Demmler GJ. Infectious Disease Society of America and Centers for Disease Control. Summary of a workshop on surveillance for congenital cytomegalovirus disease. *Rev Infect Dis.* 1991;13:315–329.
20. Lipitz S, Yagel S, Shalev E, et al. Prenatal diagnosis of fetal primary cytomegalovirus infection. *Obstet Gynecol.* 1997;89:763–767.
21. Lynch L, Daffos F, Emanuel D, et al. Prenatal diagnosis of fetal cytomegalovirus infection. *Am J Obstet Gynecol.* 1991;165:714–718.
22. Donner C, Liesnard C, Content J, et al. Prenatal diagnosis of 52 pregnancies at risk for congenital cytomegalovirus infection. *Obstet Gynecol.* 1993;82:481–486.
23. Conboy TJ, Pass RF, Stagno S, et al. Intellectual development in school-aged children with asymptomatic congenital cytomegalovirus infection. *Pediatrics.* 1986;77:801–806.
24. Becroft DMO. Prenatal cytomegalovirus infection: epidemiology, pathology and pathogenesis. *Perspectives in Pediatric Pathology.* 1981;6:203–241.
25. Gehrz RC, Leonard TE. Cytomegalovirus (CMV): specific lymphokine production in congenital CMV infection. *Clin Exp Immunol.* 1985;62:507–514.
26. Gehrz RC, Marker SC, Knorr SO, et al. Specific cell-mediated immune defect in active cytomegalovirus infection of young children and their mothers. *Lancet.* 1977;2:884–887.
27. Donner C, Liesnard C, Brancart F, et al. Accuracy of amniotic fluid testing before 21 weeks' gestation in prenatal diagnosis of congenital cytomegalovirus infection. *Prenat Diagn.* 1994;14:1055–1059.
28. van der Meer JT, Drew WL, Bowden RA, et al. Summary of the International Consensus Symposium on Advances in the Diagnosis,

Treatment and Prophylaxis and Cytomegalovirus Infection. *Antiviral Research* 1996;32:119–140.

29. Zhou XJ, Gruber W, Demmler G, et al. Population pharmacokinetics of ganciclovir in newborns with congenital cytomegalovirus infections. NIAID Collaborative Antiviral Study Group. *Antimicrobial Agents & Chemotherapy*. 1996;40:2202–2205.

30. Trang JM, Kidd L, Gruber W, et al. Linear single-dose pharmacokinetics of ganciclovir in newborns with congenital cytomegalovirus infections. NIAID Collaborative Antiviral Study Group. *Clin Pharmacol Ther*. 1993;53:15–21.

31. Nigro G, Scholz H, Bartmann U. Ganciclovir therapy for symptomatic congenital cytomegalovirus infection in infants: a two-regimen experience. *J Pediatr*. 1994;124:318–322.

32. Brown ZA, Berry S, Vontver LA. Genital herpes simplex virus infections complicating pregnancy: natural history and peripartum management. *J Reprod Med*. 1986;31:420–425.

33. Baldwin S, Whitley RJ. Intrauterine herpes simplex virus infection. *Teratology*. 1989;39:1–10.

34. Stagno S, Whitley RJ. Herpes virus infections of pregnancy: part II Herpes simplex virus and varicella-zoster infections. *N Engl J Med*. 1985;313:1327–1330.

35. Hutto C, Arvin A, Jacobs R, et al. Intrauterine herpes simplex virus infections. *J Pediatr*. 1987;110:97–101.

36. Karesh JW, Kapur S, MacDonald M. Herpes simplex virus and congenital malformations. *South Med J*. 1983;76:1561–1563.

37. Monif GR, Kellner KR, Donnelly WH Jr. Congenital herpes simplex virus type II infection. *Am J Obstet Gynecol*. 1985;152:1000–1002.

38. Brown ZA, Vontver LA, Benedetti J, et al. Effects on infants of a first episode of genital herpes during pregnancy. *N Engl J Med*. 1987;317:1246–1251.

39. Prober CG, Corey L, Brown ZA, et al. The management of pregnancies complicated by genital infections with herpes simplex virus. *Clin Infect Dis*. 1992;15:1031–1038.

40. Whitley R, Arvin A, Prober C, et al. Predictors of morbidity and mortality in neonates with herpes simplex virus infections. *N Eng J Med*. 1991;324:450–454.

41. Brown ZA, Benedetti J, Ashley R, et al. Neonatal herpes simplex virus infection in relation to asymptomatic maternal infection at the time of labor. *N Engl J Med*. 1991;324:1247–1252.

42. Nahmias AJ, Josey WE, Naib ZM, et al. Perinatal risk associated with maternal genital herpes simplex virus infection. *Am J Obstet Gynecol*. 1971;110:825–837.

43. Libman MD, Dascal A, Kramer MS, et al. Strategies for the prevention of neonatal infection with herpes simplex virus: a decision analysis. *Rev Infect Dis*. 1991;13:1093–1104.

44. Randolph AG, Washington AE, Prober CG. Cesarean delivery for women presenting with genital herpes lesions: efficacy, risks and cost. *JAMA*. 1993;270:77–82.

45. Chuang TY. Neonatal herpes: incidence, prevention and consequences. *Am J Prev Med*. 1988;4:47–53.

46. Light IJ, Linnermann CC Jr. Neonatal herpes simplex infection following delivery by cesarean section. *Obstet Gynecol*. 1974;44:496–499.

47. Sullivan-Bolyai J, Hull HF, Wilson C, et al. Neonatal herpes simplex virus infection in King County, Washington: increasing incidence and epidemiologic correlates. *JAMA*. 1983;250:3059–3062.

48. Whitley RJ, Corey L, Arvin A, et al. Changing presentation of herpes simplex virus infection in neonates. *J Infect Dis*. 1988;158:109–116.

49. Fleisher G, Bologonese R. Epstein-Barr virus infections in pregnancy: a prospective study. *J Pediatr*. 1984;104:374–379.

50. Hunter K, Stagno S, Capps E, et al. Prenatal screening of pregnant women for infections caused by cytomegalovirus, Epstein-Barr virus, herpesvirus, rubella, and *Toxoplasma gondii*. *Am J Obstet Gynecol*. 1983;145:269–273.

51. Chang RS, Seto DS. Perinatal infection by Epstein-Barr virus. *Lancet*. 1979;2:201.

52. Chang RS, Blankenship W. Spontaneous in vitro transformation of leukocytes from a neonate. *Proc Soc Exp Biol Med*. 1973;144:337–339.

53. Joncas J, Boucher J, Granger-Julien M, et al. Epstein-Barr virus infection in the neonatal period and in childhood. *Can Med Assoc J*. 1974;110:33–37.

54. Goldberg GN, Fulginiti VA, Ray CG, et al. In utero Epstein-Barr virus (infectious mononucleosis) infection. *JAMA*. 1981;246:1579–1581.

55. Joncas JH, Alfieri C, Leyritz-Wills M, et al. Simultaneous congenital infection with Epstein-Barr virus and cytomegalovirus. *N Eng J Med*. 1981;304:1399–1403.

56. Brown ZA, Stenchever MA. Infectious mononucleosis and congenital anomalies. *Am J Obstet Gynecol*. 1978;131:108–109.

57. Ornoy A, Dudai M, Sadovsky E. Placental and fetal pathology in infectious mononucleosis: a possible indicator for Epstein-Barr virus teratogenicity. *Diagn Gynecol Obstet*. 1982;4:11–16.

58. Balducci J, Rodis JF, Rosengren S, et al. Pregnancy outcome following first trimester varicella infection. *Obstet Gynecol*. 1992;79:5–6.

59. Enders G, Miller E, Cradock-Watson J, et al. Consequences of varicella and herpes zoster in pregnancy: prospective study of 1739 cases. *Lancet*. 1994;343:1548–1551.

60. Hanngren K, Grandien M, Granstrom G. Effect of zoster immunoglobulin for varicella prophylaxis in the newborn. *Scand J Infect Dis*. 1985;17:343–347.

61. Brazin SA, Simkovich JW, Johnson WT. Herpes zoster during pregnancy. *Obstet Gynecol*. 1979;53:175–181.

62. Klauber GT, Flynn FJ Jr, Altman BD. Congenital varicella syndrome with genitourinary anomalies. *Urology*. 1976;8:153–156.

63. Webster MH, Smith CS. Congenital anomalies and herpes zoster. *Br Med J*. 1977;2:1193.

64. Gratacos E, Torres PJ, Vidal J, et al. The incidence of human parvovirus B19 infection during pregnancy and its impact on perinatal outcome. *J Infect Dis* 1995;171:1360–1363.

65. Public Health Laboratory Service Working Party on Fifth Disease. Prospective study of human parvovirus (B19) infection in pregnancy. *BMJ* 1990;300:1166–1170.

66. Rodis JF, Quinn DL, Gary W Jr, et al. Management and outcomes of pregnancies complicated by human B19 parvovirus infection: a prospective study. *Am J Obstet Gynecol*. 1990;163:1168–1171.

67. Woernle CH, Anderson LJ, Tatternsall P, et al. Human parvovirus B19 infection during pregnancy. *J Infect Dis*. 1987;156:17–20.

68. Samra JS, Obhrai MS, Constantine G. Parvovirus infection in pregnancy. *Obstet Gynecol*. 1989;73:832–834.

69. Boxall E, Skidmore S, Evans C, et al. The prevalence of hepatitis B and C in an antenatal population of various ethnic origins. *Epidemiol Infect*. 1994;113:523–528.

70. Darwish MA, Raouf TA, Rushdy P, et al. Risk factors associated with a high seroprevalence of hepatitis C virus infection in Egyptian blood donors. *Am J Trop Med Hyg*. 1993;49:440–447.

71. Alter MJ. Epidemiology of hepatitis C in the West. *Semin Liver Dis*. 1993;15:5–14.

72. Conry-Cantilena C, VanRaden M, Gibble J, et al. Routes of infection, viremia, and liver disease in blood donors found to have hepatitis C virus infection. *N Eng J Med*. 1996;334:1691–1696.

73. Alter MJ, Margolis HS, Krawczynski K, et al. The natural history of community-acquired hepatitis C in the United States. The Sentinel Counties Chronic non-A, non-B Hepatitis Study Team. *N Eng J Med*. 1992;327:1899–1905.

74. Esteban JI, Lopez-Talavera JC, Genesca J, et al. High rate of infectivity and liver disease in blood donors with antibodies to hepatitis C virus. *Ann Intern Med*. 1991;115:443–449.

75. Novati R, Thiers V, Monforte AD, et al. Mother-to-child transmission of hepatitis C virus detected by nested polymerase chain reaction. *J Infect Dis*. 1992;165:720–723.

76. Thaler MM, Park CK, Landers DV, et al. Vertical transmission of hepatitis C virus. *Lancet.* 1991;338:17–18.

77. Moriya T, Sasaki F, Mizui M, et al. Transmission of hepatitis C virus from mothers to infants: its frequency and risk factors revisited. *Biomed Pharmacother.* 1995;49:59–64.

78. Hunt CM, Carson KL, Sharara AI. Hepatitis C in pregnancy. *Obstet Gynecol.* 1997;89:883–890.

79. Ohto H, Terazawa S, Sasaki N, et al. Transmission of hepatitis C virus from mothers to infants. The Vertical Transmission of Hepatitis C Virus Collaborative Study Group. *N Engl J Med.* 1994;330: 744–750.

80. Lin HH, Kao JH, Hsu HY, et al. Possible role of high- titer maternal viremia in perinatal transmission of hepatitis C virus. *J Infect Dis.* 1994;169:638–641.

81. Resti M, Azzari C, Lega L, et al. Mother-to-infant transmission of hepatitis C virus. *Acta Paediatr.* 1995;84:251–255.

82. Maggiore G, Ventura A, De Giacomo C, et al. Vertical transmission of hepatitis C. *Lancet.* 1995;345:1122.

83. Nakashima K, Ikematsu H, Hayashi J, et al. Intrafamilial transmission of hepatitis C virus among the population of an endemic area of Japan. *JAMA.* 1995;274:1459–1461.

84. Zanetti AR, Tanzi E, Paccagnini S, et al. Mother-to-infant transmission of hepatitis C virus. Lombardy Study Group on Vertical HCV Transmission. *Lancet.* 1995;345:289–291.

85. Modlin JF. Perinatal echovirus and group B coxsackie infections. *Clin Perinatol.* 1988;15:233–246.

86. Sever JL, Huebner RJ, Castellano GA. Serologic diagnosis "en masse" with multiple antigens. *Am Rev Respir Dis.* 1963;88:342.

87. Brown GC, Karunas RS. Relationship of congenital anomalies and maternal infection with selected enteroviruses. *Am J Epidemiol.* 1972;95:207–217.

88. Brown GC, Evans TN. Serologic evidence of Coxsackievirus etiology of congenital heart disease. *JAMA.* 1967;199:183–187.

89. Burch GE, Sun SC, Chu KC, et al. Interstitial and coxsackie B myocarditis in infants and children: a comparative histologic and immunofluorescent study of 50 autopsied hearts. *JAMA.* 1968;203:1–8.

90. Korones SB. Uncommon virus infections of the mother, fetus and newborn: influenza, mumps and measles. *Clin Perinatol.* 1988;15:259–272.

91. Siegel M. Congenital malformations following chickenpox, measles, mumps and hepatitis: results of a cohort study. *JAMA.* 1973;226:1521–1524.

92. Lindsay MK, Nesheim SR. Human immunodeficiency virus infection in pregnant women and their newborns. *Clinics in Perinatology.* 1997;24:161–180.

93. European Collaborative Study. Children born to women with HIV-1 infection: natural history and risk of transmission. *Lancet.* 1991;337:253–260.

94. Rogers MF, Ou CY, Rayfield M, et al. Use of the polymerase chain reaction for early detection of the proviral sequences of human immunodeficiency virus in infants born to seropositive mothers. The New York City Collaborative Study of Maternal HIV Transmission and Montefiore Medical Center HIV Perinatal Transmission Study Group. *N Eng J Med.* 1989;320:1649–1654.

95. Viscarello RR, Copperman AB, DeGennaro NJ. Is the risk of perinatal transmission by human immunodeficiency virus increased by the intrapartum use of spiral electrodes or fetal scalp pH sampling? *Am J Obstet Gynecol.* 1994;170:740–743.

96. European Collaborative Study. Risk factors for mother-to-child transmission of HIV-I. *Lancet.* 1992;339:1007–1012.

97. Gabiano C, Tovo PA, de Martino M, et al. Mother-to-child transmission of human immunodeficiency virus type 1: risk of infection and correlates of transmission. *Pediatrics.* 1992;90:369–374.

98. St. Louis ME, Kamenga M, Brown C, et al. Risk for perinatal HIV-1 transmission according to maternal immunologic, virologic, and placental factors. *JAMA.* 1993;269:2853–2859.

99. Connor EM, Sperling RS, Gelber R, et al. For the Pediatric AIDS Clinical Trials Group Protocol 076 Study Group. Reduction of maternal-infant transmission of human immunodeficiency virus type 1 with zidovudine treatment. *N Engl J Med.* 1994;331:1173–1180.

100. Mofenson LM. The role of antiretroviral therapy in the management of HIV infection in women. *Clin Obstet Gynecol.* 1996;39: 361–385.

101. Viscarello RR, Cullen MT, DeGennaro NJ, et al. Fetal blood sampling in human immunodeficiency virus-seropositive women before elective midtrimester termination of pregnancy. *Am J Obstet Gynecol.* 1992;167:1075–1079.

102. Brossard Y, Aubin JT, Mandelbrot L, et al. Frequency of early in utero HIV-1 infection: a blind DNA polymerase chain reaction study on 100 fetal thymuses. *AIDS* 1995;9:359–366.

103. Jovaisas E, Koch MA, Schafer A, et al. LAV/HTLV-III in a 20 week fetus (letter). *Lancet.* 1985;2:1129.

104. Mundy DC, Schinazi RF, Gerver AR, et al. Human immunodeficiency virus isolated from amniotic fluid. *Lancet.* 1987;2:459–460.

105. Borkowsky W, Krasinski K, Pollack H, et al. Early diagnosis of human immunodeficiency virus infection in children less than 6 months of age: comparison of polymerase chain reaction, culture, and plasma antigen capture techniques. *J Infect Dis.* 1992;166:616–619.

106. Krivine A, Yakudima A, Le May M, et al. A comparative study of virus isolation, polymerase chain reaction, and antigen detection in children of mothers infected with human immunodeficiency virus. *J Pediatr.* 1990;116:372–376.

107. Mofenson LM. A critical review of studies evaluating the relationship of mode of delivery to perinatal transmission of human immunodeficiency virus. *Pediatr Infect Dis J.* 1995;14:169–176.

108. Dunn DT, Newell ML, Ades AE, et al. Risk of human immunodeficiency virus type 1 transmission through breastfeeding. *Lancet.* 1992;340:585–588.

109. Bryson YJ, Luzuriaga K, Sullivan J, et al. Proposed definitions for in utero versus intrapartum transmission of HIV-1. *N Engl J Med.* 1992;327:1246–1247.

110. Duliege AM, Amos CI, Felton S, et al. Birth order, delivery route, and concordance in the transmission of human immunodeficiency virus type 1 from mothers to twins. *J Pediatr.* 1995;126:625–632.

111. European Collaborative Study: caesarean section and risk of vertical transmission of HIV-1 infection. *Lancet.* 1994;343:1464–1467.

112. Kuhn L, Stein ZA, Thomas PA, et al. Maternal-infant HIV transmission and circumstances of delivery. *Am J Pub Health.* 1994;84:1110–1115.

113. Tovo PA, de Martino M, Gabiano C, et al. Prognostic factors and survival in children with perinatal HIV-1 infection. *Lancet.* 1992;339:1249–1253.

114. Gabiano C, Tovo PA, de Martino M, et al. Mother-to-child transmission of human immunodeficiency virus type 1: risk of infection and correlates of transmission. *Pediatrics.* 1992;90:369–374.

115. Hutto C, Parks WP, Lai SH, et al. A hospital-based prospective study of perinatal infection with immunodeficiency virus type 1. *J Pediatr.* 1991;118:347–353.

116. Landesman SH, Kalish LA, Burns DN, et al. Obstetrical factors and the transmission of human immunodeficiency virus type 1 from mother to child. The Women and Infants Transmission Study. *N Engl J Med.* 1996;334:1617–1623.

117. Mandelbrot L, Mayaux MJ, Bongain A, et al. Obstetric factors and mother-to-child transmission of human immunodeficiency virus type 1: the French perinatal cohorts. *Am J Obstet Gynecol.* 1996;175:661–667.

118. Nair P, Alger L, Hines S, et al. Maternal and neonatal characteristics associated with HIV infection in infants of seropositive women. *J Acquir Immune Defic Syndr.* 1993;6:298–302.

119. Minkoff H, Burns DN, Landesman S, et al. The relationship of

the duration of ruptured membranes to vertical transmission of human immunodeficiency virus. *Am J Obstet Gynecol*. 1995;173:585–589.

120. Biggar RJ, Miotti PG, Taha TE, et al. Perinatal intervention trial in Africa: effect of a birth canal cleansing intervention to prevent HIV transmission. *Lancet*. 1996;347:1647–1650.

121. Boyer PJ, Dillon M, Navaie M, et al. Factors predictive of maternal-fetal transmission of HIV-1. *JAMA* 1994;271:1925–1930.

122. Marion RW, Wiznia AA, Hutcheon G, et al. Human T-cell lym-photrophic virus type III (HTLV-III) embryopathy: a new dysmorphic syndrome associated with intrauterine HTLV-III infection. *Am J Dis Child*. 1986;140:638–640.

123. Marion RW, Wiznia AA, Hutcheon G, et al. Fetal AIDS syndrome score. Correlation between severity of dysmorphism and age at diagnosis of immunodeficiency. *Am J Dis Child*. 1987;141:429–431.

124. Iosub S, Bamji M, Stone RK, et al. More on human immunodeficiency virus embryopathy. *Pediatrics*. 1987;80:512–516.

EXPOSURE TO IONIZING RADIATION DURING PREGNANCY

Daniela Koch / Arie Drugan

INTRODUCTION

Medical imaging has made rapid and impressive advances in the past 20 years. However, prenatal exposure of the fetus to ionizing radiation is an anxiety-provoking and often misunderstood issue, more than virtually any other environmental teratogen to which women are exposed during pregnancy.[1] Sources of ionizing radiation are high energy X-rays used for diagnosis or for therapy, naturally occurring radioactive materials (e.g., radium, radon), nuclear reactors, cyclotrons, linear accelerators, alternating gradient synchrotrons, and radioactive materials used in medicine and industry (such as sealed cobalt and cesium). The low levels of background radiation on the earth and in the atmosphere have no detectable effects.[2]

Man-made radiation accounts for about 15% of the total radiation burden in the United Kingdom, almost all of it (97%) being related to diagnostic medical exposure.[3] In the United States, CT now accounts for 13% of all examinations, thus contributing approximately 30% of the collective dose.[4] Although needed and beneficial to the patient, the potential for radiation-induced injury from these procedures clearly exists.[5]

The aim of this chapter is to provide physicians with a concise, up-to-date view of current diagnostic procedures and their implications on the pregnant woman and her fetus. The information is intended to help the physician and the patient make an informed choice before planned exposure to ionizing radiation or after inadvertent ones.

RADIOBIOLOGY

Ionizing radiation consists of either electromagnetic waves, which are ionizing indirectly (x-rays and gamma rays), or particulates, which are directly ionizing (alpha and beta particles, protons, and neutrons). Because all types of radiation initiate damage by ionization, differences are quantitative rather than qualitative. Ionizing radiation damages tissue either directly or by secondary reaction, as it initiates a chain of chemical reactions that may ultimately result in radiation damage. These include *physical damage* caused by ionization (takes approximately 10^{-12} seconds), *physiochemical damage* caused by production of free radicals (takes approximately 10^{-10} seconds) and *chemical damage* to DNA and RNA structure (takes approximately 10^{-6} seconds). The *biologic damage* caused from radiation may be expressed minutes to years later and may last a lifetime.[6] Genetic or somatic effects depend on total dose and dose rate (radiation dose/unit of time), amount of body area exposed, and distribution of the dose within the body.[2] Other factors affecting patient's doses include beam energy, filtration, collimation, patient's size, image processing, and source-to-skin and patient-to-image intensifier distances.[4]

Linear Energy Transfer (LET) is a measure of the density of ionization along a radiation beam. Higher LET radiation (alpha particles, protons, and neutrons) produce greater damage in a biologic system than lower LET radiation (electrons, gamma rays, and X-rays). Thus, tissue damage depends not only on the amount of energy transferred, but also on the penetrating ability of the specific type of emission.[6]

NOMENCLATURE USED IN QUANTIFICATION OF RADIATION

Exposure is the most common measure to determine the amount of radiation delivered to an area. The conventional unit is *roentgen* (R) and the Systeme Internationale (SI) unit is coulomb (C) per kilogram of air (C/kg). The exposure decreases inversely to the square of the distance from the radiation source.[7]

The human body absorbs approximately 90% of the diagnostic radiation to which it is exposed. *Absorbed dose* is defined as the mean energy absorbed by radiation per unit mass in the human body tissue. The conventional unit is the *rad* and the SI units is the Gray (Gy):

$$1 \text{ Gy} = 100 \text{ rad} = 1 \text{ J/kg} = 10{,}000 \text{ erg/g.}[8]$$

The *integral dose* is the total amount of energy absorbed in the body. It is determined not only by absorbed dose values, but also by the total mass of the tissue exposed. The conventional unit is the gram-rad ($=100$ ergs of absorbed energy) and the SI unit is the Joule (J):

$$1 \text{ J} = 10^7 \text{ erg} = 100{,}000 \text{ gram-rad}$$

As not all types of radiation have the same biologic impact, there are 2 methods of quantification associated with biologic impact: *dose equivalent* (H) and *relative biological effect* (RBE). The conventional unit of H is the *rem* and the SI unit is the Sievert (Sv). One Sv equals 100 rem. H (rem) is dependent of the dose (rad) as well as of the quality of the radiation beam, including some modifying coefficients.

The RBE is a comparison of the biologic effect of a given radiation to that of X-ray. Thus, RBE equals D X-ray / D radiation. The RBE of X-rays is 1.[6]

At present, there is an evolving consensus that the volume CT dose index (CTDIvol), the dose-length product (DLP) and the effective dose (E, in mSv units) are the most relevant parameters for estimating radiation exposure and risk. The CT dose index is defined as the integral of the dose profile along the Z-axis (patient longitudinal axis) normalized to the chosen section collimation. The weighted CTDI (CTDIw) is derived from measurements at the center and periphery of phantoms of 16 cm for the head and 32 cm for the body. It provides an estimate for the average dose to the head or body, and corrects for influences of kVp setting and prefiltering. CTDIvol = CTDIw/P. P is the pitch (table feed/total width of active collimation). CTDIvol corrects for the influence of pitch on patient dose. The dose-length product *(DLP)* is a measure of the total scan dose delivered to a patient. DPL = CTDIvol × length of scan.[9]

The radiation dose to patients are about 30–50% greater with multislice CT scanners, as a result primarily of scan overlap, positioning the X-ray tube closer to the patient, and possibly increased scattered radiation with wider X-ray beams. Using a large number of thin adjacent CT slices increases image quality, yet results in 30–50% increase in radiation dose (CTDIvol).[9] According to the EUR 16262 guidelines the recommendations are: CTDIw = 30, DLP = 650 for chest and abdominal CT.[10] There are various methods to reduce patient radiation dose, such as by decreasing the mAs, increasing the pitch, using adaptive filtering.

FETAL DOSE ESTIMATE

An estimation of fetal dose in diagnostic radiology requires knowledge of the output intensity of the X-ray equipment, entrance exposure for fluoroscopic procedures, number of views taken, beam-on time, location, and orientation in relation to the X-ray tube, half-value layer (to determine beam permeability) and published dose conversion factors / scatter factors / depth-dose and tissue-air ration tables.

Direct (inside field of view) *exposure* includes studies of the abdomen, pelvis, and lumbar spine. The fetus is directly exposed to primary beam radiation, resulting in the highest fetal doses. A shield is usually of limited value, because it cannot cover the area being imaged. *Indirect* (outside field of view) *exposure* includes examinations of the skull and head, cervical spine, chest, and extremities, and a mammography. The exposure received is from indirect scattered radiation from the maternal tissue (therefore a lead shield has a limited value). The fetal dose is low and depends on the distance between the fetus and the primary X-ray field. However, when fluoroscopy is incorporated, the fetal dose can vary greatly.[5]

PATHOPHYSIOLOGY

There are several mechanisms that may mediate the biologic effects of radiation[6]:

1. The *indirect theory* assumes that the effect of radiation on target molecules is mediated through free radicals produced by ionization. Radical formation requires the presence of water. Free radical reactions include ionization reactions (as primary event) and radical reactions (where OH and H are free radicals). LET, oxygen, and radiopro-

tectors (scavengers of free radicals such as cystamine) will modify aqueous radiochemical reactions. Aqueous radicals usually produce organic radicals by abstraction of hydrogen atoms. Free radicals may break up CH, CO, CN, CS, and C = C bonds. Organic radicals may undergo repair (recombination with hydrogen radical) or react with another organic radical. Combination with oxygen results in an abnormal (damaged) molecule.

2. *Effects on DNA:* Specific base degradation (pyrimidine or purine) occurs as well as disruption of sugar-phosphate bonds with release of base from polynucleotide chain, leading to apurinic or apyrimidinic sites in DNA and single- or double-strand breaks.

3. *Energy* from initial ionization may be transferred by several chemical reactions to a target molecule (i.e., different intermediate organic radicals are formed).

Cellular radiosensitivity and damage is related to the degree of cell differentiation and of mitotic activity. Differentiated cells (such as nerve cells and hepatocytes) are less sensitive to radiation than undifferentiated cells (e.g., erythroblasts and myeloblasts). Thus, the order of cellular radio-sensitivity is from nerve cells <intestinal crypt cells <granulocytes <T-lymphocytes <B-lymphocytes <erythroblasts and myeloblasts.

Cells are most radiosensitive when they are in mitosis (M phase) or in RNA synthesis phase (G2 phase). Cells are relatively radioresistant in the later part of the DNA synthesis phase (S phase). Pathways of mammalian cells repair include rejoining breaks in DNA strands, excision, and synthesis of damaged DNA bases and post-replication repair.[6]

The potential harmful effects of ionizing radiation can be classified into 2 broad categories: stochastic effects and deterministic effects.[11]

Effects in which the probability of occurrence increases with radiation exposure are considered *stochastic*. Examples are carcinogenesis and genetic aberrations. An important property of these effects is that the probability (but not the severity) of the endpoint condition is related to the dose of radiation.

There is legitimate reason to be concerned about stochastic effects, since they have no known dose threshold. This implies that even the smallest amount of radiation exposure may increase the probability of the induction of a stochastic effect. However, the most common stochastic effects have a fairly high spontaneous incidence, so there may be a radiation dose below which further reduction in radiation dose does not reduce the likelihood of producing the effect. Since such "negligible risk" levels have not been determined, the conservative approach is to assume that *all radiation exposure is potentially harmful.*

Deterministic (nonstochastic) effects are associated with a threshold radiation dose below that the effect is not observed. Above the threshold dose, the probability that the effect will occur is virtually 100%, and the severity of the effect is dose related. Examples of deterministic effects are skin responses (e.g., erythema, epilation, or desquamation), cataracts, fibrosis, and hematopoietic damage.

Supporting the theory that a negligible risk radiation threshold might exist is the fact that biologic repair mechanisms of radiation injury do exist. The threshold dose for prolonged radiation exposure (spread over time) is higher than that for acute exposure, due to the ability of cells to repair nonlethal radiation damage. At low dose rates, repair mechanisms may be able to keep up with radiation damage. There are studies that even state a protective effect of low levels of radiation, with a relative reduction of the risk of malignancy. At higher rates of radiation, repair mechanisms may be overwhelmed, and significant injury may occur.[11]

Precise information about the late effects of low-dose radiation is difficult to obtain since probability of occurrence is low, latency time may be long and late effects can also occur from natural (ambient) radiation. Dose response models have been developed to predict the risk in humans. The most conservative model is the basis of the concept of ALARA (As Low As Reasonably Achievable), which refers to aiming for minimal radiation dose with each exposure.[7]

The latency time for cancer induction from X-ray exposure in the dose ranges used in Computed Tomography (CT) is estimated to be 10–30 years.[4] Although the absolute likelihood of cancer induction is low, the risks of CT should not be considered negligible. Attempts to link the occurrence of cancer to past radiation exposure, for example, breast cancer in women after exposure to several thoracic CTs,[4,12] might be based on similar links of cancer to environmental carcinogens (e.g., remote asbestos exposure). Litigation efforts regarding remote asbestos exposure were successfully reinforced in some cases. It is estimated that delivery of 1 rad to the breast in women less than 35 years old increases the risk of breast cancer by about 14% over the spontaneous rate in the general population—3.5 additional cancers per 1 million irradiated women per year per rad.[11,13] In women over 35 years old, there are 7.5 additional breast cancer cases per 1 million irradiated women per year per rad. Thus, radiation-induced breast carcinoma is a lifetime risk with cumulative carcinogenic effect related to age. Each chest CT exposes the woman breast to 2–5 rads (Table 15-1). It is recommended that patients should receive written and verbal information about the estimated cancer risks associated with CT. Such information and documentation of the patient's full knowledge would help avoid unnecessary legal confrontations in the future, if the patient develops cancer.[4]

HEREDITARY EFFECTS OF RADIATION

The gonads are very sensitive to harmful effects of ionizing radiation. Ovarian irradiation may induce sterility as well as chromosomal breakage and mutations, which may be transmitted to future generations. Some effect on fetal growth restriction and an increased risk of childhood cancer has also been reported for progeny of fathers exposed to gonadal irradiation prior to conception.[14,15] From studies in small animals, acute

TABLE 15-1	ESTIMATED AVERAGE EXPOSURE DOSE FROM COMMON DIAGNOSTIC PROCEDURES (MATERNAL EXPOSURE)
Imaging Procedure	*Maternal Exposure (mrads)*
Skull, PA	250
Chest X-ray, PA (grid)	20
Chest X-ray, LAT	75
Dental	14–290
Mammography	300 (each breast)
Scintigraphy	<1000
Femur, AP	200
Abdomen, AP	300–500
Lumbar Spine, AP	500–750
Lumbo-Sacral Spine, Lat	1500
Thoracic spine AP	23
Cervical spine AP	13
Upper GI	400–600
Barium Enema	800–1500
Intravenous Pyelography	800–1500
Abdominal CT scan	2000–5000
Thoracic CT scan	2000–5000
Head CT scan	3000–7000
Low dose chest CT	200–400
Pelvis PA, Hip joint	500
Abdominal angiography	3700
Neuro angiography	1700
Ribs	75–100

Adapted from references 4, 5, 9.

X-rays exposure to 200 rad or more can result in reduction in sperm production. Radiation doses used in cancer therapy are usually in the range of 4000–7000 cGy, that is, $10^{\sim4}$–$10^{\sim5}$ times the level in diagnostic radiology. Maximum permissible doses for whole body radiation workers are 5 rem/year, and for whole body of nonradiation worker with infrequent exposure 0.5 rem/year.[16]

The increase in risk of genetic disorders, birth defects or of childhood cancer following parental exposure to irradiation of the gonads is probably extremely small, and has been estimated as 6–20 per million live births per 0.01 Gy.[17] This conclusion is supported by studies among atomic bomb survivors and by those performed by the National Cancer Institute among women who were treated with high radiation to the ovaries. Thus, in most instances, survivors of cancer should *not* be discouraged from having children. However, to reduce the likelihood of an adverse fetal outcome after radiation therapy, it is advisable to delay pregnancy for 12 months.

EFFECTS OF IONIZING RADIATION IN PREGNANCY

The damage caused by radiation to cell chromatin may be expressed clinically both in the mother and in the fetus. In the mother, the carcinogenic effect of radiation may appear after moderate to high doses of radiation (50–600 rem), depending on the area exposed. The face and neck are usually most sensitive to damage,[18] as well as the female breast during thoracic CT. The latency period for cancer induction is shortest for myeloblastic disorders (e.g., leukemia)—about 2–5 years. Solid tumors such as in the breast, thyroid, skin and brain may appear 10–30 years after exposure to radiation.[19]

Fetal compromise associated with radiation exposure in utero differs at various stages of gestation. Adverse effects include death, neuropathology, malformations, growth retardation, and cancer, such as leukemia.

Following fetal exposure to radiation doses over 10 rad, the relative risk for all childhood cancer is 1.4. The relative risk for tumors of the central nervous system and for leukemia is 1.5 and 1.7, respectively.[20] The developing fetus in the second and third trimesters of pregnancy may be more sensitive to the carcinogenic effect of ionizing radiation. After organogenesis and rapid neuron development (105 days after conception and until delivery), fetal exposure to more than 10 rads is associated with an increased frequency of childhood cancer, usually manifested in the first decade of life.

Data published in the 1950s by the Oxford Survey of Childhood Cancer (OSCC) suggests a 50% increase in cancer risk for children exposed to significant radiation before birth. In 1980, data suggested that the fetus exposed in utero to 1 rad during the first trimester would be 3.5 times more likely to develop childhood cancer. In the unexposed population the frequency of childhood cancer is 0.07% (1 in 1500). Thus, exposure to 1 rad in utero during the first trimester will cause an increase in risk of 0.25%, which is quite low. The probability that the exposed fetus will *not* develop childhood cancer is 99.75%.[4] Still, these studies suggest that the developing fetus may be more sensitive to the carcinogenic effect of ionizing radiation, than are children irradiated postnatally.[20] It should be noted that the risk for childhood leukemia is significantly increased (RR 3.6) when the pregnant mother also smokes.[21]

Possibly the greatest concern of clinicians with regard to maternal exposure to radiation during pregnancy is the risk of fetal malformations. In utero exposure to radiation at Hiroshima resulted in microcephaly, mental retardation, and growth retardation.[22] Severe mental retardation was observed at 16–25 weeks after fetal exposure to more than 50 rads.[4] Offspring born to patients receiving radiation therapy for various conditions exhibited growth retardation, eye malformations, and CNS defects, with microcephaly being the most common anomaly observed following high dose exposure in utero.[23]

Prior to implantation (first 9 days postconception) the embryo is susceptible only to the lethal effects of radiation ("all or none response")—either the embryo is lost, or there is no effect and the embryo recovers completely.[24] Thus, women undergoing diagnostic imaging in the luteal phase of the menstrual cycle, before they know that they are pregnant, may be at increased risk of pregnancy loss. Indeed, animal experiments have demonstrated an increase in the spontaneous abor-

tion rate after doses as low as 5–10 rad delivered during the preimplantation period.[25] Continuation of pregnancy is recommended at all levels of radiation exposure less than 14 days after fertilization.[4]

The fetus is most sensitive to the teratogenic effects of ionizing radiation in the period of organogenesis (2–15 weeks postconception).[26] The critical period for induction of cataracts, microphtalmia, or skeletal defects is at 4–8 weeks of gestation. The CNS remains the most sensitive organ to the effects of ionizing radiation, even at later stages of gestation. Cell death and inhibition of cell migration is described in experimental animals.[27] Radiation induced mental and growth retardation and microcephaly may be observed after in utero exposure over 10 rad, between 4–25 weeks of gestation.[16] The risk for childhood cancer may persist until birth. Small head size, seizures, and decline in IQ points (25 points/100 rad were observed with fetal dose over 10 rads in the gestational stage of rapid neuron development and migration (56–105 days after conception).

The risk of major malformations is apparently not increased by in-utero exposure to less than 5 rad or by monthly exposure of less than 50 mrad.[24] The National Council on Radiation Protection (NCRP) set guidelines for occupational exposure limits. The maximum permissible monthly occupational dose limit for pregnant radiation workers has been set at 0.5 milliSieverts = 50 millirem.[16] This implies that most diagnostic X-ray exposure should not be considered an indication for termination of pregnancy (Table 15-2). Fetal exposure to doses of 5 rad and higher during organogenesis should probably

TABLE 15-2 | ESTIMATED AVERAGE DOSE OF FETAL EXPOSURE FROM COMMON DIAGNOSTIC PROCEDURES

Imaging Procedure	Fetal Exposure (mrads)
Skull X-ray	0.05
Chest X-ray, PA	0.02–0.07
Dental	0.2
Mammography	7–20
Cholecystogram	5
Femur, AP	103–213
Femur + Hip	120–300
Abdomen, AP	100–245
Lumbar Spine AP	50–400
Thoracic Spine AP	11
Cervical Spine	<0.5
Lumbo-Sacral Spine LAT	640–720
Upper GI	100–170
Barium Enema	820–1000
Intravenous Pyelography	690–1400
Head CT	<0.5
Chest CT	16–20
Abdominal CT scan	1000–3000
Pelvimetry/HCG	1000–2000

Adapted from references 4, 9.

be considered a teratogenic risk, and pregnancy termination should be offered in selected cases. However, continuation of pregnancy should be recommended in all cases of radiation exposure after 15 weeks' gestation.

The Ionizing Radiation (POPUMET) Regulations[28] require all concerned to reduce unnecessary exposure of patients to radiation, the source commonly being medical and dental diagnostic radiation (standard X-ray imaging, CT, MRI, SPECT, PET, and other radionuclide imaging). It is estimated that some 20–40% of medical X-ray procedures are unnecessary.[29] Thus, the recommendation should be that although most X-ray diagnostic imaging procedures do not expose the fetus to potentially harmful levels, these should be done in pregnancy only after carefully weighing the benefits from the procedure and, when possible, with appropriate shielding of the uterus and the fetus.

MAGNETIC RESONANCE IMAGING (MRI)

MRI does not use ionizing radiation and is capable of imaging in multiple planes. Like ultrasound, it would seem that MRI should be considered an ideal tool for fetal imaging. However, fetal movements during the procedure may be problematic. Moreover, the safety of MRI for the unborn fetus has not yet been established. The concern is that exposure of the fetus to the strong magnetic field and electromagnetic radiation may be potentially harmful, especially in the first trimester.[11,30] Studies in rats suggest an effect of MRI exposure on fetal growth and on the rate of craniofacial malformations.[31,32] Furthermore, intravenous contrast agents used for magnetic resonance imaging have been shown to cross the placenta readily. Administration to pregnant women is ill advised because contrast agents may have a negative effect on the fetus and pregnancy, although no such effect has been proven in human.[9,33] Therefore, except for emergency situations (i.e., spinal cord compression) MRI is not routinely recommended for pregnant women.[11]

In the clinical setup MRI has also been used as an adjunct to ultrasonography for further delineation of fetal brain anomalies[34,35] or in the evaluation of the patient with third-trimester bleeding caused by placental anomalies (i.e., placenta acretta or placental separation).[36,37] Recently, the use of MRI instead of X-ray pelvimetry has been advocated.[38] With modern machinery, the use of anesthetics for the mother or curare for the fetus is obviated. Thus, it is possible that as its spatial resolution and fast scan technology advances, MRI may become useful for the diagnosis of abnormalities of the fetus or of the pregnancy.

RADIONUCLIDE EXAMINATIONS

Radiopharmaceuticals represent an internal source of exposure for the developing embryo. Radiation dose depends on the specific radionuclide, its energy emission and half-life, the dose used, the distribution in the maternal system and the permeability of the placenta. Radiopharmaceuticals that do not cross the placenta irradiate the fetus by the emission of penetrating radiation (mainly gamma rays and X-rays). Those that do cross the placenta may be distributed in the body of the fetus and, sometimes, may be concentrated locally in the target organ of the fetus.

The recent release of the pregnant female phantom series and its incorporation into the MIRDOSE 3 computer software has made possible the estimation of absorbed doses from radionuclides in the body to the fetus in early pregnancy and at 3, 6, and 9 months of gestation.[39]

A ventilation perfusion lung scan using ^{99m}Tc and ^{133}Xe emits a fetal dose of 10–37 mrad and is, therefore, certainly indicated and clinically acceptable when maternal pulmonary embolism is suspected in pregnancy.[41] In contrast, ^{125}I readily crosses the placenta and is accumulated in the fetal thyroid starting from the 8th gestational week. Iodide is volatile, increasing the potential for internal uptake. Moreover, the fetal thyroid appears to bind iodine more avidly than the thyroid gland of the mother. The calculated fetal dose is 2 rads. ^{131}I used for thyroid cancer is also associated with high exposure. Thus, volatile radioactive iodine should not be used in pregnancy for ablation of maternal thyroid activity. The use of ^{125}I for diagnostic purposes should probably be avoided as well, especially after the first 2 months of pregnancy.

High-activity sealed sources, such as ^{192}Ir and ^{137}Cs, should be of concern specifically to the pregnant radiology worker/X-ray technologist. A lead apron is most effective only for lower energy radionuclides, such as, ^{99m}Tc or ^{201}Tl. A 0.5 mm lead equivalent apron will stop about two thirds of gamma radiation from ^{99m}Tc and about 90% of the radiation from ^{201}Tl. However, a lead shield will not provide the pregnant worker protection from ^{111}In or ^{131}I.

The U.S.A. Nuclear Regulatory Commission and the NCRP (National Council on Radiation Protection and Measurements) published standards for protection against radiation, including maximum permissible dose levels and instructions concerning prenatal radiation (10CFR20, Regulatory guide 8.13).[27,40]

RADIOTHERAPY

Malignant disease is diagnosed in 1 of 1000 pregnancies. Cancers that may require radiation therapy involve the breast, brain, head and neck, uterine cervix, and the hematopoietic system (lymphoma and Hodgkin's). Radiation doses used in cancer therapy are usually in the range of 4000–7000 cGy, that is, 10^4–10^5 times the level in diagnostic radiology.[42] High doses of radiation during pregnancy may induce fetal anomalies, impaired growth, and mental retardation.[43] Thus, when cancer is diagnosed late in pregnancy, it is advisable to treat with combination chemotherapy until fetal viability is reached and to postpone radiation therapy until delivery.[44] It should be noted, however, that radiation therapy for supra-diaphragmatic disease in pregnancy is not an absolute contraindication if the fetus is adequately shielded.[45,46]

When radiotherapy is necessary for tumor control, a risk-benefit assessment should be presented to the patient by the oncologist, radiation oncologist, and a medical physicist. Special attention should be paid to whether adjuvant chemotherapy can be safely administered, to postpone radiotherapy until after delivery.[42]

SAFETY MEASURES

If exposure to radiation is inevitable:

1. Always check the possibility of pregnancy in women in their reproductive years.
2. When pregnancy is documented:
   a. Adhere to maximum permissible dose levels–below 5 rad exposure or below 50-mrad monthly occupational exposure of the pregnant worker.
   b. The patients' abdomen and pelvis should be shielded with a 0.5-mm lead equivalent apron (if the type of procedure permits).
   c. Fluoroscopy time should be limited. Limit views to the minimum necessary.
   d. In CT, use fewer & thicker slices without overlap, position the X-ray tube further away from the patient, decrease mAs, increase pitch to greater than 1:0, use adaptive filtering.
   e. Document total calculated fetal dose exposure before and after performing examinations. Keep records of all examinations performed.
   f. Avoid using intravenous MRI contrast material in the first 10 weeks postconception.
   g. Avoid using iodine as contrast material on CT.
   h. Consider postponing radiotherapy until the fetus is at a later gestational age or after delivery.
   i. In radiotherapy, decrease leakage from radiation machines, lower target dose, use smaller radiation fields, and greater distance of the edges of the radiation fields from the fetus. Avoid using wedge and lead blocks, which increase external scatter to the fetus.
   j. Shield radioactive sources by using syringe shields or lead containers for the vials.
   k. The risk-benefit assessment should be presented to the patient, and there should be documentation of her informed consent.

SUMMARY

Radiation damage to the fetus can be classified into 2 principal types—*teratogenic* (during organogenesis) and *carcinogenic* (in the second and third trimesters). For most prenatal diagnostic imaging examinations, the risk of fetal malformations, of growth or mental retardation, of death, or of childhood cancer is probably very small. Precautions should be taken especially during major organogenesis and with radiation doses exceeding 5 rads (or monthly occupational dose above the limit set

of 50 mrad). Every healthy woman has a 3–6% background risk for birth defects. According to the present state of knowledge, there is no significant risk of genetic damage from *most* radiological procedures. At any stage in gestation, prenatal exposure to diagnostic irradiation does not usually represent a valid reason to recommend therapeutic abortion.

Every effort should be made to reduce radiation exposure to the patient and, especially, to her fetus. Every female patient in her reproductive years should be asked whether she might be pregnant, before diagnostic examination with ionizing radiation is to be performed. If the patient is pregnant or could reasonably be pregnant (e.g., symptoms of nausea, vomiting, fatigue, breast tenderness), the examination should not be performed, unless the expected benefit outweighs its risks. Alternative diagnostic procedures (e.g., ultrasound) or postponing the examination to a later stage in gestation (>105 days) should be considered.

If a radiological procedure must be performed, the risks and benefits of the procedure should be discussed with the patient and documented extensively in her chart. It is always important to carefully evaluate the dose absorbed by the fetus and the mother and to correctly inform the patient about possible radiation-induced risks. In addition, technical parameters should be adjusted in the radiology or radiation-oncology departments. Such adjustments include limiting as much as possible the field of view and the number of views/scans, limiting fluoroscopy time, or using abdominal shield.

References

1. Garcia PM. Radiation injury. In: Gleicher N, ed. *Principles and Practice of Medical Therapy in Pregnancy*. 3rd ed. Stamford, CT: Appleton & Lange; 1998:277–280.
2. Beers MH, Berkow R. *The Merck Manual of Diagnosis and Therapy*. 17th ed. Whitehouse Station, NJ: Merck Research Laboratories; 1999:2443–2447.
3. Royal College of Radiologists. *Making the Best Use of a Department of Clinical Radiology-guidelines for Doctors*. 3rd ed. London: 1995:10–11.
4. Nickoloff EL, Alderson PO. Radiation exposures to patients from CT: reality, public perception and policy. *AJR*. 2001;177:285–287.
5. Parry RA, Glaze SA, Archer BR. Typical patient radiation doses in diagnostic radiology. *RadioGraphics*. 1999;19:1289–1302.
6. Weissleder R, Rieumont MJ, Wittenberg J. *Primer of Diagnostic Imaging*. 2nd ed. St Louis: Mosby, Inc; 1997:922–927.
7. Yochum TR, Haug JV, Rowe LJ. *Radiology Study Guide*. Baltimore: Williams & Wilkins; 1998:41.
8. Selman J. *The Fundamentals of X-Ray and Radium Physics*. Springfield, IL: Charles C Thomas Publisher; 1994:504.
9. International Consensus Conference on Dose in Computed Tomography. Nurnberg; 2001.
10. EUR 16262, Commission of the European Community. Quality criteria for computed tomography, 1999.
11. Katz DS, Math KR, Groskin SA. *Radiology Secrets*. Philadelphia: Hanley & Belfus, Inc; 1998:6–9,23.
12. Hopper KD, King SH, Lobell ME, et al. The breast: in-plane x-ray protection against diagnostic thoracic CT-shielding with bismuth radioprotective garments. *Radiology*. 1997;205:853–858.

13. Dahnert W. *Radiology Review Manual*. 4th ed. Philadelphia: Lippincott, Williams & Wilkins; 2003:555.

14. Shu XO, Reaman GH, Lampkin B, et al. Investigators of the Children Cancer Group. Association of paternal diagnostic x-ray exposure with risk of infant leukemia. *Cancer Epidemiol Biomarkers Prev*. 1994;3:645–653.

15. Shea KM, Little RE. The ALSPAC Study Team; Avon Longitudinal Study of Pregnancy and Childhood. Is there an association between preconception paternal x-ray exposure and birth outcome? *Am J Epidemiol*. 1997;145:546–551.

16. National Council on Radiation Protection and Measurements (NCRP) Report. Bethesda, MD: NCRP Publications;

17. Russel JGB. Diagnostic radiation, pregnancy and termination. *Br J Radiol*. 1989;62:92.

18. Shore RE. Radiation epidemiology: old and new challenges. *Environ Hlth Perspect*. 1989;81:153.

19. Edwards FM. Risks of medical imaging. In: Putman CE, Ravin CE, eds. *Textbook of Diagnostic Imaging*. Philadelphia: WB Saunders; 1994;91.

20. Rodvall Y, Pershagen G, Hrubek Z, et al. Prenatal x-ray exposure and childhood cancer in Swedish twins. *Int. J Cancer*. 1990;46:362–365.

21. Stjernfeldt M, Berglund K, Lindsten J, et al. Maternal smoking and irradiation during pregnancy as risk factors for child leukemia. *Cancer Detect Prev*. 1992;16:129–135.

22. Wood JW, Johnson KG, Omori Y. In utero exposure to the Hiroshima atomic bomb: an evaluation of head size and mental retardation: twenty years later. *Pediatrics*. 1967;39:385–392.

23. Miller RW, Mulvihill JJ. Small head size after atomic irradiation. *Teratology*. 1976;14:255–258.

24. Brent RL. Radiation teratogenesis. *Teratology*. 1980;21:281–298.

25. Bushberg JD, Seibert JA, Leidholdt EM, et al. *The Essential Physics of Medical Imaging*. Baltimore: Williams & Wilkins; 1994: 695–705.

26. Brent RL. The effects of embryonic and fetal exposure to x-ray, microwave and ultrasound. *Clin Perinatol*. 1986;13:615.

27. Ferrer I, Xumetta A, Santamaria J. Cerebral malformations induced by prenatal X-ray radiation: an autoradiographic and Golgi study. *J Anat*. 1984;138:81–93.

28. The ionizing radiation (Protection of Persons Undergoing Medical Examinations or Treatment—POPUMET) regulations, 1988.

29. Brown RF, Shaver JW, Lamel DA. Selection of patients for x-ray examinations. Center for Devices and Radiological Health, HSS publication (FDA) 80-8104. Washington DC: Government Printing Office; 1984.

30. LaBan MM, Viola S, Williams DA, et al. Magnetic resonance imaging of the lumbar herniated disc in pregnancy. *Am J Phys Med Rehabil*. 1995;74:59–61.

31. Hashemi RH, Bradley WG. *Essentials of MRI Physics*. Baltimore: Williams & Wilkins; 1996.

32. Tyndall DA. MRI effects on craniofacial size and crown rump length in C57BL/6J mice in 1.5T fields. *Oral Surg Oral Med Oral Pathol*. 1993;76:655–660.

33. Tyndall DA, Sulik KK. Effects of magnetic resonance imaging on eye development in the C57BL/6J mouse. *Teratology*. 1991;43:263–275.

34. Garel C, Sebag G, Brisse H, et al. Magnetic resonance imaging of the fetus: contribution to antenatal diagnosis. *Presse Med*. 1996;25:452–456.

35. Revel MP, Pons JC, Lelaidier C, et al. Magnetic resonance imaging of the fetus: a study of 20 cases performed without curarization. *Prenat Diagn*. 1993;13:775–799.

36. Kay HH, Spritzer CE. Preliminary experience with magnetic resonance imaging in patients with third trimester bleeding. *Obstet Gynecol*. 1991;78:424–429.

37. Amano Y. The usefulness of MRI for the diagnosis of abnormal pregnancies. *Nippon Ika Daigaku Zasshi*. 1994;61:9–16.

38. Tukeva TA, Aronen HJ, Karjalainen PT, et al. Low field MRI pelvimetry. *Eur Radiol*. 1997;7:230–234.

39. Russell JR, Stabin MG, Sparks RB, et al. Radiation absorbed dose to the embryo/fetus from radiopharmaceuticals. *Health Phys*. 1997;73:756–769.

40. U.S.A. Nuclear Regulatory Commission. *Standards for Protection Against Radiation*: Code of Federal Regulations—energy, part 20, title 10 (10CFR20). Washington, DC: Office of the Federal Register, U.S. Government Printing Office Superintendent of Documents;

41. Boiselle PM, Reddy SS, Villas PA, et al. Pulmonary embolus in pregnant patients: survey of ventilation-perfusion imaging policies and practices. *Radiology*. 1998;207:201–206.

42. Sharma SC, Williamson JF, Khan FM, et al. Measurement and calculation of ovary and fetus dose in extended field radiotherapy for 10 MV x-rays. *Int J Radiat Oncol Biol Phys*. 1981;7:843–846.

43. Arnon J, Meirow D, Lewis-Roness H, et al. Genetic and teratogenic effects of cancer treatments on gametes and embryos. *Hum Reprod Update*. 2001;7:394–403.

44. Gwyn KM, Theriault RL. Breast cancer during pregnancy. *Curr Treat Options Oncol*. 2000;1:239–243.

45. Fenig E, Mishaeli M, Kalish Y, et al. Pregnancy and radiation. *Cancer Treat Rev*. 2001;27:1–7.

46. Nuyttens JJ, Prado KL, Jenrette JM, et al. Fetal dose during radiotherapy: clinical implementations and review of the literature. *Cancer Radiother*. 2002;6:352–357.

CHEMOTHERAPY IN PREGNANCY

Ralph L. Kramer / Baruch Feldman / Yuval Yaron / Mark I. Evans

The development of potent chemotherapeutic agents has resulted in significantly improved outcome for patients afflicted with a variety of different neoplasms. Prior to their development, the only available treatment options had been radiation or surgery. Previously fatal malignancies such as choriocarcinoma, the lymphomas, and leukemia, are now medically curable. Adjuvant chemotherapy has become a standard modality following local treatment of breast cancer as well as other malignancies that affect women during their reproductive years. Not unexpectedly, many of the currently used antineoplastic agents may have significant impact on pregnancy outcome as well as on ovarian function and fertility.

The effect of administration of any chemotherapeutic agent in pregnancy will depend on several factors. Administration from the time of fertilization until the end of the second gestational week should theoretically not result in fetal malformation as this is before the establishment of an effective embryonic circulation. Exposure restricted to the second through the fifth gestational weeks may cause severe damage to the blastocyst, resulting in spontaneous abortion or may cause no anomalies at all. Organogenesis occurs between the 5th and 10th gestational weeks. Exposure to chemotherapeutic agents during this time period may result in congenital anomalies. Whether malformation results is also influenced by drug dose, the concomitant use of radiation, or other agents, the duration of use, the frequency of administration, the route of administration, as well as the genetic makeup of the embryo/fetus. Generally the timing of administration in pregnancy is the major determinant of congenital malformation for a given agent.

While chemotherapeutic agents may impact on pregnancy, the physiologic changes of pregnancy may have significant effects on the pharmacokinetics of antineoplastic agents. Glomerular filtration and plasma volume are significantly increased in pregnancy. The increased volume of distribution may lead to a decrease in peak concentrations. Plasma albumin is decreased in pregnancy that may lead to an increase in the concentration of the unbound drug. Hepatic clearance of drugs may be increased or decreased.

Data regarding the long-term follow-up of offspring, which were exposed to chemotherapeutic agents in utero, or were conceived after maternal exposure to such agents, is limited to case reports and retrospective series. Information regarding subtle alterations, such as abnormalities of physical growth, intellectual and neurologic function, reproductive function, as well as long-term transplacental carcinogenesis is even more limited. Prospective, randomized trials to evaluate the effects of chemotherapeutic agents on pregnancy outcome have not been done nor are they likely to be performed, in light of obvious ethical considerations.

Accurate assessment of the risk of any chemotherapeutic agents on pregnancy or ovarian function is also confounded by the concomitant use of other agents as well as radiation therapy. Anecdotal reports describing pregnancy outcome after the use of single agent chemotherapy frequently report doses that would frequently be considered suboptimal by today's standards. It is difficult to extrapolate from these case reports in assessing the effect of current antineoplastic protocols. Bearing these limitations in mind however, it is the intent of the current chapter to review the reproductive risks associated with the use of the more commonly used antineoplastic agents for the treatment of neoplasms most commonly seen during pregnancy.

CLASSIFICATION OF CHEMOTHERAPEUTIC AGENTS

The agents utilized in cancer chemotherapy are numerous and diverse. It is useful to classify them according to the scheme described in *Goodman & Gilman's The Pharmacologic Basis of Therapeutics.*[1]

1. Alkylating agents including nitrogen mustards (mechlorethamine, cyclophosphamide, ifosfamide, melphalan, chlorambucil) ethylemimines and methylmelamines (hexamethylmelamine, thiotepa), alkyl sulfonates (busulfan), nitrosoureas (carmustine [BCNU], lomustine [CCNU], semustine [methyl-CCNU], streptozotcin) and the triazenes (dacarbazine or DTIC).
2. Antimetabolites including folic acid analogs (methotrexate), pyrimidine analogs (5-flurouracil, floxuridine, cytarabine, mercaptopurine), purine analogs (mercaptopurine, thioguanine, pentostatin).
3. Natural products including the vinca alkaloids (vinblastine and vincristine), epidophyllotoxins (etoposide, teniposide), antibiotics (dactinomycin, daunorubicin, doxorubicin, bleomycin, plicamycin, mitomycin), the enzyme L-asparaginase, and the biological response modifiers, interferon-alfa and interleukin-2.
4. Miscellaneous agents including the platinum containing compounds (cisplatin and carboplatin), mitoxantrone, hydroxyurea, porcarbazine, and the adrenocortical suppressants (miotane, aminoglutethimide).
5. Hormones and antagonists including adrenocorticosteroids (prednisone and equivalent preparations), progestins (hydroxyprogesterone caproate, medroxyprogesterone acetate, megestrol acetate), estrogens (diethylstilbestrol, ethinyl estradiol), the antiestrogen tamoxifen, androgens (testosterone proprionate, fluoxymesterone), the antiandrogen flutamide, and the gonadotropin releasing hormone analog leuprolide.

Chemotherapeutic agents tend to be more effective when used in combination as synergy may result from their interaction. The aim of combination chemotherapy is to minimize toxicity and to avoid the combination of drugs that share mechanisms of resistance. Hence the majority of chemotherapeutic regimens currently in use today are composed of multiple drugs. Therefore this chapter will review the effects of various chemotherapeutic regimens utilized in the treatment of the more commonly seen neoplasms in pregnancy. For those interested in the effects of individual agents in pregnancy, there are several excellent reviews to which the reader is referred.[2–4]

BREAST CANCER

Breast cancer is the most common cancer diagnosed during pregnancy with an estimated incidence of 1 in 1360 to 1 in 3200 pregnancies.[5] As an increasing number of women delay childbearing, the frequency of diagnosis during pregnancy is likely to increase. Adjuvant chemotherapy is the standard of care for premenopausal patients with node-positive disease, significantly decreasing a patient's risk of recurrence and death. Benefit appears to persist for at least 20 years after initial surgery.[6] Nonetheless, firm data upon which to make clinical decisions regarding the use of multiagent chemotherapy in this group of patients is extremely limited. Mulvihill reviewed 133 pregnancies in 66 women, 1 of whom received multiagent chemotherapy for breast cancer diagnosed before pregnancy.[7] This patient received cyclophosphamide, melphalan, methrotrexate, and 5-fluorouracil. Pregnancy ended in spontaneous abortion, the time of which is not specified. It is not stated when in pregnancy this patient received her chemotherapy, only that she had 3 months of therapy. Zemlickis et al. describe 3 patients with breast cancer all of whom had first trimester exposure but only 2 of which were treated with multiagent therapy.[8] One of these patients received cyclophosphamide, methrotrexate, and 5-fluorouracil and had a spontaneous abortion. The other received cyclophosphamide, methrotrexate, 5-fluorouracil, vincristine, and tamoxifen and reportedly had a "live birth, alive and well." It should be noted that the antimetabolites, methotrexate, and aminopterin, have been more frequently associated with congenital anomalies than any other agents. When these drugs are administered in the first trimester of pregnancy, there is an associated reported risk of fetal malformation of 24%.[4] The reported risk of congenital malformation associated with these agents drops to less than 1% if they are administered in the second and third trimesters.[4]

More recently, Berry et al. reported on the M.D. Anderson experience involving 24 patients spanning 8 years, beginning in 1989.[9] Twenty-two patients had primary breast cancer and 2 had recurrent disease. Modified radical mastectomy was performed in 18 patients, 14 of whom underwent the procedure during pregnancy. Four of the 14 patients underwent operation during the first trimester; there were no reported miscarriages. Chemotherapy consisting of fluorouracil (1,000 mg/m^2), doxorubicin (50 mg/m^2), and cyclophosphamide (500 mg/m^2) was administered every 3–4 weeks beginning after the first trimester, continuing through week 37. Three patients delivered before term. One infant had a birthweight less than the 10th percentile for gestational age. No malformations were observed. One infant developed transient leukopenia without infectious complications. Based on this study of 24 patients, these authors conclude that primary and recurrent breast cancer can be treated during pregnancy without demonstrable harm to the fetus, utilizing a standardized protocol, which included surgery

and chemotherapy. Other authors would be less sanguine with respect to the use of doxorubicin in pregnancy.[10] Only recently are the long-term effects of doxorubicin administered in childhood being reported. Lipschultz et al. conclude that doxorubicin therapy in childhood impairs myocardial growth in a dose-related fashion, resulting in a progressive increase in left ventricular afterload.[11] Whether doxorubicin exerts a comparable effect on children who have been exposed in utero remains to be seen.

When breast cancer is diagnosed during pregnancy, treatment may often be delayed because of perceived risk to the fetus. Nettleton et al. quantified the risk of delaying treatment using a mathematical model.[12] These authors analyzed the data of Silverstein et al.[13] and found a linear relationship between the natural log of the average tumor size and the percent positive axillary dissections. They subsequently derived an equation to determine the increased risk of axillary nodal metastasis attributable to an n-day delay in treatment. For tumors with a doubling time of 130 days, the daily increased risk of axillary metastasis is 0.028%. For tumors with a 65-day doubling time, the figure is 0.057%. Utilizing this model, a 1-month delay in treatment for a breast cancer with a 130-day doubling time, increases the risk of axillary node involvement by 0.9%. A 3-month delay would increase the risk by 2.6%; a 6-month delay by 5.1%. For a more aggressive tumor with a 65-day doubling time, the corresponding figures would be 1.8%, 5.2%, and 10.2%. This information would be helpful to women who are diagnosed with breast cancer during pregnancy.

Until this point the focus of the discussion has been on the effect of breast cancer on pregnancy outcome. The question of the effect of pregnancy on the course of breast cancer must also be raised. Zemlickis et al. examined a cohort of women who were pregnant within 9 months before and 3 months after their first cancer treatment.[14] These women had been registered in their data base between 1958 and 1987. One hundred eighteen women with breast cancer during pregnancy (119 pregnancies) were matched with 269 nonpregnant control subjects. Matching criteria included TNM breast cancer stage at diagnosis, age (controls were within 2 years of age at the time of diagnosis), and time of treatment (controls had diagnosis or first treatment within 2 calendar years of the matched case). The mean age of pregnant patients diagnosed with breast cancer was 32.9 ± 5.13 at the time of diagnosis. Of the 119 pregnancies, 14 women were diagnosed before conception, 42 during pregnancy, and 55 after delivery or pregnancy termination. Only 5 fetuses were exposed in utero to cancer chemotherapy, 3 during embryogenesis. The latter 3 women elected pregnancy termination. These authors observed a statistically increased risk (2.5-fold) among pregnant women of being diagnosed with Stage IV disease compared with the nonpregnant controls. Not unexpectedly, pregnant women were less likely to be diagnosed with Stage I disease. The authors ascribe this delay in diagnosis to the physiologic changes of pregnancy, specifically breast engorgement that could make the physical exam less sensitive in detecting breast cancer. Despite the difference in stage at presentation, no significant difference in survival was detected between pregnant and nonpregnant women. Given that young women, pregnant or not, usually have estrogen receptor-negative tumors[15], these authors plausibly hypothesize that the hormonal stimulation of pregnancy should not, therefore, affect the course of breast cancer.

In summary, breast cancer tends to be diagnosed at a later stage in pregnancy when compared to women who are not pregnant. When the diagnosis is made, pregnant women can be treated with both surgery and adjuvant chemotherapy, utilizing the regimen of fluorouracil, doxorubicin, and cyclophosphamide administered every 3 to 4 weeks, beginning after the first trimester. It must be acknowledged however, that this recommendation is based on relatively small numbers with little follow-up into adulthood. Alternatively, if a woman elects to delay the initiation of adjuvant chemotherapy until after delivery, she needs to be informed of the calculated increased risk of axillary node involvement with potential effect on long-term survival.

LEUKEMIA

The incidence of leukemia in pregnancy is comparable to that observed in the general female population at about 1 case per 100,000 women per year.[16–18] Therefore, even at large referral centers, experience with management of leukemia in pregnancy will probably be limited.

The most common leukemias diagnosed in pregnancy are acute myelocytic leukemia (AML) and acute lymphoblastic leukemia (ALL). Combination chemotherapy is the standard in the management of these hematologic malignancies. Chemotherapeutic regimens generally include the nitrogen mustard, cyclophosphamide, the folic acid analog, methotrexate, the pyrimidine analog, cytarabine, the purine analogs, mercaptopurine and thioguanine, the vinca alkaloids, vincristine and vinblastine, the anthracycline antibiotics, doxorubicin and daunorubicin, the enzyme, L-Asparaginase, and the corticosteroid, prednisone. Chronic myelogenous leukemia (CML) constitutes 90% of chronic leukemia seen in pregnancy.[16] The mainstay of treatment of CML is the alkyl sulfonate, busulfan.

For most pregnant women facing the prospect of chemotherapy, the concern of fetal malformation is paramount. Caligiuri and Mayer summarize the effects of combination chemotherapy in the treatment of 58 women with either ALL or AML reported in the English literature between 1975 and 1988.[16] Thirteen fetuses were exposed to chemotherapy during the first trimester. Eight fetuses were born prematurely, 2 of which were stillborn. Two fetuses were born at term, 2 were aborted electively, and 1 was aborted spontaneously. None of these fetuses had evidence of malformation. Forty-five fetuses were exposed during the second and third trimesters. Twenty-three infants in this latter group were born before term. There was 1 spontaneous abortion. Three preterm infants were stillborn. Twenty-one infants were born at term, 1 with an ocular abnormality and another with polydactyly, an anomaly previously noted in other family members. More detailed

information is provided on 18 of these 58 pregnancies in the review article by Wiebe and Sipila.[2]

In an extensive review of the literature, Wiebe and Sipila provide detailed information on the outcomes of 65 pregnancies complicated by leukemia, 55 of which were acute.[2] Among 50 infants born to women treated for acute leukemia in pregnancy, 3 exhibited evidence of major malformation. All 3 women who delivered infants with major malformations had been exposed to chemotherapy during the first trimester. One woman received cyclophosphamide and prednisone, 1 received ARA-C, and the third received 6-thioguanine. One minor malformation was noted (cornea fused to iris) in an infant exposed from week 23 on. One phenotypically normal infant had evidence of gaps and rings on cytogenetic evaluation. There was 1 neonatal death associated with severe preeclampsia at 29 weeks. Fourteen living infants were delivered before 36 weeks gestation. One woman underwent elective abortion at 21 weeks while another had a spontaneous abortion at 18 weeks.

Among the 13 women with chronic leukemia, 1 woman delivered an infant with multiple anomalies. She had been exposed to busulfan, 6-mercaptopurine, and radiation beginning in the first trimester. This woman died 2 months post-partum. The remaining 12 women received busulfan as a single, at least 6 of whom began treatment either prior to conception or during the first trimester. There was 1 spontaneous abortion in this latter group at 4 months gestation. One infant was born at 34 weeks, the remainder at term.

Hematologic abnormalities have been observed in newborns exposed to chemotherapeutic regimens utilized in the treatment of acute leukemia. In the review articles by Wiebe and Sipila and Ebert et al.,[19] 9 newborns out of 96 pregnancies exhibited evidence of hematologic abnormality or bone marrow hypoplasia. None of these infants had abnormal phenotypes. These mothers were treated with multiagent chemotherapeutic regimens including cytarabine, vincristine, purine analogs, cyclophosphamide, anthracycline antibiotics, methrotrexate, and prednisone. Two of the 9 newborns died of infectious complications within 4 weeks of delivery.

In summary, the majority of infants exposed to the chemotherapeutic agents used in the treatment of leukemia will exhibit no evidence of malformation. Although malformations have been observed, there is no characteristic pattern that has been discerned. There is no substantial evidence suggesting chromosome damage as a result of treatment with these agents. Some infants will exhibit evidence of bone marrow suppression, something that can be readily identified in the newborn period.

LYMPHOMA

The age-specific incidence of Hodgkin disease is bimodal with the earlier peak occurring in the third decade.[19] Hodgkin disease is the most common hematologic malignancy diagnosed in pregnancy.[20] Non-Hodgkin lymphoma is generally seen later in life with a mean age of presentation of 42.[21]

For many years, pregnancy was thought to adversely affect the outcome of Hodgkin disease. This was refuted in a large retrospective study by Barry et al.[22] Among a total of 347 women of childbearing age, 84 women with 112 pregnancies were analyzed. Pregnancy did not affect mean survival or exacerbate disease. Gelb et al. reached a similar conclusion 34 years later.[23]

Hodgkin disease is classified histologically into 4 types: nodular sclerosis, mixed cellularity, lymphocyte predominance, and lymphocyte depletion. Nodular sclerosis is the most common type and occurs most frequently in young adults. Hence this is the subtype most often seen in pregnancy.

The staging classification proposed in Cotswolds, England, a modification of the Ann Arbor classification, is the most commonly used classification today.[24] Depending on the stage of the disease, Hodgkin disease is treated with either radiation alone, or radiation in conjunction with chemotherapy. Staging requires a history and physical exam, biopsy, blood chemistry (including CBC, erythrocyte sedimentation rate, and renal and hepatic function), imaging of the chest, abdomen, and pelvis (CT or MRI), lymphangiography, and bone marrow aspiration. Staging laparotomy including splenectomy, and liver and various lymph node biopsies are required unless percutaneous liver biopsy is positive.

In the absence of bulky disease, radiation alone is the treatment for Stage I and II disease. Bulky disease is usually treated with a combination of chemotherapy and radiation. Stage III and IV disease is treated with combination chemotherapy of which there are numerous regimens. Current regimens include MOPP (mechlorethamine, vincristine, procarbazine, and prednisone), ABVD (doxorubicin, bleomycin, vinblastine, and dacarbazine), ChIVPP (chlorambucil, vinblastine, procarbazine, and prednisone), MOPP/ABVD in alternating cycles, and MOPP/ABV.[20]

Before the development of the regimens described above, cyclophosphamide alone or in conjunction with radiation or with other antineoplastic agents was administered with probable adverse effects on the fetus, when administered in the first trimester. In their review of antineoplastic agents in pregnancy, Wiebe and Sipila cite 3 cases of Hodgkin disease treated with cyclophosphamide in pregnancy.[2] A normal infant was born to a woman when treatment was started at 18 weeks gestation.[25] This patient received a regimen of cyclophosphamide, vincristine, procarbazine, and prednisone. In 2 earlier case reports, one by Greenberg and Tanaka[26] and another by Toledo et al.,[27] infants were exposed to cyclophosphamide during the first trimester of pregnancy and both were born with multiple anomalies. In the latter case, the mother had received radiation as well.

The multidrug regimens described above may also be teratogenic when administered during the first trimester of pregnancy. In their review article, Wiebe and Sipila report 4 cases of fetuses so exposed. One fetus was exposed to vinblastine and nitrogen mustard and was born at 24 weeks with multiple anomalies.[2] Another fetus exposed to the MOPP regimen during the first trimester and aborted at 92 days, exhibited renal and cardiac anomalies at autopsy. Another fetus exposed to

vinblastine, vincristine, and procarbazine throughout pregnancy appeared dysmature at 26 weeks with an atrial septal defect noted at autopsy. Zemlickis et al. report the outcome of 3 infants exposed to the MOPP regimen during the first trimester. One woman aborted spontaneously, 1 underwent therapeutic abortion, and a third delivered an infant with hydrocephalus that died 4 hours after birth.[8] Not unexpectedly, exposure after the first trimester would appear to reduce the likelihood of malformation. Wiebe and Sipila report 4 infants exposed to multi-agent regimens beginning in the second trimester that exhibited no anomalies.[2]

More recently, Gelb et al. report on 17 women diagnosed with Hodgkin disease from 1987–1995, 8 of whom were diagnosed and followed at Stanford University Medical Center.[23] The remainder were followed at the referring institutions. Of the 17 patients, only 5 received chemotherapy in the antepartum period. The remainder was treated either with chemotherapy or radiation or a combination of the 2 in the postpartum period. Of the women who received chemotherapy in the antepartum period, 1 woman received only vincristine, another received MOPP, ABV (doxorubicin, bleomycin, vinblastine), COP (cyclophosphamide, vincristine, and prednisone), and radiation therapy, another received CHOP (cyclophosphamide, doxorubicin, vincristine, prednisone) and radiation therapy, 1 received MOPP/ABV, and 1 received CHOP. The patient receiving MOPP/ABV underwent therapeutic abortion; the remainder was delivered at term of normal infants.

Non-Hodgkin lymphoma (NHL) is the 5th leading cause of death from cancer among women aged 15 to 34.[28] NHL's are clonal neoplasms arising from the cellular constituents of lymph nodes. Most patients present with painless lymphadenopathy. NHL is commonly classified according to the Working Formulation[29] that subdivides NHL into low-, intermediate-, and high-grade subgroups depending on their natural history. The prognosis is divided into favorable, intermediate, and poor. Prognostic variables include subgroup, stage, response to treatment, time to and duration of remission. Staging is performed as it is for Hodgkin disease with modification depending on the Working Formulation histologic grade. In general, early-stage low-grade NHL is treated with radiation therapy. Most Stage II and all Stage III and IV tumors are treated with combination chemotherapy. Low-grade lymphoma has been treated with single alkylating agents such as cyclophosphamide or chlorambucil or combinations such as CVP or CHOP. Additional agents have been added to CHOP for the treatment of intermediate grades such as bleomycin, methotrexate, procarbazine, nitrogen mustard, cytosine arabinoside, and etoposide. High-dose methotrexate, L-asparaginase, and intrathecal methotrexate may be added to CHOP in the treatment of high-grade lymphoma.[29] Overall, the prognosis of NHL is worse than that for Hodgkin disease and consequently treatment must be more aggressive.[20] Delay in treatment can rarely be justified.

In their exhaustive review article, Ebert et al. cite 8 studies summarizing the outcomes of 29 patients who underwent multiagent chemotherapy for NHL.[19] There were only 2 abortions in this series, 2 spontaneous and 1 induced. There were no reported congenital anomalies despite the fact that 10 of these fetuses were exposed during the first trimester.

Eighteen of the cases cited by Ebert et al. were originally reported by Aviles et al.[30] These authors examined 43 children born to mothers with hematologic malignancies, 18 of whom had NHL. Nine of the 18 fetuses were exposed to chemotherapeutic agents beginning in the first trimester. Two mothers with NHL died during induction chemotherapy with resultant fetal loss and were not included in the study. Neither of these fetuses showed evidence of anomalies. Chemotherapeutic regimens included CHOP, CHO-bleomycin, CHOP-etoposide-methotrexate, CHOP-methotrexate-cytosine arabinoside, CHOP-cyclophosphamide-methotrexate-etopiside-dexamethasone, and CHOP-bleomycin-cytosine arabiniside-methotrexate-etopiside. All children had physical examination as well as chromosome studies. The children's schools were visited and all children underwent intelligence testing. Three children were pancytopenic at birth. All children, ages 3–18 at the time of exam, exhibited normal growth and development. All had normal chromosomes and none had evidence of congenital anomalies. Seven mothers had died of their disease at the time of this study.

In summary, based on available case reports and series, it appears that the currently utilized chemotherapeutic regimens used in the treatment of Hodgkin disease and NHL do not significantly increase the risk of fetal anomalies if administered after the period of organogenesis. The risk of congenital anomalies appears to be increased when these agents are administered during the first trimester although the results are conflicting. The magnitude of this increase appears to be small. It is readily acknowledged, however, that these conclusions are based on small numbers. Clearly the decision to administer chemotherapeutic agents must ultimately be individualized and the limitations of our knowledge acknowledged.

OVARIAN CANCER

Invasive gynecologic neoplasms treated in pregnancy with chemotherapeutic agents are largely ovarian in origin. Germ cell tumors tend to be more common in younger pregnant patients while epithelial lesions are more common at the older end of the reproductive spectrum. Despite being the second most common gynecologic malignancy occurring in pregnancy, the estimated incidence of malignant ovarian neoplasms is between 1 case per 17,000 to 1 per 38,000 term deliveries.[31] Consequently, as with other cancers, the experience of any 1 center will inevitably be limited.

Indications for adjuvant chemotherapy in cases of ovarian cancer are the same for pregnant patients as for nonpregnant patients. Low-grade, early-stage epithelial malignancies as well as those of low malignant potential can be treated surgically. Germ cell tumors (with the exception of dysgerminoma, which tends to be acutely radiosensitive) are highly lethal. Survival has been dramatically improved with the use of adjuvant chemotherapeutic agents. Because these tumors

may grow rapidly, DiSaia and Creasman suggest that delaying the institution of adjuvant chemotherapy may be harmful.[32] When germ cell tumors are diagnosed in more advanced stages, chemotherapy may be the only hope of survival and delays in treatment are probably not warranted.[32]

As with other cancers, the experience of any one institution with the treatment of ovarian cancer in pregnancy tends to be limited. Consequently, most information is provided in the form of case reports. In 1979, Weed et al. reported treatment of recurrent endodermal sinus tumor with vincristine, actinomycin-D, and cyclophosphamide (VAC). Treatment was begun in the second trimester, resulting in the delivery of a normal infant at 33 weeks.[33] A similar successful outcome in cases of endodermal sinus tumors in pregnancy have been described by Kim and Parke.[34] Metz and colleagues successfully treated a patient with endodermal sinus tumor with cyclophosphamide, vincristine, and doxorubicin from gestational week 17. The woman was delivered of a normal infant at term.

Christman et al. report a case of treatment of an immature ovarian teratoma in pregnancy using cisplatin, vinblastine, and bleomycin with delivery of a normal infant at term.[36] Horbelt et al. describe the use of cisplatin, etoposide, and bleomycin instituted in the second trimester in the treatment of a mixed germ cell tumor.[37] The infant exhibited no evidence of anomalies. Malone et al. describe the use of vinblastine, bleomycin, and cisplatin in the treatment of an endodermal sinus tumor diagnosed at 25 weeks gestation.[38] The infant was delivered at 32 weeks gestation with no evidence of congenital anomalies.

Adjuvant chemotherapy has also been used in the treatment of epithelial carcinoma in pregnancy. King et al. and Malfetano and Goldkrand each reported a case of papillary serous cystadenocarcinoma of the ovary treated with surgery and adjuvant cisplatin and cyclophosphamide.[39,40] Treatment was begun in the second trimester. Both women were delivered of infants without evidence of congenital anomalies—1 preterm, 1 term. Zemlickis et al. cite a case of "ovarian carcinoma" treated with cyclophosphamide, doxorubicin, and cisplatin during the third trimester with delivery of a normal infant at term.[8]

In summary, the use of chemotherapeutic agents in the treatment of ovarian cancer in pregnancy is the same as in the nonpregnant state. The situation becomes appreciably more difficult in the case of the malignant germ cell tumors where combination chemotherapy has markedly improved survival. These tumors may grow rapidly and often recur within months when chemotherapeutic agents are withheld.[32] Thus, if a germ cell malignancy is diagnosed in the first trimester, particularly at a more advanced stage, the woman is put in the difficult position of having to weigh the conflicting risks of fetal malformation versus reduction in cure rate of her cancer. Obviously, this decision must be individualized.

MELANOMA

Melanoma affects adults of all ages. The most important prognostic factor is stage at the time of presentation.[41] Five-year survival when disease is localized (Stage I and II) is about 85%, decreasing to 15–20% with Stage III disease when 4 or more lymph nodes are involved. Five-year survival with Stage IV disease (disseminated) is less than 5%. Improved survival in younger women when compared to older women as well as men of all ages has been documented, particularly in advanced disease.[42] It has been hypothesized that this may be related to the role of sex steroids in melanoma progression.[43] Most recent studies have found no survival difference between pregnant and nonpregnant patients although pregnant women may have a shorter disease-free interval, thought to reflect a shortened time to nodal metastasis.[44–47]

Current treatment for melanoma is surgical excision in Stages I, II, and III after biopsy.[48] In patients with Stage IV disease, excision may be performed for palliation but is not intended to be curative. Lymph node dissection is performed in patients with Stage III and IV disease. Adjuvant chemotherapy is not the standard of care in patients with Stage and IIa melanoma.[48] In patients with Stage IIb and III disease, patients are currently treated with combination chemotherapy regimens including tamoxifen, carmustine, nimustine, cisplatin, and dacarbazine, with or without the addition of intereukin-2 or interferon alfa.[49–51] Total response rate (partial plus total) varies from 25–55% with these newer regimens[49–51] although long-term survival remains uncommon. We were only able to find a single case describing the use of multiagent chemotherapy in the treatment of metastatic melanoma in pregnancy.[52] The patient described was treated with a regimen of tamoxifen, carmustine, cisplatin, and dacarbazine beginning in week 23. The patient was delivered at 30 weeks gestation of an apparently normal infant. There have been no reported cases of the use of the biological response modifiers, interferon alfa and interleukin-2. It is readily apparent that there is insufficient evidence to support or refute the use of adjuvant chemotherapy in the treatment of malignant melanoma in pregnancy.

COLON CANCER

Colon cancer is an uncommon cancer in pregnancy. Several hundred cases in pregnancy are diagnosed annually in the United States.[53] Most patients present late in pregnancy with advanced disease and have a poor prognosis.[54] Surgery is the only curative modality for colorectal cancer.[55] The goal of chemotherapy and radiotherapy is to prolong survival, reduce the risk of recurrence, and hopefully to improve the quality of life.[55,56] Currently, 6 months of fluorouracil (5-FU) plus leucovorin (folinic acid) is considered the standard of care.[55] One case report of colon cancer in pregnancy where 5-FU was utilized was identified.[56] In this case reported in 1980, a 41-year-old mother underwent radiological evaluation in the diagnosis of colon cancer with a reported fetal radiation exposure of less than 5 rads. She received 5-FU during gestational weeks 11 and 12, followed by pregnancy termination at 16 weeks. The fetus exhibited multiple anomalies including bilateral radial aplasia, absent thumbs and fingers, hypoplastic aorta, pulmonary hypoplasia, hypoplastic thymus, esophageal aplasia, aplasia of

the first part of the duodenum, biliary hypoplasia, absent appendix, imperforate anus, common bladder and rectum, and renal dysplasia with a plastic ureters. It is difficult to assess the individual roles of radiation, maternal age, and 5-FU. Given the limited role of adjuvant chemotherapy in colon cancer and the documented teratogenicity of the antimetabolites when administered during the first trimester[4] it is probably reasonable to avoid the administration of 5-FU in the first trimester when colon cancer is diagnosed in pregnancy.

SUMMARY

Fortunately, cancer in pregnancy is generally an uncommon to rare event, depending on the neoplasm. We present data on some of the more commonly seen neoplasms in pregnancy.

The number of available antineoplastic agents is large and is expanding rapidly. On the other hand, the aggregate experience with multiagent chemotherapy, much less the experience of a single institution is generally quite small. As noted in the introduction, information is almost exclusively anecdotal in human beings, and is unlikely to be otherwise, for obvious reasons (with the exception of computer simulations). With that said, however, it is fair to say that obvious congenital malformations are relatively uncommon when chemotherapy is administered beginning in the second or third trimester. This does not address the issue of more subtle alterations. Generally speaking, offspring found to be normal at birth tend to remain so during follow-up.[58] For most cancers, chemotherapy can be safely delayed until the second or third trimester with the possible exception of the non-Hodgkin lymphomas and some of the germ cell tumors of the ovary. Delay in the initiation of treatment of breast cancer may, however, increase the likelihood of nodal involvement.[12]

In summary, decisions regarding the use of antineoplastic agents in pregnancy are difficult because of the limited nature of the data on which to base these decisions. The optimal decision can be made only in the context of frank and detailed discussion, where these limitations are openly acknowledged.

References

1. Brunton L, Lazo J, Parker K, et al. *Goodman & Gilman's The Pharmacologic Basis of Therapeutics.* 11th ed. New York: McGraw-Hill Text: 2006.
2. Ring AE, Smith IE, Jones A, et al. Chemotherapy for breast cancer during pregnancy: an 18 year experience from five London teaching hospitals. *J Clin Oncol* 2005;23:4192–4197.
3. Melrow D, Levron J, Eldar-Geva T, et al. Pregnancy after transplantation of crypreserved ovarian tissue in a patient with ovarian failure after chemotherapy. *NEJM* 2005.
4. Lobo R. Potential options for preservation of fertility in women. *NEJM* 2005;353:64–73.

5. Partridge A, Schapira L. Pregnancy and breast cancer: epidemiology, treatment, and safety issues. *Oncology* 2005;19:693–697.

6. Bonadonna G, Valagussa P, Moliterni A, et al. Adjuvant cyclophosphamide, methotrexate, and fluorouracil in node-positive breast cancer: the results of 20 years of follow-up. *N Engl J Med.* 1995; 332:901–906.

7. Mulvihill JJ, McKeen EA, Rosner F, et al. Pregnancy outcome in cancer patients: experience in a large cooperative group. *Cancer.* 1987;60:1143–1150.

8. Zemlickis D, Lishner M, Degendorfer P, et al. Fetal outcome after in utero exposure to cancer chemotherapy. *Arch Intern Med.* 1992;152:573–576.

9. Berry DL, Theirault RL, Holmes FA, et al. Management of breast cancer during pregnancy using a standardized protocol. *J Clinical Oncol.* 1999;17:855–861.

10. Petrek JA. Breast cancer in pregnancy. *Cancer.* 1994;74:518–527.

11. Lipschultz SE, Colan SD, Gelber RD, et al. Late cardiac effects of doxorubicin therapy for acute lymphoblastic leukemia in childhood. *N Engl J Med.* 1991;324:808–815.

12. Nettleton J, Long J, Kuban D, et al. Breast cancer during pregnancy: quantifying the risk of treatment delay. *Obstet Gynecol.* 1996;87:414–418.

13. Silverstein MJ, Gierson ED, Waisman JR, et al. Axillary lymph node dissections for T1a breast carcinoma—is it indicated? *Cancer.* 1994;73:664–667.

14. Zemlickis DZ, Lishner M, Degendorfer P, et al. Maternal and fetal outcome after breast cancer in pregnancy. *Am J Obstet Gynecol.* 1992;166:781–787.

15. Nugent P, O'Connell TX. Breast cancer and pregnancy. *Arch Surg.* 1985;120:1088–1090.

16. Caligiuri MA, Mayer RJ. Pregnancy and leukemia. *Semin Oncol.* 1989;16:388–396.

17. Roy V, Gutteridge CN, Nysenbaum A, et al. Combination chemotherapy with conservative obstetric management in the treatment of pregnant patients with acute myeloblastic leukemia. *Clin Lab Haemat.* 1989;11:171–178.

18. Hass VA. Pregnancy in association with a newly diagnosed cancer: a population-based epidemiologic assessment. *Int J Cancer.* 1984;34:229–235.

19. Ebert U, Loffler H, Kirch W. Cytotoxic therapy and pregnancy. *Pharmacol Ther.* 1997;74:207–220.

20. Peleg D, Ben-Ami M. Lymphoma and leukemia complicating pregnancy. *Obstet Gynecol Clin North Amer.* 1998;25:365–383.

21. Orr JW, Shingleton HM. Cancer in pregnancy. *Curr Probl Cancer.* 1983;8:1–50.

22. Barry RM, Diamond HD, Craver LF. Influence of pregnancy on the course of Hodgkin's disease. *Am J Obstet Gynecol.* 1962;84:445–454.

23. Gelb AB, van de Rijn M, Warnke RA, et al. Pregnancy-associated lymphomas: A clinic pathologic study. *Canc.* 1996;78:304–310.

24. Lister TA, Crowther D, Sutcliffe SB, et al. Report of a committee convened to discuss the evaluation and staging of patients with Hodgkin's disease: Cotswolds meeting. *J Clin Oncol.* 1989;7:1630–1636.

25. Daly H, McCann SR, Hanratty TD, et al. Successful pregnancy during combination chemotherapy for Hodgkin's disease. *Acta Haematol.* 1980;64:154–156.

26. Greenberg LH, Tanaka KR. Congenital anomalies probably induced by cyclophosphamide. *J Am Med Assoc.* 1964;188:423–426.

27. Toledo TM, Harper RC, Moser RH. Fetal effects during cyclophosphamide and irradiation therapy. *Ann Intern Med.* 1971;74:87–91.

28. Boring CC, Squires TS, Tong T, et al. Cancer statistics, 1994. *CA Cancer J Clin.* 1994;44:7–26.

29. Freedman AS, Nadler LM. Malignant lymphomas. In: Isselbacher KJ, Braunwald E, Wilson JD, Martin JB, Kasper DL, eds. *Harrison's Principles of Internal Medicine.* 13th ed. New York: McGraw-Hill, Inc; 1994:1774–1788.

30. Aviles A, Diaz-Maqueo JC, Talvera A, et al. Growth and development of children of mothers treated with chemotherapy during pregnancy: current status of 43 children. *Am J Hematol.* 1991;36:243–248.

31. Jolles C. Gynecologic cancer associated with pregnancy. *Semin Oncol.* 1989;16:417–424.

32. DiSaia PJ, Creasman WT. Cancer in pregnancy. In: DiSaia PJ, Cressman WT, Dinh T, et al. *Clinical Gynecologic Oncology,* 6th ed. St. Louis: Mosby; 2003;502–544.

33. Weed JC, Roh RA, Mendenhall HW. Recurrent endodermal sinus tumor during pregnancy. *Obstet Gynecol.* 1979;54:653–656.

34. Kim DS, Park MI. Maternal and fetal survival following surgery and chemotherapy of endodermal sinus tumor of the ovary during pregnancy: a case report. *Obstet Gynecol.* 1989;73:503–507.

35. Metz SA, Day TG, Pursell SH. Adjuvant chemotherapy in a pregnant patient with endodermal sinus tumor of the ovary. *Gynecol Oncol.* 1989;32:371–374.

36. Christman JE, Teng NNH, Lebovic GS, et al. Delivery of a normal infant following cisplatin, vinblastine and bleomycin (PVB) chemotherapy for malignant teratoma of the ovary during pregnancy. *Gynecolo Oncol.* 1990;37:292–295.

37. Horbelt D, Delmore J, Meisels R, et al. Mixed germ cell malignancy of the ovary concurrent with pregnancy. *Obstet Gynecol.* 1984;84:662–665.

38. Malone JM, Gershenson DM, Creasy RK, et al. Endodermal sinus tumor of the ovary associated with pregnancy. *Obstet Gynecol.* 1986;68:86S–89S.

39. King LA, Nevin PC, Williams PP, et al. Treatment of advanced epithelial ovarian carcinoma in pregnancy with cisplatin-based chemotherapy. *Gynecol Oncol.* 1991;41:78–80.

40. Malfetano JH, Goldkrand JW. Cis-platinum combination chemotherapy during pregnancy for advanced epithelial ovarian carcinoma. *Obstet Gynecol.* 1990;75:545–547.

41. Sober AJ, Koh HK. Melanoma and other pigmented skin lesions. In: Isselbacher KJ, Braunwald E, Wilson JD, Martin JB, Fauci AS, Kasper DL, eds. *Harrison's Principles of Internal Medicine.* 13th ed. New York: McGraw-Hill; 1994:1867–1871.

42. Kemeny MM, Busch E, Stewart AK, et al. Superior survival of young women with malignant melanoma. *Am J Surg.* 1998;175:437–444.

43. Richardson B, Price A, Wagner M, et al. Investigation of female survival benefit in metastatic melanoma. *Br J Canc.* 1999; 80:2025–2033.

44. Reintgen DS, McCarty KS, Vollmer R, et al. Malignant melanoma and pregnancy. *Cancer.* 1985;55:1340–1344.

45. McManamny DS, Moss ALH, Pococock PV, et al. Melanoma and pregnancy: a long-term followup. *Br J Obstet Gynecol.* 1989; 96:1419–1423.

46. Wong JH, Sterns EE, Kopald KH, et al. Prognostic significance of pregnancy in stage I melanoma. *Arch Surg.* 1989;124:1227–1231.

47. Slinghuff CL, Reintgen DS, Vollmer RT, et al. Malignant melanoma arising during pregnancy: a study of 100 patients. *Ann Surg.* 1990;211:552–559.

48. Duran F, Garcia E, Santolaya R, et al. Treatment of malignant melanoma. *Ann Pharmacotherapy.* 1999;33:730–738.

49. Yamazaki N, Yamamoto A, Wada T, et al. Dacarbazine, nimustine hydrochloride, cisplatin and tamoxifen combination chemotherapy for advanced malignant melanoma. *J Dermat.* 1999;26:489–493.

50. Rosenberg SA, Yang JC, Schwartzentruber DJ, et al. Prospective randomized trial of the treatment of patients with metastatic melanoma using chemotherapy with cisplatin, dacarbazine, and tamoxifen alone or in combination with interleukin-2 and interferon alfa-2b. *J Clin Oncol.* 1999;17:968–975.

51. Dorval T, Negrier S, Chevreau C, et al. Randomized trial of treatment with cisplatin and interleukin either alone or in combination

with interferon-alpha-2a in patients with metastatic melanoma: a Federation Nationale des Centres de Lutte Ckontre le Cancer Multicenter, parallel study. *Cancer*. 1999;85:1060–1066.

52. DiPaola RS, Goodin S, Tatzell M, et al. Chemotherapy for metastatic melanoma in pregnancy. *Gynecol Oncol*. 1997;66:526–530.

53. Cappell MS. Colon cancer during pregnancy: the gastroenterologist's perspective. *Gastroenterol Clin N Amer*. 1998;27:225–256.

54. Walsh C, Fazio VW. Cancer of the colon, rectum and anus during pregnancy: the surgeon's perspective. *Gastroenterol Clin N Amer*. 1998;27:257–267.

55. Peeters M, Haller DG. Therapy for early-stage colorectal cancer. *Oncol*. 1999;13:307–315.

56. van Cutsem E, Peeters M, Verslype C, et al. The medical treatment of colorectal cancer: actual status and new developments. *Hepato-Gastroenterol*. 1999;46:709–716.

57. Stephens JD, Golbus MS, Miller TR, et al. Multiple congenital anomalies in a fetus exposed to 5-fluorouracil during the first trimester. *Am J Obstet Gynecol*. 1980;137:747–749.

58. Garber JE. Long-term follow-up of children exposed in utero to antineoplastic agents. *Sem Oncol*. 1989;16:437–444.

Ultrasound Diagnosis & Screening

OVERVIEW OF THE COMPREHENSIVE ULTRASOUND EXAMINATION: AN APPROACH TO DIAGNOSIS AND MANAGEMENT OF FETAL ANOMALIES

Edith D. Gurewitsch / Frank A. Chervenak

ULTRASOUND DIAGNOSIS OF FETAL ANOMALIES

Antenatal ultrasound scanning at about 18–20 weeks of gestation permits the detection of most major fetal structural anomalies.[1-7] Since a large number of women carrying a fetus with a congenital anomaly have no identifiable risk factor, it is encumbent upon all sonographers who scan pregnant women to perform at least a minimum evaluation of the fetal anatomy. Ultrasound examinations that are restricted to the documentation of fetal life, fetal number, fetal presentation, gestational age, growth assessment, amniotic fluid volume assessment, and placental localization are considered incomplete.

The employment of a systematic approach to the evaluation of the fetal anatomy is of paramount importance. This is usually accomplished by the sequential study of the distinct regions of the fetal anatomy: the head, spine, thorax, abdomen, and extremities. Examination of the fetal head is most often performed with transverse views at a minimum of 3 levels: the lateral ventricle, the biparietal diameter, and the cerebellum. At these planes, the fetal skull can be assessed. It should be elliptical with the cranium ossified and intact. The ventricular system should be studied by assessing the atrium of the lateral ventricle. In the posterior fossa, the cerebellar hemispheres should be visualized and the cisterna magna evaluated. The spine should be viewed in its entirety in a saggital plane. This is then complemented by a series of transverse sonograms to identify normal anterior and posterior ossification elements. The position of the heart within the thorax should be noted and an attempt should be made to obtain a 4 chambered view. Atria and ventricles should be of equal and appropriate sizes and the interventricular septum should be intact. Examination of the fetal outflow tracts increases the detection of heart anomalies. In the region of the abdominal cavity, the fetal stomach, and bladder should be visualized by 14 weeks of gestation; kidneys should be visualized by 16 weeks. A view of the umbilical cord insertion site is mandatory to determine whether the anterior abdominal wall is intact. The long bones of at least the lower extremitites should be visualized. Although not considered part of the *minimum* anatomical survey, examination of all areas of the anatomy, including face, genitalia, all four extremities with their digits, and measurement of nuchal skinfold thickness, is desirable.

Sonographic examination of fetal anatomy is often more detailed when it is targeted to look for a certain anomaly. However, there are general clues to the existence of a fetal anomaly to which the alert sonographer can be attuned during every examination. Many fetal anomalies can be grouped into the following categories based on the nature of the dysmorphology that permits sonographic detection:

- Absence of a structure normally present;
- Dilatation behind an obstruction;
- Herniation through a structural defect;
- Abnormal location or contour of a normal structure;
- Presence of an additional structure;
- Abnormal fetal biometry; and
- Absent or abnormal fetal motion.

ABSENCE OF A STRUCTURE NORMALLY PRESENT

A dramatic example of the absence of a structure normally detected by ultrasound is anencephaly, the absence of calvaria and forebrain. In these cases, ultrasound clearly reveals the absence of echogenic skull bones and the presence of a heterogeneous mass of cystic tissue, called the area cerebrovasculosa, which replaces well-defined cerebral structures (Fig. 17-1). In 1972, anencephaly was the first fetal anomaly to be diagnosed with sufficient certainty to support a decision to terminate a pregnancy.[8]

Alobar holoprosencephaly is characterized by the absence of midline cerebral structures, which results from incomplete cleavage of the primitive forebrain. This is noted ultrasonographically when the midline echo in the fetal head that is normally generated by acoustic interfaces of the interhemispheric fissure is absent (Fig. 17-2a). However, absence of a midline echo is not specific to alobar holoprosencephaly. To confirm the diagnosis, an additional sonographic sign should be sought, which may include hypotelorism, nasal anomalies, and facial clefts[9] (Fig. 17-2b).

The neuropathology of the Dandy-Walker malformation is characterized by the complete or partial absence of the cerebellar vermis and a posterior fossa cyst continuous with the fourth ventricle (Fig. 17-3). Theories on pathogenesis include atresia of the foramina of Luschka and Magendie and hypoplasia or gross alteration of the cerebellum. Dandy-Walker cysts appear on ultrasound as echo-spared areas in the posterior fossa. The cerebellar vermis, a bright echogenic midline structure caudal to the fourth ventricle, is absent or defective.

The kidneys are normally seen as bilateral, ovoid, paraspinal masses with echospared renal pelves. When not visualized, the diagnosis of renal agenesis should be suspected. Severe oligohydramnios and an inability to visualize the bladder support the diagnosis. Although antenatal diagnosis of renal agenesis is possible, false-positive and false-negative diagnoses can occur from inadequate visualization due to the presence of oligohydramnios and simulation of the sonographic appearance of kidneys by hypertrophied adrenal glands.[10]

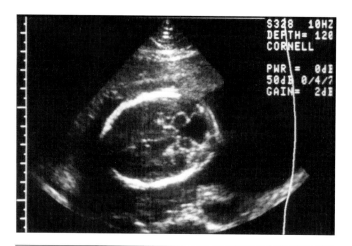

FIGURE 17-1 Coronal sonogram of fetal head demonstrating anencephaly with absence of the bony calvarium above the level of the orbits. The amorphous material above the orbits is the area cerebrovasculosa.

FIGURE 17-3 Sonogram of the Dandy-Walker malformation demonstrating the enlarged cisterna magna, splaying of the cerebellar hemispheres in the posterior fossa and absence of the cerebellar vermis.

DILATATION BEHIND AN OBSTRUCTION

In this class of anomalies, the structural defect itself is rarely seen. Rather, what is observed is the distention of structures behind a defect. Such dilatation may be caused by obstruction to the normal flow of cerebrospinal fluid, urine, or swallowed amniotic fluid.

Hydrocephalus is characterized by a relative enlargement of the cerebroventricular system with an accompanying increase of pressure of the cerebrospinal fluid within the fetal head. Hydrocephalus is suggested by a lateral ventricular atrial width greater than 10 mm,[11-13] a dangling choroid plexus,[12] and an asymmetric appearance of the choroid plexus[13,14] (Fig. 17-4). The location of the obstruction may be determined by observing which portions of the ventricular system are enlarged. There is frequently an association between fetal hydrocephalus and other anomalies, especially spina bifida.[15]

Fetal small bowel obstruction may cause dilatation proximal to the area of obstruction. Duodenal atresia has been observed to produce a characteristic "double bubble" sign, consisting of enlarged duodenum and stomach with narrowing at the pylorus and duodenum (Fig. 17-5). Duodenal atresia can be associated with Down syndrome.[16,17] Obstruction in the lower gastrointestinal tract (eg, imperforate anus) is generally not detected on antenatal ultrasound unless there is an associated lesion.

Obstructions to urinary flow can result in proximal dilatation of the renal pelvis, ureter or bladder (Fig. 17-6a, 17-6b). Ureteropelvic or ureterovesical obstructions are

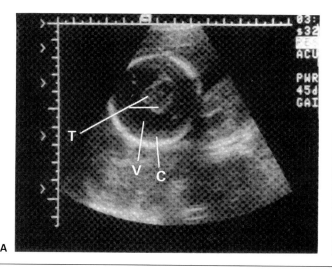

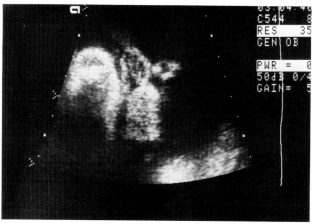

FIGURE 17-2 (**A**) Cranial sonogram demonstrating alobar holoprosencephaly (V—common ventricle; T—prominent fused thalamus; C—compressed cerebral cortex). (**B**) Coronal sonogram through the lips and nose of a fetus with cebocephaly. Note the normally placed nose with a single nostril.

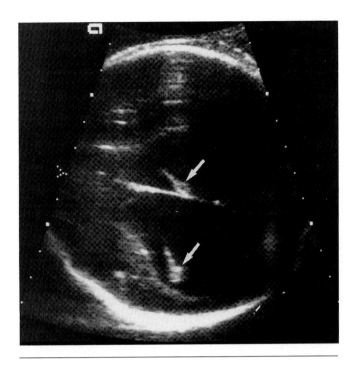

FIGURE 17-4 Transverse sonogram of fetal head demonstrating hydrocephalus (arrows point to the dangling choroid plexus).

commonly unilateral defects, whereas obstruction at the urethra from posterior urethral valves characteristically produces bilateral dilatation of the ureters and renal pelves.[18–20] When a posterior urethral valve produces a complete obstruction, renal dysplasia from increased hydrostatic pressure and pulmonary hypoplasia secondary to oligohydramnios may result.

HERNIATION THROUGH STRUCTURAL DEFECTS

A common theme in the development of the fetus is the formation of compartments containing vital structures, which is accomplished by a series of folding and midline fusion. Incom-

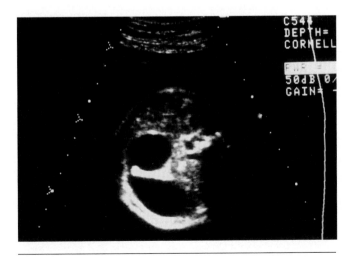

FIGURE 17-5 Transverse sonogram through the abdomen demonstrating the "double bubble" sign in a fetus with duodenal atresia.

plete fusion in a variety of locations leads to defects through which herniations of contained structures can occur.[21]

The neural tube and overlying mesoderm begin their closure in the region of the fourth somite, with fusion extending both rostrally and caudally during the fourth week of fetal life.[21] Incomplete closure at the rostral end produces cephaloceles, with herniations of meninges and, frequently, of brain substance through a defect in the cranium[22] (Fig. 17-7). Failed fusion at the caudal end produces spina bifida with protruding meningoceles and meningomyeloceles (Fig. 17-8). Sonographic diagnosis of each of these anomalies depends on the demonstration of a defect in the normal structure of the cranium or spine and of a protruding sac, often containing tissue.[23,24]

Omphaloceles result from failure of the intestines to retract from their temporary location in the umbilical cord and the subsequent herniation of other abdominal contents, including both hollow and solid structures contained within a peritoneal sac (Fig. 17-9). Insertion of the umbilical cord into the sac helps to differentiate an omphalocele from gastroschisis, which has no covering membrane (Fig. 17-10). Nonetheless, distinguishing these 2 entities may be difficult.[25]

The diaphragm forms from 4 separate structures that fuse to separate the pleural and peritoneal cavities. When a diaphragmatic hernia is present, abdominal contents may be visualized within the chest on transverse sonographic scanning. A disruption in this development of the diaphragm may be seen in the sagittal plane[26,27] (Fig. 17-11).

ABNORMAL LOCATION OR CONTOUR OF A NORMAL STRUCTURE

At times, a congenital anomaly that may normally be characterized by one of the other categories cannot be seen easily. In these instances, clues to the existence of such an anomaly come from changes in the location or contour of other normal structures. These changes are produced by the underlying defect.

Most, if not all, cases of spina bifida are complicated by the Arnold-Chiari malformation, an anomaly of the hindbrain that has 2 components. The first is a variable displacement of a tongue of cerebellar tissue into the spinal canal. The second is a similar caudal dislocation of the medulla and fourth ventricle.[28] The Arnold-Chiari malformation can serve, therefore, as an important marker for spina bifida. Two characteristic sonographic signs (the "lemon" and the "banana") of the Arnold-Chiari malformation have been described. Scalloping of the frontal bones produced by the caudal displacement of the cranial contents within a pliable skull can give a lemon-like configuration to the skull of an affected fetus when viewed in axial section (Fig. 17-12). Similarly, as the cerebellar hemispheres are displaced into the cervical canal, they are flattened rostrocaudally and the cisterna magna is obliterated, thus producing a flattened, centrally curved, banana-like sonographic appearance. In extreme instances, the cerebellar hemispheres may be absent from view during fetal head scanning[29] (Fig. 17-13).

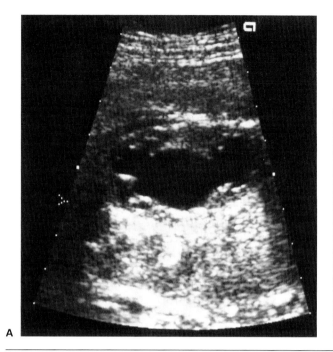

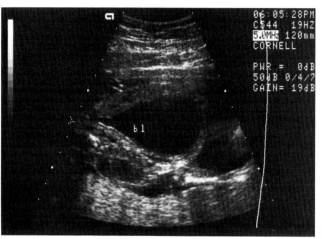

FIGURE 17-6 (**A**) Longitudinal sonogram of a fetus with an obstruction at the ureteropelvic junction resulting in marked unilateral hydronephrosis of the affected side. (**B**) Sonogram of a fetus with posterior urethral valves demonstrating the "keyhole" shape of the dilated bladder (b1).

The corpus callosum is the great commisural plate of nerve fibers interconnecting the cortical hemispheres. Agenesis of the corpus callosum can be somewhat difficult to detect since the corpus callosum itself cannot be seen on transverse scans. Therefore, it is necessary to search for anatomic alterations produced by its absence. These include lateral displacement of the bodies of the lateral ventricles, enlargement of the atria and occipital horns producing a characteristic "teardrop" shape and enlargement or upward displacement of the

third ventricle (Fig. 17-14). Agenesis of the corpus callosum can occur as an isolated anomaly, but 80% of cases will be associated with other anomalies such as hydrocephalus, Dandy-Walker syndrome, Arnold-Chiari malformation, and holoprosencephaly.

PRESENCE OF AN ADDITIONAL STRUCTURE

Small areas of cystic dilatation may be noted in the choroid plexus of the lateral ventricles of 1–2% of all fetuses (Fig. 17-15). These lesions are usually transient and lack clinical significance. Generally, they resolve before the end of the

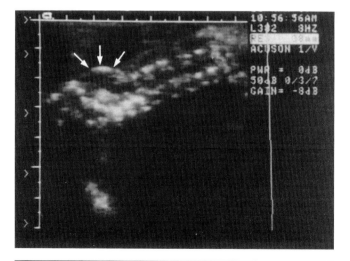

FIGURE 17-7 Occipital encephalocele (outlined by arrows, LV = dilated lateral ventricle).

FIGURE 17-8 Longitudinal sonogram of fetal spine with arrows pointing to meningomyelocele.

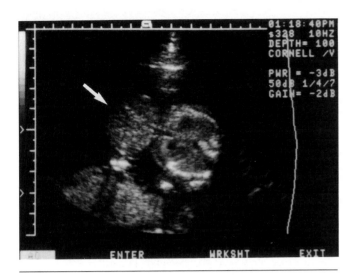

FIGURE 17-9 Sonogram of a fetus with omphalocele. Herniated contents covered by a membrane (arrow) are demonstrated at the level of the umbilical cord insertion site.

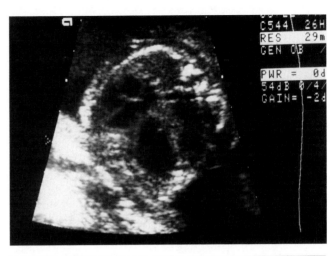

FIGURE 17-11 Transverse sonogram through the thorax of a fetus with a congenital diaphragmatic hernia demonstrating the presence of the stomach bubble within the chest causing displacement of the heart.

second trimester. Approximately 5%, however, will be associated with trisomy 18 and another 1% will have other karyotypic abnormalities.[30] Many of these fetuses will have other structural abnormalities that can be detected by ultrasound.

A typical antenatal intracranial hemorrhage is seen as an echogenic mass in the region of the germinal matrix or within the lateral ventricles (Fig. 17-16a). Porencephaly describes a condition wherein a portion of the cerebral cortex is absent and replaced by a cystic cavity. Such a cavity may be in communication with the subarachnoid space, a ventricle (Figure 17-16b), neither or both. It is thought that areas of prior hemorrhage or tissue necrosis resorb, leaving behind porencephalic cysts. Sonographically, porencephalic cysts appear as solitary or multiple echo-spared areas of variable size and location within the brain.

Fetal cystic hygromas are fluid-filled masses of the fetal neck which arise from abnormal lymphatic development. They are generally anechoic, have scattered septations, and/or a midline septum arising from the nuchal ligament (Fig. 17-17). If the lymphatic disorder causing the hygromas is widespread, it may produce fetal hydrops and intrauterine death[31,32] (Fig. 17-18).

Masses that distort normal fetal anatomy can be readily identified with ultrasound. Fetal teratomas are the most common neoplasms of fetuses. They are derived from pluripotent cells and thus they are composed of a variety of tissue types,

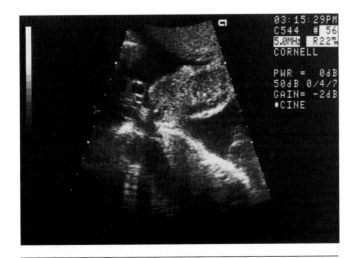

FIGURE 17-10 Sonogram of a fetus with gastroschisis demonstrating free-floating loops of bowel within the amniotic cavity.

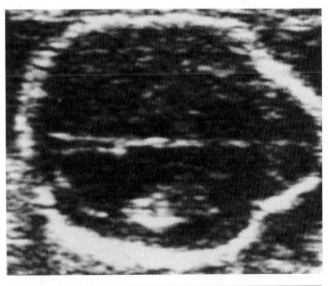

FIGURE 17-12 Transverse section of fetal head at level of cavum septi pellucidi in a fetus with open spina bifida showing the "lemon" sign. (Reprinted with permission from Nicolaides KM, Campbell S, Gabbe SG, Guidetti R. Ultrasound screening for spina bifida: cranial and cerebellar signs. *Lancet*. 1986;2:72.)

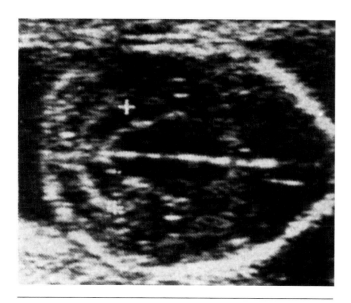

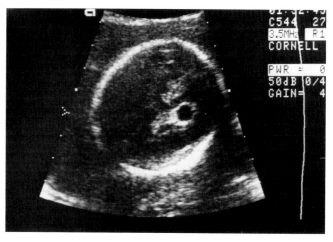

FIGURE 17-15   Sonogram of a choroid plexus cyst.

FIGURE 17-13   Suboccipital bregmatic view of the head in a fetus with open spina bifida, demonstrating "banana" sign (+). (Reprinted with permission from Nicolaides KM, Campbell S, Gabbe SG, Guidetti R. Ultrasound screening for spina bifida: cranial and cerebellar signs. *Lancet*. 1986;2:72.)

usually foreign to the anatomic site in which they arise. They may be visualized as distortions of fetal contour, often in the sacrococcygeal area or along the fetal midline. The internal sonographic appearance, characterized by irregular cystic and solid areas and occasional calcifications, helps to identify the lesion[33] (Fig. 17-19).

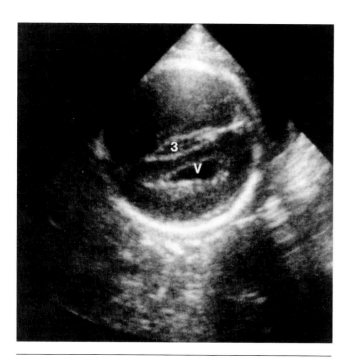

FIGURE 17-14   Sonogram of a fetus with agenesis of the corpus callosum demonstrating laterally-diplaced, "tear drop" lateral ventricle (V) and a high-riding third ventricle (3) (normally not seen in this plane of view).

ABNORMAL FETAL BIOMETRY

Several fetal anomalies are best diagnosed not by observing alterations in shape or consistency, but by determining abnormalities in size. The science of fetal biometry has generated many nomograms defining normal values for parts of the fetal anatomy at various gestational ages.[34]

Fetal microcephaly is usually the result of an underdeveloped brain. Although commonly associated with cerebral structural malformations, microcephaly may be produced by a brain that is normal in configuration but merely small. The accurate diagnosis of microcephaly has proved challenging because compressive forces within the uterus may distort the shape of the fetal head. The best correlation between microcephaly diagnosed in utero and neonatal microcephaly is made when multiple parameters are measured and suggest a small head.[35,36]

When interorbital distances are inconsistent with gestational age, hypotelorism, or hypertelorism may be suggested. Abnormal distance between the orbits may serve as a clue to several malformation syndromes, such as alobar holoprosencephaly[9] and median cleft face syndrome.[37]

The internal architecture of the kidneys may be difficult to assess in the presence of oligohydramnios, which may be caused by a renal abnormality. The diagnosis of polycystic kidneys, for example, can thus be aided by renal measurement. In addition to being echogenic, polycystic kidneys are usually enlarged and display an abnormally increased kidney circumference to abdominal circumference ratio.[38,39]

A variety of skeletal dysplasias may affect the growth of long bones. Measurement may suggest a particular skeletal dysplasia, depending on which bones are foreshortened. The shape of these bones, their density, the presence of fractures, or the absence of specific bones may aid in differentiating the various bony abnormalities (Fig. 17-20).

Although usually not significant for a true functional or anatomical deficit, some more subtle forms of abnormal measurement have been validated as markers for fetal aneuploidy, particularly Down syndrome. Examples include increased nuchal skin fold thickness,[40] renal pyelectasis,[41] hypoplasia

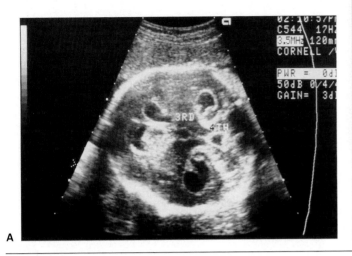

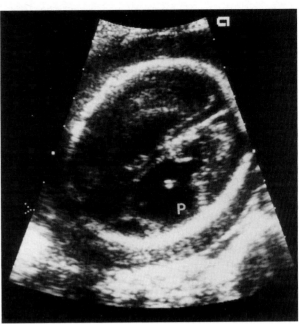

FIGURE 17-16 (A) Sonogram of a fetus with an intracranial hemorrhage demonstrating the echogenic clot within the lateral ventricle. (B) Sonogram of a porencephalic cyst (P) seen here to be communicating with the lateral ventricle.

of the middle phalynx of the fifth digit,[42] or disproportionate shortening of the femur.[43]

ABSENT OR ABNORMAL FETAL MOTION

Abnormalities in fetal motion may suggest a malformation that does not otherwise have a distinctly identifiable defect.

Although the fetus normally can assume contorted positions in utero, the persistence of such an unusual posture over time may suggest an orthopedic or neurologic anomaly such as clubfoot[44] (Fig. 17-21) or arthrogryposis.[45] A clenched hand with overlapping digits can be suggestive of trisomy 18 (Fig. 17-22).

The fetal heart is the most conspicuously dynamic part of the fetus. Real-time ultrasound is invaluable in diagnosing most fetal cardiac anomalies. In cases of a suspected fetal arrythmia, atrial and ventricular rates can be determined.[46-51]

An important principle in the overall approach to the diagnosis of fetal anomalies is that the discovery of one anomaly raises the suspicion for other associated anomalies. Therefore, once a congenital anomaly is diagnosed, careful search for a second and even third or fourth anomaly is necessary before management options can be considered. Echocardiography and karyotype determination usually should be part of this evaluation. Copel et al. have shown that 23% of fetuses referred for echocardiography because of an extracardiac anomaly had congenital heart disease.[52] Approximately one third of fetuses with structural anomalies have a chromosomal disorder.[53-55] This additional information is invaluable to define fetal

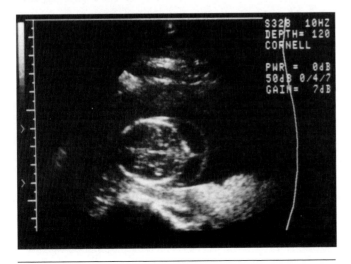

FIGURE 17-17 Sonogram demonstrating a nuchal cystic hygroma divided by a midline septum.

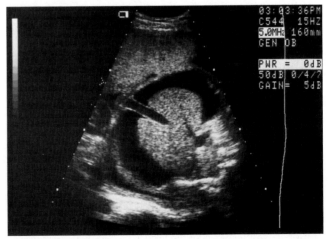

FIGURE 17-18 Transverse sonogram through fetal abdomen demonstrating fetal ascites.

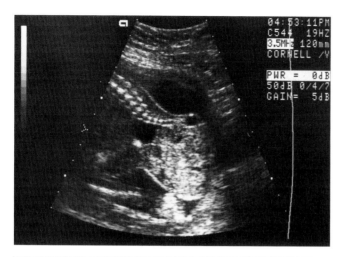

FIGURE 17-19 Sonogram of sacrococcygeal teratoma protruding beneath the base of the fetal spine.

prognosis. For example, the prognosis for isolated hydrocephalus is substantially better than that for hydrocephalus associated with alobar holoprosencephaly or trisomy 13. Amniocentesis is the most widely utilized technique for determination of fetal karyotype when an ultrasonically diagnosed anomaly is detected, but fetal blood sampling or placental biopsy may be necessary if a rapid result is required.

MANAGEMENT OF A PREGNANCY COMPLICATED BY AN ULTRASONOGRAPHICALLY DIAGNOSED FETAL ANOMALY

Once a congenital anomaly is diagnosed and the fetal evaluation is completed, the certainties and uncertainties of fetal prognosis should be explained to the prospective parents. At

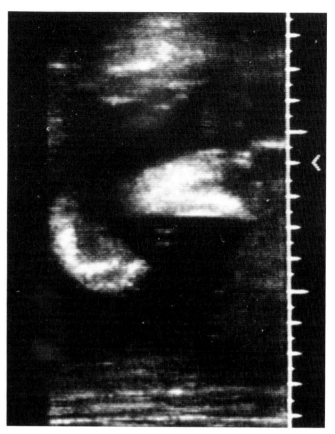

FIGURE 17-21 Sonogram demonstrating clubfoot.

the same time, when an initial second trimester scan fails to reveal an abnormality, it is important to appreciate that even a thorough ultrasound evaluation during the second trimester will not detect all structural malformations. Such anomalies as hydrocephalus, duodenal atresia, microcephaly, achondroplasia, and polycystic kidneys may not manifest until the third trimester, when the degree of anatomic distortion is sufficient

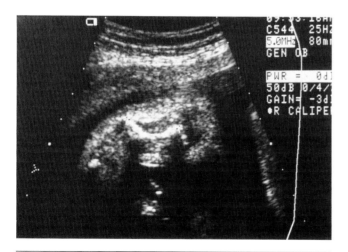

FIGURE 17-20 Sonogram of the femur of a fetus with osteogenesis imperfecta demonstrating the markedly shortened and bowed femur.

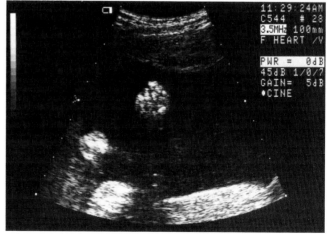

FIGURE 17-22 Sonogram demonstrating the clenched fist with overlapping digits suggestive of Trisomy 18.

to be sonographically detectable. The disclosure requirements of the informed consent process obligate the physician to be objective when presenting information about the range of available management options. That is, the physician is not justified in withholding information about available management options to which he or she might object for reasons of personal conscience.[56] Depending on the timing of the diagnosis and the severity of the abnormality, management options may include termination of pregnancy, nonaggressive management, cephalocentesis, and aggressive management.[57]

TERMINATION OF PREGNANCY

Prior to fetal viability, abortion of any pregnancy—regardless of the presence or absence of an anomaly or its severity—is a woman's right as established by *Roe v. Wade*.[58]

After fetal viability there is limited legal access in the United States to termination of pregnancy for a fetal anomaly. Ethically, the option of terminating third trimester pregnancies complicated by fetal anomalies has been defended when there is (1) certainty of diagnosis and (2) either (a) certainty of death as an outcome; or, (b) in some cases of short-term survival, certainty of the absence of cognitive developmental capacity. Anencephaly is a clear example of a sonographically diagnosed anomaly that meets these criteria,[59] whereas Trisomy 21 is a clear example of an anomaly that does not.[60]

NONAGGRESSIVE MANAGEMENT

There are circumstances where termination of pregnancy is not an option. These include when there is a personal or religious objection, when a severe anomaly is diagnosed after fetal viability but the rather restrictive criteria for termination of pregnancy for fetal anomalies during the third trimester are not met, or when termination is not possible legally even if ethical criteria for third trimester termination of pregnancy are met. Non-aggressive management is the determination to exclude any or all obstetric interventions that would normally be undertaken to benefit the fetus, such as fetal surveillance, tocolysis, cesarean delivery, or delivery in a referral center. The option of nonaggressive management for third trimester pregnancies complicated by fetal anomalies has been defended when there is (1) a very high probability of a correct diagnosis and (2) either (a) a very high probability of death as an outcome or (b) a very high probability of severe irreversible deficit of cognitive developmental capacity.[61]

CEPHALOCENTESIS

In cases of fetal hydrocephalus causing macrocephaly of a degree that would preclude vaginal delivery and where a posture of nonaggressive management is otherwise an appropriate option, there may be a role for cephalocentesis, which is the transabdominal or transvaginal aspiration of cerebrospinal fluid to avoid cesarean delivery. Because of the very high rate of mortality, cephalocentesis should be considered a destructive procedure. Therefore, since advances in modern medicine have greatly improved the prognosis for some cases of hydrocephalus, the decision to perform cephalocentesis must respect the heterogeneity of fetal hydrocephalus, which includes isolated fetal hydrocephalus, hydrocephalus associated with severe anomalies (such as alobar holoprosencephaly), and hydrocephalus with other associated anomalies (such as arachnoid cyst or spina bifida)[62,63] (Fig. 17-23).

AGGRESSIVE MANAGEMENT

Certain anomalies are amenable to therapeutic interventions, either prenatal or postnatal. To optimize fetal outcome, there should be an interdisciplinary approach, including specialists in maternal-fetal medicine, neonatology, genetics, pediatric surgery, and pediatric cardiology.[64–66] Social work services may provide important support to the family before as well as after birth. Such a team approach is best equipped to address the role of invasive fetal therapy as well as the important questions of where, when, and how the infant should be delivered.

Rarely, an invasive approach during the antenatal period may be considered to optimize outcome when there is a sonographically diagnosed anomaly. This should only be considered when the natural history of the anomaly diagnosed is dismal and a relatively simple intrauterine correction is possible. The sonographic and karyotypic evaluation described above is especially important before an invasive approach can be considered.

The most common form of invasive fetal therapy has been intrauterine shunt placement. The purpose of such a shunt is to drain fluid that is under high pressure from the affected fetal organ to the lower pressure of the amniotic cavity. Such a shunt may have a role in the treatment of a complete bladder outlet obstruction, which would be expected to eventually result in renal and pulmonary failure.[67,68] Analysis of fetal urine after bladder aspiration may help to define which fetuses are candidates for this vesico-amniotic shunt.[69,70] Intrauterine aspiration or shunt placement may also be of value in cases of isolated pleural effusions.[71–73] In fetal hydrocephalus, however, current experience does not demonstrate a clear benefit to ventriculo-amniotic shunt placement and should be avoided.[67,74,75]

The San Francisco group has pioneered open fetal surgery to manage such conditions as congenital diaphragmatic hernia and complete bladder obstruction. In such cases, there is hysterotomy and exteriorization of the fetus then repair, replacement, and continuation of the pregnancy.[64,76] At this time it is not possible to make a final judgment concerning the place of this fascinating modality in fetal therapy because more clinical experience is needed to better define the benefits to the fetus and the harms to the mother.

The disclosure requirements of the informed consent process necessitate that the experimental nature of many invasive fetal therapies and the potential harms to the fetus and the mother be carefully explained. It is generally agreed that such an approach after 32 weeks of gestation offers no clear advantage over delivery and neonatal treatment. Given the risk of inflicted premature delivery as well as the experimental nature of these procedures, a normal coincident twin is also considered to be a relative contraindication to such an approach.[64,65,67]

**RESOLUTION STRATEGIES FOR
MORAL CONFLICTS IN THE INTRAPARTUM MANAGEMENT OF
HYDROCEPHALUS WITH MACROCEPHALY**

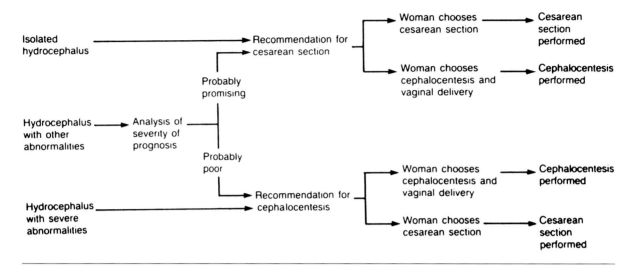

FIGURE 17-23 Resolution strategies for conflicts in the intrapartum management of hydrocephalus with macrocephaly. (Reprinted with permission from Chervenak FA, McCullough LB. Ethical challenges in perinatal medicine: The intrapartum management of pregnancy complicated by fetal hydrocephalus with macrocephaly. *Seminars Perinat.* 1987;11:232–239.)

Delivery at term is optimal for most fetal anomalies. For some anomalies, however, such as hydrocephalus, delivery as soon as fetal lung maturation has occurred may be advisable to expedite corrective neonatal surgery.[77] Rarely, because of the risk of imminent fetal death, an anomaly such as progressive fetal hydrops may necessitate delivery prior to fetal lung maturity.[65] Most infants with anomalies are best delivered in a referral center with a neonatal intensive care unit experienced in caring for such infants. In such a setting there is immediate access to diagnostic and therapeutic medical and surgical interventions.

Most fetuses with anomalies can be delivered vaginally. Cesarean delivery may be necessary to avoid dystocia if certain conditions are present, such as a sacrococcygeal teratoma or conjoined twins. For other anomalies, such as spina bifida, cesarean delivery may be recommended in order to minimize trauma to fetal tissues.[78]

SUMMARY

There is a wide range of fetal anomalies currently diagnosable in the prenatal period by ultrasonography, and the number is increasing rapidly with new advances in ultrasound technology. The incidence of congenital malformations in the general population is between 2% and 3%, with the majority of women carrying an anomalous fetus having no identifiable risk factors. It is for this reason that we believe that routine ultrasound should be offered to all pregnant women, although this stance is still hotly debated. Regardless of whether women are scanned routinely or as indicated, it is encumbent upon all who perform prenatal ultrasonography to look carefully for anomalies and make appropriate referrals when the diagnosis is in question. Once an anomaly is detected, the patient should be advised of the full range of diagnostic procedures and management options.

References

1. Sabbagha R (ed.). Diagnostic Ultrasound Applied to Obstetrics and Gynecology. Philadelphia: J P Lippincott; 1994.
2. Chervenak FA, Isaacson G, Campbell S (eds.). Ultrasound in Obstetrics and Gynecology. Philadelphia: Little, Brown; 1994.
3. Manning FA. The anomalous fetus. In: Manning FA (ed.). *Fetal Medicine. Principles and Practice.* Norwalk, CT: Appleton & Lange; 1995.
4. McGahan JP, Porto M (eds.). *Diagnostic Ultrasound.* Philadelphia: Lippincott; 1994.
5. Callen P (ed.). Ultrasonography in Obstetrics and Gynecology, 3rd ed. Philadelphia: WB Saunders; 1994.
6. Romero R, Pilu G, Jeanty P, et al. *Prenatal Diagnosis of Congenital Anomalies.* Norwalk, CT: Appleton & Lange; 1988.
7. Nyberg DA, Mahoney BS, Pretorius DH (eds.). *Diagnostic Ultrasound of Fetal Anomalies. Text and Atlas.* Chicago: Year Book; 1990.
8. Campbell S, Johnstone FD, Hold EM, et al. Anencephaly: early ultrasonic diagnosis and active management. *Lancet.* 1972;ii:1226.
9. Chervenak FA, Isaacson G, Mahoney MJ, et al. The obstetric significance of holoprosencephaly. *Obstet Gynecol.* 1984;63:115.
10. Romero R, Cullen M, Grannum P, et al. Antenatal diagnosis of renal anomalies with ultrasound. III. Bilateral renal agenesis. *Am J Obstet Gynecol.* 1985;151:38.

11. Cardoza JD, Goldstein RB, Filly RA. Exclusion of fetal ventriculomegaly with a single measurement: the width of the lateral ventricular atrium. *Radiology*. 1988;169:711.

12. Cardoza JD, Filly RA, Podarsky AE. The dangling choroid plexus: a sonographic observation of value in excluding ventriculomegaly. *Am J Rad*. 1988;151:767–770.

13. Benaceraff BR, Birnholz JC. The diagnosis of fetal hydrocephalus prior to 22 weeks. *J Clin Ultrasound*. 1987;15:531–536.

14. Benacerraff BR. Fetal hydrocephalus: Diagnosis and significance. *Radiology*. 1988;169:858–859.

15. Chervenak FA, Duncan C, Ment LR, et al. The outcome of fetal ventriculomegaly. *Lancet*. 1984;ii:179–182.

16. Lees RF, Alford BA, Brenbridge NAG, et al. Sonographic appearance of duodenal atresia in utero. *Am J Roentgenol*. 1978;131:701–705.

17. Romero R, Jeanty P, Pilu, et al. The prenatal diagnosis of duodenal atresia. Does it make any difference? *Obstet Gynecol*. 1988;71:739.

18. Hobbins JC, Romero R, Grannum P, et al. Antenatal diagnosis of renal anomalies with ultrasound. I. Obstructive uropathy. *Am J Obstet Gynecol*. 1984;148:868.

19. Corteville JE, Gray DL, Crane JP. Congenital hydronephrosis: correlation of fetal ultrasonographic findings with infant outcome. *Am J Obstet Gynecol*. 1991;165:384.

20. Mandell J, Blyth B, Peters CA, et al. Structural genitourinary defects detected in utero. *Radiology*. 1991;178:193.

21. Arey LB. Developmental Anatomy. Philadelphia: WB Saunders; 1974:245–262, 465–499.

22. Chervenak FA, Isaacson G, Mahoney MJ, et al. The diagnosis and management of fetal cephalocele. *Obstet Gynecol*. 1984;64:86.

23. Hobbins JC, Venus I, Tortora M, et al. Stage II ultrasound examination for the diagnosis of fetal abnormalities with an elevated amniotic fluid alpha-fetoprotein concentration. *Am J Obstet Gynecol*. 1982;142:1026.

24. Platt LD, Feuchtbaum L, Filly R, et al. The California maternal serum alpha-fetoprotein screening program: the role of ultrasonography in the detection of spina bifida. *Obstet Gynecol*. 1992;166:1328.

25. Nakayama DK, Harrison RM, Gross BH, et al. Management of the fetus with an abdominal wall defect. *J Pediatr Surg*. 1984;19:408.

26. Marwood RP, Dawson MR, Gross BH, et al. Antenatal diagnosis of diaphragmatic hernias. *Br J Obstet Gynecol*. 1981;88:71.

27. Sharlane GK, Lockhart SM, Heward AJ, et al. Prognosis in fetal diaphragmatic hernia. *Am J Obstet Gynecol*. 1992;166:9.

28. McIntosh R. The incidence of congenital malformations: a study of 5964 pregnancies. *Pediatrics*. 1954;14:505.

29. Nicolaides KM, Campbell S, Gabbe SG, et al. Ultrasound screening for spina bifida: cranial and cerebellar signs. *Lancet*. 1986;ii:72.

30. Nicolaides KM, Rodeck CH, Gosden CM. Rapid karyotyping in nonlethal malformations. *Lancet*. 1986;1:283.

31. Chervenak FA, Isaacson G, Blakemore KJ, et al. Fetal cystic hygroma: cause and natural history. *N Engl J Med*. 1984;309:822.

32. Johnson MP, Johnson A, Holzgreve W, et al. First trimester cystic hygromas: cause and outcome. *Am J Obstet Gynecol*. 1993;168:156.

33. Chervenak FA, Isaacson G, Touloukian R, et al. The diagnosis and management of fetal teratomas. *Obstet Gynecol*. 1984;149:94.

34. Deter RL, Harrist RB, Birnholz JC, et al. *Quantitative Obstetrical Ultrasonography*. New York: Churchill Livingstone; 1986.

35. Chervenak FA, Jeanty P, Cantraine F, et al. The diagnosis of fetal microcephaly. *Am J Obstet Gynecol*. 1984;149:512.

36. Chervenak FA, Rosenberg J, Brigthman RC, et al. A prospective study of the accuracy of ultrasound in predicting fetal microcephaly. *Obstet Gynecol*. 1987;69:908.

37. Chervenak FA, Tortora M, Mayden K, et al. Antenatal diagnosis of median cleft face syndrome: sonographic demonstration of cleft lip and hypotelorism. *Am J Obstet Gynecol*. 1984;149:94.

38. Grannum P, Bracken M, Silverman R, et al. Assessment of fetal kidney size in normal gestation by comparison of ratio of kidney circumference to abdominal circumference. *Am J Obstet Gynecol*. 1980;136:249.

39. Romero R, Cullen M, Jeanty P, et al. The diagnosis of congenital renal anomalies with ultrasound. II. Infantile polycystic kidney disease. *Am J Obstet Gynecol*. 1984;150:259.

40. Benacerraf BR, Barss VA, Laboda LA. A sonographic sign for the detection in the second trimester of the fetus with Down syndrome. *Am J Obstet Gynecol*. 1985;151:1078.

41. Benacerraf BR, Mandell J, Estroff JA, et al. Fetal pyelectasis: a possible association with Down syndrome. *Obstet Gynecol*. 1990;76:58–60.

42. Goldstein I, Gomez K, Copel JA. Fifth digit measurement in normal pregnancies: a potential sonographic sign of Down syndrome. *Ultrasound Obstet Gynecol*. 1995;5:34–37.

43. Benacerraf BR, Gelman R, Frigoletto FD. Sonographic identification of second-trimester fetuses with Down syndrome. *N Engl J Med*. 1987;317:1371.

44. Chervenak FA, Tortora MN, Hobbins JC. Antenatal sonographic diagnosis of clubfoot. *J Ultrasound Med*. 1985;4:49.

45. Goldberg JD, Chervenak FA, Lipman RA, et al. Antenatal sonographic diagnosis of arthrogryposis multiplex congenita. *Prenatal Diagnosis*. 1986;6:45.

46. Allan LD, Crawford DC, Anderson RH, et al. Echocardiographic and anatomical correlation in fetal congenital heart disease. *Brit Heart J*. 1984;52:542.

47. Copel JA, Pilu G, Green J, et al. Fetal echocardiographic screening for congenital heart disease: the importance of the four-chamber view. *Am J Obstet Gynecol*. 1987;157:648.

48. Gertgesell HP (ed.). Symposium of Fetal Echocardiography. *J Clin Ultrasound*. 1985;13:227.

49. Devore G. Fetal echocardiography. In Chervenak FA, Isaacson G, Campbell S (eds.), Ultrasound in Obstetrics and Gynecology. Boston: Little, Brown; 1994:199.

50. Reed KL, Anderson CF, Shenker L. *Fetal Echocardiography: an Atlas*. New York: Alan R. Liss;1988.

51. Klerman CS, Copel JA. Fetal cardiac dysrhythmias: diagnosis and therapy. In: Chervenak FA, Isaacson G, Campbell S, eds. *Ultrasound in Obstetrics and Gynecology*. Boston: Little, Brown; 1994:195.

52. Copel JA, Pilu G, Kleinmann CS. Congenital heart disease and extracardiac anomalies: associations and indications for fetal echocardiography. *Am J Obstet Gynecol*. 1986;154:1121.

53. Palmer CG, Miles JH, Howard-Peebles PN, et al. Fetal karyotype following ascertainment of fetal anomalies by ultrasound. *Prenat Diagn*. 1987;7:551.

54. Platt LD, DeVore GR, Lopez E, et al. Role of aminocentesis in ultrasound-detected fetal malformations. *Obstet Gynecol*. 1986;68:153.

55. Williamson RA, Weiner CP, Patil S, et al. Abnormal pregnancy sonogram: selective indication for fetal karyotype. *Obstet Gynecol*. 1987;69:15.

56. Chervenak FA, McCullough LB. Does obstetric ethics have any role in the obstetrician's response to the abortion controversy? *Am J Obstet Gynecol*. 1990;163:1425.

57. Chervenak FA, McCullough LB. An ethically justified, clinically comprehensive management strategy for third-trimester pregnancies complicated by fetal anomalies. *Obstet Gynecol*. 1990;75:311.

58. *Roe v. Wade*. Supreme Court of the United States, 1973, 410 US 113.

59. Chervenak FA, Farley MA, Walters L, et al. When is termination of pregnancy during the third trimester morally justifiable? *N Engl J Med*. 1984;310:501.

60. Chervenak FA, McCullough LB, Campbell S. Is third trimester abortion justified? *Brit J Obstet Gynecol*. 1995;102:434.

61. Chervenak FA, McCullough LB. Nonaggressive obstetric management. An option for some fetal anomalies during the third trimester. *JAMA*. 1989;261:3439.

62. Chervenak FA, McCullough LB. Ethical challenges in perinatal medicine: the intrapartum management of pregnancy complicated by fetal hydrocephalus with macrocephaly. *Seminars Perinat.* 1987;11:232.

63. Chervenak FA, McCullough LB. Fetal destructive procedures in operative obstetrics. In: O'Grady JP, Gimovsky ML, McIlhargie LJ, eds. *Operative Obstetrics.* Baltimore: Williams & Wilkins; 1995: 34.

64. Harrison M, Golbus M, Filly R. *The Unborn Patient*, 2nd ed. New York: Grune & Stratton; 1991.

65. Seeds JW, Azizkhan RG. Congenital Malformations. Antenatal Diagnosis, Perinatal Management, and Counseling. Rockville, MD: Aspen Publishers; 1990.

66. Romero R, Oyarzun E, Sirtori M, et al. Detection and management of anatomic congenital anomalies. *Obstet Gynecol Clin N Amer.* 1988;15:215–236.

67. Manning FA, Harrison MR, Rodeck C, et al. Catheter shunts for fetal hydronephrosis and hydrocephalus. Special Report. *N Engl J Med.* 1986;315:336.

68. Manning FA. The anomalous fetus. In: Manning FA, ed. Fetal Medicine. Principles and Practice. Norwalk, CT: Appleton & Lange; 1995:451.

69. Albar H, Manning FA, Harman CR. Treatment of urinary tract and CNS obstruction. In: Harman CR, ed. *Invasive Fetal Testing and Treatment.* Cambridge, UK: Blackwell Scientific; 1995:19:259.

70. Anderson RL, Golbus MS. Bladder aspiration. In: Chervenak FA, Isaacson G, Campbell S, eds. *Textbook of Ultrasound in Obstetrics and Gynecology.* Boston: Little, Brown; 1994.

71. Rodeck CH, Fisk NM, Fraser DI, et al. Long-term in utero drainage of fetal hydrothorax. *N Engl J Med.* 1988;319:1135–1138.

72. Nicolaides KH, Azar G. Thoracoamniotic shunting. In: Chervenak FA, Isaacson G, Campbell S, eds. *Textbook of Ultrasound in Obstetrics and Gynecology.* Boston: Little, Brown; 1994:1289.

73. Vaughn JI, Fisk NM, Rodeck CM. Fetal pleural effusions. In: Harman CR, ed. *Fetal Testing and Treatment.* Cambridge, Blackwell Scientific; 1995:19:219.

74. Clewell WH, Johnson ML, Meier PR, et al. A surgical approach to the treatment of fetal hydrocephalus. *N Engl J Med.* 1982;306:1320.

75. Clewell W. Current status of ventriculo-amniotic shunt placement. In: Chervenak FA, Isaacson G, Campbell S, eds. *Textbook of Ultrasound in Obstetrics and Gynecology.* Boston, Little, Brown; 1994:1283–1287.

76. Harrison MR, Adzick NS, Longaker MT, et al. Successful repair in utero of a fetal diaphragmatic hernia after removal of herniated viscera from the left thorax. *N Engl J Med.* 1990;322:1582.

77. Chervenak FA, Berkowitz RL, Tortora M, et al. The management of fetal hydrocephalus. *Am J Obstet Gynecol.* 1985;151:933–942.

78. Luthy DA, Wardinsky T, Shurtleff DB, et al. Cesarean section before the onset of labor and subsequent motor function in infants with open spina bifida. *N Engl J Med.* 1991;162:662.

CHAPTER 18

IMAGING THE FETAL BRAIN

Ana Monteagudo / Ilan E. Timor-Tritsch

INTRODUCTION

Congenital anomalies of the fetal heart are considered the most common malformations affecting the developing human fetus. Anomalies of the fetal central nervous system are a close second. Understanding embryology and the developmental changes of the human fetal brain are necessary to be able to time the brain scans to detect the greatest number of anomalies. Screening ultrasound at 15–18 weeks with a follow scan at 21–23 weeks can improve the detection rate of anomalies. But we must realize that all technology has its limitations and be aware of the fact that 100% detection rates of malformations *at present* is something we all hope for, but in reality is just a dream.

EQUIPMENT: TRANSABDOMINAL VS. TRANSVAGINAL PROBES

Several factors limits the fetal neuroscan even when continuous development and improvement of ultrasound equipment and transducers are taken into consideration. Factors such as the size of the fetal brain, (i.e., the gestational age), the available surface or the window through which the transducer can achieve the best image, the fetal presentation and position, and last but not least, the thickness of the maternal abdominal wall. Imaging of the fetal brain ultimately depends on the penetration of the sound wave as well as the acoustic impedance of the tissues. As gestational age advances there is an increasing acoustic impedance, for example the thickening of the fetal skull as the gestation progresses, this will significantly affect which types of ultrasound probes should be employed during the examination. If all this is understood, it is clear that a variety of transducers with different frequencies and frequency ranges can and should be used and alternated to obtain the best images.

Two basic ultrasound probes are used in obstetrical scanning namely the transabdominal and the transvaginal ultrasound probes. Generally, transabdominal probes use lower frequencies and the transvaginal ultrasound probes use higher ultrasound frequencies. The transabdominal probes will operate with frequencies of 3.5 to maximum of 5–6 MHZ whereas transvaginal ultrasound probes operate typically at frequencies from 5–9 MHZ. In contrast to the transabdominal transducers, the increased frequencies of the transvaginal probes result in higher resolution, at the expense of decreased penetration.

During the first half of the pregnancy, high-frequency transvaginal probes can be used. If the fetus is in a vertex any time during the pregnancy, there is absolutely no need to relinquish the transvaginal approach. However, if the fetal head cannot be "reached" through the transvaginal route, transabdominal probes will have to be employed. The more advanced the gestational age, the lower the frequencies to be used in order to penetrate the skull bones. By the end of the pregnancy the fetal cranial vault has significant amounts of deposited calcium presenting an ever increasing impedance, nearly 7 times greater than that of the water or soft tissues of the fetal body. It should be remembered, that even at the very end of the pregnancy, the fetal brain can adequately be imaged through the fontanelle as an "acoustic window," using the transvaginal ultrasound probe, provided the fetus presents as vertex (Fig. 18-1). We found it valuable to perform or at least try to perform external cephalic version in order to better be able to study a suspected anomaly.

TECHNIQUE OF FETAL NEUROSONOGRAPHY: TRANSVAGINAL APPROACH

The transabdominal scanning technique is well known and employed in all centers and by all the sonographers and sonologists, therefore, we will refrain from describing this technique.

However, the transvaginal sonographic examination of the brain that is slowly gaining its well-deserved place among the scanning options for the fetus, will be emphasized, since still in many centers around the world is not used routinely. The transvaginal scan of the fetal brain relies heavily on the experience gained from the transfontanelle examination of the neonatal brain.[1–9] Similarly, to the neonatal brain scan the transvaginal approach to image the fetal brain uses high-frequency ultrasound probes.[10–26]

Fetal neuroscan using the transvaginal technique is simple.[16,20,22,23,27] The probe is prepared as usual for transvaginal scanning, its tip covered with a clean condom or placed inside a digit of a surgical rubber glove. Recently, specially manufactured pre-gelled vinyl covers have been made available (no need to worry about latex allergies), which make the preparation of the probe easier. The patient is then placed in the lithotomy position and the tip of the probe is slowly advanced to reach the anterior cervical lip. It is easier to perform fetal neuroscan when the patient's bladder is empty in order to facilitate the presenting part, the vertex, to come close to the tip of the probe. At times, it is necessary to use the examiner's free hand abdominally to maneuver the head into the most convenient position. By twisting and turning as well as tilting the vaginal probe, the best possible images in each of the coronal and sagittal planes are sought. The abdominally placed second hand of the operator has an important task: stabilizing the fetal head or maneuvering it into the desired position for a clear ultrasound picture.

The ultrasound machine chosen to perform transvaginal fetal brain scanning should have an "end-firing" transducer. This means that there will be a symmetrical picture on both sides of the scanning axis, or in other words, the scanning

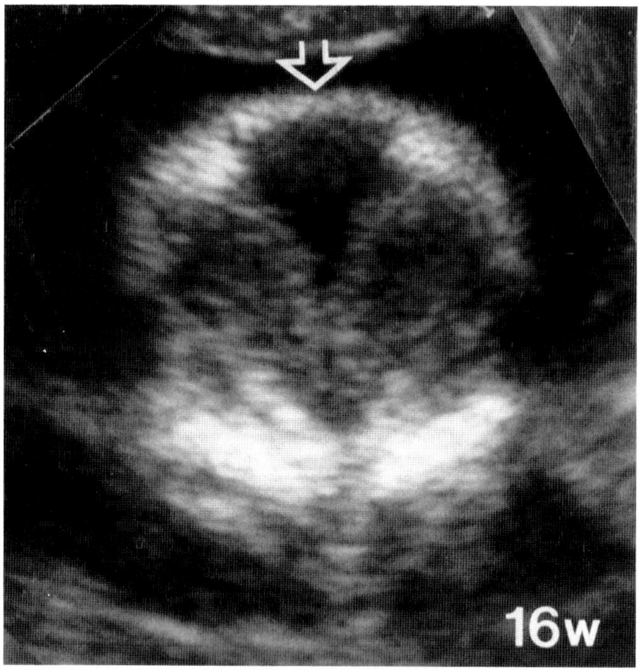

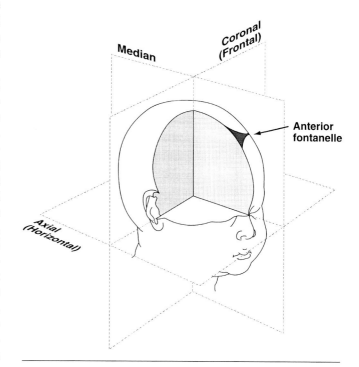

FIGURE 18-1 A transvaginal view of the anterior and metopic suture in a 16-week fetus. Note the large size of the fontanelle, which is used as an acoustic window.

axis and the straight axis of the probe are identical. If a non-end-firing-out-of-axis vaginal probe is used to scan the fetal brain, a symmetrical image of the brain in the coronal planes is cumbersome to acquire, since the probe itself has to be constantly twisted and tilted into a position to yield the desired symmetrical ultrasound picture.

Dependent upon whether transabdominal or transvaginal sonography is used, the sections and the planes will yield different information if fetuses of extremely young ages, that is, dates to approximately 11 weeks or more mature fetuses are scanned. The latter is because the head follows well-defined and continuing deflection from 7 to approximately 11–12 weeks. Scanning the brain before the 12th postmenstrual week is dependent upon the size of the fetus and the resolution of the ultrasound probe. Both the above determine the "slice thickness" hence the number of sections and the quality of the picture obtained. Scanning at or around 7–8 postmenstrual weeks, one should expect that the only possible "slice thickness" includes almost the entire width of the head, due to the relatively thick imaging slice. At and after the 9th postmenstrual week due to the somewhat larger head size, it is possible to obtain several diagnostic quality "slices," or sections. The clear and pretty pictures obtained by Blaas et al.,[18,19] who studied the brain structures with extremely high frequency transvaginal probes from 7–9 weeks, attest to the feasibility and the importance of fine and resolution-rich slices. Using such techniques, they were able to show that structures previously described only in embryological studies were readily recognized and imaged. As knowledge and the quality of the ultrasound equipment improves, in the future, it may be possible to detect deviant devel-

opment as early as the normal anatomy of the brain is available for sonographic scrutiny.

As pregnancy progresses and reaches 12–13 postmenstrual weeks, the thickening skull bones will progressively attenuate the sound waves and special approaches as well as lower transducer frequencies are necessary to successfully image the brain. As said before, due to fetal position, the transabdominal sonography is mainly used to achieve the classical axial/horizontal planes. These sections are extremely important since the measurements, which constitute the "gold standard" for determining the size of the lateral ventricles, are performed using these sections. However, if the fetal position enables the transvaginal approach, pictures of extreme resolution and clarity can be obtained. Imaging of the brain structures with high-frequency transvaginal probes is usually done through the anterior fontanelle as an acoustic window. It is very rare to obtain axial or horizontal sections using the transvaginal probe. This may be achieved only if the fetal head is not engaged, and readily moveable. Usually and classically, the transvaginal probes will achieve coronal and sagittal planes due to their restricted maneuverability and range of motion determined by the constraints of the introitus and the vagina. It is therefore virtually impossible to obtain *classical* coronal and sagittal sections as used in our anatomic sections by computer tomography or magnetic resonance imaging where the consecutive sections are parallel to each other (Fig. 18-2). Luckily,

FIGURE 18-2 The "classical" planes: median, coronal (frontal) and axial (horizontal) are depicted. These planes are hard to obtain in the fetus using transvaginal sonography due to the progressive thickening of the fetal cranium as gestation progresses. Therefore in the transvaginal approach through the anterior fontanelle is used as an acoustic window, similarly to the neonatal head scan.

however, the planes or sections obtained by the transvaginal approach are not only similar but identical to those obtained by the neonatal transfontanelle imaging of the fetal brain.[3,4,8,28,29] The similarities between the fetal and the neonatal scanning planes and sections have a practical advantage when prenatal and neonatal brain images have to be compared or a serial follow-up of pathology is compared.

Lately an important diagnostic tool was added to the diagnostic armamentarium of fetal neuroscan, namely three dimensional ultrasound. Scrolling through an acquired brain volume from side to side in the septal plane, from front to back in the coronal plane, and from the base of the skull to the top of the head is possible. Such a detailed scrutiny of the brain in the multiplanar coordinates enables localization of a brain lesion and evaluating its extent and nature.

Three dimensional scanning of the fetal brain is possible using dedicated transabdominal as well as transvaginal ultrasound probes.

EMBRYOLOGY: THE DEVELOPING BRAIN

Using present ultrasound technology, the developing fetal brain can be imaged from very early in gestation. The first sonographic images of the central nervous system are a series of sonolucencies detected within the head of the embryo around the seventh postmenstrual weeks. At this gestational age, the size of the embryo is about 7–8 mm. The coronal scan of the dorsal aspect of the embryos yield a parallel lines of hyperechoic dots representing the future vertebral column. Blaas et al.[18,19] have described in detail the development cerebral hemispheres using high-frequency transvaginal ultrasound probes. Starting from the 7th postmenstrual weeks, the transvaginal transducers using high frequencies can discern between the relatively large rhombencephalon, the diencephalon, and the 2 tiny cerebral hemispheres. During the eighth postmenstrual week of development, structures such as the cavities and the flexures of the brain appear clearer and better defined (Fig. 18-3). Toward the ninth postmenstrual week and several days past it, several sagittal and coronal sections of the head can be obtained. These sections of the brain show the mesencephalon, the rhombencephalon, the budding choroid plexus, the telencephalic vesicles, and the 2 major flexures: the cephalic and the pontine flexures of the head around which the ventricles are arranged.[30–32] The falx cerebri, will become detectable at around the 9th week and will continue to present throughout the remainder of the life of the fetus and subsequent neonate.

By the time the fetus reaches the 10th postmenstrual weeks, several axial, sagittal, and coronal sections can be obtained and by doing this, we can mentally recreate a 3-dimensional picture of the developing fetal brain. At 11–12 postmenstrual weeks, the horizontal section or axial section has a typical appearance produced by the symmetrically hyperechoic choroid plexus.

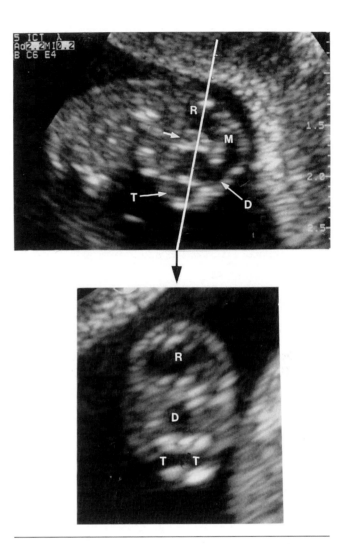

FIGURE 18-3 Embryo at 8 weeks and 2 days showing the development of the brain. The lower picture was generated along the white on the sagittal image. The arrow point to the pontine flexure. R—rhombencephalon; M—mesencephalon; D—diencephalon; T—telencephalon.

The third ventricle appears as a slit-like sonolucent ovoid structure "squeezed" between the 2 thalami in the midline.

An important clinical hint to remember when scanning the fetal brain between the 11th to almost 15th postmenstrual weeks, is that the normal frontal areas of the anterior horns of the lateral ventricles are drastically prominent and appear as large sonolucent free spaces (Fig. 18-4). This is the end result of the unremitting "migration" of the choroid plexus from the anterior horn into their final position, in the atria of the lateral ventricles. This gradual change leaves for a period of approximately 2–3 weeks, the anterior horns relatively large. Eventually the concomitant growth of the brain parenchyma will result in the almost slit-like width of the anterior horns.

Around 14–16 postmenstrual weeks, the fetal cranial vault is becoming increasingly thick which in turn prevents the high-frequency sound waves from traveling through and

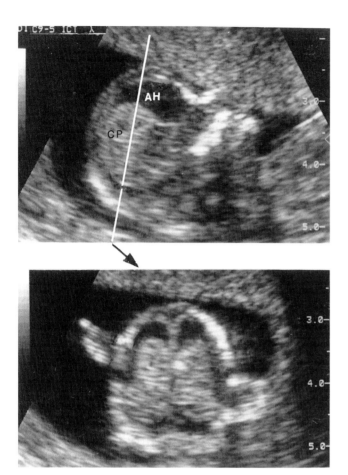

FIGURE 18-4 At 13 weeks and 2 days of gestation the anterior horns (AH) of the lateral ventricles are still prominent. Since the cortical mantle is thin. The lower picture was generated along the white line on the sagittal image. CP—choroid plexus.

clearly imaging the fetal brain. At this time, the anterior fontanelle becomes an ever increasing important acoustic window into the fetal brain. Using conventional transvaginal ultrasound probes, the sonographic sections generated through the anterior fontanelle, radiate in a fan-like fashion from the narrow triangular-shaped membranous area, which is the fontanelle. In contrast, analyzing brain sections obtained by three dimensional transvaginal ultrasound probes, the sonographic sections will be displayed in a parallel fashion much alike the CT or MRI images.

The last major fetal brain structures to develop are the corpus callosum and cavum septi pellucidi. The corpus callosum is a centrally located hypoechoic, semilunar midline structure located above the sonolucent cavum septi pellucidi. It starts developing from about the 12th postmenstrual week, and reaching completion at or around the 18th postmenstrual week.[33,34] It becomes sonographically obvious by 18–20 weeks and achieves the adult appearance by 22–28 weeks gestation. The corpus callosum grows forward and backward, in a C shape, as the primitive cerebral hemispheres grow laterally and then posteriorly.[35,36] The corpus callosum

is composed of 4 parts: *the rostrum*/beak, *genu* (knee), *trunk* and *splenium* (tail), and the *splenium* (posterior). The development of the cavum septi pellucidi parallels the corpus callosum, and is located between the lateral ventricles, in the midline. Sonographically the cavum septi pellucidi appears as 2 sheets of tissue, which extend from the corpus callosum and separate the lateral ventricles from the cavum. It is important to note that the cava (cavum septi and cavum vergae) are not part of the ventricular system and do not communicate with it.

Between the 28th–30th postmenstrual weeks of gestation, the fetal brain undergoes significant growth spurts, which results in the formation of many new gyri and sulci.[37,38] Transforming the smooth surface of the cerebral hemispheres of the first and second trimester to one with an increasingly complex pattern of echodense lines covering the cerebral surfaces.

Now that developmental highlights have been described we will turn our attention once again to imaging. The scanning planes, which are unique to fetal neurosonography, will be described in the next section.

SCANNING PLANES AND ANATOMY: TRANSVAGINAL FETAL NEUROSONOGRAPHY

Recently, we have attempted to standardize the planes and sections obtained by two dimensional transvaginal fetal neurosonography by adapting a new nomenclature. This nomenclature takes into consideration the fact that the transfontanelle approach is unable to create all the desired classical sections (true coronal and sagittal) which are parallel to each other. The first important fact, when using this approach, is that the planes and sections generated are not parallel to each other, but oblique. Therefore they do not comply with the definitions of the classical planes used in imaging the fetal head. To be able to realize this, the following paragraph will describe the classical planes with their definitions borrowed from the Nomina Anatomica.[39]

The *classical planes* consist of 2 vertical (sagittal and coronal) and 1 horizontal (axial) planes (Fig. 18-2). In the coronal plane, all sections from the back of the head (occipital) to the anterior pole of the head (frontal) are parallel to each other. The coronal planes can also be called frontal planes. In the sagittal plane, there are differences in the terminology of the specific planes. The "mid-sagittal" plane is called the median, on each of the 2 sides of the median, there are right and left paramedian planes. These can be multiple. The term "parasagittal" is incorrect.

The planes portrayed by the transvaginal probe diverge in a fan-shaped fashion from a central point which is at the anterior fontanelle (Figs. 18-5 and 18-6). It is therefore incorrect to talk about sagittal planes and coronal planes in the classical sense. Only 1 section is in the "classical" coronal and only 1 section is in the "classical" sagittal plane; the rest are really oblique planes. For better understanding and more realistic description,

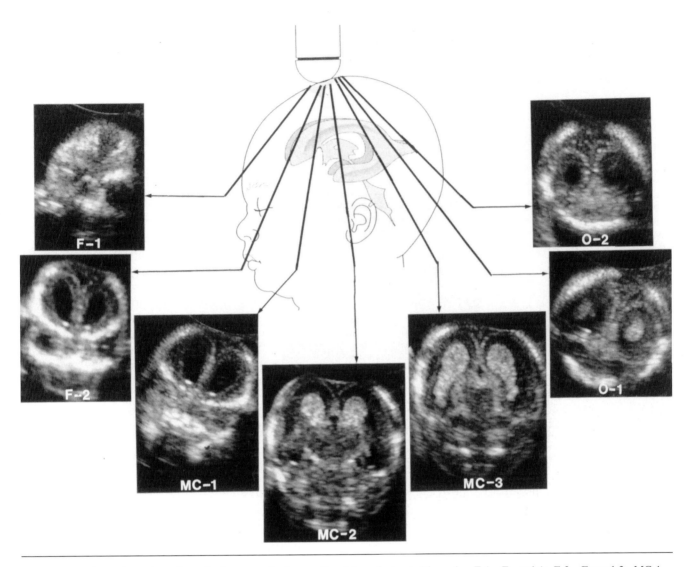

FIGURE 18-5 Several sections through the coronal planes of a fetus of about 16 weeks. F-1—Frontal-1; F-2—Frontal-2; MC-1—Mid-coronal-1; MC-2—Mid-coronal-2; MC-3—Mid-coronal-3; O-1—Occipital-1; O-2—Occipital-2.

a new nomenclature was therefore proposed.[24] The definition of each of these newly proposed sections landmark anatomic structures were selected and had to be present in each of these planes. The combination of the specific landmark structures define every plane.

The landmark structures proposed were: (1) the orbit; (2) the meninges; the falx, and the tentorium cerebelli; (3) ventricles and their connections: the lateral, third and fourth ventricle, the interhemispheric foramina, the choroid plexus, and the tela choroidea; (4) mid-brain structures such as the corpus callosum, the head of the caudate nucleus, the cavum septi pellucidi, and the thalami; (5) infratentorial structures: the cerebellar hemispheres, the vermis, and the cerebello-peduncular cistern (cisterna magna).

The newly proposed planes described in Table 18-1 and Figures 18-5 and 18-6 their anatomy and the important structures that each contain will be described in the following sections.

THE CORONAL PLANES: FRONTAL, MID-CORONAL AND OCCIPITAL

The two sections of the frontal group are: (1) *Frontal-1*, shaped like a "steer head," in which the orbits and some facial structures are seen. Only the homogeneous and symmetric brain parenchyma is imaged during the latter part of the second and the third trimester, however, if the scanning is performed before the 16th post-menstrual week, the frontal most part of anterior horns are still visible using this section. Later in gestation, if they are imaged in this section ventriculomegaly or hydrocephalus has to be suspected. (2) *In frontal-2* the orbits and the frontal most part of the anterior horns as well as the falx cerebri are displayed.

The mid-coronal group consists of three sections: (1) *Coronal-1* which contains the bodies of the lateral ventricles, the cavum septi pellucidi, corpus callosum, and the head of the caudate nucleus. (2) *Mid-coronal-2* is distinguished by the fact that the lateral ventricles contains the choroid plexus as it enters

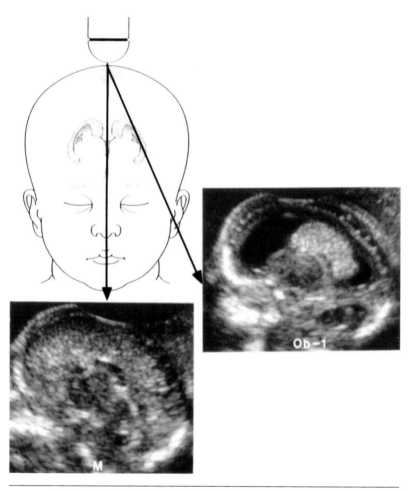

FIGURE 18-6 The clinically useful sections through the sagittal plane (M—Median; Ob-1—Oblique-1) as seen in the same fetus as Figure 18-5.

verse diameter of 8.2 mm. at term, however, it is unclear whether the choroid plexus is or is not included at the time of the measurement.[40] The bilateral and narrow intraventricular foramina (of Monro) can be seen because the hyperchoic choroid plexus passes through them from the lateral ventricle into the third ventricle. Sonographic imaging of the cerebral aqueduct (of Sylvius) which connects between the third and the 4th ventricle, were not described using conventional scanning techniques. (3) *Mid-coronal-3 structures*: the lateral ventricles (atrium) with their choroid plexus, the corpus callosum, and the thalamus.

The occipital group of sections are: (1) *Occipital-1* in which posterior horns of the lateral ventricles, cerebellar hemispheres, the vermis, and at times the fourth ventricle are imaged. (2) *Occipital-2* contains the cerebellar hemispheres, cerebellar vermis, tentorium, and cisterna magna. At times, depending on the angle, the posterior tips of the peaked posterior horns can still be detected.

The *posterior fossa* and the upper spinal cord can be the target of transvaginal ultrasound. The posterior fossa is composed of those structures below the tentorium of the cerebellum, namely the cerebellum and the vermis, and the cisterna magna (Figs. 18-7 and 18-8). The cortex of the cerebellum is hyperechoic due to the fine duplications of the pia mater into the cerebellar gyri, which densely populate the surface of the cerebellum. At times it is necessary to gently manipulate the fetal head into a desirable position through which sound waves can reach the posterior fossa easily. The usual measurements to be taken here are the bicerebellar measurement[41,42] and that of the cisterna magna, measurements usually taken on a horizontal section. The infratentorial cerebello-medullary cistern (cisterna magna) is probably the most important of the cisterns of the fetal brain as far as imaging is concerned. At times, the supratentorial quadrigeminal cistern found above the cerebellum and the quadrigeminal plate has importance, since a large percentage of arachnoid cysts arise from this area. It is important to know the shape and size of the cisterna magna since its enlargement may lead to detection of pathologies such as the Dandy-Walker malformation or even trisomies. It is considered to be normal when its size is between 3–8 mm with a mean value of 4.5 mm.[43]

into the third ventricle through the foramina interventricularis (Monro), the corpus callosum, and the thalamus. The third ventricle is rarely imaged in the late second and third trimester due to its narrow transverse diameter, however, it can readily be depicted in the late first and early second trimesters. It was suggested that the third ventricle may reach trans-

THE SAGITTAL PLANES: MEDIAN, OBLIQUE-1 AND OBLIQUE-2

The median ("mid-sagittal") section images the entire corpus callosum (before the 18th to 20th week only parts of this can be seen), cavum septi pellucidi, head of the caudate nucleus, thalamus, tela choroidea, mid-brain structures such as the

TABLE 18-1	THE TRANSVAGINALLY OBTAINED BRAIN SECTIONS: NEW NOMENCLATURE	
Classical Sections	*New Nomenclature*	
Coronal	Frontal	Frontal-1
		Frontal-2
	Mid-coronal	Mid-coronal-1
		Mid-coronal-2
		Mid-coronal-3
	Occipital	Occipital-1
		Occipital-2
Sagittal	Median	
	Oblique-1	
	Oblique-2	

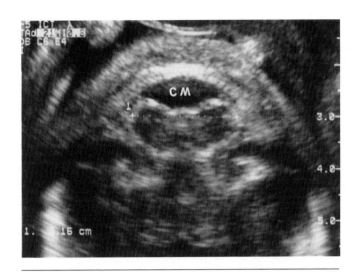

FIGURE 18-7 A conventional transabdominal picture of the normal posterior fossa at 21 weeks through the "posterior/occipital horizontal approach." The bi-cerebellar distance is 21.6 mm (CM—cisterna magna).

corpora quadrigemina, the vermis, tectum, and cisterna magna, and the fourth ventricle (Fig. 18-6). The cavum septi pellucidi and cavum vergae are not part of the ventricular system, since they do not have connections with the lateral ventricles. They are easily recognizable fluid-filled midline structures that can be found below the corpus callosum and above the nuclei of the midbrain. Their importance hinges in the fact that they develop parallel with the corpus callosum, and pathology in their development or the lack of their clear imaging may be associated with extensive developmental pathology of the brain. The corpus callosum is probably the most important midline structure connecting the right and left hemispheres (Fig. 18-9).

The fourth ventricle is usually imaged on the median plane with the transvaginal technique or on axial sections through an occipital approach. On such a plane, the hyperechoic vermis can also be appreciated.

The right and left oblique-1 ("para-sagittal") contains the lateral ventricles (anterior horn, atrium and posterior horn) with the choroid plexus like a cap over the thalami. The inferior horns should not be visible through these sections because they are lateral to them. The inferior horn extends from the atrium laterally into the temporal lobe. After 16 weeks, in a normal fetal brain, the oblique sections through the anterior and occipital horns do not include the inferior horn, which is found slightly lateral to this plane. Based on our experience, if after 16–18 postmenstrual weeks the anterior, posterior, and inferior horns are imaged on this section, ventriculomegaly should seriously be suspected.

The choroid plexus is gaining importance in fetal neurosonography. At times this importance may be slightly exaggerated. Practical all choroid plexuses present in the brain reside in the lateral ventricles and are the major source of the cerebrospinal fluid. The sonographic appearance, of the choroid plexus is "light" and appear as cotton-like structures with irregular borders filling the available space of the lateral ventricles (e.g., the antrum). The choroid plexus has a rich blood supply that can be imaged with color. As mentioned previously, the choroid plexus of the lateral ventricles assumes its final position at around 18–20 postmenstrual weeks of gestation. If they become thin and dangling, they are considered to be sensitive markers of ventriculomegaly. At times, sonography may detect cystic structures within a choroid plexus. These choroid plexus cysts will be discussed in the section of pathology of the brain. The tela choroidea is a thin layer of choroid plexus covering the thalami, and can be best imaged on a median section.

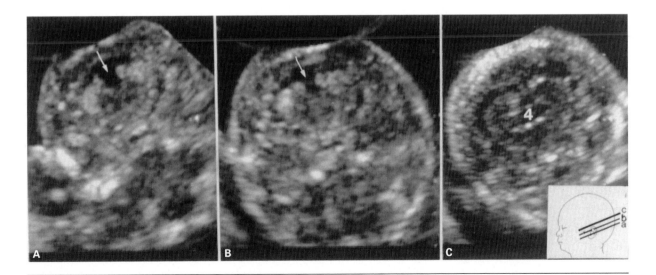

FIGURE 18-8 The more detailed scrutiny of the posterior fossa using a transvaginal ultrasound probe demonstrates the normal cisterna magna and its connection (foramen Magendie) marked by an arrow the 4th ventricle (4). These are three consecutive sections through the horizontal plane C—cerebellar hemispheres.

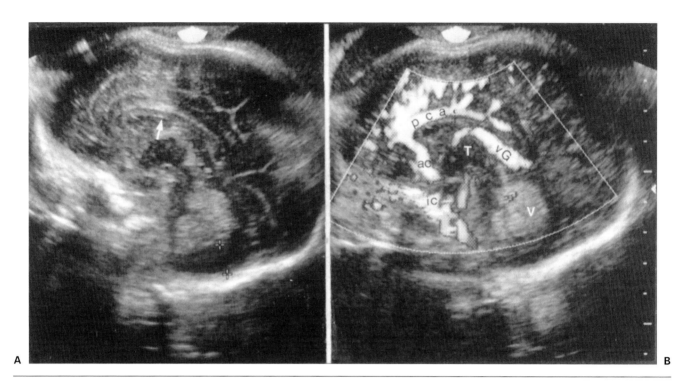

FIGURE 18-9 At 32 weeks on the median section using a transvaginal probe the corpus callosum (arrow) and some of the gyri and sulci can be seen. Using the amplitude mode the color flow picture reveals arteries and veins on the same plane. PCA—pericallosal artery; AC—anterior cerebral; IC—internal carotid artery; VG—vein of Galen; V—vermis of the cerebellum; T—thalamus.

The lateral ventricle-to-hemisphere ratio decreases in from about 70% at 18–20 postmenstrual weeks to about 30% at around 28–29 postmenstrual weeks and then remains relatively stable to the end of the pregnancy. One of the problems of measuring the ventricular system by transabdominal sonography is that the hemisphere close to the transducer is usually "blurred." The graphs and tables as well as nomograms to measure the distance from the medial wall of the lateral ventricle to its lateral wall are widely recognized and available.[44-47]

Cardoza et al.[48] measured the width of the lateral ventricular atrium as a function of increasing fetal age however the value of 7.6 ± 0.6 ml remained relatively constant throughout gestation. This article suggests that the width of the lateral ventricular atrium above 10 ml, which represents 4 times the standard deviation, should trigger the suspicion of ventriculomegaly.

Campbell[49] suggested measuring the anterior horn-hemispheric widths ratio. This ratio decreases from 60% at 14 postmenstrual weeks to 40% at 21 postmenstrual weeks. The same author proposed that the measurement of the distance between the falx to lateral wall of the atrium is a sensitive indicator of abnormality. This ratio decreases from 60% to 30% from 15–24 postmenstrual weeks.[49] From 27 postmenstrual weeks to term, this same ratio remains constant at 0.56 to 0.51.[50]

Dilatation of the posterior horn (colpocephaly) is probably the most sensitive indicator of ventriculomegaly. If the transvaginal imaging method is used, it is easy to measure the posterior horn[23] and using the constructed nomograms.[51]

Right and left oblique-2 demonstrates mostly homogenous texture of the brain tissue with a V-shaped lateral sulcus (the apex of the V-points toward the occiput). The upper arm of the V arises from the temporal lobe, and is called parietal operculum. The lower arm of the V is the temporal operculum. These 2 structures enclose between them area called the insula. The insula is "buried" and disappears toward term into the depth through the 2 closing opercula.

We felt that we made only a very slight deviation from the rigid and classical "anatomic rule" and believe that the clinically applicable gain of this adjustment is well worth the slight bending of the classical rules. Once the meaning of the definitions is known and consensus is reached, clinical applications may prove entirely useful.

The importance of each of the proposed 10 sections has to be stressed. If the landmarks of each of these sections are known, possible pathology can easily be defined and localized. If, for instance, in the mid-trimester, the frontal-1 section reveals the anterior horns and the occipital-2 show the dilated posterior horn, one could with good reason, suspect a dilatation of the lateral ventricles. In a normal brain none of these sections should contain the anterior and the posterior tips of the lateral ventricles. If, for example, an arachnoid cyst is suspected, this can be precisely localized by the use of all the described sections. If, on the oblique-1 section, all 3 horns of the lateral ventricles are seen, dilatation of the lateral ventricles can be diagnosed with great certainty. The different parts of the corpus callosum and their integrity can be followed on the frontal 2 mid-coronal-1, -2, and -3 sections. There are several other examples, however, we are sure that those listed make the necessary point.

We are convinced, that because the systematic way of imaging the fetal brain and because its simplicity as well as the logic behind it, this method of describing the fetal brain scanned by transvaginal sonography has the potential to become generally accepted as a scanning method. *Once again, we have to stress the fact that it emulates the neonatal scanning, therefore the pediatric neurologists and neurosurgeons may be the first to understand its usefulness.*

THE CEREBRAL CORTEX: GYRI, SULCI, AND FISSURES

The gyri and sulci can be imaged on a median section when the flat interhemispheric surface is tangentially scanned. In this section the cingulate gyrus and sulcus, the parieto-occipital fissure and calcarine fissure can be imaged (Fig. 18-10).[52]

The cerebral cortex, where most of the sensory, motor, and intellectual functions are performed, has fascinated imaging specialists for a long time. Based on pathological developmental studies, at 22 postmenstrual weeks, the cerebral hemispheres are smooth and the lateral sulci on both sides are widely open. By 24 postmenstrual weeks, the lateral sulcus deepens and the cingulate sulcus is also detectable. On the medial surface, the parieto occipital sulcus and the calcarine fissure (calcar avis) are also present. Beyond 26 postmenstrual weeks, deepening of these fissures and the sulci occur. The biggest increase in the number and the depth of the sulci and gyri take place between 28 and 30 postmenstrual weeks. Slagle et al.[53] describe the developmental steps in the formation of the cingulate gyrus and sulcus in preterm infants and pointed out that this sulcus first becomes continuous and later some of its pri-

mary and then secondary branches appear. Finally, during the last weeks of the gestation other sulci and gyri develop, rendering the median surface of the hemisphere a "cobblestone appearance."

Our group studied the development of the cingulate sulcus and gyrus as well as the parieto-occipital and the calcarine fissure in the normal fetuses from 14–40 postmenstrual weeks and came to the following conclusion: the developmental maturation of the normal fetal brain follows a predictable timetable, and that this maturation can be followed by ultrasonography.[26] The sonographic appearance of the fissures, the gyri and sulci, using transvaginal sonographic imaging, lagged behind their anatomic appearance. The greatest discrepancy was regarding the cingulate gyrus, which in the anatomical studies was present by 18 postmenstrual weeks and in our sonographic study was only seen after the 26th postmenstrual week. The callosal sulcus was seen at 14 postmenstrual weeks, both in the sonographic and anatomical studies. We concluded that the recognition of specific structures of the cortical map is possible, and that transvaginal sonography may be used to image the developing cortical surface. This can later on form the basis of clinical application in the diagnosis of certain diseases of the cortical development.

FETAL CEREBRAL CIRCULATION

The fetal brain similarly to the adult brain is supplied by an *anterior* and a *posterior* circulation. The anterior circulation originates from the internal carotid arteries whereas the posterior circulation stems from the vertebral arteries which join to form a single basilar artery in the median plane. Then, they once again give rise to 2 branches which in turn form the connections with the anterior circulation at the basis of the hemisphere. This hexagon-shaped ring of vessels is known as the circulus arteriosus or hexagon of Willis. It is beyond the scope of this chapter to describe all the arteries and venus drainages of the fetal central nervous system. The interested reader is referred to the classic textbooks or the more targeted anatomic atlases containing details of the circulation of the brain.[54] (Fig. 18-11).

As far as the sonographic appearance of the cerebral blood vessels are concerned, it should be stated from the outset that the earliest documented discreet pulsations of the brain vessels can be obtained at and immediately after the eighth postmenstrual week.[55] These pulsations are visualized with high frequency transvaginal ultrasound probes. The middle cerebral artery becomes visible in 71% of the cases at 9 postmenstrual weeks, and finally at 11 postmenstrual weeks, in every case, the cerebral circulation can be depicted.[56]

On the horizontal or axial section, the circulus arteriosus of Willis can be sonographically visualized. This hexagonal structure is formed by the posterior cerebral arteries, the posterior communicating arteries, the middle cerebral arteries, the anterior cerebral arteries, and finally the anterior communicating artery, as we proceed from occipital to frontal direction.

The median plane is probably one of the most revealing and clinically important sections to be imaged. On this plane,

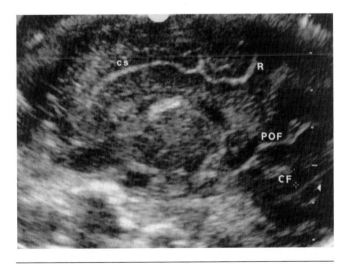

FIGURE 18-10 Some of the gyri and sulci can be scanned using the median plane obtainable by transvaginal ultrasonography. The cingulate sulcus (CS) and its branches (R—ramus) as well as the more posterior parieto-occipital fissure (POF) and calcarine fissure (CF) are imaged at 32 weeks.

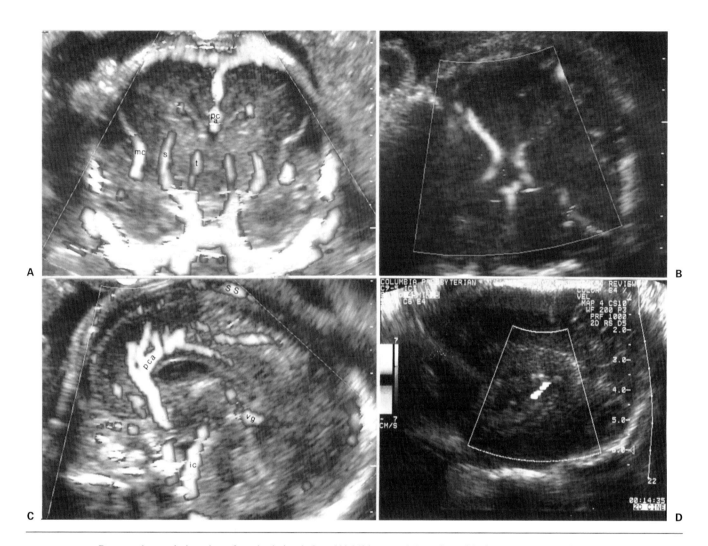

FIGURE 18-11 Power color angio imaging of cerebral circulation. **(A)** Mid-coronal-1 section with the cross-section of the pericallosal arteries (PCA) as well as the middle cerebral artery (MC) and its branches to the corpus striatum (S) and the thalamus (T). **(B)** On a low horizontal section the circle of Willis is imaged. **(C)** On the median section the internal carotid (IC) branching into the pericallosal (PCA). The superior sagittal sinus (SS) and the vein of Galen (VG) are also seen. **(D)** On a lateral Oblique-2 section the insula with the middle cerebral artery are located.

we are able to follow the internal carotid artery leading to the anterior cerebral artery. The 2 main branches of the latter are the pericallosal artery and the calloso-marginal arteries. These develop together with the corpus callosum and their presence or absence are good indicators of the size and the development of the corpus callosum. Other vessels seen on this plane are: the superior sagittal and the central draining vein—the vein of Galen.

If a "coronal plane" is sought, the most revealing may be the Midcoronal-2 section on which the internal carotid, the mid-cerebral artery and its small ventriculo striate arteries, the cross-section of the pericallosal artery, the arteries of the choroid plexus, and the superior sagittal sinus are evident.

Studies of the middle cerebral arteries with regard to measuring blood flow to the brain of normal as well as grown fetuses can be performed by using transabdominal ultrasound Doppler techniques. During the third trimester, a constant but low resistance flow in the fetal brain is present.[57] Wladimiroff

et al. detected diastolic frequencies in 75% of the fetuses at 18 weeks and in all fetuses after 34 postmenstrual weeks.[58] It was found that the PI of the middle cerebral artery was higher than that of the internal carotid artery or the anterior cerebral artery.[59] Also, the posterior cerebral artery had a lower resistance index than that of the middle and anterior cerebral arteries.[60] After 34–36 weeks, there may be a redistribution of fetal circulation with decreased impedance to the flow to the fetal brain, probably to compensate for the progressive decrease in fetal blood pO_2.[61–63] The low cerebral vascular impedance-to-blood-flow at the end of the pregnancy was attributed to the increasing metabolic requirements.[64] Meerman et al.[65] published longitudinal studies of fetal and neonatal cerebral blood flow velocities assessed in the middle cerebral artery explaining some of the changes which occur throughout gestation and as transition to the neonatal period.

It is known that several physiological variables affect the cerebral blood flow in normal pregnancies. These variables among others are the fetal heart rate, breathing movements, fetus behavioral states, glucose concentration, head compression, and last but not least, the labor and delivery. Fetal cerebral blood flow was also studied extensively in pathological states such as fetal anemia, elevated placental restriction in the intrauterine growth restricted fetus, discordant multifetal pregnancies, and increased intracranial pressure.

A detailed discussion of the ultrasonography of the fetal and neonatal cerebral circulation as well as Doppler measurements in various arteries of the fetal brain were eloquently dealt with by Degani et al.[66]

The knowledge of the anatomic location of the major arteries and the venous drainage is important to assess normal development of certain structures—the corpus callosum—or to be able to correctly determine the exact location of the space occupying lesions such as arachnoid cysts. The normal development of the corpus callosum from 12–18 weeks can be closely followed by the developing pericallosal artery. If by 18 weeks, the entire length of the pericallosal artery or for that matter, the corpus callosum, is not seen, the diagnosis of partial or total lack of development of the corpus callosum can be made easier.

The clinical importance of sonographic imaging of the venous system is not well established. Very few anomalies short of that of the vein of Galen were described. Fetal neurosonography is an extremely informative imaging modality that is relatively inexpensive and is definitely noninvasive. Understanding the normal development and the sonoanatomy of the fetal brain, we have an easier task to detect deviant development or pathology and it is easier to localize the lesion using the newly proposed sections of the brain in the sagittal and coronal planes. As stated previously, the transfer of the information to the pediatrician neonatal neurologist and neurosurgeon becomes easier, more fluent, and obviously it is to the advantage of the fetus with brain pathology.

MALFORMATIONS OF THE FETAL BRAIN: DIAGNOSIS BY PRENATAL SONOGRAPHY

Of all the fetal brain malformations amenable to prenatal diagnosis those that the geneticist deals with most commonly, on a daily basis, are those of the neural tube. Thus, this section deals predominantly with the sonographic appearance of neural tube defects. A "selected" group of other, pertinent malformations will also be described.

NEURAL TUBE DEFECTS: ANENCEPHALY, INIENCEPHALY, AND DYSRAPHIA (CRANIAL AND SPINAL)

The normal neural tube starts developing at approximately 20 days after conception. Fusion of the neural tube starts in the lower caudal area of the embryo and proceeds cranially. The completion of this neural tube formation occurs at or slightly prior to 32 post-conception. The defect of the neural tube (NTD) result from a failure of this tube to close. A closure defect in the area of the anterior neuropore results in anencephaly, closure defects in the cervical and thoracic region of the spine will result in the iniencephaly sequence and defects of this closure in the lower mid or caudal neural groove can result in meningomyeloceles.[67]

The incidence of NTDs in the United States is about 2 in 1000 births but this risk increases significantly if there is a family history of a NTD. The recurrence rate for a family in which the parents are normal and have 1 affected child is between 3–5%. If 1 of the parents has a NTD the risk to the offspring is around 5% and if 2 previous children are affected this risk increases to as high as 6–10%.[68–70]

Recently, the US Public Health Service has recommended that all pregnant women take folic acid to prevent NTD since clinical trials demonstrated that up to 70% of NTDs can be prevented by folic acid supplementation in early pregnancy; the remaining NTDs are resistant to folate. It appears that folic acid does not work by correcting a nutritional deficiency, but that a metabolic defect is responsible for the NTDs and that this defect or defects can be corrected by a sufficiently large dose of folic acid.[71] Mills et al.[71] have recently demonstrated that homocysteine metabolism is likely to be the critical pathway affected by folic acid. They found a significantly higher homocysteine levels in women carrying affected fetuses than in control women. These findings suggest that 1 of the enzymes responsible for homocysteine metabolism is likely to be abnormal in affected pregnancies. Greene and Copp[72] have recently shown that a second vitamin, myo-inositol, is capable of significantly reducing the incidence of spinal NTDs in curly tail mice, a genetic model of folate-resistant NTDs. Their findings suggest the possible efficacy of combined treatment with folate and inositol in overcoming the majority of human NTDs.

ANENCEPHALY

The anencephaly sequence is a malformation in which the fetal cranium is absent. This absence can be of various degrees. This condition is lethal, and almost three fourths of the fetuses are stillborn. Such NTDs are complex developmental malformations affecting the production of the mesenchyme.[73,74] Müller and O'Rahilly[75,76] have described 3 phases in the development of anencephaly. The first is dysraphia, or a failure of the region of the calvarium to close. The second is exencephaly, in which the developing brain is not surrounded by the cranial bones, even during the embryonic period. The third and last phase is anencephaly which appears due to the total disintegration of the exposed brain. Bronshtein et al.[77] reported on the development of anencephaly from exencephaly which they followed looking at several anencephalic fetuses from early gestation. Exencephaly and anencephaly can be detected reliably from about the 10th or 11th postmenstrual weeks (Figs. 18-12 and 18-13).[78]

Our group made similar observations when, following amniocentesis done in anencephalic fetuses, free floating neuronal cells were detected in the amniotic fluid supporting the

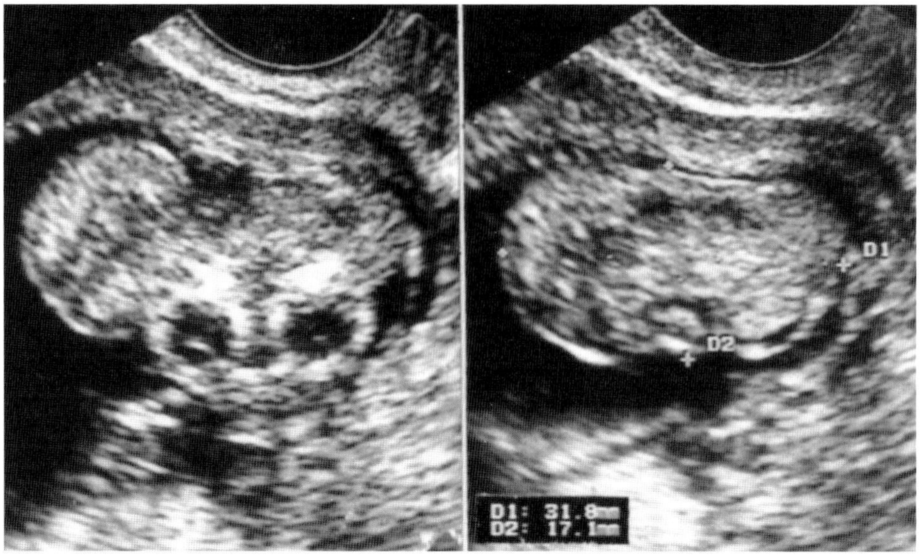

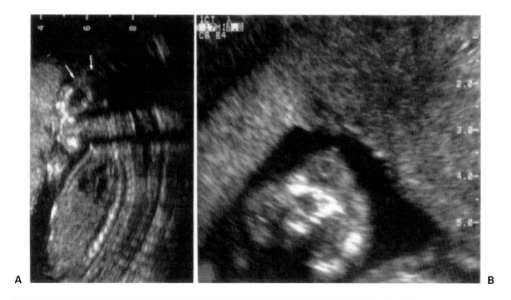

FIGURE 18-12 The typical "Mickey Mouse" appearance of an exencephalic fetus (acrania) on the coronal and horizontal planes is depicted at 12 weeks.

theory of "rubbing-off" brain tissue in a fetus previously having acrania.[79]

Anencephaly as well as exencephaly is relatively easy to detect with prenatal sonography. Of historical interest, the first fetal malformation detected by transabdominal and transvaginal ultrasound was anencephaly.[78,80] Usually, if the fetus is scanned at around 11 or 12 postmenstrual weeks, the typical picture of exencephalic/anencephalic fetus is that of a fetal head is much wider than usual and the crown rump length lags several millimeters behind the expected measurement at the specific gestational age. Two types of anencephalies can be

present: *Holoacrania* in which the entire calvarium is missing. This is the easiest to recognize sonographically. Various degrees of spinal rachischisis spanning over several vertebrae may be present. The second type is termed *meroacrania* in which there is partial or incomplete median cranial defect with parts of the brain uncovered by the skull. Polyhydramnios is a commonly associated finding.

INIENCEPHALY

Iniencephaly is a lethal and complex malformation. It is characterized by the following features: a defect in the foramen

FIGURE 18-13 The sagittal (**A**) and the coronal (**B**) sections through the upper pole of an anencephalic fetus at 18 weeks and 5 days is shown. No cranium or brain tissue is seen above the orbits.

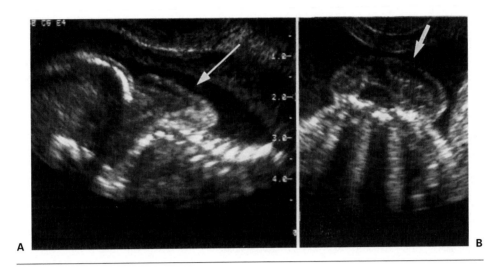

FIGURE 18-14 Iniencephalus (open type) showing a cervical meningomyelocele. (**A**) On the sagittal plane the short neck as well as the bulging neural tissue is seen (arrow). (**B**) On a coronal section the exposed brain tissue is evident (arrow).

magnum and the occiput, spinal retroflection with a short neck and trunk, defects of the thoracic cage, anterior spina bifida, diaphragmatic defects with or without hernia, and hypoplasia of the lung and/or heart.[67] There are 2 subtypes: an open and closed type. Its association with open malformation is as high as 84%. In iniencephaly as well as in anencephaly, most of the affected fetuses are female. The reported incidence is from 1–6 in 10,000 births.[81,82]

The sonographic diagnosis is relatively simple, and it is based on imaging the head in fixed retroflection, and the spine in a lordotic position (Fig. 18-14). Various degrees of posterior cephalocele or protrusion of brain tissue in the occipital area are seen as well as other anomalies such as rachischises and omphalocele.[83,84] Using TVS, iniencephaly has been diagnosed as early as the 12th postmenstrual week of gestation.[85] Malformations such as hydrocephalus, microcephaly, agenesis of various parts of the brain, and deformities of the thorax, the face, and the abdominal wall are found.

DYSRAPHIA: CRANIAL AND SPINAL

Cephaloceles are bulges of the fetal brain that has herniated through a cranial defect pushing the meninges in front of the brain tissue. At times, only the meninges are bulging, which is termed meningocele. If the defect contains brain tissue, it is called meningo-encephalocele. The incidence is 1 in 9,000 births.[86] The cephalocele may emerge from the occipital, ethmoidal, temporal, and parietal regions of the fetal head, geographical or regional differences in their incidence were described.[87–95] Occipital cephalocele: these occur more commonly in females than in males. Using TVS, occipital cephaloceles have been diagnosed as early as 12 weeks of gestation.[91] Their sizes may range from extremely small to the size of the fetal skull. The majority of cephalocele are isolated lesions, but a small number may be associated with syndromes. Of these, Meckel syndrome (or Meckel-Gruber) is the most

significant. Meckel syndrome is an autosomal recessive condition characterized by occipital cephalocele (present in 80%), bilateral polycystic kidneys and post-axial polydactyly.[90,92] The locus for the Meckel-Gruber syndrome has been mapped to 17q21–q24.[96] Other associated brain abnormalities in nonsyndromic cephalocele include hydrocephalus (85–95%), agenesis of the corpus callosum and Dandy-Walker syndrome.[97,98] Microcephaly may be also present in cases of cephalocele.

Spina bifida is characterized by an open spinal lesion with protrusion of its contents through the bony defect. The development of myelomeningocele is probably around the 4th week of gestation at the time of closure of the posterior neural tube. Myelocele and myelomeningocele develop similarly, but the term myelocele refers to a midline plaque of neural tissue (neural placode) that is flush with the surface, and is not covered by skin. In contrast the myelomeningocele is a bulging defect in which the elevated neural plate and meninges are contiguous laterally with the subcutaneous tissue. The incidence of myelomeningocele in the United States is 0.2–0.4 per 1,000 live births.[99] Ten to 15% of spinal dysraphic defects are closed and normal skin covers the bony defect. In approximately 80% of the lesions occur in the lumbar, thoraco-lumbar, or lumbo-sacral areas of the spine and the balance in the cervical and sacral areas.[100]

The sensitivity of antenatal sonography to detect myelomeningocele is reported to be between 80 and 90% and even higher prior to the knowledge of the MSAFP results.[101–103] When scanning the fetal spine to rule out the presence of a defect all 3 scanning planes must be employed. In the sagittal view of the spine irregularities of the bony spine, a bulge within the posterior contour of the fetal back or an obvious disruption of the fetal skin contours can be detected. On the axial or transverse sections the open spine has a U-shape and in the coronal section the affected bony segment show a

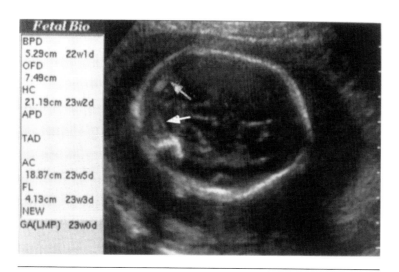

FIGURE 18-15 A 23-week fetus. Horizontal section of the brain demonstrating the banana shaped cerebellum (arrow) in the posterior fossa and the lemon-shaped cranium.

divergent configuration replacing the normal parallel lines of the normal vertebral arches (Fig. 18-14). Determining the site and the extent of the spinal lesion is important because it correlates with the neurologic outcome of the fetus. The higher and the larger the lesion, the more severe the neurologic dysfunction the neonate will have.

Over the past decade important sonographic findings have facilitated the detection of spinal defects namely the *lemon*, and the *banana sign* as well as *hydrocephaly*. The lemon sign refers to a deformity of the frontal bone and the banana sign refers to an abnormal shape of the flattened cerebellum which obliterates the cisterna magna (Fig. 18-15). Blumenfeld et al.[104] reported on the diagnosis of neural tube defects between 12–17 weeks by using the banana and the lemon signs. They found that the earliest appearance of the lemon and banana sign is at 14 weeks. Therefore, from the early second trimester these indirect cranial findings may be used to enhance the detection of open neural tube defects. Since these findings may be subtle at 14–15 weeks a follow-up scan later on the second trimester may be indicated in cases at risk. The lemon sign is present in virtually all cases between 16–24 postmenstrual weeks, but after 24 weeks of gestation the lemon sign is a less reliable marker and is present in only 13–50% of the fetuses with spinal defects.[105-108] Cerebellar abnormalities with obliteration of the cisterna magna is present all through gestation in 95–100% of the cases of spinal dysraphism although after 24 weeks cerebellar absence is more commonly seen than the banana sign.[105,108-110] When hydrocephalus accompanies a thoracolumbar, lumbar, or lumbosacral myelomeningocele is termed the *Arnold-Chiari II malformation* and is present in almost every case. The hydrocephalus most likely is the result of the hindbrain malformation that blocks the flow of cerebrospinal fluid through the 4th ventricle or posterior fossa or from aqueductal stenosis that may be present in 40–75% of the cases.[111]

MIDLINE ANOMALIES: HOLOPROSENCEPHALY, AGENESIS OF THE CORPUS CALLOSUM, AGENESIS OF THE CAVUM SEPTI PELLUCIDI, AND DANDY-WALKER MALFORMATION

Holoprosencephaly

Holoprosencephaly is a malformation sequence that results from failure of the prosencephalon to differentiate into the cerebral hemispheres and lateral ventricles during the 4th to 8th week of gestation. Holoprosencephaly is presumed to be associated with high percentage of earlier midtrimester pregnancy loss, therefore ultrasound scans performed at these early gestational ages may encounter this anomaly more frequently.[112] In abortuses the incidence has been reported to be 0.4 per 1,000 with a lower incidence in live births of 0.06 per 1,000.[87] Holoprosencephaly may occur as an isolated anomaly, however, at times is associated with chromosomal abnormalities such as trisomy 13 and 18 as well as a variety of other structural chromosomal aberrations. Over 60% of the infants with trisomy 13 also have holoprosencephaly. Conversely, 20% of the cases of holoprosencephaly are associated with trisomy 13.[113] Autosomal dominant transmission as well as its association with syndromes was also described. In the autosomal dominant form a gene located at 7q36 and designated as HPE3[114] has been described.

By their appearance and anatomic presentation, holoprosencephaly may be classified as *alobar*, *semilobar*, and *lobar holoprosencephaly*.[115-117] The sonographic diagnosis of holoprosencephaly was reported as early as 12 weeks and was based on the lack of development of the falx and the fusion of the thalami.[113] Microcephaly may be present in all 3 types of holoprosencephalies.[118] However, at times, if hydrocephalus is also present, there may be head enlargement present. At times, lipomas of the corpus callosum can be detected.[119]

Holoprosencephaly is often associated with facial anomalies. Therefore, it is important to note at this point that no fetal brain scan should be considered complete unless the fetal face has been adequately imaged. In 1964, DeMyer et al.[118] reported on the importance of the facial anomalies when faced with children with holoprosencephaly. He stated that "the face predicts brain." Hence, the children with the most dysmorphic facial features also have the most severe type of holoprosencephaly, namely alobar holoprosencephaly.

Alobar holoprosencephaly is the most severe of the 3 types of holoprosencephalies. It is characterized by a completely absent interhemispheric fissure and corpus callosum, the thalami are fused in the midline and there is an absence of the third ventricle. The anomaly consists of a single ventricle, small cerebrum, fused thalami, agenesis of the corpus callosum, and falx cerebri[120] (Fig. 18-16). Sonographic findings of alobar holoprosencephaly include absence of midline structures (falx cerebri, interhemispheric fissure, absence of the corpus callosum), mono-ventricular cavity with communicating dorsal

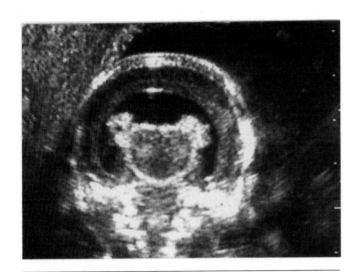

FIGURE 18-16 A 19-week fetus with alobar holoprosencephaly. Note the fused thalami and the lack of the falx as the semicircular mantle of brain (pancake-type holoprosencephaly).

cyst, fused thalami, and facial dysmorphism. Facial dysmorphism may be variable and include such abnormalities as cyclopia (single eye or partially divided eye in a single orbit), ethmocephaly (orbital hypotelorism, but separate orbits), cebocephaly (ocular hypotelorism and blind-ended, single nostril nose), hypotelorism, and other midline facial defects may be present.[87,118,121–123] The most severe facial dysmorphism, cyclopia, ethmocephaly, and cebocephaly, are usually present with alobar holoprosencephaly.[118]

In the *semilobar type*, some cleavage of the brain has occurred, there are the 2 cerebral hemispheres are partially split

or separated above which there is a singular ventricular cavity. In addition, a separation of the hemispheres in the occipital area and a partial development of the posterior and the inferior horns is also seen. This configuration renders the ventricles into a teardrop shape on the axial section.[120]

Lobar holoprosencephaly is the most subtle of the 3 types of holoprosencephalies. The sonographic findings include the presence of the interhemispheric fissure, the fused frontal horns have a flat roof and communicate freely with the third ventricle, the septum pellucidum is always absent, the corpus callosum may be absent, hypoplastic or normal and there may be midline fusion of the cingulate gyrus. Pilu et al.[124] have described an echogenic linear structure running within the third ventricle as a specific sign of fetal lobar holoprosencephaly. In the midcoronal plane, this structure appears as a small, round, solid structure approximately in the mid-portion of the third ventricle. It is believed that this echogenic linear structure demonstrates the abnormally fused fornices in the midline.[123,124] The face in semilobar and lobar holoprosencephaly may show ocular hypotelorism or hypertelorism, unilateral or bilateral cleft lip, or other mild facial dysmorphic features.[123]

The sonographic prenatal diagnosis of lobar holoprosencephaly is quite difficult and it is usually based on the absence of a septum pellucidum and the communication between the frontal horns and the third ventricle as well as the wedge-shaped separation of the thalami. The differential diagnosis of lobar holoprosencephaly is septo-optic dysplasia, which is quite a rare anomaly characterized by the absence of the septum pellucidum and the hypoplasia of the optic disks. The antenatal picture of septo-optic dysplasia is almost identical to that of lobar holoprosencephaly (Fig. 18-17). The definitive diagnosis

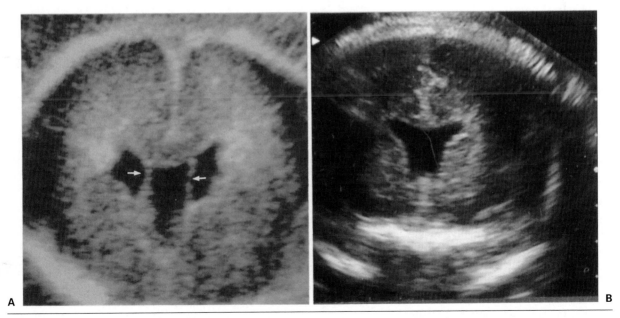

FIGURE 18-17 Comparison between a mid-coronal-1 section of a fetal brain with normal anatomy (**A**) and the mid-coronal-1 section of a fetus at 33 weeks gestation (**B**) with absent septum pellucidum. Note the prominent box-like central sonolucent structure that represents the lateral ventricle and third ventricle joined. There is absence of the sheets of tissue seen on A—marked by arrows—which form the outer wall of the cavum septum.

is usually made after birth when the vision of the newborn can be tested. If visual problems, blindness, and/or diabetes insipidus is observed, the diagnosis of septo-optic dysplasia can be confirmed.[113]

Agenesis of the Corpus Callosum

The corpus callosum is situated in the midline with its 4 segments (rostrum, genu, body, and splenium) constitutes the largest collection of fibers connecting the different areas of the cerebral cortex situated in the opposite hemispheres. Total or partial lack in the development of this midline structure is termed agenesis of the corpus callosum (ACC) or partial agenesis of the corpus callosum (PACC) depending on the extent of the missing part. If PACC is the case, usually the splenium and part of the body is missing.

The incidence in the general population is thought to be 0.3–0.7%,[116,117] however, there is a higher incidence in the neurologically impaired patient population.[125] Agenesis of the corpus callosum in the majority of cases occurs as an sporadic malformation. However, ACC has many genetic causes and has been associated with chromosomal rearrangements such as del(4)(p16), autosomal dominant and autosomal recessive syndrome and X-linked forms.[126] Chromosomal anomalies are often (about 20%) present in cases of ACC.[34] The most encountered chromosomal aneuploidies are trisomy 18, 13, and 8. In addition, part of more than 20 autosomal malformation syndromes such as Miller-Dieker, Rubenstein-Taybi, acrocallosal, and Joubert's.[127,128] In addition, some cases of ACC as well as X-linked hydrocephalus, MASA syndrome and X-linked spastic paraplegia have been known to be due to mutations in the gene for the neural cell adhesion molecule L1.[129–133] Recently, the term CRASH syndrome (the acronym for corpus callosum, retardation, adducted thumbs, spasticity, and hydrocephalus) has been proposed to refer to this clinical syndrome.[134]

Agenesis of the corpus callosum can be complete or partial depending on the stage of development at which growth was arrested. Agenesis of the corpus callosum can occur as an isolated anomaly but 80% of the cases have other associated malformations.[35,135–137] Partial agenesis of the corpus callosum usually involves the posterior portion, since embryologically it develops in a cranial-caudal fashion and may also be associated with other malformations.[128] Transvaginal sonography allows the corpus callosum to be easily imaged on a median sagittal section (Fig. 18-9).[137–142] In agenesis of the corpus callosum the gyri and sulci appear to be radiating in a perpendicular fashion from the dilated third ventricle in a "sunburst" pattern (Fig. 18-18).[34,35,137] The cavum septum pellucidum in most cases of complete agenesis of the corpus callosum is absent or severely distorted.[34,143] On

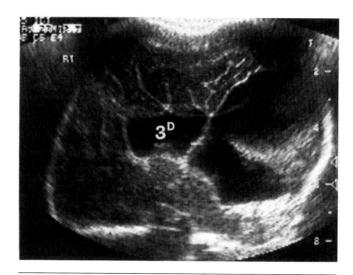

FIGURE 18-18 Median section of a fetal brain at 34 weeks demonstrating the upward displacement of the third ventricle and the "sunburst" appearance of the radiating gyri and sulci.

a oblique section the frontal horns appear narrow and laterally displaced, and the atria and occipital horn appear slightly dilated.[137] The coronal section demonstrates a wide interhemispheric fissure within which the falx cerebri is present, the lateral ventricles are widely separated and have a distinctive configuration similar to a "Viking helmet" and lastly the thalami are widely separated due to the dilated third ventricle (Fig. 18-19).[144]

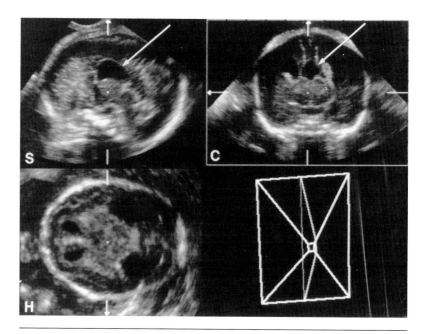

FIGURE 18-19 Three-dimensional volume scan of the fetal brain using a transvaginal 3D scanhead (Medison) depicts the median sagittal (S), the coronal (C) and the horizontal (H) planes simultaneously. The arrows indicate the pathology in this 20-week fetus. In this case the diagnosis of agenesis of the corpus callosum was made based upon the cranially displaced third ventricle and the tear drop-shaped lateral ventricles.

The sonographic diagnosis in the fetus is based on the total or partial (usually posterior) lack of the sonolucent structure connecting the hemispheres in the midline. On coronal sections, the lateral ventricles appear separated and displaced upward because the horizontal fibers of the corpus callosum are missing. It appears that the third ventricle is directly communicating with the unusually wide interhemispheric fissures. On an axial section, due to the more prominent dilatation of the occipital horns (colpocephaly) compared to those of the anterior horns, a teardrop configuration of the lateral ventricles result. The walls of the frontal horns may be so close to each other that a peculiar parallel double line appears which is termed "railroad tracks." On the median section, the normal appearance of the cavum septi pellucidi flanked from above by the C-shaped corpus callosum and cingulate sulcus, cingulate gyrus and the pericallosal artery (on color-coded flow studies) are absent. Instead, the high position of the third ventricle and the radial (sunburst) appearance of the gyri and sulci become relatively easily diagnosed. At times, lipomas were observed to appear at the location of the corpus callosum.[119] They appear as echogenic structures, however, it is rare to see them in the second trimester. Another useful way to make the diagnosis is to follow the semi-circular course of the pericallosal artery. Normally this artery follows the superior surface of the corpus callosum. If the entire corpus callosum or parts of it are missing, the artery will also be shorter indicating the extent of the anomaly.[34,145]

The diagnosis of total or partial agenesis of the corpus callosum is not hard if a targeted fetal neuroscan is performed. It should, however, be noted that on axial scans, the diagnosis is significantly harder to make than on coronal or median scanning planes. It is therefore, stressed here that if any suspicion of this developmental disorder arises, TVS should be performed. We found it worthwhile to vert fetuses from breech to vertex presentation to be able to apply the coronal and the sagittal planes to rule out or to establish the diagnosis.

Dandy-Walker Malformation

Barkovich et al.[136] suggested that the Dandy-Walker malformation, Dandy-Walker variant, and mega-cisterna magna are a continuum of posterior fossa developmental anomalies and suggested the name of Dandy-Walker complex. This classification of DWM was introduced based on postnatal neuroimaging studies. In this classification DWM is separated into the classic malformation, the Dandy-Walker variant (small defect in the cerebellar vermis without dilatation of the cisterna magna) and mega-cisterna magna (large cisterna Magna without cerebellar abnormalities).[113,146] The diagnosis of the more severe malformation—the Dandy-Walker malformation (DWM)—is made based on an enlarged cisterna magna, a significant hypoplasia of the cerebellum, absence of the cerebellar vermis, enlarged 4th ventricle, and, at times, is associated with various degrees of ventriculomegaly of the lateral ventricles and/or agenesis of the corpus callosum and even holoprosencephaly (Fig. 18-20a,b). The diagnosis of the less severe form—the Dandy-Walker variant (DWV)—demonstrates mild dilatation of the cisterna magna and a small defect in the cerebellar vermis

without dysplastic cerebellar hemispheres. It is customary to make the diagnosis of DWM if the posterior fossa, the 4th ventricle, and the cerebellar hemispheres are normal, but the 4th ventricles visibly communicates with the cerebello-peduncular cistern. The diagnosis of Dandy-Walker Complex can be reliably made starting the 14th week, however, it was detected even earlier using TVS. A cisterna magna of 10 mm or more should trigger serious investigation.

The incidence of DWM at birth is about 1 in 38,000 live births, however, it may be present in as many as 12% of all cases of infants with hydrocephalus.[147] The pathogenesis of DWM is not yet fully elucidated. One of the theories is that of an imbalance in the production of the CSF between structures below and above the aqueduct (of Sylvius).[148]

In Dandy-Walker complex there appears to be both genetic and etiologic heterogenity. Abnormalities associated with DWM include autosomal recessive diseases such as Walker-Warburg syndrome, Ellis-van-Creveld syndrome, Meckel-Gruber syndrome; X-linked dominant syndromes such as Aicardi's syndrome; numerous chromosomal abnormalities; environmental abnormalities, such as infections, alcohol, and diabetes; multifactorial abnormalities, such as neural tube defects; and congenital heart disease. DWM symptoms may occur sporadically as in holoprosencephaly, deLange's syndrome, kidney, facial and digital abnormalities, and Goldenhar syndrome, among others. Recurrence risk is high when DWM is the result of a single gene defect such as the autosomal recessive Warburg and Meckel-Gruber syndrome. But the recurrence risk is low (1–5%) if not part of a mendelian disorder.[149]

Mortality rates are reported to be high in infants; however, due to the low incidence of this anomaly, only limited series were published. The mental capacity of survivors is low in the majority of the cases.[147,149–151] Ulm et al.[152] studied 14 fetuses with DWM or DWV diagnosed before 21 weeks and 14 with the diagnosis made after 21 weeks. In the early group 8 in 14 (57%) had other anomalies, and 7 in 14 (50%) had chromosomal anomalies compared with 5 in 14 (36%), and 1 in 14 (7%). They concluded that antenatal diagnosis made before 21 weeks of gestation had a worse prognosis than when the diagnosis was made later in gestation.

HYDROCEPHALY AND VENTRICULOMEGALY

Ventriculomegaly refers to a dilatation of the lateral ventricles in the presence of normal intraventricular pressure of the cerebro-spinal-fluid (CSF). In contrast, hydrocephaly is more than just ventriculomegaly, since there is an increased amount of pressure exerted by the CSF causing increasing fetal head size and thinning of the brain tissue (Fig. 18-21). The incidence of hydrocephaly in live births is 0.5–3/1,000.[153] Hydrocephaly can be divided into 2 general groups namely noncommunicating and communicating hydrocephaly. The etiologies of noncommunicating hydrocephaly are aqueductal stenosis, Dandy-Walker malformation, or various space-occupying masses exerting pressure on the aqueduct. Communicating hydrocephaly, can occur as a result of or in

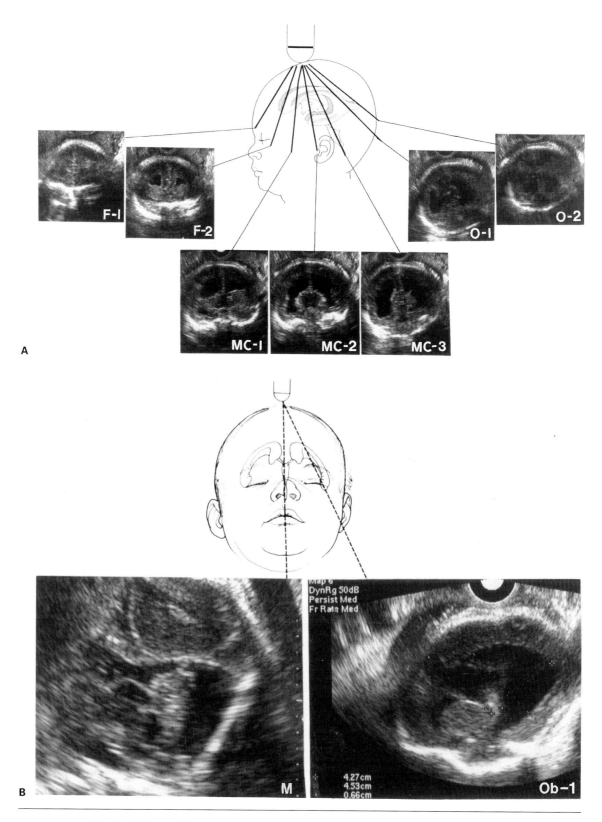

FIGURE 18-20 Dandy Walker malformation in a 36-week fetus with a mosaic trisomy karyotype. **(A)** The 7 sections through the "coronal" planes (F—frontal; MC—mid-coronal; O—occipital). **(B)** The median an oblique-1 sections (M—Median; OB—oblique).

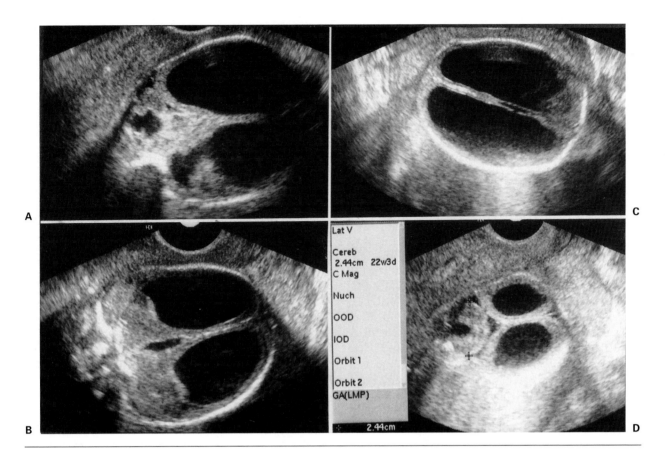

FIGURE 18-21 Severe oligohydramnios and communicating hydrocephalus at 22 weeks and 3 days in a 16-year, class C diabetic mother. At 26 weeks intrauterine fetal demises was noted. **(A)**, **(B)**, and **(D)** are coronal sections obtained transvaginally. **(C)** is a horizontal section.

association with Arnold-Chiari malformation, encephalocele, congenital absence of arachnoid granulations, inflammatory processes, and lissencephaly.[154,155]

Aqueductal stenosis may develop around 15–18 postmenstrual weeks of gestation. In almost three fourths of the cases, the reason for the obstruction of the flow through the aqueduct can be found. In about 2% of all cases, the disease may be inherited—an X-linked recessive disorder affecting males transmitted through female carriers.[156,157] There are several mutations in the gene encoding for the cell adhesion molecule L1CAM located at Xq28 reported in families with X-linked hydrocephaly (see agenesis of the corpus callosum).[158]

Early diagnosis of ventriculomegaly or hydrocephalus is and probably will remain a challenge to the ultrasonographer.[20,23,51,159,160] At the beginning of the second trimester in a normal fetus the size of the lateral ventricle is relatively large. But, as gestation progresses, the ratio of the hemispheric width to the ventricular width progressively diminishes and at around 28 weeks, it stabilizes and occupies about one third of this distance.

Sonography has made it possible to actually measure the size of the lateral ventricles within the fetal brain. Using ultrasonography they can be either assessed qualitatively or quantitatively.[20,23,48,51,159–162]

Qualitative assessment is highly subjective and an experienced sonologist or sonographer can detect ventriculomegaly by either of the following approaches:

1. *The gestalt* approach, whereby the sonographer and the sonologist appraise the degree of dilatation by relying on their experience and the appearance of the anomaly.

2. *Using indirect signs of dilatation of the ventricles.* Some of these indirect signs are the shape of the lateral ventricles, the thickness of the surrounding brain parenchyma, and the mobility of structures or parts of the lateral ventricle. These can be appreciated on sections that do not normally demonstrate the described pathological pictures—detection of the temporal horn on an oblique scan, which usually has to contain only the anterior and the posterior horns.

3. *Observing the appearance and the mobility of the choroid plexus.* If the choroid plexus is extremely thin and if it is seen "dangling" or "floating" freely within the dilated ventricle, this signifies a significant dilatation.[160,162]

4. *Observing and measuring the third ventricle.* Any time this structure is seen on an axial or a mid-coronal section, the suspicion of its dilated nature should be raised.

5. *Looking at the shape of the fetal cranium.* If the diagnosis is Arnold-Chiari Type II malformation, developing at a time when the cranium is still pliable, the bitemporal depression will create the "lemon shaped" skull. The herniation of the cerebellum in the posterior fossa will result in its banana-shaped deformity (Fig. 18-15).

Obviously quantitative methods hinge upon actual measurements of the fetal lateral ventricles.[23,48,161] Classically, measuring the size of the lateral ventricles have been performed on an axial section of the fetal head. In this section, the distance between the midline and the inner bony skull representing the hemispheric widths (HW) is compared to the measurement from the midline to the lateral wall of the lateral ventricles (LVW). As said before, this ratio decreases from about 70% at 20 weeks to about 28–30% at around 30 weeks gestational age. Thereafter it is extremely stable to term.

The average LVW/HW ratio at 15 weeks is about 71% and by 37 weeks, it is 29%, this reflects the rapid growth of the cerebral hemispheres as pregnancy progresses. The diagnosis of fetal hydrocephalus relies upon a BPD greater than 11 cm or a head circumference to abdominal circumference ratio (HC/AC) greater than 2.0. Nomograms for evaluation of the lateral ventricular width to the hemispheric width ratio are available.

It is possible with transabdominal sonography to measure the anterior horn of the lateral ventricles as well as the portion of the anterior horn found anterior to the interventricular foramen. Its relative size is decreasing with advanced gestational age. Nomograms of the cerebral-to-frontal horn distance throughout the pregnancy are also available and may indicate a ventriculomegaly.

The atrium of the lateral ventricles can also be measured on the axial plane used for the measurement of the BPD. This can be recognized by the echogenic choroid plexus within it. Measurements such as the cerebral atrial distance, the atrial width/hemispheric width ratio, and the atrial width/cerebral atrial distance ratio throughout pregnancy were determined and are available. These measurements can be considered an indication of the dilatation of the lateral ventricles in the fetus.

The increase in the size of the posterior occipital horn of the lateral ventricles may be the most indicative of ventriculomegaly. These can be imaged on a horizontal plane that is normally used for the measurement of the BPD.

Our group developed 9 nomograms to define the lateral ventricles between 14 and 40 weeks gestation using transvaginal sonography. A total of 7 measurements of the fetal lateral ventricles were used to generate these nomograms.[23,51]

The earliest changes in the size of the lateral ventricle during the formation of the ventriculomegaly or hydrocephaly are the dilatation of the posterior horns and the compression or the thinning of the choroid plexus. The change in size or the increase in the posterior horn can be detected on the longitudinal and coronal sections of the ultrasound picture. When a fetus suspected of having ventriculomegaly is scanned using TVS, the most useful and efficient section to obtain is the right or the left Oblique-1 section, from which the thickness of the choroid plexus as well as the size of the posterior horn can be easily measured. The ratio of the choroid plexus-to-the height of the posterior horn is the most sensitive measure of the colpocephaly or dilatation of the posterior horns.

If prenatal diagnosis of ventriculomegaly and hydrocephaly are made, this should prompt a careful sonographic evaluation of the fetus as well as chromosomal studies to rule out or to make a diagnosis of diseases associated with chromosomal anomalies. Approximately 70–80% of fetuses with hydrocephaly will have associated structural anomalies. Approximately 60% of these are extra-cranial, cardiac, or renal anomalies. The association of hydrocephaly with chromosomal abnormalities has been reported to range between 4% and 28%.

Several articles have dealt with the long-term outcome of fetal hydrocephaly. In Table 18-2, seven recent articles dealing with long-term follow-up shows that anywhere between 20–59% of fetus with hydrocephaly will have a good outcome. McCullogh et al.[163] studied the outcome of shunted hydrocephaly and found that 32 of 37 (86%) attempts resulted in success with 17 infants having an IQ >80 and in 6 with an IQ between 65–80. In another study from the University of Washington the IQ ≥80 was found in 16 of 19 infants.[164] Sutton et al[165] studied the outcome of neonatal hydrocephaly

TABLE 18-2 | **LONG TERM OUTCOME OF FETAL HYDROCEPHALUS**

Author	Year	Number	Follow Months/Year	Good Outcome No. (%)	Comments
Vintzileos[223]	1989	9	18 months	4/9 (44%)	
Drugan[171]	1989	26	28 months	8/26 (31%)	
Anhoury[224]	1991	20	2 months	4/20 (20%)	
Hanigan[225]	1991	14	18 months	4/14 (29%)	All aqueductal stenosis
Hudgins[168]	1988	22	3.5 years	13/22 (59%)	Non-progressive
Rosseau[226]	1992	32	2.5–4 years	15/32 (47%)	Non-progressive
Kirkinen[227]	1996	24	10 years	9/24 (38%)	

TABLE 18-3 | **NEONATAL OUTCOME OF FETUSES WITH MINIMAL FETAL LATERAL VENTRICULOMEGALY (MFLVM)**[a]

Author	No. With F/u	Abnormal Karyotype	Other Malformations	Abortion/ Fetal Demise/ Neonatal Demise	Survivors Normal Development	Survivors Abnormal Development	Comments
Goldstein[172]	13	1/13 (7%)	—	5/13 (38%)	6/8 (75%)	2 (25%)	—
	42	5/42 (16%)	42/42 (100%)	35/42 (83%)	3/7 (43%)	4 (57%)	
Drugan[171]	5	—	—	—	5 (100%)	—	Borderline
	6	—	—	—	3 (60%)	2 (40%)	Isolated
Bromley[173]	44	5/44 (11%)	17/44 (39%)	8/44 (18%)	26/36 (74%)	10/36 (26%)	30% Polyhydramnios
Achiron[174]	8	2/8 (25%)	2/8 (25%)	4/8 (50%)	3/4 (75%)	1/4 (25%)	—
Patel[175]	28	—	—	—	22/28 (65%)	6/28 (35%)	If 10–11 mm 90% were normal
Mahoney[170]	20	1/20 (5%)	—	8/20 (40%)	8/12 (66%)	4/12 (34%)	—
Hudgins[170]	22	—	—	3/22 (14%)	13/19 (68%)	6/19 (32%)	Isolated
	25	—	25	25/25 (100%)	—	—	
Total	213	14/213 (6.5%)	61/213 (40%)	66/213 (41%)	89/124 (72%)	48/124 (28%)	

[a] Best documented articles 1988–1994.

by measuring the thickness of the cortical mantle. In 10 infants followed by CT with virtual absence of cerebral tissue 5 showed no improvement after shunting. However, in 5 infants with severe hydrocephaly and some anterior horn tissue there was a remarkable improvement after shunting, with normal or slightly delayed neurological outcome.

Outcome statistics for fetal hydrocephaly shows a long-term survival rate of 50–90% with 30–60% of the infants having normal mental development.[166–168] Mortality rates for all cases of hydrocephaly is around 60–70%. Gupta et al.[169] found 21 reports in the English literature with a total of 360 cases of isolated fetal ventriculomegaly. Of these 81 has additional anomalies not diagnosed prenatally with a survival rate of 23% of which only 3% were normal. Of the 279 with isolated ventriculomegaly 63% survived and of the survivors 63% were normal and 27% had severe motor delay.

Recently an increasing concern over the significance of borderline or mild fetal ventriculomegaly (MFVM) has emerged. Mild dilation of the fetal ventricles is defined as a ventricle measuring 10–15 mm[168,170–175] on the "classical" axial section of the fetal head. Table 18-3 lists the best documented articles dealing with MFLVM between 1988 and 1994. Using these articles to make several generalizations, we find that in this group of fetuses with MFVM the incidence of other malformations is about 40%, and that of chromosomal aneuploidy is approximately 7%. In addition, a large number of pregnancies approximately 40% will result in abortion, fetal demise, or neonatal death. Of the survivors, about 70% will develop normal, and approximately 30% will have developmental problems.

In conclusion, the most important determinants in fetal ventriculomegaly or hydrocephalus are the presence of associated malformation or aneuploidy.

CYSTIC BRAIN LESIONS: CHOROID PLEXUS CYSTS, ARACHNOID CYSTS, PORENCEPHALY/SCHIZENCEPHALY

Choroid plexus cysts are among the most common sonographic findings during the second trimester of pregnancy with an approximate incidence of 0.95%. Choroid plexus cysts are typically benign and asymptomatic and disappear by the 24th postmenstrual week, and may be associated with an abnormal fetal karyotype. Various associations of the choroid plexus cysts were described and published including chromosomal aneuploidies.[176–185] We defer from discussing these aspects of the choroid plexuses. Their sonographic appearance is simple: a sonolucent structure of various sizes, unilateral or bilateral and have various shapes (Fig. 18-22). Choroid plexus cysts can be detected using TVS as early as the 11th–12th weeks of the gestation.

Arachnoid cysts are most commonly located above the tentorium of the cerebellum, however, they may also occur below the tentorium. Similarly, to the choroid plexus cysts, they consist of cerebrospinal (CSF) filled spaces. Arachnoid cysts are space occupying lesions of various sizes and are benign in nature. They do not connect with the cerebral ventricles. Sonographically, their borders are smooth and the content is sonolucent. The left side of the brain is more commonly affected. More than half are located in the middle cranial fossa, approximately 10% are in a potentially dangerous area namely the suprasellar cistern, about 10% grow in the quadrigeminal cistern, only 5–10% are seen in the posterior fossa.[186] Those cysts in the posterior fossa have to be differentiated from the DWM. At times, the differential diagnosis of arachnoid cysts present problems: large choroid plexus cysts, porencephalic cysts, and vein of Galen malformations must be considered. Its association with chromosomal syndromes is rare, however arachnoid

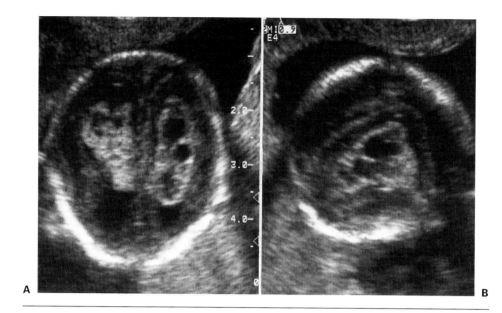

FIGURE 18-22 Multiple bilateral choroid plexus cysts were imaged using transvaginal ultrasound probe. (**A**) horizontal section; (**B**) sagittal section.

cysts may occur with other CNS or non-CNS anomalies. If the cyst is "strategically" located to block CSF circulation, it may cause hydrocephaly. The long-term outcome of arachnoid cysts is dependent on its location, however, it is generally considered good. If they are located on the convexity of the brain (e.g., temporal lobe) or between the hemispheres (Fig. 18-23) the outcome is considered good.[187] The treatment is surgical: excision, shunting, or creating an escape for the fluid in the cyst into the arachnoid space.[188] As in any other CNS anomaly, genetic counseling, and testing should be offered to the patient.

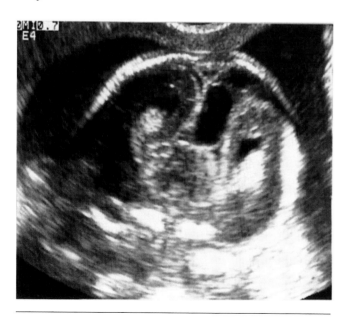

FIGURE 18-23 Interhemispheric left sided arachnoid cyst at 17 post-menstrual weeks.

Porencephaly refers to a sonolucent cystic structure amidst the substance of the fetal brain that likely results from an extensive destruction of the brain, communicating with the ventricles. Porencephalic cysts may be solitary or multiple and usually have irregularly shaped walls as well as some "debris" within the cavity (Fig. 18-24). Neurological deficit in the newborn or infant is usually the rule.

Porencephaly may be the end result of fetal intracranial hemorrhage. Intracranial hemorrhage rarely occurs in utero. Grant et al.,[189] published the transformation of hemorrhage in the intraparenchymal brain tissue into porencephalic cysts. They may be caused by hypoxemia, congenital vascular defects, blood clotting defects, ingestion of drugs, maternal complications, and thrombosis of the umbilical cord or its entanglement.[190–195] At times, trauma may also result in intracranial hemorrhage.[159,160] Periventricular hemorrhage may also occur in utero, however, its incidence is not known.

The neurodevelopmental prognosis of fetuses with intracranial hemorrhages is grossly unknown and it is related to the severity and the location of the hemorrhage. Intracerebellar hemorrhage was also reported[189,196] and are said to appear as echogenic masses in the posterior fossa, namely the area of the cerebellum. Their differential diagnosis is a tumor in the posterior fossa. Unfavorable outcome of all the cases published in the literature is evident. Subdural hemorrhages have been reported and connected to trauma sustained during the prenatal period.[197,198]

Schizencephaly is a CNS malformation in which the lateral brain ventricles communicate with the subarachnoid space and are lined with gray matter covered with pia-ependymal layer. In contrast to the arachnoid cyst, which does not connect to other structures and the porencephaly with connection only to the ventricles, *schizencephaly* appears wedge-shaped with

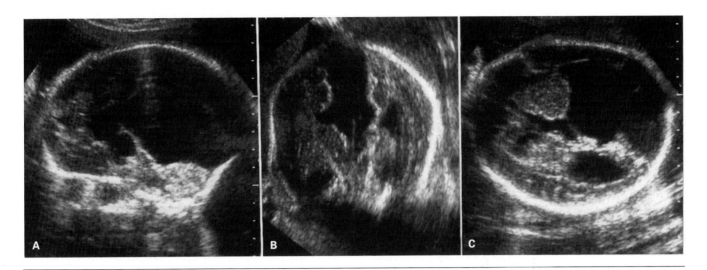

FIGURE 18-24 Porencephalic cyst of a fetus at 34 weeks. **(A)** Median section; **(B)** Coronal section; **(C)** Horizontal section.

their apex pointing toward the periphery. They may be uni-lateral or bilateral and appear along the course of the middle cerebral artery—the lateral sulcus. The occlusion of this artery may play a role in the generation of this cleft.[199] The differential diagnosis includes holoprosencephaly arachnoid cysts (bilateral) and hydranencephaly, and can be associated with ventriculomegaly, AGCC, absent cavum septi pellucidi, and septo-optic dysplasia. The prognosis is dependent on the type and the extent of the lesion.

FETAL BRAIN TUMORS

At birth, fetal brain tumors represent less than 1% of all fetal tumors. Most are teratomas, craniopharyngiomas, and hemangioblastomas.[200] The teratomas of the fetal brain usually arise from the pineal gland and distort the third ventricle. Hydrocephaly is the rule, since the space occupying lesion obliterates the flow of the CSF. Sonographically, they may appear as cystic with hyperechoic areas or foci.

Intracranial teratomas have been prenatally diagnosed.[201–208] At times, it is hard to identify the structures in general or the midline structures which usually present the point of reference in the localization of pathological structures in the brain. This is due to the distortion created by the tumor. In addition, distortion of the cranium, the face, and the orbits may also be seen. Fetal hydrops and high-output cardiac failure are also described.[207] The prognosis for the fetus as well as the neonate is not good. For the neonate prognosis depends on the size of the tumor, the extent of brain destruction, the degree of hydrocephalus, and other associated effects of the tumor itself. Some infants with intracranial teratomas have survived up to 1.5 years of age, but are severely neurologically impaired and subsequent demise is unavoidable.

Choroid plexus papillomas are rare and benign tumors of the choroid plexus.[209,210] However, this tumor may cause hydrocephaly due to its space-occupying nature or overproduction of the CSF. Sonographic examination is usu-

ally able to localize and therefore determine the nature of the lesion originating from within the ventricles.

In-Utero Infection: Effects on the Fetal Brain

Maternal infection usually reaches the fetal CNS through transplacental passage. Toxoplasmosis, rubella, cytomegalovirus, and herpes—the TORCH infections—are the most common and documented infections. Sonographic findings resulting from infections include microcephaly, hydrocephaly, intracranial hyperechogenicities (? calcifications ?), cerebellar hypoplasia, an enlarged cerebello-penducular cistern, periventricular cysts, and ischemic destructive sequelae, such as porencephaly, hydranencephaly, and polymicrogyria.[211–217] It is important to note that these intracranial, hyperechoic foci, or calcifications do not cast an acoustic shadow.[218]

In-utero diagnosis of *cytomegalo virus (CMV) infection* needs to rely on a combination of diagnostic tests such as serology, amniotic fluid, cultures, and ultrasonography. Although sonographic diagnosis is feasible, this may not be obvious before the second trimester at which time, lesions within the liver should also be looked for.

The sonographic findings of fetal intracranial *toxoplasmosis* include the intracranial calcifications, hydrocephaly, microcephaly, brain atrophy, and hydranencephaly.[219] Hydrocephaly may be present in almost 75% of the cases, however, intracranial calcifications are present in a minority of the cases (less than 20%). If intracranial calcifications are present, they are multifocal and located in the periventricular area, the white matter, the cortex, and the basal ganglia. One may consider other extracranial sonographic findings such as a thick placenta, liver echogenicities, hepatomegaly, ascites, and pericardial or pleural effusion.[217,220]

Rubella infections create subtle changes in the fetal brain tissue, in which case, high-frequency transducers—TVS—may be beneficial. Rubella may also cause sonographically detectable pathology in the fetal brain. These are subependymal-dependent cysts in the caudate nucleus, echogenic foci in the basal ganglia, and microcephaly.[221,222] Other indirect signs, such as dilatation of the ventricles or microcephaly, can be detected using high TAS.

CONCLUSION

The field of prenatal diagnosis exists largely due to ultrasound. Ultrasound, a noninvasive, relative inexpensive, and easy-to-master tool has allowed prenatal diagnosis to develop into an important specialty. Both transabdominal and transvaginal sonography yield a tremendous amount of information about the developing human fetus in general and recently about the fetal brain, in particular. We feel that fetal neurosonography at all ages should be part of the structural evaluation of the fetus.

References

1. Babcock DS, Han BK, LeQuesne GW. B-mode gray scale ultrasound of the head in the newborn and young infant. *Am J Roentg.* 1980;134:457–468.
2. Johnson ML, Rumack CM. Ultrasonic evaluation of the neonatal brain. *Radiol Clin N Am.* 1980;18:117–131.
3. Ben-Ora A, Eddy L, Hatch G, et al. The anterior fontanelle as an acoustic window to the neonatal ventricular system. *J Clin Ultrasound.* 1980;8:65–67.
4. Dewbury KC, Aluwihare AP. The anterior fontanelle as an ultrasound window for study of the brain: a preliminary report. *Br J Radiol.* 1980;53:81–84.
5. Grant EG, Schellinger D, Borts FT, et al. Real-time sonography of the neonatal and infant head. *Am J Roentg.* 1981;136:265–270.
6. Slovis TL, Kuhns LR. Real-time sonography of the brain through the anterior fontanelle. *AJR. Am J Roentg.* 1981;136:277–286.
7. Edwards MK, Brown DL, Muller J, et al. Cribside neurosonography: real-time sonography for intracranial investigation of the neonate. *Am J Roentg.* 1981;136:271–275.
8. Richardson J, Grant E. Scanning techniques and normal anatomy. In: Grant E, ed. *Neurosonography of the Pre-term Neonate.* New York: Springer-Verlag; 1986.
9. Naidich TP, Yousefzadeh DK, Gusnard DA. Sonography of the normal neonatal head: supratentorial structures: state-of-the-art imaging. *Neuroradiol.* 1986;28:408–427.
10. Timor-Tritsch IE, Farine D, Rosen MG. A close look at early embryonic development with the high-frequency transvaginal transducer. *Am J Obstet Gynecol.* 1988;159:676–681.
11. Kushnir U, Shalev J, Bronshtein M, et al. Fetal intracranial anatomy in the first trimester of pregnancy: transvaginal ultrasonographic evaluation. *Neuroradiol.* 1989;31:222–225.
12. Timor-Tritsch IE, Monteagudo A, Warren WB. Transvaginal ultrasonographic definition of the central nervous system in the first and early second trimesters. *Am J Obstet Gynecol.* 1991;164:497–503.
13. Warren WB, Timor-Tritsch I, Peisner DB, et al. Dating the early pregnancy by sequential appearance of embryonic structures. *Am J Obstet Gynecol.* 1989;161:747–753.
14. Timor-Tritsch IE, Peisner DB, Raju S. Sonoembryology: an organ-oriented approach using a high-frequency vaginal probe. *J Clin Ultrasound.* 1990;18:286–298.
15. Timor-Tritsch I, Blumenfeld Z, Rottem S. Sonoembryology. In: Timor-Tritsch I, Rottem S, eds. *Transvaginal Sonography.* New York: Chapman & Hall; 1991.

16. Timor-Tritsch IE, Monteagudo A. Transvaginal sonographic evaluation of the fetal central nervous system. *Obstet Gynecol Clin N Am.* 1991;18:713–748.
17. Achiron R, Achiron A. Transvaginal ultrasonic assessment of the early fetal brain. *Ultrasound Obstet Gynecol.* 1991;1:336–344.
18. Blaas HG, Eik-Nes SH, Kiserud T, et al. Early development of the forebrain and midbrain: a longitudinal ultrasound study from 7 to 12 postmenstrual weeks of gestation. *Ultrasound Obstet Gynecol.* 1994;4:183–192.
19. Blaas HG, Eik-Nes SH, Kiserud T, et al. Early development of the hindbrain: a longitudinal ultrasound study from 7 to 12 weeks of gestation [see comments]. *Ultrasound Obstet Gynecol.* 1995;5:151–160.
20. Monteagudo A, Reuss ML, Timor-Tritsch IE. Imaging the fetal brain in the second and third trimesters using transvaginal sonography. *Obstet Gynecol.* 1991;77:27–32.
21. Blaas HG, Eik-Nes SH, Kiserud T, et al. Three-dimensional imaging of the brain cavities in human embryos [see comments]. *Ultrasound Obstet Gynecol.* 1995;5:228–323.
22. Monteagudo A, Timor-Tritsch I, Reuss M, et al. Transvaginal sonography of the second and third trimester fetal brain. In: Timor-Tritsch I, Rottem S, eds. *Transvaginal Sonography.* New York: Chapman & Hall; 1991.
23. Monteagudo A, Timor-Tritsch IE, Moomjy M. Nomograms of the fetal lateral ventricles using transvaginal sonography. *J Ultrasound Med.* 1993;12:265–269.
24. Timor-Tritsch IE, Monteagudo A. Transvaginal fetal neurosonography: standardization of the planes and sections used by anatomic landmarks. *Ultrasound Obstet Gynecol.* 1996;8:42–47.
25. Malinger G, Zakut H. The corpus callosum: normal fetal development as shown by transvaginal sonography. *AJR. Am J Roentg.* 1993;161:1041–1043.
26. Monteagudo A, Timor-Tritsch I. Development of fetal gyri, sulci and fissures: a transvaginal sonographic study. *Ultrasound Obstet Gynecol.* 1997;9:422–428.
27. Monteagudo A, Timor-Tritsch I. Transvaginal fetal neurosonography: the second and third trimesters of pregnancy. In: Chervenak F, Kurjak A, Comstock C, eds. *Ultrasound and the Fetal Brain.* New York: Parthenon; 1995.
28. Cohen H, Ziprkowski M. New diagnostic insight in pediatric neurosonography. *Diagn Imag.* 1991;3:142–146.
29. Grant E, Richardson J. Infant and neonatal neurosonography technique and normal anatomy. In: Taveras J, ed. *Diagnosis Imaging Intervention.* Vol 3. Philadelphia: Lippincott; 1994.
30. O'Rahilly R, Muller F. Ventricular system and choroid plexuses of the human brain during the embryonic period proper. *Am J Anat.* 1990;189:285–302.
31. O'Rahilly R, Muller F. Embryonic length and cerebral landmarks in staged human embryos. *Anatomical Record.* 1984;209:265–271.
32. Westergaard E. The lateral cerebral ventricles of human fetuses with a crown-rump length of 26–178 MM. *Acta Anat.* 1971;79:409–421.
33. Lemire R, Loeser J, Leech R, et al. *Normal and Abnormal Development of the Human Nervous System.* New York: Harper & Row; 1975.
34. Pilu G, Sandri A, Perolo A, et al. Sonography of fetal agenesis of the corpus callosum: a survey of 35 cases. *Ultrasound Obstet Gynecol.* 1993;3:318–329.
35. Hernanz-Schulman M, Dohan FC Jr, Jones T, et al. Sonographic appearance of callosal agenesis: correlation with radiologic and pathologic findings. *Am J Neuroradiol.* 1985;6:361–368.
36. Babcock DS. The normal, absent, and abnormal corpus callosum: sonographic findings. *Radiology.* 1984;151:449–453.
37. Chi JG, Dooling EC, Gilles FH. Gyral development of the human brain. *Ann Neurol.* 1977;1:86–93.
38. Dorovini-Zis K, Dolman CL. Gestational development of brain. *Arch Pathol Lab Med.* 1977;101:192–195.

39. Nomina Anatomica. N. Authorized by the 12th International Congress of Anatomists. London, 1985. Edinburgh: Churchill Livingstone, 1989.

40. Denkhaus H, Winsberg F. Ultrasonic measurement of the fetal ventricular system. *Radiology.* 1979;131:781–787.

41. Goldstein I, Reece EA, Pilu G, et al. Cerebellar measurements with ultrasonography in the evaluation of fetal growth and development. *Am J Obstet Gynecol.* 1987;156:1065–1069.

42. Hill LM, Guzick D, Fries J, et al. The transverse cerebellar diameter in estimating gestational age in the large for gestational age fetus. *Obstet Gynecol.* 1990;75:981–985.

43. Laing F, Stamler C, Jeffrey B. Ultrasonography of the fetal subarachnoid space. *J Ultrasound Med.* 1983;2:29–32.

44. Goldstein I, Reece E, Pilu G, et al. Sonographic evaluation of the normal developmental anatomy of the fetal cerebral ventricles: The frontal horn: part I. *Obstet Gynecol.* 1988;72:588–592.

45. Pilu G, Reece EA, Goldstein I, et al. Sonographic evaluation of the normal developmental anatomy of the fetal cerebral ventricles: The atria: part II. *Obstet Gynecol.* 1989;73:250–256.

46. Goldstein I, Reece E, Pilu G, et al. Sonographic evaluation of the normal developmental anatomy of the fetal cerebral ventricles: the posterior horn: part IV. *Am J Perinatol.* 1990;7:79–83.

47. Goldstein I, Reece EA, Pilu G, et al. Sonographic assessment of the fetal frontal lobe: a potential tool for prenatal diagnosis of microcephaly. *Am J Obstet Gynecol* 1988;158:1057–1062.

48. Cardoza JD, Goldstein RB, Filly RA. Exclusion of fetal ventriculomegaly with a single measurement: the width of the lateral ventricular atrium. Radiology 1988;169:711–714.

49. Campbell S. Diagnosis of fetal abnormalities by ultrasound. In: Milunsky A, ed. *Genetic Disorders of the Fetus.* New York: Plenum Press; 1979.

50. Hadlock FP, Deter RL, Park SK. Real-time sonography: ventricular and vascular anatomy of the fetal brain in utero. *AJR. Am J Roentg.* 1981;136:133–137.

51. Monteagudo A, Timor-Tritsch IE, Moomjy M. In utero detection of ventriculomegaly during the second and third trimesters by transvaginal sonography. *Ultrasound Obstet Gynecol.* 1994;4:193–198.

52. Monteagudo A, Timor-Tritsch I. Sonographic evaluation of fetal cortical maturation. *J Ultrasound Med.* 1996;15:69.

53. Slagle TA, Oliphant M, Gross SJ. Cingulate sulcus development in preterm infants. *Pediatr Res.* 1989;26:598–602.

54. Martin J. *Neuroanatomy: Text and Atlas.* New York: Elsevier; 1989.

55. Predanic M, Zudenigo D, Funduk-Kurjak B, et al. Assessment of early normal pregnancy. In: Kurjak A, ed. *An Atlas of Transvaginal Color Doppler: The Current State of the Art.* London: Parthenon, 1994.

56. van den Wijngaard JA, Groenenberg IA, Wladimiroff JW, et al. Cerebral Doppler ultrasound of the human fetus. *Br J Obstet Gynecol.* 1989;96:845–849.

57. Wladimiroff JW, van den Wijngaard JA, Degani S, et al. Cerebral and umbilical arterial blood flow velocity waveforms in normal and growth-retarded pregnancies. *Obstet Gynecol.* 1987;69:705–709.

58. Vyas S, Nicolaides KH, Bower S, et al. Middle cerebral artery flow velocity waveforms in fetal hypoxemia. *Br J Obstet Gynecol.* 1990;97:797–803.

59. Mari G, Moise KJ Jr, Deter RL, et al. Doppler assessment of the pulsatility index in the cerebral circulation of the human fetus. *Am J Obstet Gynecol.* 1989;160:698–703.

60. Hata K, Hata T, Makihara K, et al. Fetal intracranial arterial hemodynamics assessed by color and pulsed Doppler ultrasound. *Internat J Gynaecol Obstet.* 1991;35:139–145.

61. Ferrazzi E, Gementi P, Bellotti M, et al. Doppler velocimetry: critical analysis of umbilical, cerebral and aortic reference values. *Eur J Obstet Gynecol Reprod Biol.* 1991;38:189–196.

62. Satoh S, Koyanagi T, Hara K, et al. Developmental characteristics of blood flow in the middle cerebral artery in the human fetus in utero, assessed using the linear-array pulsed Doppler method. *Early Human Dev.* 1988;17:195–203.

63. Veille JC, Hanson R, Tatum K. Longitudinal quantitation of middle cerebral artery blood flow in normal human fetuses. *Am J Obstet Gynecol.* 1993;169:1393–1398.

64. Mari G, Deter RL. Middle cerebral artery flow velocity waveforms in normal and small-for-gestational-age fetuses [see comments]. *Am J Obstet Gynecol.* 1992;166:1262–1270.

65. Meerman RJ, van Bel F, van Zwieten PH, et al. Fetal and neonatal cerebral blood velocity in the normal fetus and neonate: a longitudinal Doppler ultrasound study. *Early Human Dev.* 1990;24:209–217.

66. Degani S, Lewinsky R. Fetal and neonatal circulation in ultrasonography of the prenatal and neonatal brain. In: Timor-Tritsch I, Monteagudo A, Cohen H, eds. *Ultrasonography of the Prenatal and Neonatal Brain.* Stamford, CT: Appleton & Lange; 1996;387–403.

67. Jones K. *Smith's Recognizable Patterns of Human Malformations.* Philadelphia: Saunders, 1997.

68. Carter CO, Evans KA, Till K. Spinal dysraphism: genetic relation to neural tube malformations. *J Med Genet.* 1976;13:434–450.

69. Carter CO, Roberts JAF. The risk of recurrence after two children with central-nervous-system malformations. *Lancet.* 1967;I:306–308.

70. ACOG TB. Alpha-fetoprotein. April, 154, 1991.

71. Mills J, Scott J, Kirke P, et al. Homocysteine and neural tube defects. *J Nutr.* 1996;126:756S–760S.

72. Greene ND, Copp AJ. Inositol prevents folate-resistant neural tube defects in the mouse [see comments]. *Nature Med.* 1997;3:60–66.

73. O'Rahilly R, Muller F. *The Nervous System: Human Embryology and Teratology.* New York: Wiley-Liss Inc; 1992.

74. Marin-Padilla M. Cephalic axial skeletal-neural dysraphic disorders: embryology and pathology. *Can J Neurol Sciences.* 1991;18:153–169.

75. Muller F, O'Rahilly R. Cerebral dysraphia (future anencephaly) in a human twin embryo at stage 13. *Teratology.* 1984;30:167–177.

76. Muller F, O'Rahilly R. Development of anencephaly and its variants. *Am J Anat.* 1991;190:193–218.

77. Bronshtein M, Ornoy A. Acrania: anencephaly resulting from secondary degeneration of a closed neural tube: two cases in the same family. *J Clin Ultrasound.* 1991;19:230–234.

78. Rottem S, Bronshtein M, Thaler, et al. First trimester transvaginal sonographic diagnosis of fetal anomalies. *Lancet.* 1989;1:444–445.

79. Timor-Tritsch I, Greenebaum E, Monteagudo A, et al. Exencephalyanencephaly sequence: proof by ultrasound imaging and amniotic fluid cytology. *J Mat Fetal Med.* 1996;5:182–185.

80. Campbell S, Johnstone F, Holt E, et al. Anencephalus: early ultrasonic diagnosis and active management. *Lancet.* 1972;2:1226.

81. Rodriguez MM, Reik RA, Carreno TD, et al. Cluster of iniencephaly in Miami. *Pediatr Pathol.* 1991;11:211–221.

82. Aleksic S, Budzilovich G, Greco MA, et al. Iniencephaly: a neuropathologic study. *Clin Neuropathol.* 1983;2:55–61.

83. Foderaro AE, Abu-Yousef MM, Benda JA, et al. Antenatal ultrasound diagnosis of iniencephaly. *J Clin Ultrasound.* 1987;15:550–554.

84. Shoham Z, Caspi B, Chemke J, et al. Iniencephaly: prenatal ultrasonographic diagnosis—a case report. *J Perinat Med.* 1988;16:139–143.

85. Bronshtein M, Timor-Tritsch I, Rottem S. Early detection of fetal anomalies. In: Timor-Tritsch I, Rottem S, eds. *Transvaginal Sonography.* New York: Chapman & Hall; 1991;327–371.

86. Salonen R, Norio R. The Meckel syndrome in Finland: epidemiologic and genetic aspects. *A J Med Genet.* 1984;18:691–698.

87. Icenogle DA, Kaplan AM. A review of congenital neurologic malformations. *Clin Pediatr.* 1981;20:565–576.

88. Hidalgo H, Bowie J, Rosenberg ER, et al. Review: in utero sonographic diagnosis of fetal cerebral anomalies. *AJR Am J Roentg.* 1982;139:143–148.

89. Chervenak FA, Isaacson G, Mahoney MJ, et al. Diagnosis and management of fetal cephalocele. *Obstet Gynecol.* 1984;64:86–91.

90. Naidich TP, Altman NR, Braffman BH, et al. Cephaloceles and related malformations. *AJNR Am J Neuroradiol.* 1992;13:655–690.

91. Fleming AD, Vintzileos AM, Scorza WE. Prenatal diagnosis of occipital encephalocele with transvaginal sonography. *J Ultrasound Med.* 1991;10:285–286.

92. Monteagudo A. Cephalocele: anterior. *Fetus.* 1992;2:4–6.

93. Brown MS, Sheridan-Pereira M. Outlook for the child with a cephalocele. *Pediatr.* 1992;90:914–919.

94. Cullen MT, Athanassiadis AP, Romero R. Prenatal diagnosis of anterior parietal encephalocele with transvaginal sonography. *Obstet Gynecol.* 1990;75:489–491.

95. Yokota A, Kajiwara H, Kohchi M, et al. Parietal cephalocele: clinical importance of its atretic form and associated malformations. *J Neurosurg.* 1988;69:545–551.

96. Paavola P, Salonen R, Weissenbach J, et al. The locus for Meckel syndrome with multiple congenial anomalies maps to chromosome 17q21–q24. *Nature Genet.* 1995;11:213–215.

97. Pretorius DH, Russ PD, Rumack CM, et al. Diagnosis of brain neuropathology in utero. *Neuroradiol.* 1986;28:386–397.

98. Fiske CE, Filly RA. Ultrasound evaluation of the normal and abnormal fetal neural axis. *Radiol Clin N Am.* 1982;20:285–296.

99. Yen IH, Khoury MJ, Erickson JD, et al. The changing epidemiology of neural tube defects: United States, 1968–1989. *Am J Dis Child.* 1992;146:857–861.

100. Welch K, Winston K. Spina bifida. In: Myrianthopoulos N, ed. *Handbook of Clinical Neurology.* Vol 6. Amsterdam: Elsevier; 1987:477–508.

101. Main DM, Mennuti MT. Neural tube defects: issues in prenatal diagnosis and counseling. *Obstet Gynecol.* 1986;67:1–16.

102. Thornton JG, Lilford RJ, Newcombe RG. Tables for estimation of individual risks of fetal neural tube and ventral wall defects, incorporating prior probability, maternal serum alpha-fetoprotein levels, and ultrasonographic examination results [see comments]. *Am J Obstet Gynecol.* 1991;164:154–160.

103. Hogge WA, Thiagarajah S, Ferguson JE, et al. The role of ultrasonography and amniocentesis in the evaluation of pregnancies at risk for neural tube defects [see comments]. *Am J Obstet Gynecol.* 1989;161:520–3, discussion 523–524.

104. Blumenfeld Z, Siegler E, Bronshtein M. The early diagnosis of neural tube defects. *Prenat Diagn.* 1993;13:863–871.

105. Thiagarajah S, Henke J, Hogge WA, et al. Early diagnosis of spina bifida: the value of cranial ultrasound markers. *Obstet Gynecol.* 1990;76:54–57.

106. Nyberg DA, Mack LA, Hirsch J, et al. Abnormalities of fetal cranial contour in sonographic detection of spina bifida: evaluation of the "lemon" sign. *Radiology.* 1988;167:387–392.

107. Penso C, Redline RW, Benacerraf BR. A sonographic sign which predicts which fetuses with hydrocephalus have an associated neural tube defect. *J Ultrasound Med.* 1987;6:307–311.

108. van den Hof MC, Nicolaides KH, Campbell J, et al. Evaluation of the lemon and banana signs in one hundred thirty fetuses with open spina bifida. *Am J Obstet Gynecol.* 1990;162:322–327.

109. Goldstein RB, Podrasky AE, Filly RA, et al. Effacement of the fetal cisterna magna in association with myelomeningocele [see comments]. *Radiology.* 1989;172:409–413.

110. Pilu G, Romero R, Reece EA, et al. Subnormal cerebellum in fetuses with spina bifida. *Am J Obstet Gynecol.* 1988;158:1052–1056.

111. Volpe J. *Neuronal Proliferation, Migration, Organization and Myelination: Neurology of the Newborn.* Philadelphia: WB Saunders; 1995.

112. Matsunaga E, Shiota K. Holoprosencephaly in human embryos: epidemiologic studies of 150 cases. *Teratology.* 1977;16:261–272.

113. Pilu G, Perolo A, David C. Midline anomalies of the brain. In: Timor-Tritsch I, Monteagudo A, Cohen H, eds. *Ultrasonography of the Prenatal and Neonatal Brain.* Stamford, CT: Appleton & Lange; 1996.

114. Jones K. *Holoprosencephaly Sequence: Smith's Recognizable Patterns of Human Malformations.* Philadelphia: Saunders; 1997.

115. Pilu G, Sandri F, Perolo A, et al. Prenatal diagnosis of lobar holoprosencephaly. *Ultrasound Obstet Gynecol.* 1992;2:88–94.

116. Grogono JL. Children with agenesis of the corpus callosum. *Dev Med Child Neurol.* 1968;10:613–616.

117. Jellinger K, Gross H, Kaltenback E, et al. Holoprosencephaly and agenesis of the corpus callosum: frequency of associated malformations. *Acta Neuropathol.* 1981;55:1–10.

118. DeMyer W, Zeman W, Palmer CG. The face predicts the brain: diagnostic significance of medial facial anomalies for holoprosencephaly (arrhinencephaly). *Pediatr.* 1964;34:256–262.

119. Mulligan G, Meier P. Lipoma and agenesis of the corpus callosum with associated choroid plexus lipomas: in utero diagnosis. *J Ultrasound Med.* 1989;8:583–588.

120. Nyberg D, Pretorius D. Cerebral malformations. In: Nyberg D, Mahoney B, Pretorius D, eds. *Diagnostic Ultrasound of Fetal Anomalies: Text and Atlas.* Chicago, IL: Year Book Medical Publishers, Inc; 1990:82–202.

121. Filly RA, Chinn DH, Callen PW. Alobar holoprosencephaly: ultrasonographic prenatal diagnosis. *Radiology.* 1984;151:455–459.

122. Babcock DS. Sonography of congenital malformations of the brain. *Neuroradiol.* 1986;28:428–439.

123. Cohen MM Jr, Sulik KK. Perspectives on holoprosencephaly: central nervous system, craniofacial anatomy, syndrome commentary, diagnostic approach, and experimental studies: part II. *J Cranio Genet Dev Biol.* 1992;12:196–244.

124. Pilu G, Ambrosetto P, Sandri F, et al. Intraventricular fused fornices: a specific sign of fetal lobar holoprosencephaly. *Ultrasound Obstet Gynecol.* 1994;4:65–67.

125. Jeret JS, Serur D, Wisniewski K, et al. Frequency of agenesis of the corpus callosum in the developmentally disabled population as determined by computerized tomography. *Pediatr Neuroscience.* 1985;12:101–103.

126. Dobyns WB. Absence makes the search grow longer [editorial; comment]. *Am J Human Genet.* 1996;58:7–16.

127. Jones K. *Smith's Recognizable Patterns of Human Malformations.* Philadelphia: Saunders; 1997.

128. Bertino RE, Nyberg DA, Cyr DR, et al. Prenatal diagnosis of agenesis of the corpus callosum. *J Ultrasound Med.* 1988;7:251–260.

129. Rosenthal A, Jouet M, Kenwrick S. Aberrant splicing of neural cell adhesion molecule L1 mRNA in a family with X-linked hydrocephalus [published erratum appears in *Nat Genet.* 1993;3:273]. *Nat Genet.* 1992;2:107–112.

130. Fransen E, Vits L, Van Camp G, et al. The clinical spectrum of mutations in L1: a neuronal cell adhesion molecule. *Am J Med Genet.* 1996;64:73–77.

131. Jouet M, Kenwrick S. Gene analysis of L1 neural cell adhesion molecule in prenatal diagnosis of hydrocephalus. *Lancet.* 1995;345:161–162.

132. Jouet M, Moncla A, Paterson J, et al. New domains of neural cell-adhesion molecule L1 implicated in X-linked hydrocephalus and MASA syndrome. *Am J Human Genet.* 1995;56:1304–1314.

133. Ruiz JC, Cuppens H, Legius E, et al. Mutations in L1-CAM in two families with X linked complicated spastic paraplegia, MASA syndrome, and HSAS. *J Med Genet.* 1995;32:549–552.

134. Fransen E, Lemmon V, van Camp G, et al. CRASH syndrome: clinical spectrum of corpus callosum hypoplasia, retardation, adducted thumbs, spastic paraparesis and hydrocephalus due to mutations in one single gene, L1 [published erratum appears in *Eur J Hum Genet.* 1996;4:126]. *Eur J Human Genet.* 1995;3:273–284.

135. Kendall BE. Dysgenesis of the corpus callosum. *Neuroradiol.* 1983;25:239–256.

136. Barkovich AJ, Norman D. Anomalies of the corpus callosum: correlation with further anomalies of the brain. *AJR Am J Roentg.* 1988;151:171–179.

137. Atlas SW, Shkolnik A, Naidich TP. Sonographic recognition of agenesis of the corpus callosum. *AJR Am J Roentg.* 1985;145:167–173.

138. Hilpert PL, Kurtz AB. Prenatal diagnosis of agenesis of the corpus callosum using endovaginal ultrasound. *J Ultrasound Med.* 1990;9:363–365.

139. Gebarski SS, Gebarski KS, Bowerman RA, et al. Agenesis of the corpus callosum: sonographic features. *Radiology.* 1984;151:443–448.

140. Lockwood CJ, Ghidini A, Aggarwal R, et al. Antenatal diagnosis of partial agenesis of the corpus callosum: a benign cause of ventriculomegaly. *Am J Obstet Gynecol.* 1988;159:184–186.

141. Vergani P, Ghidini A, Mariani S, et al. Antenatal sonographic findings of agenesis of corpus callosum. *Am J Perinatol.* 1988;5:105–108.

142. Meizner I, Barki Y, Hertzanu Y. Prenatal sonographic diagnosis of agenesis of corpus callosum. *J Clin Ultrasound.* 1987;15:262–264.

143. Leech RW, Shuman RM. Holoprosencephaly and related midline cerebral anomalies: a review. *J Child Neurol.* 1986;1:3–18.

144. Poe L, Coleman L, Mahmud F. Congenital central nervous system anomalies. *Radiographics.* 1989;9:801–826.

145. Baarsma R, Martijn A, Okken A. The missing pericallosal artery on sonography: a sign of agenesis of the corpus callosum in the neonatal brain? *Neuroradiol.* 1987;29:47–49.

146. Barkovich AJ, Kjos BO, Norman D, et al. Revised classification of posterior fossa cysts and cystlike malformations based on the results of multiplanar MR imaging. *AJR. Am J Roentg.* 1989;153:1289–1300.

147. Osenbach R, Menezes A. Diagnosis and management of the Dandy-Walker malformation: 30 years of experience. *Pediatr Neurosurg.* 1991;18:179.

148. Gardner E, O'Rahilly R, Prolo D. The Dandy-Walker and Arnold-Chiari malformations: clinical, developmental, and teratological considerations. *Arch Neurol.* 1975;32:393–407.

149. Murray JC, Johnson JA, Bird TD. Dandy-Walker malformation: etiologic heterogeneity and empiric recurrence risks. *Clin Genet.* 1985;28:272–283.

150. Sawaya R, McLaurin RL. Dandy-Walker syndrome: clinical analysis of 23 cases. *J Neurosurg.* 1981;55:89–98.

151. Hirsch JF, Pierre-Kahn A, Renier D, et al. The Dandy-Walker malformation prenatal sonographic diagnosis and its clinical significance. *J Neurosurg.* 1984;61:515.

152. Ulm B, Deutinger J, Bernaschek G. Dandy-Walker malformation diagnosed before 21 weeks gestation: associated malformations and chromosomal abnormalities. *Ultrasound Obstet Gynecol.* 1997;10:167–170.

153. Habib Z. Genetics and genetic counseling in neonatal hydrocephalus. *Obstet Gynecol Surv.* 1981;36:529–534.

154. Mealey J Jr, Gilmor RL, Bubb MP. The prognosis of hydrocephalus overt at birth. *J Neurosurg.* 1973;39:348–355.

155. Burton BK. Recurrence risks for congenital hydrocephalus. *Clin Genet.* 1979;16:47–53.

156. Friedman JM, Santos-Ramos R. Natural history of X-linked aqueductal stenosis in the second and third trimesters of pregnancy. *Am J Obstet Gynecol.* 1984;150:104–106.

157. Brocard O, Ragage C, Vilbert M, et al. Prenatal diagnosis of X-linked hydrocephalus. *J Clin Ultrasound.* 1993;21:211–214.

158. Van Camp G, Vits L, Coucke P, et al. A duplication in the L1CAM gene associated with X- linked hydrocephalus. *Nat Genet.* 1993;4:421–425.

159. Benacerraf BR, Birnholz JC. The diagnosis of fetal hydrocephalus prior to 22 weeks. *J Clin Ultrasound.* 1987;15:531–536.

160. Bronshtein M, Ben-Shlomo I. Choroid plexus dysmorphism detected by transvaginal sonography: the earliest sign of fetal hydrocephalus. *J Clin Ultrasound.* 1991;19:547–553.

161. Pretorius DH, Drose JA, Manco-Johnson ML. Fetal lateral ventricular ratio determination during the second trimester. *J Ultrasound Med.* 1986;5:121–124.

162. Cardoza JD, Filly RA, Podrasky AE. The dangling choroid plexus: a sonographic observation of value in excluding ventriculomegaly. *AJR. Am J Roentg.* 1988;151:767–770.

163. McCullough DC, Balzer-Martin LA. Current prognosis in overt neonatal hydrocephalus. *J Neurosurg.* 1982;57:378–383.

164. Shurtleff DB, Foltz EL, Loeser JD. Hydrocephalus: a definition of its progression and relationship to intellectual function, diagnosis and complications. *Am J Dis Child.* 1973;125:688–693.

165. Sutton LN, Bruce DA, Schut L. Hydranencephaly versus maximal hydrocephalus: an important clinical distinction. *Neurosurg.* 1980;6:34–38.

166. Pretorius DH, Davis K, Manco-Johnson ML, et al. Clinical course of fetal hydrocephalus: 40 cases. *AJR. Am J Roentg.* 1985;144:827–831.

167. Nyberg DA, Mack LA, Hirsch J, et al. Fetal hydrocephalus: sonographic detection and clinical significance of associated anomalies. *Radiology.* 1987;163:187–191.

168. Hudgins RJ, Edwards MS, Goldstein R, et al. Natural history of fetal ventriculomegaly. *Pediatr.* 1988;82:692–697.

169. Gupta JK, Bryce FC, Lilford RJ. Management of apparently isolated fetal ventriculomegaly. *Obstet Gynecol Surv.* 1994;49:716–721.

170. Mahony BS, Nyberg DA, Hirsch JH, et al. Mild idiopathic lateral cerebral ventricular dilatation in utero: sonographic evaluation. *Radiology.* 1988;169:715–721.

171. Drugan A, Krause B, Canady A, et al. The natural history of prenatally diagnosed cerebral ventriculomegaly. *JAMA.* 1989;261:1785–1788.

172. Goldstein RB, La Pidus AS, Filly RA, et al. Mild lateral cerebral ventricular dilatation in utero: clinical significance and prognosis. *Radiology.* 1990;176:237–242.

173. Bromley B, Frigoletto FD Jr, et al. Mild fetal lateral cerebral ventriculomegaly: clinical course and outcome. *Am J Obstet Gynecol.* 1991;164:863–867.

174. Achiron R, Schimmel M, Achiron A, et al. Fetal mild idiopathic lateral ventriculomegaly: is there a correlation with fetal trisomy? *Ultrasound Obstet Gynecol.* 1993;3:89–92.

175. Patel MD, Filly AL, Hersh DR, et al. Isolated mild fetal cerebral ventriculomegaly: clinical course and outcome. *Radiology.* 1994;192:759–764.

176. Nadel AS, Bromley BS, Frigoletto FD Jr, et al. Isolated choroid plexus cysts in the second-trimester fetus: is amniocentesis really indicated? *Radiology.* 1992;185:545–548.

177. Gabrielli S, Reece EA, Pilu G, et al. The clinical significance of prenatally diagnosed choroid plexus cysts. *Am J Obstet Gynecol.* 1989;160:1207–1210.

178. Achiron R, Barkai G, Katznelson MB, et al. Fetal lateral ventricle choroid plexus cysts: the dilemma of amniocentesis. *Obstet Gynecol.* 1991;78:815–818.

179. Chinn DH, Miller EI, Worthy LM, et al. Sonographically detected fetal choroid plexus cysts: frequency and association with aneuploidy [see comments]. *J Ultrasound Med.* 1991;10:255–258.

180. Gross SJ, Shulman LP, Tolley EA, et al. Isolated fetal choroid plexus cysts and trisomy 18: a review and meta-analysis. *Am J Obstet Gynecol*. 1995;172:83–87.

181. Hertzberg BS, Kay HH, Bowie JD. Fetal choroid plexus lesions: relationship of antenatal sonographic appearance to clinical outcome. *J Ultrasound Med*. 1989;8:77–82.

182. Kupferminc MJ, Tamura RK, Sabbagha RE, et al. Isolated choroid plexus cyst(s): an indication for amniocentesis. *Am J Obstet Gynecol*. 1994;171:1068–1071.

183. Porto M, Murata Y, Warneke LA, et al. Fetal choroid plexus cysts: an independent risk factor for chromosomal anomalies. *J Clin Ultrasound*. 1993;21:103–108.

184. Platt LD, Carlson DE, Medearis AL, et al. Fetal choroid plexus cysts in the second trimester of pregnancy: a cause for concern [see comments]. *Am J Obstet Gynecol*. 1991;164:1652–5, discussion 1655–1656.

185. Sarno AP Jr, Polzin WJ, Kalish VB. Fetal choroid plexus cysts in association with cri du chat (5p-) syndrome. *Am J Obstet Gynecol*. 1993;169:1614–1615.

186. Osborn A. *Miscellaneous Tumors, Cysts and Metastases: Diagnostic Neuroradiology*. St. Louis: Mosby-Year Book; 1994.

187. Richard KE, Dahl K, Sanker P. Long-term follow-up of children and juveniles with arachnoid cysts. *Child Nerv System*. 1989;5:184–187.

188. Marinov M, Undjian S, Wetzka P. An evaluation of the surgical treatment of intracranial arachnoid cysts in children. *Child Nerv System*. 1989;5:177–183.

189. Fogarty K, Cohen HL, Haller JO. Sonography of fetal intracranial hemorrhage: unusual causes and a review of the literature. *J Clin Ultrasound*. 1989;17:366–370.

190. Martin R, Roessmann U, Fanaroff A. Massive intracerebellar hemorrhage in low-birth-weight infants. *J Pediatr*. 1976;89:290–293.

191. Zalneraitis EL, Young RS, Krishnamoorthy KS. Intracranial hemorrhage in utero as a complication of isoimmune thrombocytopenia. *J Pediatr*. 1979;95:611–614.

192. Jackson JC, Blumhagen JD. Congenital hydrocephalus due to prenatal intracranial hemorrhage. *Pediatr*. 1983;72:344–346.

193. Lustig-Gillman I, Young BK, Silverman F, et al. Fetal intraventricular hemorrhage: sonographic diagnosis and clinical implications. *J Clin Ultrasound*. 1983;11:277–280.

194. Achiron R, Pinchas OH, Reichman B, et al. Fetal intracranial hemorrhage: clinical significance of in utero ultrasonographic diagnosis [see comments]. *Br J Obstet Gynecol*. 1993;100:995–999.

195. Hadi HA, Finley J, Mallette JQ, et al. Prenatal diagnosis of cerebellar hemorrhage: medicolegal implications. *Am J Obstet Gynecol*. 1994;170:1392–1395.

196. Portman MA, Brouillette RT. Fatal intracranial hemorrhage complicating amniocentesis. *Am J Obstet Gynecol*. 1982;144:731–733.

197. Rotmensch S, Grannum PA, Nores JA, et al. In utero diagnosis and management of fetal subdural hematoma. *Am J Obstet Gynecol*. 1991;164:1246–1248.

198. Kawabata I, Imai A, Tamaya T. Antenatal subdural hemorrhage causing fetal death before labor. *Internat J Gynaecol Obstet*. 1993;43:57–60.

199. Messer J, Haddad J, Casanova R. Transcranial Doppler evaluation of cerebral infarction in the neonate. *Neuro Pediatr*. 1991;22:147–151.

200. Wakai S, Arai T, Nagai M. Congenital brain tumors. *Surgical Neurology*. 1984;21:597–609.

201. Hoff NR, Mackay IM. Prenatal ultrasound diagnosis of intracranial teratoma. *J Clin Ultrasound*. 1980;8:247–249.

202. Kirkinen P, Suramo I, Jouppila P, et al. Combined use of ultrasound and computed tomography in the evaluation of fetal intracranial abnormality. *J Perinat Med*. 1982;10:257–265.

203. Paes BA, deSa DJ, Hunter DJ, et al. Benign intracranial teratoma—prenatal diagnosis influencing early delivery. *Am J Obstet Gynecol*. 1982;143:600–601.

204. Smith WL, Menezes A, Franken EA. Cranial ultrasound in the diagnosis of malignant brain tumors. *J Clin Ultrasound*. 1983;11:97–100.

205. Cappe IP, Lam AH. Ultrasound in the diagnosis of choroid plexus papilloma. *J Clin Ultrasound*. 1985;13:121–123.

206. Ferreira J, Eviatar L, Schneider S, et al. Prenatal diagnosis of intracranial teratoma: prolonged survival after resection of a malignant teratoma diagnosed prenatally by ultrasound: a case report and literature review. *Pediatr Neurosurg*. 1993;19:84–88.

207. Sherer DM, Abramowicz JS, Eggers PC, et al. Prenatal ultrasonographic diagnosis of intracranial teratoma and massive craniomegaly with associated high-output cardiac failure. *Am J Obstet Gynecol*. 1993;168:97–99.

208. Ulreich S, Hanieh A, Furness ME. Positive outcome of fetal intracranial teratoma. *J Ultrasound Med*. 1993;12:163–165.

209. Gradin WC, Taylon C, Fruin AH. Choroid plexus papilloma of the third ventricle: case report and review of the literature. *Neurosurg*. 1983;12:217–220.

210. Hawkins JC. Treatment of choroid plexus papilloma in children: a brief analysis of twenty year's experience. *Neurosurg*. 1980;6:380.

211. Shackelford GD, Fulling KH, Glasier CM. Cysts of the subependymal germinal matrix: sonographic demonstration with pathologic correlation. *Radiology*. 1983;149:117–121.

212. Mittelmann-Handwerker S, Pardes JG, Post RC, et al. Fetal ventriculomegaly and brain atrophy in a woman with intrauterine cytomegalovirus infection: a case report. *J Reprod Med*. 1986;31:1061–1064.

213. Butt W, Mackay RJ, de Crespigny LC, et al. Intracranial lesions of congenital cytomegalovirus infection detected by ultrasound scanning. *Pediatr*. 1984;73:611–614.

214. Twickler DM, Perlman J, Maberry MC. Congenital cytomegalovirus infection presenting as cerebral ventriculomegaly on antenatal sonography. *Am J Perinatol*. 1993;10:404–406.

215. Tassin GB, Maklad NF, Stewart RR, et al. Cytomegalic inclusion disease: intrauterine sonographic diagnosis using findings involving the brain. *AJNR. Am J Neuroradiol*. 1991;12:117–122.

216. Achiron R, Pinhas-Hamiel O, Lipitz S, et al. Prenatal ultrasonographic diagnosis of fetal cerebral ventriculitis associated with asymptomatic maternal cytomegalovirus infection. *Prenat Diagn*. 1994;14:523–526.

217. Hohlfeld P, MacAleese J, Capella-Pavlovski M, et al. Fetal toxoplasmosis: ultrasonographic sings. *Ultrasound Obstet Gynecol*. 1991;1:241–244.

218. Fakhry J, Khoury A. Fetal intracranial calcifications: the importance of periventricular hyperechoic foci without shadowing. *J Ultrasound Med*. 1991;10:51–54.

219. Becker LE. Infections of the developing brain. *AJNR: Am J Neuroradiol*. 1992;13:537–549.

220. Blaakaer J. Ultrasonic diagnosis of fetal ascites and toxoplasmosis. *Acta Obstet Gynecol Scand*. 1986;65:653–654.

221. Osborn A. *Infections of the Brain and Its Linings: Diagnostic Neuroradiology*. St. Louis, MI: Mosby-Year Book; 1994.

222. Yamashita Y, Matsuishi T, Murakami Y, et al. Neuroimaging findings (ultrasonography, CT, MRI) in 3 infants with congenital rubella syndrome. *Ped Radiol*. 1991;21:547–549.

223. Vintzileos AM, Campbell WA, Weinbaum PJ, et al. Perinatal management and outcome of fetal ventriculomegaly. *Obstet Gynecol*. 1987;69:5–11.

224. Anhoury P, Andre M, Droulle P, et al. Dilatation of the cerebral ventricles diagnosed in utero. 85 case reports. *J de Gynecologie, Obstetrique et Biologie de la Reproduction*. 1991;20:191–197.

225. Hanigan WC, Morgan A, Shaaban A, et al. Surgical treatment and long-term neurodevelopmental outcome for infants with idiopathic aqueductal stenosis. *Child Nerv System*. 1991;7:386–390.

226. Rosseau GL, McCullough DC, Joseph AL. Current prognosis in fetal ventriculomegaly. *J Neurosurg*. 1992;77:551–555.

227. Kirkinen P, Serlo W, Jouppila P, et al. Long-term outcome of fetal hydrocephaly. *J Child Neurol*. 1996;11:189–192.

CHAPTER 19

HEART AND VASCULAR MALFORMATIONS

Joshua A. Copel / Charles S. Kleinman

Although congenital cardiac malformations constitute the most common lethal congenital malformations, and carry a tremendous burden of disability for patients, their families, and society, the fetal cardiovascular system was the last major organ system to be subjected to detailed examination in the fetus. Through the past two decades, however, fetal cardiac imaging has become increasingly common and has led to the development of fetal cardiology as a new discipline within pediatric cardiology and maternal-fetal medicine.

The dynamic nature of the tiny fetal heart and its complex anatomy, both when normal and in the presence of congenital cardiac malformations, made complete examination virtually impossible prior to the development of high-resolution real-time ultrasound equipment with dynamic focusing. In 1964 Wang and Xiao used M-mode echocardiography to evaluate fetal cardiac motion against time.[1] The first similar publication in English appeared in 1972 by Winsberg.[2] These first applications of human fetal echocardiography evaluated fetal life. Winsberg attempted to estimate fetal cardiac output, and suggested that this technology could be used to evaluate cardiac pump function. He went on to suggest that it was unlikely that abnormalities of fetal cardiac structure could be evaluated due to the complexity of the cardiac anatomy.

During the past two decades detailed evaluation of both normal and abnormal fetal cardiac anatomy has become a reality.[3-6] The more recent additions of pulsed- and color-flow Doppler have made it possible to evaluate fetal flow physiology within the central circulation and within the vascular system. These studies can be performed throughout the second and third trimesters of pregnancy and have even been applied in the first trimester utilizing transvaginal-imaging techniques.[7-15]

The information gleaned from prenatal cardiac studies may have important practical applications for the management of pregnancy, delivery, and the neonatal period.

FETAL ECHOCARDIOGRAPHIC IMAGING TECHNIQUES

The mainstay in the diagnosis of normal and abnormal fetal cardiac anatomy is the two-dimensional study of the heart, which provides structural information. In performing these studies we apply the same imaging principles that form the foundation of postnatal echocardiography. We reserve M-mode echocardiography for the analysis of cardiac arrhythmias and for the analysis of ventricular function. We only occasionally use M-mode to measure the cardiac walls and interventricular septum in cases that are at risk for cardiomyopathies (e.g., diabetics).[4,16,17]

Examinations may be performed utilizing either sector, linear, or curvilinear array transducers. Higher frequency transducers provide better resolution than do more powerful lower frequency transducers. We use the highest possible frequency transducer that provides adequate penetration to the depth of the heart. More recently, high-frequency vaginal transducers have provided 4-chamber imaging during the late first trimester of pregnancy and complex structural anomalies have been diagnosed as early as the 10th week of gestation.[12,14,15]

The simplest and most important single view of the fetal heart to obtain is the 4-chamber view (Fig. 19-1) that shows the atria and ventricles with the interposed interatrial and interventricular septa, and the atrioventricular valves. One can thus visualize the inflow, or posterior, aspect of the interventricular septum, the central fibrous body of the heart, the interatrial septum, and the integrity of the atrioventricular valves. This view is best obtained by first finding the cross-sectional image of the fetal abdomen that demonstrates the stomach and the hook of the umbilical vein in the liver, that is, the section that is used to measure the fetal abdominal circumference. Angling the transducer cephalad will then bring the 4-chamber view of the heart into view. The 4-chamber view is especially useful for assessing relative cardiac chamber sizes, and for assessing the structure of the central fibrous portion of the fetal heart, and may also be used to detect pericardial effusions.

By specifying that one starts with a view of the fetal abdomen to obtain the 4-chamber view, it is implicit that the sonographer or sonologist must also analyze the situs of the fetal abdomen and heart. It is usually a simple matter to find the fetal stomach on the left and the rightward hook of the umbilical vein in the liver, and to compare them to the position of the fetal spine in conjunction with the lie of the fetus to determine the right and left sides of the fetus. The cardiac apex should normally be on the same side of the fetus as the stomach. The inferior vena cava should be on the right side of the fetal abdomen and should be traced into the morphologic right atrium. If there is abdominal situs inversus the stomach will be found on the right side of the fetal abdomen and the inferior vena cava will be on the left entering the morphologic fetal right atrium, which in this case is left sided (but should also be anterior to the left atrium). The inferior vena cava is a marker of position of the fetal right atrium. The inferior vena cava only rarely crosses the midline to enter a morphologic right atrium on the opposite side of the fetus, in which case the cardiac apex will be to the right, that is, concordant with the position of the fetal stomach.

When the fetal stomach and heart are not on the same side of the fetal body there is a high likelihood of complex cardiac malformations. Such fetuses often have visceral heterotaxia and may have critical forms of congenital heart disease, often involving abnormalities of spleen formation (either asplenia or polysplenia) and intestinal malrotation. Most, but not all, such fetuses have defects of atrioventricular septation and may have abnormalities of pulmonary venous drainage and possible arterial transposition with associated pulmonary outflow tract obstruction. It is important to identify these fetuses prior to birth, since sophisticated neonatal cardiac management may be required. In our experience an increasing number of fetuses

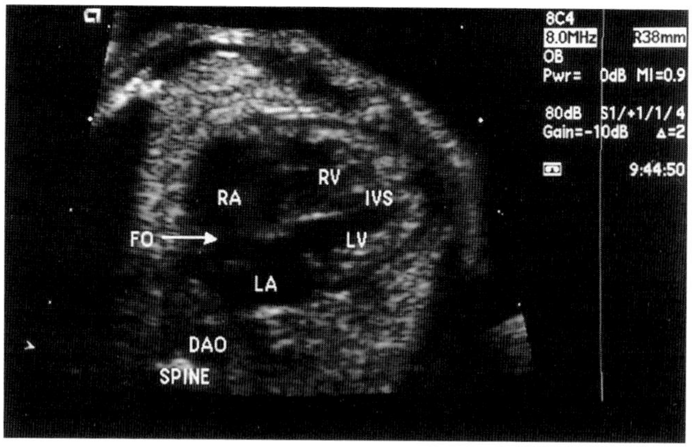

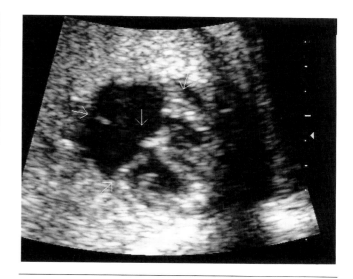

FIGURE 19-1 Normal 4-chamber view. The fetal spine is on the lower left with the descending aorta (DAO) anterior to it. Immediately anterior to the aorta is the left atrium (LA) which communicates with the right atrium (RA) via the foramen ovale. The right and left ventricles (RV, LV) are separated by the interventricular septum (IVS). Note that the atria are of approximately equal size, as are the ventricles, and that the tricuspid valve inserts on the IVS slightly closer to the apex of the heart than does the mitral valve.

FIGURE 19-2 Atrioventricular septal defect. Four-chamber view with apex of the heart in lower left. Arrow in center of heart indicates absent lower atrial septal tissue. Two arrows at either side of heart point to insertions of the common atrioventricular valve. Note that it forms a straight line between the arrows, without the usual apical displacement of the tricuspid valve.

have been determined to have congenital heart disease after basic sonograms have identified abnormal visceral or cardiac situs.

In looking at the 4-chamber view, the posterior atrial chamber, that is the one closest to the fetal spine, is the left atrium. It contains the flap valve of the foramen ovale (the septum primum of the atrial septum), which appears to undulate within the left atrium. This movement reflects the position of the atrial septum primum in a unidirectional right-to-left stream of blood entering the left atrium from the ductus venosus. The left atrium, on close inspection, can be seen to have irregular walls posteriorly and laterally, due to the entrance of the pulmonary veins. Flow into the left atrium from the pulmonary veins can be demonstrated with color flow Doppler or power Doppler imaging if the settings are adjusted to detect the relatively low flow velocities of these veins.

The anterior atrium is the right atrium, which should contain the entrance of the inferior vena cava, close to the foramen ovale. This position is important as it allows the highly oxygenated umbilical venous blood flowing from the ductus venosus to enter the left atrium and from there the left ventricle and ascending aorta. The smaller superior vena cava may also be visible in the same paramedian view of the thorax that demonstrates the inferior vena cava. On the 4-chamber view, however, neither of these will be visible. It is important to note that the right and left atria are approximately equal in size.

The more anterior ventricular chamber, the right ventricle, has a more coarsely trabeculated wall than does the posterior ventricle. A thick muscle bundle, called the moderator band, at the apex of the ventricle and a papillary muscle inserting into the interventricular septum together identify this as the mor-

phologic right ventricle. The two atrioventricular valves insert close to the center of the heart, at the junction of the atrial and ventricular septa. However, the tricuspid valve (right atrioventricular valve) inserts slightly closer to the apex of the heart than does the mitral valve. This is another way to distinguish the right and left sides of the heart. If the two atrioventricular valves appear to insert on the septum at the same level, an atrioventricular septal defect, also known as an atrioventricular canal defect (Fig. 19-2), or an endocardial cushion defect, may be present.

The long-axis view, of the fetal heart is obtained by orienting the tomographic imaging plane between the fetal left hip and right shoulder. This view demonstrates the origin of the aorta from the left ventricle (Fig. 19-3). The anterior wall of the aorta should be seen in continuity with the interventricular septum, and the aorta should arise completely from the left ventricle. The mitral valve is also seen in continuity with the posterior wall of the aorta. This view provides visualization of the anterior portion of the interventricular septum and is useful for the detection of conoventricular, or malalignment, defects within the septum leading to over-riding aorta or double-outlet right ventricle (Fig. 19-4).

Further rotation of the transducer provides the pulmonary artery/ductus view, which demonstrates the pulmonary artery arising from the right ventricle and then appearing to dive posteriorly to cross over the aorta (Fig. 19-5). This vessel then bifurcates into the pulmonary artery and the ductus arteriosus, which in turn continues into the descending aorta. The pulmonary artery subsequently divides into smaller right and left pulmonary arteries. The apparent crossing of the aorta and pulmonary artery is important to identify, since in transposed

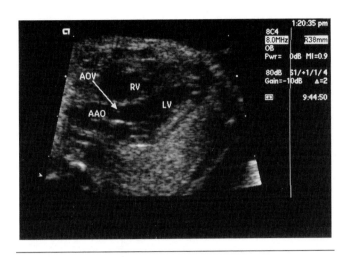

FIGURE 19-3 Long axis view of left ventricle. The interventricular septum can be seen separating the right and left ventricles (RV, LV). The ascending aorta (AAO) leaves the left ventricle with clear continuity between its anterior wall and the septum. AOV: aortic valve.

ventriculoarterial connections the two arteries run parallel to one another. The curved sweep of the ductus arteriosus into the descending aorta can be confused with the aortic arch if one is not careful to recognize that the aortic arch is the origin of the 3 great arterial branches (innominate, left carotid, and left subclavian), which should be identified easily, while the pulmonary artery bifurcates into two branches.

Further rotation of the transducer, into a position at right angles to the long-axis view, provides the short-axis view. Slight caudal orientation provides a short-axis cross-sectional view of the fetal ventricles, demonstrating the interventricular septum between the two ventricles and often demonstrating the two

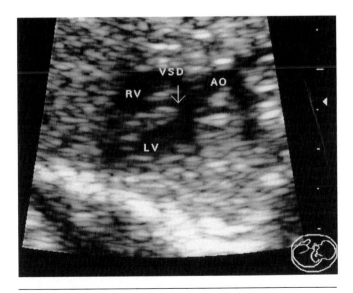

FIGURE 19-4 Overriding aorta. The arrow indicates the ventricular septal defect (VSD) caused by the discontinuity between the anterior wall of the aorta (AO) and the interventricular septum. RV: Right Ventricle; LV: Left Ventricle

small papillary muscles attached to the mitral valve. Slight cephalad orientation in the transducer demonstrates the great arteries in cross-section. In this view the aorta, seen in cross-section, appears as a small circular structure surrounded posteriorly by the atria and anteriorly by the right atrium, and the curve of the right ventricular outflow tract, leading into the pulmonary trunk.

FETAL CARDIAC FUNCTION

The fetal right ventricle acts as a relatively volume-overloaded chamber when compared with the fetal left ventricle. This has been suggested based on the fetal interventricular septum appearing to bow into the left ventricular cavity during diastole.[3,6] Pulsed Doppler flow studies have also demonstrated the fetal right ventricle to have an output exceeding that of the left by a ratio of approximately 55% to 45%.[18-21] This contrasts with fetal lamb blood flow studies during the last third of pregnancy showing a 66% to 33% relationship between the ventricles.[22,23] Doppler estimates of relative ventricular output correlate well with simultaneous measurements utilizing the radionuclide microsphere and flow-probe techniques in the fetal lamb model.[23] It is likely that the decreased ratio of right versus left ventricular output in the human compared with the lamb reflects the proportionately larger fetal brain in the human, which requires more left ventricular output.

Fetal echocardiographic studies must be interpreted in the context of the unique properties of the fetal circulation. These include the parallel circuitry of the fetal heart, with communications between the atria through the foramen ovale, and between the great arteries across the ductus arteriosus. Perturbations in the fetal circulation are likely to have an impact on the structure of the fetal heart. Understanding these alterations can help in our understanding of fetal adaptation to structural heart disease, plan neonatal management for a smoother transition to the postnatal circulatory pattern. For example, when prenatal evaluation has suggested that the neonate will be dependent upon persistent patency of the ductus arteriosus for adequate pulmonary or systemic blood flow, the neonate may benefit from prostaglandin E_1 therapy to maintain ductal patency, while plans for surgery can be completed. This should help avoid severe hypoxemia or ischemia as the presenting sign of congenital cardiac disease.[24]

INDICATIONS FOR FETAL ECHOCARDIOGRAPHIC STUDY

Despite the fact that universal fetal echocardiography might increase the number of cases of congenital heart disease diagnosed prenatally, performing the requisite number of studies would be difficult to justify in this era of shrinking resources.

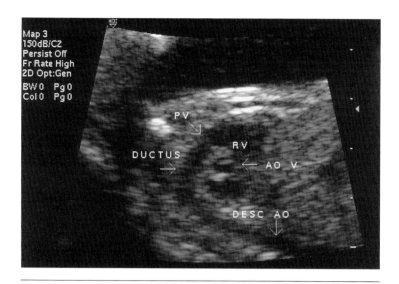

FIGURE 19-5 Right ventricular outflow and ductus arteriosus. The pulmonic artery leaves the right ventricle (RV) via the pulmonic valve (PV) and continues into the ductus arteriosus and then to the descending aorta (DESC AO). The normal course of the pulmonic artery and ductus around the aortic valve (AOV) can be seen.

A recent study from Austria[25] has suggested that routine detailed fetal echocardiographic screening of all fetuses could identify up to 86% of all congenital heart disease. Similar results have also been reported by Yagel, who found that 89% of fetuses with structural heart disease could be detected with a full echocardiogram protocol.[26] An editorial accompanying the Austrian paper suggested that to accomplish screening by using a full echocardiogram in Britain alone would require at least 400 more specialists.[27] That approach also contradicts the underlying assumption of a screening test, which must be accomplished rapidly with tools or skills easily available to all practitioners.

Offering full fetal echocardiograms must be limited to populations defined as having risk factors that place the pregnancy at higher risk for significant congenital heart disease than average. The overall population risk is approximately 8 cases of congenital heart disease per 1,000 births. Only about half of these (4 in 1,000 births) have anomalies that are severe enough to require postnatal medical and/or surgical therapy, and which are severe enough to be potentially identifiable prenatally. The risk factors that serve as indications for fetal echocardiography can be grouped into fetal, maternal, and familial factors.

Over the 8 years from 1984 to 1991, we performed fetal echocardiograms on 3513 fetuses at the Yale Fetal Cardiovascular Center and we diagnosed 213 cases of congenital heart disease (6.1%). The most common indication for cardiac scan during this period was a familial or maternal history of congenital heart disease. Cardiac abnormalities were found in slightly less than 2% of this group. We believe that the small positive yield in this group does not detract from the cost effectiveness and social effectiveness of the sonograms. The

important psychological impact that negative studies have on families, especially when parental levels of anxiety regarding possible recurrent heart disease are high, is often immeasurable. Considerably higher positive yields were found among fetuses that were referred for specific fetal risk factors, including fetal extracardiac malformations, fetal chromosome abnormalities, nonimmune hydrops, and a suspicion of structural heart disease based on a basic ultrasound study.

The association of structural heart disease with nonimmune hydrops has remained a consistent source of major congenital heart disease. We previously reported that fetal hydrops was frequently associated with congenital or functional heart disease.[28] Subsequent studies utilizing Doppler flow have demonstrated a high incidence of severe atrioventricular valve regurgitation in fetuses with structural heart disease and hydrops.[29,30] Studies of the intrinsic properties of fetal ventricular myocardium[31] demonstrated that passive tension is higher than in the adult, suggesting lower compliance in fetal myocardium. In addition, at any given preload, fetal myocardium generates less tension than adult myocardium. These studies explain why fetal hearts have limited diastolic, as well as systolic, reserve in the presence of several ventricular outlet obstruction and/or semilunar or atrioventricular valve regurgitation, and how this results in the rapid development of fetal edema probably secondary to systemic venous hypertension.

IMPORTANCE OF THE 4-CHAMBER VIEW

In a study we performed between 1984 and 1986 we evaluated 1,193 fetal echocardiograms from 991 women who carried a total of 1,022 fetuses,[32] including 31 sets of twins. Gestational ages at the time of examination varied from 18 weeks to term. Seventy-four of the fetuses had structurally abnormal hearts (7.2%), and 3 additional abnormalities were identified postnatally. In 71 of the prenatally recognized abnormals (96%), the 4-chamber view of the heart suggested that there was an abnormality. Examination of the 4-chamber view had a sensitivity of 92% and a 99.7% specificity for predicting the existence of congenital heart disease. The positive predictive value was 95.8% and the negative predictive value was 99.4%. We concluded that a 4-chamber screening view of the heart should be included as part of all routine obstetric ultrasound examinations. We emphasized at that time that the 4-chamber view of the heart could not offer a comprehensive study of cardiac structure, but rather might stand as an effective initial screen. It also must be emphasized that the study was retrospective, knowing that congenital heart disease existed in the fetuses that were being examined, and that the investigators were particularly experienced in fetal echocardiography. This could not be considered a screening study of low-risk pregnancies performed by relatively inexperienced observers. Our hope was that once 4-chamber cardiac screening became common in laboratories performing fetal ultrasound, additional tomographic views of the heart and great arteries could also become part of the ultrasound surgery, which would further improve sensitivity.

The much lower sensitivity of fetal 4-chamber screening reported by the RADIUS study[33] and studies carried out in Rotterdam,[34] Trieste,[35] and Trondheim[36] must be looked on as significantly more accurate estimates of the efficacy of 4-chamber screening studies in a low-risk population. A recent study from the Piemonte region of Italy showed similarly low sensitivity (15%), and reviewed the data of 11 prior screening studies. There was an overall sensitivity of 23% in a screened population of 108,182, and a 5.8/1000 rate of congenital heart disease in follow-up.[37]

It is quite clear that a rather protracted learning curve will need to take place before such examinations can be considered routine and reasonably sensitive. Therefore, while the American Institute of Ultrasound in Medicine, the American College of Obstetrics and Gynecology, and the American College of Radiology have recommended that 4-chamber screening views be included as a part of any basic fetal ultrasound study it is too early to consider a failure to identify fetal heart disease during a screening study to be a breach of the standard of care. We hope that such examinations will improve our ability to identify previously unsuspected cases of congenital heart disease, and offer greater reassurance regarding normality as well. The addition of an abnormal cardiac axis as a predictor of congenital heart disease recently may further improve the sensitivity in future screening studies.[38,39]

The fact that some congenital heart disease will be missed by 4-chamber screening alone should not discourage us from including this view in general fetal examinations. The alternative to 4-chamber screening, that is not attempting to assess the heart, must necessarily result in an even lower sensitivity than the disappointing results reported from some screening studies.

The most common significant diagnoses that are missed with full fetal echocardiograms in our experience, include transposition of the great arteries, aortic coarctation, and ventricular septal defect with or without valvar pulmonic stenosis. Recent false-positive diagnoses have included an incorrect identification of an overriding aorta, a case of suspected subaortic tunnel obstruction, and a case of aortic coarctation. It is important to recognize that even in a relatively experienced laboratory such as our own occasional errors are still made, although errors have been extremely rare in the past decade of our experience, and have been limited primarily to missed cases of small ventricular septal defect. We tend to avoid making the diagnosis of isolated ventricular septal defect, unless the defects are extremely large, involve great arterial malalignment or abnormalities of the inflow atrioventricular septum, or have been visualized in multiple imaging planes at multiple examining sessions.

Review of the correct diagnoses established in our laboratory during the past 10 years demonstrates a relatively high incidence of major abnormalities affecting 4-chamber anatomy. In many cases this is due to direct identification of the structural abnormality, for example septal defects and atrioventricular valve abnormalities in atrioventricular septal defects, ventricular hypoplasia, and atrioventricular valve atresia with absent atrioventricular valve connections, atrial and ventricular dilation in the Ebstein malformation of the tricuspid valve. In others the abnormality of the 4-chamber view occurs secondary to flow perturbations which, in turn, are due to structural anomalies outside the 4-chamber tomographic view, for example right atrial dilation and right ventricular hypertrophy secondary to tricuspid valve regurgitation in severe pulmonic stenosis, or right ventricular dilation in cases of double outlet right ventricle.

FETAL HEART DISEASE AND CHROMOSOME ABNORMALITIES

Pediatric series have reported a 5–10% frequency of chromosomal abnormalities in infants with congenital heart disease.[40] The association between congenital heart disease and chromosomal anomalies is even stronger among fetuses. We reported the results of 594 echocardiograms performed on 520 fetuses varying in age from 18 weeks gestation to term and with indications as described above.[41] We excluded 18 patients who were referred after aneuploidy syndromes had already been diagnosed. Thirty-four of the 502 fetuses with previously unknown chromosomal status had congenital cardiac malformations (6.8%). Eleven of these 34 fetuses (32%) also had abnormal chromosomes. This marked difference from the pediatric data may relate to nonviable fetuses identified in utero who escape pediatric case identification. Based on this study we concluded that all fetuses with congenital heart disease merit chromosome analysis. Similar findings were reported by Berg,[42] who extrapolated back from pediatric experience using Hook's data on expected losses of chromosomally abnormal fetuses[43] to estimate that approximately one third of midtrimester fetuses with congenital heart disease could be expected to have chromosome abnormalities.

Further study in our lab between 1984 and 1994 included 300 mothers identified to have fetuses with congenital heart disease who were routinely offered karyotyping. Two hundred and seventy-seven karyotypes were obtained and 85 aneuploid fetuses were identified (28.5%).[44] The single most common karyotype abnormality was trisomy 18 (28 cases) followed closely by trisomy 21 (27 cases), with an additional 13 cases of trisomy 13. In addition, there were 11 cases of Turner syndrome,[45] with left heart outlet obstruction including aortic coarctation and hypoplastic left heart syndrome (Fig. 19-6), often in association with cystic hygromas. The remainder of the aneuploidy syndromes were rare abnormalities. As one might expect, the incidence of aneuploidy was highest among

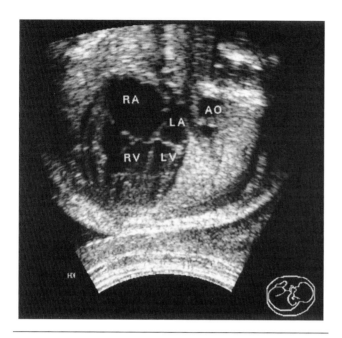

FIGURE 19-6 Disproportion in ventricular sizes. In this 4-chamber view there is a discrepancy in the sizes of the right and left ventricles (RV, LV), and in the sizes of the atria (RA, LA). The right ventricle is beginning to dominate at the apex of the heart. This appearance may be due to a coarctation of the aorta, or, if further disproportion in ventricular sizes develops, a hypoplastic left heart. This view alone is insufficient to make a definitive diagnosis, and further imaging of the aortic arch, as well as serial fetal echocardiograms to evaluate progression of the lesion, may be required.

fetuses who were noted to have multiple congenital anomalies (approximately 30%), but the incidence of aneuploidy among fetuses with isolated congenital heart disease, generally involving ventricular septal defects, was also significant (15%). We believe that a karyotype should be offered to the parents regardless of the stage of pregnancy at which the congenital heart disease is detected. Even when abortion is no longer an option, or for families who would not select abortion, abnormal results may result in formulation of a management strategy involving much less aggressive neonatal resuscitation, or may avert a cesarean section for delivery of a nonviable infant. For nonviable fetuses (e.g., Trisomy 13 or 18) the option of labor without fetal monitoring can be offered to the parents.

The family of lesions known as conotruncal malformations includes aortic override of the interventricular septum in lesions such as tetralogy of Fallot, double outlet right ventricle, truncus arteriosus, and aortic arch interruption. The etiology of these lesions includes the important contribution of cell migration from the neural crest to form the outflow portion of the interventricular septum, participate in septation of the truncus arteriosus, and contribute to embryonic organs deriving from the 4th and 5th pharyngeal pouches. Neonates with these lesions may also be found to have the diGeorge syndrome which includes anomalies of thymic T-cell, parathyroid, and thyroid

function. A related syndrome, encoded in the same area, referred to as the velocardiofacial syndrome (Schprintzin syndrome) includes these cardiac defects and abnormalities of the palate, and unusual facies, with frequent ear infections, speech abnormalities, and later development of psychological problems including psychosis. It has recently been demonstrated in two laboratories[45,46] that both these syndromes are associated with microdeletions in the 11 region of the long arm of chromosome 22 (22q11). For this reason patients with malalignment interventricular septal defects (Fig. 19-4) are now offered both standard karyotyping and fluorescent in situ hybridization testing for the 22q11 microdeletion syndrome.

We can speculate that, as our understanding of the molecular genetic encoding of cardiac malformations is enhanced, additional molecular diagnoses will become available for structural heart disease diagnosed both before and after birth. This knowledge may help us identify families at extremely high risk of recurrent heart disease with genetic abnormalities, and others at substantially lower risk lacking identifiable genetic causes.

IMPACT OF FETAL ECHOCARDIOGRAPHY ON OBSTETRIC MANAGEMENT

Regardless of the potential of 4-chamber screening studies to identify fetal heart disease, there will always be a need for detailed fetal echocardiograms to be performed in a referral setting. This should generally involve a cooperative effort of experts in fetal ultrasound and in congenital heart disease. Patients with specific risk factors for fetal heart disease will continue to require these studies, because the sensitivity of screening studies is, by definition, always imperfect, and screening is therefore inappropriate in those with clearly increased risks of disease. Since the greatest number of fetal cardiac abnormalities still occurs among fetuses that have not been identified to have risk factors by patient history alone, many cardiac anomalies will be identified during obstetric scanning for other purposes. This can be anticipated to become increasingly common, especially as fetal cardiac screening becomes an accepted standard part of general fetal ultrasound scans, and as general fetal sonologists and sonographers become more acquainted with fetal anatomy, and include outflow views of the heart to 4-chamber screening views. The total impact of these diagnoses is complex to evaluate.

Some anomalies will be incompatible with postnatal survival, for example structural heart disease associated with severe non-immune hydrops fetalis. If these are found early in gestation the parents may choose to terminate the pregnancy, removing the pregnancy from any comparison with postnatal outcomes. Even when diagnoses are made so late that pregnancy termination is no longer an option, or when the parents are opposed to pregnancy interruption, important benefits may still accrue by allowing the formulation of management plans that take parental wishes for noninterventive approaches to be accommodated. To do that, specific signs associated with an especially poor prognosis need to be understood.

One specific sign that is associated with a poor outcome is early-onset cardiomegaly. Hornberger reported that the heart should not occupy more than approximately one third of the chest area.[47] She found that when atrioventricular valve regurgitation was associated with marked cardiomegaly and the heart occupies more than 40–50% of the area of the chest in the mid-trimester there was a high incidence of pulmonary hypoplasia. This can be understood as being the result of the same factors that lead to similar outcomes in fetuses with congenital diaphragmatic hernia, and with congenital cystic adenomatoid malformation of the lung. The enlarged heart leads to pulmonary hypoplasia which may preclude surgery for the congenital heart disease, even for lesions that are theoretically amenable to surgery.

Another poor prognostic sign is fetal hydrops. This may be present at the time of diagnosis, and frequently develops in the presence of atrioventricular valve regurgitation.[48] The combination of structural heart disease and fetal hydrops is virtually always fatal. Fetuses with atrioventricular valve regurgitation should be followed with serial fetal echocardiography to assess cardiac function and to seek early signs of hydrops, such as polyhydramnios or an increasing pericardial effusion. As the third trimester progresses, especially in the presence of documented fetal lung maturity, elective delivery may be helpful if hydrops is thought to be developing. Atrioventricular valve regurgitation does not occur solely as the result of atrioventricular valve abnormalities. It is frequently seen with pulmonic stenosis and atresia.

Fetal noncardiac anomalies and aneuploidies have already been discussed. Even a cardiac lesion that is generally considered amenable to surgical treatment may be considered inoperable in the presence of a more severe extracardiac anomaly (e.g., anencephaly). Counseling of families must be highly individualized, and take into account all of the findings from the ultrasound examination.

Many cardiac diagnoses are made late in pregnancy. This often reflects referral due to suspicious-appearing hearts noted during obstetric sonography, and due to the identification of extracardiac anomalies with associated heart disease. In such cases, accurate prenatal diagnosis permits honest counseling for parents and adequate medical planning for delivery and neonatal management (e.g., insuring that prostaglandin E_1 is prepared for administration after delivery of a fetus who is dependent upon persistent patency of the ductus arteriosus to provide adequate pulmonary or systemic blood flow). Delivery of these infants in an institution equipped to provide comprehensive neonatal cardiac and cardiac surgical therapy may be expected to improve outcome in some cases.

Chang suggested that in severe left heart outlet obstruction, prenatal diagnosis and transfer for delivery at the institution where definitive therapy could be afforded resulted in a lower morbidity, including a lower incidence of acidosis, presurgical cardiac arrest, shorter postsurgical hospitalization, and a tendency toward improved survival (despite a lack of statistically significant improved survival). While an important preliminary study, the design of the study prevents drawing firm conclusions.[49]

A similar study, undertaken in our laboratory over the last 5 years, looking at all forms of congenital heart disease, rather than specifically at left heart outlet obstruction produced slightly different results.[50] We compared infants with a prenatal diagnosis to a group that were diagnosed only within the first 48 hours postnatally. We found that infants requiring eventual single ventricle repair did no better if diagnosed prenatally, which may be a function of the severity of these lesions, and which may have been responsible for the referral for fetal echocardiography. Postnatal surgery was refused in significantly more cases in the postnatal group. This suggests that the prenatal diagnosis group were self-selected to include patients predisposed to surgical management, with others opting for abortion or delivery with compassionate care. Shorter hospital stays were found in the postnatal group partly as a function of parents declining surgery, after which the infant either died or went home for supportive care.

In a similar study comparing 15 fetuses with critical left heart obstruction to 45 similar neonates, Eapen has reported less acidosis and hemodynamic instability among those diagnosed prenatally.[51] Episodes of major organ dysfunction, especially renal dysfunction and seizures or intraventricular hemorrhage, were less common among the prenatal diagnosis group. Mortality was not significantly improved overall, including no deaths among 5 prenatal and 14 postnatal diagnoses of coarctation. Surgery was not attempted for 2 prenatal and 9 postnatal diagnoses, essentially. In the group with attempted Norwood repairs there were 6 deaths in 7 prenatally diagnosed patients, and 8 deaths in 19 postnatally diagnosed patients. Although this is not statistically significant, Fisher exact test comes close to significance (p = 0.08).

In the group amenable to biventricular surgical management, we found significantly better survival in the prenatally diagnosed group (96% versus 76% in the postnatally diagnosed group, p < 0.05). Hospitalizations were significantly shorter, and the cost of hospitalization was also less, although the latter difference fell slightly short of statistical significance.

With continuing surgical advances cardiac abnormalities that were considered hopeless only a few years ago are undergoing surgical correction today. For example, both neonatal cardiac transplantation and the Norwood procedure have been offered for neonates with the hypoplastic left heart syndrome.[52,53] When infants are delivered at community hospitals with these lesions, complex support must be provided until the neonate is transported to a center offering definitive diagnostic and surgical management. We believe that this argues for delivery to be accomplished at an institution capable of providing comprehensive maternal and neonatal care. It is also important to allow parents adequate time to consider their options. Our impression from talking to parents is that "informed consent" for surgery may be difficult in the best of circumstances, but with a critically ill neonate it may be an impossibility.

Parents also often say in retrospect that prenatal diagnosis and a longer period of time to develop an understanding of the nature of the underlying defect and the proposed surgery had an important impact on their level of informed consent and their comfort with their decisions. Education of patients at 1 or more prenatal visits is, therefore, essential for their active participation in decision making, for example regarding expectant management versus transplantation or the Norwood procedure for infants with the hypoplastic left heart syndrome. Recent data indicate that neonatal surgery involving cardiopulmonary bypass make significant effects on neurodevelopmental outcome.[54] This makes it important for us to develop good long-term follow-up studies to be able to provide accurate counseling for parents.

PRENATAL SURGICAL THERAPY

In considering the prenatal diagnosis and management of congenital heart disease, we must take into account the potential for prenatal therapy. This includes in utero cardiac surgery, catheter therapies such as balloon valvuloplasty, and pacemaker therapy.

Harrison pioneered in the field of prenatal fetal surgery, including developing techniques of fetal exteriorization for the treatment of urinary tract obstruction, diaphragmatic hernia, cystic adenomatoid malformation of the lung, and sacrococcygeal teratoma.[55] The frustration of dealing with infants who were already compromised at birth, due to structural abnormalities that could conceivably have been corrected if addressed earlier in gestation provided some impetus, as did the identification of such abnormalities, often by chance alone, during routine ultrasound examinations of the fetus.

Harrison has emphasized the importance of refraining from potentially dangerous (to the mother and fetus) intervention until the natural history of the untreated condition is understood, and until the pathophysiology of the disease is more fully elucidated. The latter information usually requires the development of an animal model.

Although the natural history of congenital heart disease in the fetus has been the subject of considerable investigation, animal models are only now being studied. Current areas of investigation include techniques for surface cooling and rewarming of the exteriorized fetus undergoing cardiopulmonary bypass. Major problems still need to be addressed using this model of heart bypass.[56]

Maxwell has reported an experience with balloon valvuloplasty performed on 4 fetuses identified to have critical left ventricular outflow obstruction with associated left ventricular fibroelastosis.[57] Only 1 surviving neonate resulted, suggesting that the fibroelastosis had rendered the fetuses unsalvageable by the time of treatment. A subsequent procedure, performed in a fetus who was not noted to have fibroelastosis also failed to result in a surviving fetus. These studies underline the importance of accurate prenatal diagnosis, as well as a knowledge of pathophysiology, before one can reasonably offer invasive

fetal treatment, regardless of how well meaning the attempt at therapy may be.

Postnatal valvuloplasty, whether performed surgically or via a catheter may result in significant valvular regurgitation, and the limited diastolic reserve of the fetal heart may make this a critical consideration. An animal model for fetal therapy is a prerequisite to further attempts in human fetuses, to avoid creating a worse problem with our treatment than is caused by the original lesion.

Restriction of the foramen ovale has been suggested as a potential cause of left heart hypoplasia. The potential for surgical or angioplasty intervention to dilate a restrictive foramen has been postulated on the assumption that improving atrial right-to-left shunting could reverse the problem. Feit[58] demonstrated that the size of the fetal foramen ovale, indexed to the size of the interatrial septum, could be used to distinguish left heart obstructive lesions (in which the foramen ovale/atrial septal ratio was smaller than in normals) from right heart obstructive lesions (in which this ratio was larger than in normals). This study found, however, that this difference was not apparent before 19 weeks gestation. In addition, several patients with left heart obstructive lesions were found to have predominantly left-to-right rather than right-to-left atrial level shunts, even in the absence of critical mitral or aortic obstruction. This suggests that a small foramen ovale size, while reflecting transatrial flow volumes, may be a secondary phenomenon rather than causal in the pathophysiology of some cases of left heart hypoplasia, and that opening the foramen would not be likely to reverse the pathologic process.

The possibility of associated chromosomal abnormalities and extracardiac malformations must be appreciated and fully evaluated before any prenatal surgical intervention. The operability of the patient is not solely dependent on a technique for palliation of the structural heart disease. It should also involve evaluation of the fetus' potential to survive postnatally without prenatal intervention. The extracardiac malformation may well rule out the potential for survival despite the provision of aggressive cardiac surgical therapy.

Another area of interest for possible prenatal cardiac treatment has been fetuses with complete heart block. About half of fetuses with heart block have structural heart disease, usually complex abnormalities of situs (left atrial isomerism), atrioventricular septal defects, or corrected transposition of the great arteries (atrioventricular discordance with ventriculoarterial discordance). This group often develops hydrops, and have a poor prognosis in that event. The other half of fetuses with heart block occur in mothers carrying the anti-Ro and/or anti-La antibodies associated with Sjogren syndrome and systemic lupus erythematosus, but also occurring in the absence of clinically apparent maternal disease.[59]

The antibodies damage the fetal conduction system causing the heart block, and also can damage the cardiac myocytes themselves, leading to a myocarditis[60] Either or both of these events may cause fetal hydrops, with its poor prognosis. While we and others have reported that high dose maternal steroid treatment, using steroids that cross the placenta such as dexamethasone, may have a beneficial effect, standard treatment postnatally has included pacemaker placement. There have been two reports of pacemaker placement in fetuses in the literature,[61,62] and we are aware of 1 other case (M. Harrison, personal communication), but none have resulted in fetal survival. All were undertaken when fetuses were extremely ill. For now, pacemaker placement cannot be recommended for several reasons. It is likely that restoration of a normal sequence atrioventricular contraction will be desirable, but that would require placement of both atrial and ventricular leads, which is not currently technically feasible short of fetal exteriorization. Any external pacemaker would also involve the potential for the lead wires to be left floating freely in the amniotic cavity, with the potential to become entangled with the fetal umbilical cord, or fetal extremities.

Despite our seemingly pessimistic outlook toward fetal cardiac surgical therapy for congenital heart disease, we are actually cautiously optimistic that such therapy will ultimately become available and desirable for a limited number of fetuses. Considerably more basic work must be completed combining diagnostic abilities, surgical skills, and knowledge of pathophysiology before these treatments can be offered. At present they should be considered purely investigational techniques, limited to institutions with special abilities in this area, and performed with appropriate institutional review board approval.

FETAL TUMORS

Fetal tumors are uncommon, but the most often reported type are teratomas, which may occur virtually anywhere, but typically appear in midline structures.[63–65] Fetal teratomas have been reported in the oropharynx, where they may obstruct swallowing of amniotic fluid, or in the mediastinum, where they may interfere with cardiac function.

The largest reported fetal teratomas are sacrococcygeal in origin. They may be anterior to the sacrum, in which case they are intraperitoneal, occupying the lower abdomen and pelvis as a heterogenous mass. More commonly, they are seen externally, as a large mass extending from the sacrum, but not disrupting the normal anatomy of the spinal canal or, more importantly, disrupting normal intracranial anatomy, as occurs with spina bifida. These tumors may be quite vascular, and dramatically increase cardiac output, leading to fetal congestive heart failure.[66] Fetal treatment strategies including administration of digitalis and open fetal surgery have been proposed,[67,68] but the safety and efficacy of these approaches remains unresolved.

The literature regarding fetal vascular malformations is sparse enough to make sweeping conclusions difficult. Intracranial arteriovenous malformations, most often involving aneurysmal dilation of the vein of Galen, has been well described.[69–71] While heart failure is a possibility, current management includes postnatal embolization rather than primary resection. Hepatic hemangiomas have also been reported.[72]

Aneurysmal dilation of the umbilical artery must be differentiated from other cysts of the umbilical cord such as persistence of the urachus, but this is easily accomplished with color or power Doppler imaging. There has been 1 report of fatal compression of the umbilical vein by an umbilical arterial aneurysm.[73] Aneurysmal dilation of the intraabdominal

portion of the umbilical vein also occurs,[74] and may, in our experience, be associated with high systolic and diastolic velocities in the aorta and intraabdominal umbilical arteries, suggestive of an arteriovenous fistula. Since both these vessels clot and regress shortly after birth, confirmation of the diagnosis with good outcomes, as we have seen, remains elusive. Other complications reported in this setting include fetal intravascular coagulopathy and thrombosis. Estroff has reported a series of 5 such umbilical vein varices.[75] The only complication was a single fetus who demonstrated transient cardiomegaly.

CONCLUSION

The prenatal diagnosis of structural heart disease is now widely available. The identification of patients with risk factors, and careful screening of those lacking identifiable risks can enable us to make prenatal diagnoses of structural heart disease and reduce the frequency of unanticipated congenital heart disease in neonates. Any pregnancy with significant risk factors for congenital heart disease should be thoroughly evaluated with a detailed fetal echocardiogram.

Particular attention should be paid to obtaining fetal echocardiograms in pregnancies found to have noncardiac structural anomalies, to diagnose a syndromes with specific inheritance patterns, which may alter neonatal management. Similarly, any fetus with structural heart disease should undergo a thorough ultrasound examination of all other organ systems. If fetal heart disease is found, even in the absence of other structural abnormalities, parental counseling should include the possibility of chromosomal abnormalities.

Complete counseling requires a team approach. The team can be composed primarily of obstetricians and pediatric cardiologists with further assistance from cardiac surgeons, genetic counselors, pediatric cardiology nursing specialists, social workers, clergymen, and even parents of other children with similar lesions, to provide information to the parents regarding realistic expectations about the care that their infants will require.

We still need further understanding of the short-term and long-term outcomes of these prenatal diagnoses, to understand the prognostic implications of our diagnoses, and whether our prenatal interventions have benefits or merely assuage our desire to do something for our fetal patients.

References

1. Wang KF, Xiao JP. Fetal echocardiography for pregnancy diagnosis. *Chinese J Obstet Gynecol.* 1964;10:267–269.
2. Winsberg F. Echocardiography of the fetal and newborn heart. *Invest Radiol.* 1972;7:152–158.
3. Kleinman CS, Hobbins JC, Jaffe CC, et al. Echocardiographic studies of the human fetus: prenatal diagnosis of congenital heart disease and cardiac dysrhythmias. *Pediatrics.* 1980;65:1059–1067.

4. Allan LD, Tynan MJ, Campbell S, et al. Echocardiographic and anatomical correlates in the fetus. *Br Heart J*. 1980;44:444–450.

5. Axel L. Real-time sonography of fetal cardiac anatomy. *Am J Roentgen*. 1983;141:283–295.

6. Sahn DJ, Lange LW, Allen HD, et al. Quantitative real-time cross-sectional echocardiography in the developing normal human fetus and newborn. *Circulation*. 1980;62:588–597.

7. Kleinman CS, Weinstein EM, Copel JA. Pulsed Doppler analysis of human fetal blood flow. In: Kisslo J, Adams D, Mark DB, eds. *Basic Doppler Echocardiography*. Churchill Livingstone; 1986: 173–185.

8. Allan LD, Chita SK, Al-Ghazali W, et al. Doppler echocardiographic evaluation of the normal human fetal heart. *Br Heart J*. 1987;57:528–533.

9. deVore GR, Horenstein J, Siassi B, et al. Fetal echocardiography VII: doppler color flow mapping: a new technique for the diagnosis of congenital heart disease. *Am J Obstet Gynecol*. 1987;156:1054–1064.

10. Huhta JC, Moise KJ, Fisher DJ, et al. Detection and quantitation of constriction of the fetal ductus arteriosus by Doppler echocardiography. 1987;75:406–412.

11. Copel JA, Morotti R, Hobbins JC, et al. The antenatal diagnosis of congenital heart disease using fetal echocardiography: is color flow mapping necessary? *Obstet Gynecol*. 1991;78: 1–8.

12. Bronshtein M, Zimmer EZ, Milo S, et al. Fetal cardiac abnormalities detected by transvaginal sonography at 12–16 weeks gestation. *Obstet Gynecol*. 1991;75:496–500.

13. Kurjak A, Zalud I, Predanic M. Transvaginal color Doppler in early pregnancy: rationale and clinical potential. *J Perinat Med*. 1994;22:475–482.

14. Gembruch U, Knopfle G, Bald R, et al. Early diagnosis of fetal congenital heart disease by transvaginal echocardiography. *Ultrasound Obstet Gynecol*. 1993;3:310–317.

15. Yagel S, Achiron R, Ron M, et al. Transvaginal ultrasonography at early pregnancy cannot be used alone for targeted organ ultrasonographic examination in a high-risk population. *Am J Obstet Gynecol*. 1995;172:971–975.

16. Allan LD, Chita SK, Sharland GK, et al. The accuracy of fetal echocardiography in the diagnosis of congenital heart disease. *Int J Cardiol*. 1989;25:279–288.

17. Kleinman CS, Santulli TV Jr. Ultrasonic evaluation of the fetal human heart. *Semin Perinatol*. 1983;7:90–101.

18. Kleinman CS, Donnerstein RL. Ultrasonic assessment of cardiac function in the intact human fetus. *J Am Coll Cardiol*. 1985;5:84S–94S.

19. Reed KL, Meijboom EJ, Sahn DJ, et al. Cardiac Doppler flow velocities in human fetuses. *Circulation*. 1986;73:41–46.

20. Reed KL, Sahn DJ, Scagnelli S, et al. Doppler echocardiographic studies of diastolic function in the human fetal heart: changes during gestation. *J Amer Coll Cardiol*. 1986;8:391–395.

21. de Smedt MCH, Visser GHA, Meijboom EJ. Fetal cardiac output estimated by Doppler echocardiography during mid- and late gestation. *Am J Cardiol*. 1987;60:338–342.

22. Rudolph AM, Heymann MA. Circulatory changes during growth in the fetal lamb. *Circ Res*. 1970;26:289–297.

23. Rudolph AM. Distribution and regulation of blood flow in the fetal and neonatal lamb. *Circ Res*. 1985;57:811–826.

24. Neutze JM, Starling MB, Elliot RB, et al. Palliation of cyanotic congenital heart disease in infancy with Type E Prostaglandin. *Circulation*. 1977;55:238–241.

25. Stumpflen I, Stumpflen A, Wimmer M, et al. Effect of detailed fetal echocardiography as part of routine prenatal ultrasonographic screening on detection of congenital heart disease. *Lancet*. 1996;348:854–857.

26. Yagel S, Weissman A, Rotstein X, et al. Congenital heart defects: natural course and in utero development. *Circulation*. 1997;96:550–555.

27. Kleinert S. Routine prenatal screening for congenital heart disease. *Lancet*. 1996;348:836.

28. Kleinman CS, Donnerstein RL, DeVore GR, et al. Fetal echocardiography in nonimmune fetal hydrops: a technique for evaluation of in utero heart failure. *N Engl J Med*. 1982;306:568–575.

29. Silverman NS, Kleinman CS, Rudolph JA, et al. Fetal atrioventricular valve insufficiency associated with nonimmune hydrops: a two-dimensional echocardiographic and pulsed-Doppler ultrasound study. *Circulation*. 1985;72: 825–832.

30. Respondek ML, Kammermeier M, Ludomirsky A, et al. The prevalence and clinical significance of fetal tricuspid valve regurgitation with normal heart anatomy. *Am J Obstet Gynecol*. 1994;171:1265–1270.

31. Friedman WF. The intrinsic physiologic properties of the developing heart. In Friedman WF, Lesch M, Sonnenblick EH, eds. *Neonatal Heart Disease*. New York: Grune & Stratton; 1973:.

32. Copel JA, Pilu G, Green J, et al. Fetal echocardiographic screening for congenital heart disease: the importance of the four-chamber view. *Am J Obstet Gynecol*. 1987;157:648–655.

33. Ewigman BG, Crane JP, Frigoletto FD, et al. Effect of prenatal ultrasound screening on perinatal outcome. RADIUS study group. *N Engl J Med*. 1993;329:821–827.

34. Buskens E, Grobee DE, Frohn-Mulder IM. Efficacy of routine fetal ultrasound screening for congenital heart disease in normal pregnancy. *Circulation*. 1996;94:67–72.

35. Rustico MA, D'Ottavio G, Maieron A, et al. Fetal heart screening in low risk pregnancies. *Ultrasound Obstet Gynecol*. 1995;6:1–7.

36. Tegnander E, Eik-Nes SH, Johansen OJ, et al. Prenatal detection of heart defects at the routine fetal examinations at 18 weeks in a non-selected population. *Ultrasound Obstet Gynecol*. 1995;5: 372–380.

37. Todros T, Faggiano F, Chiappa E, et al. Accuracy of routine ultrasonography in screening heart disease prenatally. *Prenat Diagn*. 1997;17:901–906.

38. Shipp TD, Bromley B, Hornberger LK, et al. Levorotation of the fetal cardiac axis: a clue for the presence of congenital heart disease. *Obstet Gynecol*. 1995;85:97–102.

39. Smith RS, Comstock CH, Kirk JS, et al. Ultrasonographic left cardiac axis deviation: a marker for fetal anomalies. *Obstet Gynecol*. 1995;85:187–191.

40. Copel JA, Pilu G, Kleinman CS. Congenital heart disease and extracardiac anomalies: associations and indications for fetal echocardiography. *Am J Obstet Gynecol*. 1986;154:1121–1132.

41. Copel JA, Cullen M, Green JJ, et al. The frequency of aneuploidy in prenatally diagnosed congenital heart disease: an indication for fetal karyotyping. *Am J Obstet Gynecol*. 1988;158:409–413.

42. Berg KA, Clark EB, Astemborski JA, et al. Prenatal detection of cardiovascular malformations by echocardiography: an indication for cytogenetic evaluation. *Am J Obstet Gynecol*. 1988;159: 477–481.

43. Hook EB. Chromosome abnormalities and spontaneous fetal death following amniocentesis: further data and associations with maternal age. *Am J Hum Genet*. 1983;35:110–116.

44. Smythe JF, Copel JA, Kleinman CS. Outcome of prenatally detected cardiac malformations. *Am J Cardiol*. 1992;69:1471–1474.

45. Wilson DI, Goodship JA, Burn J, et al. Deletions within chromosome 22q11 in familial congenital heart disease. *Lancet*. 1992;340:573–575.

46. Driscoll DA, Salvin J, Sleeinger B, et al. Prevalence of 22q11 deletions in DiGeorge and velocardiofacial syndromes: implications for genetic counseling and prenatal diagnosis. *J Med Genet*. 1993;30: 813–817.

47. Hornberger LK, Sahn DJ, Kleinman CS, et al. Tricuspid valve disease with significant tricuspid insufficiency in the fetus: diagnosis and outcome. *J Am Coll Cardiol.* 1991;17:167–173.

48. Silverman NH, Schmidt KG. Ventricular volume overload in the human fetus: observations from fetal echocardiography. *J Am Soc Echocardiogr.* 1990;3:20–29.

49. Chang AC, Huhta JC, Yoon GY, et al. Diagnosis, transport and outcome in fetuses with left ventricular outflow tract obstruction. *J Thorac Cardiovasc Surg.* 1991;102:841–846.

50. Copel JA, Tan AS, Kleinman CS. Does a prenatal diagnosis of congenital heart disease alter short-term outcome? *Ultrasound Obstet Gynecol.* 1997;10:237–241.

51. Eapen RS, Rowland DG, Franklin WH. Effect of prenatal diagnosis of critical left heart obstruction on perinatal morbidity and mortality. *Am J Perinatol.* 1998;15:237–242.

52. Bailey LL, Gundry SR, Rozyacek AJ, et al. Bless the babies: one hundred fifteen late survivors of heart transplantation during the first year of life. *J Thorac Cardiovasc Surg.* 1993;105:805–814.

53. Norwood WI, Lang P, Castaneda AR, et al. Experience with operations for hypoplastic left heart syndrome. *J Thorac Cardiovasc Surg.* 1981;82:511–519.

54. Bellinger DC, Jonas R, Rappaport LA, et al. Developmental and neurological status of children after heart surgery with hypothermia, circulatory arrest, or low flow cardiopulmonary bypass. *N Engl J Med.* 1995;332:549–555.

55. Harrison MR, Golbus MS, Filly RA, eds. *The Unborn Patient.* 2nd ed. Philadelphia, PA: WB Saunders; 1991.

56. Verrier ED, Vlahakes GJ, Hanley FL, et al. Experimental fetal cardiac surgery. In: Harrison MR, Golbus MS, Filly RA, eds. *The Unborn Patient: Prenatal Diagnosis and Treatment.* Philadelphia, PA: WB Saunders; 1991:548–556.

57. Maxwell D, Allan L, Tynan MJ. Balloon dilatation of the aortic valve in the fetus: a report of two cases. *Br Heart J.* 1991;65:256–261.

58. Feit L, Copel JA, Kleinman CS. Foramen ovale size in the normal and abnormal fetal heart: an indicator of transatrial flow physiology. *Ultrasound Obstet Gynecol.* 1991;1:313–319.

59. Schmidt KG, Ulmer HE, Silverman NH, et al. Perinatal outcome of fetal complete atrioventricular block: a multicenter experience. *J Am Coll Cardiol.* 1991;17:1360–1366.

60. Litsey SE, Noonan JA, O'Connor WN, et al. Maternal connective tissue disease and congenital heart block: demonstration of immunoglobulin in cardiac tissue. *N Engl J Med.* 1985;312:98–100.

61. Carpenter RJ, Strasburger JF, Garson A, et al. Fetal ventricular pacing secondary to complete heart block. *J Am Coll Cardiol.* 1986;8:1434–1436.

62. Walkinshaw SA, Welch CR, McCormack J, et al. In utero pacing for fetal congenital heart block. *Fetal Diagn Ther.* 1994;9:183.

63. Pringle KC, Weiner CP, Soper RT, et al. Sacrococcygeal teratoma. *Fetal Therapy.* 1987;2:80–87.

64. Holzgreve W, Miny P, Anderson R, et al. Experience with 8 cases of prenatally diagnosed sacrococcygeal teratomas. *Fetal Therapy.* 1987;2:88–94.

65. Kuhlmann RS, Warsof SL, Levey DL, et al. Fetal sacrococcygeal teratoma. *Fetal Therapy.* 1987;2:95–100.

66. Schmidt KG, Silverman NH, Harrison MR, et al. High-output cardiac failure in fetuses with large sacrococcygeal teratoma: diagnosis by echocardiography and Doppler ultrasound. *J Pediatr.* 1989;114:1023–1028.

67. Langer JC, Harrison MR, Schmidt KG, et al. Fetal hydrops and death from sacrococcygeal teratoma: rationale for fetal surgery. *Am J Obstet Gynecol.* 1989;160:1145–1150.

68. Hecher K, Hackeloer B-J. Intrauterine endoscopic laser surgery for fetal sacrococcygeal teratoma. *Lancet.* 199;347:470.

69. Doren M, Tercanli S, Holzgreve W. Prenatal diagnosis of a vein of Galen aneurysm: relevance of associated malformations for timing and mode of delivery. *Ultrasound Obstet Gynecol.* 1995;6:287–289.

70. Sepulveda W, Platt CC, Fisk NM. Prenatal diagnosis of cerebral arteriovenous malformation using color Doppler ultrasonography: case report and review of the literature. *Ultrasound Obstet Gynecol.* 1995;6:282–286.

71. Chisholm CA, Kuller JA, Katz VL, et al. Aneurysm of the vein of Galen: prenatal diagnosis and perinatal management. *Am J Perinatol.* 1996;13:503–506.

72. Abuhamad AZ, Lewis D, Inati MN, et al. The use of color Doppler in the diagnosis of fetal hepatic hemangioma. *J Ultrasound Med.* 1993;12:223–226.

73. Siddiqi TA, Bendon R, Schultz DM, et al. Umbilical artery aneurysm. *Obstet Gynecol.* 1992;80:530–533.

74. Moore L, Toi A, Chitayat D. Abnormalities of the intra-abdominal fetal umbilical vein: reports of four cases and a review of the literature. *Ultrasound Obstet Gynecol.* 1996;7:21–25.

75. Estroff JA, Benacerraf BR. Fetal umbilical vein varix: sonographic appearance and postnatal outcome. *J Ultrasound Med.* 1992;11:69–73.

NORMAL AND ABNORMAL FINDINGS OF THE FETAL ABDOMEN AND ANTERIOR WALL

Wayne H. Persutte / John C. Hobbins

INTRODUCTION

An evaluation of the continuity of the abdomen and the intraabdominal contents is a standard component of the obstetrical ultrasound examination performed in the United States. Although many abdominal abnormalities are obvious because of their unusual appearance, there is considerable variability in the appearances of both normal and abnormal abdominal anatomy. In some cases, overtly abnormal anatomy may look normal: conversely, normal anatomy can appear strikingly unusual. As a result, it is important to: (1) obtain a clear and accurate sonographic impression of the true state of fetal anatomy; (2) understand the constellation of normal and abnormal sonographic appearances; and (3) recognize that some apparently abnormal images may result from the dynamic nature of organs and organ systems. Serial evaluations are often necessary to determine the extent and severity of abnormalities.

The following chapter is intended to provide a review of normal fetal abdominal anatomy (excluding the genitourinary system), anomalies of specific organ systems, multiple anomaly complexes involving the abdomen, and other pathologies associated with significant abdominal findings.

GENERAL CONSIDERATIONS REGARDING THE FETAL ABDOMEN

EMBRYOLOGY

The primitive gut is divided into 3 sections: the foregut, the midgut, and the hindgut.[1] The gut begins formation at approximately 4 weeks after the last menstrual period. The foregut develops into the esophagus, stomach, duodenum, pharynx (structures that extend from the buccopharyngeal membrane to the duodenum), liver, pancreas, and lower respiratory tract.

From that time, the stomach can immediately be recognized as a fusiform dilatation of the caudal foregut. It continues to enlarge and broaden ventrodorsally and at approximately 6 weeks it ascends into the abdomen. By 11 weeks, the muscles within the walls of the stomach are capable of contracting. The stomach slowly rotates clockwise 90 degrees as a result of differential growth of the dorsal and ventral borders of the greater curvature of the stomach. Finally, it acquires its adult shape and it settles into place into the left upper quadrant of the abdomen.

The midgut forms the largest portion of the GI tract and it remains connected to the yolk sac via the vitelline and omphalomesenteric ducts to the posterior intestinal portal until 10–12 weeks' gestation. At that time the anterior abdominal wall of the fetus can be observed sonographically to close.

Thereafter the bowel is identifiable within the fetal abdomen. Lastly, the hindgut forms the distal gastrointestinal tract and is closely associated with genitourinary tract formation. The hindgut forms into the posterior intestinal portal to the cloacal membrane.

THE EXPECTATION OF THE ULTRASOUND EXAMINATION

In 2002, the American Institute of Ultrasound in Medicine published their revised standard for the constituents of a routine prenatal ultrasonographic examination.[2] In this standard, they suggest the assessment of the fetal abdomen should include:

"The abdominal circumference should be determined on a true transverse view, preferably at the level of the left and right portal sinuses . . . the study should include, but not necessarily be limited to, assessment . . . stomach . . . fetal umbilical cord insertion site and intactness of the interior abdominal wall . . . . While not considered part of the minimum examination . . . it is desirable to examine other areas of the *anatomy.*"

These requirements are fundamentally similar to those standards endorsed by the American Colleges of Radiology, and Obstetrics and Gynecology. Many physicians consider these guidelines to be minimum "Standard of Care" in the performance and evaluation of the routine ultrasound examination. These guidelines should be followed in order to minimize the potential for malpractice liability.

NORMAL APPEARANCE AND ABNORMALITIES OF THE GASTROINTESTINAL TRACT

OVERVIEW OF GASTROINTESTINAL ABNORMALITIES

Generally, fetuses with gastrointestinal abnormalities have shorter pregnancies, are of lower birth weight, and have increased postnatal mortality, compared with their uncomplicated counterparts.[3] Fitzimmons et al. studied the length of the gastrointestinal tract and its constituents in both normal fetal autopsies and those that were associated with fetal abnormalities[4] including omphalocele, congenital heart disease, and fetal chromosomal abnormalities. They reported that fetuses with abnormalities were found to have significantly shorter overall gastrointestinal tract lengths, compared with autopsy specimens that had no major structural abnormalities.

A recent report from Ireland suggested that ingestion and gastrointestinal absorption of the amniotic fluid plays an important role in fetal nutrition. Amniotic fluid is found to favorably contribute to fetal growth. This contribution is thought to increase with advancing gestational age. Surana and Puri report that fetuses with gastrointestinal tract abnormalities have poor fetal growth when compared with unaffected fetuses: the higher the GI tract obstruction the more pronounced the fetal growth impairment.[5]

Muller and associates showed that the examination of the amniotic fluid digested enzymes (gamma-glutamyl-transpeptidase and intestinal alkaline phosphatase) was useful in confirming the presence of a gastrointestinal obstruction. However, these enzymes were not very useful in determining the etiology of the abnormality.

LARNYX AND PHARNYX

Normal

Both the fetal larynx and pharynx can be observed with ultrasound from approximately 14 weeks of pregnancy. The oropharynx and laryngopharynx appear as fluid-filled structures and therefore can be seen frequently when attempted.[6] The best view to investigate the pharynx is from a transverse axial plane through the upper neck of the fetus. However, longitudinal views, which can be harder to obtain, depict the structures in a more anatomical position. In this plane, both the continuity of the pharyngeal cavities and the relationship between the larynx and pharynx can be discerned. The detailed anatomy that can sometimes be depicted include the pyriform sinuses, valleculae, and glottis. Active pharyngeal movement can be seen during swallowing.

Abnormalities

Very few reports of abnormalities of the gastrointestinal system proximal to the hypopharynx have been reported in the prenatal literature. However, when present they can provide significant information of use to neonatologists in the immediate postpartum period. The importance of this information can be measured in terms of impaired neurologic function. Further, these abnormalities can result in difficulty of ventilation and resuscitation in the neonate.

ASTOMIA

The most devastating congenital maldevelopment of the oral cavity and upper gastrointestinal tract is astomia, or absence of the mouth. This is usually the result of a developmental field defect and is commonly associated with other abnormalities of first pharyngeal arch development. As such, it is often accompanied by agnathia, a congenital absence of the mandible, or the constellation of abnormalities that constitute the Aagnatia malformation complex.[7] Agnathia is a very rare and lethal abnormality.

LARYNGEAL ATRESIA

Laryngeal atresia is also very rare and is a universally lethal defect of the upper respiratory tract. It has been prenatally diagnosed only 6 times; once in a fetus of a twin pair and another associated with chondrodysplasia punctata.[8-11]

LARYNGEAL PALSY

Laryngeal palsy, paralysis of the larynx, has been reported in many infants with brain abnormalities (including ventriculomegaly, and Arnold Chiari Type II malformation) and in association with meningomylocele. Although the recognition of this entity has never been reported in the fetus, current sonographic techniques should allow for its diagnosis. Prenatal presence or absence of laryngeal palsy in affected cases may provide a more accurate method of determining the magnitude of neurologic impairment.

TERATOMA

The prenatal diagnosis of pharyngeal teratoma has been described as a discretely complex mass in posterior oral cavity.[12]

ESOPHAGUS

Normal

The middle and distal esophagus can be seen from the mid-second trimester in 90% and 30% of cases, respectively.[13] The proximal esophagus is difficult to visualize and can be seen in less than 19% of cases. However, when visualized, the proximal esophagus may be useful in assessing for esophageal atresia.[14] The esophagus can be seen in longitudinal, coronal, and transverse axial planes and it can appear as a fluid filled hypoechoic structure anterior to the descending thoracic aorta.

Abnormal

With the exception of the last category, when isolated, all abnormalities of the esophagus are surgically correctable and the prognosis is generally excellent. Complications from surgery may require long-term care. Mortality associated with surgical correction is closely related to the magnitude of coexisting abnormalities or growth retardation.

CONGENITAL ISOLATED ESOPHAGEAL ATRESIA

Congenital esophageal atresia is a rare nonlethal (except when untreated) birth defect usually identified in the immediate neonatal period. Clinical symptoms include excess salivation, regurgitation, and obstruction of the esophageal tract. The incidence of congenital esophageal atresia is 1 in 32,000 births.

In 1995, Satoh et al. reported the prenatal sonographic appearances of 8 cases of congenital esophageal atresia. In addition to polyhydramnios and a small stomach, a transient anechoic area in the fetal neck was seen in all cases. They suggest that this finding should be a significant indicator of this abnormality. Half of all cases of congenital esophageal atresia have other congenital abnormalities. In descending order of frequency, these abnormalities include congenital heart disease, other gastrointestinal abnormalities, genitourinary abnormalities, skeletal abnormalities, and facial clefting. Congenital esophageal atresia has been associated with an unexplained elevated amniotic fluid alpha-fetoprotein.[15] It has also been associated with trisomy 21. One third of cases of esophageal atresia are delivered prematurely (likely due to polyhydramnios).

CONGENITAL ESOPHAGEAL DUPLICATION

Congenital Esophageal Duplication, along with esophageal cyst and neurenteric cyst, is a rare abnormality of the upper gastrointestinal tract. Occasionally associated with other duplications of the gastrointestinal tract, the rate of occurrence in the general population is unknown.[16] Only 2 reports of the prenatal sonographic features of esophageal duplication can be found in the literature.

ESOPHAGEAL STENOSIS

Esophageal stenosis, diverticulum, and achalasia have not been described prenatally. These are unlikely to be described because they are not associated with significant gastrointestinal obstruction, which results in polyhydramnios or dilatation of the gastrointestinal tract. It is likely that sufficient amniotic fluid will make its way into the fetal stomach such that a small stomach would not tip off the observer to suspect an abnormality.

ESOPHAGEAL ATRESIA ASSOCIATED WITH TRACHEOESOPHAGEAL FISTULA

Esophageal atresia associated with tracheoesophageal fistula is more common than isolated esophageal atresia (prevalence of 1 in 3000–5000 and 1 in 32,000, respectively). The most common site of fistula formation is in the distal esophagus (85% of cases). Esophageal atresia with tracheoesophageal fistula is also more commonly associated with other fetal abnormalities (≈70% of cases). The most common of these abnormalities

include congenital heart defect, other gastrointestinal abnormalities, imperforate anus, and Vater association. It has been suggested that esophageal atresia with tracheoesophageal fistula may have an autosomal recessive mode of inheritance.

STOMACH

Normal

Sonographically, the fetal stomach appears as a hypo-echogenic, elliptical structure in the left upper quadrant of the fetal abdomen. Goldstein et al. reported the identification of the fetal stomach as early as 9 weeks in gestation, and they reported that it should be seen consistently from 10 weeks.[17] Recognizable anatomy of the stomach should include the greater and lesser curvatures, the fundus, the body, and the pylorus. These structures should be consistently identified from 14 weeks of pregnancy.[18] Later, an echogenic structure can be identified in the lesser curvature of the stomach; the incisura angularis ventriculi. Fluid in the fetal stomach is imbibed as a result of the swallowing of the amniotic fluid after 16 weeks. At the inferior margin of the stomach, the pylorus marks the confluence between the stomach and the duodenum. It can be recognized in the left upper quadrant of the fetal abdomen. The position of the stomach may distinguish it from the gall bladder, which also may appear as a hypoechoic or anechoic in the fetal abdomen, the gall bladder appears more anterior to the abdominal wall and to the right of midline.

The typical size of the fetal stomach for gestational age has been reported (Fig. 20-1).[19–21] However, Zimmer and associates recently reported that variability caused by dynamic filling and emptying of the stomach make its measurement unreliable.[22]

Abnormalities

Marked dilatation of the fetal stomach is usually overt and easily recognized. Dilatation is commonly observed with proximal intestinal atresias.[23] Conversely, nonvisualization of the

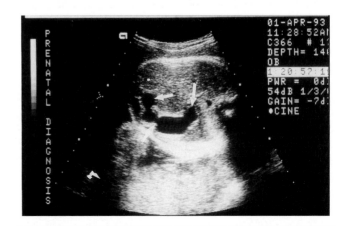

FIGURE 20-1 *Normal Ultrasonographic Appearance of the Upper Gastrointestinal Tract.* This transverse image of the fetal abdomen at 24 weeks shows a fluid-filled stomach (arrow), pyloris (arrow), and proximal duodenum (arrow).

TABLE 20-1	CAUSES OF NONVISUALIZATION OF THE FETAL STOMACH

Esophageal atresia
Oligohydramnios
Impaired swallowing
    CNS abnormalities
    Facial clefts
    Neuromuscular disorders
Abnormal location
    Congenital diaphragmatic hernia
    Situs inversus

From Hertzberg B. Sonography of the fetal gastrointestinal tract: anatomic variants, diagnostic pitfalls, and abnormalities. *AJR* 1994;162:1175–1182.

fetal stomach may be associated with esophageal atresia, tracheoesophageal fistula, or central nervous system anomalies resulting from aberrant fetal swallowing.

Absent or small fetal stomach is a nonspecific finding (Table 20-1), primarily because the size of the stomach can be highly variable, and even when observed as small, it may be a normal size in as little as 20 minutes. There are only two circumstances that can result in an identifiable stomach in the face of a nonpatent esophagus. First, in the case of a tracheoesophageal fistula inferior to esophageal atresia, fluid can access the fetal stomach through the trachea and via the fistula. Second, esophageal atresia without tracheoesophageal fistula in addition to an atresia of the proximal small bowel can cause gastric secretions from the stomach to accumulate within the gastric lumen. When the stomach is absent after 19 weeks, Pretorius et al. reported an abnormal outcome in 100% of cases.[24] Millener et al. found abnormal outcomes occurred in 48% of those who were found to have no demonstrable stomach after 14 weeks of gestation.[25,26]

Although the determination of smallness of the stomach is based on subjective criteria alone, McKenna et al. reported inter and intra-observer agreement in the ultrasonographic measurement of the fetal stomach to be admirable (93% and 100%, respectively).

The rate of abnormal karyotype is approximately 38% with a very small or absent fetal stomach.[26] In absent stomach, McKenna and associates reported trisomy 18 to complicate approximately 75% of these cases and trisomy 21 to complicate approximately 25%.[26] All aneuploid fetuses had other morphologic abnormalities detectable on ultrasound. The prognosis in small or absent fetal stomach is dependent upon the type and severity of concomitant abnormalities. When other findings are seen, the survival rate is only 33%; whereas when isolated, the survival rate is 96%. Polyhydramnios is seen in 36% of cases with either an absent or a small stomach. Thirty-one percent of these have esophageal atresia.

Sometimes echogenic foci or debris can be seen within the stomach; *gastric pseudomasses* (Fig. 20-2).[27] Since this more frequently occurs after an invasive procedure such as amniocentesis, it is thought to result from a concentration of red blood cells which may have been swallowed with amniotic

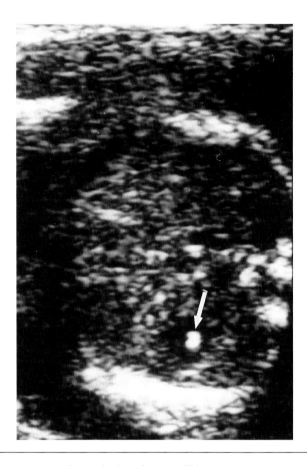

FIGURE 20-2 *Stomach Pseudomass.* This transverse ultrasonographic image of the fetal abdomen at 19 weeks shows a *pseudomass* in the stomach (arrow). These masses are usually benign and of no clinical significance.

fluid. This is usually a transient finding and many have reported this to be of no clinical significance.[28]

CONGENITAL DUPLICATION OF THE STOMACH

Congenital duplication of the stomach or a duplication cyst (congenital diverticulum) is a very rare occurrence. This is usually a solitary finding, but occasionally may be associated with other duplications of gastrointestinal organs. More common in females (8:1), congenital duplication of the stomach can result in postnatal rupture and subsequent peritonitis, sepsis, and autodigestion. When recognized early, surgical incision is the usual treatment. Small remnant cysts may persist undetected until later in life when an increased risk of carcinoma has been observed.

The prenatal sonographic visualization of congenital duplication of the stomach has been described in a few reports. In 1986, Bidwell and Nelson described congenital stomach duplication to appear as a cystic mass in the right upper quadrant of the fetal abdomen with peristaltic activity.[29,30]

CONGENITAL AGASTRIA

Congenital agastria remained unreported until 1987 when Dorney et al. described this finding.[31] In a single case, investigators could find no stomach (including a rudimentary stomach or pylorus) and the esophagus was observed to directly communicate with the duodenum. This case was also complicated by microagnathia. Although this rare finding has not been identified before birth, it should be considered when an absent fetal stomach is seen consistently without polyhydramnios.

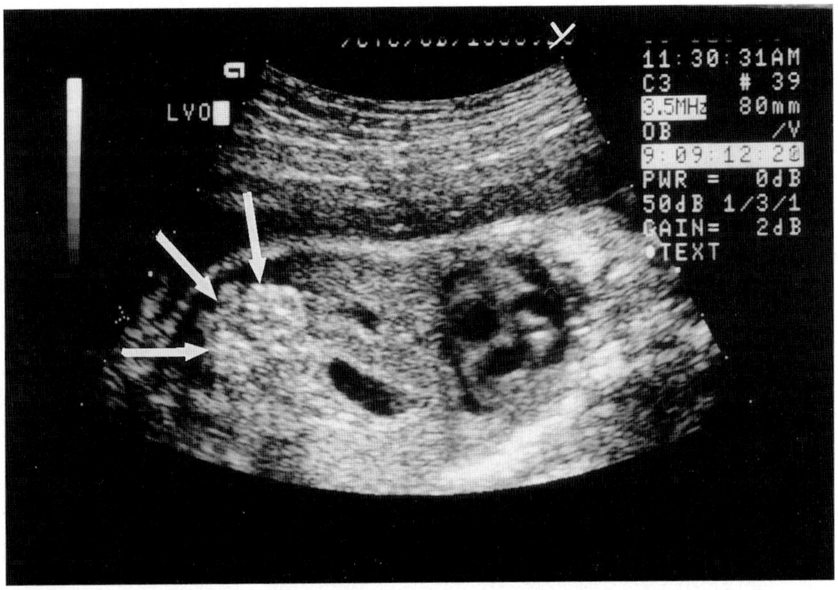

MICROGASTRIA

Congenital microgastria, also known as hypoplasia of the stomach, is a result of the failure of rotation of the stomach without sectional differentiation (i.e., fundus, body, and pyloris). Most effected patients have limited longevity associated with chronic poor health. This finding is not associated with concomitant abnormalities. Only 1 known case of the prenatal diagnosis of microgastria exists. In 1994, Hill presented a case of congenital microgastria that had no discernable stomach associated with normal amounts of amniotic fluid.[32]

PYLORIC ATRESIA

Pyloric atresia results from an error in recanalization of the gastric lumen. It is characterized by a dilated stomach and is usually first recognized in the neonatal period with vomiting. Pyloric atresia appears very rarely (1:1 million) and it accounts for only 1% of all gastrointestinal atresias. The association between pyloric atresia and epidermalysis bulosa has been established.[33] A dilated fetal stomach seen in combination with polyhydramnios should tip off the prenatal investigator to suspect pyloric atresia (Fig. 20-3).

Pyloric atresia has an autosomal recessive mode of inheritance and is associated with trisomy 21. Reported cases suggest a familial predisposition. Peled et al. was able to prenatally diagnose pyloric atresia in a patient with a strong suspicion based on a positive family history.[34]

Rizzo et al. found color and pulsed Doppler of the gastroesophogeal junction to be useful in the diagnosis of pyloric atresia.[35] They demonstrated that biphasic fluid flow (apparently consistent with gastroesophogeal reflux) confirmed the diagnosis of atresia.

FIGURE 20-3 *Small Intestines.* The ultrasonographic appearance of fetal small bowel is a complex structure in the lower abdomen of the abdomen (arrow). In this sagittal image the bowel appears typical, albeit somewhat more echogenic because of mild abdominal ascites.

SMALL INTESTINE

Normal

The intestine may appear highly varied during the prenatal period with ultrasonography.[36] The fetal small intestine can be seen sonographically as early as 12 weeks of gestation. In the early second trimester, the bowel appears as homogenous, mildly echogenic, and ill defined in the lower abdomen of the fetus (Fig. 20-4).[37] Meconium accumulates in the small bowel from the early second trimester. As pregnancy progresses, the bowel becomes more heterogenic and well defined with echogenic lumen and hypoechogenic (muscular wall) constituents. Peristalsis within the fetal bowel can be seen as early as 18 weeks of gestation. Goldstein et al. graded peristaltic movements in the small intestine, but the usefulness of this technique is equivocal.[38] Late in pregnancy, discrete fluid-filled loops of bowel can be seen in virtually all fetuses. The serosa is more echogenic than the muscularus.

Abnormalities

Corteville and associates investigated the prenatal and postnatal findings in a large series of fetuses with small bowel pathology.[39] They found ultrasound to be 100% sensitive and had a positive predictive value of 73% in the identification of the fetus with small bowel atresia. In comparison, the sensitivity of ultrasound in the identification of large bowel lesions was only 8% and the positive predictive value was 18%. A pattern of increasing bowel dilatation in the 3rd trimester in hyperperistalsis was helpful in predicting small bowel obstruction. They concluded that wide variability in ultrasound appearance of bowel abnormalities exists.

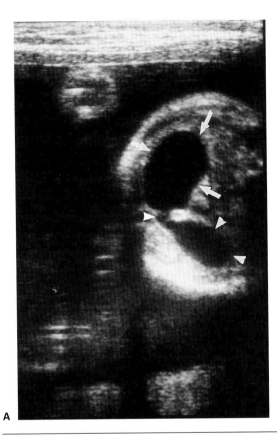

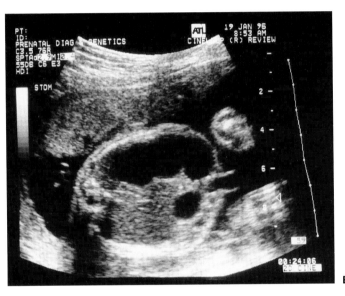

FIGURE 20-4 *Duodenal Atresia.* Transverse ultrasonographic image of the fetal abdomen shows the stomach, pyloris, and dilated duodenum (arrows).

Duodenal Atresia/Stenosis

Duodenal atresia or stenosis occurs in approximately 1 in 10,000 live births. Most cases are diagnosed in the first days of life. An annular pancreas or small bowel malrotation is associated with 20–30% of these cases. In 80% of affected patients, the atresia/stenosis occurs immediately distal to the pyloris. Fifty percent of affected infants are growth retarded or deliver preterm and one third of all cases of duodenal atresia have trisomy 21. Congenital heart disease occurs in 20 percent of cases. Although duodenal atresia is usually sporadic, at least 1 case of autosomal recessive inheritance has been reported.

Many cases of the prenatal diagnosis of duodenal atresia have been reported. The hallmark of duodenal atresia is the classic double-bubble sign (Fig. 20-5). Actually, it may be better described as a dilated hour glass configuration on transverse, oblique section. In this image, the stomach and duodenum can appear as dilated and the pyloris is narrowed, creating an hourglass shape. The importance of sonographically "connecting" the stomach and duodenum is underscored when one considers other cystic masses that can be identified in

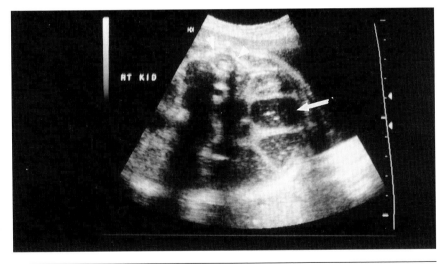

FIGURE 20-5 *Pyloric Stenosis.* Dilated fetal stomach without proximal duodenal dilatation is characteristic of pyloric stenosis.

the abdomen (none of which can be connected to the stomach, Table 20-2).

Jejunal Atresia/Stenosis

Jejunal atresia/stenosis is slightly more common than duodenal atresia (1 in 3,000–5,000 versus 1 in 5,000, respectively). In descending order of frequency, mid-bowel atresias are found

TABLE 20-2	CAUSES OF PSEUDO-DOUBLE-BUBBLE SIGN ON ULTRASONOGRAPHY
Bisection of normal stomach	
Choledochal cyst	
Renal cyst	
Splenic cyst	
Bowel duplication cyst	
Ovarian cyst	
Hepatic cyst	
Omental or mesenteric cyst	

From Hertzberg B. Sonography of the Fetal Gastrointestinal Tract: Anatomic Variants, Diagnostic Pitfalls, and Abnormalities. *AJR* 1994;162:1175–1182.

in the distal ileum (36%), proximal jejunum (31%), distal jejunum (20%), and proximal ileum (13%).[40,41,42] Jejunal atresias are thought to develop as a result of a vascular accident during organogenesis.[43] Further, jejunal atresias have been associated with esophageal atresia and anal rectal atresia in 10% of cases.[44]

Like other proximal GI atresias, both jejunal atresia and ileum atresia are detected based on dilated proximal gastrointestinal organs. It may also be associated with polyhydramnios. The sensitivity of ultrasound in the identification of these types of atresias are likely to be low, since some of these cases, especially those that are more distal, may have only subtle or no demonstrable accompanying sonographic findings.

Vulvulous

Vulvulous, an intestinal obstruction due to knotting or twisting of the bowel, may occur if embryological fixation occurs abnormally. In the first trimester, the bowel normally herniates and rotates in position, thereafter the bowel grows to become affixed to the retroperitoneum. If this does not occur appropriately, a vulvulous can result.

Meconium Ileus

Meconium ileus is used to describe the condition of impacted, sticky or thick meconium in the distal ileum. Almost all neonates with meconium ileus are found to have cystic fibrosis; an autosomal recessive disorder affecting 1 in 2,000 Caucasian births. However, of those with cystic fibrosis, only 10–15% will have meconium ileus.[45] Inspissated meconium can temporarily obstruct the colon.

Sonographically, a dilated ileum, normal jejunum, and an empty or collapsed colon characterize meconium ileus.[41] Bowel can appear as dilated and meconium appear echogenic in meconium ileus after 26 weeks. Polyhydramnios usually accompanies this finding.

Ileal Atresia

Ileal atresia has been prenatally described in many cases. Typically, multiple distended loops of dilated bowel can be seen with strong peristaltic movements. The stomach may also be distended.[46]

Echogenic Bowel

Echogenic bowel has received a great deal of attention in prenatal literature (Fig. 20-6). Traditionally, echogenic bowel has been closely associated with meconium peritonitis from ileus. More recently, it has been further associated with many fetal abnormalities (primarily Trisomy 21) and adverse perinatal outcome.[47,48] Nyberg suggested the location of the echogenicity (small bowel versus colon), gestational age, and magnitude of echogenicity, may be significant factors in diagnosis and prognosis. He speculated that echogenic bowel is likely the result of decreased water concentration or inspissation of meconium.

The association between echogenic bowel and fetal aneuploidy has been clearly established.[49–57] Dicke and Crane found an association between echogenic bowel and cystic fibrosis, perinatal death (17% versus 4% in controls) and growth retardation (23% versus 2% in matched controls).[58] In regard to the latter, Sepulveda et al. demonstrated a 4-fold increased risk for intrauterine growth retardation and lower birth weight with no increased risk for preterm delivery with isolated echogenic bowel.[59] Both Hill et al. and Muller et al. also reported an association between echogenic bowel and both cytomegalovirus and parvovirus.[60]

Recommendations in regard to echogenic bowel include enhanced ultrasonographic surveillance, consideration of screening for cystic fibrosis and infectious disease, and fetal genetic testing (depending on the recognition of other ultrasonographic findings) and amniotic fluid digestive enzymes.[61] New data seem to suggest that concerns regarding echogenic bowel should surround the increased risk for pregnancy complications. Echogenic bowel combined with an elevated MSAFP has been shown to be a significant indicator as adverse perinatal outcome. Achiron et al. called this combination ominous.[62] They reported a small series of 6 fetuses with echogenic bowel and high elevated MSAFP: all of whom died perinatally (4 before birth and 2 after). Secondarily, considerations regarding cystic fibrosis should be made. In fact, Sepulveda and associates suggest that echogenic bowel is only associated with cystic fibrosis in those cases with a significant family history.[63] A linear relationship has been observed between the magnitude of echogenic bowel and the risk for aneuploidy and cystic fibrosis. Multiple grading systems for echogenic bowel have been recently proposed.[64] A universal scoring system should be recognized and adopted.

LARGE INTESTINE

Normal

The large bowel is not clearly recognizable with prenatal sonography until the early third trimester (Fig. 20-7a). Thereafter, it becomes increasingly easy to visualize. The contents of the colon are usually hypoechoic: thus, the normal colon can be erroneously considered dilated small bowel. The identification of hofstral folds should allow small bowel to be distinguished from colon (Fig. 20-7b). Large bowel can be seen ascending on the right side of the fetal abdomen to the hepatic flexure,

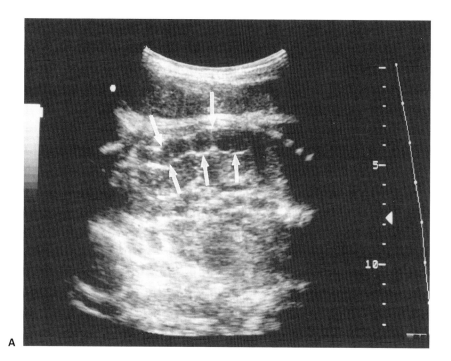

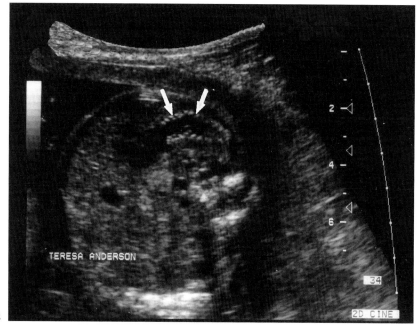

FIGURE 20-6 *Large Bowel.* (**A**) The large bowel appears sonographically as linear abdominal echogenicities (arrows) in which the Hofstral folds (**B**) may be identified. The contents of the bowel usually appear as hypoechogenic.

transverse to the splenic flexure and inferior to the sigmoid and rectum.

Abnormalities

Colon Atresia

Vascular injury to the inferior mesenteric artery results in segmental colon atresia with normal rectum and perineum. This occurs in approximately 1 in 1,500-20,000 live births. Only 1

case of the prenatal diagnosis of atresia of the colon has been reported. Anderson et al. observed dilated transverse colon at approximately 32 weeks with colon atresia.[65]

Anal Rectal Atresia

While anal rectal atresia has only rarely been recognized prenatally, Harris and associates in 1987 retrospectively reviewed their experience of 12 cases with anal rectal atresia.[66] They found that 42% had sonographically identifiable dilated bowel. While this was the only distinguishing sonographic feature, 92% had other demonstrable fetal anomalies; most of which were overt and severe.

Colon Duplication

Duplication of the colon results from abortive occult twinning and is usually (approximately 90%) accompanied by duplication of the external genitalia, anus, bladder, or urethra. Duplication of the colon accounts for 30% of all alimentary duplications.

LIVER

Normal

Interest in the human fetal liver has arisen from the observation that in many pathologic conditions the liver is thought to be first and most severely affected. These conditions include intrauterine growth retardation, fetal macrosomia, and Rh sensitization.[67] High-resolution ultrasonography now allows for the prenatal investigation of the margins of the liver quite clearly.

The abdominal circumference is a standard component of every routine ultrasound examination. Since the abdominal circumference is a direct representation of the fetal nutritional status and it is largely affected by fetal liver size, many have concluded that the fetal abdominal circumference is most notably affected by fetal liver size. Unfortunately, liver size can not be used to predict fetuses at risk for IUGR.[68] Sonographic measurement of the fetal liver has been reported in numerous studies (Fig. 20-8).[69] The optimal method of determining the size of the fetal liver is with linear measurements, in both longitudinal and transverse planes (Table 20-3). These measurements have been shown to be both accurate and reproducible. Proportionally, the size of the fetal liver is larger in the fetus than at any other time in

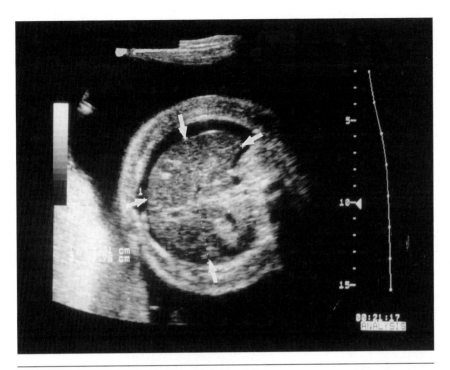

FIGURE 20-7 *Liver.* Fetal liver measurement can be obtained in both the anterior-posterior and the transverse dimensions. These measurements are illustrated (arrows) in this fetus with *hydrops fetalis* (anasarca and abdominal ascites).

this finding occurs in conjunction with multiple and severe fetal abnormalities.

SPLEEN

Normal

Although technically the spleen is not a gastrointestinal organ, for the purpose of comprehension we will include it here. Prenatally, the spleen arises from an aggregation of reticular mesenchyme size in the dorsal mesentery of the fetal stomach between 6 and 7 weeks of pregnancy. The spleen acquires its typical shape shortly thereafter and it begins its role as a hematopoitic organ by 12 weeks. Bounded superiorly by the diaphragm, laterally by the ribs, medially by the stomach and posteriorly by the diaphragm and kidney, the spleen can be accurately visualized in a transverse plane from approximately 16 weeks. The spleen is isoechogenic to the liver. The normal measurement of the fetal spleen has been described.[73,74]

human development. In the second trimester of pregnancy, the liver can comprise 10% of the overall weight of the fetus.

Abnormalities

Vintzileos and associates obtained fetal liver measurements in normal pregnancies in 1985.[70] Roberts and associates found a relationship between liver length and both fetal hemoglobin level (R = 4.79, P < 0.001) and the reticulocyte count (R = 0.72, P < 0.001). Fetal liver length was reported to be a useful indicator in the degree of anemia in isoimmunized pregnancies.[71] In a small series, Roberts et al. found women with diabetic pregnancies to have significantly larger liver measurements than controls.[72] These differences were found to increase with advancing gestational age.

Calcifications in the liver bowel and omentum often accompany congenital infection. These masses usually appear as multiple highly echogenic foci in the fetal abdomen (Fig. 20-9a,b).

Accessory Lobe of the Liver

Supernumerary lobes of liver occur in various size and shapes. Accessory lobes are frequently associated with omphalocele. Although the prenatal recognition of an accessory lobe of the liver has not been described, it seems reasonable that it may be recognized in the future.

Agenesis of the Liver

Complete agenesis of the liver is incompatible with life and has been reported in second and third trimester abortuses. Usually,

Abnormal

Oepkes et al. investigated the relationship between the ultrasonographic ascertained fetal spleen size and fetal hemoglobin levels.[75] They attempted to determine the predictive value of splenomegaly in estimating the severity of fetal hemolytic anemia. They found a significant positive correlation between the spleen perimeter and hemoglobin deficit. Splenomegaly was present in 94% of severely anemic fetuses and the authors suggest that this technique is a useful adjunctive tool in the management of severe red blood cell-alloimmunized pregnancies. Our experience with a case of severe anemia resulting from a 'silent' fetomaternal bleed suggests that splenomegaly is more a reflection of hemolysis than hematopoesis.

GALLBLADDER

Normal

For many years, the identification of the fetal gall bladder was thought to be inconsequential. Located in the right upper quadrant of the fetal abdomen, the gall bladder can be seen routinely on transverse section of the fetal abdomen. Normally, the gall bladder is anechoic. Normal fetal gallbladder growth and development has been described.[76] Rarely, the gall bladder can be seen to contain echogenic debris or foci. These echoes are thought to represent cholelithiasis or sludge.[77]

Abnormal

Gall Bladder Agenesis

Isolated agenesis of the gall bladder occurs in 0.08% of the general population of the United States. In 70% of these

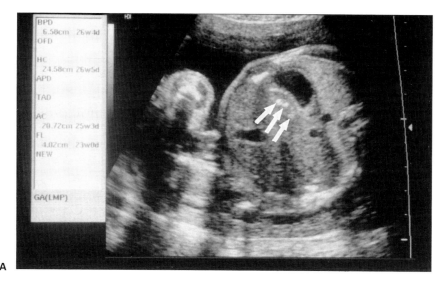

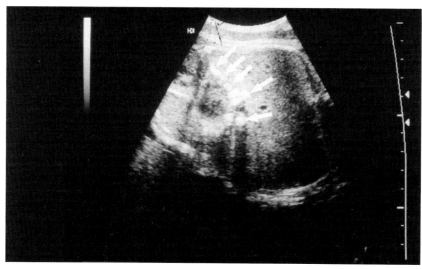

FIGURE 20-8 *Calcifications.* **(A)** Hepatic calcifications can be seen on this transverse ultrasonographic image of the fetal abdomen anterior to the stomach in the left lobe of the liver. **(B)** Similarly, peritoneal calcifications can appear in the omentum or appose the bowel.

cases, they are associated with clinical neonatal signs and symptoms. Twenty-one percent of children with gall bladder agenesis (and without bile duct atresia) have associated anomalies, including ventricular septal defects (13%), imperforate anus (13%), duodenal malrotation (12%), renal agenesis (9%), syndactyly (9%), horseshoe kidney (7%), and duodenal atresia (6%). This finding is also strongly associated with trisomy 13 and triploidy.

Pancreas

Although difficult to determine the margins of the pancreas, it can be recognized in transverse plane.[78,79] The pancreas lies posterior to the stomach and it appears as a broad band of tissue between the splenic vein and the superior mesenteric artery, and the posterior gastric wall.

OVERVIEW OF ABDOMINAL WALL DEFECTS

Defects of the fetal anterior abdominal wall can be either isolated; occur in association with other apparently unrelated defects (such as congenital heart defects or neurocranial abnormalities); occur as a feature of a syndromic condition (as in Pentalogy of Cantrell or Beckwith-Weidemann syndrome); or occur as a part of a developmental field defect (limb body-wall anomaly or cloacal extrophy). The two most common anterior abdominal wall defects are omphalocele (which often occurs in association with other fetal abnormalities) and gastroschisis (which is usually an isolated defect). In the current discussion, we will focus on these abnormalities; however, it is important to recognize that there is a wide variety of other abnormalities of the anterior fetal abdomen. These should be considered differentially in diagnosis, including abnormalities of the

| TABLE 20-3 | NORMAL RANGE OF FETAL LIVER LENGTH[a] |

Menstrual Age (wks)	Liver Length (cm)		
	−2SD	Predicted Value	+2SD
15	0.9	1.7	2.4
16	1.1	1.9	2.6
17	1.3	2.0	2.8
18	1.5	2.2	3.0
19	1.7	2.4	3.2
20	1.9	2.7	3.4
21	2.1	2.8	3.6
22	2.3	3.0	3.8
23	2.5	3.2	4.0
24	2.7	3.4	4.2
25	2.9	3.6	4.4
26	3.1	3.8	4.6
27	3.3	4.0	4.8
28	3.5	4.2	5.0
29	3.6	4.4	5.2
30	3.8	4.6	5.3
31	4.0	4.8	5.5
32	4.2	5.0	5.7
33	4.4	5.1	5.9
34	4.5	5.3	6.0
35	4.7	5.4	6.2
36	4.8	5.6	6.3
37	5.0	5.7	6.5
38	5.1	5.9	6.6
39	5.2	6.0	6.7
40	5.3	6.1	6.8

[a]Liver length was measured in a longitudinal plane from the hemidiaphragm to the tip of the right lobe. Liver length $= 0.165 + 0.00858$ (Menstrual Age)^2 − 0.000122 (MA)^3, SD$_R^a = 0.3778$. From Senoh D, Hata T, Kitao M: Fetal liver length measurement does not provide a superior means for prediction of a small for gestational age fetus. *Am J Perinatology* 1994;11(5):334–344.

| TABLE 20-4 | NORMAL RANGE OF FETAL SPLEEN LENGTH[a] |

Menstrual Age (wks)	Spleen Measurements		
	Splenic Length[b](cm)	Splenic Circumference (cm)	Splenic Area(cm²)
20	1.5 (1.0–2.0)[c]	4.2 (2.9–5.5)	1.0 (*–2.2)
21	1.7 (1.2–2.2)	4.7 (3.4–6.0)	1.3 (0.1–2.4)
22	1.9 (1.4–2.4)	5.2 (3.9–6.4)	1.5 (0.4–2.7)
23	2.1 (1.6–2.6)	5.6 (4.4–6.9)	1.8 (0.7–3.0)
24	2.2 (1.8–2.7)	6.1 (4.8–7.4)	2.2 (1.0–3.3)
25	2.4 (1.9–2.9)	6.6 (5.3–7.8)	2.5 (1.3–3.7)
26	2.6 (2.1–3.1)	7.0 (5.7–8.3)	2.8 (1.7–4.0)
27	2.8 (2.3–3.3)	7.4 (6.2–8.7)	3.2 (2.0–4.4)
28	2.9 (2.4–3.4)	7.9 (6.6–9.1)	3.6 (2.4–4.7)
29	3.1 (2.6–3.6)	8.3 (7.0–9.6)	3.9 (2.8–5.1)
30	3.2 (2.8–3.7)	8.7 (7.4–10.0)	4.3 (3.2–5.5)
31	3.4 (2.9–3.9)	9.1 (7.8–10.4)	4.7 (3.8–5.9)
32	3.5 (3.0–4.0)	9.5 (8.2–10.7)	5.2 (4.0–6.3)
33	3.7 (3.2–4.2)	9.9 (8.6–11.1)	5.6 (4.4–6.8)
34	3.8 (3.3–4.3)	10.2 (9.0–11.5)	6.0 (4.9–7.2)
35	3.9 (3.4–4.4)	10.6 (9.3–11.9)	6.5 (5.3–7.7)
36	4.0 (3.5–4.5)	11.0 (9.7–12.2)	7.0 (5.8–8.1)
37	4.1 (3.6–4.6)	11.3 (10.0–12.6)	7.5 (6.3–8.6)
38	4.2 (3.7–4.6)	11.6 (10.4–12.9)	8.0 (6.8–9.1)
39	4.2 (3.7–4.7)	12.0 (10.7–13.2)	8.5 (7.3–9.6)
40	4.3 (3.8–4.8)	12.3 (11.0–13.6)	9.0 (7.9–10.2)
41	4.3 (3.8–4.8)	12.6 (11.3–13.9)	9.6 (8.4–10.7)

[a]From Aoki S, Hata T, Kitao M: Ultrasonographic assessment of fetal and neonatal spleen. *Am J Perinatology* 1992;9:361–367.

[b]In a transverse view of the upper fetal abdomen, the spleen can be visualized as a well-circumscribed triangular-shaped structure posterior to the stomach. The splenic length is the maximal anterior to posterior dimension; circumference and area are calculated using this plane of view.

[c](−2SD)-(+2SD).

omphalomesenteric duct, allantoic duct/urachus, or umbilical cord.

Historically, the incidence of omphalocele is approximately twice that of gastroschisis (1:3000–5000 vs. 1:10,000, respectively). However, a recently released investigation calls into question these incidences. Tan et al. reviewed the incidence of abdominal wall defects in England and Wales between 1987 and 1993.[80] They found the overall incidence of abdominal wall defects to be 2.15/10,000 with 1043 affected pregnancies (539 cases of gastroschisis and 448 cases of omphalocele). During the study period, the authors found the incidence of gastroschisis to have doubled from 1987–1991 (from .65 in 10,000 live births to 1.35 in 10,000) and the incident of omphalocele decreased (from 1.13 in 10,000 to .77 in 10,000). Others have recently corroborated these findings.[81,82]

Prenatal ultrasonography is an invaluable tool in the identification of fetal abnormalities, however it is not infallible.

Several recent studies suggest that, in the second and third trimesters of pregnancy, only 60–75% of anterior abdominal wall abnormalities are identified prospectively in an unselected population.[83–86] When abdominal wall defects fail to be recognized with ultrasonography, it is often due to the small size of the anomaly, or the presence of multiple congenital anomaly, intrauterine fetal demise, multiple gestation, or late gestation.

OMPHALOCELE

The *omphalocele* or *exomphalos* is a rare congenital abnormality of the anterior abdominal wall. An omphalocele results when the lateral ectomesodermal folds fail to fuse at approximately 4 weeks of pregnancy. In the second and third trimester, it is characterized as a solid mass near the ventral wall of the fetus at the umbilical cord insertion site. This extra-abdominal mass is covered by an amnioperitoneal membrane and the umbilical cord can be observed to insert into its apex. Visceral organs encased in this mass often include bowel, liver, and stomach.

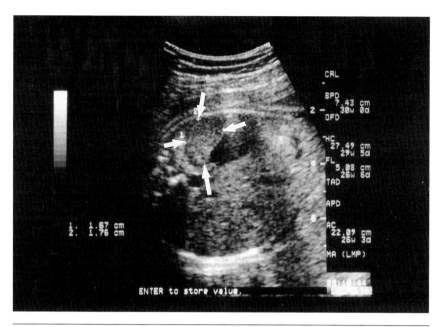

FIGURE 20-9 *Spleen.* The fetal spleen can be identified in a transverse plane posterior to the stomach.

Fetal omphalocele occurs in 1 in 5,000 live births. Unusually, this anomaly occurs sporadically and the recurrence risk is low (<1%). However, sex-linked or autosomal patterns of inheritance have been suggested. In one report, 5 consecutive pregnancies of a single family were complicated by isolated omphalocele.[87] Several other familial cases have been reported suggesting an environmental teratological effect.[88,89]

Since routine ultrasonography is not considered standard of care in the United States, *Maternal Serum Triple Evaluation* or *Maternal Serum Alpha-Fetoprotein (MSAFP) Evaluation* forms the basis for widespread screening for fetal anterior abdominal wall defects. Although unconjugated estriol and human chorionic gonadotropin are of no value in screening for these abnormalities, alpha-fetoprotein is essential.[90] Most prenatally identified cases of fetal omphalocele are either identified serendipitously with ultrasonography or are identified because of a heightened index of suspicion from an elevated MSAFP.

The ultrasonographic diagnosis of omphalocele is based on the identification of a distinct mass anterior and apposed to the ventral wall of the fetus (Fig. 20-10). Close ultrasound assessment, often made easier by the utilization of color and power Doppler technologies, will reveal the fetal end of the umbilical cord to insert into the apex of the mass and the membranous covering. A tremendous burden rests on the examiner to determine whether the defect is isolated or is associated with other abnormalities, which occur relatively commonly in association with omphalocele (27–59%).[80,84,91] Abnormalities not related to the gastrointestinal tract and ventral wall occur more frequently in fetuses with omphalocele. Significant associations have been described between omphalocele and, congenital heart disease (24–47% of cases), renal defects, and neural tube defects.[94] The prognosis of the affected fetus is largely dependent on the presence or absence of additional significant findings. Overall, the survival rate is 85%.[92] This finding and the fetal age at delivery seem to be the greatest contributors to assessing long-term prognosis. Preterm delivery, when it occurs, is often the result of preterm labor associated with polyhydramnios.

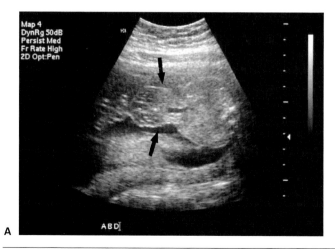

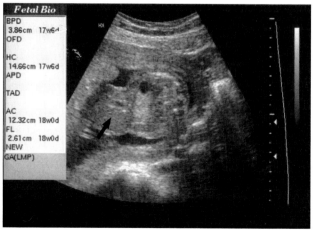

FIGURE 20-10 *Omphalocele*-Sonographic images of the transverse view of the fetal abdomens at the level of the umbilical cord insertion. (A) This image shows a small bowel-only omphalocele (commonly associated with fetal aneuploidy). (B) This image shows a larger omphalocele that contains fetal liver. Both images are in fetuses less than 20 weeks of gestation.

Chromosomal abnormalities also occur relatively frequently with omphalocele. The incidence of aneuploidy has been reported to range from 10–60% in fetuses with omphalocele.[93,94] Interestingly, the assessment of the contents of the extra-abdominal mass is an important predictor of risk for aneuploidy.[95] If fetal liver is contained in the omphalocele, then the risk of aneuploidy is low; conversely, if liver is not in the mass, the risk is high. Regardless of this observation, fetal genetic testing should be offered to all women with affected pregnancies. Although the risk of aneuploidy is low when liver is found in the omphalocele (18%), the risk of mortality is much higher (52%).[94]

After the initial diagnosis of omphalocele and a detailed search for concomitant fetal defects, many researchers suggest that serial ultrasound examinations are indicated to evaluate fetal growth and the fetal condition. Ascites, seen both intra-abdominally and in the extra-abdominal mass, is a common development. Polyhydramnios may also occur as a result of gastrointestinal obstruction.

A great deal of controversy remains regarding the optimal timing, mode, and place of delivery. In isolated omphalocele, only rarely do circumstances arise which necessitate premature pregnancy intervention. Passionate debate continues in the international literature regarding the optimal mode of delivery. The efficacy of elective cesarean section either before the onset of labor or following spontaneous onset, or spontaneous vaginal delivery are debated. Proponents of the former cite work done by Lenke and Hatch that suggests a significant advantage of empiric cesarean section.[96] Proponents of the latter cite two independent reports, which suggest that there is no significant medical advantage to cesarean section. Most agree that delivery should occur at a center equipped to the special neonatal intensive care and surgical needs of affected children.

Dunn and Foukalsrud investigated the neonatal care needs of children with omphalocele.[97] While acknowledging many improvements in surgical management of omphalocele, they state that the mortality rate in recent decades has remained stable at approximately 10%.[97] They summarize ". . . results following surgical repair of omphalocele defects depend on the degree of visceroabdominal disproportion and on the severity of associated anomalies. The operative mortality for staged omphalocele repair with limited evaluation of intra-abdominal pressure is low and long-term quality of life is good."

GASTROSCHISIS

In contrast to the omphalocele, which is a midline defect with membranous covering, the *gastroschisis* is a para-umbilical defect of the ventral wall without covering (Fig. 20-11). Gastroschisis appears as an apparent evisceration of the bowel into the amniotic cavity. Only rarely does the extra-abdominal organs include the fetal liver and stomach. With advancing gestational age and prolonged inflammation (secondary to irritants in the amniotic fluid), exposed structures can become diffusely thickened and matted.

Gastroschisis is thought to result from a vascular accident involving either the omphalomesenteric artery or right umbil-

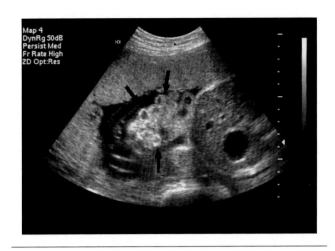

FIGURE 20-11 *Gastroschisis.* In fetal gastroschisis, bowel can be identified free-floating and uncovered in the amniotic fluid. The umbilical cord can be observed to insert adjacent to the defect. This ultrasonographic example is typical of gastroschisis.

ical vein early in fetal development. Abnormal involution of the right umbilical vein has also been offered as a possible explanation for the defect.[92,98] Recently established associations between gastroschisis and salicylates, pseudoephedrine, and phenylpropanoline, which are vasoactive, support the hypothesis of vascular disruption in the etiology of gastroschisis.[99]

Pregnancies complicated by fetal gastroschisis occur in approximately .3 to 2 per 10,000 live births. This anomaly usually occurs sporadically, but familial cases have been reported. In these instances, both autosomal recessive and autosomal dominant with variable expression modes of inheritance were suggested. Recent reports also suggest that environmental factors may play a significant role.[100] Fetal gastroschisis typically occurs in young, socially disadvantaged mothers with a history of substance abuse.[101,102]

Like omphalocele, pregnancies complicated by gastroschisis are often identified as a result of abnormal MSAFP screening or an abnormal ultrasound performed for "low-risk" indications. In addition to the distinctions between omphalocele and gastroschisis mentioned above, the extra-abdominal mass associated with the omphalocele tends to be smooth in contour (from the membranous covering), whereas the margins of the mass in gastroschisis are irregular and often characterized as cauliflower-like. The defect usually occurs to the right of a normal fetal umbilical cord insertion site. This mass is usually freely floating and mobile. It may be complex in echogenicity with both hyperechoic and hypoechoic components. Color and power Doppler allow easy identification of the umbilical cord insertion site.

Historically, gastroschisis is thought usually to be an isolated defect. However, recent reports suggest associated non-gastrointestinal anomalies can occur frequently (in 5–25% of cases).[80,92,91] Undescended testes are commonly observed in association with gastroschisis.[103] Complications secondary to gastroschisis, such as bowel adhesions, malrotation, enterocolitis, perforations, atresia, or stenosis, occur in 25%

of cases.[105,106] Further, 25–48% of affected fetuses have intrauterine growth retardation.[98,104]

Ultrasonographic estimations of fetal weight tends to underpredict actual birth weight. Raynor and Richards found the mean *estimated* fetal weight for their infants with gastroschisis to be 2079 g; significantly less than their *actual* birth weight of 2331 g.[104] Therefore, they concluded that estimated fetal weight from ultrasound tended to over-predict intrauterine growth retardation (predicted incidence of IUGR—43% and actual incidence of IUGR—23%). Although the rare case has been reported, gastroschisis is not associated with fetal chromosomal anomalies. No gender predilection has been observed in gastroschisis.[105,106]

Following identification of the affected fetus, serial ultrasound examinations are often indicated to monitor fetal growth and development. The utility of sonographic assessment of the appearance and size of the fetal bowel has been thoroughly discussed in the literature, but no conclusions are clear. Several references are available in the literature which suggest that bowel dilatation in gastroschisis is associated with poorer perinatal outcome.[107–110] Brun et al. reported 67% of fetuses with bowel dilatation >17 mm had intestinal atresia.[111] Cusick et al. found that the single most significant prognostic indicator of outcome in gastroschisis is the presence or absence of small bowel stenosis or atresia.[112] In that series of 63 cases of gastroschisis, of 6 fetuses who died, 4 (67%) had atresia or stenosis. Only 4 (<0.7%) of the surviving 57 cases had atresia or stenosis. Alsulyman et al. recently argued that bowel dilation was not related to perinatal outcome. They found no significant difference in (1) length of time to oral feeding, (2) length of hospital stay, or (3) need for bowel resection when gastroschisis fetuses with dilated bowel were compared with those who had no dilated bowel.[113]

Assessment of the amniotic fluid volume should also be performed at the time of follow-up examination. Polyhydramnios is a frequent complication of gastroschisis. Fetuses with gastroschisis seem to be at risk for later intrauterine demise. Thirteen percent of cases result in stillbirth.[114] As such, many have stressed the importance of routine weekly or biweekly nonstress testing.[115,116] In 1 series, 7 of 18 fetuses with gastroschisis had highly abnormal or preterminal nonstress testing.[117]

Delivery of the fetus with gastroschisis should occur at a center equipped to handle the immediate and secondary needs of the neonate. Fetuses with gastroschisis have better perinatal outcomes when delivered at a tertiary care center.[118] The mean age and weight of the fetus with gastroschisis is 36.3 weeks and 2500 g.[106] The same issues that complicate the discussion regarding omphalocele similarly complicate this discussion regarding the optimal mode of delivery. Some claim that birth trauma associated with vaginal delivery will result in untoward affects on the exposed bowel, while others report no medical advantage to empiric operative delivery.

Ninety-four percent of neonates with gastroschisis survive and this rate has dramatically risen in recent years.[119,120] The primary sources of mortality are sepsis, inadequate perioperative resuscitation, and prolonged gastrointestinal dysfunction.[92] Davies and Stringer assessed the long-term survival in children more than 1 year of age born with gastroschisis. Among 23 children evaluated, 22 were characterized as being in good health with appropriate growth. However, 35% had required additional pediatric surgery for small bowel obstruction and adhesions. Davies and Stringer state, "Most gastroschisis survivors can expect normal growth and good health." In a similar study, Tunell et al. re-evaluated affected children somewhat later (mean age of 14.2 year) and found 80% of patients were without long-term complications.[121]

References

1. Pansky B. *Review of Medical Embryology*. New York: MacMillan Publishing; 1982.
2. American Institute of Ultrasound in Medicine. Guidelines for second and third trimester sonography. *JUM* 1996;15:186–189.
3. Penninccky F. Treatment of intestinal atresia. *Acta Chirurgica Velgica*. 1988;88:17–20.
4. FitzSimmons J, Chinn A, Shepard TH. Normal length of the human fetal gastrointestinal tract. *Pediatric Pathology*. 1988;8:633–641.
5. Surana R, Puri P. Small intestinal atresia: affect on fetal nutrition. *J Pediatr Surg*. 1994;250–291.
6. Filly RA. Sonographic anatomy of the normal fetus. In: *The Unborn Patient*. Harrison MR, Golbus MS, Filly RA, eds. 2nd ed. Philadelphia: W.B. Saunders; 1984:114–118.
7. Persutte WH, Yeasting RA, Kurczynski TW, et al. The agnathia malformation complex associated with a cystic distention of the oral cavity and hydranencephaly. *J Craniofac Genet and Development Biol*. 1990;10:391–397.
8. Tang PT, Meagher SE, Khan AA, et al. Laryngeal atresia: antenatal diagnosis in a twin pregnancy. *Ultrasound in Obstetrics and Gynecology*. 1996;7:371–373.
9. Dolkart LA, Reimero FT, Wertheimer IS, et al. Prenatal Diagnosis of larengeal atresia. *J Ultrasound Med* 1992;11:496–498.
10. Strom W, Fasse M: Laryngeal Atresia in an Infant with Chondrodysplasia Punctata, Monastsschrift Kunderkeilkunde, 1991;139:629–631.
11. Kalache KD, Chaoui R, Tennstedt C, et al. Prenatal diagnosis of laryngeal atresia in two cases of congenital airway obstruction syndrome. *Prenatal Diagnosis*. 1997;17:577–581.
12. Moriarty AJ, McEvans IP. Pharyngeal teratoma. *Anesthesia*. 1993; 48:792–794.
13. Avini EF, Rypens F, Milarie J. Fetal esophagus: normal sonographic appearance. *JUM*. 1994;13:175–180.
14. Satoh S, Takashima T, Takeuchi H, et al. Antenatal sonographic detection of the proximal esophageal segment: specific evidence for esophageal atresia. *JCU*. 1995;23:419.
15. Seppala M. Elevated alpha-fetoprotein in amniotic fluid associated with a congenital esophageal atresia of the fetus. *Obstet Gynecol*. 1973;42:613–614.
16. Jacquemarda F, Palaric JC, Herve D, et al. Antenatal diagnosis of abdominothoracic elementary tract duplication: a case report. *Surgical and Radiologic Anatomy*. 1991;13:53–57.
17. Goldstein I, Reece EA, Yarkoni S, et al. Growth of the fetal stomach in normal pregnancies. *Obstet Gynecol*. 1987;70:641–644.
18. Hertzberg BS, Bowie JD. Fetal gastrointestinal abnormalities. *Radiologic Clinics in North America*. 1990;28:101–114.
19. Vandenberghe K, deWolf F. Ultrasonic assessment of fetal stomach function: physiology and clinic. In: Kurjak A, ed. *Recent Advances in Ultrasound Diagnosis*. 2. Amsterdam: Exerpta Medica; 1980:275.

20. Nagata S, Koyanagi T, Fukushima S, et al. Change in the three-dimensional shape of the stomach in the developing human fetus. Early Human Development. 1994;37:27–38.

21. Nagata S, Koyanagi T, Horimoto N, et al. Chronological development of the fetal stomach assessed using real time ultrasound. *Early Human Development*. 1990;22:15.

22. Zimmer EZ, Chao CR, Abramovich G, et al. Fetal stomach measurements: not reproducible by the same observer. *Journal of Ultrasound in Medicine*. 1992;11:663–665.

23. Bovicelli L, Rizzo N, Orsini LF, et al. Prenatal diagnosis and management of fetal GI abnormalities. *Seminars in Perinatology*. 1983;7:109.

24. Pretorius DH, Gosink BB, Clautice-Engle I, et al. Sonographic evaluation of the fetal stomach: significance of nonvisualization. *AJR*. 1988;151:987–989.

25. Millener PB, Anderson NG, Chrisolm RJ. Prognostic significance of nonvisualization of the fetal stomach by sonography. *AJR*. 1993; 160:827–830.

26. McKenna KM, Goldstein RB, Stringer MD. Small or absent fetal stomach: prognostic significance. *Radiology*. 1995;197:729–733.

27. Daly-Jones E, Sepulveda W, Hollingsworth J, et al. Fetal intraluminal gastric masses after second trimester amniocentesis. *JUM*. 1994;13:963–966.

28. Daly-Jones E, Sepulveda W, Hollingsworth J, et al. Fetal intraluminal gastric masses after second trimester amniocentesis. *JUM*. 1994;13:963–966.

29. Bidwell JK, Nelson A. Prenatal ultrasonographic diagnosis of congenital duplication of the stomach. *JUM*. 1986;5:589–591.

30. Richards DS, Langham MR, Anderson DC. The prenatal sonographic appearance of enteric duplication cysts. *Ultrasound in Obstet Gynecol*. 1996;7:17–20.

31. Dorney SF, Middleton AW, Kozlowski K, et al. Congenital agastria. *Journal of Pediatric Gastroenterology & Nutrition*. 1987;6:307–310.

32. Hill L. Congenital microgastria: absence of the fetal stomach and normal third trimester amniotic fluid volume. *JUM*. 1994;13:894–896.

33. Nazzaro V, Nicolini U, DeLuca L, et al. Prenatal diagnosis of junctional epidermalosis bulosa associated with pyloric atresia. *J Med Genetics*. 1990;27:244–248.

34. Peled Y, Hod M, Friedman S, et al. Prenatal diagnosis of familial congenital pyloric atresia. *Prenatal Diagnosis*. 1992;12:151–154.

35. Rizzo G, Capponi A, Arduini D, et al. Prenatal diagnosis of gastrointestinal reflux by color and pulsed Doppler ultrasound in a case of congenital pyloric atresia. *Ultrasound in Obstet Gynecol*. 1995;6:290–292.

36. Parulekar SG. Sonography of normal fetal bowel. *J Ultrasound Med*. 1991;10:211–220.

37. Nyberg DA, Mac LA, Patten RM, et al. Fetal bowel: normal sonographic findings. *JUM*. 1987;6:3–6.

38. Goldstein I, Lockwood C, Hobbins JC. Ultrasonographic assessment of fetal intestinal development in the evaluation of gestational age. *Obstet Gynecol*. 1987;70:682–686.

39. Corteville JE, Gray DL, Langer JC. Bowel abnormalities in the fetus—correlation of prenatal ultrasonographic findings with outcome. *Am J Obstet Gynecol*. 1996;175:724–729.

40. Nyberg DA. Intra-abdominal abnormalities. In: Nyberg DA, Mahony BS, Pretorius DH, eds. *Diagnostic Ultrasound of Fetal Anomalies*. Chicago: Year Book Medical Publishers; 1990:355–359.

41. Gray SW, Skandalakis JE. The small intestines. In: *Embryology for Surgeons*. Philadelphia: WB Saunders Co; 1972:129–186.

42. Nixon HH, Tawes R. Etiology and treatment of small intestinal atresia: analysis of a series of 127 jejunoileal atresias and comparison with 62 duodenal atresia. *Surgery*. 1971;69:41–51.

43. Touloukian RJ. Intestinal atresia. *Clin Perinatology*. 1978;5:3–18.

44. De Lorimier AA, Fonkalsrud EW, Hays DM. Congenital atresia and stenosis of the jejunum and ileum. *Surgery*. 1969;65:819–827.

45. Park RW, Grand RJ. Gastrointestinal malformations of cystic fibrosis: a review. *Gastroenterology*. 1981;81:1143–1161.

46. Kgoller M, Holm-Neilsen G, Meiland H, et al. Prenatal obstruction of the illius diagnosed by ultrasound. *Prenatal Diagnosis*. 1985;5:427–430.

47. Persutte WH. Second trimester abdominal hyperechogenicity in the lower abdomen of two fetuses with trisomy 21: is there a correlation? *J. Clin. Ultrasound*. 1990;18:425–428.

48. Hill LM, Fries J, Hecker J, et al. Second trimester small bowel: increased risk for adverse perinatal outcome. *Prenat Diagnosis*. 1994;14:845–850.

49. Dicke JM, Crane JP, Sciosia AL, et al. Second trimester echogenic bowel in chromosomal abnormalities. *Am J Obstet Gynecol*. 1992;167:889–894.

50. Sipes SL, Weiner CP, Wenstrom KD, et al. Fetal echogenic bowel on ultrasound: is there clinical significance? *Fetal Diagnosis & Therapy*. 1994;9:38–43.

51. Bromley B, Doubilet P, Frigoletto FD, et al. Is Fetal Hyperechogenic Bowel on Second Trimester Sonogram an Indication for Amniocentesis? *Obstet Gynecol*. 1994;83:647–651.

52. Sepulveda W, Hollingsworth J, Bower S, et al. Fetal Hyperechogenic Bowel Following Intraamniotic Bleeding. *Obstet Gynecol*. 1994;83:947–950.

53. Sepulveda W, Reid R, Nicolaidis P, et al. Second Trimester Echogenic Bowel and Intraamniotic Bleeding: association Between Fetal Bowel Echogenicity and Amniotic Fluid at Spectroscopy 414NM. *Am J Obstet Gynecol* 1996;174:839–842.

54. Seoud MA, Alley DC, Smith DL, et al. Prenatal Sonographic Findings in Trisomy 13, 18, 21, and 22. A Review of 46 Cases. *J Repro Med*. 1994;39:781–787.

55. Sepulveda W, Bower S, Fisk NM: Third Trimester Hyperechoic Bowel in Down Syndrome. *Am J Obstet Gynecol*. 1995;192:210–211.

56. Slotnick RN, Abuhamad AZ.: Prognostic implications of fetal echogenic bowel. *Lancet*. 1996;347:85–87.

57. Hamada H, Okuno S, Fujiki Y, et al. Fetal echogenic bowel in the third trimester associated with trisomy 18. *European J Obstet Gynecol and Repro Biol*. 1996;67:65–67.

58. Dicke JM, Crane JP: Sonographically detected hyperechogenic fetal bowel: significance and implications for pregnancy. *Obstet Gynecol*. 1992;80:778–782.

59. Sepulveda W, Nicolaidis P, Mai AM, et al. Is isolated second trimester hyperechogenic bowel a predictor of suboptimal fetal growth? *Ultrasound in Obstetrics & Gynecology*. 1996;7:104–107.

60. Muller F, Dommergues M, Aubry MC, et al. Hyperechogenic fetal bowel: an ultrasound marker for adverse fetal and neonatal outcome. *Am J Obstet Gynecol*. 1995;173:508–513.

61. MacGregor SN, Tamura R, Sabbagha R, et al. Isolated hyperechoic fetal bowel: significance and implications for management. *American Journal of Obstetrics & Gynecology*. 1995;173:1254–1258.

62. Achiron R, Seidman DS, Horowitz A, et al. Hyperechogenic fetal bowel and elevated serum AFP: a poor fetal prognosis. *Obstet Gynecol*. 1996;88:368–371.

63. Sepulveda W, Leung KY, Robertson NE, et al. Prevalence of cystic fibrosis mutations in pregnancies with fetal echogenic bowel. *Obstet Gynecol*. 1996;87:103–106.

64. Slotnick RN, Abuhamad AZ. Prognostic implications of fetal echogenic bowel. *Lancet*. 1996;347:85–87.

65. Anderson N, Malpas T, Robertson R. Prenatal diagnosis of colon atresia. *Pediatric Radiology*. 1993;23:63–64.

66. Harris RD, Nyberg DA, Mack LA, et al. Anal rectal atresia: prenatal sonographic diagnosis. *AJR*. 1987;147:395–400.

67. Gimondo P, LaBella A, Messina G, et al. Sonographic estimation of fetal liver weight: an additional biometric parameter for assessment of fetal growth. *J Ultrasound in Medicine*. 1995;14:327–333.
68. Senoh D, Hata T, Kitao M. Fetal liver length measurement does not provide a superior means for the prediction of a small for gestational age fetus. *Am J Perinatology*. 1994;11:344–347.
69. Murao F. Measurements of fetal liver size, hormonal level and pregnancy outcome. *Gynecol Obstet Invest*. 1991;32:153–156.
70. Vintzileos AM, Neckles S, Campbell WA, et al. Fetal liver ultrasonographic measurements during pregnancy. *Obstet Gynecol*. 1985;66:477–480.
71. Roberts AB, Mitchell JM, Pattison NS. Fetal liver length in normal and isoimmunized pregnancies. *Am J Obstet Gynecol*. 1989;161:42–46.
72. Roberts AD, Mitchell J, Murphy C, et al. Fetal liver length in diabetic pregnancy. *Am J Obstet Gynecol* 1994;170:1308–1312.
73. Schmidt W, Yarkoni S, Jeanty P, et al. Sonographic measurement of the fetal spleen: clinical implications. *J Ultrasound in Med*. 1985;4:667–672.
74. Aoki S, Hata T, Kitao M. Ultrasonographic assessment of fetal and neonatal spleen. *Am J Perinatology*. 3:361–367.
75. Oepkes D, Meerman RH, Vandenbussche FP, et al. Ultrasonographic fetal spleen measurements in red blood cell-alloimmunized pregnancies. *Am J Obstet Gynecol*. 1993;169:121–128.
76. Chan L, Rao BK, Jiang Y, et al. Fetal gallbladder growth and development during gestation. *J Ultrasound in Medicine*. 1995;14:421–425.
77. Petrikovsi B, Klein B, Holstein N. Sludge in the fetal gall bladder: natural history and neonatal outcome. *British J Radiol*. 1996;69:1017.
78. Hata K, Hata T, Kitao M. The ultrasonographic identification and measurement for the fetal pancreas in utero. *Int J Gynaecol Obstet*. 1989;26:61–64.
79. Hill LM, Peterson C, Ribello D, et al. Sonographic detection of the fetal pancreas. *J Clin Ultrasound*. 1989;17:475–479.
80. Tan KH, Kilby MD, Beattie BR, et al. Congenital anterior abdominal wall defects in England and Wales 1987–1993: a retrospective analysis of OPCS data. BMJ 1996;313:903–906.
81. Puffinbarger NK, Taylor DV, Stevens RJ, et al. Gastroschisis: a birth defect seen in increasing numbers in Oklahoma. *Journal of Oklahoma State Medical Association*. 1995;88:291–294.
82. Nicholls EA, Ford WD, Barnes KH, et al. A decade of gastroschisis in the era of antenatal ultrasound. *Aust N Z J Surg*. 1996;66:366–368.
83. Walkinshaw SA, Renwick M, Hebisch G, et al. How good is ultrasound in the detection and evaluation of anterior abdominal wall defects? *Br J Radiol*. 1992;65:298–301.
84. Chen CP, Liu FF, Jan SW, et al. Prenatal diagnosis and perinatal aspects of abdominal wall defects. *Am J Perinatology*. 1996;13:355–361.
85. Dillon PW, Cilley RE: Newborn surgical emergencies. Gastrointestinal anomalies, abdominal wall defects. *Pediatric Clinics of North America*. 1993;40:1289–1314.
86. Dillon E, Renwick M. The antenatal diagnosis and management of abdominal wall defects: the northern region experience. *Clin Radiol*. 1995;50:855–859.
87. Pryde PG, Greb A, Lsada NB, et al. Familial omphalocele: considerations in genetic counseling. *Am J Med Genet*. 1992;44:624–627.
88. Chun K, Andrews HG, White JJ. Gastroschisis in successive siblings: further evidence of an acquired etiology. *J Pediatr Surg*. 1993;28:838–839.
89. Reece A, Thornton J, Stringer MD. Genetic factors in the etiology of gastroschisis: a case report. *Eur J Obstet Gynecol Reprod Biol*. 1997;73:127–128.

90. Saller DN Jr, Canick JA, Palomaki GE, et al. Second trimester maternal serum alpha-fetoprotein, unconjugated estriol and hCG levels in pregnancies with ventral wall defects. *Obstet Gynecol*. 1994;84:852–855.
91. Heydanus R, Raats MA, Tibboel D, et al. Prenatal diagnosis of fetal abdominal wall defects: a retrospective analysis of 44 cases. *Prenat Diagn*. 1996;16:411–417.
92. Chang PV, Yeh ML, Shew JC, et al. Experience with treatment of gastroschisis and omphalocele. *J Formos Med Assoc*. 1992;91:447–451.
93. Chen CP, Liu FF, Jan SW, et al. Prenatal diagnosis and perinatal aspects of abdominal wall defects. *Am J Perinatol*. 1996;13:355–361.
94. St-Vil D, Shaw KS, Lallier M, et al. Chromosomal anomalies in newborns with omphalocele. *J Pediatr Surg*. 1996;31:831–834.
95. De Veciana M, Major CA, Porto M. Prediction of an abnormal karyotype in fetuses with omphalocele. *Prenat Diagn*. 1994;14:487–492.
96. Lenke RR, Hatch EI. Fetal gastroschisis: a preliminary report advocating the use of cesarean section. *Obstet Gynecol*. 1986;67:395–398.
97. Dunn JC, Fonkalsrud EW. Improved survival of infants with omphalocele. *Am J Surg*. 1997;173:284–287.
98. Fries MH, Filly RA, Callen PW, et al. Growth retardation in prenatally diagnosed cases of gastroschisis. *J Ultrasound Med*. 1993;12:583–588.
99. Werler MM, Mitchell AA, Shapiro S. First trimester maternal medication use in relation to gastroschisis. *Teratology*. 1992;45:361–367.
100. Yang P, Beaty TH, Khoury MJ, et al. Genetic-epidemiologic study of omphalocele and gastroschisis: evidence for heterogeneity. *Am J Med Genet*. 1992;44:668–675.
101. Torfs CP, Velie EM, Oechsli FW, et al. A population-based study of gastroschisis: demographic, pregnancy, and lifestyle risk factors. *Teratology*. 1994;50:44–53.
102. Werler MM, Mitchell AA, Shapiro S. Demographic, reproductive, medical and environmental factors in relations to gastroschisis. *Teratology*. 1992;45:353–360.
103. Levard G, Laberge JM. The fate of undescended testes in patients with gastroschisis. *Eur J Pediatr Surg*. 1997;7:163–165.
104. Raynor BD, Richards D. Growth retardation in fetuses with gastroschisis. *J Ultrasound Med*. 1997;16:13–16.
105. Novotny DA, Klein RL, Boeckman CR. Gastroschisis: an 18 year review. *J Pediatr Surg*. 1993;28:650–652.
106. Haddock G, Davis CF, Raine PA. Gastroschisis in the decade of prenatal diagnosis: 1983–1993. *Eur J Pediatr Surg*. 1996;6:18–22.
107. Lenke RR, Persutte WH, Nemes JM. Ultrasonographic assessment of intestinal damage in fetuses with gastroschisis: is it of clinical value? *Am J Obstet Gynecol*. 1990;163:995–998.
108. Babcook CJ, Hedrick MH, Goldstein RB, et al. Gastroschisis: can sonography of the fetal bowel accurately predict postnatal outcome. J Ultrasound Medicine. 1994;13:701–706.
109. Langer JC, Khanna J, Caco C, et al. Prenatal diagnosis of gastroschisis: development of objective sonographic criteria for predicting outcome. *Obstetrics & Gynecology*. 1993;81:53–56.
110. Adra AM, Landy HJ, Nahmias J, et al. The fetus with gastroschisis: impact of route of delivery and prenatal ultrasonography. *Am J of Obstet Gynecol*. 1996;174:540–546.
111. Brun M, Grignon A, Guibaud L, et al. Gastroschisis: are prenatal ultrasonographic findings useful for assessing the prognosis? *Pediatr Radiol*. 1996;26:723–726.
112. Cusick E, Spicer RD, Beck JM. Small-bowel continuity: a crucial factor in determining survival in gastroschisis. *Pediatr Surg Int*. 1997;12:34–37.
113. Alsulyman OM, Monteiro H, Ouzounian JG, et al. Clinical significance of prenatal ultrasonographic intestinal dilatation

in fetuses with gastroschisis. *Am J Obstet Gynecol.* 1996;175:982–984.

114. Adair CD, Rosnes J, Frye AH, et al. The role of antepartum surveillance in the management of gastroschisis. *Int J Gynaecol Obstet.* 1996;52:141–144.

115. Burge DM, Ade-Ajayi N. Adverse outcome after prenatal diagnosis of gastroschisis: the role of fetal monitoring. *J Pediat Surg.* 1997;32:441–444.

116. Crawford RA, Ryan G, Wright VM, et al. The importance of serial biophysical assessment of fetal well-being in gastroschisis. *Br J Obstet Gynecol.* 1992;99:899–902.

117. Ingamells S, Saunders NJ, Burge D. Gastroschisis and reduced fetal heart-rate variability. *Lancet.* 1995;345:1024–1025.

118. Quirk JG Jr, Fortney J, Collins HB II, et al. Outcomes of newborns with gastroschisis: the effects of mode of delivery, site of delivery and interval from birth to surgery. *Am J Obstetr Gynecol.* 1996;174:1134–1138, discussion 1138–1140.

119. Brun M, Grignon A, Guibaud L, et al. Gastroschisis: are prenatal ultrasonographic findings useful for assessing the prognosis? *Pediatr Radiol.* 1996;26:723–726.

120. Blakelock RT, Harding JE, Kolbe A, et al. Gastroschisis: can morbidity be avoided. *Pediatr Surg Int.* 1997;12:276–282.

121. Tunell WP, Puffinbarger NK, Tuggle DW, et al. Abdominal wall defects in infants: survival and implications for adult life. *Ann Surg.* 1995;221:525–558, 528–530.

GENITO-URINARY TRACT ABNORMALITIES

Marjorie C. Treadwell / Mark P. Johnson

Urinary tract abnormalities continue to constitute a large portion of prenatally diagnosed congenital abnormalities, making up almost 50% of anomalies diagnosed with ultrasound.[1] The ability to reliably identify urinary tract structures allows diagnosis early in pregnancy. The fetal bladder can be seen at 10 weeks gestation and inability to visualize this in the second trimester with accompanying oligohydramnios suggests a lethal abnormality of the fetal urinary tract.[2] With transvaginal ultrasound 92% of fetal kidneys will be identified by 13 weeks gestation.[3] Between 14–18 weeks gestation, 0.33% of fetuses will be identified as having renal abnormalities.[4] This percentage becomes higher as gestation advances as some abnormalities do not manifest until later in pregnancy. There is a familial influence, 14% of the parents of a fetus with a renal abnormality will themselves have a urinary tract abnormality.[4] This finding may not be isolated and 24% of fetuses will have associated abnormalities, sometimes a component of a genetic syndrome.

In addition to detecting structural abnormalities, prenatal ultrasound is able to offer some degree of assessment of urinary function based on evaluation of amniotic fluid volume and bladder dynamics. Invasive testing may be appropriate to further define prognosis, facilitate counseling, and in some cases provide therapy. This information is critical for determining management of labor and delivery.

This chapter will review genitourinary tract abnormalities that can be diagnosed on prenatal ultrasound and discuss the evaluation and prognosis for these disorders.

AGENESIS

Bilateral renal agenesis is associated with early onset oligohydramnios and can be diagnosed with ultrasound at 14–16 weeks' gestation. Failure to identify the renal structures along with an empty fetal bladder and oligohydramnios is key.[5] Prenatal detection of unilateral and bilateral renal agenesis may not be straightforward, as adrenal tissue occupying the renal fossa may appear to be kidney. Doppler assessment of the renal arteries may help differentiate renal from adrenal tissue. Cases of abnormal kidneys that have involuted and not been detected postnatally have been described.[6]

The prognosis for bilateral renal agenesis is dismal with no long-term survival due to pulmonary hypoplasia. Compression abnormalities, flattening of the facies and clubfeet, along with pulmonary hypoplasia comprise the Potter's sequence of deformities. When bilateral renal agenesis is diagnosed, extensive counseling of parents regarding this lethal condition should be conducted. Delivery should be undertaken for any maternal indication and termination of pregnancy should be offered at diagnosis if legal. In patients continuing to term, discussion should include the route of delivery as a high

percentage of these fetuses may present in breech presentation at the time of delivery[7] or with fetal heart rate abnormalities in labor. Cesarean section should be reserved for maternal indications only. Avoiding continuous intrapartum monitoring of the fetus may prevent operative delivery for fetal indications.

Unilateral agenesis, much more common than bilateral, has a much better prognosis and is usually associated with normal bladder and amniotic fluid volume. The prenatal diagnosis may be missed when fetal position causes shadowing of one kidney.[8] After ruling out associated anomalies, these patients are managed with routine prenatal care.

The recurrence risk for bilateral or unilateral renal agenesis is higher than the general population risk and there appears to be a multifactorial inheritance pattern. Parents and siblings are also at increased risk for genitourinary tract abnormalities. There is a 9% rate of asymptomatic renal malformations in parents and siblings of fetuses with renal agenesis or dysgenesis, 4.5% will have unilateral renal agenesis.[9]

HORSESHOE AND PELVIC KIDNEYS

The prenatal detection of fetal pelvic kidneys has been reported in case series. Based on reports of necropsy data, it would be expected in 1 in 1120 prenatal ultrasound examinations.[10,11] Ectopic kidneys may be mistaken for renal agenesis if the structure is not recognized outside the renal pelvis. Because of the incidence of associated abnormalities, careful ultrasound is extremely important. Associated abnormalities most frequently involve the genitourinary or gastrointestinal tracts but may include cardiovascular, central nervous system, or skeletal anomalies with postnatal series describing an incidence of associated abnormalities as high as 85%.[12] The increased incidence of genital tract abnormalities in the female fetus may not be appreciated prenatally or immediately after birth but parents should be aware of the association. In addition to concerns over associated anomalies, pelvic kidneys are more likely to be associated with obstruction than are normal kidneys.[11] Observing these patients prenatally for the development of hydronephrosis is appropriate.

Horseshoe kidney is less frequently diagnosed in the prenatal period with limited case reports.[13] The ultrasound appearance may be symmetric or asymmetric with a band of fibrous tissue identified between the two renal structures. A single transverse plane of the kidneys may fail to identify the abnormality.[14] There is up to a 30% rate of associated anomalies, with a 25% rate of associated genitourinary tract abnormalities.[15]

Prenatal management of both pelvic and horseshoe kidneys is uncomplicated when normal amniotic fluid is present and additional anomalies absent. The recommendation for karyotype is based on associated anomalies. Serial ultrasound to monitor for the development of hydronephrosis, most often due to ureteropelvic junction obstruction, is indicated.[16]

Early intervention is indicated only if oligohydramnios develops.

URINARY TRACT DILATATION OR OBSTRUCTION

There are a wide variety of fetal obstructive uropathies involving both the upper and lower urinary tracts. Differentiation of the different entities may be difficult but is important for appropriate management and counseling. One of the largest series of prenatally diagnosed obstructive uropathies included 987 patients.[17] Fifty percent of the infants who died had associated anomalies with an aneuploidy rate of 12%. In their series, they found 77% concordance of the prenatal and postnatal diagnosis.[17]

URETERAL PELVIC JUNCTION OBSTRUCTION

Pyelocaliceal retention secondary to ureteropelvic junction (UPJ) obstruction is one of the more common etiologies of obstructive uropathy, occurring in approximately 50% of prenatally detected upper tract dilatations[18] and is also the most common cause of postnatal hydronephrosis. The ability to make an antenatal diagnosis has facilitated the postnatal management with early relief of severe obstructions postnatally seeming to improve ultimate creatinine clearance[19] and possibly limiting the 3.5–20% risk of renal deterioration in the postnatal period.[20] The prenatal ultrasound findings, including pyelocaliceal distention without megaureter, are bilateral in 21–36% of cases.[18] The false positive rate for prenatal diagnosis is less than 3%.[19]

Guys et al.[19] reported spontaneous resolution in 5 of 47 prenatally diagnosed cases (11%). There was bilateral obstruction in 12 cases. Follow-up extending 2–6 years after birth showed 3 kidneys requiring nephrectomy, 50 kidneys were operated on; 90% of the cases had reduction of renal pelvis dilatation, and normal kidney function.[19] The degree of dilatation does seem to correlate with postnatal function. Fasolato et al.[21] confirmed abnormalities after birth in 18% of infants with upper tract dilatation; all had renal pelvis diameters greater than 15 mm in the prenatal period. In their series, all infants with less than 10 mm dilatation had resolution of the upper tract dilatation during the first postnatal year.

There is also a familial association with ureteropelvic obstruction. Fifty-five percent of families identified had siblings with uropathology. Abnormalities identified most frequently included reflux with a male:female distribution of 4 to 1 in the proband group and 1.8 to 1 in the sibling group suggesting that the sex difference is less marked within the families with uropathology.[22]

URETEROVESICOJUNCTION

Ureterovesicojunction abnormalities are recognized by megaureter in the absence of enlarged bladder. Characteristic ultrasound findings are dilatation of the distal ureter more so than the upper collecting system. Hyperparastalsis of the lower ureter and adynamic segments of the distal portion have been described.[23] Prenatal diagnosis may prompt earlier identification with earlier intervention, ideally before severe renal parenchymal compromise occurs.[23] The condition is also much more common in males and although usually sporadic, may be familial with 32% of asymptomatic siblings of patients with reflux exhibiting reflux.[24] Causes of megaureter other than reflux include obstruction or bladder dysfunction; primary megaureter from fibrosis or stenosis of the valves[25] or benign primary megaureter that is congenital.[26] The latter requires no prenatal intervention. Ultrasound findings include the dilated peristaltic ureter with or without dilated renal pelvis.[26] Duplicated collecting systems may also result in megaureter and is a common urinary tract abnormality.[27] Ectopic ureteroceles may be associated with the duplication and if present, occurs bilaterally in 15%.

Management of these patients revolves around amniotic fluid volume and expectant management is appropriate if normal fluid is present.

POSTERIOR URETHRAL VALVE

There are many etiologies of obstruction of the proximal urethra. This is most frequently seen in the male fetus and usually involves posterior urethral valves, prune belly syndrome, or urethral atresias. In the female fetus a complex cloacal abnormality is much more likely and may be associated with a more complicated genetic syndrome. Because a chromosomal abnormality may be associated with any of the above findings a karyotype is indicated, especially if the ultrasound findings are not isolated to the genitourinary tract.

The findings of an enlarged bladder, with a thickened bladder wall and the keyhole sign (Fig. 21-1) are classic for posterior urethral valves. As the pregnancy progresses, usually past 14–16 weeks oligohydramnios may accompany the bladder findings. Without intervention these findings would be expected to be lethal with neonatal demise more common than

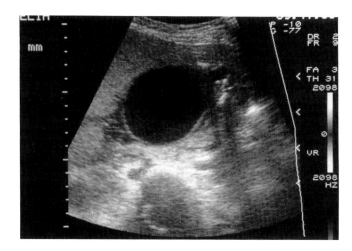

FIGURE 21-1 Enlarged fetal bladder demonstrating the keyhole sign.

| TABLE 21-1 | ABILITY OF SELECTED BIOCHEMICAL VALUES TO PREDICT THE ABSENCE OF RENAL DYSPLASIA | | |

	Value	*Positive Predictive Value*	*Negative Predictive Value*
Sodium	<100 mg/dl	0.56	0.88
Calcium	<8 mg/dl	0.43	1.00
Osmolality	<200 mOsm/L	0.71	0.90
B-2 Microglobulin	<4 mg/L	1.00	0.44
Total protein	<20 mg/dl	0.80	0.83

intrauterine demise. Amniotic fluid is required for the transition from cannicular to alveolar development to occur in the fetal lung, between 18–24 weeks. The failure of pulmonary development resulting from oligohydramnios is the leading cause of mortality in obstructive uropathies. Pulmonary hypoplasia accounts for the 45% mortality seen with posterior urethral valves.[28] This mortality rate may exceed 90% when the oligohydramnios presents in the early second trimester.[29]

Management of the fetus requires ultrasound to exclude other etiologies of the oligohydramnios and dilated bladder. Prevention of pulmonary hypoplasia requires correction of the oligohydramnios. Interventions, which potentially could improve neonatal survival, are most appropriately reserved for those fetuses that have evidence of renal function in the absence of associated anomalies.

If thorough ultrasound evaluation and karyotype are consistent with isolated genitourinary tract abnormalities, then invasive testing of the urinary tract is appropriate. Assessment of renal function is accomplished through sampling of fetal urine, vesicocentesis. Measurements of serial urinary electrolytes and proteins along with documentation of progressive hypotonicity seem to identify fetuses with an improved prognosis (Table 21-1).[30] The use of serial sampling is important to accurately assess current renal function.[30] There is also a strong correlation between final urine values and patterns of hypertonicity in predicting the presence or absence of significant renal damage.[31] If urinary measurements are consistent with normal function vesicoamniotic shunt placement is appropriate. The use of endoscopy to further define pathology and perhaps treat the conditions in utero is an exciting area for further study. Although this procedure involves considerable risk to the fetus it may allow more appropriate selection of patients for shunts and allows in utero ablation of valves in fetuses with this pathology.

An area that is less certain is the role of shunting in patients that do not have oligohydramnios. Pulmonary hypoplasia is not a concern in these patients. The question remains as to whether shunting the bladder prior to development of oligohydramnios prevents some of the permanent renal damage. Given the 45% complication rate associated with vesicoamniotic shunt placement, and the relatively low (47%) survival after intervention,[32]

this procedure should be reserved for fetuses exhibiting oligohydramnios until further research dictates otherwise.

The prognosis for these infants depends on the gestational age at diagnosis, the severity of the blockage (is it a complete obstruction versus a partial obstruction), and associated abnormalities. Overall, outcome is most closely related to gestational age at delivery and whether renal function was spared. Prenatal care of patients who have had in utero shunt placement involves serial ultrasounds to confirm shunt placement, amniotic fluid volume, and evaluation of the renal tissue. The remainder of their prenatal care is routine with anticipation of vaginal delivery at term if the shunt continues to function. Recurrence risk for subsequent pregnancies is extremely small.

CLOACAL ANOMALIES

Many of the features of cloacal exstrophy should be detectable by prenatal ultrasound. The ventral defect is wide and occupies most of the abdomen below the level of the cord insertion. The pelvis may appear small and ascites may be present. An associated single umbilical artery is common. A distinct bladder may be identified and polyhydramnios has been described (Fig. 21-2).[33] Associated lower urinary tract abnormalities are frequent as are genital tract abnormalities which are unlikely to be seen on prenatal ultrasound such as vaginal or uterine duplication or atresias.[34] The prognosis is related to the degree of the abnormality and associated abnormalities. Initially, infection is a large risk for these patients. Surgery initially is geared towards decompression to prevent further organ damage. Definitive therapy is usually postponed until the child is out of the neonatal period.[35]

RENAL PELVIS DILATION

There has been much attention in the literature over the past decade concerning fetal pyelectasis detected on ultrasound, primarily due to an association with Trisomy 21.[36] Certainly renal pelvis dilatation serves as a marker and prompts further investigation for ultrasound markers of Trisomy 21 or offering

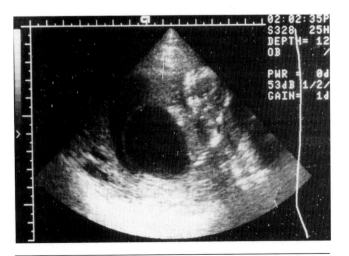

FIGURE 21-2 Early gestation fetus with a cloacal anomaly.

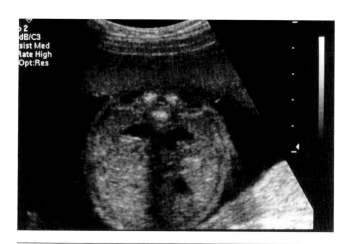

FIGURE 21-3 Bilateral renal pelvis dilatation.

fetal karyotype (Fig. 21-3). In the presence of a normal karyotype and no other anomalies noted on ultrasound, renal pelvis dilatation still serves as a marker for potential problems in the fetus. Measurements used in the literature variably recognize the increasing diameter frequently seen with advancing gestational age and range from greater than 4 mm at less than 32 weeks to greater than 8 mm regardless of gestational age if accompanied by transverse and longitudinal measurements of 11 and 14 mm respectively.[37,38] In one of the less conservative studies, defining renal pelvis as greater than 5 mm independent of gestational age, the diagnosis was made in 0.59% of the population. Of 100 patients diagnosed with dilatation, 64% had postnatal hydronephrosis at 1 and/or 6 weeks after delivery, the most common anomaly being vesico-ureteric reflux.[39] The high rate of vesico-ureteric reflux has been confirmed in other studies, even when regression of the prenatal renal pelvis dilatation has been noted.[37] Due to five cases (10%) of patients with regression of prenatal dilatation requiring surgical intervention, a careful follow-up of these infants may be appropriate.[37]

RENAL CYSTIC DISEASE

Multicystic Dysplastic Kidney

Multicystic dysplastic kidneys encompass a wide range of clinico-pathological entities.[40] Etiologies range from obstruction to an inherited familial dysplasia, with the overwhelming majority due to obstruction.[41] The incidence of associated urological malformations is high, found in 51% of patients[42] especially for vesicoureteric reflux.[43] The presence of dysplasia implies irreversible renal damage. The hallmark of a kidney with multicystic dysplasia is identification of multiple peripheral cysts seen on ultrasound. The presence of interfaces between the cysts and the nonmedial location of the cysts are helpful to differentiate the fluid seen from a dilated renal calyx.[44] The presence of cortical cysts is 100% predictive of multicystic dysplasia in the fetus with an obstructive lesion. Unfortunately, the absence of cysts is much less accurate. Increased echogenicity may be related to the presence of small cysts, detectable

only on histology. Assessment of renal echogenicity and the degree of hydronephrosis seen have limited value in assessing the presence of dysplastic changes due to their less frequent occurrence. Only 41% of dysplastic kidneys in a series of 34 patients had significant hydronephrosis.[45] Although multicystic kidneys usually appear enlarged, they may become smaller with time and eventually be undetectable grossly, a pattern detected in the pre- and postnatal course.[46] By 2 years post-natal life, 7 of 33 disappear completely, 20 of 33 regressed in size.[47]

The prenatal management is dictated by the location of the dysplastic changes. The lesion is most often unilateral (75% on the left)[48] with 1 normal kidney and normal amniotic fluid volume; routine prenatal care is indicated. When bilateral lesions are present, the condition may be lethal and assessment of the fetus for pulmonary hypoplasia and/or compression deformities if oligohydramnios is long standing is appropriate. Evaluation for associated anomalies may include a karyotype analysis.

Recurrence risk is small as most of the lesions are secondary to obstruction but further assessment regarding the anomaly is indicated to diagnose familial patterns and allow appropriate counseling.

Infantile Polycystic Kidney

The ultrasound appearance of infantile polycystic kidney disease is typically of echogenic kidneys that are enlarged although they retain their normal shape (Fig. 21-4). A series of 10 patients reported describes no false positive diagnosis but one false negative in a fetus with a less severe form of the disease.[49] We have identified a patient with enlargement of the fetal kidneys preceding oligohydramnios by as much as 10 weeks in an affected fetus. Enlarged kidneys alone may not be associated with pathology but increased echogenicity and decreased amniotic fluid volume along with absence of fluid in the fetal

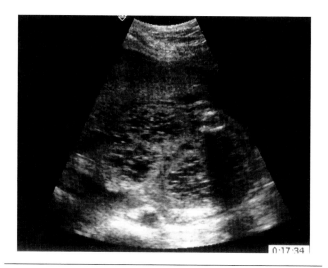

FIGURE 21-4 Bilateral infantile polycystic kidneys filling the fetal abdomen.

bladder and enlarged kidneys are classic for infantile polycystic kidneys. There is no prenatal therapy proven to benefit these fetuses. Antedotal reports of amnioinfusion to prevent lung hypoplasia or other complications have no proven efficacy.

Management after the diagnosis requires thorough counseling regarding the poor renal function expected with this diagnosis. The development of pulmonary hypoplasia is directly related to the gestational age at which oligohydramnios develops and this correlates with immediate neonatal survival.

This is an autosomal recessive disorder and parents have a 25% recurrence risk with subsequent pregnancies. Unfortunately, there is variable expression of the disorder and normal prenatal ultrasounds do not guarantee the disorder has not been inherited. Postnatal expression of the abnormality may be associated with cystic changes in the liver and biliary duct hyperplasia, as well as portal hypertension.

Prenatal management of patients at risk includes serial ultrasound to potentially diagnose the condition. In an affected fetus, the gestational age at which anhydramnios developed correlates with pulmonary hypoplasia. These fetuses are at increased risk of abdominal dystocia because of the increased abdominal girth and may require cesarean section if they progress to term.

RENAL TUMORS

The most common renal tumor seen in the neonatal period is congenital mesoblastic nephroma[50] and prenatal diagnosis has been reported.[51,52] The ultrasound findings include a solid mass contiguous with the kidney resembling normal renal tissue (Fig. 21-5). This may markedly increase the size of the fetal abdomen and soft tissue dystocia may be a concern if the abdomen is excessively large. Polyhydramnios has been described associated with the renal mass. The prenatal course may be complicated by premature labor secondary to polyhydramnios but prenatal care is otherwise unremarkable. Surgical resection of the tumor is necessary after birth but the lesions are operable. The prognosis for these fetuses is excellent. There is no increased recurrence risk.

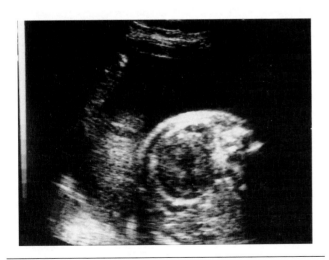

FIGURE 21-5 Fetus with polyhydramnios and congenital mesoblastic nephroma.

References

1. Helin I, Persson PH. Prenatal diagnosis of urinary tract abnormalities by ultrasound. *Pediatrics*. 1986;78:879–883.
2. Brumfield CG, Guinn D, Davis R, et al. The significance of non-visualization of the fetal bladder during an ultrasound examination to evaluate second trimester oligohydramnios. *Ultrasound Obstet Gynecol*. 1996;8:186–191.
3. Rosati P, Guariglia L. Transvaginal sonographic assessment of the fetal urinary tract in early pregnancy. *Ultrasound Obstet Gynecol*. 1996;7:95–100.
4. Bronshtein M, Bar-Hava I, Lightman A. The significance of early second trimester sonographic detection of minor fetal renal anomalies. *Prenat Diagn*. 1995;15:627–632.
5. Romero R, Cullen M, Peter Grannum P, et al. Antenatal diagnosis of renal anomalies with ultrasound: bilateral renal agenesis. *Am J Obstet Gynecol*. 1985;151:38–43.
6. Hitchcock R, Burge DM. Renal agenesis: an acquired condition? *J Pediatr Surg*. 1994;29(3):454–455.
7. Ratten GJ, Beischer NA, Fortune DW. Obstetric complications when the fetus has Potter's syndrome: clinical considerations: part I. *Am J Obstet Gynecol*. 1973;115:890–896.
8. Sherer DM, Thompson HO, Armstrong B, et al. Prenatal sonographic diagnosis of unilateral fetal renal agenesis. *J Clin Ultrasound*. 1990;18:648–652.
9. Roodhooft AM, Birnholz JC, Holmes LB. Familial nature of congenital absence and severe dysgenesis of both kidneys. *N Engl J Med*. 1984;310:1341–1344.
10. Hill LM, Peterson CS. Antenatal diagnosis of fetal pelvic kidneys. *J Ultrasound Med*. 1987;6:393–396.
11. Meizner I, Yitzhak M, Levi A, et al. Fetal pelvic kidney: a challenge in prenatal diagnosis? *Ultrasound Obstet Gynecol*. 1995;5:391–393.
12. Malek RS, Kelalis PP, Burke EC. Ectopic kidney in children and frequency of association with other malformations. *Mayo Clinic Proc*. 1971;46:461–467.
13. Kovo-Hasharoni M, Machiach R, Levy S, et al. Prenatal sonographic diagnosis of horseshoe kidney. *J Clin Ultrasound*. 1997;25:405–407.
14. King KL, Koofinas AD, Simon NV, et al. Antenatal ultrasound diagnosis of fetal horseshoe kidney. *J Ultrasound Med*. 1991;10:643–644.
15. Campbell MF. Anomalies of the kidney. In Campbell MF, Harrison JH, eds. *Urology*. 5th ed. Philadelphia: WB Saunders; 1986:1165–1705.
16. Donahue PK, Hendren WH. Pelvic kidney in infants and children: experience with 16 cases. *J Pediatr Surg*. 1980;15:486–495.
17. Cusick EL, Didier F, Droulle P, et al. Mortality after an antenatal diagnosis of foetal uropathy. *J Pediatr Surg*. 1995;30:463–466.
18. Reddy PP, Mandell J. Prenatal diagnosis: therapeutic implications. *Urol Clin North Am*. 1998;25:171–180.
19. Guys JM, Borella F, Monfort G. Ureteropelvic junction obstructions: prenatal diagnosis and neonatal surgery in 47 cases. *J Pediatr Surg*. 1988;23:156–158.
20. Freedman ER, Rickwod AMK. Prenatally diagnosed pelvi-ureteric junction obstruction: a benign condition? *J Pediatr Surg*. 1994;29:769–772.
21. Fasolato V, Poloniato A, Bianchi C, et al. Feto-neonatal ultrasonography to detect renal abnormalities: evaluation of 1 year screening program. *Am J Perinatol*. 1998;15:161–164.
22. Dwoskin JY. Ureteropelvic junction obstruction and sibling uropathology. *Urology*. 1979;13:153–154.

23. Wood BP, BenAmi T, Teele RL, et al. Ureterovesical obstruction and megaloureter: Diagnosis by real-time US. *Radiology*. 1985;156:79–81.

24. Jerkins GR, Noe HN. Familial vesicoureteral reflux: a prospective study. *J Urol*. 1981;128:774–778.

25. Tokunaka S, Koyanagi T. Morphologic study of primary non-reflux megaureters with particular emphasis on the role of ureteral sheath and ureteral dysplasia. *J Urol*. 1981;128:399–402.

26. Dunn V, Glasier CM. Ultrasonographic antenatal demonstration of primary megaureters. *J Ultrasound Med*. 1985;4:101–103.

27. Jeffrey RB, Laing FC, Wing VW, et al. Sonography of the fetal duplex kidney. *Radiology*. 1984;153:123–124.

28. Nakayama DK, Harrison MR, de Lorimier AA. Prognosis of posterior urethral valves presenting at birth. *J Pediatr Surg*. 1986;21:43–45.

29. Mahoney BS, Callen PW, Filly RA. Renal urethral obstruction: ultrasound evaluation. *Radiology*. 1985;157:221–224.

30. Johnson MP, Bukowski TP, Reitleman C, et al. In utero surgical treatment of fetal obstructive uropathy: a new comprehensive approach to identify appropriate candidates for vesicoamniotic shunt therapy. *Am J Obstet Gynecol*. 1994;170:1770–1779.

31. Quereshi F, Jacques SM, Seifman B, et al. In utero fetal urine analysis and renal histology do correlate with outcome in fetal obstructive uropathies. *Fetal Diagn Ther*. 1996;11:306–312.

32. Coplen DE. Prenatal intervention for hydronephrosis. *J Urol*. 1997;157:2270–2277.

33. Meizner I, Bar-Ziv J. Prenatal ultrasonic diagnosis of cloacal exstrophy. *Am J Obstet Gynecol*. 1985;153:802–803.

34. Jaramillo D, Lebowitz RL, Hendren WH. The cloacal malformation: radiologic findings and imaging recommendations. *Radiology*. 1990;177:441–448.

35. Allen TD, Husmann DA. Cloacal anomalies and other urorectal septal defects in female patients: a spectrum of anatomical abnormalities. *J Urol*. 1991;145:1034–1039.

36. Benacerraf BR. Identification of second trimester fetuses with autosomal trisomy by use of a sonographic scoring index. *Radiology*. 1994;193:135–140.

37. Lepercq J, Beaudoin S, Bargy F. Outcome of 116 moderate renal pelvis dilatations at prenatal ultrasonography. *Fetal Diagn Ther*. 1998;13:79–81.

38. Gotoh H, Massuzzaki H, Fukuda H, et al. Detection and assessment of pyelectasis in the fetus: relationship to postnatal renal function. *Obstet Gynecol*. 1998;92:226–231.

39. Dudley JA, Haworth JM, McGraw ME, et al. Clinical relevance and implications of antenatal hydronephrosis. *Arch Dis Child*. 1997;76:31–34.

40. Bernstein J. The morphogenesis of renal parenchymal maldevelopment (renal dysplasia). *Pediatr Clin North Am*. 1971;18:395–407.

41. Sanders RC, Nussbaum AR, Solez K. Renal dysplasia: sonographic findings. *Radiology*. 1988;167:623–626.

42. Atiyeh B, Husmann D, Baum M. Contralateral renal abnormalities in multicystic-dysplastic kidney disease. *J Pediatr*. 1992;121:65–67.

43. Gough DCS, Postlethwaite RJ, Lewis MA, et al. Multicystic renal dysplasia diagnosed in the antenatal period: a note of caution. *Brit J Urol*. 1995;76:244–248.

44. Stuck KJ, Koff SA, Silver TM. Ultrasonic features of multicystic-dysplastic kidney: expanded diagnostic criteria. *Radiology*. 1982;143:217–221.

45. Mahoney BS, Filly RA, Callen PW, et al. Fetal renal dysplasia: sonographic evaluation. *Radiology*. 1984;152:143–146.

46. Strife JL, Souza AS, Kirks DR, et al. Multicystic-dysplastic kidney in children: US follow-up. *Radiology*. 1993;186:785–788.

47. Heymans C, Breysem L, Proesmans W. Multicystic kidney dysplasia: a prospective study on the natural history of the affected and the contralateral kidney. *Eur J Pediatr*. 1998;156:673–675.

48. Akl K. Multicystic-dysplastic kidney and contralateral urologic abnormalities. *J Pediatr*. 1993;122:501.

49. Romero R, Cullen M, Jeanty P, et al. The diagnosis of congenital renal anomalies with ultrasound. *Am J Obstet Gynecol*. 1984;130:259–262.

50. Bolande RP. Congenital and infantile neoplasia of the kidney. *Lancet*. 1974;2:1497.

51. Ehman RL, Nicholson SF, Machin GA. Prenatal sonographic detection of congenital mesoblastic nephroma in a monozygotic twin pregnancy. *J Ultrasound Med*. 1983;2:555–557.

52. Geirsson RT, Ricketts NEM, Taylor DJ, et al. Prenatal appearance of a mesoblastic nephroma associated with polyhydramnios. *J Clin Ultrasound*. 1985;13:488–490.

SKELETAL DYSPLASIA

Jana K. Silva / Lawrence D. Platt / Deborah Krakow

The skeletal dysplasias encompass a group of disorders characterized by generalized abnormalities in skeletal growth and development. Of the 150 well-described entities, approximately 40% may be clinically apparent at birth.[1] In one large study, the prevalence of skeletal dysplasias recognizable in the perinatal period was 2.3 per 10,000 births; however under registration of cases suggested a real value of approximately twice that amount.[2] The wide range of disorders and variability in prognoses command early and accurate prenatal identification. Unfortunately, the number of cases identifiable in the antepartum period is exceedingly small, and remains a challenge even to the most experienced.

Advances in high-resolution ultrasound technology has improved prenatal diagnosis for many of the skeletal dysplasias.[3] In turn, the number of case reports on the sonographic features of potentially diagnosable conditions has grown.[4] Thanatophoric dysplasia, achondrogenesis, achondroplasia, and osteogenesis imperfecta however, continue to be the 4 disorders most commonly reported, though the actual incidence of these disorders are rare.[5] Since most skeletal dysplasias are uncommon, the potential lethality of some warrants immediate diagnosis since the prenatal implications for pregnancy termination or nonheroic measures are substantial. This chapter is a partial survey of the skeletal dysplasias currently amenable to prenatal diagnosis, reproductive risk assessment, and antenatal management. The most common occurring skeletal dysplasias will be covered, as will some dysostoses followed by brief discussion of less common disorders identified prenatally as reported in the literature.

NORMAL SKELETAL DEVELOPMENT

By the end of the embryonic period (10 menstrual weeks) the fetal extremities have developed into structures with relative arrangement and configuration identical to those of an adult.[6] This period also marks the beginning of endochondral ossification of long bones,[7] joint development, and fetal muscular activity.[8] The remainder of gestation and early postnatal development is subsequently devoted to increases in size and complexity of the fetal musculoskeletal system.

Fetal skeletal ossification occurs in an orderly manner. The clavicle and mandible are the earliest to ossify at 8 menstrual weeks, followed 3–4 weeks later by the appendicular long bones, phalanges, ileum and scapula. The metacarpals and metatarsals ossify at between 12 and 16 weeks, and by the twentieth to twenty-fourth week, the pubis, talus, and calcaneus begin to undergo ossification. Carpal tarsal ossification and (pubic) ossification however, are not complete until after birth.[5]

Secondary ossification is a third trimester event wherein centers appear at 28–35 weeks in the distal femur, followed by the proximal tibia, and proximal humerus.[5] Sequential development of these secondary ossification centers has proved helpful in the estimation of gestational age. Identification of the distal femoral epiphysis predicts a gestational age of at least 33 weeks, the presence of a proximal tibial epiphysis, a gestational age of 35 weeks, and the late appearing proximal humeral epiphysis, a gestational age of at least 38 weeks.[9] Identification of the epiphysis may be useful in differentiating some skeletal dysplasias though this is only relevant in the third trimester.

LONG BONE MEASUREMENTS

The lengths of the fetal extremities are easily measured by ultrasound from about the eleventh–thirteenth week of gestation.[10–12] Standard curves exist for most limb bone measurements, however, the ossified femoral diaphysis is the easiest to measure with reproducibility,[13] correlates well with gestational age,[14] and assists in the prediction of fetal skeletal growth disturbances.[15–18] The second and third trimester screening ultrasound examination therefore, includes femur length as part of the standard assessment.

The estimation of gestational age from extremity length measurements should use gestational age as the independent variable.[18] When evaluating the fetus for skeletal dysplasia however, the extremity length must be compared with other parameters of gestational age assessment such as biparietal diameter,[21–22] abdominal circumference, or cerebellar diameter. It is critical that all the available long bones be measured. These include the femur, humerus tibia, fibula, radius, and ulna. In most skeletal dysplasias the follow-up in growth of the long bones is uniform and symmetric.

CLASSIFICATION OF SKELETAL DYSPLASIAS

Classification of skeletal dysplasias is based primarily on descriptive findings of clinical, radiographic features, and molecular information when available.[23] Disorders have been classified according to the part of the skeleton involved (eg, epiphyseal disorders are resultant from epiphyseal abnormalities), by Greek terms describing the appearance of bone (eg, diastrophic dysplasia describes twisted bones) or by the course of disease (eg, thanatophoric "death bringing" dysplasia), by terms describing the pathogenesis of the condition (eg, osteogenesis imperfecta abnormal bone development).[23] More specifically, some skeletal dysplasias are also sub-classified based on the segment of long bone affected. Rhizomelic (proximal segment), mesomelic (middle segment), acromelic (distal segment), and micromelic (all segments) shortening, are terms widely used to describe the extent of long bone involvement.[23] While this classification is particularly helpful in narrowing the diagnostic possibilities, definitive diagnoses are best obtained through thorough systematic ultrasonographic evaluation of fetal anatomy.

SONOGRAPHIC APPROACH TO SKELETAL ABNORMALITIES

Skeletal dysplasias are frequently ascertained when a patient with a previously affected child or affected parent with a skeletal dysplasia seeks prenatal diagnosis, however the majority of cases are evaluated when abnormal extremities are noted incidentally on routine ultrasound examination.[24] Since many of the skeletal dysplasias occur as a result of a sporadic or autosomal dominant mutation, screening ultrasound is the method by which many of these disorders are usually first detected.[1,8,12,16,17] Any fetus with long bones measuring less than 2 standard deviations below the mean for gestational age, must be considered at risk for a skeletal dysplasia.[15,17] These patients should be followed with thorough fetal anatomic evaluation and close scrutiny of skeletal structure, mineralization, pattern of involvement, and interval growth. The presence of other structural anomalies, polyhydramnios,[27] or positive family history for skeletal dysplasia further validates the diagnosis of a skeletal dysplasia. However fetuses with long bones in the third percentile and normal interval growth are usually small for gestational age, resultant from maternal factors or other fetal genetic alterations.

The fetal skeletal survey should focus on the degree and location of bone shortening patterns of ossification, and the presence or absence of fractures or bowing.[8] Dependent on gestational age, the shape of the vertebral bodies,[28] focal loss of extremity bone, altered calvarial contour, small thoracic size, extra digits, and impaired fetal mobility and posture, provide additional clues to the presence of a skeletal disorder.[8] The most important goal is to determine a lethal skeletal dysplasia from a nonlethal skeletal dysplasia. Fetal thoracic circumference measurements taken at the level of the 4-chamber heart view, may easily identify a lethal dysplasia.[29–31] Measurements below the fifth percentile for gestational age, are often associated with pulmonary hypoplasia and neonatal death.[29–30] The fortunate sonographic manifestation of lethal short limb dysplasias before 24 weeks gestation helps distinguish them from non lethal syndromes.[5] Early diagnosis in turn, facilitates termination prior to viability, and prevents unnecessary institution of futile heroic measures at the time of delivery. However, even without a small chest circumference and lethality assumed, diagnosis should be attempted because many nonlethal skeletal dysplasias are associated with significant medical complications. It is critical that postmortem or neonatal radiographs be taken along with appropriate histomorphology samples to confirm the diagnosis. Ultrasonogra-

phy has not been proven to be effective in making definitive diagnoses necessary for appropriate genetic counseling.[1]

THE SKELETAL DYSPLASIAS

THANATOPHORIC DYSPLASIA

Definition: First described by Maroteaux in 1967.[32] Most commonly diagnosed lethal short-limbed congenital chondrodysplasia. Two types: type I and type II.[32]
Epidemiology: Estimated frequency of 0.28–0.60 in 10,000 births;[2] 1 in 20,000–40,000 live births.[33,34]
Pathology: Disorganization of endochondral bone formation[32] secondary to disordered and deficient chondrocyte formation and maturation (abnormal growth plate).[24] Membranous bone is unaffected resulting in disproportionate growth of the two bone types thereby explaining some of the phenotypic features seen.[35]

Common Sonographic Features

When Detectable: Reports suggest that most cases are detectable by 24 weeks gestation,[4] with definitive diagnosis reported as early as 19.7 weeks however diagnosis can be made earlier than that.[36]

Type I

Growth: Severe growth deficiency.[37]
Behavior: Decreased fetal movement,[33] hypotonia.[32,38]
Craniofacial: Large head with frontal bossing, narrow foramen magnum, hydrocephalus. Intact normally ossified bony cranium. Flat nasal bridge.[32–36,38,39]
Thorax: Small narrow chest and short ribs, with relative abdominal prominence but normal trunk length[32–36,38,39] (see Fig. 22-1).

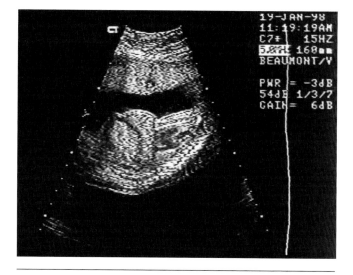

FIGURE 22-1 Ultrasound of a lateral chest view of a fetus with thanatophoric dysplasia exhibiting a short ribs with abdominal prominence.

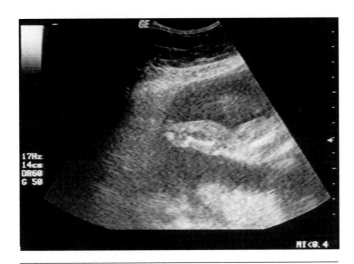

FIGURE 22-2 Lower extremities of a thanatorphic fetus demonstrating rhizo and mesomelia of the lower limb.

Spine: Short with shortened intervertebral distance and significantly flattened vertebral bodies.[12,39,40]

Extremities: Severe rhizomelia with bowed limbs and sometimes "telephone receiver" femurs.[33,38,39,41] Short stubby widely spaced fingers[33] (see Fig. 22-2).

Other Associated Findings: Redundant soft tissue.[39] Polyhydramnios.[33,39]

Type II

Differentiated from type I by: Straight femora, taller vertebral bodies, and cloverleaf skull.[32]

Inheritance

Autosomal dominant with all cases representing new mutations. Associated with higher paternal age, and a higher maternal—paternal age difference.[41]

Type I

All cases due to mutations in the fibroblast growth factor receptor 3 (FGFR3) gene.[32,34] Most of the mutations occur in the extracellular domain portion of the protein.

Type II

Many are a result of Lys650Glu residue change in the tyrosine kinase domain of FGFR3,[32,34] however other mutations have been identified.

Recurrence Risk: Negligible.[42]

Prognosis: Lethal shortly after birth. Cause of death is most often respiratory distress due to small thorax.[38] Cases of prolonged survival in neonates mechanically ventilated at birth demonstrate profound developmental delay and growth failure[37] with extensive central nervous system abnormalities.[43]

Testing: Molecular testing is available for FGFR3. However not all the mutations will be screened for and a negative result does not rule the disorder out.[34]

Management: Pregnancy termination should be offered when the diagnosis is made prior to viability. Since severe polyhydramnios and preterm labor are known complications,[33,44] and breech personation and cephalopelvic disproportion typical,[33,44] a plan for nonintervention for diagnoses established prior to delivery, is appropriate.[33]

Achondrogenesis

Definition: First described by Donnath and Vogl in 1925. Coined in 1952 by Fraccaro.[32] Second most common diagnosed lethal osteochondrodysplasia. Two types: type I and type II. Type I, previously known as Parenti–Fraccaro, actually represents two radiographically and histopathologically distinct disorders now recognized as types IA and IB.[32] Type II: Langer–Saldino Achondrogenesis–Hypochondrogenesis is actually a spectrum of the same disorder, with the slightly milder phenotype classified as hypochondrogenesis though it is lethal.[32]

Epidemiology: Rare, occurring in approximately 1 in 40,000 births.[2] Type I (A and B) represents 20% of cases. Type II represents 80% of cases.

Pathology: Failure of endochondral bone growth[45] with minimal chondrocyte proliferation at the epiphyseal growth plate.[46]

Type IA

Normal appearing cartilage with hypervascular matrix and increased cellular density. Chondrocytes contain round cytoplasmic inclusion bodies.

Type IB

Sparse cartilage matrix with deficiency of cartilage fibers. Chondrocytes are large with central round nuclei.[32]

Type II

Decreased secretion of type II collagen.[47]

Common Sonographic Features

When Detectable: Earliest diagnosis reported in the first trimester at 13–14 weeks.[33,47]

Type IA

Growth: Growth deficiency

Craniofacial: Enlarged cranium with frontal bossing and diminished calvarial ossification.[5,33,46] Low nasal bridge, micrognathia.[32]

Thorax: Short trunk. Thin short ribs with multiple fractures.[32,33]

Spine: Markedly diminished vertebral ossification[5,32,33,46] particularly in the lumbar spine[33] enabling clear sonographic visualization of the spinal column on longitudinal views. Only 2 vertebral ossification centers per spinal segment are seen in the transverse plane[5] (see Fig. 22-3).

Extremities: Severe micromelia.[5,32,33,46]

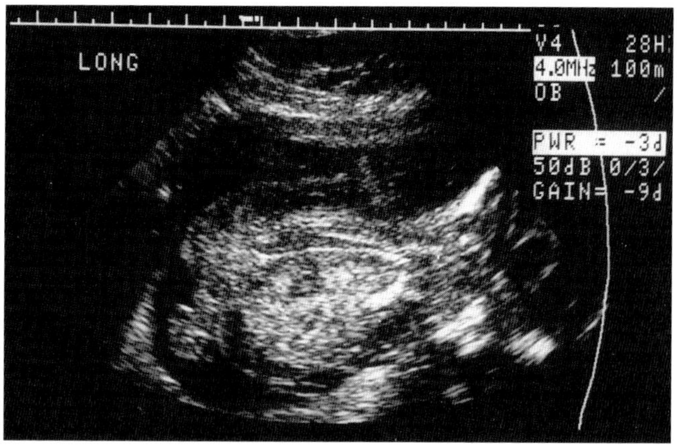

FIGURE 22-3 Achondrogenesis II: ultrasound of the fetal spine showing an absence ossification of the vertebral processes.

Other Associated Findings: Nuchal thickening and polyhydramnios.[33]

Type IB

Differentiated from type IA by: Absence of rib fractures.[32]

Type II

Differentiated from type IA and IB by: Normal calvarial ossification. Most cases are characterized by diminished and/or absent vertebral ossification. As a group, type II achondrogenesis is more often associated with cystic hygroma, polyhydramnios, hydrops and cleft soft palate, although the latter may not be easily seen on ultrasound. Rib fractures are also not present in any of the type II prototypes.[5,45]

Inheritance

Type IA and IB: Autosomal recessive disorders.[32,48] In type IB, mutations are identified in the gene for diastrophic dysplasia which encodes a sulfate transporter (DTDST).[32,49] Achondrogenesis and diastrophic dysplasia are therefore allelic disorders.[32] The gene defect for types IA is not known.

Type II

Molecular studies demonstrate heterozygous mutations in the COL2A1 gene encoding type II collagen.[32,47]

Recurrence Risk: Twenty-five percent for types IA and IB. For Achondrogenesis type II, the recurrence risk is less than 1%, however cases of gonadal mosaicism exist.

Prognosis: Most infants are stillborn or die shortly after birth due to pulmonary hypoplasia, although one child survived to 3 months of life.[32]

Testing: Since most cases of Achondrogenesis II are sporadic, molecular testing is not available. In cases of Achondrogenesis IB, linkage analysis for the DTDST is available if there is a previously affected fetus and DNA is available.[49]

Management: Pregnancy termination should be offered whenever the diagnosis is confirmed prior to viability.

ACHONDROPLASIA

Definition: Initially described by Parrot in 1878.[50] Two types: Heterozygous and homozygous. Heterozygous achondroplasia is the most common nonlethal osteochondrodysplasia. Homozygous achondroplasia, which occurs when both parents have achondroplasia is rare.

Epidemiology: Achondroplasia occurs in 1 in 15,000–30,000 births.[5,32]

Pathology: Quantitative decrease in the rate of endochondral ossification with normal membranous bone formation.[33,50]

Common Sonographic Features

When Detectable: Diagnosis may be suspected when the femur length—biparietal diameter ratio is < 1%.[10] Most cases are detected between 21 and 27 weeks, with the majority of diagnoses made after 24 weeks gestation.[26,33] Homozygous achondroplasia manifests very similarly to thanatorphic dysplasia. One cannot exclude achondroplasia on the basis of a normal femur length before 27 weeks gestation.[15,26]

Growth: Usually normal until 24 weeks.

Craniofacial: Megalocephaly, small foramen magnum, and frontal bossing. Hydrocephalus may also occur,[4,10,32] but is more pronounced in the homozygous condition, and can be associated with a cloverleaf skull.[5,10] Flat nasal bridge.

Thorax: *Heterozygous:* Relatively small.[33] *Homozygous:* Extremely small.[4]

Spine: Small spine width may be seen.[33]

Extremities: *Heterozygous achondroplasia:* Progressive third trimester rhizomelic limb shortening.[10,26,33] *Homozygous achondroplasia:* Severe progressive micromelia beginning in the mid to late second trimester and appears very similar to thanatophoric dysplasia.[4,5]

Other Associated Findings: Polyhydramnios. Large abdomen relative to trunk size.[33]

Inheritance: Autosomal dominant with 100% penetrance. Approximately 80–90% represent new spontaneous mutations[5,32,33] in the transmembrane domain of the gene encoding fibroblast receptor growth factor 3 (FGFR3) gene. Ninety-eight percent of cases demonstrate a substitution for a glycine residue at position 380 of the mature protein.[52] Nonfamilial cases are associated with advanced paternal age.[32]

Recurrence Risk: *Heterozygous achondroplasia:* Small if parents are normal stature though cases of gonadal mosaicism have been reported. For offspring of an affected parent: 50%.

Prognosis: *Heterozygous achondroplasia:* Normal intelligence and life span is usual, however affected individuals may be at risk for spinal cord compression, and obstructive sleep apnea.[32,33,50]

Homozygous dominant achondroplasia: Uniformly lethal with stillbirth or early neonatal death due to respiratory failure.[4,5,33]

Testing: DNA molecular analysis for the FGFR3 mutation.

Management: Late manifestation of long bone shortening may preclude elective termination of pregnancy. The presence of a large head, narrow foramen magnum, and risk of spinal cord compression, warrants cesarean section for atraumatic delivery. Obstetric management is otherwise routine.[33]

OSTEOGENESIS IMPERFECTA

Definition: Clinically Heterogeneous group of inherited connective tissue disorders characterized by bone fragility and deformation. There are 4 types identified: I–IV, based on clinical, radiographic and biochemical data.[5,54] Type II is lethal.
Epidemiology: As a group, the incidence is approximately 1.6–3.5 of 100,000 births.[33]
Pathology: Defective type I collagen synthesis.[4,5,32,33]

Common Sonographic Features

When Detectable: Lethal type II osteogenesis imperfecta has been identified as early as 13.5–15 weeks gestation.[5] Types III and IV may be seen in the third trimester secondary to a bowing or fracture of a long bone.

Type I

The identification of fractures may assist in the diagnosis of approximately 5% of cases.[8] Decreased ossification and bone length may also be detected in some cases,[55] however in general, the antenatal diagnosis of type I is exceedingly difficult.

Type II

The majority of cases detected in the antenatal period are type II.[33,56,57]
Growth: Intrauterine growth restriction is common.[58]
Behavior: Hypotonia[32] with decreased fetal movement.[57]
Cranium: The head is easily compressible. Clear visualization of intracranial structures and absence of skull reverberations, are classic features of type II.
Thorax: The chest is extremely small. Rib fractures are common. Most ribs have a beaded appearance due to multiple healed fractures (see Fig. 22-4).
Spine: Flattened vertebrae may be seen.
Extremities: Differential shortening of the extremities and limb thickening as a result of fractures and callus formation.[5,32]

Type III

Characterized by moderate shortening of the femur with multiple rib and long bone fractures, and decreased bone echogenicity.[8] Macrocephaly and intrauterine growth restriction are not uncommon.[32]

Type IV

Sonographic features are similar to type I and therefore antenatal diagnosis is difficult, but fractures may be seen.
Other Associated Findings: Polyhydramnios in type II.[33]
Inheritance:
Type I: Autosomal dominant with marked variability in expression resulting from mutations in COL1AI, leading to decreased production of type I collagen.[32]
Types II, III and IV: The majority of cases are due to sporadic mutations in one of the two type I collagen genes, COL1A1

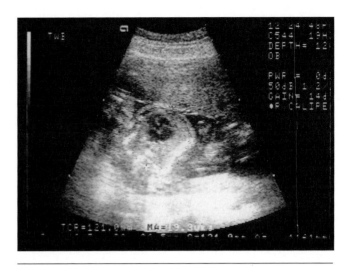

FIGURE 22-4 Osteogenesis Imperfecta II: ultrasound findings of an affected fetus demonstrating a small misshapen chest due to repeated fractures.

or COL1A2 which encode the proα1(I) and proα2(I) chains of type I collagen.[32,59,60] A rare autosomal recessive variety of type III osteogenesis imperfecta has been described in South Africa.[32]
Recurrence Risk: If a parent is affected then the recurrence risk for types I, III, and IV is 50%. New dominant mutations in type II are associated with a 6% recurrence rate due to parental gonadal mosaicism.
Prognosis: In general, prognosis depends on the severity of the specific phenotype.[33]
Types I and IV: Good prognosis with decreasing fracture potential noted with age.[4,32] If fractures appear before walking age however, there is a 30% chance that the child will be wheelchair bound.[33] *Type II:* Uniformly lethal due to stillbirth or respiratory compromise in the neonatal period.[32,33]
Type III: Not lethal at birth, but many die in infancy or early childhood due to cardiorespiratory complications.[4]
Testing: Cultured amniotic fluid fibroblasts in 85% of cases demonstrate abnormal type I procollagen synthesis in types II, III, and IV.[4] The diagnosis may be refined if the precise abnormality in a particular family is known. In this circumstance, chorionic villus samples may also be analyzed for the mutation.[33]
Management: Standard obstetric management for all types except type II which is lethal at birth. Pregnancy termination for diagnoses established prior to viability, or nonintervention for cases diagnosed thereafter, is appropriate.[33]

SHORT RIB POLYDACTYLY SYNDROME

Definition: Lethal skeletal dysplasia with at least 4 types described in the literature. Type I (Saldino–Noonan Type), type II (Majewski), Type III (Verma–Naumoff),[61,62,63] and type IV (Beemer).[63]
Epidemiology: Rare.

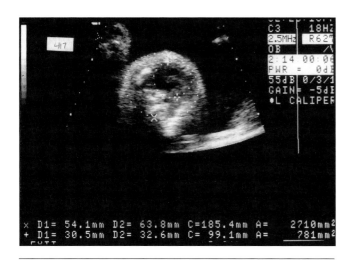

FIGURE 22-5 Short Rib Polydactyly Sydrome type I: Small chest without fractures. Note the abnormal cardiac circumference to thoracic circumference ratio.

Pathology: Defective maturation of chondrocytes with reduced and disorganized columnization resulting in growth plate disorganization and broad short trabeculae.[64]

Common Sonographic Features

When Detectable: Diagnoses reported between 16 and 19 weeks.[65,66]

Type I (Saldino–Noonan)

Growth: Intrauterine growth restriction.
Thorax: Short horizontal ribs with a narrow thorax.[5,32] (See Fig. 22-5)
Spine: Flat vertebrae with poor ossification and wide intervertebral disc spaces.[4,64]
Extremities: Severely shortened limbs with postaxial polydactyly of the hands and or feet.[4,5] Underossified phalanges.[32] Metaphyseal narrowing is characteristic, but may not be evident on ultrasound.[5,32]
Cardiac: Transposition of the great vessels, double-outlet right ventricle, double-outlet left ventricle, endocardial cushion defect, and hypoplastic right heart have all been identified.[32]
Genitourinary: Polycystic kidneys.[4,5,32] Cystic renal dysplasia.[4,5]
Other Associated Findings: Absent bladder, oligohydramnios,[4] and rarely penile hypoplasia with sex reversal (phenotypic females with 46XY karyotype).[32]

Type II (Majewski)

As in type I, but differentiated by micrognathia, a small nose, low-set ears, disproportionately short tibiae, and cleft lip and or palate.[4,5,32,63] Small cerebellar vermis, persistent left superior vena cava, polyhydramnios and hydrops have been reported.[32] Polydactyly may be either preaxial or postaxial and may include 7 digits.[67]

Type III (Verma–Naumoff)

Larger vertebral bodies, frontal bone prominence, and metaphyseal spurs are characteristic.[63] Although long bones are better formed, type III may be part of a specturm of the same disease, and as such may be difficult to distinguish from type I.[63]

Type IV (Breemer)

Very similar to type II, however mild platyspondyly, and bowing of long bones with a tibia longer than the fibula is characteristic and polydactyly is absent.[68]
Inheritance: All forms are autosomal recessive inheritance.
Recurrence Risk: Twenty-five percent recurrence risk.
Prognosis: All cases lethal with stillbirth or death soon after birth secondary to pulmonary hypoplasia and respiratory insufficiency.[4,32]
Testing: Sex reversal in the presence of other typical sonographic findings may provide clues to a diagnosis, however, this is extremely rare. The gene defect is not known at this time, but is thought to be either 4g13 or 4p16.
Management: Since this disorder is uniformly lethal, pregnancy termination is recommended.

CAMPOMELIC DYSPLASIA

Definition: A disorder characterized by bowing deformities of the femur and tibia.[33] Earliest reports of this skeletal dysplasia date back to the 1950s, however, the syndrome was not widely recognized until the 1970s when Springer and Maroteaux coined the term "camptomelique" (bent limb) to describe this disorder.[32]
Epidemiology: Rare, occurring with a frequency of approximately 1 in 150,000 births.[5]
Pathology: Retarded osseous maturation,[32] but the growth plate is normal.

Common Sonographic Features

When Detectable: Mid second trimester, at about 17 weeks.[4,33]
Growth: Intrauterine growth restriction.[32]
Craniofacial: Macrocephaly, venticulomegaly, hypotelorism, severe micrognathia, cleft palate, flat nasal bridge, and malformed and or low-set ears.[32,33,69–71]
Thorax: Small narrow thorax[4,5,69–71] with slender and or decreased number of ribs.[32,70]
Spine: Short flat vertebrae.[5,32]
Extremities: Severe bowing of the tibiae, fibulae, and femora.[32,33,69–71] Scapulae may be absent or hypoplastic.[5,69–71]
Other Associated Findings: Ambiguous genitalia[33] with sex reversal,[4,72–74] polyhydramnios, cardiac defects,[32,33] and varying degrees of renal calyceal dilitations[5,33,69] are seen.
Inheritance: Heterozygous mutations in the SOX9 gene located at chromosome 17q24.[32,73] This gene is presumed to be involved in bone formation and control of testicular development but not proven.[73]

Recurrence Risk: Negligible, though cases of reoccurrence based on gonadal mosaicism have been reported.

Prognosis: Usually lethal in the neonatal period. Survival for up to 17 years has been reported.[32] Length of survival is related to the degree of respiratory compromise[33] which is often substantial at birth.

Testing: DNA molecular analysis for the SOX9 mutation.

Management: When the diagnosis is established prior to viability, pregnancy termination may be offered. Preterm labor secondary to polyhydramnios is not uncommon, however, there are no benefits to prolonging the pregnancy. A plan for nonintervention is appropriate when the diagnosis is certain.[33]

DIASTROPHIC DYSPLASIA

Definition: Short-limbed skeletal dysplasia with wide variability of phenotypic expression[75] initially described in 1960 by Lamy and Maroteaux.[32]

Epidemiology: Rare, though more common in some populations.

Pathology: Chondrocyte degeneration[64] with undersulfation of proteoglycans in the cartilage matrix.[32,76]

Common Sonographic Features

When Detectable: First detectable at about 13 weeks[33] with most cases diagnosed between 16 and 20 weeks gestation.[77,78]

Growth: Early onset intrauterine growth restriction.[79]

Behavior: Flexion deformities of the elbows, knees, and hips[5,33] may impair fetal movement.

Craniofacial: Micrognathia, and cleft lip and or palate are characteristic features.[4,5,32,33] The hypertrophied articular cartilage unique to this disorder is not seen until the early neonatal period.[32]

Thorax: Relatively normal size.

Spine: Cervical kyphoscoliosis if present in utero is very subtle.[33]

Extremities: Severe micromelia.[5,33] Abducted and proximally inserted "hitchhiker" thumbs[4,5,32,33,77,78] and great toe, talipes equinovarus, and flexion deformities of the elbows, knees, and hips are characteristic features.[5,33] Ulnar deviation of the hands with short phalanges and limited finger joint movement may also be apparent.[5,33]

Other Associated Findings: Polyhydramnios.[33]

Inheritance: Autosomal recessive. The gene which encodes a novel sulfate transporter maps to chromosome 5q 31–34[33,79,80] and this disorder is allelic with achondrogenesis IB.

Recurrence Risk: Approximately 25%.

Prognosis: Wide variability in phenotypic expression with prognoses ranging from lethal to normal life expectancy. Death secondary to laryngeal obstruction is common in the lethal variant.[33] Increased infant mortality is usually secondary to respiratory complications.[5,32,33] Those who survive infancy, have a normal life span if the progressive kyphoscoliosis does not compromise neurologic[32] or cardiopulmonary function.[5] Intelligence is normal.[5,32]

Testing: DNA linkage disequilibrium mapping is available for at-risk families.[80]

Management: Lethal variants which justify termination before viability, must be excluded before developing a management plan. Preterm labor is not uncommon and should be treated. The presence of micrognathia may complicate intubation of these infants and should be anticipated and prepared for.[33]

CHONDROECTODERMAL DYSPLASIA (ELLIS-VAN CREVELD SYNDROME)

Definition: Short-limb osteochondrodysplasia originally described by Ellis and van Creveld in 1940.[32]

Epidemiology: One in 200,000 births with a higher prevalence in the Amish community.[5]

Pathology: Chondrocyte disorganization in the epiphyseal growth zone.[81]

Common Sonographic Features

When Detectable: Diagnosis reported as early as 17 weeks gestation.[82]

Growth: Intrauterine growth restriction.[32]

Thorax: Small narrow thorax with short poorly developed ribs represent a lethal form of this disorder that may be present in 50% of cases.[4,32]

Extremities: Disproportionally shortened extremities[32] with postaxial polydactyly of the fingers, and occasionally the toes.[5]

Cardiac: Approximately 50% of cases are associated with cardiac defects, most of which are atrial septal defects, often with a single atrium.[4,5,32]

Other Associated Findings: Dandy-Walker malformation, talipes equinovarus and renal agenesis may also be present.[32] Genital hypoplasia and multiple cervical and thoracic fusion defects characterize a possible variant of this disorder.[83]

Inheritance: Autosomal recessive[4,5,32,81,82] and linkage has been established to chromosome 4p.[108]

Recurrence Risk: Approximately 25%.

Prognosis: Fifty percent die in early infancy secondary to pulmonary hypoplasia and cardiorespiratory complications.[32] Normal intelligence for those who survive.[32]

Testing: Linkage may be available for certain facilities.

Management: Termination of pregnancy is an option for cases diagnosed prior to viability. Routine obstetric care should otherwise be offered.

ASPHYXIATING THORACIC DYSTROPHY (JEUNE SYNDROME)

Definition: Osteochondrodysplasia with variable expressivity initially described by Jeune in 1955.[5,32]

Epidemiology: One in 70,000 births.[5]

Pathology: The histopathologic changes are similar to that found in chondroectodermal dysplasia,[63] and may be an allelic disorder.

Common Sonographic Features

When Detectable: Diagnosis reported at 17–18 weeks gestation.[84,85]

Thorax: Small thin horizontal ribs with small thorax.[4,5,32,84,85]

Extremities: Mild to moderate rhizomelic shortening[4,5,84,85] is characteristic, however the fibulae and ulnae may also be short.[4,32] Bowing of the long bones can be seen and needs to be differentiated from campomelic dysplasia.[4]

Renal: Cystic tubular dysplasia.[4,5,32]

Other Associated Findings: Postaxial polydactyly of the hands and feet are present in approximately 14% of cases.[5,32] Situs inversus.[32]

Inheritance: Autosomal recessive.[4,5,32,84,85]

Recurrence Risk: Twenty-five percent.[84,85]

Prognosis: Neonatal death due to respiratory failure with or without pneumonia occurs in approximately 70% of cases.[4,5,32,84,85] Chronic nephritis with renal insufficiency and failure may be evident by age 2.[32] Progressive hepatic dysfunction with early cirrhosis may also contribute to the poor long-term prognosis, although survival to the fourth decade has been reported.[32,86]

Testing: The gene defect is unknown.

Management: When identified prior to viability, termination of pregnancy may be a viable option for lethal cases with a marginal thoracic circumference. Routine obstetric care is otherwise indicated.

SPONDYLOEPIPHYSEAL DYSPLASIA CONGENITA

Definition: Usual nonlethal osteochondrodysplasia originally described by Spranger and Weidemann in 1966. Due to mutations in the gene encoding type II collagen.[32]

Epidemiology: Rare.

Pathology: Delayed ossification of the epiphyses.[87]

Common Sonographic Features

When Detectable: Earliest diagnosis reported at between 17 and 20 weeks gestation.[87]

Growth: Intrauterine growth restriction is common,[32] although normal birth weight for gestational age has been reported.[87]

Behavior: Diminished joint mobility at elbows, knees, and hips.[32]

Craniofacial: Flat facies[32] may be evident in coronal view. Cleft palate and micrognathia may also be seen.[4,32]

Thorax: Short trunk with narrow thoracic circumference.[87]

Spine: Delayed ossification with short flattened vertebrae.[32]

Extremities: Shortened femur, humerus, radius and ulna.[4,87]

Other Associated Findings: Talipes equinovarus and polyhydramnios are sometimes found.[32]

Inheritance: Autosomal dominant with a variety of alterations identified in the COL2A1 gene encoding type II collagen.[32] Gonadal mosaicism has been documented.

Recurrence Risk: Fifty percent if there is an affected parent.

Prognosis: Hypotonic weakness may contribute to late onset of walking. High-grade myopia vitreous degeneration is common and may lead to retinal detachment in 50% of cases.[32] Normal intelligence and life span are characteristic[87] unless complicated by poor chest wall growth and respiratory failure.

Testing: Deletions, duplications, and single base substitutions may be identified in the COL2A1 gene.[32]

Management: Standard obstetric management and support, although elective termination may be offered in cases diagnosed prior to viability.

CONGENITAL HYPOPHOSPHATASIA (PERINATAL LETHAL TYPE)

Definition: Lethal inborn error of metabolism with abnormal bone mineralization initially described by Rathburn in 1948 and 4 forms have been identified.[88] Only the prenatally diagnosed lethal form will be discussed.

Epidemiology: Incidence of approximately 1 in 100,000 births.[89]

Pathology: Deficient activity of the tissue nonspecific isoenzyme of alkaline phosphatase results in severe deficiency of tissue and serum alkaline phosphatase and impaired skeletal calcification.[4,5,32,89−95]

Common Sonographic Features

Poor skeletal ossification is characteristic.

When Detectable: First trimester biochemical analysis of cases at risk have been reported,[89−91] although sonographic findings may not be apparent until the second trimester and needs to be differentiated from osteogenesis imperfecta type II.[90,92]

Growth: Intrauterine growth restriction.[33]

Behavior: Hypotonia may be detected in utero.[32]

Craniofacial: Inability to identify the fetal calvarium at 16 weeks gestation is suggestive of a diagnosis.[4,91,92] Skull is easily deformable.[4]

Thorax: Short beaded ribs with a small thoracic cage.[32]

Spine: Abnormal vertebral bodies with varying shapes and poor ossification of posterior elements.[32]

Extremities: Moderate to severe micromelia with thin delicate bowed lower extremities.[4,5]

Other Associated Findings: Polyhydramnios[32] and hydrops[33] may be seen.

Inheritance: Autosomal recessive with marked variability of expression.[32] The gene for hypophosphatasia has been mapped to chromosome 1p36.1–p34.[95] The disease gene is liver/bone/kidney Alkaline Phosphatase (ALPL).[95]

Recurrence Risk: Twenty-five percent.

Prognosis: Uniformly lethal due to respiratory insufficiency.[32]

Testing: Measurement of the liver-bone-kidney isoenzyme of alkaline phosphatase in chorionic villus samples or amniotic fluid using monoclonal antibodies demonstrate low levels of the isoenzyme.[90] Linkage analysis may also be performed in informative families.

Management: The lethal prognosis warrants offering of pregnancy termination for cases diagnosed prior to viability.

Nonintervention with expectant management for polyhydramnios, hydrops, or preterm labor is appropriate when diagnosed after the legal age for termination.

FIBROCHONDROGENESIS

Definition: Neonatal lethal short-limbed chondrodysplasia initially described by Lazzaroni-Fossati in 1978.[32,96]
Epidemiology: Exremely rare.
Pathology: Interwoven fibrous septa with fibroblastic dysplasia of chondrocytes[96] and fibrosis of growth plate cartilage.[32]

Common Sonographic Features

When Detectable: Prenatal diagnosis reported in twins at 24 weeks gestation though changes can be seen earlier in gestation.[96]
Growth: Impaired.
Craniofacial: Protuberant eyes, low-set malformed ears,[32] and hypoplastic nose with flat nasal bridge.[32,96]
Thorax: Short, thin ribs with small chest.[32]
Spine: Posterior vertebral hypoplasia with flattened vertebrae.[32]
Extremities: Rhizomelic shortening[96] with metaphyseal flaring, fifth finger clinodactyly and short fibulae.[32]
Other Associated Findings: Omphalocele and hydrops may be present.[32,96]
Inheritance: Occurrence in siblings and consanguinity of parents suggest autosomal recessive inheritance.[32,96]
Recurrence Risk: Twenty-five percent for the autosomal recessive condition.
Prognosis: Lethal.[32]
Testing: None available at present.
Management: Nonintervention for cases diagnosed prior to delivery. If a diagnosis is confirmed prior to viability, elective termination is a viable option. Important to differentiate this disorder from thanatophoric dysplasia and lethal metatropic dysplasia which may be difficult via ultrasound.

SPONDYLOCOSTAL DYSPLASIA TYPE I (JARCHO-LEVIN SYNDROME)

Definition: First described in 1938 by Jarcho and Levin[32] and compromised by a heterogenous group of vertebral segmentation defects. It is not a generalized skeletal dysplasia, but a dysostosis.
Epidemiology: Rare, however increased in some populations.

Common Sonographic Features

When Detectable: Prenatal diagnosis reported at 17–23 weeks gestation.[8,97]
Craniofacial: Prominent occiput.
Thorax and Spine: Short thorax with "crab-like" chest[32] secondary to vertebral and rib disorganization.[8]
Extremities: Normal.[8,32,97]
Other Associated Findings: Cleft palate, hydronephrosis, and CNS abnormalities.[32]
Inheritance: Autosomal recessive and autosomal dominant patterns of inheritance.[32,97]

Recurrence Risk: 0–25%.[97]
Prognosis: Although survival to 11 years of age has been reported, the disorder is frequently lethal in the neonatal period due to respiratory insufficiency and or recurrent pulmonary infection.[32]
Testing: None available.
Management: Elective termination may be offered in cases diagnosed prior to viability. Supportive care with expectant management is otherwise indicated.

CLEIDOCRANIAL DYSPLASIA

Definition: Osteochondrodysplasia with generalized dysplasia of osseous and dental tissues described in 1897 by Marie and Sainton.[32]
Epidemiology: Rare with a prevalence of approximately 1 per million.[98]

Common Sonographic Features

When Detectable: Diagnosis reported at 15–20 weeks gestation.[99]
Craniofacial: Brachycephaly, frontal bossing, low nasal bridge, and hypertelorism are frequent but not constant features of this disorder.[32,99]
Thorax: Small thorax with short ribs.[32] Hypoplasia or absence of one or both clavicles is characteristic.[32,99]
Spine: Normal.
Extremities: No significant abnormalities detected on ultrasound. Subtle hand abnormalities may be seen on radiograph.
Other Associated Findings: Micrognathia, cleft palate, and absence of the pubic bone have been reported.[32]
Inheritance: Autosomal dominant with complete penetrance and wide variability of expression.[32,98] The gene for this disorder is CBFA1.[32,98,110]
Recurrence Risk: 50% if there is an affected parent.
Prognosis: Good.
Testing: Linkage analysis.[98,100]
Management: Routine obstetric management.

LANGER MESOMELIC DYSPLASIA

Definition: Initially described by Brailsford in 1935, and classified as a distinct disorder in 1967 by Langer.[32]
Epidemiology: Rare.
Pathology: Chondrocyte degeneration and disorganization of the epiphyseal growth plate.[101]

Common Sonographic Features

When Detectable: Can be identified in the second trimester by disproportionate mesomelic limb shortness.[101]
Craniofacial: Micrognathia.[32,101]
Thorax: Normal.
Spine: Normal.
Extremities: Mesomelia with hypoplasia of the tibia, fibula, ulna, and radius.[32,101]
Inheritance: Probable homozygosity for the autosomal dominant dyschondrosteosis gene, but this has not been proven.[32]

Recurrence Risk: At least 25% recurrence risk for the homozygous phenotype.
Prognosis: Good with normal intelligence.[32]
Testing: None available.
Management: Routine obstetric care.

ROBERTS-SC PHOCOMELIA

Definition: Initially described by Roberts in 1919; not a skeletal dysplasia but a dysostoses.
Epidemiology: Rare.

Common Sonographic Features

When Detectable: Diagnosis reported as early as 19 weeks gestation.[3]
Growth: Profound intrauterine growth restriction.[32]
Behavior: Flexion contractures of knees, ankles, wrists, and/or elbows[32] may limit intrauterine movement.
Craniofacial: Microcephaly, hypertelorism, micrognathia, malformed ears, and cleft lip with or without cleft palate have been identified.[4,32,102,103]
Thorax and Spine: Normal.
Extremities: Hypomelia of varying degrees ranging from tetraphocomelia to lesser degrees of limb reduction.[3,4,32,102,103]
Other Associated Findings: Renal dysplasia, oligohydramnios,[3] frontal encephalocele, and cardiac defects are common.[4]
Inheritance: Autosomal recessive with variability of expression.[32,103]
Recurrence Risk: Approximately 25%.
Prognosis: Most are stillborn or die in early infancy. Marked growth deficiency with varying degrees of mental deficiency are seen in survivors.[32]
Testing: Chromosome analysis of cultured aminiocytes under certain conditions may reveal the characteristic centromeric splitting and puffing.[4,32]
Management: Pregnancy termination option for cases diagnosed prior to viability. Supportive obstetric care when diagnosed prior to delivery.

HOLT-ORAM SYNDROME

Definition: Syndrome of skeletal and cardiovascular anomalies initially described by Holt and Oram in 1960.[32]
Epidemiology: Rare.
Pathology: Detect in the TBX5 gene[112] though there is evidence for genetic heterogeneity.[104]

Common Sonographic Features

When Detectable: As early as 14 weeks in individuals at risk.[104]
Cardiovascular: Ventricular septal defects and ostium secundum atrial septal defects with or without conduction disturbances and PDA are most commonly described.[32,104]
Skeletal: Upper limb abnormalities of varying degrees.[32,104] Thumbs and radii may be hypoplastic or absent.[104] Syndactyly may be detected between the thumb and index finger.[32] The left upper extremity is usually more involved than the right.[8]

Other Associated Findings: Hypertelorism, pulmonic stenosis, postaxial, and central polydactyly,[32] polyhydramnios.[104]
Inheritance: Autosomal dominant with 100% penetrance and variable expression.[32,104] The responsible gene is TBX5,[111] though there is evidence for genetic heterogeneity.
Recurrence Risk: At least 50% risk of recurrence, if there is an affected parent.
Prognosis: Depends on the type and extent of skeletal and cardiovascular involvement.
Testing: Linkage analysis available in informative families.
Management: Elective termination may be offered for severe phenotypes diagnosed prior to viability. Routine obstetric management with careful planning of the timing of delivery may be necessary for optimal cardiac intervention.

RADIAL APLASIA-THROMBOCYTOPENIA SYNDROME

Definition: Described in 1956 by Gross, Groh, and Weippl.[32]
Epidemiology: Rare.

Common Sonographic Features

When Detectable: Prenatal diagnosis reported at 19 weeks gestation.[105]
Skeletal: Bilateral absence of the radius.[4,32,105,106] Ulnar abnormalities detected in 70%[4] with hypoplasia seen in 100%, bilateral absence of the ulna in 20%, and unilateral absence of the ulna in 10%.[32] Abnormal humerus is seen in 50% with bilateral absence detected in 5–10%.[32] The thumbs are always present.[32] Fibula may also be absent.[32]
Hematologic: Severe thrombocytopenia, "leukemoid" granulocytopenia, eosinophilia, and anemia are seen in early infancy.[32,106]
Other Associated Findings: Congenital heart defects consisting mainly of tetralogy of Fallot, and atrial septal defects.[32] Brachycephaly, micrognathia, neural tube defects and renal anomalies may be associated.[32]
Inheritance: Autosomal recessive.
Recurrence Risk: Twenty-five percent.
Prognosis: Forty percent of those affected die in early infancy as a result of hemorrhage or intracranial bleeding. With advancing age, the severity of the hematologic disorder is less profound. Delayed motor development may be apparent.
Testing: Umbilical cord sampling may be performed to detect thrombocytopenia.[4]
Management: Pregnancy termination of cases diagnosed prior to viability. Cesarean section with atraumatic delivery is indicated to avoid neonatal hemorrhage.

SUMMARY

This review is by no means an exhaustive review of prenatally diagnosable skeletal dysplasias and dysostoses. Radiographic and postnatally defined features that are not usually seen on ultrasound were intentionally omitted, and emphasis placed on prenatal sonographic features instead. Prenatal diagnosis of skeletal dysplasias has historically been by radiography. Many of the skeletal and other structural abnormalities seen in the skeletal dysplasias are not detectable by ultrasound. There are concentrated ultrasound findings that may aid in differentiating the skeletal dysplasias, especially focused on the issue of lethality versus nonlethality. We believe the critical role of the ultrasonographer is to determine potential lethality not in making a precise diagnosis in these rare conditions.

With this in mind, the importance of postnatal diagnosis and radiographic correlation cannot be overemphasized.[108] If a fetus is terminated, intact delivery is extremely helpful to accomplish this task, as are the collection of appropriate tissue samples for histomorphology, biochemical analyses, or molecular genetic studies.[33] Accurate diagnosis of the proband and application to future offspring is paramount; along with progressive improvement in ultrasound technology, such measures can only serve to strengthen the scope of prenatal diagnosis in the future.

References

1. Lachman RS, Rappaport V. Fetal imaging in the skeletal dysplasias. *Clin Perinat.* 1991;17:703–722.
2. Orioli IM, Castilla EE, Barbosa-Neto JG. The birth prevalence ratios for the skeletal dysplasias. *J Med Genet.* 1986;23:328–332.
3. Hobbins JC, Bracken MB, Mahony M. Diagnosis of fetal skeletal dysplasias with ultrasound. *Am J Obstet Gynecol.* 1982;142:306–312.
4. Donnenfeld AE, Mennuti MT. Second trimester diagnosis of fetal skeletal dysplasias. *Obstet Gynecol Surv.* 1987;42:199–217.
5. Mahony BS. Ultrasound evaluation of the fetal musculoskeletal system. In Callen PW (ed.): Ultrasonography in obstetrics and gynecology. WB Saunders Co; Philadelphia: 1994.
6. Garn SM, Burd AR, Babler WJ, et al. Early prenatal attainment of adult metacarpal-phalangeal rankings and proportions. *Am J Phys Anthrop.* 1975;43:327.
7. O'Rahilly R, Gardner E. The initial appearance of ossification in staged human embryos. *Am J Anat.* 1972;134:291.
8. Mahony BS. The extremities. In: Nyberg DA, Mahony BS, Pretorius DH, eds. *Diagnostic Ultrasound of fetal anomalies: text and atlas.* Mosby Year Book; Chicago: 1990:492–562.
9. Chinn DH, Bolding DB, Callen PW, et al. Ultrasonographic identification of fetal lower extremity epiphyseal ossification centers. *Radiology.* 1983;147:815–818.
10. Filly RA, Golbus MS. Ultrasonography of the normal and pathologic fetal skeleton. *Radiol Clin North Am.* 1982;20:311–323.
11. Goldstein RB, Filly RA, Simpson G. Pitfalls in femur length measurements. *J Ultrasound Med.* 1987;6:203–207.
12. Pretorius DH, Rumack CM, Manco-Johnson ML, et al. Specific skeletal dysplasias in utero: sonographic diagnosis. *Radiology.* 1986;159:237–242.
13. Queenan JT, O'Brien GD, Campbell S. Ultrasound measurement of fetal limb bones. *Am J Obstet Gynecol.* 1980;138:297–302.
14. Hadlock FP, Harrist RB, Deter RL, et al. Fetal femur length as a predictor of menstrual age: sonographically measured. *AJR.* 1982;138:875–878.
15. Filly RA, Golbus MS, Carey JC, et al. Short-limbed dwarfism: ultrasonographic diagnosis by mensuration of fetal femoral length. *Radiology.* 1981;138:653–656.
16. Hegge FN, Prescott GH, Watson PT. Utility of a screening examination of the fetal extremities during obstetrical sonography. *J Ultrasound Med.* 1986;5:639–645.
17. Kurtz AB, Needleman L, Wapner R, et al. Usefulness of a short femur in the in utero detection of skeletal dysplasias. *Radiology.* 1990;177:197–200.
18. Deter RL, Rossavik IK, Hill RM, et al. Longitudinal studies of femur growth in normal fetuses. *J Clin Ultrasound.* 1987;15:299–305.
19. Mercer BM, Sklar S, Shanatmadar A, et al. Fetal foot length as a predictor of gestational age. *Am J Obstet Gynecol.* 1987;156:350–355.
20. Campbell J, Henderson A, Campbell S. The fetal femur/foot length ratio: a new parameter to assess dysplastic limb reduction. *Obstet Gynecol.* 1988;72:181–184.
21. Wolfson RN, Peisner DB, Chik LL, et al. Comparison of biparietal diameter and femur length in the third trimester: effects of gestational age and variation in fetal growth. *J Ultrasound Med.* 1986;5:145–149.
22. Merz E, Kim-Kein M, Pehl S. Ultrasonic mensuration of fetal limb bones in the second and third trimesters. *J Clin Ultrasound.* 1987;15:175–183.
23. Sillence DO, Rimoin DL, Lachman RS. Neonatal dwarfism. *Pediatr Clin North Am.* 1978;25:453–483.
24. Romero R, Pilu G, Jeanty P, et al. Skeletal dysplasias. In Prenatal diagnosis of congenital anomalies. Norwalk, CT: Appleton & Lange; 1988:311–384.
25. Golbus MS, Hall BD. Failure to diagnose achondroplasia in utero. *Lancet.* 1974;i:629.
26. Kurtz AB, Filly RA, Wapner RJ, et al. In utero analysis of heterozygous achondroplasia: variable time of onset as detected by femur length measurements. *J Ultrasound Med.* 1986;5:137–40.
27. Wong WS, Filly RA. Polyhydramnios associated with fetal limb abnormalities. *AJR.* 1983;140:1001–1003.
28. Rouse GA, Filly RA, Toomey F, et al. Short-limb skeletal dysplasias: evaluation of the fetal spine with sonography and radiography. *Radiology.* 1990;174:177–180.
29. Nimrod C, Danes D, Iwanicki S, et al. Ultrasound prediction of pulmonary hypoplasia. *Obstet Gynecol.* 1986;68:495–498.
30. Nimrod C, Nicholson S, Davies D, et al. Pulmonary hypoplasia testing in clinical obstetrics. *Am J Obstet Gynecol.* 1988;158:277–280.
31. Fong K, Ohlson A, Zalev A. Fetal thoracic circumference: a prospective cross-sectional study with real time ultrasound. *Am J Obstet Gynecol.* 1988;158:1154–1160.
32. Jones KL. *Smiths recognizable patterns of human malformation.* Philadelphia: WB Saunders; 1997.
33. Sanders RC, Blackman LR, Hogge WA, et al. *Structural fetal anomalies: the total picture.* St. Louis: Mosby; 1996.
34. Tavormina PL, Shiang R, Thompson LM, et al. Thanatophoric dysplasia (types I and II) caused by distinct mutations in fibroblast growth factor receptor 3. *Nature Genet.* 1995;9:321–328.
35. Isaacson G, Blakemore KJ, Chervenak FA. Thanatophoric dysplasia with cloverleaf skull. *Am J Dis Child.* 1983;137:896–898.
36. Burrows PE, Stannard MW, Pearrow J, et al. Early antenatal sonographic recognition of thanatophoric dysplasia with cloverleaf skull deformity. *AJR.* 1984;143:841–843.
37. MacDonald IM, Hunter AJ, MacLeod PM, et al. Growth and development in thanatophoric dysplasia. *Am J Med Genet.* 1989;33:508–512.
38. Kaufman RL, Rimoin DL, McAlister WH, et al. Thanatophoric dwarfism. *Am J Dis Child.* 1970;120:53–57.
39. Cremin BJ, Shaff MI. Ultrasonic diagnosis of thanatophoric dwarfism utero. *Radiology.* 1977;124:479–480.

40. Mahony BS, Filly RA, Callen PW, et al. Thanatophoric dwarfism with the cloverleaf skull: a specific antenatal sonographic diagnosis. *J Ultrasound Med.* 1985;4:151–154.

41. Martinez-Frias ML, Ramos-Arroyo MA, Salvador J. Thanatophoric dysplasia: an autosomal dominant condition? *Am J Med Genet.* 1988;31:815–820.

42. Weiner CP, Williamson RA, Bonsib SM. Sonographic diagnosis of cloverleaf skull and thanatophoric dysplasia in the second trimester. *J Clin Ultrasound.* 1986;14:463–465.

43. Wongmongkolrit T, Bush M, Roessmann U. Neuropathological findings in thanatophoric dysplasia. *Arch Pathol Lab Med.* 1983;107:132–135.

44. Thompson BH, Parmley TH. Obstetric features of thanatophoric dwarfism. *Am J Obstet Gynecol.* 1971;109:396–401.

45. Whitley CB, Gorlin RJ. Achondrogenesis: new nosology with evidence of genetic heterogeneity. *Radiology.* 1983;148:693–698.

46. Meizner I, Barnhard Y. Achondrogenesis type I diagnosed by transvaginal ultrasonography at 13 weeks gestation. *Am J Obstet Gynecol.* 1995;173:1620–1622.

47. Godfrey M, Hollister DW. Type II achondrogenesis-hypochondrogenesis: identification of abnormal type II collagen. *Am J Hum Genet.* 1988;43:904–913.

48. Glenn LW, Teng SSK. In utero sonographic diagnosis of achondrogenesis. *J Clin Ultrasound.* 1985;13:195–198.

49. Superti-Furga A, Hastbacka J, Wilcox WR, et al. Achondrogenesis type IB is caused by a mutation in the diastrophic dysplasia sulfate transporter gene. *Nat Genet.* 1996;12:100–102.

50. Rimoin DL. Cervicomedullary junction compression in infants with achondroplasia: when to perform neurosurgical decompression. *Am J Hum Genet.* 195;56:824–827.

51. Le Merrer M, Rousseau F, Legeai-Mallet L, et al. A gene for achondroplasia-hypochondroplasia maps to chromosome 4p. *Nature Genetics.* 1994;6:318–321.

52. Shiang R, Thompson LM, Zhu YZ, et al. Mutation in the transmembrane domain of FGFR3 cause the most common genetic form of dwarfism, achondroplasia. *Cell.* 1994;78:335–342.

53. Brinkman G, Schlitt H, Zorowka P, et al. Cognitive skills in achondroplasia. *Am J Med Genet.* 1993;47:800–804.

54. Byers PH, Wallis GA, Willing MC. Osteogenesis imperfecta: translation of mutation to phenotype. *J Med Genet.* 1991;28:433–442.

55. Chervenak FA, Romero R, Berkowitz RL, et al. Antenatal sonographic findings of osteogenesis imperfecta. *Am J Obstet Gynecol.* 1982;143:228–230.

56. Merz E, Goldhofer W. Sonographic diagnosis of lethal osteogenesis imperfecta in the second trimester: case report and review. *J Clin Ultrasound.* 1986;14:380–383.

57. Shapiro JE, Phillips JA, Byers PH, et al. Prenatal diagnosis of lethal perinatal osteogenesis imperfecta (OI Type II). *J Pediatr.* 1982;100:127–133.

58. Elias S, Simpson JL, Griffin LP. Intrauterine growth retardation in osteogenesis imperfecta. *JAMA.* 1978;239:23.

59. Sykes B, Ogilvie D, Wordsworth P, et al. Consistent linkage of dominantly inherited osteogenesis imperfecta to the type I collagen loci: COL1A1 and COL1A2. *Am J Hum Genet.* 1990;46:293–307.

60. Byers PH, Tsipouras P, Bonadio JF, et al. Perinatal lethal osteogenesis imperfecta (OI Type II): a biochemically heterogeneous disorder usually due to new mutations in the genes for type I collagen. *Am J Hum Genet.* 1988;42:237–248.

61. Meizner I, Bar-Ziv J. Prenatal ultrasonic diagnosis of short-rib polydactyly syndrome (SRPS) type III: A case report and a proposed approach to the diagnosis of SRPS and related conditions. *J Clin Ultrasound.* 1985;13:284–287.

62. Naumoff P, Young LW, Mazer J, et al. Short rib-polydactyly syndrome type 3. *Radiology.* 1977;122:443–447.

63. McAlister WH, Herman TE. Osteochondrodysplasias, dysostoses, chromosomal aberrations, mucopolysaccharidoses, and mucolipi-

doses. In: Resnik D, ed. *Diagnosis of bone and joint disorders.* Philadelphia: WB Saunders Co.; 1995:4163–4244.

64. Rimoin DL, Lachman RS. The chondrodysplasias. In: Emery AE, Rimoin DL, Sofaer JA. eds. *Principles and practice of medical genetics.* Edinburgh: Churchill Livingstone; 1990.

65. Richardson MM, Beaudet AL, Wagner ML, et al. Prenatal diagnosis of recurrence of Saldino—Noonan dwarfism. *J Pediatr.* 1977;91:467–471.

66. Gembruch U, Hansmann M, Fodisch HJ. Early prenatal diagnosis of short rib-polydactyly (SRP) syndrome type I Majewski by ultrasound in a case at risk. *Prenat Diagn.* 1985;5:357.

67. Lungarotti MS, Martello C, Martinelli I, et al. Lethal short rib syndrome of the Beemer type without polydactyly. *Pediatr Radiol.* 1993;23:325.

68. Cooper CP, Hall CM. Lethal short-rib polydactyly syndrome of the Majewski type: a report of three cases. *Radiology.* 1982;144:513–517.

69. Sanders RC, Greyson-Fleg RT, Hogge WA, et al. Osteogenesis imperfecta and campomelic dysplasia: difficulties in prenatal diagnosis. *J Ultrasound Med.* 1994;13:691–700.

70. Hall BD, Spranger JW. Campomelic dysplasia: further elucidation of a distinct entity. *Am J Dis Child.* 1980;134:285–289.

71. Balcar I, Bieber FR. Sonographic and radiologic findings in campomelic dysplasia. *AJR.* 1983;141:481–482.

72. Kim MR, Qazi QH, Anderson VM, et al. A genetic male infant with female phenotype: a possible relationship to exposure to oral contraceptives during pregnancy. *Am J Obstet Gynecol.* 1995;172:1042–1043.

73. Foster JW, Domiguez-Stelich MA, Guioli S, et al. Campomelic dysplasia an autosomal sex reversal caused by mutations in an SRY-related gene. *Nature.* 1994;372:525–530.

74. Mansour S, Hall CM, Pembrey ME, et al. A clinical and genetic study of campomelic dysplasia. *J Med Genet.* 1995;32:415–420.

75. Horton WA, Rimoin DL, Lachman RS, et al. The phenotypic variability of diastrophic dysplasia. *J Pediatr.* 1978;93:609–613.

76. Hastbacka J, Kaitila I, Sistonen P, et al. Diastrophic dysplasia gene maps to the distal long arm of chromosome 5. *Proc Natl Acad Sci USA.* 1990;87:8056–8059.

77. Gollop TR, Eigier A. Brief clinical report: prenatal ultrasound diagnosis of diastrophic dysplasia at 16 weeks. *Am J Med Genet.* 1987;27:321–324.

78. Mantagos S, Weiss RR, Mahony M, et al. Prenatal diagnosis of diastrophic dwarfism. *Am J Obstet Gynecol.* 1981;139:111–113.

79. O'Brien GD, Rodek C, Queenan JT. Early prenatal diagnosis of diastrophic dwarfism by ultrasound. *Br Med J.* 1980;280:1300.

80. Hastbacka J, de la Chapelle A, Mahtani MM, et al. The diastrophic dysplasia gene encodes a novel sulfate transporter: positional cloning by fine-structure linkage disequilibrium mapping. *Cell.* 1994;78:1073–1087.

81. Qureshi F, Jaques SM, Evans MI, et al. Skeletal histopathology in fetus with chondroectodermal dysplasia (Ellis-van Creveld syndrome). *Am J Med Genet.* 1993;45:471–476.

82. Mahony MJ, Hobbins JC. Prenatal diagnosis of chondroectodermal dysplasia (Ellis-van Creveld syndrome) with fetoscopy and ultrasound. *N Engl J Med.* 1977;297:258–260.

83. Fryns JP, Moerman P. Short limbed dwarfism, genital hypoplasia, sparse hair, and vertebral anomalies: a variant of Ellis-van Creveld syndrome? *J Med Genet.* 1993;30:322–324.

84. Schnizel A, Savoldelli G, Briner J, et al. Prenatal sonographic diagnosis of Jeune syndrome. *Radiology.* 1985;154:777–778.

85. Skiptunas SM, Weiner S. Early prenatal diagnosis of asphyxiating thoracic dysplasia (Jeune's syndrome) value of fetal thoracic measurement. *J Ultrasound Med.* 1987;6:41–43.

86. Hidgins L, Rosengren S, Treem W, et al. Early cirrhosis in survivors with Jeune thoracic dystrophy. *J Pediatr.* 1992;120:754–756.

87. Kirk JS, Constock CH. Antenatal sonographic appearance of spondyloepiphyseal dysplasia congenita. *J Ultrasound Med.* 1990; 9:173–175.

88. Shohat M, Rimoin DL, Gruber HE, et al. Perinatal lethal hypophosphatasia: clinical, radiologic, and morphologic findings. *Pediatr Radiol.* 1991;21:421–427.

89. Rattenbury JM, Blau K, Sandler M, et al. Prenatal diagnosis of hypophosphatasia. *Lancet.* 1976;i:306.

90. Warren RC, Rodeck CH, Brock DJ, et al. First trimester diagnosis of hypophosphatasia with a monoclonal antibody to the liver/bone/kidney isoenzyme of alkaline phosphatase. *Lancet.* 1985;ii:856–858.

91. Koussef BG, Mulivor RA. Prenatal diagnosis of hypophosphatasia. *Obstet Gynecol.* 1981;57:9s–12s.

92. Rudd NL, Miskin M, Hoar DI, et al. Prenatal diagnosis of hypophosphatasia. *N Engl J Med.* 1976;295:146–148.

93. Henthorn PS, Raducha M, Fedde KN, et al. Different missense mutations at the tissue-nonspecific alkaline phosphatase gene locus in autosomal recessively inherited forms of mild and severe hypophosphatasia. *Proc Natl Acad Sci USA.* 1992;89:9924–9928.

94. Chodirker BN, Evans JA, Seargeant LE, et al. Hyperphosphatemia in infantile hypophosphatasia for carrier diagnosis and screening. *Am J Hum Genet.* 1990;46:280–285.

95. Greenberg CR, Evans JA, McKendry-Smith S, et al. Infantile hypophosphatasia: localization within chromosome region 1p36.1-34 and prenatal diagnosis using linked DNA markers. *Am J Hum Genet.* 1990;46:286–292.

96. Bankier A, Fortune D, Duke J, et al. Fibrochondrogenesis in male twins at 24 weeks gestation. *Am J Med Genet.* 1991;38:95–98.

97. Romero R, Ghidini A, Eswara MS, et al. Prenatal findings in a case of spondylocostal dysplasis type I (Jarcho-Levin syndrome). *Obstet Gynecol.* 1988;71:988–991.

98. Mundlos S, Mulliken JB, Abramson DL, et al. Genetic mapping of cleidocranial dysplasia and evidence of a microdeletion in one family. *Hum Molec Genet.* 1995;4:71–75.

99. Hammer LH, Fabbri EL, Browne PC. Prenatal diagnosis of cleidocranial dysostosis. *Obstet Gynecol.* 1994;83:856–857.

100. Ramesar RS, Greenberg J, Martin R, et al. Mapping of a gene for cleidocranial dysplasia in the historical Cape Town (Arnold) kindred and evidence for locus homogeneity. *J Med Genet.* 1996;33:511–514.

101. Evans MI, Zador IE, Qureshi F, et al. Ultrasonographic prenatal diagnosis and fetal pathology of Langer mesomelic dwarfism. *Am J Med Genet.* 1988;31:915–920.

102. Holmes-Siedle M, Seres-Santamaria A, Crocker M, et al. A sibship with Roberts/SC phocomelia syndrome. *Am J Med Genet.* 1990;37:18–22.

103. Van Den Berg D, Francke U. Roberts syndrome: a review of 100 cases and a new rating system for severity. *Am J Med Genet.* 1993;47:1104–1123.

104. Muller LM, De Jong G, Van Heerden KM. The antenatal ultrasonographic detection of the Holt-Oram syndrome. *S Afr Med J.* 1985;68:313–315.

105. Luthy DA, Mack L, Hirsch J, et al. Prenatal ultrasound diagnosis of thrombocytopenia with absent radii. *Am J Obstet Gynecol.* 1981;141:350–351.

106. Hall JG. Thrombocytopenia and absent radius (TAR) syndrome. *J Med Genet.* 1987;24:79–83.

107. Wladimiroff JW, Niermeijer MF, Laar J, et al. Prenatal diagnosis of skeletal dysplasia by real-time ultrasound. *Obstet Gynecol.* 1984;63:360–364.

108. Francomano CA, Ortez deLuna RI, Ide SE, et al. The gene for the Ellis-van Creveld syndrome maps to chromosome 4p16 (Abstract). *Am J Hum Genet.* 1995;57(supp.):A191.

109. Basson CT, Bachinsky DR, Lin RC, et al. Mutations in human cause limb and cardiac malformation in Holt-Oram syndrome. *Nature Genet.* 1997;15:30–35.

110. Mundlos S, Otto F, Mundlos C, et al. Mutations involving the transcription factor CBFA1 cause cleidocranial dysplasia. *Cell.* 1997;89:773–779.

BIOCHEMICAL SCREENING

Mark I. Evans / James N. Macri / Robert S. Galen / Arie Drugan

INTRODUCTION

For decades in obstetrics and gynecology there have been 2 areas of nearly universally accepted screening procedures. The first was for cervical cancer via the Papanicolau smear. The second was for fetuses with neural tube defects, and later chromosome abnormalities such as Down syndrome by alpha-fetoprotein, and later other biochemical and sometimes biophysical markers.

Identifying individuals with disease usually involves tests or procedures performed on persons who for whatever reason were felt to be at increased risks, which is a small portion of the population. Investigations come in many forms. They may be clinical examination, laboratory testing, and minor invasive procedures, such as obtaining blood, or even major surgical investigations. Particularly for genetic disorders, there are often population subgroups known to be at particularly high risk, whether it be advanced maternal age and Down syndrome, Ashkenazi Jewish heritage and Tay-Sachs disease, African heritage and sickle cell disease, or numerous others.[1] However, for some of these disorders, while the risk for any given individual in the high-risk category is certainly higher than for those in the low-risk category, if the high-risk category is small enough, the majority of affected individuals may actually come from a low-risk group.[1] Particularly with the advent of molecular technologies and the application of knowledge from the Human Genome Project, we will now have the ability to look for literally thousands of potential disorders in any individual who may be totally asymptomatic.[2]

PRINCIPLES OF SCREENING TESTS

We will first review some of the key issues underlying the fundamental principles of screening. The foundation of screening for any disease process requires a fundamental understanding of the differences between diagnostic and screening tests. Diagnostic tests are designed to give a definitive answer to the question: Does the patient have this particular problem? Diagnostic tests are generally complex and require sophisticated analysis and interpretation. The tests tend to be expensive, and they are usually only performed on patients felt to be "at risk." Conversely, screening tests are generally performed on healthy patients and are often offered to the entire relevant population. They therefore should be cheap, easy to use, and interpretable by everyone; their function is only to help define who, among the low-risk group is in fact at high risk (Table 23-1).

Screening test results are, by definition, not pathonomonic for the disease,[1] but rather delineate who needs further testing. Fortunately the concept of screening tests is certainly not new to obstetrics and gynecology, having been pioneered decades ago with the development of the Pap smear for cervical cancer screening.

With regard to genetic diseases, for example, asking a patient "how old are you?" is nothing more than a cheap screening test. Using maternal age 35 as a cutoff, 25–30% of chromosomal abnormalities, such as Down syndrome, can be detected because that is the percentage that occurs to women over age 35 and who, in the United States, have been routinely offered invasive testing based on that criterion.

There are 4 key measures used in the evaluation of screening tests: sensitivity, specificity, positive predictive value, and negative predictive value (Fig. 23-1). Sensitivity and specificity fundamentally address the question from an epidemiologic viewpoint. For example of all the people with the disease, what percentage was identified by the test? This is the definition of sensitivity. Conversely, of all the people who do not have the disease, what percentage of the patients test negative? This is specificity. Physicians are generally more interested in different questions, however, because only after a positive test does the patient usually become interested. Of all patients who have a positive test, what percentage of them actually have the disease? This is the positive predictive value. The negative predictive value is just the opposite—of all the people who have a negative test, what percentage of them are actually negative?

A key point to remember is that, in general, sensitivity and specificity do not vary as a function of prevalence; unless there is an influence of other factors on the equation. However, positive and negative predictive values do. In low risk populations, even great screening tests will have low positive predictive values. This has particular relevance, for example, to the mid 1980s when HIV testing first became a subject of public debate. One of the suggestions of the Reagan White House was to have mandatory testing of (heterosexual) couples about to marry. In a population in which the prevalence is very low, the proportion of positives that will be false positive will be much higher than in a population in which the prevalence is very high. In the latter case, the vast majority of positives will, in fact, be true positives. In both high and low prevalence areas, the sensitivity and specificity of the tests should be the same, however, the positive and negative predictive values will be widely different. A test is absolutely useless if predictive value after the test is the same as the population risk before the test. Some tests have even been worse than that, ie, the chance of them determining the correct outcome was less than a coin flip.

For example, consider a very high-risk population of HIV testing, such as that of a sexually transmitted disease clinic in a large city with a large homosexual population. In a hypothetical example of 1,000 patients, illustrated here, there are 180 positives, 20 false positives, 20 false negatives, and 780 true negatives (Fig. 23-2). Thus, here the sensitivity is 180/180 + 20, or 200, going vertically, using the formula A/A + C. These numbers give a sensitivity of 90%. The positive predictive value is likewise 180/200, but this time going horizontally, A/A + B, and again gives a positive predictive value of 90%. Historically, a screening test is considered

TABLE 23-1	SCREENING TESTS VS. DIAGNOSTIC TESTS

Diagnostic Tests
 Performed only on "at risk" population
 Commonly expensive
 Commonly have risk
 Give definitive answer
Screening Tests
 Offered to general population of patients
 Healthy patients
 Cheap
 Easy
 Reliable
 Quick
 Define "at risk" population
 Do not give definitive answer

excellent if the sum of these 2 numbers equals at least 150. So, at 180, this would be considered a superb screening test.

If one moves the scenario to a very rural, conservative area, where prevalence of HIV is 20 per 1,000 rather than 200 per 1,000, then the implication can be quite different. In this example, (Fig. 23-3) the sensitivity will now be 18/18 + 2, or 20—again, vertically A/A + C. The proportion stays the same because the fact that patients are false negative is a function of the disease, not of the laboratory test. However, the 20 false positives, which are a function of the laboratory test and not the disease will still be there. The positive predictive value is now 18/18 + 20, or 38, or 47% going horizontally—A/A + B. Thus, from a clinical perspective in the examples just defined, the true likelihood that a patient who has a positive test will, in fact, have HIV can double depending on whether the patient is a rural or inner-city high risk. This is why national standards and national statistics for certain tests can be very problematic.

The past few years have seen continued advancement in attempts to refine the sensitivity and specificity of chromosomal screening, and to reduce the overall costs of the screening

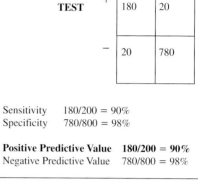

Sensitivity   180/200 = 90%
Specificity   780/800 = 98%

Positive Predictive Value   180/200 = 90%
Negative Predictive Value   780/800 = 98%

FIGURE 23-2 Table for sensitivity and predictive values in high-risk population.

programs in particular.[3,4] The goal is to reduce the need for expensive costs of invasive testing that follow a positive screening, and also, although not commonly mentioned, to reduce the cost of the care of abnormal newborns who might, as a result of screening, be detected and terminated at the wishes of the parents.[1,3–6] Work surrounding such screening and reducing the incidence of birth defects falls into 4 categories:

1. the use of preconceptual and early pregnancy folic acid to reduce the incidence of neural tube defects,
2. the use of biochemical and ultrasound markers in the second trimester to increase the detection of Down syndrome,
3. expansion of biochemical markers into the first trimester to allow for screening at earlier gestational ages, and
4. the development of biophysical-ultrasonic characteristics of fetal structure in both the first and second trimesters.

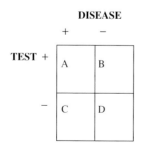

Sensitivity   A/A+C
Specificity   D/B+D

Positive Predictive Value   A/A+B
Negative Predictive Value   D/C+D

FIGURE 23-1 Table of disease and tests.

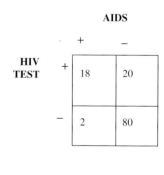

Sensitivity   18/20 = 90%
Specificity   780/800 = 98%

Positive Predictive Value   18/38 = 47%
Negative Predictive Value   780/782 = ~100%

FIGURE 23-3 Table for sensitivity and predictive values in low-risk population.

NEURAL TUBE DEFECTS

Nearly 3 decades ago, Brock and Sutcliffe[7] first described the use of alpha-fetoprotein in amniotic fluid, and later in maternal serum,[8] for the prenatal detection of neural tube defects. Since the mid-1970s, routine prenatal screening became accepted in the United Kingdom, and since the mid-1980s in the United States. Evaluation of the impact of such screening has clearly shown that the birth rate of children with neural tube defects (NTDs) has declined from 1.3 per 1,000 births in 1970, to 0.6 per 1,000 births in 1989.[9] The decline was even more dramatic in some sections of the United States such as the southeast, which had higher than average rates. Since the introduction of folic acid fortification of breads and grains in the United States in 1998, the decline of NTDs as evidenced by birth registry data has been approximately 20%[10] and by high maternal serum alpha fetoprotein levels, the decline is over 30%.[11] The successful application of folic acid has been a dramatic public health success story and is deserving of its own chapter.[12-22]

Several changes in the epidemiologic characteristics of NTDs have also been observed. (1) The proportion of spina bifida cases has increased. (2) The proportion of neural tube defects combined with other unrelated defects has increased. (3) The incidence of NTDs in the white population has decreased relative to the incidence in other races. (4) The incidence of isolated NTDs in females has decreased.[9,10]

All of the above findings are consistent with increased utilization of maternal serum alpha-fetoprotein screening, particularly in the white population. A similar study in South Australia by Chan et al.[23] from 1966 to 1991, found that the overall prevalence of neural tube defects (including prenatally diagnosed cases) had not varied between the 2 years. However, there was an 84% reduction in NTD births from 2.29 per 1,000 in 1966 to 0.35 per 1,000 in 1991. The fall was 96% for anencephaly and 82% for spina bifida. Approximately 85% of defects, both open and closed, were detected before 28 weeks gestation by either alpha-fetoprotein or ultrasound.

It has long been appreciated that there are racial, geographic, and ethnic variations in the incidence of neural tube defects, and that there are patients at increased risk based on other medical conditions. For example, diabetics are known to have an increased risk of neural tube defects, as are women taking antiepileptic drugs.[24] Conversely, a 1992 study concluded that patients undergoing ovulation induction do not have higher than the general population background rates of neural tube defects.[25]

SCREENING FOR CHROMOSOME ABNORMALITIES

In 1984, Merkatz et al. studied the association of low maternal serum alpha-fetoprotein with an increased risk of chromosome abnormalities, particularly Down syndrome.[26] In subsequent years there was a gradual acceptance of the association, as well as an eventual understanding that Down syndrome is not the only aneuploid condition association with low maternal serum

alpha-fetoprotein. For example, Trisomy 18 usually has even lower alpha-fetoprotein values.[27]

The adoption of widespread screening with maternal serum alpha-fetoprotein effectively doubled the potential detection of chromosome abnormalities in the population. Before the massive explosion of infertility therapies, only about 20% of Down syndrome babies were born to women over age 35. More recent data suggest that the proportion of births to women over 35 has gone from about 5% to nearly 15%, and the proportion of Down syndrome cases in women over 35 years old is now more than 30%.[28] The addition of a well-coordinated maternal serum alpha-fetoprotein screening program as developed in the late 1980s could detect approximately 30% of the 75% of cases that are born to women under age 35. The detailed mechanics of biochemical screening—with adjustments for gestational age, race, diabetic status, multiple gestation status, maternal weight, and adjustments via a different database or correction factors for maternal race—have been published previously and will not be repeated here.[29]

In 1988, Wald et al. suggested that a combination of parameters including alpha-fetoprotein (AFP), beta human chorionic gonadotrophin (β-hCG), and unconjugated estriol (uE3) could significantly increase the detection frequency of Down syndrome to approximately 60% of the total incidence[30] (Fig. 23-4). Multiple studies have corroborated the increased efficacy of multiple marker screening as opposed to AFP alone in detecting chromosome abnormalities, particularly Down syndrome.[31-36] The improvements in detection by screening can be tabulated using Figures 23-1–23-3. In fact, both of the HIV examples of population incidences for screening tests are far higher than that actually observed. The 2×2 model in Figures 23-1–23-3 can be used in AFP screening for Down syndrome, which is known to occur in approximately 1/800 births

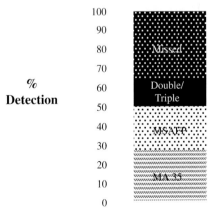

Screening for Chromosomal Abnormalities

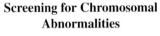

FIGURE 23-4 Maternal age 35 identifies about 20% of Down syndrome pregnancies. Low AFP brings the total to about 50%. Double or triple screening raises that number to about 60% of the total which is about half of the 80% of cases occurring to women under 35.

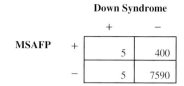

		Down Syndrome	
		+	−
MSAFP	+	5	400
	−	5	7590

Sensitivity   5/10 = 50%
Specificity   7590/7990 = 95%

Positive Predictive Value   5/405 = 1.2%
Negative Predictive Value   7590/7595 = ~100%

FIGURE 23-5 Table application for low MS AFPs.

(Fig. 23-5). For example, for every 8,000 cases screened, 10 are positive for Down syndrome. Screening Down syndrome with AFP alone will detect approximately 50% of all the cases. Historically for all patients who underwent an amniocentesis because of a low MSAFP, an abnormality was detected in approximately 1 in every 90 procedures.[3,4] So, thus applying the same 2 × 2 grid for low MSAFP, one would see 5 cases detected and 5 cases missed (false negatives). There would be approximately 400 false positives to find the 5 cases of Down syndrome and 7,590 true negatives. This results in a sensitivity of 50%, and a positive predictive value of approximately 1.2%. With the shift to double, triple, or even quadruple screening, in which case approximately 60–70%% of all cases were detected, there was an abnormal result in approximately 1 of every 50 procedures performed. The table thus now shifts to 6 cases detected, 4 cases missed, for a sensitivity of 60%, and 6 positive Down syndrome cases found out of 300 amnios, for a positive predictive value of only approximately 2% (Fig. 23-6).

Despite overwhelming data and recommendations of national organizations such as the American College of Obstetricians and Gynecologists that multiple numbers be offered, in 2000 only 20% of patients in the United States were screened for AFP alone.[37]

hCG is widely accepted as the most important parameter in NTD screening, with AFP and uE3 being the second most important. However, since AFP was already used in America

and much of Western Europe for the detection of NTDs, many question whether adding uE3 as a third parameter is cost beneficial, considering its reduced detection levels compared with AFP and hCG.[38]

The debate over the use of uE3—double screening versus triple screening—has increased over the years. Those in favor of double screening believe that the studies as a whole suggest that there is no real cost effectiveness of adding the third marker. Furthermore, since 1991 when Crossley et al. first proposed the β-HCG to AFP ratio be used as a marker, the question of how the data are interpreted has been added into the overall equation of sensitivity and specificity.[39–42] Other studies suggest that the wide variability is the result of higher coefficients of variability among uE3 assays than for the other parameters.[43] This variation may, in part, explain the incongruity among studies.

Cuckle raised the question of whether screening should be offered to all patients, or for example only to those age 27 or greater, and showed that if screening were offered only to women over age 27, more than 50% of the population would be excluded, and there would be an approximate 9% lower detection of affected pregnancies.[44] While not reaching the conclusion that this was cost beneficial, he stated that such rationing of services can be considered when resources are scarce.

Many important questions about the utilization of health care resources, patient autonomy, and maximization of cost effectiveness have been raised. Gardosi and Mongelli have suggested that the problem of inaccurate dating as a cause of abnormal biochemical screening can be addressed by limiting the use of ultrasounds those patients at the greatest likelihood of having their dates changed.[36] Gardosi and Mongelli use data from 20,000 computer-simulated cases, up to maternal age 40, to conclude that of 14% of high-risk women, only 30% would be identified as high risk following the ultrasound, making them candidates for amniocentesis.

Palomaki et al. investigated the influence of cigarette smoking and levels of maternal serum AFP, β-HCG, and uE3.[45] They concluded that AFP was reduced by 3%, uE3 by 3%, and β-HCG by 23%. However the statistical impact on screening was small, and given the uncertainty over the effects of cigarette smoking on Down syndrome, such adjustments are unjustified. More recently Spenser et al. concluded that corrections would only have minor impact and thus, are unnecessary.[46]

Evans, et al. investigated many of the "dogmas" of biochemical screening and found that many of these are no longer valid. We believe that the wide variance in results reported from around the world is largely due to differences in laboratory methodologies.[40,41,43] For example, the controversy over double versus triple screening can be attributed to the lack of standardization in assays among labs particularly affects the wide coefficient of variance estriol.[43] Most discrepancies in the literature disappear with standardization, and the diabetic correction factor becomes unnecessary with proper accounting for the fact that diabetic patients are of higher maternal weight,[40] and maternal weight correction continues to be important.[41,42]

		Down Syndrome	
		+	−
Double/ Triple	+	6	300
	−	4	7690

Sensitivity   6/10 = 60%
Specificity   7690/7990 = 96%

Positive Predictive Value   6/306 = 2%
Negative Predictive Value   7690/7694 = ~100%

FIGURE 23-6 Table application for double and triple screening.

A number of papers in the past several years have looked at the various constituents in the marker regimen, focusing the use of free β-HCG as opposed to the intact β-HCG. Wald et al. reported in 1993 that the use of free β-HCG as compared to total β-HCG would increase the detection frequency by about 4% for a given false-positive rate used in conjunction with maternal age, AFP, and uE3.[47] Other studies have suggested that, particularly at earlier gestational ages (e.g., 14 and 15 weeks) that free β has better sensitivity and specificity than the intact molecule.

Numerous papers have also attempted to refine methodologies of sample collection[48,49] and more precisely explore the impact of various factors such as more precise dating or the efficacy of Down syndrome detection rates.[50] Similarly, with an ever-increasing proportion of pregnancies resulting from infertility therapies, many question whether modifications of risk or screening strategies are required.[51,52]

Several other markers have been investigated, come, and gone over the past few years. Cole et al. have found increased effectiveness in using "nicked" β (a structurally abnormal form), but the molecule is relatively labile.[53] For the research assay to be usable as a clinical screening test, stability has to be increased. The urea-resistant fraction of neutrophil alkaline phosphatase has also shown promising results.[54] Its manual assay first proposed by Cuckle was too cumbersome for practical use, but automated methods have been developed to make it practical.[55]

Studies on hyperglycosylated hCG have been conflicting, with huge variation in reported sensitivities and specificities.[56–61] Hyperglycosylated hCG tests have the potential advantage of being urine based, which could ease collection issues in technologically deprived areas.

A number of papers have suggested dimeric inhibin A as an excellent marker that may raise the sensitivity by 3–7% for a given screen positive rate.[62–66] Out of this data has come calls for "quadruple" screening, and various combinations of biochemical and biophysical (ultrasound) data. There are also paradigms that include different parameters at different times. While preliminary data suggest a high sensitivity with improved specificity, hiding[64,67,68] results from patients for up to a month which is "required" for integrated screening is ethically problematic in our opinion. No doubt multiple screening approaches will emerge, creating even less standardization. The use of first trimester combined screening is a very large topic that is reported in chapter 22b.

Another promising marker is the search for fetal cells in maternal circulation. Studies over the past 15 years suggest that isolation and analysis of fetal cells or free fetal DNA may, in fact, become practical and useful as a screening test.[69–71] The current state of screening is the result of 2 decades of process evolution, since Hertzenberg et al. first demonstrated detection and enrichment by fluorescent activated cell sorting.[72] Much of the past 2 decades has focused on ways to improve the efficacy of detection methods focusing on the need to increase enrichment of fetal cells from the maternal blood circulation, with an estimated prevalence of 1 in 10,000,000 cells.[73–75]

Three types of fetal cells have been sought extensively in the past several years—trophoblast, lymphocytes, and nucleated fetal red cells. Trophoblasts are the most obvious candidates because they are purely fetal, however, the huge variability in their passage through the maternal circulation creates frustration and leads to disappointing results.[69] Lymphoblasts have the advantage of being much more stable, in fact, they are commonly too stable. There is documentation of lymphocytes persisting in the maternal circulation literally decades after a woman's last pregnancy and from pregnancy to pregnancy in cases of a recent miscarriage followed by another pregnancy.

The cell type most likely to be successful nucleated red blood cells. Bianchi et al. (1990) were the first to use slow sorting to isolate nucleated fetal erythrocytes using an antibody to the transfer interceptor.[73] In the late 1990s, studies focused on 2 general approaches that using fluorescent activated cell sorting (FACS) and those using magnetic activated cell sorting (MACS).[69,75] Trisomic concepti subsequently confirmed by invasive testing were found by both methods.[76–78] Analysis of progress through the millennium suggests that the MACS approach is better able than FACS to isolate fetal cells, and that the overall sensitivity of fetal cells was not an improvement over current screens, but that the specificity of fetal cells might be much better. If this is the case, then a 2-step approach might emerge in which a higher percentage of patients—perhaps 10% using double or triple testing—would be positive to raise the sensitivity to around 80%. Then these 10% would undergo fetal cell testing to reduce that risk group to 2–3% (Fig. 23-7). Fetal cells are described in Chapter 46.

Another area of potential applicability of fetal cells in maternal blood is for the isolation of molecular diagnosis of Mendelian disorders. Lo et al. were able to determine fetal Rh status in women known to be sensitized and married to heterozygous men.[79] By 2005, fetal cell/DNA analysis was already being offered commercially for Rh determination and sex selection.

The next several years will ultimately determine how successful fetal cell sorting is as a screening test. It was originally hoped that it could be a diagnostic test and replace the need for invasive testing; however, as of this writing, fetal karyotypes cannot be obtained from cells that are isolated, and therefore only fluorescent in situ hybridization (FISH) related results are possible. While such is as good as a screening test for aneuploidy, approximately one third of

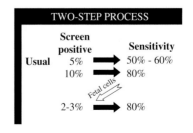

FIGURE 23-7 Two-step approach to fetal cell analysis.

abnormal karyotypes seen in prenatal diagnosis programs are, in fact, not detected by the standard probes for chromosomes 13, 18, 21, X, and Y.[80] Until and unless complete karyotypes can be obtained, fetal cells will not replace invasive testing, but may potentially be an important addition to the armamentarium of screening technologies. Fortunately, look at from the other direction, with a normal ultrasound and normal FISH, the residual risk of aneuploidy is considerably lower than 170.

INTEGRATED TESTING

Another two-step approach is the "integrated" test,[67,68,69] which is a combination of first trimester blood and ultrasound. The first trimester results are not communicated to the patient, who then waits for second trimester blood results before a risk assessment is completed. Two studies, the SURUSS trial and the FASTER trial suggest a reduced false-positive rate for comparable sensitivity; however, the trade off is the need for patients to wait as much as 6 weeks for results.[67,68] For patients who do not particularly care about the results, the delay may be fine, but our experience suggests that many anxious patients would find such delay intolerable.[81-84]

As reproductive techniques have dramatically increased the proportions of multiple pregnancies (Chapter 51), questions about the efficacy of screening tests have emerged. We and others have debated the data of biochemical screening of twins and multiple births.[56,85-90] We continue to be concerned about the accuracy of screening tests in multiple births and believe that biophysical data are more likely to be accurate.[56,85-90]

FIRST TRIMESTER

The future of screening for Down syndrome (and other anomalies) lies in the first trimester. Substantial evidence shows that free βHCG is reliably elevated and PAPP-A is diminished in Down syndrome pregnancies.[82-84] Data from multiple labs have been consistent in suggesting 70% to even 90% detection rates. In combination with ultrasound nuchal translucency measurements (described in Chapter 24). Almost all publications in which the ultrasound component was performed in a technically sound fashion have shown at least a 70% sensitivity.

Several large-scale studies—particularly the King College group in London and the NICHD-funded BUN and FASTER trials—confirmed that first trimester data will be at least equal to routine second trimester double or triple screening.[68,90]

Why then hasn't first trimester screening already replaced the second trimester testing? The answers are complex, but can be divided into several categories. First, many patients do not come for prenatal care until the second trimester. It is well known that there are universal correlation between socioeconomic status and gestational age at first visit for prenatal care. No matter how good a first trimester test is, it does no good for a patient first seen at 24 weeks.

Second, even as late as 2001 with numerous articles and college opinions touting multiple markers since the early to mid 90's, 20% of patients were still getting the 1980s model of AFP alone.[37] Significant professional education will be needed to initiate widespread use of first trimester screening.

Third, until immediate invasive testing is readily available and accepted, first trimester screening results are ineffective if the patient then had to wait a month to have an amniocentesis for a definitive answer. We see this as very problematic for the "integrated" test that combines first and second trimester lab results and ultrasound. CVS has long since proven to be safe and effective in experienced hands. As the so-called limb reduction defect scare has been shown to be false at appropriate gestational ages (see Chapter 34) hopefully the availability and acceptability of CVS will swing the pendulum back toward the desire for first trimester screening. We actually expect the concept of maternal age as a stand-alone variable to be phased out over the next several years.

TRISOMY 18

Although screening has generally focused on Trisomy 21, data suggest a varied pattern of anomalies detected by screening.[92] A different pattern of analyte levels has been observed in Trisomy 18. The values of AFP, hCG, and uE3 appear to be very low.[93] This suggests a different pathophysiology than for Down syndrome. In Down syndrome, the low AFP and uE3, and high hCG can be explained as reflecting inappropriate immaturity or dysmaturity of the fetus—all values are consistent with a younger gestational age. In Trisomy 18 however, this explanation is invalid.[94] We have previously shown that there are different patterns of genomically directed intrauterine growth retardation in different aneuploidies.[92] How this translates into serum markers is unclear. Nevertheless some reports have shown that an algorithm can be used to identify the majority of Trisomy 18 cases while adding about 0.75% to the population being offered amniocentesis.[94]

ALGORITHMIC QUESTIONS

The equations used to generate the Gaussian curves have been a source of debate for several years. Analysis of the equations suggest that they are needlessly complex, and that considerable simplification would produce equivalent results.[3,4] Our group has analyzed the mathematical bases upon which these equations were generated, and has several concerns, relating in part to the normalcy of the distribution curves, and assumptions made thereof. Logrhythmic transformations of the data do not completely satisfy these concerns. We have tried several approaches in large studies to reanalyze the act of mathematical alterations on screening efficacy, and in publications have shown that the use of discriminant function analysis and/or logistic regression analysis can potentially improve the sensitivity and specificity. Furthermore, analysis of actual outcomes in large series of data, both that of patient populations predominantly in the New York metropolitan area and in Romford, England have shown that new equations can be generated that fit the data curves far better than those published and used in most algorithmic equations.[3,4]

The impact of altered equations is such that the likelihood ratios magnify the errors in the curves, creating substantial variance between computed risk rates and what experience suggests the real risks are. We believe that quoting patients' risk of considerably under 1 in 2,000 is fraught with inaccuracies, and that the high end of the risk spectrum that average risks quoted to patients are probably half that of reality.[1,3] Studies show that abnormalities were detected in approximately 1 in every 85 taps patients who had amniocentesis because of a low AFP, for double and triple screening the number was about 1 in 45.

In a published series of 25,000 patients, we found that for triple screening, the threshold risk was approximately 1 in 180, the mean risk was approximately 1 in 10, the median risk was approximately 1 in 75, and the observed risk was 147.[3] No wonder everybody was confused. We are gradually evolving, hopefully into a re-engineered mathematics of biochemical screening that can give more accurate results, and ultimately reduce the costs of such screening.

There are also mathematical issues surrounding the shift to first trimester screening. First, if a large proportion of abnormalities are detected in the first trimester and the pregnancy is terminated, then the number of abnormalities still remaining in the population by the time of second trimester screening are diminished. As illustrated in the HIV example at the beginning of the chapter, the positive predictive value of an abnormal screening could be significantly reduced. New cut-off points would have to be generated.

Also, the apparent sensitivity of first trimester screening is probably too high because of "hidden mortality issues." If "missed" cases spontaneously abort, they will not be recognized as being missed.[95] Data suggest that 7–20% of Down syndrome cases may fall into this category. Thus an 80% first trimester dictation is probably mathematically comparable to a 60–70% second trimester rate.[67,95] However, the clinical benefits of first trimester diagnosis are still very significant (see Chapter 34).

PUBLIC POLICY AND ETHICAL ISSUES

The efficacy of multiple marker biochemical screening in detecting chromosome abnormalities such as Down syndrome has ignited policy and ethical debates on both sides of the Atlantic. Several studies have shown that in women over age 35, nearly 90% of Down syndrome fetuses can be detected while reducing the number of invasive procedures by perhaps approximately half.[67,91] From purely public health and mathematical perspectives, denying access to women over age 35 whose biochemical screens do not meet a risk level sufficiently high enough to warrant expenditure of resources might seem appropriate.[44] However, such screening would require a re-orientation of philosophy and a removal of patient autonomy

over such issues. When autonomy and public dollars come into conflict, it is reasonable to expect disagreements over the appropriate utilization of these resources.

Over the years, many arguments have emerged over the high cost of choice for both younger and older women, and that Down syndrome is not sufficiently enough of a problem to warrant screening in the first place.[96] In a pluralistic society, clearly there are a variety of opinions. Likewise, Marteau et al. have called for increased study of the psychological sequelae of screening, believing that this important characteristic has been far too little studied.[97] Stratham and Green have concluded that the way in which serum screening is being implemented does not always meet the needs of women with positive results.[98] They recommend that appropriate support measures be available for all patients. Connor has argued for biochemical screening to be available for all pregnant women who want it, and that the cost is justified considering the majority of women who have abnormal fetuses will choose to terminate, providing subsequent savings in health care expenditures.[99] Waldron and Williams have emphasized the often overlooked point that informed consent for screening is still necessary.[100]

Czeizel et al. have summarized the data on what proportion of congenital abnormalities could be detected and prevented.[101] They believe that approximately 51 of 73 congenital abnormality types (70%) could be evaluated. The birth prevalence of all congenital anomalies could, therefore, be reduced from about 65 to 26 per 1,000. Thus, 39 per 1,000 or 60% are preventable. The authors caution, however, that while many congenital abnormalities can be prevented, they do not represent a single pathological category, and there is no single appropriate strategy for their prevention.

MacNaughton and MacNaughton Dunn have argued that while termination of pregnancy following the diagnosis of a congenital abnormality should be available, that patients should be counseled against termination of pregnancy in minor anomalies.[102] The ethical issues surrounding this theory are discussed in Chapter 63.

TIME TO ABANDON "ADVANCED MATERNAL AGE"

The association of advanced maternal age (AMA) with increasing risks of chromosomal abnormalities particularly Down syndrome has existed for decades. In the 1960s, with varying degrees of counseling to prospective parents such an association was about the extent of medical knowledge provided, and there were certainly no preventative strategies other than abstinence from pregnancy. The demographics were also such that most women over 40 becoming pregnant were having their last of multiple children after many years of marriage.

The 1970s saw the beginnings of use of technology for prenatal diagnosis. Ultrasound documentation of fetal anomalies was first reported in 1972 by Campbell, and amniocentesis was beginning to be offered to patients in the highest risk situations for aneuploidy—initially those with a previous abnormality or at least 40 years of age.[29] There were few physicians capable of performing the procedure and even fewer laboratories able to analyze the samples. By the middle of the decade, amniocentesis was clearly being utilized by a growing proportion of the high-risk population, and pressure from both patients and physicians was forcing the AMA standard down from 40 to 38 and eventually 35.

The choice of age 35 was an arbitrary compromise determined in part by lack of data. Cohorts of Down syndrome risk were usually reported in 5-year groupings, and there was clearly a big jump from the 30–34 to 35–39 age group. It was only later when data were reported on a year age specific curve that the slope of the curve was shown to be changing before age 35. Furthermore, the difference from one year to the next was obviously not nearly as dramatic as it appeared only when using 5-year cohorts.[29]

Another dramatic development of the 1970s was changing laws in the United States concerning a woman's right to end a pregnancy. New York and California were among the first states to repeal laws that made abortion virtually impossible to obtain legally. In 1973 the US Supreme Court in 2 related cases, *Roe v. Wade*, and *Doe v. Bolton*, ruled that in the first trimester a state had very little rights to interfere with a woman's defined right of privacy in terminating a pregnancy.[103,104] In the second trimester the state's interests were primarily only in ensuring the safety of the procedure. It was only the third trimester that the state could exert a compelling interest in protecting the "rights" of the fetus over the mother's wishes.

The combination of new technology and the ability to terminate abnormal pregnancies led to a surge of interest in prenatal diagnosis. As with most new technologies, utilization was initially highest among patients of upper socioeconomic status who had the knowledge of the availability of the technology as well as the means to travel to far off centers to obtain such services.[105]

In the 1980s came the widespread physician recognition that the majority of babies born with Down syndrome and some other aneuploid conditions such as Trisomy 18 were actually born to more women under age 35.[1,2] Obstetrical screening for fetal abnormalities pioneered in the 1970s with elevated maternal serum alpha fetoprotein (MSAFP) for neural tube defects was being extended to Down syndrome with low MSAFPs.[26,29] As the quality of ultrasound examinations was being enhanced, patients' behaviors were also changing. Visualization of the fetal form on ultrasound was shown to accelerate the bonding process of both mothers and fathers to the fetus.[106] In some cases the contemplation of termination of an otherwise wanted pregnancy following the diagnosis of a serious fetal anomaly was made that much more difficult after seeing the image of the fetus. Thus, there were pressures to try to move prenatal diagnosis into the first trimester. Likewise, with the election of President Ronald Reagan in 1980, there was an acceleration of political efforts to curtail the availability of abortions—particularly those late in pregnancy—a disproportionate share of which were for genetic reasons.

First trimester testing with CVS was begun in the early 1980s, and following several years of National Institutes of Health and other's sponsored testing, became an increasing popular form of prenatal diagnosis. At many large centers, CVS surpassed amniocentesis as the primary mode of genetic testing.[107]

In the 1990s, the limb reduction defect scare surrounding CVS (now completely disproved for CVS as generally used in the US) severely halted the move to the first trimester. Furthermore, the election of Bill Clinton slightly reduced the concerns about abortion becoming illegal again, which also slowed the "need" to move everything as early in pregnancy as possible.

Expanding data on the advantages of multiple markers screening using AFP, hCG, with or without estriol showed multiple markers to be far superior to AFP alone. Multiple studies were showing detection rates for Down syndrome approaching 60–70%, and there were initial calls to replace AMA criteria with required prior second trimester screening before being allowed (ie, the government or insurance company paying) to have amniocentesis.[29,30,32] Such a system became commonplace in European communities, and mediCal in California began to offer the "option" of screening to patients ≥35. However, if a patient had a "negative" screen, she could no longer still have an amniocentesis.

Data from the United Kingdom suggested an improved overall sensitivity for Down syndrome detection, yet approximately 10–15% of Down cases in women ≥35 were missed. There were further concerns raised about the legal exposure for patients who refused invasive testing and then had a false-negative screen. A massive shift in culture would be necessary to learn to accept the increased risk of cases in women ≥35 that would be potentially missed as the "price" for an overall increase in sensitivity. There was no widespread movement to attempt to create such a culture shift in the United States.

Other objections to mandatory screening in the 1990s included the fact that the option of first trimester diagnosis by CVS would not be available. Anecdotally, the debates often were between epidemiology and public health trained nonphysicians who emphasized sensitivity and specificity as the primary driver of their conclusions. The debate was with front-line obstetricians and geneticists who were more concerned about the ability of the patient to choose her desired method of screening or diagnosis. The general position was that until screening was available in the first trimester, that AMA should be the controlling variable to offer first trimester diagnosis. In the second trimester, it became reasonable to offer but not require serum and/or ultrasound screening to modify risks and patient's choices. There will continue to be wide differences among patients as to whether they are more concerned about detection rate, avoiding procedures, or early answers.[108–110]

Clearly, first trimester screening followed by first trimester diagnosis by CVS can bring about a substantially higher sensitivity and specificity within the same time frame as AMA offered CVS. The question thus reduces to how and when to update the accepted "culture" in the United States to be consistent with the current scientific knowledge base.

Cultures and behaviors evolve with technology, but there has been no simple or predictable time table for adoption of new ways of thinking. The reality is that asking a patient "how old are you" is merely a cheap and ineffective screening test. Until there is a general perception of age as merely a screening test and not a fixed generator of rights to a test because of risks inherent in age, it will be difficult to gain widespread acceptance from the general population for a shift. As Danny DiVito's character in the movie *Ruthless People* pointed out, when cars began to replace horse driven carriages, the number of companies making "buggy whips" gradually declined. At the end, there was only 1 company left, and it made the best buggy whips possible at the time. Yet, the technology changed, and there was no longer a use for buggy whips. Age, as a standalone variable, will likewise meet this fate.

As our culture has become very accustomed to the coming and goings of new technologies, fax machine, cell phones, and endless generations of computers, the concept of a change in technology should be more acceptable. Yet, age has been the foundation of risk perception for over 40 years. The sophisticated concept of a greater overall detection having the price of some cases missed will have to be internalized in American medical culture.

To achieve the switch, a number of steps are necessary. First, there has to be a scientific consensus. Data from all over the world are showing that the combination of first trimester ultrasound and biochemistry are better determinants than age. Other methodologies that use first and second trimester tests are not in competition with this concept but merely provide another method for achieving higher sensitivity and specificity than the current system. Patients will have to make complex decisions about risks to have an answer in the first trimester, versus the second trimester, versus waiting until birth.

There has to be the understanding that age is not being discarded, but will merely become 1 of a number of variables that can be assessed to give the most accurate assessment of risk possible. With education, the ultrasound portion of the equation will become more standardized to laboratory levels of quality assurance. Nonprofit organizations such as the Fetal Medicine Foundation in London, and the Fetal Medicine Foundation of America as well as others will help coordinate the transition and training needed to make such a reality.

Similarly, extensive literature explaining the change in the legal standards in the United States is necessary. Undoubtedly, a flurry of lawsuits will emerge for cases in women ≥35 that are missed because of negative screens with "experts" contending that the standards have not changed, and that it is never permissible to remove a "right" once given. While such suits can not be stopped, they can be won.

It is also not realistic to expect a shift of "standards" and practice to change on a single day. Thus, there will have to be a short phase during which both approaches are acceptable. However, it is also reasonable to expect that the insurance companies who will have to pay for such to vociferously and clearly articulate to their subscribers and physicians, that they are not about to vastly increase the numbers of patients having tests. Thus, the right will be likely the "right" to pay out of one's own pocket for testing for AMA in particular.

It is time for advance maternal age, as a standalone criterion, for having invasive testing to go the way of the buggy whip. The principal objection to screening as entry to testing has been removed. It can all now be done in the first trimester. The science has evolved. It is now time for the culture and the standards to follow.

SUMMARY

In sum, the past years have seen considerable progress in the area of biochemical screening. Increasing data has now clearly shown the advantages of multiple markers, particularly β-hCG over AFP alone. There continues to be considerable controversy over the best mathematical algorithm and which markers are best (eg, for β-HCG, uE3, etc). There appears to be a plateau of detection frequencies at about 65–70% with current second trimester methodologies. Much further work needs to be done however, including some new approaches, if there is to be substantial improvement of screening sensitivity. The combination of biochemical with biophysical parameters as discussed in another chapter represents the next level of sophistication in the attempt to identify the highest proportion of abnormalities with the fewest false positives.

References

1. Evans MI, Krivchenia EL, Yaron Y. Screening in Evans MI and Bui: genomic revolution and obstetrics and gynecology. *Baillieres Clin Obstet Gynaecol*. 2002;16:645–658.
2. Evans MI, Wapner RJ, Bui TH. Future directions in genomic revolution and obstetrics and gynecology. *Baillieres Clin Obstet Gynaecol*. 2002;16:757–759.
3. Evans MI, Chik L, O'Brien JE, et al. MOMs and DADS: improved specificity and cost effectiveness of biochemical screening for aneuploidy with DADS. *Am J Obstet Gynecol*. 1995;172:1138–1147.
4. Evans MI, Chik L, O'Brien JE, et al. Logistic regression generated probability estimates for Trisomy 21 outcomes from serum AFP and BHCG: simplification with increased specificity. *J Mat Fetal Med*. 1996;5:1–6.
5. Evans MI, Sobecki MA, Krivchenia EL, et al. Parental decisions to terminate/continue following abnormal cytogenetic prenatal diagnosis: "what" is still more important than "when." *Am J Med Genet*. 1996;61:353–355.
6. Pryde PG, Odgers AE, Isada NB, et al. Determinants of parental decision to abort or continue for non-aneuploid ultrasound detected abnormalities. *Obstet Gynecol*. 1992;80:52–56.
7. Brock DJ, Stucliffe RG. Alpha-fetoprotein in the antenatal diagnosis of anencephaly and spina bifida. *Lancet*. 1972;2:197.
8. Brock DJ, Bolton AE, Monaghan JM. Prenatal diagnosis of anencephaly through maternal serum alpha-fetoprotein measurements. *Lancet*. 1973;2:923–924.
9. Yen IH, Khoury MJ, Erickson JD, et al. The changing epidemiology of neural tube defects: United States, 1968–1989. *Am J Contact Dermat*. 1992;146:857–861.

10. Honein MA, Paulozzi LJ, Matthews TJ, et al:. Impact of folic acid fortification of the US food supply on the occurrence of neural tube defects. *JAMA*. 2001;285:2981–2986.

11. Evans MI, Llurba E, Landsberger EJ, et al. Impact of folic acid supplementation in the United States: markedly diminished high maternal serum AFPs. *Obstet Gynecol*. 2004;103:474–479.

12. Shane B, Stokstad EL. Vitamin B12 folate interrelationships. *Ann Rev Nutr*. 1985;5:115.

13. Shoiania AM. Folic acid and vitamin B12 deficiency in pregnancy and the neonatal period. *Clin Perinatol*. 1984;11:433.

14. Smithells RW, Sheppard S, Schorah CJ. Vitamin deficiencies and neural-tube defects. *Arch Dis Child*. 1976;51:944.

15. Smithells RW, Sheppard S, Schorah CJ, et al. Possible prevention of neural-tube defects by periconceptional vitamin supplementation. *Lancet*. 1980;1:339.

16. Smithells RW, Seller MJ, Harris R, et al. Further experience of vitamin supplementation for prevention of neural-tube defect recurrences. *Lancet*. 1983;1:1027.

17. Smithells RW, Sheppard S, Wild L, et al. Prevention of neural-tube defect recurrences in Yorkshire: final report. *Lancet*. 1989;2:498.

18. Steegers-Theunissen RP, Coers GH, Trijbels JM, et al. Neural-tube defects and derangement of homocysteine metabolism. *N Engl J Med*. 1991;324:199.

19. Yates JR, Ferguson-Smith MA, Shenkin A, et al. Is disordered folate metabolism the basis for the genetic predisposition to neural-tube defects? *Clin Genet*. 1987;31:279.

20. Wald J, Schorah CJ, Sheldon TA, et al. Investigation of factors influencing folate status in women who have had a neural tube defect—affected infant. *Br J Obstet Gynaecol*. 1993;100:546–549.

21. Holmes-Siedle M, Dennis J, Lindenbaum RH, et al. Long term effects of periconceptional multivitamin supplements for prevention of neural tube defects: a seven to 10 year follow up. *Arch Dis Child*. 1992;67:1436–1441.

22. From the Centers for Disease Control and Prevention, Leads from the Morbidity and Mortality Weekly Report, Atlanta, GA. Recommendations for use of folic acid to reduce number of spina bifida cases and other neural-tube defects. *JAMA*. 1993;69:1233–1238.

23. Chan A, Robertson E, Haan EA, et al. Prevalence of neural-tube defects in South Australia, 1966–91: effectiveness and impact of prenatal diagnosis. *Br Med J*. 1993;307:703–705.

24. Steegers-Theunissen RP, Smithells RW, Eskes TK. Update of new risk factors and prevention of neural-tube defects. *Obstet Gynecol Surv*. 1993;48:287–293.

25. Van Loon K, Besseghir K, Eshkol A. Neural tube defects after infertility treatment: a review. *Fertil Steril*. 1992;58:875–884.

26. Merkatz IR, Nitowsky FM, Macri JN, et al. An association between low maternal serum alpha-fetoprotein and fetal chromosome abnormalities. *Am J Obstet Gynecol*. 1984;148:886–894.

27. Nyberg DA, Kramer D, Resta RG, et al. Prenatal monographic findings of trisomy 18: review of 47 cases. *J Ultrasound Med*. 1993;2:103–113.

28. Martin JA, Hamilton BE, Ventura SJ, et al. Births: final data for 2001. *National Vital Statistics Report 51*. No 2. Hyattsville, MD: National Center for Health Statistics; 2002.

29. Evans MI, Dvorin E, O'Brien JE, et al. Alpha-fetoprotein and biochemical screening. In: Evans MI, ed. *Reproductive Risks and Prenatal Diagnosis*. Norwalk, CT: Appleton & Lange;1992:223–235.

30. Wald NJ, Cuckle HS, Densem JW, et al. Maternal serum screening for Down syndrome in early pregnancy. *Br Med J*. 1988;297:883–887.

31. Cheng EY, Luthy DA, Zebelman AM, et al. A prospective evaluation of a second trimester screening test for fetal Down syndrome using maternal serum alpha-fetoprotein, hCG and unconjugated estriol. *Obstet Gynecol*. 1993;81:72–77.

32. Aitken DA, McCaw G, Crossley JA, et al. First trimester biochemical screening for fetal chromosome abnormalities and neural tube defects. *Prenat Diagn*. 1993;13:681–683.

33. Rodriguez L, Sanchez R, Hernandez J, et al. Results of 12 years' combined maternal serum alpha-fetoprotein screening and ultrasound fetal monitoring for prenatal detection of fetal malformations in Havana City, Cuba. *Prenat Diagn*. 1997;17:301–304.

34. Wald N, Densem J, Stone R, et al. The use of free hCG in antenatal screening for Down syndrome. *Br J Obstet Gynaecol*. 1993;100:550–557.

35. Goodburn SF, Yates JR, Raggatt PR, et al. Second trimester maternal serum screening using alpha-fetoprotein, human chorionic gonadotrophin, and unconjugated estriol: experience of a regional program. *Prenat Diagn*. 1994;14:391–402.

36. Gardosi J, Mongelli M. Risk assessment adjusted for gestational age in maternal serum screening for Down syndrome. *Br Med J*. 1993;306:1509–1511.

37. Evans MI. Unpublished data.

38. Yaron Y, Hamby DD, O'Brien JE, et al. The combination of elevated maternal serum alpha-fetoprotein and low estriol is highly predictive of anencephaly. *Am J Med Genet*. 1998;75:297–299.

39. Crossley JA, Aitken DA, Connor JM. Prenatal screening for chromosome abnormalities using maternal serum chorionic gonadotrophin, alphafetoprotein and age. *Prenat Diagn*. 1991;11:83–101.

40. Evans MI, Harrison HH, O'Brien JE, et al. Correction for insulin dependent diabetes in maternal serum alpha fetoprotein testing has outlived its usefulness. *Am J Obstet Gynecol*. 2002;187:1084–1086.

41. Evans MI, Harrison HH, O'Brien JE, et al. Maternal weight correction for alpha fetoprotein: mathematical truncations revisited. *Genetic Testing*. 2002;6:221–223.

42. Spencer K, Bindra R, Micolaides KH. Maternal weight correction of maternal serum PAPP-A and free beta-hCG MOM when screening for trisomy 21 in the first trimester pregnancy. *Prenat Diagn*. 2003;23:851–855.

43. Evans MI, O'Brien JE, Dvorun E, et al. Standardization of methods reduces variability: explanation for the historical discrepancies in biochemical screening. *Genetic Testing*. 2003;7:81–83.

44. Cuckle HS. Maternal serum screening policy for Down syndrome. *Lancet*. 1992;340:799.

45. Palomaki GE, Knight GJ, Haddow JE, et al. Cigarette smoking and levels of maternal serum alpha-fetoprotein, unconjugated estriol and hCG: impact on Down syndrome screening. *Obstet Gynecol*. 1993;81:675–678.

46. Spencer K, Bindra R, Cacho AM, et al. The impact of correcting for smoking status when screening for chromosomal anomalies using maternal serum biochemistry and fetal nuchal translucency thickness in the first trimester of pregnancy. *Prenat Diagn*. 2004;24:169–173.

47. Wald NJ, Hackshaw A. Antenatal screening for Down syndrome. *Br Med J*. 1993;306:1198–1199.

48. Krantz DA, Hallahan TW, Orlandi F, et al. First-trimester Down syndrome screening using dried blood biochemistry and nuchal translucency. *Obstet Gynecol*. 2000;96:207–213.

49. Spencer K. The influence of different sample collection types on the levels of markers used for Down syndrome screening as measured by the Kryptor Immunoassay system. *Ann Clin Biochem*. 2003;40(pt 2):166–168.

50. Spencer K, Crossley JA, Aitken DA, et al. Temporal changes in maternal serum biochemical markers of trisomy 21 across the first and second trimester of pregnancy. *Ann Clin Biochem*. 2002;39(pt 6):567–576.

51. Ghisoni L, Ferrazzi E, Castagna C, et al. Prenatal diagnosis after ART success: the role of early combined screening tests in counseling pregnant patients. *Placenta*. 2003; Suppl B:99–103.

52. Donnenfeld AE, Icke KV, Pargas C, et al. Biochemical screening

for aneuploidy in ovum donor pregnancies. *Am J Obstet Gynecol.* 2002;187:1222–1225.

53. Cole LA, Kardana A, Park SY, et al. The deactivation of hCG by nicking and disassociation. *J Clin Endocrinol Metab.* 1993;76:704–710.

54. Cuckle HS, Iles RK, Chard T. Urinary β-core human chorionic gonadotrophin: a new approach to Down syndrome screening. *Prenat Diagn.* 1994;14:953–958.

55. Tafas T, Evans MI, Cuckle HS, et al. An automated image analysis method for the measurement of neutrophil alkaline phosphatase in the prenatal screening of Down syndrome. *Fetal Diagn Ther.* 1996;11:254–260.

56. Weinans MJ, Butler SA, Mantingh A, et al. Urinary hyperglycosylated hCG in first trimester screening for chromosomal abnormalities. *Prenat Diagn.* 2000;20:976–978.

57. Davies S, Byrn F, Cole LA. Human chorionic gonadotrophin testing for early pregnancy viability and complications. *Clin Lab Med.* 2003;23:257–264.

58. Cole LA, Khanlian SA, Sutton JM, et al. Hyperglycosylated hCG (invasive trophoblast antigen, ITA) a key antigen for early pregnancy detection. *Clin Biochem.* 2003;36:647–655.

59. Sutton JM, Cole LA. Sialic acid-deficient invasive trophoblast antigen (sd-ITA): a new urinary variant for gestational Down syndrome screening. *Prenat Diagn.* 2004;24:194–197.

60. Spencer K, Talbot JA, Abushoufa RA. Maternal serum hyperglycosylated human chorionic gonadotrophin (HhCG) in the first trimester of pregnancies affected by Down syndrome, using a single a sialic acid-specific lectin immunoassay. *Prenat Diagn.* 2003;23:176–178; author reply 178.

61. Cuckle HS, Canick JA, Kellner LH. Collaborative study of maternal urine beta-core human chorionic gonadotrophin screening for Down syndrome. *Prenat Diagn.* 1999;19:911–917.

62. Canick JA, Saller DN Jr, Lambert-Messerlian GM. Prenatal screening for Down syndrome: current and future methods. *Clin Lab Med.* 2003;23:395–411.

63. Silver HM, Lambert-Messerlian GM, Reis FM, et al. Mechanism of increased maternal serum total activin a and inhibin a in preeclampsia. *J Soc Gynecol Investig.* 2002;9:308–312.

64. Wald NJ, Huttly WJ, Hackshaw AK. Antenatal screening for Down syndrome with the quadruple test. *Lancet.* 2003;8:835–836.

65. Benn PA, Fang M, Egan JF, et al. Incorporation of inhibin-A in second trimester screening for Down syndrome. *Obstet Gynecol.* 2003;102:413; author reply 413–414.

66. Spencer K, Liao AW, Ong CY, et al. Maternal serum levels of dimeric inhibin A in pregnancies affected by trisomy 21 in the first trimester. *Prenat Diagn.* 2001;21:441–444.

67. Malone F, et al.: Faster trial. *N Engl J Med.* (In press) 2005.

68. Wald NJ, Rodeck C, Hackshaw AK, et al. First and second trimester antenatal screening for Down syndrome: the results of the Serum, Urine and Ultrasound Screening Study (SURUSS). *J Med Screen.* 2003;10:56–104.

69. Elias S, Simpson JL. Prenatal Diagnosis. In: Rimoin DL, Connor JM, Pyeritz PE, eds. *Emery and Rimoin's Principles and Practice of Medical Genetics.* 3rd ed. New York, NY: Churchill Livingstone; 1997.

70. Elias S, Simpson JL. Prospects for prenatal diagnosis by isolating fetal cells from maternal blood. *Contemp Rev Obstet Gynecol.* 1995;7:135–139.

71. Lewis DE, Schober W, Murrell S, et al. Rare event selection of fetal nucleated erythrocytes in maternal blood by flow cytometry. *Cotymetry.* 1996;23:218–227.

72. Herzenberg LA, Bianchi DW, Schroder J. Fetal cells in the blood of pregnant women: detection and enrichment by fluorescence-activated cell sorting. *Proc Nat Acad Sci USA.* 1979;76:1453–1455.

73. Bianchi DW, Flint AF, Pizzimenti MF, et al. Isolation of fetal DNA from nucleated erythrocytes in maternal blood. *Proc Natl Acad Sci USA.* 1990;87:3279–3283.

74. Bianchi DW, Klinger KW. Prenatal diagnosis through the analysis of fetal cells in the maternal circulation. In: Milunsky A, ed. *Genetic Disorders and the Fetus.* 3rd ed. Baltimore, MD: Johns Hopkins University Press; 1992:759.

75. Ganshirt-Ahlert D, Borjesson-Stoll R, Burschyk M, et al. Detection of fetal trisomies 21 and 18 from maternal blood using triple gradient and magnetic cell sorting. *Am J Reprod Immunol.* 1994;30:194–201.

76. Elias S, Price J, Dockter M, et al. First trimester prenatal diagnosis of trisomy 21 in fetal cells from maternal blood. *Lancet.* 1992;34:1033.

77. Ganshirt D, Borjesson-Stoll R, Burschyk M, et al. Noninvasive prenatal diagnosis: isolation of fetal cells from maternal circulation. In: Zakuk H, ed. *Seventh International Conference on Early Prenatal Diagnosis.* Bologna: Monduzzi Editore;1994:19.

78. Bianchi DW, Simpson JL, Jackson LG, et al. Fetal gender and aneuploidy detection using fetal cells in maternal blood: analysis of NIFTY I data. *Prenat Diagn.* 2002;22:609–615.

79. Lo YM, Bowell PJ, Selinger M, et al. Prenatal determination of fetal RhD status by analysis of peripheral blood of rhesus negative mothers. *Lancet.* 1993;341:1147–1148.

80. Evans MI, Henry GP, Miller WA, et al. International, collaborative assessment of 146,000 prenatal karyotypes: expected limitations if only chromosome-specific probes and fluorescent in situ hybridization were used. *Hum Reprod.* 1999;14:1213–1216.

81. Souter VL, Nyberg DA, Benn PA, et al. Correlation of second trimester sonographic and biochemical markers. *J Ultrasound Med.* 2004;23:505–511.

82. Cusick W, Buchanan P, Hallahan TW, et al. Combined first trimester versus second trimester serum screening for Down syndrome: a cost analysis. *Am J Obstet Gynecol.* 2003;188:745–751.

83. Muller F, Benattar C, Audibert F, et al. First trimester screening for Down syndrome in France combining fetal nuchal translucency measurement and biochemical markers. *Prenat Diagn.* 2003;23:833–836.

84. Nicolaides KH, Bindra R, Heath V, et al. One-stop clinic for assessment of risk of chromosomal defects at 12 weeks of gestation. *J Matern Fetal Neonatal Med.* 2002;12:9–18.

85. Crossley JA, Aitken DA, Cameron AD, et al. Combined ultrasound and biochemical screening for Down syndrome in the first trimester: a Scottish multicentre study. *Br J Obstet Gynaecol.* 2002;109:667–676.

86. Drugan A, O'Brien JE, Dvorin E, et al. Multiple marker screening in multifetal gestations: prediction of adverse pregnancy outcomes. *Fetal Diagn Ther.* 1996;11:16–19.

87. O'Brien JE, Dvorin E, Yaron Y, et al. Differential increases in AFP, HCG and uE3 in twin pregnancies: impact upon attempts to quantify Down syndrome screening calculations. *Am J Med Genet.* 1997;73:109–112.

88. Wald N, Cuckle H, Wu TS, et al. Maternal serum unconjugated estriol and human chorionic gonadotrophin levels in twin pregnancies: implications for screening for Down syndrome. *Br J Obstet Gynaecol.* 1991;98:905–908.

89. Cuckle H. Down syndrome screening in twins. *J Med Screen.* 1998;5:3–4.

90. Wald NJ, Rish S, Hackshaw AK. Combining nuchal translucency and serum markers in prenatal screening for Down syndrome in twin pregnancies. *Prenat Diagn.* 2003;23:588–592.

91. Wapner R, Thom E, Simpson JL, et al. First trimester maternal serum biochemistry and fetal nuchal translucency screening (BUN) study group: First trimester screening for trisomies 21 and 18. *N Engl J Med.* 2003;349:1405–1413.

92. Johnson MP, Barr M Jr, Qureshi F, et al. Symmetrical intrauterine growth retardation is not symmetrical: the ontogeny of organ specific gravimetric deficits in midtrimester and neonatal trisomy 18. *Fetal Diagn Ther*. 1990;4:110–119.

93. Drugan A, Dvorin E, Koppitch FC, et al. Counseling for low maternal serum alpha-fetoprotein should emphasize all chromosome anomalies, not just Down syndrome! *Obstet Gynecol*. 1989;73:271–274.

94. Palomaki GE, Haddow JE, Knight GJ, et al. Risk-based prenatal screening for trisomy 18 using alpha-fetoprotein, unconjugated estriol and human chorionic gonadotrophin. *Prenat Diagn*. 1995;15:713.

95. Leporrier N, Herrou M, Morello R, et al. Fetuses with Down syndrome detected by prenatal screening are more likely to abort spontaneously than fetuses with Down syndrome not detected by prenatal screening. *Br J Obstet Gynaecol*. 2003;110:18–21.

96. Elkins TE, Brown D. The cost of choice: a price too high in the triple screen for Down syndrome. *Chin Obstet Gynecol*. 1993;36:532–540.

97. Marteau TM. Psychological consequences of screening for Down syndrome. *Br Med J*. 1993;307:146–147.

98. Statham H, Green J. Serum screening for Down syndrome: some women's experiences. *Br Med J*. 1993;307:174–176.

99. Connor M. Biochemical screening for Down syndrome: the NHS should provide it for all pregnant women who want it. *Br Med J*. 1993;306:1705.

100. Waldron G, Williams ES. Serum screening for Down syndrome: informed consent is vital. *Br Med J*. 1993;307:500–502.

101. Czeizel AE, Intody Z, Modell B. What proportion of congenital abnormalities can be prevented? *Br Med J*. 1993;306:499–502.

102. MacNaughton M, MacNaughton DP. Ethical aspects of termination of pregnancy following prenatal diagnosis. *Int J Gynecol Obstet*. 1992;39:1–2.

103. US Supreme Court. *Roe v. Wade*. 410 US, 1973;113.

104. US Supreme Court. *Doe v. Bolton*. 410 US, 1973;179.

105. Evans MI, Hanft RS. The introduction of new technologies. *ACOG clinical seminars*. 1997;2:1–3.

106. Fletcher JC, Evans MI. Maternal bonding in early fetal ultrasound examinations. *N Engl J Med*. 1983;308:392–393.

107. Evans MI, Drugan A, Koppitch FC, et al. Genetic diagnosis in the first trimester: the norm for the 1990s. *Am J Obstet Gynecol*. 1989;160:1332–1339.

108. Mulvey S, Zachariah R, McIiwaine K, et al. Do women prefer to have screening tests for Down syndrome that have the lowest screen positive rate or the highest detection rate? *Prenat Diagn*. 2003;23:828–832.

109. Spencer K. Age related detection and false positive rates were screening for Down syndrome in the first trimester using fetal nuchal translucency and maternal serum free beta hCG and PAPP-A. *Br J Obstet Gynaecol*. 2001;108:1043–1046.

110. DeVore GR, Romero R. Genetic sonography: an option for women of advanced maternal age with negative triple-marker maternal serum screening results. *J Ultrasound Med*. 2003;22:1191–1199.

CHAPTER 24

FIRST TRIMESTER ULTRASOUND SCREENING WITH NUCHAL TRANSLUCENCY

Jon Hyett / Kypros Nicolaides

INTRODUCTION

The phenotypic features of Trisomy 21 were first described by Langdon Down in 1866 and included the observation *that* "the skin appears to be too large for the body, the nose is small and the face is flat."[1] In the last decade it has become possible to observe these features by ultrasound examination at 11^{+0} to 13^{+6} weeks gestation and there is extensive evidence that effective screening for major chromosomal abnormalities can be provided at this early stage of pregnancy. Prospective studies involving over 200,000 pregnancies, including 871 fetuses with Trisomy 21, have demonstrated that increased nuchal translucency (NT) can identify 77% of fetuses with Trisomy 21 for a false positive rate (FPR) of 4.2%. More recently, several prospective studies have also demonstrated that approximately 70% of fetuses affected by Trisomy 21 have an absent nasal bone at the same gestational age.

As well as being associated with Trisomy 21 and other chromosomal abnormalities, increased NT is associated with fetal death, a wide range of fetal defects and with many genetic syndromes. Several groups have reported on the outcome of fetuses with increased NT and a normal karyotype and these data should be used to develop an approach to counsel parents and to manage ongoing pregnancies appropriately.

PATIENT-SPECIFIC RISKS FOR CHROMOSOMAL ABNORMALITY

The association between Down syndrome and increased maternal age was first described by Shuttleworth in 1909. He examined 350 affected infants and concluded that "in a considerable proportion—from one half to one third—the mothers were at the time of gestation approaching the climacteric period."[2] The risk of Trisomy 21 is now well-recognized as increasing with maternal age.[3] This can be used most simply to define a fixed maternal age cut-off at which diagnostic tests for chromosomal abnormalities will be offered to pregnant women. As a screening test, this has the advantage of being inexpensive, readily accessible, and clearly defined, but the test has poor sensitivity and a low positive predictive value. In the 1970s, approximately 5% of women were over the age of 35 years, including 30% of pregnancies affected by Trisomy 21.[4] In other words, 70% of affected pregnancies were born to younger women, traditionally considered to be at low risk. Although the sensitivity of maternal age has recently been reported to be much higher, this is primarily due to the demographic change seen in most western populations, as an increasing proportion of women conceive at a later stage of their reproductive life. In the United Kingdom, the sensitivity of a 35-year-old maternal age cut-off has increased to 53% by the start of this millennium, but this is associated with a 3-fold increase in the screen positive rate to 15%, that has significant implications in terms of pregnancy loss and financial cost.[5] One final concern over screening based on maternal age is that 50% of women would prefer to avoid invasive testing, and this benchmark provides no means for reassurance that this is a reasonable option.[6]

An alternative to screening by a fixed maternal age cut-off is to calculate an individualized level of risk for every woman. This approach allows us to take additional factors, such as the gestational age of the pregnancy and the outcome of previous pregnancies, into account. Fetuses with chromosomal abnormalities are more likely to die in utero than normal fetuses, so the risk for chromosomal abnormality decreases with advancing gestation (Table 24-1).[7–9]

Original estimates of the maternal age-related risk for Trisomy 21 at birth were based on surveys with almost complete ascertainment of the affected patients.[3] During the last decade, with the introduction of maternal serum biochemistry and ultrasound screening for chromosomal abnormalities at different stages of pregnancy, it has become necessary to establish maternal age and gestational age-specific risks for chromosomal abnormalities. These estimates were derived by comparing the birth prevalence of Trisomy 21 to the prevalence in women undergoing second-trimester amniocentesis or first-trimester chorionic villus sampling (CVS).[10] The rates of fetal death in Trisomy 21 between 12 weeks (when NT screening is carried out) and 40 weeks is about 30% and between 16 weeks (when second trimester serum biochemistry is carried out) and 40 weeks is about 20%.[11] In trisomies 18 and 13, the rate of fetal death between 12 weeks and 40 weeks is about 80% (Table 24-1).[9]

The risk for trisomies in women who have had a previous fetus or child with a trisomy is higher than that expected on the basis of their age alone. In a study of 2,054 women who had a previous pregnancy with Trisomy 21, the risk of recurrence in the subsequent pregnancy was 0.75% higher than the maternal and gestational age related risk for Trisomy 21 at the time of testing. A similar increase in risk was found for women who had a previous pregnancy affected by Trisomy 18, but while the risk increased for a pregnancy affected by Trisomy 18, the risk for Trisomy 21 did not change.[12] Thus, for a 35-year-old woman at 12 weeks gestation who has had a previous pregnancy affected by Trisomy 21, the risk increases from 1 in 249 (0.40%), based on maternal and gestational age, to 1 in 87 (1.15%) including the previous history.

Risks based on maternal age, gestational age, and pregnancy history can be combined with the findings of ultrasound or maternal serum biochemical tests to provide patient-specific risks for chromosomal abnormalities. The background (a priori) risk, based on maternal age, gestational age and pregnancy history is adjusted by the likelihood ratio, a statistical measure of the chance of a particular test result being normal or abnormal to give a new risk. Different screening tests can be applied

TABLE 24-1	ESTIMATED RISK FOR TRISOMIES 21, 18, AND 13 IN RELATION TO MATERNAL AGE AND GESTATION											
Maternal Age (yrs)	**Trisomy 21**				**Trisomy 18**				**Trisomy 13**			
	Gestation (wks)				**Gestation (wks)**				**Gestation (wks)**			
	12	**16**	**20**	**40**	**12**	**16**	**20**	**40**	**12**	**16**	**20**	**40**
20	1,068	1,200	1,295	1,527	2,484	3,590	4,897	18,013	7,826	11,042	14,656	42,423
25	946	1,062	1,147	1,352	2,200	3,179	4,336	15,951	6,930	9,778	12,978	37,567
30	626	703	759	895	1,456	2,103	2,869	10,554	4,585	6,470	8,587	24,856
31	543	610	658	776	1,263	1,825	2,490	9,160	3,980	5,615	7,453	21,573
32	461	518	559	659	1,072	1,549	2,114	7,775	3,378	4,766	6,326	18,311
33	383	430	464	547	891	1,287	1,755	6,458	2,806	3,959	5,254	15,209
34	312	350	378	446	725	1,047	1,429	5,256	2,284	3,222	4,277	12,380
35	249	280	302	356	580	837	1,142	4,202	1,826	2,576	3,419	9,876
36	196	220	238	280	456	659	899	3,307	1,437	2,027	2,691	7,788
37	152	171	185	218	354	512	698	2,569	1,116	1,575	2,090	6,050
38	117	131	142	167	272	393	537	1,974	858	1,210	1,606	4,650
39	89	100	108	128	208	300	409	1,505	654	922	1224	3544
40	68	76	82	97	157	227	310	1139	495	698	927	2683
41	51	57	62	73	118	171	233	858	373	526	698	2020
42	38	43	46	55	89	128	175	644	280	395	524	1516

Data from references 7 to 9.

sequentially provided they are independent of each other. After each likelihood ratio is applied, the new risk is used as the a priori risk for the next test. If the tests are not independent of each other then more sophisticated techniques, involving multivariate statistics, can be used to calculate the combined likelihood ratio.

MEASURING FETAL NUCHAL TRANSLUCENCY THICKNESS

The process of risk assessment described in the previous section involves the development of a likelihood ratio as a statistical representation of the test result. Accuracy of measurement is therefore essential to ensure that an accurate likelihood ratio is used in calculating a new level of risk. Although processes of quality assurance are well described in chemical pathology, they have not previously been universally applied to imaging techniques. The Fetal Medicine Foundation (FMF), which is a UK-registered charity, has established a process of training and quality assurance for the appropriate introduction of NT screening into clinical practice.[13] Training is based on a theoretical course and practical instruction on how to obtain the appropriate image and make the correct measurement of NT. A logbook of images is submitted to demonstrate that the NT is measured in the appropriate manner. Ongoing quality assurance is based on assessment of the distribution of fetal NT measurements and examination of a sample of images obtained by each sonographer involved in screening.[14–16] The distribution of measurements from each sonographer and each center are compared to those established by a major multicentre study coordinated by the FMF.[17] The services of the FMF, including Certification, the software for calculation of risk and quality assurance are provided free of charge. The variation in mea-

surements is reduced considerably after an initial earning phase and after feedback to the sonographers. Additional evidence in favor of appropriate training of sonographers and adherence to a standard technique for the measurement of NT is provided by Monni et al., who reported that, by modifying their technique of measuring NT in accordance with the guidelines established by the FMF, their detection rate of Trisomy 21 improved from 30–84%.[18]

The optimal gestational age for measurement of fetal NT is 11^{+0} weeks to 13^{+6} weeks, which corresponds to a crown–rump length of 45 mm to 84 mm. The lower gestational limit allows sufficient embryological development to detect most major anatomical defects. For example the diagnosis or exclusion of acrania and therefore anencephaly, cannot be made before 11 weeks because sonographic assessment of ossification of the fetal skull is not reliable before this gestation. At 8–10 weeks all fetuses demonstrate herniation of the midgut that is visualized as a hyperechogenic mass in the base of the umbilical cord, and it is therefore unsafe to diagnose or exclude exomphalos at this gestation.[19–22] In addition, in the early 1990s it was appreciated that chorionic villous sampling (CVS) before 10 weeks was associated with transverse limb reduction defects, so NT screening between 11^{+0} and 13^{+6} weeks gestation provides risk assessment at a gestation where invasive testing can be immediately offered.[23,24]

NT measurement becomes more difficult from 14 weeks onward because the fetus is often in a vertical position.[25,26] The incidence of abnormal accumulation of nuchal fluid in chromosomally abnormal fetuses also decreases beyond 14 weeks, and these factors have led to the selection of 13^{+6} weeks gestation as the upper limit for screening.[27–30] In

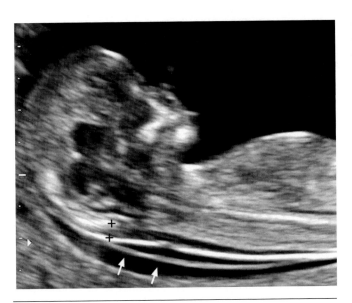

FIGURE 24-1 Ultrasound picture of a chromosomally 12-week fetus with normal nuchal translucency thickness and present nasal bone.

addition, this ceiling provides women with affected fetuses the option of an earlier and safer form of termination.

Clear images and accurate measurements of nuchal translucency are best obtained with a high-resolution ultrasound machine that has a video-loop function and calipers that provide measurements to one decimal point. Fetal NT can be measured successfully by transabdominal ultrasound examination in about 95% of cases; in the others, it is necessary to perform transvaginal sonography. The results from transabdominal and transvaginal scanning are similar.[31] A good sagittal section of the fetus, as for measurement of fetal crown–rump length, should be obtained and the NT should be measured with the fetus in the neutral position.[29] The image should be magnified so that only the fetal head and upper thorax are included and so that each slight movement of the calipers produces only a 0.1 mm change in the measurement. Care must be taken to distinguish between fetal skin and amnion because, at this gestation, both structures appear as thin membranes (Fig. 24-1).[29] This is achieved by waiting for spontaneous fetal movement away from the amniotic membrane; alternatively, the fetus is bounced off the amnion by asking the mother to cough and/or by tapping the maternal abdomen.

Precise caliper placement is another key part of the process of measurement standardization. The maximum thickness of the subcutaneous translucency between the skin and the soft tissue overlying the cervical spine should be measured.[29] The calipers should be placed on the lines that define the NT thickness—the crossbar of the caliper

should be such that it is hardly visible as it merges with the white line of the border and not in the nuchal fluid. Reducing the gain and removing harmonics prevents the edge of the nuchal space being blurred, which leads to underestimation of the nuchal measurement.[32] During the scan, more than one measurement must be taken and the maximum one should be used for risk assessment.

Other factors that can cause the nuchal measurement to be inaccurate include hyperextension of the fetal neck that can artificially increase the NT measurement by 0.6 mm or flexion that can decrease the measurement by 0.4 mm.[33] The umbilical cord may be round the fetal neck in 5–10% of cases and this finding may produce a falsely increased NT, adding about 0.8 mm to the measurement.[34,35] In such cases, the measurements of NT above and below the cord are different and, in the calculation of risk, it is more appropriate to use the average of the 2 measurements.[35] There are no clinically relevant effects on NT measurements by ethnic origin,[36,37] parity or gravidity,[38] cigarette smoking,[39,40] diabetic control,[41] conception by assisted reproduction techniques,[42–45] bleeding in early pregnancy[46] or fetal gender.[47–49] The intra-observer and inter-observer differences in measurements of fetal NT are less than 0.5 mm in 95% of cases.[50–52]

NUCHAL TRANSLUCENCY THICKNESS AND RISK FOR CHROMOSOMAL ABNORMALITIES

The largest prospective study examining the association between increased NT and chromosomal abnormalities was coordinated by the FMF. It involved 100,311 singleton pregnancies examined by 306 appropriately trained sonographers in 22 UK centers.[17] Fetal NT and crown–rump length were measured in all cases and individual patient-specific risks, based on maternal age, gestational age and fetal NT were calculated. Follow-up was obtained from 96,127 cases, including 326 with Trisomy 21 and 325 with other chromosomal abnormalities (Table 24-2). The median gestation at the time of screening

TABLE 24-2	MULTICENTER STUDY COORDINATED BY THE FETAL MEDICINE FOUNDATION. NUMBER OF PREGNANCIES WITH NUCHAL TRANSLUCENCY (NT) THICKNESS ABOVE THE 95th PERCENTILE AND AN ESTIMATED RISK FOR TRISOMY 21, BASED ON MATERNAL AGE AND FETAL NUCHAL TRANSLUCENCY AND CROWN-RUMP LENGTH, OF 1 IN 300 OR MORE		

Fetal Karyotype	*N*	*NT >95th Percentile*	*Risk ≥1 in 300*
Normal	95,476	4,209 (4.4%)	7,907 (8.3%)
Trisomy 21	326	234 (71.2%)	268 (82.2%)
Trisomy 18	119	89 (74.8%)	97 (81.5%)
Trisomy 13	46	33 (71.7%)	37 (80.4%)
Turner syndrome	54	47 (87.0%)	48 (88.9%)
Triploidy	32	19 (59.4%)	20 (62.5%)
Other[a]	64	41 (64.1%)	51 (79.7%)
Total	96,127	4,767 (5.0%)	8,428 (8.8%)

Data from reference 17.

[a]Deletions, partial trisomies, unbalanced translocations, sex chromosome aneuploidies.

TABLE 24-3	PROSPECTIVE SCREENING STUDIES FOR TRISOMY 21 BY MEASUREMENT OF FETAL NUCHAL TRANSLUCENCY (NT) THICKNESS. IN SOME OF THE STUDIES. A CUT-OFF IN NT WAS USED TO DEFINE THE SCREEN POSITIVE GROUP, AND IN OTHERS THE FETAL MEDICINE FOUNDATION SOFTWARE WAS USED TO ESTIMATE PATIENT-SPECIFIC RISKS BASED ON MATERNAL AGE, GESTATIONAL AGE, AND FETAL NT (SEE TABLE 24-4)

Author	Gestation (wks)	N	Successful Measurement	NT Cut-off	FPR	DR Trisomy 21
Pandya et al. 1995[53]	10–13^{+6}	1,763	100.0%	2.5 mm	3.4%	3/4 (75.0%)
Schwarzler et al. 1999[54]	10–13^{+6}	4,523	100.0%	2.5 mm	2.7%	8/12 (66.7%)
Schuchter et al. 2001[55]	10–12^{+6}	9,342	100.0%	2.5 mm	2.1%	11/19 (57.9%)
Wayda et al. 2001[56]	10–13^{+0}	6,841	100.0%	2.5 mm	4.1%	17/17 (100.0%)
Panburana et al. 2001[57]	10–13^{+6}	2,067	100.0%	2.5 mm	2.9%	2/2 (100.0%)
Snijders et al. 1998[17]	10–13^{+6}	96,127	100.0%	95th percentile	4.4%	234/326 (71.8%)
Theodoropoulos et al. 1998[58]	10–13^{+6}	3,550	100.0%	95th percentile	2.3%	10/11 (90.9%)
Zoppi et al. 2001[59]	10–13^{+6}	10,111	100.0%	95th percentile	5.1%	52/64 (81.3%)
Gasiorek-Wiens et al. 2001[60]	10–13^{+6}	21,959	100.0%	95th percentile	8.0%	174/210 (82.9%)
Brizot et al. 2001[61]	10–13^{+6}	2,492	100.0%	95th percentile	6.4%	7/10 (70.0%)
Comas et al. 2002[62]	10–13^{+6}	7,345	100.0%	95th percentile	4.9%	38/38 (100.0%)
Chasen et al. 2003[63]	11–13^{+6}	2,248	100.0%	95th percentile	3.4%	9/12 (75.0%)
Szabo et al. 1995[64]	9–12^{+6}	3,380	100.0%	3.0 mm	1.6%	27/30(90.0%)
Taipale et al. 1997[65]	10–13^{+6}	6,939	98.6%	3.0 mm	0.7%	4/6 (66.7%)
Pajkrt et al. 1998+1998[66,67]	10–13^{+6}	3,614	100.0%	3.0 mm	4.2%	32/46 (69.6%)
Audibert et al. 2001[68]	10–13^{+6}	4,130	95.5%	3.0 mm	1.7%	7/12 (58.3%)
Rosenberg et al. 2002[69]	12–14^{+0}	6,234	98.6%	3.0 mm	2.8%	13/21 (61.9%)
Economides et al. 1998[70]	11–14^{+6}	2,256	100.0%	99th percentile	0.4%	6/8 (75.0%)
Whitlow et al. 1999[71]	11–14^{+6}	5,947	100.0%	99th percentile	0.7%	15/23 (65.2%)
Total		200,868	99.8%		4.2%	669/871 (76.8%)

FPR—false positive rate; DR—detection rate.

was 12 weeks (range 10–14 weeks) and the median maternal age was 31 years. The estimated risk for Trisomy 21 was above 1 in 300 in 7,907 (8.3%) of the normal pregnancies, in 268 (82.2%) of those with Trisomy 21 and in 253 (77.8%) with other chromosomal abnormalities. For a screen-positive rate of 5%, the detection rate was 77% (95% confidence interval 72–82%).[17]

The results of this study are supported by other prospective studies that have examined the implementation of NT screening in clinical practice (Tables 24-3 and 24-4).[17,54–75] In some of these studies the screen positive group was defined by a cut-off in fetal NT (Table 24-3) while others used a combined risk derived from the maternal age and deviation in fetal NT from the normal median for fetal crown-rump length (Table 24-4). Collectively, these studies demonstrate that fetal NT can be successfully measured in more than 99% of cases and the combined data of more than 200,000 pregnancies, including more than 900 fetuses with Trisomy 21, demonstrates that fetal NT screening identifies more than 75% of fetuses with Trisomy 21 and other major chromosomal abnormalities for a false positive rate of 5%. Alternatively, a detection rate of about 60% can be achieved with a false positive rate of 1%.

In comparison to these studies reporting the implementation of NT screening programs (Table 24-3 and 24-4), there are other observation studies, that perform less well (Table 24-5).[76–80] Successful measurement of NT was achieved in more than 99% of cases in the interventional studies (Table 24-3), but in only 75% of cases in the observational studies (Table 24-5). Furthermore in the interventional studies there was increased NT in 76.8% of the Trisomy 21 and 4.2% of the chromosomally normal fetuses, compared to the respective rates of 38.4% and 5.0% in the observational studies. The results of these studies differ as the scans were often carried out at inappropriate gestations by sonographers who were either inadequately trained or not sufficiently motivated to measure NT. These studies demonstrate the importance of training, standardization of measurement, and ongoing quality control.

COMBINED FIRST TRIMESTER SCREENING

Trisomic pregnancies are associated with altered maternal serum concentrations of various feto-placental products. At 10^{+3}–13^{+6} weeks gestation, the maternal serum concentration of free ß-hCG is increased and PAPP-A is decreased in pregnancies affected by Trisomy 21.[82–87] These biochemical markers have no significant association between fetal NT in either Trisomy 21 or chromosomally normal pregnancies and

| TABLE 24-4 | PROSPECTIVE SCREENING STUDIES FOR TRISOMY 21 AT 10–14 WEEKS USING THE FETAL MEDICINE FOUNDATION SOFTWARE TO ESTIMATE PATIENT-SPECIFIC RISKS BASED ON MATERNAL AGE, GESTATIONAL AGE, AND FETAL NUCHAL TRANSLUCENCY THICKNESS |

| | | | Screen Positive | | |
| Author | Mean Maternal Age (yrs) | Cut-off | Normal | Chromosomal Abnormalities | |
				Trisomy 21	Other
Snijders et al. 1998[17]	31	1 in 300	7,907/95,476 (8.3%)	268/326 (82.2%)[a]	253/325 (77.8%)
Theodoropoulos et al. 1998[58]	29	1 in 300	151/3,528 (4.3%)	10/11 (90.9%)	11/11 (100.0%)
Thilaganathan et al. 1999[72]	29	1 in 300	762/9,753 (7.8%)	17/21 (81.0%)[a]	25/28 (89.3%)
Schwarzler et al. 1999[54]	29	1 in 270	212/4,500 (4.7%)	10/12 (83.3%)	8/11 (72.7%)
O'Callaghan et al. 2000[73]	32	1 in 300	59/989 (6.0%)	6/8 (75.0%)	3/3 (100.0%)
Brizot et al. 2001[61]	28	1 in 300	183/2470 (7.4%)	9/10 (90.0%)	9/12 (75.0%)
Gasiorek-Wiens et al. 2001[60]	33	1 in 300	2,800/21,475 (13.0%)	184/210 (87.6%)	239/274 (88.2%)
Sau et al. 2001[74]	28	1 in 100	61/2,600 (2.3%)	8/8 (100%)	5/7 (71.4%)
Zoppi et al. 2001[59]	33	1 in 300	887/10,001 (8.9%)	58/64 (90.6%)	39/46 (84.8%)
Prefumo, Thilaganathan 2002[75]	31	1 in 300	565/11,820 (4.8%)	22/27 (81.5%)	—
Chasen et al. 2003[63]	33	1 in 300	169/2,216 (7.5%)	10/12 (83.3%)[a]	15/20 (75.0%)
Total			13,756/164,828 (8.3%)	602/709 (84.9%)	607/737 (82.4%)

[a] In three studies the detection rate at a fixed 5% false positive rate was estimated. In the combined data on a total of 359 cases of trisomy 21 it was estimated that 278 (78.4%) would have been detected.

therefore the ultrasonographic and biochemical markers can be combined to provide more effective screening than either method individually.[84–88] In a retrospective study of 210 singleton pregnancies with Trisomy 21 and 946 chromosomally normal controls, matched for maternal age, gestation, and sample storage time, we estimated that the detection rate for Trisomy 21 by a combination of maternal age, fetal NT, maternal serum PAPP-A, and free ß-hCG would be about 90% for a screen-positive rate of 5%.[88]

Six prospective screening studies have confirmed the feasibility and effectiveness of combining fetal NT and maternal serum free ß-hCG and PAPP-A (Table 24-6).[89–94] The study of Bindra et al, also reported the detection rates for fixed false positive rates between 1% and 5% (Table 24-7), and the false positive rates for fixed detection rates between 60% and 90% (Table 24-8) of screening for Trisomy 21 by maternal age alone, maternal age and fetal NT, maternal age and serum free ß-hCG

and PAPP-A and by maternal age, fetal NT, and maternal serum biochemistry.[90] Thus, for a 5% false positive rate the detection rate of Trisomy 21 by the first trimester combined test was 90%, which is superior to the 30% achieved by maternal age and 65% by second trimester biochemistry. Alternatively, the detection rate of 65% achieved by second trimester biochemical testing at a 5% false positive rate, can be achieved by first trimester combined testing with a false positive rate of only 0.5%.[90]

In trisomies 18 and 13 maternal serum free β-hCG and PAPP-A are decreased.[95,96] In cases of sex chromosomal anomalies maternal serum free ß-hCG is normal and PAPP-A is low.[97] In diandric triploidy maternal serum free ß-hCG is greatly increased, whereas PAPP-A is mildly decreased.[98] Digynic triploidy is associated with markedly decreased maternal serum free ß-hCG and PAPP-A.[98] Screening by a combination of fetal NT and maternal serum PAPP-A and free ß-hCG

| TABLE 24-5 | RESULTS OF OBSERVATIONAL STUDIES ON THE EFFECTIVENESS OF NUCHAL TRANSLUCENCY (NT) PROVIDING DATA ON GESTATION AT SCREENING, NUMBER OF PATIENTS RECRUITED, AND NUMBER OF THOSE WITH SATISFACTORY MEASUREMENTS OF NT, FALSE POSITIVE RATE (FPR) AND DETECTION RATE OF TRISOMY 21 |

Author	Gestation (wks)	N	Successful Measurement	NT Cut-off	FPR	Detection Rate
Roberts et al. 1995[76] Bewley et al. 1995[77]	8–13[+6]	1,704	66.1%	3.0 mm	6.2%	1/3 (33.3%)
Kornman et al. 1996[78]	8–13[+6]	923	58.2%	3.0 mm	6.3%	2/4 (50.0%)
Haddow et al. 1998[79]	9–15[+6]	4,049	83.0%	95th centile	5.0%	18/58 (31.0%)
Crossley et al. 2002[80]	10–14[+6]	17,229	72.9%	95th centile	5.0%	18/37 (48.6%)
Wald et al. 2003[81]	6–16[+6]	47,053	76.6%[a]	95th centile	5.0%	29/75 (38.7%)
Total		70,958	75.1%		5.0%	68/177 (38.4%)

[a] Satisfactory images at 10–14 weeks.

| TABLE 24-6 | **PROSPECTIVE FIRST-TRIMESTER SCREENING STUDIES BY FETAL NUCHAL TRANSLUCENCY (NT) AND MATERNAL SERUM FREE ß-HCG AND PAPP-A PROVIDING DATA ON THE DETECTION RATE FOR TRISOMY 21 AT A 5% FALSE POSITIVE RATE** |

Author	*Gestation (wks)*	*N*	*Detection Rate*
Krantz et al. 2000[89]	10–13[+6]	5,809	30/33 (90.9%)
Bindra et al. 2002[90]	11–13[+6]	14,383	74/82 (90.2%)
Spencer et al. 2000;[91] 2003[92]	10–13[+6]	11,105	23/25 (92.0%)
Schuchter et al. 2002[93]	10–13[+6]	4,802	12/14 (85.7%)
Wapner et al. 2003[94]	10–13[+6]	8,514	48/61 (78.7%)
Total		44,613	187/215 (87.0%)

can identify about 90% of all these chromosomal abnormalities for a screen positive rate of 1%.

SCREENING MULTIPLE PREGNANCIES

The prenatal diagnosis of chromosomal abnormalities in multiple pregnancies is potentially complicated by a number of factors. Chorionicity can be determined reliably by ultrasonography in early pregnancy.[99,100] In counseling parents it is possible to give more specific estimates of one and/or both fetuses being affected depending on chorionicity. Thus in monochorionic twins the parents can be counseled that both fetuses would be affected and this risk is similar to that in singleton pregnancies. If the pregnancy is dichorionic, then the parents can be counseled that the risk of discordancy for a chromosomal abnormality is about twice that in singleton pregnancies whereas the risk that both fetuses would be affected can be derived by squaring the singleton risk ratio. This is in reality an oversimplification, since, unlike monochorionic pregnancies that are always monozygotic, only about 90% of dichorionic pregnancies are dizygotic.

Both CVS and amniocentesis can be performed in twin pregnancies, but in some circumstances, may be associated with higher risks of miscarriage and of uncertain diagnosis.[101–104] If twins are discordant for an anomaly, one of the options for the subsequent management may be selective feticide, with risks of spontaneous abortion or severe preterm delivery that have an inverse correlation with the gestation at fetocide.[105]

The effectiveness of NT as a means of screening for Trisomy 21 was examined in a series of 448 twin pregnancies that found that NT thickness was above the 95th percentile in 7 of 8 (87.5%) fetuses with Trisomy 21.[106] Although the false positive rate was only 5.4% in dichorionic pregnancies, it was increased to 8.4% in monochorionic pregnancies, a finding confirmed in other studies.[107,108] The increase in the false positive rate in monochorionic twins occurs because increased NT is an early manifestation of twin-to-twin transfusion syndrome.[108,109]

In dichorionic twins, NT can be used as an effective means of screening for chromosomal abnormalities. This allows earlier prenatal diagnosis and therefore safer selective feticide for parents with an affected fetus that choose this option. An important advantage of using fetal NT to assess risk for chromosomal abnormality is that when there is discordance for a chromosomal abnormality, the presence of a sonographically detectable marker helps to ensure the correct identification of the abnormal twin should the parents choose selective termination.

In monochorionic twins, which are almost always of identical chromosomal constitution, the numbers of cases with discordant NT measurements are too small to draw definite conclusions about counseling for the risk of chromosomal abnormalities. The risk of twin-twin transfusion syndrome should also be considered and if there are no other ultrasound features of aneuploidy, one option may be to delay invasive testing until a later stage, once other features of twin-twin transfusion syndrome can also be assessed.

The first trimester biochemical markers free ß-hCG and PAPP-A are also increased in pregnancies affected by Trisomy 21 and can be combined with the measurement of NT to screen for chromosomal abnormality.[110] In a study of 159 twin pregnancies, the average free ß-hCG was 2.1 and the PAPP-A 1.9 times greater than in 3,466 singleton pregnancies. Using statistical modeling techniques it was predicted that at a 5% false positive rate screening by a combination of fetal NT and maternal serum biochemistry would identify about 80% of

| TABLE 24-7 | **DETECTION RATES FOR DIFFERENT FIXED FALSE POSITIVE RATES IN SCREENING FOR TRISOMY 21 BY THE COMBINATION OF MATERNAL AGE, FETAL NUCHAL TRANSLUCENCY, AND MATERNAL SERUM FREE ß-HCG AND PAPP-A. IN THIS POPULATION OF 14,383 PREGNANCIES THERE WERE 82 CASES OF TRISOMY 21** |

| | *Fixed False Positive Rate* | | | | |
Method of Screening	*1%*	*2%*	*3%*	*4%*	*5%*
Maternal age (MA)	9 (11.0%)	14 (17.1%)	19 (23.2%)	23 (28.0%)	25 (30.5%)
β-hCG and PAPP-A	22 (26.8%)	33 (40.2%)	39 (47.6%)	42 (51.2%)	49 (59.8%)
Nuchal translucency (NT)	53 (64.6%)	60 (73.2%)	62 (75.6%)	64 (78.0%)	65 (79.3%)
NT and β-hCG and PAPP-A	63 (76.8%)	65 (79.3%)	69 (84.1%)	72 (87.8%)	74 (90.2%)

Data from reference 90.

TABLE 24-8	**FALSE POSITIVE RATES FOR DIFFERENT FIXED DETECTION RATES IN SCREENING FOR TRISOMY 21 BY THE COMBINATION OF MATERNAL AGE, FETAL NUCHAL TRANSLUCENCY, AND MATERNAL SERUM FREE ß-HCG AND PAPP-A. IN THIS POPULATION THERE WERE 14,240 NORMAL AND 82 TRISOMY 21 PREGNANCIES**						

	Fixed Sensitivity						
Method of Screening	*60%*	*65%*	*70%*	*75%*	*80%*	*85%*	*90%*
Maternal age (MA)	1,993 (14.0%)	2,724 (19.1%)	3,577 (25.1%)	3,939 (27.7%)	4,782 (33.6%)	6,603 (46.4%)	7,537 (52.9%)
β-hCG and PAPP-A	723 (5.1%)	815 (5.7%)	1,002 (7.0%)	1,433 (10.1%)	1,866 (13.1%)	2,167 (15.2%)	2,594 (18.2%)
Nuchal translucency (NT)	80 (0.6%)	140 (1.0%)	193 (1.4%)	367 (2.6%)	874 (6.1%)	1,299 (9.1%)	2,276 (16.0%)
NT and ß-hCG and PAPP-A	37 (0.3%)	68 (0.5%)	91 (0.6%)	128 (0.9%)	305 (2.1%)	432 (3.0%)	718 (5.0%)

Data from reference 90.

Trisomy 21 pregnancies.[111] In a prospective screening study in 206 twin pregnancies the false positive rate was 9.0% (19 of 206) of pregnancies and 6.9% of fetuses (28 of 412) and the detection rate of Trisomy 21 was 75% (3 of 4).[112]

ABSENT NASAL BONE AND SCREENING FOR CHROMOSOMAL ABNORMALITY

As the first trimester scan has become more established, the technique has developed to include sequential examination of fetal systems rather than being restricted to NT measurement. Several other markers for chromosomal abnormality have been noted. In his original description of the phenotypic features of infants affected by Trisomy 21, Down noted that a common characteristic was a small nose.[1] An anthropometric study in 105 patients with Down syndrome at 7 months to 36 years of age reported that the nasal root depth was abnormally short in 49.5% of cases.[113] In the combined data from 4 post mortem radiological studies in a total of 105 aborted fetuses with Trisomy 21 at 12–25 weeks of gestation there was absence of ossification of the nasal bone in 32.4% and nasal hypoplasia in 21.4% of cases.[114–117] Sonographic studies at 15–24 weeks of gestation reported that about 65% of Trisomy 21 fetuses have absent or short nasal bone.[118–122]

The fetal nasal bone can be visualized by sonography at 11^{+0}–13^{+6} weeks of gestation.[123] This examination requires that the image is magnified so that the head and the upper thorax only are included in the screen (Fig. 24-2). A mid-sagittal view of the fetal profile is obtained with the ultrasound transducer held in parallel to the longitudinal axis of the nasal bone. The angle of insonation is crucial as the nasal bone will almost invariably not be visible when the longitudinal axis of the bone is perpendicular to the ultrasound transducer. In the correct view there are 3 distinct lines. The first 2, which are proximal to the forehead, are horizontal and parallel to each other, resembling an "equal sign." The top line represents the skin and the bottom one, which is thicker and more echogenic than the overlying skin, represents the nasal bone. A third line, almost in continuity with the skin, but at a higher level, represents the tip of the nose. When the nasal bone line appears as a thin line, less echogenic than the overlying skin, it suggests that the nasal bone is not yet ossified, and it is therefore classified as absent.

A study investigating the necessary training of 15 sonographers with experience in measuring fetal NT to become competent in examining the fetal nasal bone at 11^{+0}–13^{+6} weeks has demonstrated that the number of supervised scans required is on average 80 with a range of 40–120.[124] Another study of 501 consecutively scanned fetuses by experienced sonographers reported that the fetal nasal bone can be successfully examined and measured in all cases without extending the length of time required for scanning.[125]

Several studies have demonstrated a high association between absent nasal bone at 11^{+0}–13^{+6} weeks and Trisomy 21, as well as other chromosomal abnormalities (Tables 24-9 and 24-10).[123,126–133] In the combined data from these studies on a total of 15,822 fetuses the fetal profile was successfully examined in 15,413 (97.4%) cases and the nasal bone was absent in 176 of 12,652 (1.4%) chromosomally normal fetuses and in 274 of 397 (69.0%) fetuses with Trisomy 21. An important

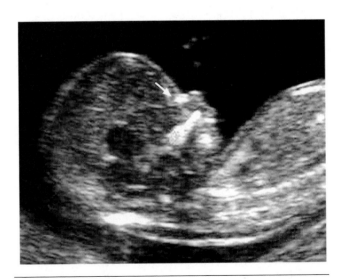

FIGURE 24-2 Ultrasound picture of a 12-week trisomy 21 fetus with increased nuchal translucency thickness and absent nasal bone.

| TABLE 24-9 | STUDIES REPORTING ON THE INCIDENCE OF ABSENT NASAL BONE IN FIRST-TRIMESTER TRISOMY 21 FETUSES | | | | | | |

Author	Type of Study	Gestation (wks)	N	Successful Examination	FPR	DR Trisomy 21
Cicero et al. 2001[123][a]	Pre-CVS	$11–13^{+6}$	701	100%	0.5%	43/59 (72.9%)
Otano et al. 2002[126]	Pre-CVS	$11–13^{+6}$	194	94.3%	0.6%	3/5 (60.0%)
Zoppi et al. 2003[127]	Screening	$11–13^{+6}$	5,532	99.8%	0.2%	19/27 (70.0%)
Orlandi et al. 2003[128]	Screening	$11–13^{+6}$	1,089	94.3%	1.0%	10/15 (66.7%)
Viora et al. 2003[129]	Screening	$11–13^{+6}$	1,906	91.9%	1.4%	8/10 (80.0%)
Senat et al. 2003[130]	Retrospective	$11–13^{+6}$	1,040	91.9%	0.4%	3/4 (75.0%)
Wong et al. 2003[131]	Pre-CVS	$11–13^{+6}$	143	83.2%	0.9%	2/3 (66.7%)
Cicero et al. 2003[132]	Pre-CVS	$11–13^{+6}$	3,829	98.9%	2.8%	162/242 (67.0%)
Cicero et al. 2004[133]	Pre-CVS	$11–13^{+6}$	5,918	98.9%	2.5%	229/333 (68.8%)
Total			15,822	97.4%	1.4%	274/397 (69.0%)

[a] Data from reference 133.

FPR—false positive rate; DR—detection rate position this first.

finding of these studies was that the incidence of absent nasal bone decreased with fetal crown-rump length, increased with NT thickness and was substantially higher in Afro-Caribbeans than in Caucasians. Consequently, in the calculation of likelihood ratios in screening for Trisomy 21 adjustments must be made for these confounding factors.[132,133]

In contrast to the above studies, Malone et al. reported that they were able to examine the fetal nose in only 75.9% of 6,316 fetuses scanned at 10–13 weeks and that the nasal bone was apparently present in all 9 of their Trisomy 21 fetuses.[134] However, the image they published to illustrate their technique reports the nasal bone at the tip rather than the base of the nose.[135] Similarly, De Biasio and Venturini, who examined retrospectively the photographs obtained for measurement of fetal NT reported that the nasal bone was present in all 5 fetuses with Trisomy 21.[136] However, all 5 images that they published were inappropriate both for the measurement of fetal NT and for examination of the nasal bone, because they were either too small or the fetus was too vertical or too oblique.

It can be concluded that at $11^{+0}–13^{+6}$ weeks the fetal profile can be successfully examined in more than 95% of cases and that the nasal bone is absent in about 70% of Trisomy 21 fetuses and 55% of Trisomy 13 fetuses. In chromosomally normal fetuses the incidence of absent nasal bone is less than 1%

| TABLE 24-10 | INCIDENCE OF ABSENT NASAL BONE AT $11–13^{+6}$ WEEKS IN CHROMOSOMALLY ABNORMAL FETUSES |

Chromosomal Abnormality	Absent Nasal Bone (%)
Trisomy 21	229/333 (68.8)
Trisomy 18	68/124 (54.8)
Trisomy 13	13/38 (34.2)
Triploidy	0/19 (0)
Turner syndrome	5/46 (10.9)
XXY, XXX, XYY	1/20 (5)
Other	8/48 (16.7)

Data from reference 133.

in Caucasian populations and about 10% in Afro-Caribbeans. Consequently, absence of the nasal bone is an important marker of Trisomy 21. However, it is imperative that sonographers undertaking risk assessment by examination of the fetal profile receive appropriate training and certification of their competence in performing such a scan.

The potential performance of combining the ultrasound markers of increased nuchal translucency and absent nasal bone with the biochemical markers ß-hCG and PAPP-A at $11^{+0}–13^{+6}$ weeks has been examined in a case-control study of 100 Trisomy 21 and 400 chromosomally normal singleton pregnancies. This estimated that the detection rate for Trisomy 21 would be 97% for a false positive rate of 5%, or 91% for a false positive rate of 0.5% (Table 24-11).[137]

INCREASED NUCHAL TRANSLUCENCY IN THE CHROMOSOMALLY NORMAL FETUS

As well as being an effective screening tool for chromosomal abnormalities, increased NT is associated with miscarriage, fetal death, and a wide range of fetal malformations and genetic syndromes. The relationship between NT thickness and poor pregnancy outcome is summarized in Table 24-1.[17,138–140]

In chromosomally normal fetuses, the prevalence of fetal death increases exponentially with NT thickness. In the combined data from 2 studies on a total of 4,540 chromosomally normal fetuses with increased NT but no obvious fetal defects, the prevalence of miscarriage or fetal death increased from 1.3% in those with NT between the 95th and 99th percentiles to about 20% for NT of 6.5 mm or more.[138,139] The majority of fetuses that die do so by 20 weeks and they usually show progression from increased NT to severe hydrops. Another study of 6,650 pregnancies undergoing NT screening, reported that in chromosomally normal fetuses the prevalence of miscarriage or fetal death was 1.3% in those with NT below the 95th percentile, 1.2% for NT between the 95th and 99th percentiles and 12.3% for NT above the 99th percentile.[140]

Several studies have reported that increased fetal NT thickness is associated with a high prevalence of major fetal

| TABLE 24-11 | INTEGRATED FIRST TRIMESTER SONOGRAPHIC AND BIOCHEMICAL SCREENING FOR TRISOMY 21. ESTIMATED DETECTION RATES FOR DIFFERENT FIXED FALSE POSITIVE RATES USING VARIOUS MARKER COMBINATIONS WITH MATERNAL AGE |

	Detection Rate (%)	
False Positive Rate (%)	*Nuchal Translucency, Free ß-hCG and PAPP-A*	*Nuchal Translucency, Nasal Bone, Free ß-hCG and PAPP-A*
0.5	70	91
1.0	75	94
2.0	80	95
3.0	84	96
4.0	86	97
5.0	89	97

Data from reference 137.

abnormalities (Table 24-2).[54,66,138–164] In the combined data of 28 studies on a total of 6,153 chromosomally normal fetuses with increased NT the prevalence of major defects was 7.3%. However, there were large differences between the studies in the prevalence of major abnormalities, ranging from 3–50%, because of differences in their definition of the minimum abnormal NT thickness, which ranged from 2 mm to 5 mm. The prevalence of major fetal abnormalities in chromosomally normal fetuses increases with NT thickness, from 1.6%, in those with NT below the 95th percentile[140] to 2.5% for NT between the 95th and 99th percentiles and exponentially thereafter to about 45% for NT of 6.5 mm or more.[138,139]

Although a wide range of fetal abnormalities have been reported in fetuses with increased NT, the prevalence of many of these may not differ from that seen in the general population. However, the prevalence of major cardiac defects, diaphragmatic hernia, exomphalos, body stalk anomaly, skeletal defects, and certain genetic syndromes, such as congenital adrenal hyperplasia, fetal akinesia deformation sequence, Noonan syndrome, Smith-Lemli-Opitz syndrome, and spinal muscular atrophy, appears to be substantially higher than in the general population and it is therefore likely that there is a true association between these abnormalities and increased NT.

The heterogeneity of conditions associated with increased NT suggests that there may not be a single underlying mechanism for this condition. Possible mechanisms include cardiac dysfunction in association with abnormalities of the heart and great arteries, venous congestion in the head and neck, altered composition of the extracellular matrix, failure of lymphatic drainage due to abnormal or delayed development of the lymphatic system or impaired fetal movements, fetal anemia or hypoproteinemia, and congenital infection.[164–173] Investigation of these mechanisms has, in part, led to a better understanding of the clinical associations between increased NT and structural abnormalities.

In pathological studies of both chromosomally abnormal and normal fetuses there is a high association between increased NT and abnormalities of the heart and great arteries.[174–178] This has also been observed clinically, and in 3 studies with a combined total of 30 fetuses with major cardiac defects diagnosed by echocardiography at 11–14 weeks, 83% had increased NT.[179–181] Similarly, in 6 studies with a combined total of 3,911 fetuses with increased NT, there was a high prevalence of cardiac defects (41.2 of 1,000) and this increased with NT thickness from 16.8 of 1,000 in those with NT of 2.5–3.4 mm to 75.2 of 1,000 in those with NT of 3.5 mm or more (Table 24-14).[182–187]

This has led several groups to investigate the screening performance of NT thickness for the detection of cardiac defects (Table 24-15).[54,140,154,188–192] In total, 67,256 pregnancies were examined and the prevalence of major cardiac defects was 2.4 per 1,000. For a false positive rate of 4.9%, the detection rate of cardiac defects was 37.5%. A meta-analysis of screening studies reported that the detection rates were about 37% and 31% for the respective NT cut-offs of the 95th and 99th percentiles.[193] It was estimated that specialist fetal echocardiography in all chromosomally normal fetuses with NT above the 99th percentile would identify one major cardiac

| TABLE 24-12 | RELATION BETWEEN NUCHAL TRANSLUCENCY THICKNESS AND PREVALENCE OF CHROMOSOMAL DEFECTS, MISCARRIAGE OR FETAL DEATH AND MAJOR FETAL ABNORMALITIES. IN THE LAST COLUMN IS THE ESTIMATED PREVALENCE OF DELIVERY OF A HEALTHY BABY WITH NO MAJOR ABNORMALITIES |

Nuchal Translucency	*Chromosomal Defects*[17]	*Fetal Death*[138–140]	*Major Fetal Abnormalities*[138–140]	*Alive and Well*
<95th percentile	0.2%	1.3%	1.6%	97%
95th–99th percentiles	3.7%	1.3%	2.5%	93%
3.5–4.4 mm	21.1%	2.7%	10.0%	70%
4.5–5.4 mm	33.3%	3.4%	18.5%	50%
5.5–6.4 mm	50.5%	10.1%	24.2%	30%
≥6.5 mm	64.5%	19.0%	46.2%	15%

TABLE 24-13 | **STUDIES REPORTING MAJOR ABNORMALITIES IN CHROMOSOMALLY NORMAL FETUSES WITH INCREASED NUCHAL TRANSLUCENCY (NT) THICKNESS. THE CUT-OFF OF INCREASED NT AND THE PREVALENCE OF ABNORMALITIES VARIED BETWEEN THE STUDIES**

Authors	Increased Nuchal Translucency Thickness		
	Cut-off	N	Abnormalities
Johnson et al. 1993[141]	2.5 mm	32	5 (15.6%)
Trauffer et al. 1994[142]	2.5 mm	32	1 (3.1%)
Shulman et al. 1994[143]	2.5 mm	72	7 (9.7%)
Schwarzler et al. 199[54]	2.5 mm	116	5 (4.3%)
Souka et al. 1998,[138] 2001[139]	95th centile	4,697	283 (6.0%)
Maymon et al. 2000[144]	95th centile	42	4 (9.5%)
Bilardo et al. 2001[145]	95th centile	140	7 (5.0%)
Michailides & Economides 2001[140]	95th centile	235	12 (5.1%)
Fukada et al. 2002[146]	95th centile	90	10 (11.1%)
Van Zalen-Sprock et al. 1992[147]	3.0 mm	13	3 (23.1%)
Ville et al. 1992[148]	3.0 mm	61	10 (16.4%)
Hewitt et al. 1993[149]	3.0 mm	10	1 (10.0%)
Salvesen and Goble 1995[150]	3.0 mm	5	2 (40.0%)
Hewitt et al. 1996[151]	3.0 mm	44	3 (6.8%)
Hernadi and Torocsik 1997[152]	3.0 mm	17	2 (11.8%)
Reynders et al. 1997[153]	3.0 mm	35	3 (8.6%)
Bilardo et al. 1998[154]	3.0 mm	47	11 (23.4%)
Pajkrt et al. 1998[66]	3.0 mm	21	1 (4.8%)
Van Vugt et al. 1998[155]	3.0 mm	63	8 (12.7%)
Hiippala et al. 2001[156]	3.0 mm	64	10 (15.6%)
Mangione et al. 2001[157]	3.0 mm	165	11 (6.7%)
Cheng et al. 2004[158]	3.0 mm	15	2 (13.3%)
Nadell et al. 1993[159]	4.0 mm	16	5 (31.3%)
Moselhi et al. 1996[160]	4.0 mm	8	3 (37.5%)
Adenkule et al. 1999[161]	4.0 mm	30	10 (33.3%)
Senat et al. 2002[162]	4.0 mm	79	30 (38.0%)
Fukada et al. 1998[163]	5.0 mm	4	2 (50.0%)
Total		6,153	451 (7.3%)

TABLE 24-14 | **PREVALENCE OF MAJOR CARDIAC DEFECTS IN FETUSES WITH INCREASED NUCHAL TRANSLUCENCY THICKNESS AT 11–13^{+6} WEEKS**

Author	N	Nuchal Translucency	Cardiac Defects
Hyett et al. 1997[182]	1,389	2.5–3.4 mm	6/1102 (5.4/1,000)
		≥3.5 mm	9/287 (31.4/1,000)
Zosmer et al. 1999[183]	1,319	2.5–3.4 mm	18/722 (24.9/1,000)
Ghi et al. 2001[184]		≥3.5 mm	42/597 (70.4/1,000)
Lopes et al. 2003[185]	275	2.5–3.4 mm	2/185 (10.8/1,000)
		≥3.5 mm	11/90 (122.2/1,000)
Galindo et al. 2003[186]	353	2.5–3.9 mm	7/131 (53.4/1,000)
		≥4.0 mm	25/222 (112.6/1,000)
McAuliffe et al. 2004[187]	177	2.5–3.4 mm	5/122 (41.0/1,000)
		≥3.5 mm	8/55 (145.5/1,000)
Total	3,911	2.5–3.4 mm	38/2262 (16.8/1,000)
		≥3.5 mm	95/1251 (75.9/1,000)

| TABLE 24-15 | SCREENING FOR MAJOR CARDIAC DEFECTS BY MEASUREMENT OF FETAL NUCHAL TRANSLUCENCY THICKNESS AT 10—13^{+6} WEEKS |

Author	N	Cardiac Defects N (/1,000)	NT Cut-off	FPR	DR
Josefsson et al. 1998[188]	1,460	13 (8.9)[a]	2.5 mm	129/1,447 (8.9%)	5 (38.5%)
Bilardo et al. 1998[154]	1,590	4 (2.5)	3.0 mm	45/1,586 (2.8%)	2 (50.0%)
Hyett et al. 1999[189]	2,9154	50 (1.7)	95th percentile	1,794/29,104 (6.2%)	28 (56.0%)
Schwarzler et al. 1999[54]	4,474	9 (2.0)	2.5 mm	115/4,465 (2.6%)	1 (11.1%)
Michailidis, Economides 2001[140]	6,606	11(1.7)	2.5 mm	231/6,595 (3.5%)	4 (36.4%)
Mavrides et al. 2001[190]	7,339	26 (3.5)	2.5 mm	254/7,313 (3.5%)	4 (15.4%)
Ovros et al. 2002[191]	3,655	20 (5.5)	3.0 mm	92/3,635 (2.5%)	9 (45.0%)
Hafner et al. 2003[192]	1,2978	27 (2.1)	95th percentile	642/12,951 (5.0%)	7 (25.9%)
Total	6,7256	160 (2.4)		3,302/67,096 (4.9%)	60 (37.5%)

[a]In this study the type of cardiac defects is not defined.

| TABLE 24-16 | FETAL ABNORMALITIES IN FETUSES WITH INCREASED NUCHAL TRANSLUCENCY THICKNESS |

Abnormality	References	Abnormality	References
Central nervous system defect		**Skeletal defect**	
Acrania/anencephaly	161	Achondrogenesis	149,220–222
Agenesis of the corpus callosum	157	Achondroplasia	152, 165
Craniosynostosis	139	Asphyxiating thoracic dystrophy	223
Dandy-Walker malformation	139,154,199	Blomstrand osteochondrodysplasia	224
Diastematomyelia	138	Campomelic dwarfism	225
Encephalocele	139	Cleidocranial dysplasia	156
Fowler syndrome	200	Hypochondroplasia	163
Holoprosencephaly	139,150,201	Hypophosphatasia	226
Hydrolethalus syndrome	202,203	Jarcho-Levin syndrome	138, 227–230
Iniencephaly	204	Kyphoscoliosis	139
Joubert syndrome	138,153	Limb reduction defect	139,142,231
Macrocephaly	161	Nance-Sweeney syndrome	232
Microcephaly	138	Osteogenesis imperfecta	233,234
Spina bifida	139,161	Roberts syndrome	235
Trigonocephaly C	138	Robinow syndrome	236
Ventriculomegaly	139,201	Short-rib polydactyly syndrome	237
		Sirenomelia	139,238
Facial defect		Talipes equinovarus	139,161
Agnathia/micrognathia	139,154	Thanatophoric dwarfism	139,157
Facial cleft	139,148,159,162,205	VACTER association	138
Microphthalmia	138		
Treacher-Collins syndrome	139	**Fetal anemia**	
		Blackfan Diamond anaemia	239
Nuchal defect		Congenital erythropoietic porphyria	240
Cystic hygroma	139,143	Dyserythropoietic anaemia	239
Neck lipoma	139	Fanconi anemia	241
		Parvovirus B19 infection	242–245
Cardiac defect		Thalassaemia-α	246
Di George syndrome	54,138–140, 154,179–194 206,207		
		Neuromuscular defect	
		Fetal akinesia deformation sequence	139,148,159,201,247
Pulmonary defect		Myotonic dystrophy	154
Cystic adenomatoid malformation	139	Spinal muscular atrophy	139,154,156, 248–250
Diaphragmatic hernia	139,155,158, 159,194,201,208		

(continued)

TABLE 24-16 | **FETAL ABNORMALITIES IN FETUSES WITH INCREASED NUCHAL TRANSLUCENCY THICKNESS (Continued)**

Abnormality	References		References
Fryn syndrome	139,209,210	**Metabolic defect**	
		Beckwith-Wiedemann syndrome	138
Abdominal wall defect		GM1 gangliosidosis	154
Cloacal exstrophy	139	Long-chain 3-hydroxyacyl-coenzyme A Dehydrogenase deficiency	251
Exomphalos	139,157,159,161,162,195, 201,204,211–213	Mucopolysaccharidosis type VII	252–254
Gastroschisis	139	Smith-Lemli-Opitz syndrome	139,291,255–258
		Vitamin D resistant rickets	232
Gastrointestinal defect		Zellweger syndrome	154, 258–260
Crohn's disease	139		
Duodenal atresia	139,155	**Other defect**	
Esophageal atresia	154,213	Body stalk anomaly	139,158,197,198,201
Small bowel obstruction	139	Brachmann-de Lange syndrome	142,262
		Charge association	201
Genitourinary defect		Deficiency of the immune system	139
Ambiguous genitalia	139	Congenital lymphedema	262
Congenital adrenal hyperplasia	214–216	EEC syndrome	154,263
Congenital nephrotic syndrome	217	Neonatal myoclonic encephalopathy	139
Hydronephrosis	139	Noonan syndrome	139,141,142,144,153, 154,156,161,264
Hypospadias	139		
Infantile polycystic kidneys	139	Perlman syndrome	265
Meckel-Gruber syndrome	139,155	Stickler syndrome	201
Megacystis	139,141,142,144,155,158, 196,201,218,219	Unspecified syndrome	139,148,156, 266–268
Multicystic dysplastic kidneys	139,147,148, 153,155,201,204	Severe developmental delay	139,155,158, 161,162
Renal agenesis	139,201		

defect in every 16 patients examined. Additionally, this analysis showed that the performance of screening by increased NT does vary with the type of cardiac defect.

The clinical implication of these findings is that increased nuchal translucency constitutes an indication for specialist fetal echocardiography. Certainly, the overall prevalence of major cardiac defects in such a group of fetuses (1–2%) is similar to that found in pregnancies affected by maternal diabetes mellitus or with a history of a previously affected offspring, which are well-accepted indications for fetal echocardiography. At present, there may not be sufficient facilities for specialist fetal echocardiography to accommodate the potential increase in demand if the 95th percentile of nuchal translucency thickness is used as the cut-off for referral. In contrast, a cut-off of the 99th percentile would result in only a small increase in workload and, in this population, the prevalence of major cardiac defects would be very high.

Other structural abnormalities are also associated with increased NT. Increased NT thickness is present in about 40% of fetuses with diaphragmatic hernia, including more than 80% of those that result in neonatal death due to pulmonary hypoplasia and in about 20% of the survivors.[194] Increased NT is observed in about 85% of chromosomally abnormal and

40% of chromosomally normal fetuses with exomphalos.[195] Similarly, megacystis, defined as a bladder diameter of 7 mm or more, is associated with increased NT, in particular Trisomy 13, which were observed in about 75% of those with chromosomal abnormalities and in about 30% of those with normal karyotype.[196] Body stalk anomaly has also been diagnosed in 25 of 106,727 fetuses screened at 10–14 weeks gestation. The major ultrasonographic features were a major abdominal wall defect, severe kyphoscoliosis, and short umbilical cord with a single artery.[197,198] Although the fetal NT was increased in 84% of the fetuses, the karyotype was normal in all cases.[197,198]

Increased NT has also been associated with a variety of genetic syndromes. As most genetic conditions are relatively rare, it is often difficult to know whether these are true associations, but the prevalence of increased NT in conditions such as congenital adrenal hyperplasia, fetal akinesia deformation sequence, Noonan syndrome, Smith-Lemli-Opitz syndrome, and spinal muscular atrophy suggest that there is a pathological association. The genetic syndromes associated with increased NT are summarized in Table 24-15. Seven studies have reported on the long-term follow up of chromosomally and anatomically normal fetuses with increased NT (Table 24-16).

TABLE 24-17	POSTNATAL FOLLOW-UP IN CHROMOSOMALLY NORMAL FETUSES WITH INCREASED NUCHAL TRANSLUCENCY (NT) THICKNESS				
Author	*Method of Assessment*	*Age (Months)*	*NT Cut-off*	*Developmental Delay*	
Van Vugt et al. 1998[155]	Questionnaire	7–75	3.0 mm	0/34	
Adekunle et al. 1999[161]	Questionnaire	12–38	4.0 mm	2/31(6.5)	
Maymon et al. 2000[144]	Telephone interview	12–36	95th percentile	0/36	
Sub-total				2/101 (2.0%)	
Brady et al. 1998[232]	Clinical examination	6–42	3.5 mm	1/89 (1.12)	
Hiippala et al. 2001[156]	Clinical examination	24–84	3.0 mm	1/50 (2.0)	
Senat et al. 2002[162]	Clinical examination	12–72	4.0 mm	3/54 (5.6)	
Cheng et al. 2004[158]	Clinical examination	8–30	3.0 mm	1/14 (7.14)	
Sub-total				6/207 (3.9%)	
Total				8/308 (2.6)	

In 3 studies, based on questionnaires to the parents, the prevalence of developmental delay was 2% in the combined total of 101 infants.[144,155,161] In 4 studies on a combined total of 207 infants that had increased NT in fetal life, clinical examination demonstrated developmental delay in 3.9% of cases.[156,158,162,232] It is difficult to assess the true significance of these findings because only 1 of the studies had a control group for comparison.[232] Brady et al. performed a clinical follow up study of 89 children that in fetal life had NT of 3.5 mm or more and 302 children whose fetal NT was less than 3.5 mm.[232] Delay in achievement of developmental milestones was observed in one of the children in each group.

CONCLUSIONS

Prospective studies in more than 200,000 pregnancies, including more than 900 fetuses with Trisomy 21, have demonstrated that NT screening can identify more than 75% of fetuses with Trisomy 21 and other major chromosomal abnormalities for a false positive rate of 5%. This is superior to the 30% detection rate achieved by maternal age and 65% by second trimester maternal serum biochemistry. Further studies, in more than 40,000 pregnancies, including more than 200 fetuses with Trisomy 21, have demonstrated that first trimester screening by a combination of fetal NT and maternal serum free ß-hCG and PAPP-A can identify 85–90% of fetuses with Trisomy 21 for a false positive rate of 5%. This method can also identify more than 90% of fetuses with trisomies 18 and 13, Turner syndrome and triploidy for a screen positive rate of 1%.

In addition to being associated with chromosomal abnormalities, increased NT is associated with a wide range of fetal malformations and genetic syndromes. The prevalence of fetal abnormalities and adverse pregnancy outcome increases exponentially with NT thickness. However, parents can be reassured that the chances of delivering a baby with no major abnormalities is more than 90% if the fetal NT is between the 95th and 99th percentiles, about 70% for NT of 3.5–4.4 mm, 50% for NT 4.5–5.4 mm, 30% for NT of 5.5–6.4 mm and 15% for NT of 6.5 mm or more. The vast majority of fetal abnormalities associated with increased NT can be diagnosed by a series of investigations that can be completed by 14 weeks of gestation.

References

1. Langdon DJ. Observations on an ethnic classification of idiots. *Clinical Lectures and Reports.* 1866;3:259–262.
2. Shuttleworth GE. Mongolian imbecility. *Br Med J.* 1909;2:661–665.
3. Hecht CA, Hook EB. The imprecision in rates of Down syndrome by 1-year maternal age intervals: a critical analysis of rates used in biochemical screening. *Prenat Diagn.* 1994;14:729–738.
4. ACOG Committee Opinion: Committee on Obstetric Practice. Down syndrome screening. *Int J Gynaecol Obstet.* 1994:186–190.
5. Wellesley D, Boyle T, Barber J, et al. Retrospective audit of different antenatal screening policies for Down syndrome in eight district general hospitals in one health region. *Br Med J.* 2002;325:15–20.
6. Benn PA, Egan JF, Fang M, et al. Changes in the utilization of prenatal diagnosis. *Obstet Gynecol.* 2004;103:1255–1260.
7. Snijders RJ, Sundberg K, Holzgreve W, et al. Maternal age and gestation-specific risk for trisomy 21. *Ultrasound Obstet Gynecol.* 1999;13:167–170.
8. Snijders RJ, Holzgreve W, Cuckle H, et al. Maternal age-specific risks for trisomies at 9–14 weeks' gestation. *Prenat Diagn.* 1994;14:543–552.
9. Snijders RJ, Sebire NJ, Cuckle H, et al. Maternal age and gestational age-specific risks for chromosomal defects. *Fetal Diag Ther.* 1995;10:356–367.
10. Halliday JL, Watson LF, Lumley J, et al. New estimates of Down syndrome risks at chorionic villus sampling, amniocentesis and live-birth in women of advanced maternal age from a uniquely defined population. *Prenat Diagn.* 1995;15:455–465.
11. Morris JK, Wald NJ, Watt HC. Fetal loss in Down syndrome pregnancies. *Prenat Diagn.* 1999;19:142–145.
12. Snijders RJ, Sundberg K, Holzgreve W, et al. Maternal age and gestation specific risk for trisomy 21: effect of previous affected pregnancy. *Ultrasound Obstet Gynecol.* submitted.

13. Down screening at 11–14 weeks. Fetal Medicine Foundation. Available at: www.fetalmedicine.com.

14. Herman A, Dreazen E, Maymon R, et al. Implementation of nuchal translucency image-scoring method during ongoing audit. *Ultrasound Obstet Gynecol*. 1999;14:388–392.

15. Wojdemann KR, Christiansen M, Sundberg K, et al. Quality assessment in prospective nuchal translucency screening for Down syndrome. *Ultrasound Obstet Gynecol*. 2001;18:641–644.

16. Snijders RJ, Thom EA, Zachary JM, et al. First trimester trisomy screening: nuchal translucency measurement training and quality assurance to correct and unify technique. *Ultrasound Obstet Gynecol*. 2002;19:353–359.

17. Snijders RJ, Noble P, Sebire N, et al. UK multicentre project on assessment of risk of trisomy 21 by maternal age and fetal nuchal translucency thickness at 10–14 weeks of gestation. *Lancet*. 1998;351:343–346.

18. Monni G, Zoppi MA, Ibba RM, et al. Results of measurement of nuchal translucency before and after training. *Lancet*. 1997;350:1631.

19. Green JJ, Hobbins JC. Abdominal ultrasound examination of the first trimester fetus. *Am J Obstet Gynecol*. 1988;159:165–175.

20. Timor-Tritsch IE, Warren W, Peisner DB, et al. First trimester midgut herniation: a high frequency transvaginal sonographic study. *Am J Obstet Gynecol*. 1989;161:831–833.

21. van Zalen-Sprock RM, van Vugt JMG, van Geijn HP. First trimester sonography of physiological midgut herniation and early diagnosis of omphalocele. *Prenat Diagn*. 1997;17:511–518.

22. Snijders RJ, Sebire NJ, Souka A, et al. Fetal exomphalos and chromosomal defects: relationship to maternal age and gestation. *Ultrasound Obstet Gynecol*. 1995;6:250–255.

23. Firth HV, Boyd PA, Chamberlain P, et al. Severe limb abnormalities after chorion villous sampling at 56–66 days' gestation. *Lancet*. 1991;337:762–763.

24. Firth HV, Boyd PA, Chamberlain PF, et al. Analysis of limb reduction defects in babies exposed to chorion villus sampling. *Lancet*. 1994;343:1069–1071.

25. Whitlow BJ, Economides DL. The optimal gestational age to examine fetal anatomy and measure nuchal translucency in the first trimester. *Ultrasound Obstet Gynecol*. 1998;11:258–261.

26. Mulvey S, Baker L, Edwards A, et al. Optimizing the timing for nuchal translucency measurement. *Prenat Diagn*. 2002;22:775–777.

27. Benacerraf BR, Gelman R, Frigoletto FD. Sonographic identification of second trimester fetuses with Down syndrome. *N Engl J Med*. 1987;317:1371–1376.

28. Nicolaides KH, Azar G, Snijders RJ, et al. Fetal nuchal edema: associated malformations and chromosomal defects. *Fetal Diagn Ther*. 1992;7:123–131.

29. Nicolaides KH, Azar G, Byrne D, et al. Fetal nuchal translucency: ultrasound screening for chromosomal defects in first trimester of pregnancy. *Br Med J*. 1992;304:867–889.

30. Comas C, Torrents M, Munoz A, et al. Measurement of nuchal translucency as a single strategy in trisomy 21 screening: should we use any other marker? *Obstet Gynecol*. 2002;100:648–654.

31. Braithwaite JM, Economides DL. The measurement of nuchal translucency with transabdominal and transvaginal sonography—success rates, repeatability and levels of agreement. *Br J Radiol*. 1995;68:720–723.

32. Edwards A, Mulvey S, Wallace EM. The effect of image size on nuchal translucency measurement. *Prenat Diagn*. 2003;23:284–286.

33. Whitlow BJ, Chatzipapas IK, Economides DL. The effect of fetal neck position on nuchal translucency measurement. *Br J Obstet Gynaecol*. 1998;105:872–876.

34. Schaefer M, Laurichesse-Delmas H, Ville Y. The effect of nuchal cord on nuchal translucency measurement at 10–14 weeks. *Ultrasound Obstet Gynecol*. 1998;11:271–273.

35. Miguelez J, Faiola S, Sachini C, et al. Nuchal cord at the 11–14 week scan: effect on nuchal translucency measurement. *Ultrasound Obstet Gynecol*. 2004.

36. Thilaganathan B, Khare M, Williams B, et al. Influence of ethnic origin on nuchal translucency screening for Down syndrome. *Ultrasound Obstet Gynecol*. 1998;12:112–114.

37. Chen M, Lam YH, Tang MH, et al. The effect of ethnic origin on nuchal translucency at 10–14 weeks of gestation. *Prenat Diagn*. 2002;22:576–578.

38. Spencer K, Ong CY, Liao AW, et al. The influence of parity and gravidity on first trimester markers of chromosomal abnormality. *Prenat Diagn*. 2000;20:792–794.

39. Spencer K, Ong CY, Liao AW, et al. First trimester markers of trisomy 21 and the influence of maternal cigarette smoking status. *Prenat Diagn*. 2000;20:852–853.

40. Niemimaa M, Heinonen S, Seppala M, et al. The influence of smoking on the pregnancy-associated plasma protein A, free beta human chorionic gonadotrophin and nuchal translucency. *Br J Obstet Gynaecol*. 2003;110:664–667.

41. Bartha JL, Wood J, Kyle PM, et al. The effect of metabolic control on fetal nuchal translucency in women with insulin-dependent diabetes: a preliminary study. *Ultrasound Obstet Gynecol*. 2003;21:451–454.

42. Liao AW, Heath V, Kametas N, et al. First trimester screening for trisomy 21 in singleton pregnancies achieved by assisted reproduction. *Hum Reprod*. 2001;16:1501–1504.

43. Wojdemann KR, Larsen SO, Shalmi A, et al. First trimester screening for Down syndrome and assisted reproduction: no basis for concern. *Prenat Diagn*. 2001;21:563–565.

44. Maymon R, Shulman A. Serial first and second trimester Down syndrome screening tests among IVF-versus naturally-conceived singletons. *Hum Reprod* 2002;17:1081–1085.

45. Orlandi F, Rossi C, Allegra A, et al. First trimester screening with free beta-hCG, PAPP-A and nuchal translucency in pregnancies conceived with assisted reproduction. *Prenat Diagn*. 2002;22:718–721.

46. de Biasio P, Canini S, Crovo A, et al. Early vaginal bleeding and first trimester markers for Down syndrome. *Prenat Diagn*. 2003;23:470–473.

47. Spencer K, Ong CY, Liao AW, et al. The influence of fetal sex in screening for trisomy 21 by fetal nuchal translucency, maternal serum free beta-hCG and PAPP-A at 10–14 weeks of gestation. *Prenat Diagn*. 2000;20:673–675.

48. Yaron Y, Wolman I, Kupferminc MJ, et al. Effect of fetal gender on first trimester markers and on Down syndrome screening. *Prenat Diagn*. 2001;21:1027–1030.

49. Larsen SO, Wojdemann KR, Shalmi AC, et al. Gender impact on first trimester markers in Down syndrome screening. *Prenat Diagn*. 2002;22:1207–1208.

50. Pandya PP, Altman D, Brizot ML, et al. Repeatability of measurement of fetal nuchal translucency thickness. *Ultrasound Obstet Gynecol*. 1995;5:334–337.

51. Schuchter K, Wald N, Hackshaw AK, et al. The distribution of nuchal translucency at 10–13 weeks of pregnancy. *Prenat Diagn*. 1998;18:281–286.

52. Pajkrt E, de Graaf IM, Mol BW, et al. Weekly nuchal translucency measurements in normal fetuses. *Obstet Gynecol*. 1998;91:208–211.

53. Pandya PP, Goldberg H, Walton B, et al. The implementation of first trimester scanning at 10–13 weeks' gestation and the measurement of fetal nuchal translucency thickness in two maternity units. *Ultrasound Obstet Gynecol*. 1995;5:20–25.

54. Schwarzler P, Carvalho JS, Senat MV, et al. Screening for fetal aneuploidies and fetal cardiac abnormalities by nuchal translucency thickness measurement at 10–14 weeks of gestation as part of routine antenatal care in an unselected population. *Br J Obstet Gynaecol*. 1999;106:1029–1034.

55. Schuchter K, Hafner E, Stangl G, et al. Sequential screening for trisomy 21 by nuchal translucency measurement in the first

trimester and maternal serum biochemistry in the second trimester in a low-risk population. *Ultrasound Obstet Gynecol.* 2001;18:23–25.

56. Wayda K, Kereszturi A, Orvos H, et al. Four years experience of first trimester nuchal translucency screening for fetal aneuploidies with increasing regional availability. *Acta Obstet Gynecol Scand.* 2001;80:1104–1109.

57. Panburana P, Ajjimakorn S, Tungkajiwangoon P. First trimester Down syndrome screening by nuchal translucency in a Thai population. *Int J Gynaecol Obstet.* 2001;75:311–312.

58. Theodoropoulos P, Lolis D, Papageorgiou C, et al. Evaluation of first trimester screening by fetal nuchal translucency and maternal age. *Prenat Diagn.* 1998;18:133–137.

59. Zoppi MA, Ibba RM, Floris M, et al. Fetal nuchal translucency screening in 12,495 pregnancies in Sardinia. *Ultrasound Obstet Gynecol.* 2001;18:649–651.

60. Gasiorek-Wiens A, Tercanli S, Kozlowski P, et al. Screening for trisomy 21 by fetal nuchal translucency and maternal age: a multicenter project in Germany, Austria and Switzerland. *Ultrasound Obstet Gynecol.* 2001;18:645–648.

61. Brizot ML, Carvalho MHB, Liao AW, et al. First trimester screening for chromosomal abnormalities by fetal nuchal translucency in a Brazilian population. *Ultrasound Obstet Gynecol.* 2001;18:652–655.

62. Comas C, Torrents M, Munoz A, et al. Measurement of nuchal translucency as a single strategy in trisomy 21 screening: should we use any other marker? *Obstet Gynecol.* 2002;100:648–654.

63. Chasen ST, Sharma G, Kalish RB, et al. First trimester screening for aneuploidy with fetal nuchal translucency in a United States population. *Ultrasound Obstet Gynecol.* 2003;22:149–151.

64. Szabo J, Gellen J, Szemere G. First trimester ultrasound screening for fetal aneuploidies in women over 35 and under 35 years of age. *Ultrasound Obstet Gynecol.* 1995;5:161–163.

65. Taipale P, Hiilesmaa V, Salonen R, et al. Increased nuchal translucency as a marker for fetal chromosomal defects. *N Engl J Med.* 1997;337:1654–1658.

66. Pajrkt E, van Lith JMM, Mol BWJ, et al. Screening for Down syndrome by fetal nuchal translucency measurement in a general obstetric population. *Ultrasound Obstet Gynecol.* 1998;12:163–169.

67. Pajrkt E, Mol BW, van Lith JM, et al. Screening for Down syndrome by fetal nuchal translucency measurement in a high-risk population. *Ultrasound Obstet Gynecol.* 1998;12:156–162.

68. Audibert F, Dommergues M, Benattar C, et al. Screening for Down syndrome using first trimester ultrasound and second trimester maternal serum markers in a low-risk population: a prospective longitudinal study. *Ultrasound Obstet Gynecol.* 2001;18:26–31.

69. Rozenberg P, Malagrida L, Cuckle H, et al. Down syndrome screening with nuchal translucency at 12(+0)−14(+0) weeks and maternal serum markers at 14(+1)−17(+0) weeks: a prospective study. *Hum Reprod.* 2002;17:1093–1098.

70. Economides DL, Whitlow BJ, Kadir R, et al. First trimester sonographic detection of chromosomal abnormalities in an unselected population. *Br J Obstet Gynaecol.* 1998;105:58–62.

71. Whitlow BJ, Chatzipapas IK, Lazanakis ML, et al. The value of sonography in early pregnancy for the detection of fetal abnormalities in an unselected population. *Br J Obstet Gynaecol.* 1999;106:929–936.

72. Thilaganathan B, Sairam S, Michailidis G, et al. First trimester nuchal translucency: effective routine screening for Down syndrome. *Br J Radiol.* 1999;72:946–948.

73. O'Callaghan SP, Giles WB, Raymond SP, et al. First trimester ultrasound with nuchal translucency measurement for Down syndrome risk estimation using software developed by the Fetal Medicine Foundation, United Kingdom—the first 2000 examinations in Newcastle, New South Wales, Australia. *Aust N Z J Obstet Gynaecol.* 2000;40:292–295.

74. Sau A, Langford K, Auld B, et al. Screening for trisomy 21: the significance of a positive second trimester serum screen in women screen negative after nuchal translucency scan. *J Obstet Gynaecol.* 2001;21:145–148.

75. Prefumo F, Thilaganathan B. Agreement between predicted risk and prevalence of Down syndrome in first trimester nuchal translucency screening. *Prenat Diagn.* 2002;22:917–918.

76. Roberts LJ, Bewley S, Mackinson AM, et al. First trimester fetal nuchal translucency: problems with screening the general population: part I. *Br J Obstet Gynaecol.* 1995;102:381–385.

77. Bewley S, Roberts LJ, Mackinson AM, et al. First trimester fetal nuchal translucency: problems with screening the general population: part II. *Br J Obstet Gynaecol.* 1995;102:386–388.

78. Kornman LH, Morssink LP, Beekhuis JR, et al. Nuchal translucency cannot be used as a screening test for chromosomal abnormalities in the first trimester of pregnancy in a routine ultrasound practice. *Prenat Diagn.* 1996;16:797–805.

79. Haddow JE, Palomaki GE, Knight GJ, et al. Screening of maternal serum for fetal Down syndrome in the first trimester. *N Engl J Med.* 1998;338:955–961.

80. Crossley JA, Aitken DA, Cameron AD, et al. Combined ultrasound and biochemical screening for Down syndrome in the first trimester: a Scottish multicenter study. *Br J Obstet Gynaecol.* 2002;109:667–676.

81. Wald NJ, Rodeck C, Hackshaw AK, et al. SURUSS Research Group. First and second trimester antenatal screening for Down syndrome: the results of the Serum, Urine and Ultrasound Screening Study (SURUSS). *Health Technol Assess.* 2003;7:1–77.

82. Macri JN, Kasturi RV, Krantz DA, et al. Maternal serum Down syndrome screening: free beta protein is a more effective marker than human chorionic gonadotrophin. *Am J Obstet Gynecol.* 1990;163:1248–1253.

83. Brambati B, Macintosh MC, Teisner B, et al. Low maternal serum level of pregnancy associated plasma protein (PAPP-A) in the first trimester in association with abnormal fetal karyotype. *Br J Obstet Gynaecol.* 1993;100:324–326.

84. Cuckle HS, van Lith JM. Appropriate biochemical parameters in first-trimester screening for Down syndrome. *Prenat Diagn.* 1999;19:505–512.

85. Brizot ML, Snijders RJ, Bersinger NA, et al. Maternal serum pregnancy associated placental protein A and fetal nuchal translucency thickness for the prediction of fetal trisomies in early pregnancy. *Obstet Gynecol.* 1994;84:918–922.

86. Brizot ML, Snijders RJ, Butler J, et al. Maternal serum hCG and fetal nuchal translucency thickness for the prediction of fetal trisomies in the first trimester of pregnancy. *Br J Obstet Gynaecol.* 1995;102:1227–1232.

87. Noble PL, Abraha HD, Snijders RJ, et al. Screening for fetal trisomy 21 in the first trimester of pregnancy: maternal serum free beta-hCG and fetal nuchal translucency thickness. *Ultrasound Obstet Gynecol.* 1995;6:390–395.

88. Spencer K, Souter V, Tul N, et al. A screening program for trisomy 21 at 10–14 weeks using fetal nuchal translucency, maternal serum free ß-human chorionic gonadotrophin and pregnancy-associated plasma protein-A. *Ultrasound Obstet Gynecol.* 1999;13:231–237.

89. Krantz DA, Hallahan TW, Orlandi F, et al. First-trimester Down syndrome screening using dried blood biochemistry and nuchal translucency. *Obstet Gynecol.* 2000;96:207–213.

90. Bindra R, Heath V, Liao A, et al. One-stop clinic for assessment of risk for trisomy 21 at 11–14 weeks: a prospective study of 15,030 pregnancies. *Ultrasound Obstet Gynecol.* 2002;20:219–225.

91. Spencer K, Spencer CE, Power M, et al. One stop clinic for assessment of risk for fetal anomalies; a report of the first year of prospective screening for chromosomal anomalies in the first trimester. *BJOG* 2000;107:1271–1275.

92. Spencer K, Spencer CE, Power M, et al. Screening for chromosomal abnormalities in the first trimester using ultrasound and maternal serum biochemistry in a one stop clinic: a review of three years prospective experience. *Br J Obstet Gynaecol.* 2003;110:281–286.

93. Schuchter K, Hafner E, Stangl G, et al. The first trimester "combined test" for the detection of Down syndrome pregnancies in 4939 unselected pregnancies. *Prenat Diagn.* 2002;22:211–215.

94. Wapner R, Thom E, Simpson JL, et al. First trimester maternal serum biochemistry and fetal nuchal translucency screening (BUN) study group: first trimester screening for trisomies 21 and 18. *N Engl J Med* 2003;349:1405–1413.

95. Tul N, Spencer K, Noble P, et al. Screening for trisomy 18 by fetal nuchal translucency and maternal serum free beta hCG and PAPP-A at 10–14 weeks of gestation. *Prenat Diagn.* 1999;19:1035–1042.

96. Spencer K, Ong C, Skentou H, et al. Screening for trisomy 13 by fetal nuchal translucency and maternal serum free beta hCG and PAPP-A at 10–14 weeks of gestation. *Prenat Diagn.* 2000;20:411–416.

97. Spencer K, Tul N, Nicolaides KH. Maternal serum free beta hCG and PAPP-A in fetal sex chromosome defects in the first trimester. *Prenat Diagn.* 2000;20:390–394.

98. Spencer K, Liao A, Skentou H, et al. Screening for triploidy by fetal nuchal translucency and maternal serum free ß-hCG and PAPP-A at 10–14 weeks of gestation. *Prenat Diagn.* 2000;20:495–499.

99. Monteagudo A, Timor-Tritsch I, Sharma S. Early and simple determination of chorionic and amniotic type in multifetal gestations in the first 14 weeks by high frequency transvaginal ultrasound. *Am J Obstet Gynecol.* 1994;170:824–829.

100. Sepulveda W, Sebire NJ, Hughes K, et al. The lambda sign at 10–14 weeks of gestation as a predictor of chorionicity in twin pregnancies. *Ultrasound Obstet Gynecol.* 1996;7:421–423.

101. Yukobowich E, Anteby EY, Cohen SM, et al. Risk of fetal loss in twin pregnancies undergoing second trimester amniocentesis. *Obstet Gynecol.* 2001;98:231–234.

102. Aytoz A, De Catte L, Camus M, et al. Obstetric outcome after prenatal diagnosis in pregnancies obtained after intracytoplasmic sperm injection. *Hum Reprod.* 1998;13:2958–2961.

103. De Catte L, Liebaers I, Foulon W. Outcome of twin gestations after first trimester chorionic villus sampling. *Obstet Gynecol.* 2000;96:714–720.

104. Brambati B, Tului L, Guercilena S, et al. Outcome of first trimester chorionic villus sampling for genetic investigation in multiple pregnancy. *Ultrasound Obstet Gynecol.* 2001;17:209–216.

105. Evans MI, Goldberg JD, Dommergues M, et al. Efficacy of second trimester selective termination for fetal abnormalities: international collaborative experience among the world's largest centers. *Am J Obstet Gynecol.* 1994;171:90–94.

106. Sebire NJ, Snijders RJM, Hughes K, et al. Screening for trisomy 21 in twin pregnancies by maternal age and fetal nuchal translucency thickness at 10–14 weeks of gestation. *Br J Obstet Gynaecol.* 1996;103:999–1003.

107. Monni G, Zoppi MA, Ibba RM, et al. Nuchal translucency in multiple pregnancies. *Croat Med J.* 2000;41:266–269.

108. Sebire NJ, Souka A, Skentou H, et al. Early prediction of severe twin-to-twin transfusion syndrome. *Hum Reprod.* 2000;15:2008–2010.

109. Sebire NJ, Hughes K, D'Ercole C, et al. Increased fetal nuchal translucency at 10–14 weeks as a predictor of severe twin-to-twin transfusion syndrome. *Ultrasound Obstet Gynecol.* 1997;10:86–89.

110. Noble PL, Snijders RJ, Abraha HD, et al. Maternal serum free beta-hCG at 10 to 14 weeks in trisomic twin pregnancies. *Br J Obstet Gynaecol.* 1997;104:741–743.

111. Spencer K. Screening for trisomy 21 in twin pregnancies in the first trimester using free beta-hCG and PAPP-A combined with fetal nuchal translucency thickness. *Prenat Diagn.* 2000;20:91–95.

112. Spencer K, Nicolaides KH. Screening for trisomy 21 in twins using first trimester ultrasound and maternal serum biochemistry in a one-stop clinic: a review of three years experience. *Br J Obstet Gynaecol.* 2003;110:276–280.

113. Farkas LG, Katic MJ, Forrest CR, et al. Surface anatomy of the face in Down syndrome: linear and angular measurements in the craniofacial regions. *J Craniofac Surg.* 2001;12:373–379.

114. Stempfle N, Huten Y, Fredouille C, et al. Skeletal abnormalities in fetuses with Down syndrome: a radiographic post-mortem study. *Pediatr Radiol.* 1999;29:682–688.

115. Keeling JW, Hansen BF, Kjaer I. Pattern of malformations in the axial skeleton in human trisomy 21 fetuses. *Am J Med Genet.* 1997;68:466–471.

116. Tuxen A, Keeling JW, Reintoft I, et al. A histological and radiological investigation of the nasal bone in fetuses with Down syndrome. *Ultrasound Obstet Gynecol.* 2003;22:22–26.

117. Larose C, Massoc P, Hillion Y, et al. Comparison of fetal nasal bone assessment by ultrasound at 11–14 weeks and by postmortem X-ray in trisomy 21: a prospective observational study. *Ultrasound Obstet Gynecol.* 2003;22:27–30.

118. Sonek J, Nicolaides KH. Prenatal ultrasonographic diagnosis of nasal bone abnormalities in three fetuses with Down syndrome. *Am J Obstet Gynecol.* 2002;186:139–141.

119. Cicero S, Sonek JD, McKenna DS, et al. Nasal bone hypoplasia in trisomy 21 at 15–22 weeks' gestation. *Ultrasound Obstet Gynecol.* 2003;21:15–18.

120. Bunduki V, Ruano R, Miguelez J, et al. Fetal nasal bone length: reference range and clinical application in ultrasound screening for trisomy 21. *Ultrasound Obstet Gynecol.* 2003;21:156–160.

121. Bromley B, Lieberman E, Shipp TD, et al. Fetal nose bone length: a marker for Down syndrome in the second trimester. *J Ultrasound Med.* 2002;21:1387–1394.

122. Gamez F, Ferreiro P, Salmean JM. Ultrasonographic measurement of fetal nasal bone in a low risk population at 19–22 gestational weeks. *Ultrasound Obstet Gynecol.* 2003;22.

123. Cicero S, Curcio P, Papageorghiou A, et al. Absence of nasal bone in fetuses with Trisomy 21 at 11–14 weeks of gestation: an observational study. *Lancet.* 2001;358:1665–1667.

124. Cicero S, Dezerega V, Andrade E, et al. Learning curve for sonographic examination of the fetal nasal bone at 11–14 weeks. *Ultrasound Obstet Gynecol.* 2003;22:135–137.

125. Kanellopoulos V, Katsetos C, Economides DL. Examination of fetal nasal bone and repeatability of measurement in early pregnancy. *Ultrasound Obstet Gynecol.* 2003;22:131–134.

126. Otano L, Aiello H, Igarzabal L, et al. Association between first trimester absence of fetal nasal bone on ultrasound and Down syndrome. *Prenat Diagn.* 2002;22:930–932.

127. Zoppi MA, Ibba RM, Axinan C, et al. Absence of fetal nasal bone and aneuploidies at first trimester nuchal translucency screening in unselected pregnancies. *Prenat Diagn.* 2003;23:496–500.

128. Orlandi F, Bilardo CM, Campogrande M, et al. Measurement of nasal bone length at 11–14 weeks of pregnancy and its potential role in Down syndrome risk assessment. *Ultrasound Obstet Gynecol.* 2003;22:36–39.

129. Viora E, Masturzo B, Errante G, et al. Ultrasound evaluation of fetal nasal bone at 11 to 14 weeks in a consecutive series of 1906 fetuses. *Prenat Diagn.* 2003;23:784–787.

130. Senat MV, Bernard JP, Boulvain M, et al. Intra- and inter-operator variability in fetal nasal bone assessment at 11–14 weeks of gestation. *Ultrasound Obstet Gynecol.* 2003;22:138–141.

131. Wong SF, Choi H, Ho LC. Nasal bone hypoplasia: is it a common finding amongst chromosomally normal fetuses of southern Chinese women? *Gynecol Obstet Invest.* 2003;56:99–101.

132. Cicero S, Longo D, Rembouskos G, et al. Absent nasal bone at 11–14 weeks of gestation and chromosomal defects. *Ultrasound Obstet Gynecol.* 2003;22:31–35.

133. Cicero S, Rembouskos G, Vandecruys H, et al. Likelihood ratio for trisomy 21 in fetuses with absent nasal bone at the 11–14 weeks scan. *Ultrasound Obstet Gynecol.* 2004.

134. Malone FD, Ball RH, Nyberg DA, et al. First trimester nasal bone evaluation for aneuploidy in an unselected general population: results from the FASTER trial. *SMFM* 2004; Abstract 58.

135. Welch KK, Malone FD. Nuchal translucency-based screening. *Clinical Obstet Gynecol*. 2003;46:909–922.

136. De Biasio P, Venturini PL. Absence of nasal bone and detection of trisomy 21. *Lancet*. 2002;13:1344.

137. Cicero S, Bindra R, Rembouskos G, et al. Integrated ultrasound and biochemical screening for trisomy 21 at 11 to 14 weeks. *Prenat Diagn*. 2003;23:306–310.

138. Souka AP, Snidjers RJ, Novakov A, et al. Defects and syndromes in chromosomally normal fetuses with increased nuchal translucency at 10–14 weeks of gestation. *Ultrasound Obstet Gynecol*. 1998;11:391–400.

139. Souka AP, Krampl E, Bakalis S, et al. Outcome of pregnancy in chromosomally normal fetuses with increased nuchal translucency in the first trimester. *Ultrasound Obstet Gynecol*. 2001;18:9–17.

140. Michailidis GD, Economides DL. Nuchal translucency measurement and pregnancy outcome in karyotypically normal fetuses. *Ultrasound Obstet Gynecol*. 2001;17:102–105.

141. Johnson MP, Johnson A, Holzgreve W, et al. First trimester simple hygroma: cause and outcome. *Am J Obstet Gynecol*. 1993;168:156–161.

142. Trauffer ML, Anderson CE, Johnson A, et al. The natural history of euploid pregnancies with first trimester cystic hygromas. *Am J Obstet Gynecol*. 1994;170:1279–1284.

143. Shulman LP, Emerson DS, Grevengood C, et al. Clinical course and outcome of fetuses with isolated cystic nuchal lesions and normal karyotypes detected in the first trimester. *Am J Obstet Gynecol*. 1994;171:1278–1281.

144. Maymon R, Jauniaux E, Cohen O, et al. Pregnancy outcome and infant follow-up of fetuses with abnormally increased first trimester nuchal translucency. *Hum Reprod*. 2000;15:2023–2027.

145. Bilardo CM, Muller MA, Zikulnig L, et al. Ductus venosus studies in fetuses at high risk for chromosomal or heart abnormalities: relationship with nuchal translucency measurement and fetal outcome. *Ultrasound Obstet Gynecol*. 2001;17:288–294.

146. Fukada Y, Amemiya A, Kohno K, et al. Prenatal course and pregnancy outcome of fetuses with a transient nuchal translucency. *Int J Gynaecol Obstet*. 2002;79:225–228.

147. van Zalen-Sprock RM, van Vugt JMG, van Geijn HP. First trimester diagnosis of cystic hygroma—course and outcome. *Am J Obstet Gynecol*. 1992;167:94–98.

148. Ville Y, Lalondrelle C, Doumerc S, et al. First trimester diagnosis of nuchal anomalies: significance and fetal outcome. *Ultrasound Obstet Gynecol*. 1992;2:314–316.

149. Hewitt B. Nuchal translucency in the first trimester. *Aust NZ J Obstet Gynaecol*. 1993;33:389–391.

150. Salvesen DR, Goble O. Early amniocentesis and fetal nuchal translucency in women requesting karyotyping for advanced maternal age. *Prenat Diagn*. 1995;15:971–974.

151. Hewitt BG, de Crespigny L, Sampson AJ, et al. Correlation between nuchal thickness and abnormal karyotype in first trimester fetuses. *Med J Aust*. 1996;165:365–368.

152. Hernadi L, Torocsik M. Screening for fetal anomalies in the 12th week of pregnancy by transvaginal sonography in an unselected population. *Prenat Diagn*. 1997;17:753–759.

153. Reynders CS, Pauker SP, Benacerraf BR. First trimester isolated fetal nuchal translucency: significance and outcome. *J Ultrasound Med*. 1997;16:101–105.

154. Bilardo CM, Pajkrt E, de Graaf IM, et al. Outcome of fetuses with enlarged nuchal translucency and normal karyotype. *Ultrasound Obstet Gynecol*. 1998;11:401–406.

155. Van Vugt JM, Tinnemans BW, Van Zalen-Sprock RM. Outcome and early childhood follow-up of chromosomally normal fetuses with increased nuchal translucency at 10–14 weeks' gestation. *Ultrasound Obstet Gynecol*. 1998;11:407–409.

156. Hiippala A, Eronen M, Taipale P, et al. Fetal nuchal translucency and normal chromosomes: a long-term follow-up study. *Ultrasound Obstet Gynecol*. 2001;18:18–22.

157. Mangione R, Guyon F, Taine L, et al. Pregnancy outcome and prognosis in fetuses with increased first trimester nuchal translucency. *Fetal Diagn Ther*. 2001;16:360–363.

158. Cheng C, Bahado-Singh RO, Chen S, et al. Pregnancy outcomes with increased nuchal translucency after routine Down syndrome screening. *Int J Gynaecol Obstet*. 2004;84:5–9.

159. Nadel A, Bromley B, Benacerraf BR. Nuchal thickening or cystic hygromas in first and early second trimester fetuses: prognosis and outcome. *Obstet Gynecol*. 1993;82:43–48.

160. Moselhi M, Thilaganathan B. Nuchal translucency: a marker for the antenatal diagnosis of aortic coarctation. *Br J Obstet Gynaecol*. 1996;103:1044–1045.

161. Adekunle O, Gopee A, El-Sayed M, et al. Increased first trimester nuchal translucency: pregnancy and infant outcomes after routine screening for Down syndrome in an unselected antenatal population. *Br J Radiol*. 1999;72:457–460.

162. Senat MV, De Keersmaecker B, Audibert F, et al. Pregnancy outcome in fetuses with increased nuchal translucency and normal karyotype. *Prenat Diagn*. 2002;22:345–349.

163. Fukada Y, Yasumizu T, Takizawa M, et al. The prognosis of fetuses with transient nuchal translucency in the first and early second trimester. *Acta Obstet Gynecol Scand*. 1998;76:913–916.

164. Hyett JA, Brizot ML, von Kaisenberg CS, et al. Cardiac gene expression of atrial natriuretic peptide and brain natriuretic peptide in trisomic fetuses. *Obstet Gynecol*. 1996;87:506–510.

165. Matias A, Gomes C, Flack N, et al. Screening for chromosomal abnormalities at 11–14 weeks: the role of ductus venosus blood flow. *Ultrasound Obstet Gynecol*. 1998;2:380–384.

166. Matias A, Huggon I, Areias JC, et al. Cardiac defects in chromosomally normal fetuses with abnormal ductus venosus blood flow at 10–14 weeks. *Ultrasound Obstet Gynecol*. 1999;14:307–310.

167. von Kaisenberg CS, Brand-Saberi B, Christ B, et al. Collagen type VI gene expression in the skin of trisomy 21 fetuses. *Obstet Gynecol*. 1998;91:319–323.

168. von Kaisenberg CS, Krenn V, Ludwig M, et al. Morphological classification of nuchal skin in fetuses with trisomy 21, 18 and 13 at 12–18 weeks and in a trisomy 16 mouse. *Anat Embryol*. 1998;197:105–124.

169. Bohlandt S, von Kaisenberg CS, Wewetzer K, et al. Hyaluronan in the nuchal skin of chromosomally abnormal fetuses. *Hum Reprod*. 2000;15:1155–1158.

170. Chitayat D, Kalousek DK, Bamforth JS. Lymphatic abnormalities in fetuses with posterior cervical cystic hygroma. *Am J Med Genet*. 1989;33:352–356.

171. von Kaisenberg CS, Nicolaides KH, Brand-Saberi B. Lymphatic vessel hypoplasia in fetuses with Turner syndrome. *Hum Reprod*. 1999;14:823–826.

172. von Kaisenberg CS, Prols F, Nicolaides KH, et al. Glycosaminoglycans and proteoglycans in the skin of aneuploid fetuses with increased nuchal translucency. *Human Reprod*. 2003;18:2544–2561.

173. Sebire NJ, Bianco D, Snijders RJ, et al. Increased fetal nuchal translucency thickness at 10–14 weeks: is screening for maternal-fetal infection necessary? *Br J Obstet Gynaecol*. 1997;104:212–215.

174. Hyett JA, Moscoso G, Nicolaides KH. First trimester nuchal translucency and cardiac septal defects in fetuses with trisomy 21. *Am J Obstet Gynecol*. 1995;172:1411–1413.

175. Hyett JA, Moscoso G, Nicolaides KH. Increased nuchal translucency in trisomy 21 fetuses: relation to narrowing of the aortic isthmus. *Human Reprod*. 1995;10:3049–3051.

176. Hyett JA, Moscoso G, Nicolaides KH. Cardiac defects in first trimester fetuses with trisomy 18. *Fetal Diagn Ther*. 1995;10:381–386.

177. Hyett JA, Moscoso G, Nicolaides KH. Abnormalities of the heart and great arteries in first trimester chromosomally abnormal fetuses. *Am J Med Genet*. 1997;69:207–216.

178. Hyett J, Moscoso G, Papapanagiotou G, et al. Abnormalities of the heart and great arteries in chromosomally normal fetuses with increased nuchal translucency thickness at 11–13 weeks of gestation. *Ultrasound Obstet Gynecol.* 1996;7:245–250.

179. Gembruch U, Knopfle G, Bald R, et al. Early diagnosis of fetal congenital heart disease by transvaginal echocardiography. *Ultrasound Obstet Gynecol.* 1993;3:310–317.

180. Achiron R, Rotstein Z, Lipitz S, et al. First trimester diagnosis of fetal congenital heart disease by transvaginal ultrasonography. *Obstet Gynecol.* 1994;84:69–72.

181. Smrcek JM, Gembruch U, Krokowski M, et al. The evaluation of cardiac biometry in major cardiac defects detected in early pregnancy. *Arch Gynecol Obstet.* 2003;268:94–101.

182. Hyett JA, Perdu M, Sharland GK, et al. Increased nuchal translucency at 10–14 weeks of gestation as a marker for major cardiac defects. *Ultrasound Obstet Gynecol.* 1997;10:242–246.

183. Zosmer N, Souter VL, Chan CSY, et al. Early diagnosis of major cardiac defects in chromosomally normal fetuses with increased nuchal translucency. *Br J Obstet Gynaecol.* 1999;106:829–833.

184. Ghi T, Huggon IC, Zosmer N, et al. Incidence of major structural cardiac defects associated with increased nuchal translucency but normal karyotype. *Ultrasound Obstet Gynecol.* 2001;18:610–614.

185. Lopes LM, Brizot ML, Lopes MA, et al. Structural and functional cardiac abnormalities identified prior to 16 weeks' gestation in fetuses with increased nuchal translucency. *Ultrasound Obstet Gynecol.* 2003;22:470–478.

186. Galindo A, Comas C, Martinez JM, et al. Cardiac defects in chromosomally normal fetuses with increased nuchal translucency at 10–14 weeks of gestation. *J Matern Fetal Neonatal Med.* 2003;13:163–170.

187. McAuliffe F, Winsor S, Hornberger L, et al. Fetal cardiac defects and increased nuchal translucency thickness. *Am J Obstet Gynecol.* 2004;189:S215.

188. Josefsson A, Molander E, Selbing A. Nuchal translucency as a screening test for chromosomal abnormalities in a routine first trimester ultrasound examination. *Acta Obstet Gynecol Scand.* 1998;77:497–499.

189. Hyett J, Perdu M, Sharland G, et al. Using fetal nuchal translucency to screen for major congenital cardiac defects at 10–14 weeks of gestation: population based cohort study. *British Medical Journal.* 1999;318:81–85.

190. Mavrides E, Cobian-Sanchez F, Tekay A, et al. Limitations of using first trimester nuchal translucency measurement in routine screening for major congenital heart defects. *Ultrasound Obstet Gynecol.* 2001;17:106–110.

191. Orvos H, Wayda K, Kozinsky Z, et al. Increased nuchal translucency and congenital heart defects in euploid fetuses: the Szeged experience. *Eur J Obstet Gynecol Reprod Biol.* 2002;101:124–128.

192. Hafner E, Schuller T, Metzenbauer M, et al. Increased nuchal translucency and congenital heart defects in a low-risk population. *Prenat Diagn.* 2003;23:985–989.

193. Makrydimas G, Sotiriadis A, Ioannidis JP. Screening performance of first trimester nuchal translucency for major cardiac defects: a meta-analysis. *Am J Obstet Gynecol.* 2003;189:1330–1335.

194. Sebire NJ, Snijders RJ, Davenport M, et al. Fetal nuchal translucency thickness at 10–14 weeks of gestation and congenital diaphragmatic hernia. *Obstet Gynecol.* 1997;90:943–947.

195. Snijders RJ, Brizot ML, Faria M, et al. Fetal exomphalos at 11–14 weeks of gestation. *J Ultrasound Med.* 1995;14:569–574.

196. Liao AW, Sebire NJ, Geerts L, et al. Megacystis at 10–14 weeks of gestation: chromosomal defects and outcome according to bladder length. *Ultrasound Obstet Gynecol.* 2003;21:338–341.

197. Daskalakis G, Sebire NJ, Jurkovic D, et al. Body stalk anomaly at 10–14 weeks of gestation. *Ultrasound Obstet Gynecol.* 1997;10:416–418.

198. Smrcek JM, Germer U, Krokowski M, et al. Prenatal ultrasound diagnosis and management of body stalk anomaly: analysis of nine singleton and two multiple pregnancies. *Ultrasound Obstet Gynecol.* 2003;21:322–328.

199. Chen SH, Lin MY, Chang FM. Prenatal diagnosis of Dandy-Walker syndrome in early pregnancy presenting with increased nuchal translucency and generalized edema at 13 weeks of gestation. *Prenat Diagn.* 2003;23:514–515.

200. Laurichesse-Delmas H, Beaufrere AM, Martin A, et al. First trimester features of Fowler syndrome (hydrocephaly-hydranencephaly proliferative vasculopathy). *Ultrasound Obstet Gynecol.* 2002;20:612–615.

201. Pandya PP, Kondylios A, Hilbert L, et al. Chromosomal defects and outcome in 1015 fetuses with increased nuchal translucency. *Ultrasound Obstet Gynecol.* 1995;5:15–19.

202. Ammala P, Salonen R. First trimester diagnosis of hydrolethalus syndrome. *Ultrasound Obstet Gynecol.* 1995;5:60–62.

203. de Ravelle TJL, van der Griendt MC, Evan P, et al. Hydrolethalus syndrome in a non-Finnish family: confirmation of the entity and early prenatal diagnosis. *Prenat Diagn.* 1999;19:279–281.

204. Cha'Ban FK, van Splunder P, Los FJ, et al. Fetal outcome in nuchal translucency with emphasis on normal fetal karyotype. *Prenat Diagn.* 1996;16:537–541.

205. Markov D, Jacquemyn Y, Leroy Y. Bilateral cleft lip and palate associated with increased nuchal translucency and maternal cocaine abuse at 14 weeks of gestation. *Clin Exp Obstet Gynecol.* 2003;30:109–110.

206. Lazanakis MS, Rodgers K, Economides DL. Increased nuchal translucency and CATCH 22. *Prenat Diagn.* 1998;18:507–510.

207. Machlitt A, Tennstedt C, Korner H, et al. Prenatal diagnosis of 22q11 microdeletion in an early second trimester fetus with conotruncal anomaly presenting with increased nuchal translucency and bilateral intracardiac echogenic foci. *Ultrasound Obstet Gynecol.* 2002;19:510–513.

208. Varlet F, Bousquet F, Clemenson A, et al. Congenital diaphragmatic hernia: two cases with early prenatal diagnosis and increased nuchal translucency. *Fetal Diagn Ther.* 2003;18:33–35.

209. Bulas D, Saal H, Allen JF, et al. Cystic hygroma and congenital diaphragmatic hernia: early prenatal sonographic evaluation of Fryn's syndrome. *Prenat Diagn.* 1992;12:867–875.

210. Hosli IM, Tercanli S, Rehder H, et al. Cystic hygroma as an early first trimester ultrasound marker for recurrent Fryn's syndrome. *Ultrasound Obstet Gynecol.* 1997;10:422–424.

211. van Zalen-Sprock RM, van Vugt JM, van Geijn HP. First trimester sonography of physiological midgut herniation and early diagnosis of omphalocele. *Prenat Diagn.* 1997;17:511–518.

212. Schemm S, Gembruch U, Germer U, et al. Omphalocele-exstrophy-imperforate anus-spinal defects (OEIS) complex associated with increased nuchal translucency. *Ultrasound Obstet Gynecol.* 2003;22:95–97.

213. Brown RN, Nicolaides KH. Increased fetal nuchal translucency: possible association with esophageal atresia. *Ultrasound Obstet Gynecol.* 2000;15:531–532.

214. Masturzo B, Hyett JA, Kalache KD, et al. Increased nuchal translucency as a prenatal manifestation of congenital adrenal hyperplasia. *Prenat Diagn.* 2001;21:314–316.

215. Fincham J, Pandya PP, Yuksel B, et al. Increased first trimester nuchal translucency as a prenatal manifestation of salt-wasting congenital adrenal hyperplasia. *Ultrasound Obstet Gynecol.* 2002;20:392–394.

216. Flores Anton B, Bonet Serra B, Adiego Burgos B, et al. Congenital adrenal hyperplasia: an association with increased fetal nuchal translucency. *An Pediatr (Barc).* 2003;58:52–54.

217. Souka AP, Skentou H, Geerts L, et al. Congenital nephrotic syndrome presenting with increased nuchal translucency in the first trimester. *Prenat Diagn.* 2002;22:93–95.

218. Sebire NJ, Von Kaisenberg C, Rubio C, et al. Fetal megacystis at 10–14 weeks of gestation. *Ultrasound Obstet Gynecol.* 1996;8:387–390.

219. Favre R, Kohler M, Gasser B, et al. Early fetal megacystis between 11 and 15 weeks of gestation. *Ultrasound Obstet Gynecol.* 1999;14:402–406.

220. Fisk NM, Vaughan J, Smidt M, et al. Transvaginal ultrasound recognition of nuchal oedema in the first trimester diagnosis of achondrogenesis. *J Clin Ultrasound.* 1991;19:586–590.

221. Soothill PW, Vuthiwong C, Rees H. Achondrogenesis type 2 diagnosed by transvaginal ultrasound at 12 weeks of gestation. *Prenat Diagn.* 1993;13:523–528.

222. Meizner I, Barnhard Y. Achondrogenesis type I diagnosed by transvaginal ultrasonography at 13 weeks' gestation. *Am J Obstet Gynecol.* 1995;173:1620–1622.

223. Ben Ami M, Perlitz Y, Haddad S, et al. Increased nuchal translucency is associated with asphyxiating thoracic dysplasia. *Ultrasound Obstet Gynecol.* 1997;10:297–298.

224. den Hollander NS, van der Harten HJ, Vermeij-Keers C, et al. First trimester diagnosis of Blomstrand lethal osteochondrodysplasia. *Am J Med Genet.* 1997;73:345–350.

225. Hafner E, Schuchter K, Liebhart E, et al. Results of routine fetal nuchal translucency measurement at weeks 10–13 in 4,233 unselected pregnant women. *Prenat Diagn.* 1998;18:29–34.

226. Souka AP, Raymond FL, Mornet E, et al. Hypophosphatasia associated with increased nuchal translucency: a report of three consecutive pregnancies. *Ultrasound Obstet Gynecol.* 2002;20:294–295.

227. Eliyahu S, Weiner E, Lahav D, et al. Early sonographic diagnosis of Jarcho-Levin syndrome: a prospective screening program in one family. *Ultrasound Obstet Gynecol.* 1997;9:314–318.

228. Lam YH, Eik-Nes SH, Tang MH, et al. Prenatal sonographic features of spondylocostal dysostosis and diaphragmatic hernia in the first trimester. *Ultrasound Obstet Gynecol.* 1999;13:213–215.

229. Hull AD, James G, Pretorius DH. Detection of Jarcho-Levin syndrome at 12 weeks' gestation by nuchal translucency screening and three-dimensional ultrasound. *Prenat Diagn.* 2001;21:390–394.

230. Clementschitsch G, Hasenohrl G, Steiner H, et al. Early diagnosis of a fetal skeletal dysplasia associated with increased nuchal translucency with 2D and 3D ultrasound. *Ultraschall Med.* 2003;24:349–352.

231. Souter V, Nyberg D, Siebert JR, et al. Upper limb phocomelia associated with increased nuchal translucency in a monochorionic twin pregnancy. *J Ultrasound Med.* 2002;21:355–360.

232. Brady AF, Pandya PP, Yuksel B, et al. Outcome of chromosomally normal live-births with increased fetal nuchal translucency at 10–14 weeks' gestation. *J Med Genet.* 1998;35:222–224.

233. Makrydimas G, Souka A, Skentou H, et al. Osteogenesis imperfecta and other skeletal dysplasias presenting with increased nuchal translucency in the first trimester. *Am J Med Genet.* 2001;98:117–120.

234. Viora E, Sciarrone A, Bastonero S, et al. Osteogenesis imperfecta associated with increased nuchal translucency as a first ultrasound sign: report of another case. *Ultrasound Obstet Gynecol.* 2003;21:200–202.

235. Petrikovsky BM, Gross B, Bialer M, et al. Prenatal diagnosis of pseudothalidomide syndrome in consecutive pregnancies of a consanguineous couple. *Ultrasound Obstet Gynecol.* 1997;10:425–428.

236. Percin EF, Guvenal T, Cetin A, et al. First trimester diagnosis of Robinow syndrome. *Fetal Diagn Ther.* 2001;16:308–311.

237. Hill LM, Leary J. Transvaginal sonographic diagnosis of short-rib polydactyly dysplasia at 13 weeks' gestation. *Prenat Diagn.* 1998;18:1198–1201.

238. Monteagudo A, Mayberry P, Rebarber A, et al. Sirenomelia sequence: first trimester diagnosis with both two- and three-dimensional sonography. *Ultrasound Med.* 2002;21:915–920.

239. Souka AP, Bower S, Geerts L, et al. Blackfan-Diamond anemia and dyserythropoietic anemia presenting with increased nuchal translucency at 12 weeks of gestation. *Ultrasound Obstet Gynecol.* 2002;20:197–199.

240. Pannier E, Viot G, Aubry MC, et al. Congenital erythropoietic porphyria (Gunther's disease): two cases with very early prenatal manifestation and cystic hydroma. *Prenat Diagn.* 2003;23:25–30.

241. Tercanli S, Miny P, Siebert MS, et al. Fanconi anemia associated with increased nuchal translucency detected by first trimester ultrasound. *Ultrasound Obstet Gynecol.* 2001;17:160–162.

242. Petrikovsky BM, Baker D, Schneider E. Fetal hydrops secondary to human parvovirus infection in early pregnancy. *Prenat Diagn.* 1996;16:342–344.

243. Markenson G, Correia LA, Cohn G, et al. Parvoviral infection associated with increased nuchal translucency: a case report. *J Perinatol.* 2000;20:129–131.

244. Smulian JC, Egan JF, Rodis JF. Fetal hydrops in the first trimester associated with maternal parvovirus infection. *J Clin Ultrasound.* 1998;26:314–316.

245. Sohan K, Carroll S, Byrne D, et al. Parvovirus as a differential diagnosis of hydrops fetalis in the first trimester. *Fetal Diagn Ther.* 2000;15:234–236.

246. Lam YH, Tang MH, Lee CP, et al. Nuchal translucency in fetuses affected by homozygous a-thalassemia-1 at 12–13 weeks of gestation. *Ultrasound Obstet Gynecol.* 1999;13:238–240.

247. Hyett J, Noble P, Sebire NJ, et al. Lethal congenital arthrogryposis presents with increased nuchal translucency at 10–14 weeks of gestation. *Ultrasound Obstet Gynecol.* 1997;9: 310–313.

248. Rijhsinghani A, Yankowitz J, Howser D, et al. Sonographic and maternal serum screening abnormalities in fetuses affected by spinal muscular atrophy. *Prenat Diagn.* 1997;17:166–169.

249. Stiller RJ, Lieberson D, Herzlinger R, et al. The association of increased fetal nuchal translucency and spinal muscular atrophy type I. *Prenat Diagn.* 1999;19:587–589.

250. de Jong-Pleij EA, Stoutenbecek P, van der Mark-Batseva NN, et al. The association of spinal muscular atrophy type II and increased nuchal translucency. *Ultrasound Obstet Gynecol.* 2002;19:312–313.

251. Tercanli S, Uyanik G, Hosli I, et al. Increased nuchal translucency in a case of long-chain3-hydroxyacyl-coenzyme A dehydrogenase deficiency. *Fetal Diagn Ther.* 2000;15:322–325.

252. van Eyndhoven HWF, Ter Brugge HG, van Essen AJ, et al. *β*-glucuronidase deficiency as cause of recurrent hydrops fetalis: the first early prenatal diagnosis by chorionic villus sampling. *Prenat Diagn.* 1998;18:959–962.

253. den Hollander NS, Kleijer WJ, Schoonderwaldt EM, et al. In utero diagnosis of mucopolysaccharidosis type VII in a fetus with an enlarged nuchal translucency. *Ultrasound Obstet Gynecol.* 2000;16:87–90.

254. Geipel A, Berg C, Germer U, et al. Mucopolysaccharidosis VII (Sly disease) as a cause of increased nuchal translucency and non-immune fetal hydrops: study of a family and technical approach to prenatal diagnosis in early and late pregnancy. *Prenat Diagn.* 2002;22:493–495.

255. Hobbins JC, Jones OW, Gottesfeld S, et al. Transvaginal sonography and transabdominal embryoscopy in the first trimester diagnosis of Smith–Lemli–Opitz syndrome, type 2. *Am J Obstet Gynecol.* 1994;171:546–549.

256. Hyett JA, Clayton PT, Moscoso G, et al. Increased first trimester nuchal translucency as a prenatal manifestation of Smith–Lemli–Opitz syndrome. *Am J Med Genet.* 1995;58:374–376.

257. Sharp P, Haant E, Fletcher JM, et al. First trimester diagnosis of Smith–Lemli–Opitz syndrome. *Prenat Diagn.* 1997;17:355–361.

258. de Graaf IM, Pajkrt E, Keessen M, et al. Enlarged nuchal translucency and low serum protein concentration as possible markers for Zellweger syndrome. *Ultrasound Obstet Gynecol.* 1999;13:268–270.

259. Christiaens GC, de Pater JM, Stoutenbeek P, et al. First trimester nuchal anomalies as a prenatal sign of Zellweger syndrome. *Prenat Diagn.* 2000;20:517–525.

260. Johnson JM, Babul-Hirji R, Chitayat D. First trimester increased nuchal translucency and fetal hypokinesia associated with Zellweger syndrome. *Ultrasound Obstet Gynecol.* 2001;17:344–346.

261. Sekimoto H, Osada H, Kimura H, et al. Prenatal findings in Brachmann-de Lange syndrome. *Arch Gynecol Obstet.* 2000; 263:182–184.

262. Souka AP, Krampl E, Geerts L, et al. Congenital lymphedema presenting with increased nuchal translucency at 13 weeks of gestation. *Prenat Diagn.* 2002;22:91–92.

263. Leung KY, MacLachlan NA, Sepulveda W. Prenatal diagnosis of ectrodactyly: the 'lobster claw' anomaly. *Ultrasound Obstet Gynecol.* 1995;6:443–446.

264. Achiron R, Heggesh J, Grisaru D, et al. Noonan syndrome: a cryptic condition in early gestation. *Am J Med Genet.* 2000;92:159–165.

265. van der Stege, van Eyck J, Arabin B. Prenatal ultrasound observation in subsequent pregnancies with Perlman syndrome. *Ultrasound Obstet Gynecol.* 1998;11:149–151.

266. Schwarzler P, Homfray T, Campbell S, et al. Prenatal findings on ultrasound and x-ray in a case of overgrowth syndrome associated with increased nuchal translucency. *Prenat Diagn.* 2001;21:341–345.

267. Prefumo F, Homfray T, Jeffrey I, et al. A newly recognized autosomal recessive syndrome with abnormal vertebral ossification, rib abnormalities, and nephrogenic rests. *Am J Med Genet.* 2003;120A:386–388.

268. Carroll SG, Hyett J, Eustace D, et al. Evolution of sonographic findings in a fetus with agenesis of the urethra, vagina and rectum. *Prenatal Diagn.* 1996;16:931–933.

CHAPTER 25

SECOND TRIMESTER SONOGRAPHIC MARKERS FOR ANEUPLOIDY

Bryan Bromley / Beryl R. Benacerraf

OVERVIEW

Sonographic evaluation of the fetus in the mid trimester of pregnancy allows for the identification of structural abnormalities, biometric inconsistencies, and variations in normal anatomy that can serve as a means of detecting fetuses with chromosomal abnormalities. Each of the major chromosomal syndromes present with a relatively distinct constellation of sonographic findings, thus allowing the sonologist to establish a tentative diagnosis (Table 25-1).

The risk of most fetal chromosomal abnormalities increases with advancing maternal age. The rate of all age-related clinically significant abnormalities considered together is approximately 5 in 1,000 at 35 years of age, 15 in 1,000 at 40 years of age and 50 in 1,000 at 45 years.[1] Second trimester sonography can detect 60–80% of mid-trimester Down syndrome fetuses with approximately a 6% false-positive rate.[2,3] The identification of fetuses affected with Trisomy 18 and Trisomy 13 has been even higher approaching 80–100%.[4–7]

TRISOMY 21: DOWN SYNDROME

Down syndrome is the most common chromosomal abnormality to result in a live birth. The trisomic etiology of syndrome was described in 1959 by Lejeune et al. and is most often due to an extra chromosome 21 resulting from nondisjunction during meiosis. Two to 3% of individuals with Trisomy 21 have the chromosome translocated to one of the D-group chromosomes [13,14,15].[8] One to 2% of all pregnant women ≥35 years of age have a second-trimester fetus with Down syndrome.[9]

NUCHAL FOLD

In 1985, we first reported a sonographic finding characterized by increased soft tissue thickness at the fetal occiput as a sign of Down syndrome in the mid trimester.[10,11] This measurement is obtained using a transverse view through the fetal head, across the thalami and angled posteriorly to include the cerebral peduncles, cerebellar hemispheres and cisterna magna as well as the occipital bone. The measurement is made from the surface of the occipital bone to the surface of the skin edge (Fig. 25-1). Care must be taken not to angle below the occiput as this will lead to spuriously large measurements. We also established normative values of nuchal skin fold thickness in a prospective series of 303 karyotypically normal fetuses scanned between 15 and 20 weeks gestation showing that normal measurements ranged from 1–5 mm and were relatively constant throughout this gestational age window.[12]

In our initial retrospective study of 904 patients undergoing amniocentesis, three of six fetuses with Down syndrome had a nuchal fold measuring ≥6 mm.[10] The significance of a thickened nuchal fold was then studied prospectively in two larger patient groups, showing that 40–50% of fetuses with Down syndrome had a nuchal fold ≥6 mm. A nuchal fold measuring ≥6 mm places the fetus at a high risk for Trisomy 21 with a false-positive rate of 0.1%.[11,13]

Numerous investigators using prospective studies have now validated the significance of a thickened nuchal fold as a maker for Down syndrome. Lynch and colleagues evaluated this finding in twin pregnancies, each of which had one fetus with Down syndrome, and found a thickened nuchal fold in 56% of affected fetuses.[14] Ginsberg et al. found a thickened nuchal fold in 44% of trisomic fetuses.[15] In a large prospective series, Crane et al. found a thickened nuchal fold in 75% of fetuses with Down syndrome as well as in 1.4% of normals, resulting in a positive predictive value of 1/13.[16] Many prospective series have now confirmed this finding, with sensitivities ranging from 16–78% and false positive rates of 0–2.1%.[17–21]

The optimal threshold for a thickened nuchal fold was reevaluated by Gray and Crane who found that between 14–18 weeks gestation a measurement of greater than or equal to 5 mm occurred in 2.9% of pregnancies and had a sensitivity of 42% for the detection of Down syndrome. Adjusted to the incidence of Down syndrome in the general population, this yielded a positive predictive value of 1 in 48. Between 19 and 24 weeks gestation the optimal threshold was increased to greater than or equal to 6 mm. This degree of nuchal thickening occurred in 3.7% of pregnancies and had an 83% sensitivity for the detection of Down syndrome with an adjusted positive predictive value of 1/38.[22]

The utility of the thickened nuchal fold as a sonographic marker appears to be independent of maternal age. We reported the utility of a thickened nuchal fold in a low-risk population and found that 33% of fetuses with this finding had an abnormal karyotype, the majority of whom had Down syndrome.[23] The resolution of a nuchal fold during the course of gestation should not be considered indicative of a normal karyotype. We have observed two cases in which a nuchal fold was identified in the early mid trimester of pregnancy and resolved spontaneously within a 1–3 week time span, each of these fetuses was subsequently identified as having Down syndrome by karyotype.[24]

NASAL BONE

Although the fetal nose has been known to be small in individuals with Down syndrome since the first report by Langdon Down in 1867,[25] the sonographic correlate of this condition in the mid trimester has only recently been described (Fig. 25-2). In a study of 239 fetuses referred to our laboratory for amniocentesis due to a risk of Down syndrome of 1 in 270 or greater, we identified 16 fetuses with Down syndrome by karyotype. Six of the 16 (37%) fetuses with Down syndrome

TABLE 25-1	**SONOGRAPHIC FINDINGS**

Trisomy 21	**Triploidy**
Nuchal fold	Assymetric IUGR
Absent/hypoplastic nasal bone	Ventriculomegaly
	Heart defects
Short long bones	3–4 Syndactyly
Heart defect	Neural tube defects
Hyperechoic bowel	Molar placenta
Echogenic intracardiac focus	
Pyelectasis	**Trisomy 13**
Ventriculomegaly	Holoprosencephaly
Hypoplasia of fifth digit	Microcephaly
Wide iliac angle	Neural tube defects
	Facial clefts
Trisomy 18	Occular anomalies
Choroid plexus cyst	Cardiac defects
Cardiac defect	Echogenic intracardiac focus
Cystic hygroma	Cystic hygroma
Omphalocele	Polydactyly
Diaphragmatic hernia	Polycystic kidneys
Neural tube defects	Intrauterine growth retardation
Rockerbottom feet	
Clenched hands	**Turner X0**
Radial ray anomalies	Septate cystic hygroma
Clubfeet	Cardiac defects
Stawberry shape skull	Renal anomalies
Intrauterine growth retardation	
Polyhydramnios	

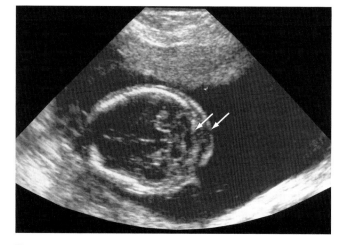

FIGURE 25-1 Down syndrome. Transverse view of the fetal head across the thalami and angled posteriorly to include the fetal peduncles, cerebellar hemispheres and cisterna magna as well as occipital bone. The thickened nuchal fold is shown by arrows.

did not have a detectable nasal bone. The absence of a nasal bone conferred a likelihood ratio of 83 for Down syndrome. Of the fetuses with a detectable nasal bone, the mean length of the nasal bone was 3.5 mm compared to the mean nasal bone length of 4.5 mm in euploid fetuses. P < .001. A receiver operator characteristic curve for the prediction of DS based on BPD/NBL reveals that a cutoff of ≥10 identified 81% of affected fetuses with an 11% false positive. If a cutoff of ≥11 was used one would identify 69% of Down syndrome fetuses with a 5% false positive.[26] Vintzileos et al. retrospectively evaluated the significance of the nasal bone in fetuses referred for genetic sonogram. There were 29 fetuses with Down syndrome that were compared to 102 euploid fetuses. These investigators found that the absence of the nasal bone was seen in 40% of fetuses with Down syndrome and none of the euploid fetuses. Adding the absence of the nasal bone to their genetic sonogram resulted in a sensitivity of 90% for the detection of Down syndrome.[27] The high sensitivity of the absent nasal bone for the detection of Down syndrome and the low false positive rate makes this one of the most significant markers for the detection of Down syndrome.

LONG BONE BIOMETRY

Femur Length

Short stature is a well-recognized feature of Down syndrome. In 1987, Lockwood et al. reported that second-trimester Down syndrome fetuses have slightly short femurs when compared with normal fetuses.[28] That same year, we developed a linear regression model of the relation between femur length and biparietal diameter (BPD) in normal fetuses. Femur lengths were measured end-to-end from the greater trochanter to the end of the distal diaphysis. The expected FL = −9.645 + 0.9338 × BPD accounted for 94% of variation in normal femur length.[29] Based on biparietal diameter, a measured-to-expected femur length ratio of ≤0.91 identified 40% of fetuses with Down syndrome, with a 5% false-positive rate and a positive predictive value of 3.1% in our high-risk population.[30] When the nuchal fold thickness was added as a criterion, 75% of fetuses with Down syndrome were identified with a 2% false-positive rate.[29] The BPD of the fetuses with Down syndrome was in agreement with the gestational age of the pregnancies based on menstrual history, and the femur lengths were smaller than anticipated suggesting that the femurs were actually short rather than that the biparietal diameter was wide.

Hill et al. found an abnormal head-to-femur length ratio in 36% of fetuses with Down syndrome and 6.6% of normal fetuses.[31] Brumfield and colleagues also found an abnormal BPD/femur length ratio of 1.8 or higher resulted in the identification of 40% of fetuses with Down syndrome and also was present in 2.2% of normals.[32] Dicke and coworkers reported that a BPD/femur length ratio of more than 1.5 SD above the mean correctly identified 18% of fetuses with Down syndrome with a false-positive rate of 4%.[33] The presence of the short femur in identifying fetuses at risk for Down syndrome has also been validated by Ginsberg et al., who reported that

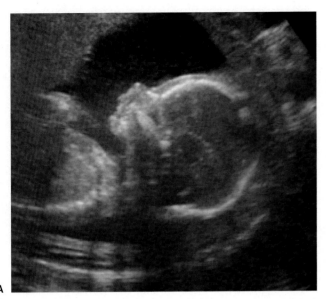
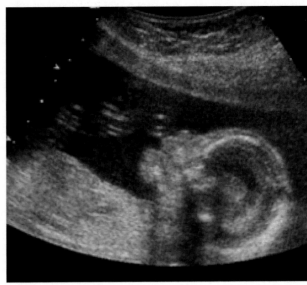

FIGURE 25-2 (**A**) Normal nasal bone in euploid fetus. (**B**) Down syndrome fetus with absent nasal bone.

using a BPD/FL ratio >1.5 SD of the control mean resulted in a sensitivity of 46% for the identification of Down syndrome.[15] Grist et al. reported that a measured femur length/expected femur length of .90 or less identified 50% of fetuses with Down syndrome, with a 6.5% false positive rate.[34]

Alternatively, LaFollette and colleagues did not find any statistically discernible deviation in femur lengths among fetuses with Down syndrome compared with normals.[35] Other investigators have also been unable to find any correlation between the diagnosis of Trisomy 21 and an abnormal BPD/FL ratio.[36,37]

Nyberg et al. also confirmed that second-trimester fetuses with Down syndrome have shorter femur lengths relative to biparietal diameter than normal fetuses but concluded that the positive predictive value of this finding was quite low thus limiting its use as a single screening parameter for Down syndrome.[38] Several other investigators have also found a significant reduction in the femur length in fetuses with Down syndrome compared with normal controls, however the magnitude of this reduction varies within laboratories and was not felt to be sufficient to permit the use of this finding as an isolated marker for Trisomy 21.[39–41]

HUMERUS

Fitzsimmons et al. reported that the long bones of Down syndrome abortuses were shorter than those of their normal counterparts on evaluation of pathologic specimens. The difference was most pronounced in the humerus, indicating that it might be more predictive of Down syndrome than femur length.[42]

In 1991, we reported the use of the humeral length in the detection of second-trimester fetuses with Down syndrome and developed a linear regression model of the relation between humeral length and biparietal diameter (BPD). The expected humeral length $= -7.9404 + 0.8492 \times$ BPD accounted for 82% of the variability in normal control fetuses. A ratio of measured-to-expected humeral length of less than 0.90 identified 50% of the fetuses with Down syndrome with a false-positive rate of 6.25%. Combining a short humeral length with a thickened nuchal fold, allowed the identification of 75% of fetuses with Down syndrome. This yielded a positive predictive value of 4.6% in women aged 35 whose a priori risk of having a fetus with Trisomy 21 was 0.4% based on advanced maternal age.[43]

Rodis et al. confirmed the utility of a shortened humerus for the detection of Down syndrome. In their study, a humeral length less than the 5th percentile had a sensitivity of 64% and specificity of 95% for the identification of Down syndrome. The positive predictive value of a short humerus was 6.8% in this population where the prevalence of Down syndrome was 1:173.[44] Rotmensch and colleagues also found that the humeral length in Down syndrome fetuses was significantly shorter than in normal controls, by showing that a ratio of 0.90 for observed/expected humeral length resulted in a sensitivity of 28% for the detection of Down syndrome with a specificity of 91%.[45]

Nyberg et al., using a measured humerus length /predicted humerus length ratio of $\leq.89$ detected 24.4% of fetuses with Down syndrome with a false positive rate of 4.5%. Fetuses with Down syndrome were 5.4 times more likely to have a short humerus than normal fetuses. The use of a measured femur length/predicted femur length ratio of $\leq.91$ also identified 24.4% of affected fetuses with a 4.7% false positive rate, similarly resulting in a 5.2 fold increased risk of Trisomy 21. The finding of both a short humerus and a short femur increased the risk of Down syndrome by 11-fold.[46]

Johnson and colleagues have shown that fetal foot length and femur length versus gestational age have a linear relationship in both normal and Down syndrome populations. Using a femur/foot length ratio of ≤0.90, they were able to identify 71% of fetuses with Trisomy 21 with a specificity of 89%. This resulted in an odds ratio of 18.3 for having an affected fetus. Using the ultrasonographic parameter of a femur + humerus length/foot length ratio of ≤1.75 these same investigators correctly identified 53% of fetuses with Trisomy 21 with a 7% false positive rate. This yielded an odds ratio of 15.3 for having an affected fetus.[47,48]

Vintzileos et al. reported a series of 515 patients scanned between 14–23 weeks gestation. Of the 515 patients, 493 had normal karyotypes and were used to derive regression equations for predicted long bone lengths on the basis of biparietal diameter measurement. Twenty-two fetuses had Trisomy 21. The sensitivity of an abnormal ultrasound, defined as the presence of 1 or more short bones, was 63.6% and the specificity was 78.5% for the identification of an affected fetus.[49]

HYDRONEPHROSIS

The majority of fetuses with mild pyelectasis are karyotypically normal; however there has been an association between pyelectasis and Down syndrome. In 1990, our laboratory described 210 fetuses with pyelectasis using the following criteria: anterior posterior dimension of the renal pelvis measuring at least 4 mm between 16–20 weeks gestation, 5 mm between 20–30 weeks and 7 mm between 30–40 weeks. The incidence of Trisomy 21 in this population was 3.3%. Among fetuses with Down syndrome, 25% have mild pyelectasis identified prenatally compared with 2.8% of normals.[50] This finding was substantiated by Corteville et al. using a similar threshold for identifying pyelectasis. These investigators found that pyelectasis was present in 17.4% of fetuses with Down syndrome versus 2% of normals. They found that the sensitivity of isolated pyelectasis for detecting Down syndrome was only 4% with a false positive rate of 2% and the predictive value of isolated pyelectasis was 1/340 for the detection of Down syndrome and therefore recommended that amniocentesis be considered only if pyelectasis was present in conjunction with other clinical or sonographic parameters.[51]

HYPERECHOIC BOWEL

Hyperechoic bowel (Fig. 25-3) is a relatively rare sonographic finding in the second trimester occurring in approximately 0.2–0.8% of the population.[52–54] Initially, many investigators reported hyperechoic bowel as a normal variant, however, in 1990, Nyberg et al. described an association between chromosomal abnormalities and second-trimester hyperechoic bowel. In a study of 94 fetuses with Down syndrome, he noted that 7% had hyperechoic bowel.[28] In a subsequent study, these same investigators found the sensitivity of hyperechoic bowel for the detection of Down syndrome to be 11.8% with a specificity of 99.3% and a positive predictive value of 14.5%. This yielded a relative risk of 16.8 (95% CI: 8.2–32.5). In a low-risk population, hyperechoic bowel carried a risk of Down syndrome of 1:47.[54]

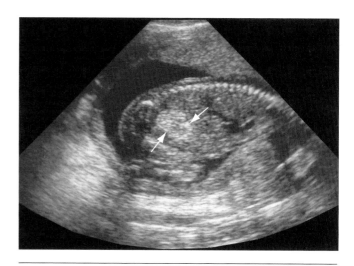

FIGURE 25-3 Down syndrome. Longitudinal view of the fetal abdomen, showing an area of bowel hyperechogenicity (arrows).

The incidence of chromosomal abnormalities in the setting of hyperechoic bowel has ranged from 3.3% to 27%.[53,55] Scioscia and colleagues identified Down syndrome in five of 19 fetuses (27%) with hyperechoic bowel. We reported on a series of 50 fetuses with hyperechoic bowel defined as bowel echogenicity comparable to bone and found that 12% of fetuses with this finding had a Down syndrome. In addition, 12.5% of fetuses with Down syndrome karyotyped by second trimester amniocentesis had hyperechoic bowel.[52] The etiology of hyperechoic bowel seen in association with aneuploidy has not been clearly established but may be related to poor bowel motility and decreased water content of meconium.[54]

ECHOGENIC INTRACARDIAC FOCUS

An echogenic intracardiac focus (Fig. 25-4) is a discrete, echogenic dot, which is as bright as, bone and which may occur in either or both ventricles (although it is most frequently seen within the left ventricle). Initially, this focus was felt to be a benign finding.[56] However, several recent reports have suggested that an echogenic intracardiac focus may be associated with autosomal trisomies.[57–59]

In 1992, Roberts and Genest showed that microcalcifications of the papillary muscle is a pathologic feature of fetuses with trisomies 21 and 13. This finding was seen in 16% of fetuses with Trisomy 21, 39% of fetuses with Trisomy 13, and 2% of normal fetuses.[60]

In 1994, Brown et al. described the sonographic finding of a fetus with an echogenic intracardiac focus and Trisomy 21. Pathologic evaluation confirmed the focus was a calcified papillary muscle.[61] In 1995, we reported a series of 1,334 second-trimester fetuses undergoing amniocentesis and found that 66 (4.9%) had an echogenic intracardiac focus (EIF). Four of 22 fetuses with Down syndrome (18%) had an EIF compared

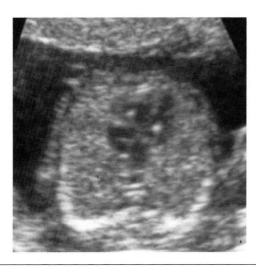

FIGURE 25-4 Down syndrome. Four-chamber view of the fetal heart, showing a bright papillary muscle in each ventricle.

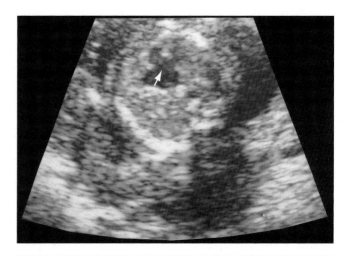

FIGURE 25-5 Down syndrome. Four-chamber view of the fetal heart in the second trimester, showing an AV canal (arrow) in diastole.

with 62 (4.7%) of the remaining 1312 fetuses without Down syndrome. The sonographic identification of an echogenic intracardiac focus was associated with a 4-fold increase in the risk of Down syndrome (risk ratio 4.3; 95% confidence interval 1.5–12.3). The sensitivity, specificity, and positive predictive value for using the presence of an echogenic intracardiac focus to identify a fetus with Down syndrome were 18.2%, 95.3%, and 6.1%, respectively. The overall incidence of Down syndrome in the study population was 1.6%.[58]

The association between an echogenic intracardiac focus and karyotypic abnormality was further confirmed by Simpson et al. who demonstrated that although the majority of fetuses with this sonographic finding were normal, there was a 1% risk of chromosomal abnormalities.[59]

MAJOR ANOMALIES

Major structural abnormalities occur in approximately one third of fetuses with Down syndrome. Nyberg et al. reported on a series of 94 fetuses with Down syndrome and found that 33% of these fetuses had sonographically detected, major structural malformations, including cardiac abnormalities (Fig. 25-5), cystic hygroma, omphalocele, and hydrops.[21] Work by our group is in agreement with this reporting major structural abnormalities in 34–35% of the Down syndrome fetuses including ventriculomegaly, cerebellar clefts, heart defects, and limb abnormalities among other findings.[2,3]

ADJUNCT FEATURES OF DOWN SYNDROME

GENDER

In 1993, Lockwood et al. first suggested an effect of fetal gender on the prediction of Down syndrome in second-trimester fetuses. Among 42 fetuses with Down syndrome, these inves-

tigators found that the observed reduction in fetal long bone lengths from the expected value for a given biparietal diameter, was greater among male fetuses than among female fetuses. Using a sonographic criteria of a thickened nuchal fold ≥6 mm or a humeral length ≥3.6 mm below the expected mean for a given BPD, they were able to identify 41.7% of female Down fetuses versus 66.7% of male Down fetuses.[62] A similar gender-specific pattern of fetal biometry was supported by Smulian.[63]

Our group however evaluated the biometric and structural sonographic features of 95 second-trimester fetuses with Down syndrome and were unable to show any statistically significant difference in the incidence of the sonographic findings when male and female fetuses with Down syndrome were compared.[64]

ILIAC LENGTH AND ANGLE MEASUREMENTS

Pelvic bone abnormalities are common in newborns with Down syndrome. A small acetabular angle, wide and low ilia and elongated tapering ischia are reported in 70–80% of newborns with Down syndrome.[65] Recently, several investigators have studied the utility of iliac length and angle measurements in the sonographic detection of Down syndrome.

In 1994, Abuhamad reported that the iliac length measurement is increased in fetuses with Down syndrome. These investigators derived a linear regression of iliac length measurement (cm) = −0.2723 + 0.0333 BPD (mm) and found that a ratio of observed/expected iliac length measurement ≥1.21 had a sensitivity of 40% and specificity of 98% for the detection of Down syndrome.[66]

Recent attention has focused on the width of the angle between the two iliac bones measured on a cross-section of the fetal pelvis. Our laboratory has reported that the mean iliac angle measurements differed significantly for fetuses affected by Down syndrome compared with normal controls. Using an iliac angle of 90 degrees or greater as abnormal, we identified 36.8% of fetuses with Down syndrome with a false positive rate of 4.3%.[67] We also noted a large variation in the angle measurement depending on the level that the image was obtained and caution that the ideal level of angle determination has yet to be established.

SONOGRAPHIC FINDINGS IN THE EXTREMITIES OF FETUSES WITH DOWN SYNDROME

Sixty percent of neonates with Trisomy 21 have hypoplasia of the middle phalanx of the fifth digit. We described the sonographic appearance of this hypoplastic middle phalanx as well as curvature of the fifth digit in fetuses with Down syndrome in 1988 when we reported this finding in 4 of 5 mid-trimester fetuses with Down syndrome.[68] This was subsequently studied in a prospective study of over 1,000 fetuses between 15 and 20 weeks gestation. The ratio of the middle phalanx of the fifth digit over the middle phalanx of the fourth digit was calculated; the median ratio for normal fetuses and Down fetuses were 0.85 and 0.59, respectively. Using a cut-off of 0.70, we identified 75% of Down syndrome fetuses; however, this finding was also present in 18% of normal fetuses. The sonographic appearance of the fetal digits was not suggested as a screening tool for Down syndrome but rather as an adjunct to other signs.[69]

A simian crease (transverse palmar crease) is present in 50% of newborns with Down syndrome as well as in 4% of the normal population. Jeanty has described the prenatal sonographic appearance of this finding in the fetus.[70]

Separation of the great toes is present in 45% of children with Down syndrome but also occurs as a normal variant. The separation is evident when amniotic fluid completely surrounds the great toe. This finding has also been reported antenatally in fetuses with Down syndrome.[71]

FETAL EAR MEASUREMENTS, FRONTAL LOBE DIMENSIONS, CEREBELLAR DIAMETER, AND HEART RATE

Diminished fetal ear length has been reported as a potential marker for Down syndrome. Lettieri et al. studied ultrasound-measured ear lengths in 14 second-trimester fetuses with aneuploidy of which 9 had Down syndrome. Seven of these 9 fetuses had ear lengths at or below the 10th percentile.[72] Birnholz and Farrel examined 15 aneuploid fetuses of which six had Trisomy 21. Three had ear lengths below 1 SD of the norm.[73] Gill et al. have also shown that there is a statistically significant difference between the ear sizes of normal and Trisomy 21 abortuses but that the wide range seen within each gestational age window makes this finding not diagnostically useful, as all the fetal ear measurements in fetuses with Down syndrome fell within 2 SD of the gestational age-specific norm.[74]

Frontal lobe dimensions have been reported to be smaller in fetuses with Down syndrome. Bahado-Singh and colleagues reported that 52% of Down syndrome fetuses between 16–21

weeks gestation had a frontothalamic distance of less than the 10th percentile. These investigators found that an observed/expected frontothalamic distance ratio of ≤ 0.84 had a sensitivity and specificity of 21.2% and 95.2% respectively for the detection of Down syndrome. This reflected a positive predictive value of 1.2% in a population with a 1 in 270 risk of Down syndrome.[75]

The cerebellum has been reported to be small in children and adults with Down syndrome. Hill et al. studied this potential marker for Trisomy 21 and found that the mean cerebellar diameter between 15–20 weeks gestation was unaffected by Down syndrome. This paradox is explained by the time period during which cerebellar development occurs. The cerebellar hypoplasia in neonates and adults with Down syndrome appears to occur after the second trimester and therefore this measurement is not useful to identify affected fetuses.[76]

Fetal heart rate abnormalities have also been reported to be more common in fetuses with Down syndrome when compared to normals. Martinez and coworkers in a preliminary study found that using a cutoff of a fetal heart rate in the fifth percentile, 63.6% of Down syndrome fetuses could be identified with a specificity of 96.2% and a positive predictive value of 17.9% in the population being studied.[77]

There have been sporadic cases of Trisomy 21 reported in fetuses with choroid plexus cysts. Choroid plexus cysts were initially part of the sonographic scoring index proposed by our laboratory in 1994.[3] In that study population, choroid plexus cysts were identified in 1 in 45 (2%) of fetuses with Down syndrome and in 2 in 106 (2%) normal control population. This finding prompted us to further evaluate the association of choroid plexus cysts and Down syndrome. In a study comparing the prevalence of choroid plexus cysts between fetuses with and without Trisomy 21, no statistically significant difference was identified. We concluded that choroid plexus cysts occur with similar frequency in fetuses with Trisomy 21 compared to fetuses in the general population and that the finding of an isolated choroid plexus cysts should not be used to increase the patient's calculated risk of having a fetus with Down syndrome.[78] Gupta and colleagues in a large study of choroid plexus cysts reported that the risk of Down syndrome in fetuses with choroid plexus cysts but no other abnormalities was 1 in 880.[79]

COMBINATIONS

Several studies have shown that the best sensitivity and specificity for the sonographic detection of Down syndrome can be achieved by using multiple markers in combination, rather than one individual finding.[2,3,80–82] In 1992, we developed a sonographic scoring index for the detection of fetuses at risk for Down syndrome using the following criteria: thickened nuchal fold = 2; major structural malformations = 2; and shortened femur, shortened humerus, and pyelectasis = 1 each.[2] We evaluated 5000 fetuses between 14 and 20 weeks gestation at the time of amniocentesis. There were 32 fetuses with Trisomy 21, 9 with Trisomy 18, and 2 with Trisomy 13. A sample of

588 consecutive, normal fetuses was compared with the 43 fetuses found to have autosomal trisomies. Using the previously published formulas and criteria described earlier in this chapter, a thickened nuchal fold was found in 69% of the Down syndrome fetuses and 0.34% of the normal fetuses. Short long bones (humerus and femur) were both identified in 53% of the Down syndrome fetuses and 4% of the normal fetuses. Applying the sonographic scoring system with a positive threshold of 2, we identified 81% of fetuses with Down syndrome, with a 4.4% false-positive rate. This suggested a 10- to 20-fold increase in the risk of Down syndrome for a fetus with an abnormal sonographic score, when compared with the initial risk based only on advanced maternal age.[2] This scoring system has been recently modified to include newer sonographic markers such as hyperechoic bowel = 1 and echogenic intracardiac foci = 1. In 1997, our group reported on a series of 53 fetuses with Down syndrome identified by karyotype and compared them to a control group of 177 non-Down fetuses. A score of ≥2 as a criterion for a positive test resulted in the identification of 75.4% of fetuses with Down syndrome, with a 5.7% false-positive rate. A score of ≥1 increased the sensitivity to 83%, with a false-positive rate of 17.5%. The scoring index was further expanded to include maternal age as a variable. Women greater than 40 years of age were assigned a score of 2, while women 35–39 were assigned a score of 1. Women under the age of 35 received no age-related points. The age-adjusted modification resulted in the identification of 86.8% of fetuses with Down syndrome with a false-positive rate of 27.1%. The false positives were noted to cluster in the women greater than 40 years of age, since 100% of these women scored ≥2 even if they had a normal sonogram[81] (Table 25-2).

TABLE
25-2 | **SONOGRAPHIC SCORING INDEX**

Sonographic Marker	*Score*
Major anomaly	2
Nuchal fold ≥6 mm	2
Short femur	1
Short humerus	1
Pyelectasis ≥4 mm	1
Hyperechoic bowel	1
Echogenic intracardiac focus	1
Score of ≥2 = positive test:	Sens: 75.4%
	False+: 5.7%

Added Age Adjustment

Age < 35 years	0
Age 35–39 years	1
Age ≥40 years	2
Score of ≥ 2 = positive test:	Sens: 86.8%
	False+: 27.1%
	Most false + patients
	are among older women

Vintzileos and colleagues evaluated 573 patients at increased risk for Trisomy 21 between 15 and 23 weeks gestation. A detailed evaluation of each fetus was performed including biometry and a search for structural abnormalities as well as pyelectasis, hyperechoic bowel, nuchal fold thickening, choroid plexus cysts, hypoplastic middle phalanx of the fifth digit, wide space between the first and second toe as well as a 2-vessel cord. Using 1 or more abnormal ultrasound markers, the sensitivity, specificity, and positive predictive values for Trisomy 21 were 92.8%, 86.7%, and 19.4% respectively. If 2 or more abnormal markers were present the corresponding values were 85.7%, 96.8%, and 48% respectively.[82]

CAN THE AGE-SPECIFIC RISK OF AUTOSOMAL TRISOMY BE REDUCED IN FETUSES OF OLDER WOMEN FOLLOWING A NORMAL SONOGRAM?

The assignment of risk for aneuploidy in older women was also addressed in our laboratory, by using the sonographic scoring index previously described for increasing the age-based risk of aneuploidy among patients with a score of 2. In older women, we defined a normal sonogram as a score of 0 (no abnormal findings), and a score of 1 or greater was the positivity criterion for an abnormal test. We combined the sonographic scores of all fetuses in the previously described scoring index studies[2,3] and calculated the sensitivity and specificity for a sonographic score of 1 or greater (this maximized the sensitivity at the expense of the specificity). The sensitivity of a sonographic score of ≥1 for identifying an autosomal Trisomy was 86%, and the specificity was 87%. The probability of an autosomal Trisomy at various maternal ages given a sonographic score of zero was calculated using Bayes's theorem. Using the lower limit of the 95% confidence interval for sensitivity and specificity, the probability of having a fetus with an autosomal Trisomy falls from 18.8 in 1,000 to 5.3 in 10,000 for a 40-year-old woman with a sonographic score of 0.[83]

Vintzileos and Egan reviewed numerous studies on the use of second-trimester sonography in the detection of fetuses with Trisomy 21 to establish the average sensitivity and specificity of multiple sonographic markers for the detection of fetuses with Down syndrome. They then used Bayes theorem to generate tables to adjust the risk of Trisomy 21 in the second trimester depending on the presence and absence of various sonographically detected markers. These authors concluded that in experienced hands, the second-trimester sonogram may be used to adjust the a priori risk of both high and low-risk women for Trisomy 21 and subsequently the need for invasive genetic testing.[80] In a further attempt to simplify screening for Down syndrome, these same authors examined the efficacy of long bone biometry (femur, humerus, tibia, fibula) in detecting fetuses with Down syndrome. The sensitivity of an abnormal ultrasound (one or more short bones) to detect Trisomy 21 was 63.6% with a specificity of 78.5%. Using Bayes theorem, they generated tables that allowed the readjustment of the risk of Down syndrome using biometry alone. If all

4 long bones were of normal length, the theoretical risk of Trisomy 21 was decreased by 64%. This potentially reduces the risk of a patient less than 40 years of age to less than 1:270, the risk level at which genetic amniocentesis is generally offered.[49] Vintzileos and colleagues also reported on the use of the "genetic" sonogram in guiding clinical management in patients at increased risk of Down syndrome. These investigators found that among patients at increased risk for Trisomy 21 (at least 1:274), the use of ultrasound in which one or more sonographic markers for Down syndrome was considered a positive test would result in the detection of 93% of affected fetuses with an amniocentesis rate of less than 20%.[82]

ULTRASOUND IN WOMEN AT INCREASED RISK OF DOWN SYNDROME DUE TO ABNORMAL SERUM MARKERS

Prenatal screening for Down syndrome in women under age 35 was first considered in 1984, when low maternal serum alpha-fetoprotein (MS-AFP) levels were noted in pregnancies with Down syndrome fetuses.[84,85] In 1988, Wald and coworkers showed that MS-AFP, unconjugated estriol (uE3) and human chorionic gonadotropin (hCG) were independent of maternal age and only weakly correlated with each other. The use of this multiple marker system allowed Wald and colleagues to detect 60% of fetuses with Down syndrome, with a 5% false-positive rate.[86,87] In 1994, Haddow and associates reported on the use of maternal serum markers in women over 35 years of age showing that the age-specific risk of aneuploidy can be re-evaluated and a more limited population of patients can be identified as being at increased risk for aneuploidy.[88]

Nyberg et al. addressed the utility of second-trimester sonography among women with maternal serum panels positive for Down syndrome in 1995. These investigators described 395 patients who underwent sonography on the basis of a triple-marker screen identifying their fetuses to be at ≥1:195 risk of Down syndrome between 15 and 18 weeks gestation. Three hundred and seventy four (94.7%) had normal karyotypes and 18 (4.5%) had Down syndrome. Three other patients had other chromosomal abnormalities. One or more sonographic abnormality was found in 9 in 18 fetuses with Down syndrome compared to 27 in 377 (7.2%) of other fetuses. An abnormal scan resulted in an increased risk of Down syndrome by 5.6-fold (25% from 4.5%) and a negative result reduced the risk by 45% (2.5% from 4.5%). These authors concluded that an abnormal sonogram increased the risk for Down syndrome among this group of patients, however, normal findings were less predictive of normalcy and they recommended that genetic amniocentesis be offered despite a normal scan in women at risk due to a positive maternal serum triple screen.[89]

Bahado-Singh et al. evaluated the use of a normal nuchal skin fold thickness (<6 mm) as a means of identifying euploid fetuses between 14 and 21 weeks gestation in 651 patients at increased risk for Down syndrome based on a serum marker risk of ≥1:270. These investigators reported that among 390

cases with a risk of Down syndrome of <1:100 based on serum markers and a normal nuchal thickness, there were no cases of Down syndrome. They concluded that a normal nuchal thickness significantly reduces the risk of Down syndrome.[90]

INDIVIDUAL RISK ASSESSMENT

An individual's a priori risk of carrying a fetus with Down syndrome can be modified using Bayes theorem and likelihood ratios (sensitivity/false positive).[91] A patient specific risk for Down syndrome can be estimated by multiplying the a priori risk by the likelihood ratio of a marker. Several groups have developed likelihood ratios (LR) for isolated markers as well as groupings of the markers.[92-94] The LR for markers overall and as isolated findings are presented in Table 25-3. The nuchal fold, absent nasal bone and short humerus carry high LR resulting in a substantial increase in the risk of Down syndrome, while other markers such as the echogenic intracardiac focus, pyelectasis, and a short femur have a reasonable sensitivity for Down syndrome but occur frequently enough in the euploid population so as to carry a minimally increased risk when identified as an isolated finding. The most remarkable feature of genetic sonography for risk assessment is that the absence of any sonographic markers yields a negative LR of between .2 and .4. This results in a 60–80% decrease in the risk of Down syndrome below the a priori risk.[92-101]

TABLE 25-3 | LIKELIHOOD RATIOS FOR SONOGRAPHIC MARKERS

Likelihood Ratios of Markers

Reference	93	94	93	94	101
Marker	Overall LR	Overall LR	Isolated LR	Isolated LR	Isolated LR
Nuchal fold	61	94.7	11	N/C	17
Humerus	15.3	23.5	5.1	5.8	7.5
Femur	6.1	10.1	1.5	1.2	2.7
Bowel	33.8	14.4	6.7	N/C	6.1
EIF	6.3	8	1.8	1.4	2.8
Pyelectasis	5.2	8.8	1.5	1.5	1.9
Anomaly		22		3.3	

Cluster of Markers

Reference	93	94
# of Marker	LR	LR
0	0.36	0.2
1	2	1.6
2	9.7	5.9
3	115.2	90.6

For example, a patient with a risk of 1:100 for Down syndrome who has a genetic sonogram in which no markers are identified (LR .4) will have at risk reduction to 1:250. A similar patient with an a priori risk of 1:100 who is identified of having an echogenic intracardiac focus (LR 1.4) will have a revised risk of at least 1:70. Although this is not a marked increase in risk above the a priori risk, the patient's individual risk has been increased when compared to the same woman whose fetus had no markers.

In low-risk women, the presence of a thickened nuchal fold or an absent nasal bone may increase the risk of Down syndrome significantly enough to offer amniocentesis should prenatal diagnosis be desired. The presence of isolated minor markers such as an echogenic intracardiac focus or short femur would tend not to increase the risk of Down syndrome above the commonly accepted threshold for offering amniocentesis and may not even need to be discussed with the patient.[102] Clusters of markers appear to have more significance than individual markers.

The benefit of the individual risk assessment is that it allows the parents to decide based on their individual risk assessment, whether or not to pursue invasive testing to obtain a definitive karyotype.

TRISOMY 18: EDWARD SYNDROME

Trisomy 18 is the second most common multiple malformation syndrome with an incidence of .64 in 1,000 in the mid trimester and 0.16 in 1,000 live births.[103] Like other trisomies, the incidence of Trisomy 18 increases with advancing maternal age. At age 35, the risk of Trisomy 18 in the mid trimester is estimated at 1 in 1,000 and increases to 3.3 in 1,000 at age 40 and up to 10.6 in 1,000 at age 45.[1]

Babies born with Edwards syndrome have a limited capacity for survival. Fifty percent of affected newborns die within the first week and only 5–10% survive beyond the first year of life. In cases where survival occurs, the individuals are severely mentally and physically handicapped.[104] Over 130 different abnormalities have been reported in individuals with Trisomy 18 and include growth deficiency, cardiac defects, abdominal wall defects, abnormalities of the extremities with clenched hands and a tendency for overlapping the index finger over the third finger and the fifth finger over the fourth finger, abnormal feet, renal abnormalities, craniofacial abnormalities such as micrognathia, as well as many other structural defects.

SONOGRAPHY

The large number of structural defects in affected individuals lends itself to sonographic identification during the mid trimester of pregnancy. (Figs. 25-6 to 25-11). In 1988, we described the sonographic features of fifteen fetuses with Trisomy 18. Twelve of these 15 fetuses (80%) had structural malformations warranting karyotypic evaluation, including diaphrag-

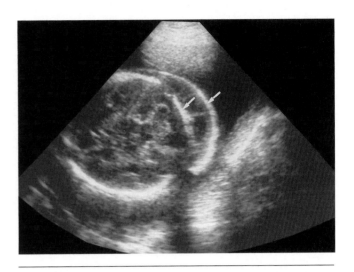

FIGURE 25-6 Trisomy 18. Modified transverse view of the fetal head, showing the posterior fossa and the nuchal area. Note the thickened nuchal fold containing multiple cystic hygromas (arrows).

matic hernias, congenital heart defects, and abnormalities of the extremities. The 3 fetuses that were not identified as being anomalous were scanned early in gestation (16–17 weeks).[5] In 1990, our group reported a series of 26 consecutive fetuses with Trisomy 18 scanned between 13.5 and 36 weeks gestation and was able to identify 20 in 26 (77%) as having major structural abnormalities suggestive of aneuploidy. The abnormalities included congenital heart defects, neural tube defects, diaphragmatic hernia, omphalocele, hydrocephalus, cystic hygroma, and abnormally fisted hands.[105] Using a sonographic scoring index with a positivity threshold of 2 (see Down syndrome discussion), we were able to detect 85–100% of fetuses with Trisomy 18.[2,3] The cases of Trisomy 18 not identified in our experience were scanned at 15 weeks gestation when a complete structural survey was not feasible.

Nyberg et al. reviewed the sonographic features of 47 consecutive fetuses with Trisomy 18. One or more structural abnormalities were identified in 39 in 47 (83%) of fetuses overall. The identification of abnormalities increased with gestational age as 72% of fetuses examined between 14–24 weeks were identified as abnormal versus 100% of fetuses examined after 24 weeks gestation. The individual abnormalities most often seen in this study included intrauterine growth retardation (51%), cardiac defects (38%), cystic hygromas/nuchal thickening (19%), prominent cisterna magna (19%), omphalocele (21%), neural tube defect (17%), renal abnormalities (15%), single umbilical artery (13%), clubbed or rocker-bottom feet (21%) and clenched hands (19%).[7]

Abnormalities of the cerebellum and cisterna magna have been reported as a feature of fetuses with Trisomy 18.[5,7,106–109] This finding appears to be related to gestational age as pointed out by Nyberg et al. in 1993, only 1 of 30 (3%) fetuses with Trisomy 18 was noted to have an "enlarged" cisterna magna (>9 mm) before 24 weeks gestation compared to 8 in

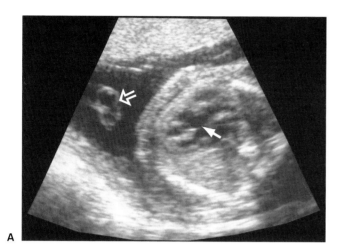
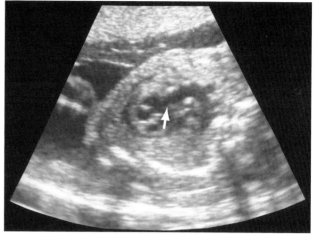

FIGURE 25-7 Trisomy 18. (**A**) Four-chamber view of the heart, showing a large VSD (arrow). Note is made also of the two-vessel cord (open arrow). (**B**) Longitudinal view of the same fetal heart, showing a large VSD (arrow) with an overriding aorta.

19 (44%) examined after 24 weeks.[7] This likely reflects increasing atrophy of the cerebellum with advancing age and may explain the conflicting reports by Watson et al., who evaluated 585 fetuses at increased risk for aneuploidy between 14–21 weeks and found that each of the 28 fetuses with aneuploidy had normal measurements of the cisterna magna.[110]

A strawberry-shaped skull (flattening of the occiput with pointing of the frontal bones) was described by Nicolaides and colleagues as a feature of Trisomy 18. They reported a group of 2,086 fetuses at high risk for aneuploidy and identified 54 fetuses with a strawberry-shaped head (plus additional malfor-

mations) and found that 81% of these fetuses had Trisomy 18. In this series, an additional 40 fetuses with Trisomy 18 did not exhibit this finding.[111]

Nyberg et al. identified a cardiac defect in 14% of fetuses with Trisomy 18 prior to 24 weeks and in 78% scanned after 24 weeks gestation.[7] Dicke et al. reported a similar experience detecting cardiac defects in trisomic fetuses, they identified 14% of heart defects before 22 weeks versus 75% after 22 weeks gestation.[112] This discrepancy of detection of cardiac defects in the second versus the third trimester indicated the difficulties in the early sonographic identification of fetuses with anomalous hearts.

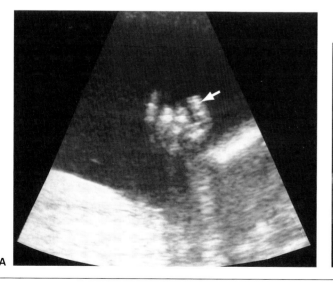
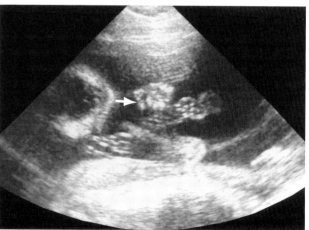

FIGURE 25-8 Trisomy 18. Two different fetuses with trisomy 18, showing the characteristic positioning of the hand with a clenched fist and overlapping index finger (arrow = index finger).

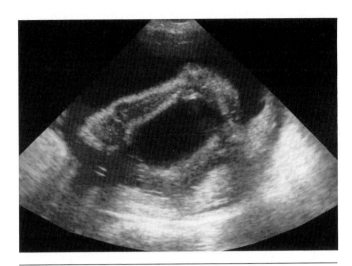

FIGURE 25-9 Trisomy 18. Longitudinal view of the lower extremities, showing a clubbed foot.

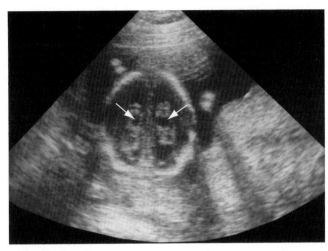

FIGURE 25-11 Trisomy 18. Transverse view of the fetal head through the level of the choroid plexes, showing multiple choroid plexus cysts (arrows) in a fetus with Trisomy 18.

Omphaloceles are a feature of Trisomy 18 and 70% of these defects were of the bowel-only type. This is consistent with other studies in the literature that have shown a higher incidence of karyotypic abnormalities omphaloceles which contain only bowel compared with those in which the liver is involved.[113,114]

Abnormalities of the hands and feet such as clenched hands, rocker-bottom feet, clubfeet, radial ray defects, and limb reduction defects have been reported with Trisomy 18.[5,7,115] Umbilical cord cysts are also associated with Trisomy 18.[116–118]

The sonographic findings observed in fetuses with Trisomy 18 vary with gestational age. As expected, cystic hygromas are seen more frequently in the early mid trimester while cardiac defects and growth retardation were more of-

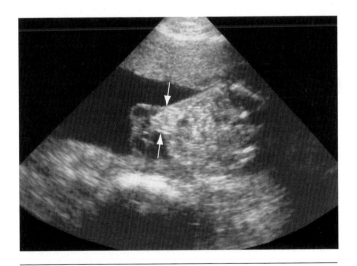

FIGURE 25-10 Trisomy 18. View of the cord insertion on the fetus, showing a small bowel-containing omphalocele (arrows).

ten a third-trimester diagnosis. In Nyberg's study, intrauterine growth retardation was seen in 28% of affected fetuses scanned at less than 24 weeks and in 89% of those evaluated in the third trimester. Growth retardation in combination with polyhydramnios was seen in 21% of fetuses with Trisomy 18.[7] Dicke and Crane reported that growth delay was evident in 59% of fetuses with Trisomy 18 in the mid trimester of pregnancy and became more pronounced with advancing gestational age.[112] In a study of 458 growth-restricted fetuses, Snijders et al. reported a 19% rate of aneuploidy. The most common chromosomal abnormality seen after 26 weeks gestation was Trisomy 18, accounting for 46% of the abnormal karyotypes.[118] Carlson et al. reported that fetal hydramnios, abnormal hand posturing, and any other anomaly were highly predictive of this autosomal trisomy.[119]

CHOROID PLEXUS CYSTS

The fetal choroid plexus are echogenic structures essentially filling the lateral ventricles and are readily visualized during second-trimester sonography. Choroid plexus cysts are thought to be the result of folding of the neuroepithelium, resulting in trapping of secretory products and desquamated cells.[120] Discrete echolucencies within the choroid plexus occur in 0.18–3.6% of the normal obstetrical population and are generally most common in the mid trimester of pregnancy, usually resolving spontaneously by 24–26 weeks gestation. These cysts usually are less than 10 mm in diameter and may be unilateral or bilateral. They are almost always asymptomatic and have been reported postnatally, frequently as an incidental finding at autopsy in all age groups.[121–140]

Chudleigh et al. first described the sonographic findings of choroid plexus cysts in the mid trimester of pregnancy in 1984 and suggested that these were benign entities that usually resolved spontaneously.[121] In 1986, Nicolaides and colleagues first demonstrated the association between choroid plexus cysts and Trisomy 18.[122] Since then, there have been multiple reports on the significance of choroid plexus cysts and recommendations for clinical management have remained controversial.[122–139]

Fitzsimmons et al. studied the brains of abortuses with Trisomy 18 and found the prevalence of choroid plexus cysts in the mid trimester was 80%. This however was an in vitro study in which the brain of each fetus was examined directly with a high frequency transducer that likely would yield a much higher incidence than that identified in a live patient during the second trimester of pregnancy.[130]

The association between choroid plexus cysts and Trisomy 18 has been clearly established in vivo as well. Choroid plexus cysts can be sonographically identified in approximately 30% of fetuses with Trisomy 18 during the mid trimester.[5,7,105] The multitude of structural abnormalities present in fetuses with Trisomy 18 leads to ready sonographic diagnosis and karyotypic evaluation is not controversial in the fetus with choroid plexus cysts other structural findings. The management of patients with isolated choroid plexus cysts has been contentious.

Our group described a series of 26 consecutive fetuses with Trisomy 18 of whom 77% were identified as having a major structural malformation. Using the incidence of choroid plexus cysts in the second-trimester fetal population as 1% and given an incidence of Trisomy 18 of 3 in 10,000, we calculated that there would be one fetus with Trisomy 18 for every 477 normal fetuses with isolated choroid plexus cysts. Thus, we concluded that if amniocentesis was done on all mid-trimester fetuses with isolated choroid plexus cysts, 2 normal fetuses would be lost for every fetus with Trisomy 18 identified.[105] Other investigators have also felt that the risk of aneuploidy is not high enough to warrant amniocentesis in cases of isolated choroid plexus cysts.[79,123,125,127,131]

On the other hand, several authors have reported that isolated choroid plexus cysts were associated with a significant risk of aneuploidy. Platt et al. reported on 7,350 women who underwent sonographic evaluation in the mid trimester of pregnancy. Fetal choroid plexus cysts were identified in 71 (0.96%) and 62 of these patients underwent genetic amniocentesis resulting in 4 (6.4%) abnormal karyotypes. Three fetuses were noted to have Trisomy 18 and 1 was found to have Trisomy 21. Despite the fact that all 4 of these fetuses had other sonographic findings in addition to the choroid plexus cysts which were correctly identified prenatally, the authors concluded that the sonographic finding in one fetus was a subtle cardiac defect and therefore offering cytogenetic analysis to patients with isolated choroid plexus cysts to detect aneuploidy was warranted.[134] Kupferminc et al. studied 9,100 women undergoing mid trimester evaluation and identified choroid plexus cysts in 102 (1.1%) fetuses. Four fetuses had other structural abnormalities, 2 of which had Trisomy 18 and 1 with an unbalanced translocation. The fourth was karyotypically normal. Of the remaining 98 fetuses with isolated choroid plexus cysts, there were 4 fetuses with abnormal karyotypes. One had Trisomy 18 and 3 had Trisomy 21. The rate of aneuploidy with isolated choroid plexus cysts in this study was 4.1% leading the authors to recommend amniocentesis for isolated choroid plexus cysts.[135] Other investigators have also felt the need to recommend karyotype in the setting of isolated choroid plexus cysts.[128,136]

In 1995, Gross et al. performed a metaanalysis on a series of patients prospectively evaluated for choroid plexus cysts in their own institution and the currently available prospective series (with >10 cases of choroid plexus cysts) to estimate the positive predictive value of isolated choroid plexus cysts for Trisomy 18. Seventy-four cases of isolated choroid plexus cysts were identified in their unit, none of which had Trisomy 18. They also identified 748 fetuses from the literature with isolated choroid plexus cysts and found two with Trisomy 18 (1/374). To derive a positive predictive value of isolated choroid plexus cysts for Trisomy 18, they reviewed the available literature and found a total of 50 fetuses with Trisomy 18 who were scanned in the mid trimester. Twelve of 50 (24%) had no other sonographic findings and of these 12, 3 had isolated choroid plexus cysts resulting in a sensitivity of 25%. The prevalence of Trisomy 18 in the mid trimester was taken from the literature to be 1 in 2,641. The prevalence of choroid plexus cysts in the population was 0.95% based on multiple studies and a positive predictive value of 1:390 was obtained. The results were similar for the metaanalysis and the calculated positive predictive value, leading these authors to conclude that the available data does not support the routine offering of invasive prenatal cytogenetic testing in cases of isolated choroid plexus cysts.[133]

Gupta and colleagues in 1995, reported a prospective study on an unselected population and identified 524 fetuses with choroid plexus cysts. These cases were then amalgamated and analyzed with 1,361 cases from prospective studies reported in the literature as well as an additional 71 unpublished cases from a 2-year prospective study done elsewhere. The mean prevalence of choroid plexus cysts in this population was 0.53%. The risk of an abnormal karyotype in the presence of choroid plexus cysts and other sonographically detected abnormalities was 1:3. In the setting of isolated choroid plexus cysts, the risk of chromosomal abnormalities was 1:150 (95% CI 1:85–1:261). The aneuploidies reported were Trisomy 18 (76%), Trisomy 21 (17%), and 7% Klinefelters or Triploidy. These authors concluded that the predictive value of isolated choroid plexus cysts for aneuploidy is low when no other abnormalities are seen and that the sonographic finding of a choroid plexus cysts should be an indication for a detailed ultrasound assessment and correlation with clinical circumstance such as results of maternal serum marker screening, age, and other factors should be considered.[79]

Some investigators have suggested that the larger cysts are more predictive of aneuploidy while others caution about not ignoring smaller cysts. Several authors have also expressed concern about the laterality of the findings and complexity of the appearance of the choroids.[138–140] Many investigators, including us have not found cyst size or laterality to be helpful in distinguishing affected fetuses from normals.[79,131,132] Importantly, resolution of choroid plexus cysts does not necessarily reflect a normal karyotype.[134]

TRISOMY 13: PATAU SYNDROME

Patau et al. first recognized Trisomy 13 as being due to an extra D1 chromosome in 1960.[141] The incidence of Trisomy 13 in liveborns is approximately 1 in 12,000.[142] As with the other Trisomy syndromes, the incidence increases with advancing maternal age. Liveborns with Trisomy 13 are fraught with a multitude of structural abnormalities and are severely retarded. Various degrees of forebrain defects are common as are ocular anomalies. Facial and heart defects as well as abnormal extremities are common. Forty-five percent of liveborns die in the first month and 90% do not survive beyond 6 months of age. Rarely survival is more long term.[143]

SONOGRAPHY

Due to the plethora of structural abnormalities that are often apparent sonographically, recent studies have reported a 91–100% detection rate for this syndrome.[3,5,6,144] (Figs. 25-12 to 25-17) In 1986, we described the sonographic features of 6 fetuses with Trisomy 13. Five of these 6 fetuses had holoprosencephaly and all 6 had severely malformed faces. The abnormalities seen included large facial clefts, hypotelorism, cyclopia, and microcephaly.[4] Subsequently we reported 9 additional cases of Trisomy 13 with similar findings as well as cardiac defects, neural tube defects, polycystic kidneys, and

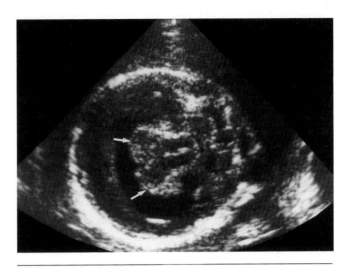

FIGURE 25-13 Trisomy 13. View of the fetal head in a late second-trimester fetus, showing holoprosencephaly. Note the fused thalami (arrows) and the monoventricle directly above it.

anomalies of the extremities such as polydactyly and clubbed feet.[5]

Lehman et al. reported a series of 33 consecutive fetuses with Trisomy 13 and found 1 or more structural abnormalities in 30 (91%). Nineteen of 33 (39%) had central nervous system abnormalities with holoprosencephaly being the most common finding, present in 13 (39%) of affected fetuses. An enlarged cisterna magna including a Dandy-Walker variant was seen in five of 33 affected fetuses (15%). Lateral ventricular enlargement (10–12 mm) was present in 9% of fetuses. Microcephaly was diagnosed by means of sonography in 4 in 33 fetuses (12%) but an additional 4 cases were diagnosed at autopsy but were

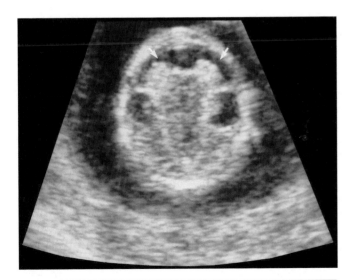

FIGURE 25-12 Trisomy 13. Coronal view through the fetal head of a late first-trimester fetus with holoprosencephaly. Note the monoventricle (arrows) and the fused thalami beneath it.

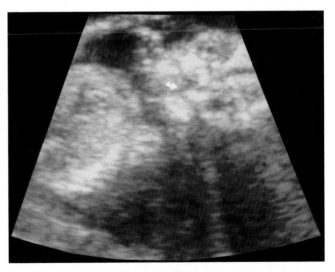

FIGURE 25-14 Trisomy 13. Coronal view of the midface of an early second-trimester fetus with a midfacial cleft (arrow) in a fetus with holoprosencephaly.

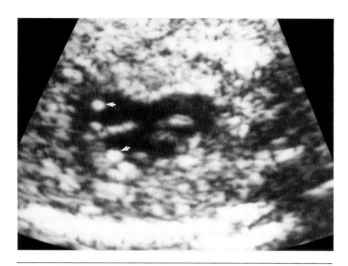

FIGURE 25-15 Trisomy 13. Long axis view of the fetal heart in the second trimester, showing a large VSD (arrow) with an overriding aorta. Note the bright papillary muscles in the ventricles.

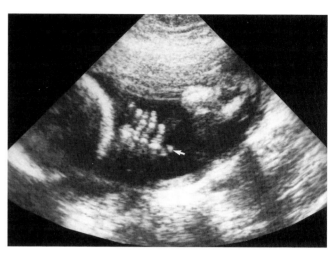

FIGURE 25-17 Trisomy 13. View of the fetal hand of a fetus with Trisomy 13, showing postaxial polydactyly (arrow).

not evident by sonography. The authors noted an association between CNS findings and a propensity for facial anomalies. Cleft lip and palate was the most common facial abnormality and was seen in 45% (15/33) of affected fetuses. Slightly greater than half of fetuses with facial clefts had midline clefts and the others had bilateral cleft lip and palate. Midfacial hypoplasia was observed in many fetuses with facial clefting. Cystic hygroma and nuchal edema were identified in 21% of affected fetuses in the study and in 28% of those examined prior to 18 weeks gestation.

Structural cardiac anomalies were identified in 48% of affected fetuses. In addition, an echogenic intracardiac focus was noted in 30% of fetuses with Trisomy 13. Renal abnormalities were identified in 33% of affected fetuses and most

often consisted echogenic renal parenchyma. The overall size of the kidney was large in a majority of fetuses with renal anomalies. Abdominal wall abnormalities were seen in 18% of fetuses and most of these were omphalocele, two thirds of which contained bowel only. Abnormalities of the extremities were seen in one third of fetuses. These included polydactyly, clubbed or rocker-bottom feet and persistently clenched hands or overlapping digits.

Growth restriction was identified in 16 in 33 fetuses (48%) including 12 in 15 (80%) examined after 20 weeks gestation. Abnormal amniotic fluid volume was seen in 28% of affected pregnancies including the unusual combination of growth retardation and polyhydramnios in 4 pregnancies.[6]

Umbilical cord cysts have also been reported as associated with Trisomy 13.[145,146]

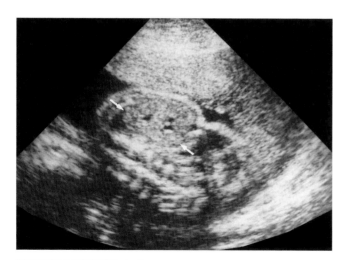

FIGURE 25-16 Trisomy 13. Longitudinal view of the fetal kidney in a fetus with Trisomy 13, showing a large and echogenic kidney (arrows).

TRIPLOIDY

Triploidy is a complete extra set of chromosomes and is estimated to occur in approximately 1–2% of conceptuses. Most triploid conceptions are spontaneously aborted. The prevalence of Triploidy between 16–20 weeks has been reported as 1:5,000 pregnancies.[147] The extra set of chromosomes is often paternally derived (73%) and most commonly occurs from a double fertilization (dispermy) although fertilization with a diploid sperm (diandry) is also seen. On occasion, Triploidy may result of fertilization of a diploid egg (digyny).[148] The extra haploid set gives a total of 69 chromosomes (XXX, XXY, XYY). Unlike trisomic fetuses, Triploidy does not seem to be associated with advanced maternal age.

The survival of a fetus with Triploidy beyond 20 weeks gestation is rare and most livebirths die within the first few days of life although survival to 10.5 months has been reported.[149,150]

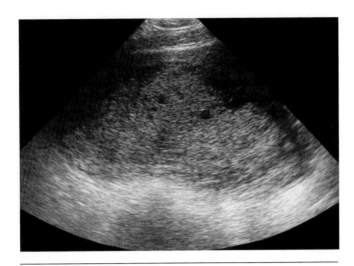

FIGURE 25-18 Triploidy. Longitudinal view of an enlarged, thickened placenta in a second-trimester pregnancy with a partial mole and a karyotype of triploidy.

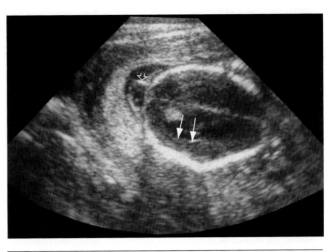

FIGURE 25-20 Triploidy. Transverse view through the fetal head, showing a posterior midline encephalocele (open arrow). The closed arrow shows the lateral wall of the lateral ventricle in this fetus with ventriculomegaly.

Fetuses with triploidy surviving into the midtrimester have a multitude of structural malformations and asymmetric growth restriction.[151–155] (Figs. 25-18 to 25-20)

Placental pathologic studies on first- and second-trimester abortuses have shown that 60–80% have hydatidiform changes.[156] Paternal triploid origin is almost always associated with these placental changes while Triploidy on the basis of digyny is usually associated with normal placentation.[148] Triploidy results in a variety of maternal complications including early onset pre-eclampsia, bilateral multicystic ovaries, hyperemesis gravidarum, and persistent trophoblastic disease.[157,158]

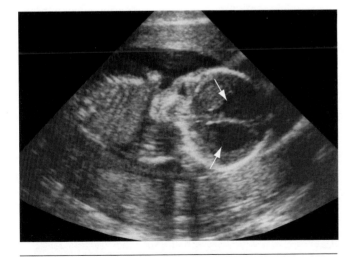

FIGURE 25-19 Triploidy. Coronal view of the fetal head and body of a fetus with triploidy, showing bilateral ventriculomegaly (arrows). Also note that the fetal body is considerably smaller than anticipated for the size of the fetal head, consistent with early, asymmetrical intrauterine growth restriction.

In 1985, Crane et al. reported on the features of three triploid fetuses. They noted early-onset fetal growth retardation, body asymmetry with relative macrocephaly and an elevated head: abdominal circumference ratio, hydrocephalus, oligohydramnios, and an abnormally large and/or hydropic placenta.[151] Jauniaux and colleagues described 70 cases of Triploidy scanned between 13 and 29 weeks gestation. Anatomic defects were found in 92.9% of cases with abnormalities of the hands being the most frequent finding occurring in 34/70 (52.3%) of cases. The majority of fetuses with abnormal hand (31/34) findings had syndactyly of the third and fourth fingers. Cerebral ventriculomegaly was identified in 24/70 cases (36.9%). Cardiac defects were detected in 22/70 fetuses (33.8%) and these were primarily atrioventricular defects. Seventeen (26.2%) of 70 fetuses had micrognathia. Placental molar changes were seen in 28.6% of affected pregnancies and amniotic fluid volume was decreased in 31/70 (44.2%). Karyotypes were XXX in 71.4% and XXY in 28.6% of triploid fetuses. Asymmetric growth restriction was seen in 45 cases (72%) with measurements available and each of these fetuses had a sonographically normal appearing placenta. An abnormally high uterine artery resistance index was found in half the cases investigated leading the authors to suggest an abnormal placentation phenomenon. Interestingly, there was no difference in uterine artery RI between triploid pregnancies with and without partial mole.[159] These same investigators addressed the timing in gestation when most fetuses with triploidy can be detected. In a large retrospective series of singleton pregnancies scanned between 10 and 14 weeks' gestation, they were theoretically able to identify 88.9% of triploidies, based on sonographic features and elevated hCG levels. Congenital abnormalities were identified in 44.4% of fetuses within this gestational age window and were major defects such as holoprosencephaly, exomphalos, and posterior fossa cysts. Almost two thirds of the fetuses (62.5%) showed evidence of early

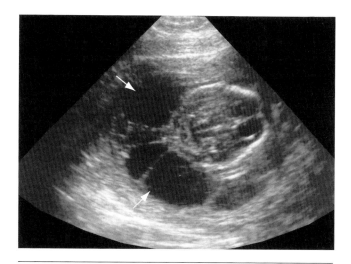

FIGURE 25-21 Turner syndrome. Transverse view through the fetal head, showing large nuchal septate cystic hygromas (arrows).

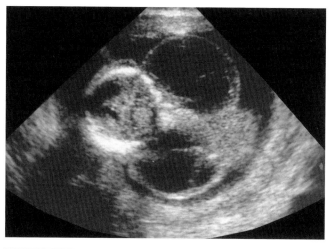

FIGURE 25-22 Turner syndrome. Coronal view of the fetal head and neck, showing the large, paired, septate cystic hygromas, bilaterally.

growth delay, and 66.7% had a fetal nuchal lucency. Thirty-three percent of fetuses had a molar placenta, and 84.6% had elevated gonadotropin levels. Interestingly, there was a similar gonadotropin distribution in molar and nonmolar triploidies.[160]

Snijders et al. in a study of 132 growth retarded fetuses scanned at less than 26 weeks gestation found 50 (38%) were karyotypically abnormal, the most common chromosomal abnormality being Triploidy (29/50) accounting for 58% of abnormal karyotypes.[118]

45 XO: TURNER SYNDROME

Turner described a syndrome of sexual infantilism, short stature, webbing of the neck, and cubitus valgus in 1938.[161] In 1959, Ford et al. recognized the 45 X chromosomal comple-ment, which is usually due to loss of the paternal X chromosome and is unrelated to maternal age.[162] Ninety-five percent of conceptuses with monosomy for the X chromosome are spontaneously aborted. Turner syndrome occurs in approximately 1:2,000 to 1:5,000 live births and 40% of those born are mosaic or have a variant chromosome pattern.[163] The lethal type of Turner syndrome seen in the mid trimester of pregnancy generally presents with large septated cystic hygromas, total body lymphedema, pleural effusions, ascites, and cardiac defects[164–167] (Figs. 25-21 to 25-24).

Fetal cystic hygromas are congenital malformations of the lymphatic system and appear as sacular septated fluid collections most often surrounding the fetal occiput and neck. Numerous studies have reported a wide range in the incidence of aneuploidy associated with cystic hygroma ranging from 46–90%.[164] Fetuses with hydrops in addition to the nuchal hygromas have the highest association with aneuploidy

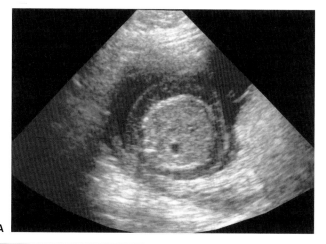

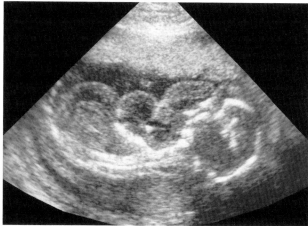

FIGURE 25-23 Turner syndrome. (**A**) Transverse view of the fetal abdomen, showing marked edema of the soft tissues, consistent with lymphangiectasia. (**B**) Longitudinal view of a fetus with severe lymphangiectasia of the body and limbs.

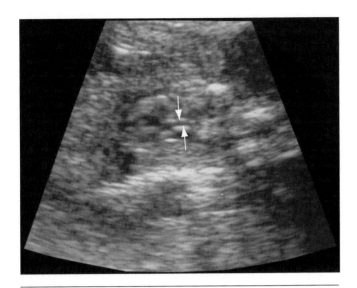

FIGURE 25-24 Turner syndrome. Long axis view of the fetal heart in a fetus with Turner syndrome showing a small aorta, consistent with coarctation of the aorta (arrow = aorta).

compared to those with isolated nuchal edema and tend to die in utero.[165]

Chervenak et al. reported a series of second-trimester fetuses with large cystic hygromas and found that 73% had karyotypes consistent with Turner syndrome.[166] Azar and coworkers reported an incidence of chromosomal defects of 75% in fetuses with bilateral dorsal septated nuchal cervical hygromata, the most common being Turner syndrome (94%).[167] Although many second-trimester fetuses with cystic hygromas have Turner syndrome, other karyotypic abnormalities including Trisomy 21, Trisomy 18, Trisomy 13, Triploidy, and Klinefelter have also been reported in association with cystic hygroma. In general, cystic hygromas in fetuses with Turner syndrome are larger than those seen with other karyotypic abnormalities and these fetuses may also have generalized lymphedema characterized by a "space suit" appearance.

Cardiac abnormalities such as coarctation of the aorta may be visualized in fetuses with Turner syndrome. Azar reported a strong association between Turner syndrome and congenital heart defects (48%). In addition, 19% of affected fetuses had renal abnormalities. Short stature is a hallmark feature of people with Turner syndrome and this same group has reported a decreased femur length to biparietal diameter ratio in 90% of affected fetuses.[167]

CONCLUSION

In the last 10 years, ultrasound has emerged as a powerful tool for identifying fetuses with certain abnormal chromosome complements. The use of a targeted ultrasound provides a unique opportunity to refine a patient's age-specific risk for aneuploidy thus allowing the detection of a greater number of karyotypically abnormal fetuses with fewer invasive procedures and subsequently the loss of fewer normal fetuses.

References

1. Hook EB, Cross PK, Schreinemachers DM. Chromosomal abnormality rates at amniocentesis and in live-born infants. *J Am Med Assoc.* 1983;249:2034–2038.
2. Benacerraf BR, Neuberg D, Bromley B, et al. Sonographic scoring index for prenatal detection of chromosomal abnormalities. *J Ultrasound Med.* 1992;11:449–458.
3. Benacerraf BR, Nadel A, Bromley B. Identification of second trimester fetuses with autosomal trisomy by use of a sonographic scoring index. *Radiology.* 1994;193:135–140.
4. Benacerraf BR, Frigoletto Jr. FD, Greene MF. Abnormal facial features and extremities in human trisomy syndromes: prenatal US appearance. *Radiology.* 1986;159:243–246.
5. Benacerraf B, Miller W, Frigoletto F. Sonographic detection of fetuses with trisomies 13 and 18: accuracy and limitations. *Am J Obstet Gynecol.* 1988;158:404–409.
6. Lehman CD, Nyberg DA, Winter III TC, et al. Trisomy 13 syndrome: prenatal US findings in a review of 33 cases. *Radiology.* 1995;194:217–222.
7. Nyberg DA, Kramer D, Resta RG, et al. Prenatal sonographic findings in trisomy 18: review of 47 cases. *J Ultrasound Med.* 1993;2:103–113.
8. Lejeune J, Turpin R, Gautier M. Le mongolisme, premier example d'aberration autosomique humaine. *Ann Genet.* 1959;1:41–49.
9. Cruikshank DP, Varner MW, Cruikshank JE, et al. Midtrimester amniocentesis: an analysis of 923 cases with neonatal follow-up. *Am J Obstet Gynecol.* 1983;146:204.
10. Benacerraf BR, Barss VA, Laboda LA. A sonographic sign for the detection in the second trimester of the fetus with Down syndrome. *Am J Obstet Gynecol.* 1985;151:1078–1079.
11. Benacerraf BR, Frigoletto Jr. FD, Laboda LA. Sonographic diagnosis of Down syndrome in the second trimester. *Am J Obstet Gynecol.* 1985;153:49–52.
12. Benacerraf BR, Frigoletto Jr. FD. Soft tissue nuchal fold in the second trimester fetus: standards for normal measurements compared to the fetus with Down syndrome. *Am J Obstet Gynecol.* 1987;157:1146–1149.
13. Benacerraf BR, Frigoletto Jr. FD, Cramer DW. Down syndrome: sonographic sign for diagnosis in the second trimester fetus. *Radiology.* 1987;163:811–813.
14. Lynch L, Berkowitz GS, Chitkara U, et al. Ultrasound detection of Down syndrome: is it really possible? *Obstet Gynecol.* 1989;73:267–270.
15. Ginsberg N, Cadkin A, Pergament E, et al. Ultrasonographic detection of the second trimester fetus with trisomy 18 and trisomy 21. *Am J Obstet Gynecol.* 1990;163:1186–1190.
16. Crane JP, Gray DL. Sonographically measured nuchal skin fold thickness as a screening tool for Down syndrome: results of a prospective clinical trial. *Obstet Gynecol.* 1991;77:533–536.
17. Grandjean H, Sarramon MF. Sonographic measurement of nuchal skin fold thickness or detection of Down syndrome in the second trimester fetus: a multicenter prospective study. The AFDPHE Study Group. Association Francaise pour le Depistage et la Prenvention des Handicaps de l'Enfant. *Obstet Gynecol.* 1995;85:103–106.
18. Watson WJ, Miller RC, Menard K, et al. Ultrasonographic measurement of fetal nuchal skin to screen for chromosomal abnormalities. *Am J Obstet Gynecol.* 1994;170:583–586.

19. Borrell A, Costa D, Martinez JM, et al. Early midtrimester fetal nuchal thickness: effectiveness as a marker of Down syndrome. *Am J Obstet Gynecol.* 1996;175:45–49.

20. Kirk JS, Comstock CH, Fassnacht MA, et al. Routine measurement of nuchal thickness in the second trimester. *J Matern Fetal Med.* 1992;1:82–86.

21. Nyberg DA, Resta RG, Luthy DA, et al. Prenatal sonographic findings of Down syndrome: review of 94 cases. *Obstet Gynecol.* 1990;76:370–377.

22. Gray DL, Crane JP. Optimal nuchal skin fold thresholds based on gestational age for prenatal detection of Down syndrome. *Am J Obstet Gynecol.* 1994;171:1282–1286.

23. Benacerraf BR, Laboda LA, Frigoletto Jr. FD. Thickened nuchal-fold in fetuses not at risk for aneuploidy. *Radiology.* 1992;184:239–242.

24. Bromley B, Benacerraf BR. The resolving nuchal fold in second trimester fetuses: not necessarily reassuring. *J Ultrasound Med.* 1995;14:253–255.

25. Down LJ. Observations on an ethnic classification of idiots. *Clinical Lectures and Reports, London Hospital.* 1866;3:259–262.

26. Bromley B, Lieberman E, Shipp T, et al. Fetal nose bone length: a marker for Down syndrome in the second trimester. *J Ultrasound Med.* 2002;21:1387–1394.

27. Vintzileos A, Walters C, Yeo L. Absent nasal bone in the prenatal detection of fetuses with trisomy 21 in a high-risk population. *Obstet Gynecol.* 2003;101:905–908.

28. Lockwood C, Benacerraf B, Krinsky A, et al. A sonographic screening method for Down syndrome. *Am J Obstet Gynecol.* 1987;157:803–808.

29. Benacerraf BR, Gelman R, Frigoletto Jr. FD. Sonographic identification of second trimester fetuses with Down syndrome. *N Engl J Med.* 1987;317:1371–1376.

30. Benacerraf BR, Cnaan A, Gelman R, et al. Can sonographers reliably identify anatomy features associated with Down syndrome? *Radiology.* 1989;173:377–380.

31. Hill LM, Guzick D, Belfar RL, et al. The current role of sonography in the detection of Down syndrome. *Obstet Gynecol.* 1989;74:620–623.

32. Brumfield CG, Hauth JC, Cloud GA, et al. Sonographic measurements and ratios in fetuses with Down syndrome. *Obstet Gynecol.* 1989;73:644–646.

33. Dicke JM, Gray DL, Songster GS, et al. Fetal biometry as a screening tool for the detection of chromosomally abnormal pregnancies. *Obstet Gynecol.* 1989;74:726–729.

34. Grist TM, Fuller RW, Albiez KL, et al. Femur length in ultrasound prediction of trisomy 21 and other chromosome abnormalities. *Radiology.* 1990;174:837–839.

35. LaFollette L, Filly RA, Anderson R, et al. Fetal femur length to detect trisomy 21. *J Ultrasound Med.* 1989;8:657–660.

36. Marquette GP, Boucher M, Desrochers M, et al. Screening for trisomy 21 with ultrasonographic determination of biparietal diameter/femur length ratio. *Am J Obstet Gynecol.* 1990;163:1604–1605.

37. Shah YG, Eckl CJ, Stinson SK, et al. Biparietal diameter/femur length ratio, cephalic index and femur length measurements: not reliable screening techniques for Down syndrome. *Obstet Gynecol.* 1990;75:186–188.

38. Nyberg DA, Resta RG, Hickok DE, et al. Femur length shortening in the detection of Down syndrome: is prenatal screening feasible? *Am J Obstet Gynecol.* 1990;162:1247–1252.

39. Hadlock FP, Harrist RB, Martinez-Poyer J. Fetal body ratios in second trimester: a useful tool for identifying chromosomal abnormalities? *J Ultrasound Med.* 1992;11:81–85.

40. Peters MT, Lockwood CJ, Miller WA. The efficacy of fetal sonographic biometry in Down syndrome screening. *Am J Obstet Gynecol.* 1989;161:297–300.

41. Grandjean H, Sarramon M. Femur/foot length ratio for detection of Down syndrome; results of a multicenter prospective study. *Am Obstet Gynecol.* 1995;173:16–19.

42. FitzSimmons J, Droste S, Shepard TH, et al. Long-bone growth in fetuses with Down syndrome. *Am J Obstet Gynecol.* 1989;161:1174–1177.

43. Benacerraf BR, Neuberg D, Frigoletto Jr. FD. Humeral shortening in second trimester fetuses with Down syndrome. *Obstet Gynecol.* 1991;77:223–227.

44. Rodis JF, Vintzileos AM, Fleming AD, et al. Comparison of humerus length with femur length in fetuses with Down syndrome. *Am J Obstet Gynecol.* 1991;165:1051–1056.

45. Rotmensch S, Luo JS, Liberati M, et al. Fetal humeral length to detect Down syndrome. *Am J Obstet Gynecol.* 1992;166:1330–1334.

46. Nyberg DA, Resta RG, Luthy DA, et al. Humerus and femur length shortening in the detection of Down syndrome. *Am J Obstet Gynecol.* 1993;168:534–538.

47. Johnson MP, Barr M, Treadwell MC, et al. Fetal leg and femur/foot length ratio: a marker for trisomy 21. *Am J Obstet Gynecol.* 1993;169:557–563.

48. Johnson MP, Michaelson JE, Barr Jr. M, et al. Combining humerus and femur length for improved ultrasonographic identification of pregnancies at increased risk for trisomy 21. *Am J Obstet Gynecol.* 1995;172:1229–1235.

49. Vintzileos AM, Egan JFX, Smulian JC, et al. Adjusting the risk for trisomy 21 by a simple ultrasound method using fetal long-bone biometry. *Obstet Gynecol.* 1996;87:953–958.

50. Benacerraf BR, Mandell J, Estroff JA, et al. Fetal pyelectasis, a possible association with Down syndrome. *Obstet Gynecol.* 1990;76:58–60.

51. Corteville JE, Dicke JM, Crane JP. Fetal pyelectasis and Down syndrome: is genetic amniocentesis warranted? *Obstet Gynecol.* 1992;79:770–772.

52. Bromley B, Doubilet P, Frigoletto, Jn. FD, et al. Is fetal hyperechoic bowel on second trimester sonogram an indication for amniocentesis? *Obstet Gynecol.* 1994;83:647–651.

53. Dicke JM, Crane JP. Sonographically detected hyperechoic fetal bowel: significance and implications for pregnancy management. *Obstet Gynecol.* 1992;80:778–782.

54. Nyberg DA, Resta RG, Mahony BS, et al. Fetal hyperechogenic bowel and Down syndrome. *Ultrasound Obstet Gynecol.* 1993;3:330–333.

55. Scioscia AL, Pretorius DH, Budorick NE, et al. Second trimester hyperechoic bowel and chromosomal abnormalities. *Am J Obstet Gynecol.* 1992;167:889–994.

56. Petrikovsky BM, Challenger M, Wyse LJ. Natural history of echogenic foci within ventricles of the fetal heart. *Ultrasound Obstet Gynecol.* 1995;5:92–94.

57. Sepulveda W, Cullen S, Nicolaides P, et al. Echogenic foci in the fetal heart: a marker of chromosomal abnormality. *Br J Obstet Gynaecol.* 1995;102:490–492.

58. Bromley B, Lieberman E, Laboda LA, et al. Echogenic intracardiac focus, a sonographic sign for Down syndrome? *Obstet Gynecol.* 1995;86:998–1001.

59. Simpson JM, Cook A, Sharland G. The significance of echogenic foci in the fetal heart: a prospective study of 228 cases. *Ultrasound Obstet Gynecol.* 1996;8:225–228.

60. Roberts DJ, Genest D. Cardiac histologic pathology characteristic of trisomies 13 and 21. *Hum Path.* 1992;23:1130–1140.

61. Brown DL, Roberts DJ, Miller WA. Left ventricular echogenic focus in the fetal heart: pathologic correlation. *J Ultrasound Med.* 1994;13:613–666.

62. Lockwood CJ, Lynch L, Ghidini A, et al. The effect of fetal gender on the prediction of Down syndrome by means of maternal serum alpha-fetoprotein and ultrasonographic parameters. *Am J Obstet Gynecol.* 1993;169:1190–1197.

63. Smulian JC, Vintzileos AM, Ciarleglio L, et al. Gender-specific patterns of second trimester femur and humerus measurements in fetuses with Down syndrome. *J Matern Fetal Med.* 1995;4:225–230.

64. Benacerraf BR, Miller WA, Nadel A, et al. Does gender have an impact on the sonographic detection of second trimester fetuses with Down syndrome? *Ultrasound Obstet Gynecol.* 1995;5:30–33.

65. Caffey J, Ross S. Mongolism (mongoloid deficiency) during early infancy—some newly recognized diagnostic changes in the pelvic bones. *Pediatrics.* 1956;17:642–651.

66. Abuhamad AZ, Kolm P, Mari G, et al. Ultrasonographic fetal iliac length measurement in the screening for Down syndrome. *Am J Obstet Gynecol.* 1994;171:1063–1067.

67. Shipp TD, Bromley B, Lieberman E, et al. The iliac angle as a sonographic marker for Down syndrome in second trimester fetuses. *Obstet Gynecol.* 1997;89:446–450.

68. Benacerraf BR, Osathanondh R, Frigoletto Jr. FD. Sonographic demonstration of hypoplasia of the middle phalanx of the fifth digit: a finding associated with Down syndrome. *Am J Obstet Gynecol.* 1988;159:181–183.

69. Benacerraf BR, Harlow B, Frigoletto Jr. FD. Hypoplasia of the middle phalanx of the fifth digit: a feature of the second trimester fetus with Down syndrome. *J Ultrasound Med.* 1990;9:389–394.

70. Jeanty P. Prenatal detection of simian crease. *J Ultrasound Med.* 1990;9:131–136.

71. Wilkins I. Separation of the great toe in fetuses with Down syndrome. *J Ultrasound Med.* 1994;13:229–231.

72. Lettieri L, Rodis JF, Vintzileos AM, et al. Ear length in second trimester aneuploid fetuses. *Obstet Gynecol.* 1993;81:57–60.

73. Birnholz JC, Farrell EE. Fetal ear length. *Pediatrics.* 1988;81:555–558.

74. Gill P, Vanhook J, Fitzsimmons J, et al. Fetal ear measurements in the prenatal detection of trisomy 21. *Prenat Diagn.* 1994;14:739–743.

75. Bahado-Singh RO, Wyse L, Dorr MA, et al. Fetuses with Down syndrome have disproportionately shortened frontal lobe dimensions on ultrasonographic examination. *Am J Obstet Gynecol.* 1992;167:1009–1014.

76. Hill LM, Rivello D, Peterson C, et al. The transverse cerebellar diameter in the second trimester is unaffected by Down syndrome. *Am J Obstet Gynecol.* 1991;164:101–103.

77. Martinez JM, Comas C, Ojuel J, et al. Fetal heart rate patterns in pregnancies with chromosomal disorders of subsequent fetal loss. *Obstet Gynecol.* 1996;87:118–121.

78. Bromley B, Lieberman E, Benacerraf BR. Choroid plexus cysts: not associated with Down syndrome. *Ultrasound Obstet Gynecol.* 1996;232–235.

79. Gupta JK, Cave M, Lilford RF, et al. Clinical significance of fetal choroid plexus cysts. *Lancet.* 1995;346:724–729.

80. Vintzileos AM, Egan JF. Adjusting the risk for trisomy 21 on the basis of second trimester ultrasonography. *Am J Obstet Gynecol.* 1995;172:837–844.

81. Bromley B, Lieberman E, Benacerraf B. The incorporation of maternal age into the sonographic scoring index for the detection at 14–20 weeks of fetuses with Down syndrome. *Ultrasound Obstet Gynecol.* 1997;10:321–324.

82. Vintzileos AM, Campbell WA, Rodis JF, et al. The use of second trimester genetic sonogram in building clinical management of patients at increased risk for fetal trisomy 21. *Obstet Gynecol.* 1996;87:948–952.

83. Nadel A, Bromley B, Frigoletto Jr. FD, et al. Can the presumed risk of autosomal trisomy be decreased in fetuses of older women following a normal sonogram? *J Ultrasound Med.* 1995;143:297–302.

84. Merkatz IR, Nitowsky HM, Macri JN, et al. An association between low maternal serum alpha-fetoprotein and fetal chromosomal abnormalities. *Am J Obstet Gynecol.* 1984;148:886–894.

85. Cuckle S, Wald NJ, Lindenbaum RH. Maternal serum alpha-fetoprotein measurement: a screening test for Down syndrome. *Lancet.* 1984;1:926–929.

86. Wald NJ, Cuckle HS, Densem JW, et al. Maternal serum screening for Down syndrome in early pregnancy. *Br Med J.* 1988;297:883–887.

87. Wald NJ, Cuckle HS, Densem JW, et al. Maternal serum unconjugated estriol as an antenatal screening test for Down syndrome. *Brit J Obstet Gynaecol.* 1988;95:334–341.

88. Haddow JE, Palomaki GE, Knight GJ, et al. Reducing the need for amniocentesis in women 35 years of age or older with serum markers for screening. *N Engl J Med.* 1994;330:1114–1118.

89. Nyberg DA, Luthy DA, Cheng EY, et al. Role of prenatal ultrasonography in women with positive screen for Down syndrome on the basis of maternal serum markers. *Am J Obstet Gynecol.* 1995;173:1030–1035.

90. Bahado-Singh RO, Goldstein I, Uerpairojkit B, et al. Normal nuchal thickness in the midtrimester indicates reduced risk of Down syndrome in pregnancies with abnormal triple-screen results. *Am J Obstet Gynecol.* 1995;173:1106–1110.

91. Ingelfinger JA, Mosteller FR, Thibodeau LA, et al. *Biostatistics in Clinical Medicine.* New York, NY: Macmillan Publishing, Inc; 1983:29–30.

92. Nyberg DA, Luthy DA, Resta RG, et al. Age-adjusted ultrasound risk assessment for fetal Down syndrome during the second trimester: description of the method and analysis of 142 cases. *Ultrasound Obstet Gynecol.* 1998;12:8–14.

93. Nyberg DA, Souter VL, El-Bastawissi A, et al. Isolated sonographic markers for detection of fetal Down syndrome in the second trimester of pregnancy. *J Ultrasound Med.* 2001;20:1053–1063.

94. Bromley B, Shipp TD, Lieberman E, et al. The genetic sonogram: a method of risk assessment for Down syndrome in the midtrimester. *J Ultrasound Med.* 2002;21:1087–1097.

95. Bahado-Singh RO, Deren O, Oz U, et al. An alternative for women initially declining genetic amniocentesis: individual Down syndrome odds on the basis of maternal age and multiple ultrasonographic markers. *Am J Obstet Gynecol.* 1998;179:514–519.

96. Bahado-Singh RO, Oz AU, Kovanci E, et al. New Down syndrome screening algorithm: ultrasonographic biometry and multiple serum markers combined with maternal age. *Am J Obstet Gynecol.* 1998;179:1627–1631.

97. Sohl B, Scioscia A, Budorick NE, et al. Utility of minor ultrasonographic markers in the prediction of abnormal fetal karyotype at a prenatal diagnostic center. *Am J Obstet Gynecol.* 1999;18:898–903.

98. Vergani P, Locatelli A, Piccoli MG, et al. Best second trimester sonographic markers for the detection of trisomy 21. *J Ultrasound Med.* 1999;18:469–473.

99. Pinette MG, Garrett J, Salvo A, et al. Normal midtrimester (17–20 weeks) genetic sonogram decreases amniocentesis rate in a high-risk population. *J Ultrasound Med.* 2001;20:639–644.

100. Devore GR. Trisomy 21: 91% detection rate using second trimester ultrasound markers. *Ultrasound Obstet Gynecol.* 2000;16:133–141.

101. Smith–Bindman R, Hosmer W, Feldstein VA, et al. Second trimester ultrasound to detect fetuses with Down syndrome: a meta-analysis. *JAMA.* 2001;285:1044–1055.

102. Filly RA, Benacerraf BR, Nuberg DA. Choroid plexus cyst and echogenic intracardial focus in women at low risk for chromosomal abnormalities. Editorial. *J Ultrasound Med.* 2004;23:447–449.

103. Hook EB, Woodbury DF, Albright SG. Rates of trisomy 18 in live births, stillbirths, and at amniocentesis. *Birth Defects.* 1979;15:81–93.

104. Jones KL. *Smith's Recognizable Patterns of Human Malformation.* 5th ed. Philadelphia, PA: WB Saunders Company; 1997:8–23, 30–31, 72–75.

105. Benacerraf BR, Harlow B, Frigoletto Jr. FD. Are choroid plexus cysts an indication for second trimester amniocentesis? *Am J Obstet Gynecol.* 1990;162:1001–1006.

106. Nyberg DA, Mahony BS, Hegge FN, et al. Enlarged cisterna magna and the Dandy-Walker malformation: factors associated with chromosome abnormalities. *Obstet Gynecol.* 1991;77:436–442.

107. Hill LM, Marchese S, Peterson C, et al. The effect of trisomy 18 on transverse cerebellar diameter. *Am J Obstet Gynecol.* 1991;165:72–75.

108. Steiger RM, Porto M, Lagrew DC, et al. Biometry of the fetal cisterna magna: estimates of the ability to detect trisomy 18. *Ultrasound Obstet Gynecol.* 1995;5:384–390.

109. Thurmond AS, Nelson DW, Lowensohn RI, et al. Enlarged cisterna magna in trisomy 18: prenatal ultrasonographic diagnosis. *Am J Obstet Gynecol.* 1989;161:83–85.

110. Watson WJ, Katz VL, Chescheir NC, et al. The cisterna magna in second trimester fetuses with abnormal karyotypes. *Obstet Gynecol.* 1992;79:734–735.

111. Nicolaides KH, Salvesen DR, Snijders RJ, et al. Strawberry-shaped skull in fetal trisomy 18. *Fetal Diagn Ther.* 1992;7:132–137.

112. Dicke JM, Crane JP. Sonographic recognition of major malformations and aberrant fetal growth in trisomic fetuses. *J Ultrasound Med.* 1991;10:433–438.

113. Nyberg D, Fitzsimmons J, Mack LA, et al. Chromosomal abnormalities in fetuses with omphalocele: significance of omphalocele contents. *J Ultrasound Med.* 1989;8:299–308.

114. Benacerraf B, Saltzman D, Estroff J, et al. Abnormal karyotype of fetuses with omphalocele: prediction based on omphalocele contents. *Obstet Gynecol.* 1990;75:317–319.

115. Sepulveda W, Treadwell MC, Fisk NM. Prenatal detection of preaxial upper limb reduction in trisomy 18. *Obstet Gynecol.* 1995;85:847–850.

116. Jauniaux E, Donner C, Thomas C, et al. Umbilical cord pseudocyst in trisomy 18. *Prenat Diagn.* 1988;8:557–563.

117. Ramirez P, Haberman S, Baxi L. Significance of prenatal diagnosis of umbilical cord cyst in a fetus with trisomy 18. *Am J Obstet Gynecol.* 1995;173:955–957.

118. Snijders RJ, Sherrod C, Gosden CM, et al. Fetal growth retardation: associated malformations and chromosomal abnormalities. *Am J Obstet Gynecol.* 1993;168:547–555.

119. Carlson D, Platt LD, Medearis AL. The ultrasound triad of fetal hydramnios, abnormal hand posturing and any other anomaly predicts autosomal trisomy. *Obstet Gynecol.* 1992;79:731–734.

120. Shuangshoti S, Roberts MP, Netsky MB. Neuroepithelial (colloid) cysts: pathogenesis and relation to choroid plexus and ependyma. *Arch Pathol.* 1965;80:214–224.

121. Chudleigh P, Pearce JM, Campbell S. The prenatal diagnosis of transient cysts of the choroid plexus. *Prenat Diagn.* 1984;4:135–137.

122. Nicolaides KH, Rodeck CH, Gosden CM. Rapid karyotyping in non-lethal fetal malformations. *Lancet.* 1986;1:283.

123. Chitkara U, Cogswell C, Norton K, et al. Choroid plexus cysts in the fetus: a benign anatomic variant or pathologic entity?: Report of 41 cases and review of the literature. *Obstet Gynecol.* 1988;72:185–189.

124. Clark SL, deVore GR, Sabey PL. Prenatal diagnosis of cysts of the fetal choroid plexus. *Obstet Gynecol.* 1988;72:585–587.

125. de Roo TR, Harris RD, Sargent SK, et al. Fetal choroid plexus cysts: prevalence, clinical significance and sonographic appearance. *Am J Roentgenol.* 1988;151:1179–1181.

126. Gabrielli S, Reece A, Pilu G, et al. The clinical significance of prenatally diagnosed choroid plexus cysts. *Am J Obstet Gynecol.* 1989;160:1207–1210.

127. Chinn DH, Miller EI, Worthy LM, et al. Sonographically detected fetal choroid plexus cysts: frequency and association with aneuploidy. *J Ultrasound Med.* 1991;10:255–258.

128. Achiron R, Barkai G, Katznelson BM, et al. Fetal lateral ventricle choroid plexus cysts: the dilemma of amniocentesis. *Obstet Gynecol.* 1991;78:815–818.

129. Benacerraf BR, Laboda LA. Cyst of the fetal choroid plexus: a normal variant? *Am J Obstet Gynecol.* 1989;160:319–321.

130. Fitzsimmons J, Wilson D, Pascoe-Mason J, et al. Choroid plexus cysts in fetuses with trisomy 18. *Obstet Gynecol.* 1989;73:257–260.

131. Thorpe-Beeston JG, Gosden M, Nicolaides KH. Choroid plexus cysts and chromosomal defects. *Br J Radiol.* 1990;63:783–786.

132. Nadel AS, Bromley BS, Frigoletto Jr. FD, et al. Isolated choroid plexus cysts in the second trimester fetus: is amniocentesis really indicated? *Radiology.* 1992;185:545–548.

133. Gross SJ, Shulman LP, Tolley EA, et al. Isolated fetal choroid plexus cysts and trisomy 18: a review and meta-analysis. *Am J Obstet Gynecol.* 1995;172:83–87.

134. Platt LD, Carlson DE, Medearis AL, et al. Fetal choroid plexus cysts in the second trimester of pregnancy: a cause for concern. *Am J Obstet Gynecol.* 1991;161:1652–1656.

135. Kupferminc MJ, Tamura RK, Sabbagha RE, et al. Isolated choroid plexus cyst(s): an indication for amniocentesis. *Am J Obstet Gynecol.* 1994;171:1068–1071.

136. Porto M, Murata Y, Warneke LA, et al. Fetal choroid plexus cysts: an independent risk factor for chromosomal anomalies. *J Clin Ultrasound.* 1993;21:103–108.

137. Fakhry J, Shecter A, Tenner MS, et al. Cysts of the choroid plexus in neonates: documentation and review of the literature. *J Ultrasound Med.* 1985;4:561–563.

138. Perpignano MC, Cohen HL, Klein VR, et al. Fetal choroid plexus cysts: beware the smaller cyst. *Radiology.* 1992;182:715–717.

139. Twining P, Zuccollo J, Clewes J, et al. Fetal choroid plexus cysts: a prospective study and review of the literature. *Brit J Radiol.* 1991;64:98–102.

140. Hertzberg BS, Kay HH, Bowie JD. Fetal choroid plexus lesions: relationship of antenatal sonographic appearance to clinical outcome. *J Ultrasound Med.* 1989;8:77–82.

141. Patau K, Therman E, Smith DW, et al. Multiple congenital anomalies caused by an extra autosome. *Lancet.* 1960;1:790–793.

142. Hook EB. Rates of 47, +13 and 46 translocation D/13 Patau syndrome in live births and comparison with rates in fetal deaths and at amniocentesis. *Am J Human Genet.* 1980;32:849–858.

143. Redheendran R, Neu RL, Bannerman RM. Long survival in trisomy 13 syndrome: 21 cases including prolonged survival in two patients, 11 and 19 years old. *Am J Med Genet.* 1981;8:167–172.

144. Nicolaides KH, Snijders RJ, Gosden CM, et al. Ultrasonographically detectable markers of fetal chromosomal abnormalities. *Lancet.* 1992;340:704–707.

145. Shipp TD, Bromley B, Benacerraf BR. Sonographically detected abnormalities of the umbilical cord. *Int J Gynecol Obstet.* 1995;48:179–185.

146. Zelante L, Dallapiccola B. Umbilical cord pseudocyst in trisomy 13. *Prenat Diagn.* 1989;9:448.

147. Fergusson-Smith MA, Yates JR. Maternal age specific rates for chromosomal aberrations and factors influencing them: report of a collaborative European study on 52,965 amniocenteses. *Prenat Diagn.* 1984;4:5–44.

148. Jacobs PA, Szulman AE, Funkhouser J, et al. Human triploidy: relationship between parental origin of the additional haploid complement and development of partial hydatidiform mole. *Ann Hum Genet.* 1982;46:223–231.

149. Doshi N, Surti U, Szulman AE. Morphologic anomalies in triploid live-born fetuses. *Hum Pathol.* 1983;14:716–723.

150. Sherard J, Bean C, Bove B, et al. Long survival in a 69 XXY triploid male. *Am J Med Genet.* 1986;25:307–312.

151. Crane JP, Beaver HA, Cheung SW. Antenatal ultrasound findings in fetal triploidy syndrome. *J Ultrasound Med.* 1985;4:519–524.

152. Benacerraf BR. Intrauterine growth retardation in the first trimester associated with triploidy. *J Ultrasound Med.* 1988;7:153–154.

153. Rubenstein JB, Swayne LC, Dise CA, et al. Placental changes in fetal triploidy syndrome. *J Ultrasound Med.* 1986;5:545–550.

154. Edwards MT, Smith WL, Hanson J, et al. Prenatal sonographic diagnosis of triploidy. *J Ultrasound Med.* 1986;5:279–281.

155. Lockwood C, Scioscia A, Stiller R, et al. Sonographic features of the triploid fetus. *Am J Obstet Gynecol.* 1987;157:285–287.

156. Szulman AE, Phillipe E, Boue JG, et al. Human triploidy: association with partial hydatidiform moles and nonmolar conceptuses. *Hum Pathol.* 1981;12:1016–1021.

157. Broekhuizen FF, Elejalde R, Hamilton PR. Early-onset preeclampsia, triploidy and fetal hydrops. *J Reproductive Med.* 1983;28:223–226.

158. Goldstein DP, Berkowitz RS. Current management of complete and partial molar pregnancy. *J Reprod Med.* 1994;39:139–146.

159. Jauniaux E, Brown R, Rodeck C, et al. Prenatal diagnosis of triploidy during the second trimester of pregnancy. *Obstet Gynecol.* 1996;88:983–989.

160. Jauniaux E, Brown R, Snijders RJ, et al. Early prenatal diagnosis of triploidy. *Am J Obstet Gynecol.* 1997;176:550–554.

161. Turner HH. A syndrome of infantilism, congenital webbed neck and cubitus valgus. *Endocrinology.* 1938;23:566.

162. Ford CE, Jones K, Polani P, et al. A sex chromosome anomaly in a case of gonadal dysgenesis (Turner syndrome). *Lancet.* 1959;1:711–713.

163. Wax JR, Blakemore KJ, Baser I, et al. Isolated fetal ascites detected by sonography: an unusual presentation of Turner syndrome. *Obstet Gynecol.* 1992;79:862–863.

164. Nicolaides K, Shawwa L, Brizot M, et al. Ultrasonographically detectable markers of fetal chromosomal defects. *Ultrasound Obstet Gynecol.* 1993;3:56–69.

165. Nadel A, Bromley BS, Benacerraf BR. Nuchal thickening or cystic hygromas in first and early second trimester fetuses: prognosis and outcome. *Obstet Gynecol.* 1993;82:43–48.

166. Chervenak FA, Isaacson G, Blakemore RJ, et al. Fetal cystic hygroma—cause and natural history. *N Engl J Med.* 1983;309:822–825.

167. Azar G, Snidjers RJ, Gosden CM, et al. Fetal nuchal cystic hygromata: associated malformations and chromosomal defects. *Fetal Diagn Ther.* 1991;6:46–57.

COLOR DOPPLER IN CONGENITAL DEFECTS

Asim Kurjak / Sanja Kupesic

The use of color Doppler ultrasound offers a novel approach for the investigation of human uteroplacental and fetal circulations. Using this modality, our understanding of the integrity of the matemo-fetal circulation has tremendously improved, allowing precise assessment of the circulatory modifications in cases of abnormal pregnancy. There is an obvious benefit from this technique in performing invasive procedures in prenatal diagnosis, particularly in identification and differentiation of the umbilical arteries and vein during the funiculocenthesis. This chapter attempts to demonstrate the role of color Doppler in the diagnosis of fetal malformations, and evaluation of the chromosomal defects.

COLOR DOPPLER IN THE DIAGNOSIS OF FETAL MALFORMATIONS

MALFORMATIONS OF THE CEPHALIC POLE

During the seventh gestational week it is already possible to observe early cerebral circulation, which is potentially helpful in the evaluation of cranial malformations and/or the degree of their effect on the central nervous system (Fig. 26-1).

Anencephaly can be diagnosed very early, from the eighth week onwards.[1-4] In these cases color Doppler studies reveal normal or even increased blood flow in carotid arteries, while the cerebral blood flow is absent (Fig. 26-2).

In patients with exencephaly, blood flow is detected arising from the circle of Willis by an aberrant route[5] (Figs. 26-3, 26-4). In normal pregnancies the pulsed Doppler waveform analysis indicates permanent diastolic flow and significantly lower impedance to flow than in other fetal vessels (Fig. 26-5). In exencephalocele vascular structures are clearly detected within the hemiated cerebral mass and show an abnormal Doppler feature: absence of diastolic flow (Figs. 26-4, 26-6). This fact permits a differential diagnosis from cystic hygroma.

Cystic hygroma is produced by a blockade of the lymphatic drainage at the level of the outlet of the jugular vein. Therefore, it is at first associated with the appearance of a bursa in the lateral aspect of the neck (Fig. 26-7), which later due to its extension occupies the posterior portion, giving rise to a septated aspect, or simply a cystic image[5] (Fig. 26-8). In many cases, when it progresses it is accompanied by ascites, generalized edema, and anasarca.

The cystic hygroma is accompanied by a frequency of chromosomopathies of between 40 and 90%: Turner syndrome being the most common followed by trisomy 21 and mosaicisms.[5] The presence of cystic hygroma, detectable during the first trimester of pregnancy necessitates amniocentesis or chorial biopsy.[6-22]

It is clearly shown that the malformation may disappear during gestation, even at the end of the first trimester.[6,9,10,14,18] Cystic hygromas never manifest vascular flow in the tumor mass. However, blood flow signals from cerebral vessels are easily obtainable (Fig. 26-9).

Intracranial cystic formations (such as cysts of arachnoid fossae, agenesis of the corpus callosum, Dandy-Walker syndrome, etc.) may affect the cerebral circulation. In these cases, color Doppler accurately differentiates between cystic and vascular origin.

It has already been reported[23-26] that aneurism of the vein of Galen demonstrates a turbulent blood flow that permits a differential diagnosis from an arachnoid cyst. Commonly, this finding is associated with other malformations of the central nervous system.

Choroid plexus cysts are very common, and occur as a consequence of vascular dilatations with an accumulation of cerebrospinal liquor, so that they do not show any blood flow alterations (Fig. 26-10). Today they are considered completely physiological and they tend to disappear spontaneously toward the 24th–26th week.[5] However, there has been a lot of discussion about their significance as indirect signs of chromosomal malformations.[27-29] Based on our experience, choroid plexus cysts do not demonstrate increased flow and do not alter blood flow in other cerebral vessels.

Hydrocephaly and hydranencephaly are among the most common malformations of the central nervous system. Their origin is associated with obstruction or stenosis of the cerebral aqueduct. In general, they tend to be bilateral, although they may appear unilateral due to obliteration of the foramen of Monro.

In hydrocephaly and hydranencephaly a progressive compression of the vessels takes place, increasing the resistance to blood flow (Figs. 26-11, 26-12). This causes hypoxia and progressive degeneration of the cerebral parenchyma.[30] In cases of unilateral hydrocephaly, a marked difference in the cerebral flow between the affected and the contralateral hemispheres has been observed.[28]

It is clearly assumed that the increase in cerebral flow resistance is a reflection of the increase in intracranial pressure, and therefore its finding in these lesions, particularly in the beginning, involves a worse prognosis. Color Doppler has a very limited application in detection of the neural tube defects since they do not modify the embryonic and fetal circulations.

MALFORMATIONS OF THE THORAX

Color Doppler may assist in detection of the malformations of the thorax. In pulmonary sequestration, color Doppler permits the identification of the aberrant origin of the systemic vascularization of the pulmonary parenchyma, allowing it to be differentiated from an adenomatoid cystic malformation. Similarly, color Doppler improves the diagnosis of all intra- or extra-cardiac malformations that are accompanied by an anomalous venous return (inferior or superior vena cava, portal vein, etc.) that can be located early with this technique.[30,31]

This method has significantly increased our diagnostic capacity in prenatal diagnosis of congenital cardiopathies. Starting from the eighth week of gestation it becomes possible to detect heart action (Fig. 26-13) and to obtain the cardiac

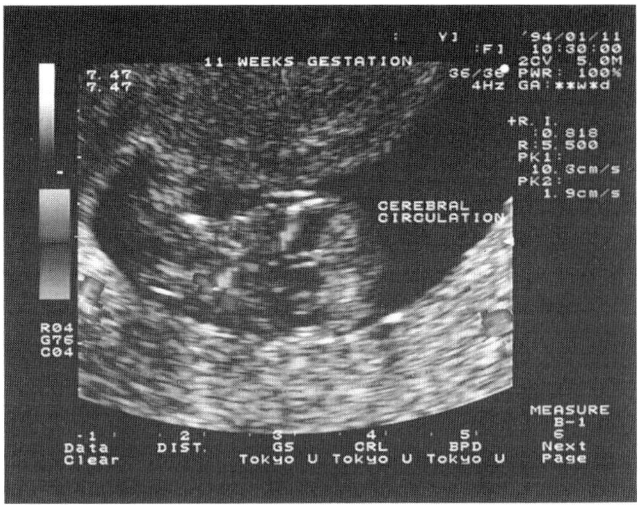

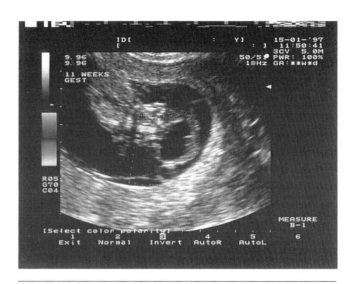

FIGURE 26-1 Transvaginal color Doppler scan of cerebral vessels at 8 weeks' gestation. Color signals are displayed from anterior, middle, and posterior cerebral arteries.

FIGURE 26-3 Exencephaly at 11 weeks of gestation. Note a cyst of the posterior fossa (Dandy-Walker syndrome).

frequency of an embryo (Fig. 26-14). It was clearly demonstrated by De Vore[32] that sudden decrease of the fetal cardiac frequency is one of the most harmful prognostic factors in the first trimester of pregnancy. Knowledge of the normal embryonic and fetal cardiovascular anatomy is significantly increased allowing rapid identification of major cardiac defects (Fig. 26-15).

Color Doppler is very useful in the first phase of the echocardiographic examination since it provides rapid identification of the great vessels, such as the aorta and the pulmonary artery, allowing for immediate orientation by the examiner.[31]

In a normal fetus, color Doppler allows evaluation of the cardiovascular hemodynamics with great simplicity.[33] Venous circulation is easily observed by identifying blood flow in the superior vena cava and inferior to the right atrium, as well as blood flow through the foramen ovale to the left atrium. The aortic arch is also identified without difficulty and the presence of an "aliasing" phenomenon in the region of the ductus often facilitates the identification of this structure.[31] In the same manner, it is possible to clearly observe the turbulent flow of the pulmonary artery and its branches. The fact that color Doppler completely opacifies these vessels greatly facilitates the measurement of their diameters.

In fetuses with congenital cardiopathies, the additional information provided by color Doppler facilitates the identification and documentation of a certain number of anomalies, especially septi, valvular regurgitation, and complex lesions.

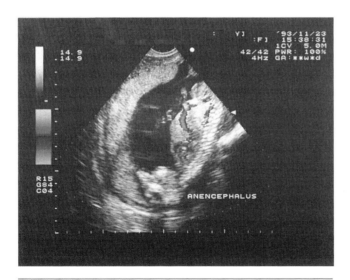

FIGURE 26-2 Anencephaly at 11 weeks of gestation. Color signals are obtained from the fetal heart, aorta, and umbilical artery.

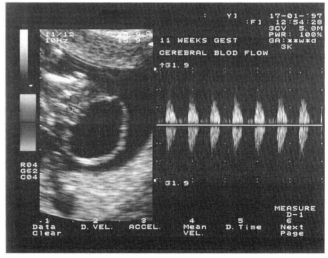

FIGURE 26-4 The same patient as in Figure 26-3. Blood flow signals obtained from the cerebral structures demonstrate absence of the diastolic flow and RI of 1.0.

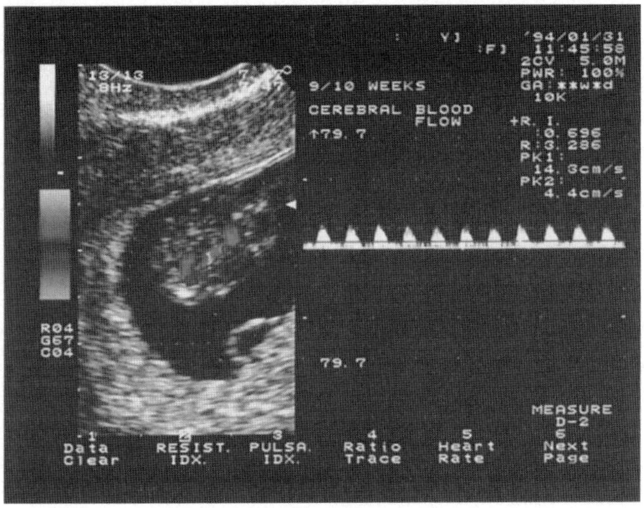

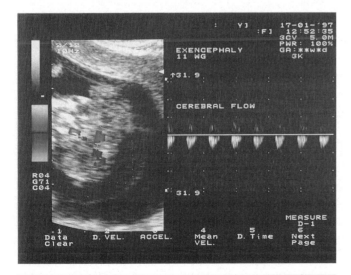

FIGURE 26-5 Starting from the tenth gestational week onward one can obtain a continuous diastolic flow in the cerebral vessels. This is an illustrative case of normal middle cerebral blood flow represented with RI of 0.70.

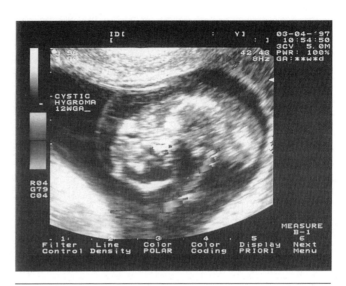

FIGURE 26-7 Hygroma colli at 12 weeks' gestation. The cephalic pole shows the typical cervical edema. Using color Doppler no vessels are detectable.

According to Coppel and colleagues[34] 20% of cardiopathies can be diagnosed in utero only with the use of color Doppler. Therefore, this technique is considered essential in these cases. In 47% of cardiopathies, the contribution of color Doppler is considered useful but not essential, and in 24%, color Doppler does not provide any additional diagnostic information than that provided by conventional echocardiography.

In general, color Doppler is essential to determine the course and direction of blood flow in the great vessels, is helpful but not essential in identifying the tiny "jets" in areas of regurgitation from the atrioventricular valves, and, finally, it is not essential in diagnosing the majority of anatomic congen-

ital cardiopathies which are generally readily identified with 2-dimensional ultrasound.[31,34] Color Doppler may be very useful in evaluation of the cardiac flow in patients with generalized nonimmune hydrops as shown in Figure 26-16.

ABDOMINAL WALL DEFECTS

Color Doppler permits the confirmation of structural pathologies that are difficult to diagnose early in pregnancy. The primitive gut is morphologically formed in the sixth week. The intestinal tract and liver grow more rapidly than the abdominal wall, and therefore the abdominal cavity becomes temporarily too small to contain the bowel, so they are displaced into

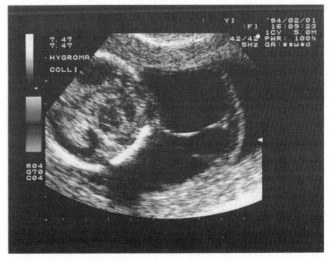

FIGURE 26-6 In a patient with exencephaly at 11 weeks' gestation blood flow signals obtained from cerebral structures demonstrate absence of diastolic flow and high vascular resistance (RI = 1.0).

FIGURE 26-8 Cystic hygroma at 13 weeks' gestation. Note avascular tiny septa extending from the posterior portion of the neck.

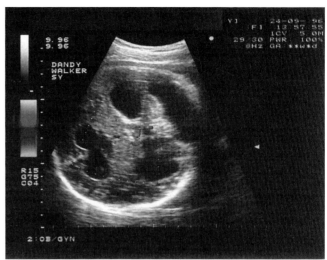

FIGURE 26-9　The same patient as in Figure 26-8. Contrary to avascular image of cystic hygroma, cerebral vascular network is easily obtainable.

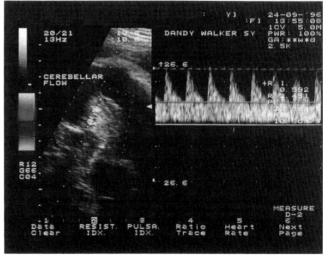

FIGURE 26-11　Transvaginal sonogram of a Dandy-Walker malformation. Note a cyst of the posterior fossa and dilatation of the fourth ventricle. A plane through the upper cerebellum demonstrates the vermis. Color signals are obtained from cerebral vessels.

the umbilical cord. Toward the eighth week, this physiological migration[35–37] is clearly visible using transvaginal ultrasound.

During the tenth week these organs return to their normal intra-abdominal position, due to the more rapid growth of the abdominal wall. During this process the midgut undergoes 270 degrees of rotation, which occurs in two stages: the first stage of 90 degrees when the midgut is herniated, and the second of 180 degrees after the return to the intra-abdominal location. The definitive intra-abdominal location is completely established in the eleventh week.

Due to this physiological herniation, it is difficult to diagnose abdominal wall defects before the eleventh week, although with experience they may be suspected.

Such defects, which occur in 1 of 5,000 living newborns,[5] include a very common group formed by omphaloceles and gastroschisis, and an exceptional second group that includes ectopia cordis, cloaca, and bladder extrophy, the limb-body wall complex, and Cantrell's pentalogy.

Apart from gastroschisis, 70% of these defects are accompanied by chromosomal abnormalities and by other severe organ malformations. Therefore, there is an obvious importance of an early diagnosis which can be carried out using

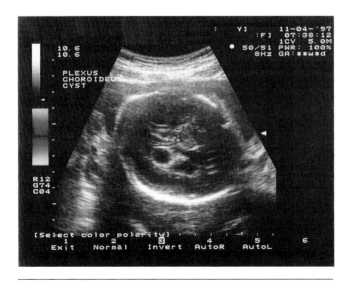

FIGURE 26-10　Transvaginal color Doppler scan of a fetus at 13 weeks' gestation. Note an avascular choroid plexus cyst and blood flow signals representing middle cerebral artery.

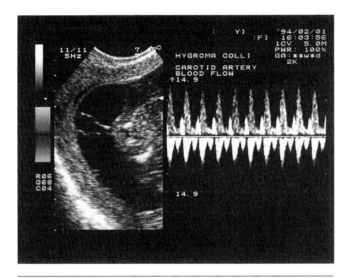

FIGURE 26-12　In the same patient as in Figure 26-11 pulsed Doppler waveform signals are obtained from the cerebellar arteries in the upper part of cerebellum. Moderate vascular resistance (RI = 0.59) is easily extracted from these arteries. At this stage there is no alteration of blood flow indicative of increased intracranial pressure.

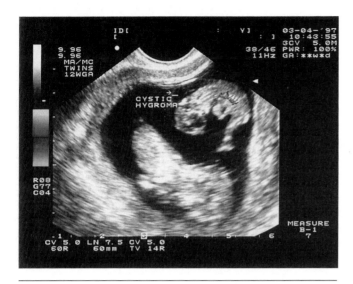

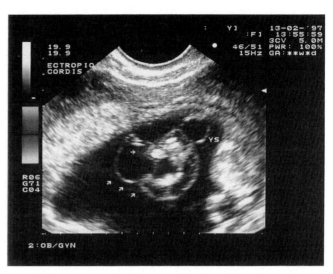

FIGURE 26-13 Transvaginal scan of a monochorionic-monoamniotic twin gestation. Note absence of cardiac activity in one embryo and regular heart action in another. In the nuchal region of the second one note cystic hygroma. The pregnancy was aborted spontaneously, and both embryos were diagnosed as Turner syndrome.

FIGURE 26-15 Transvaginal color Doppler facilitates detection of the major congenital defects such as ectopia cordis. The heart is located outside the fetal body.

transvaginal ultrasound coupled with color flow imaging. Using this technique one can observe the displacement of the entire hepatic vascular map into the interior of the defect in the case of gastroschisis, or the vascular absence in the omphalocele and visualization of the mesenteric vessels at the base of the defect (Figs. 26-17, 26-18).

MALFORMATIONS OF THE GENITO-URINARY TRACT

Renal and urinary tract anomalies represent 40–50% of all malformations diagnosed with sonography.[38] Although the kid-

neys are formed in the tenth week[39] and the existence of urine production is known from the twelfth week on,[38] it is difficult to diagnose these anomalies prior to the sixteenth week.[5]

Color Doppler has been used to confirm the diagnosis of renal genesis, poly-micro-, and macrocystic kidneys and obstructive uropathies.[5,31,40–43] In cases of renal agenesis, the existence of normal flow in the aorta and umbilical cord has been observed,[40] with no visualization of the renal arteries. In renal ectopias the displaced renal vessels have been observed with normal velocimetric indices.[41,42]

In cases of multicystic renal dysplasia Bonilla et al.[5] observed renal flow with normal indices which, as the gestation advanced and the lesion progressed, became highly pathological. Figs. 26-19 and 26-20 show the correlation between the

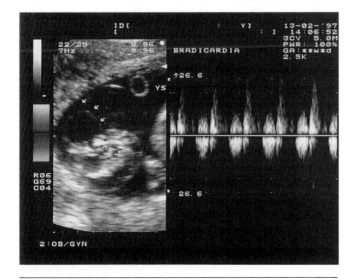

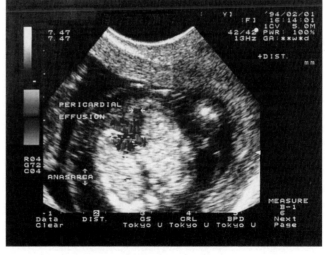

FIGURE 26-14 Decreased cardiac frequency in an embryo of 7–8 weeks' gestation. Spontaneous abortion occurred two days after bradicardia has been detected using color Doppler technique.

FIGURE 26-16 Heart action depicted by color flow mapping in a patient with anasarca and pericardial effusion.

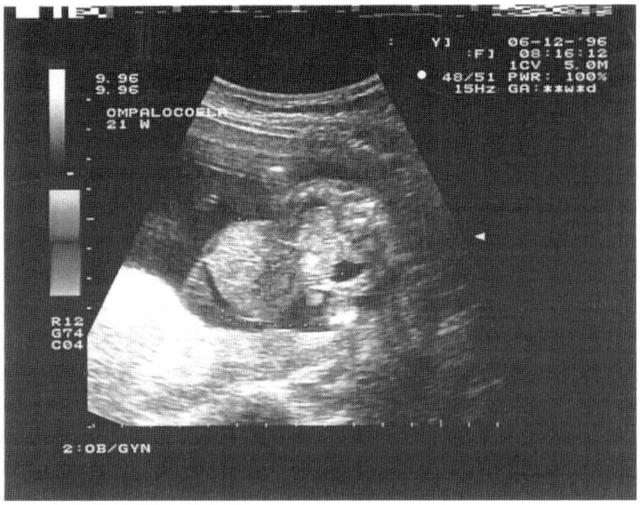

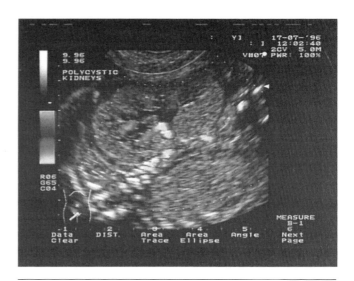

FIGURE 26-17 Omphalocoele at 21 weeks' gestation. Note mesenteric vessels at the base of the abdominal wall defect.

fetal aorta blood flow and polycystic kidney disease. The abnormal kidney tissue changes the vessels' diameter increasing the resistance to flow (expressed through RI and PI). These alterations initially have few consequences on the fetal systemic circulation but affects the function of the renal parenchyma, increasing the oligohydramnios and furthering the hemodynamic consequences. Color Doppler serves to establish a neonatal prognosis[43] as well as to determine whether 1 or both kidneys are involved.

OTHER ABDOMINAL TUMORS

Transvaginal color Doppler also may be used for identification of the intra-abdominal cystic lesions.[44] They are easily identified by their lack of blood flow using this modality. In cases of vascularized cystic tumors one can differentiate their origin

FIGURE 26-19 Polycystic kidneys. Renal artery and fetal aorta are clearly visible using color Doppler facilities.

due to location and vascular relationship with kidneys, ovaries or intestines (Figs. 26-21, 26-22). In cases with obstructive uropathy color Doppler can detect local circulatory changes (Figs. 26-23, 26-24) and may be used for follow-up of the functional changes produced by the lesion. Furthermore, it may facilitate the visualization of minor lesions such as pyelectasia, which is a well-known phenotypic marker of chromosomal defects.

OTHER MALFORMATIONS

In contrast to cystic hygroma, nonimmune edema produces a loosening of the neck and back skin, and is not accompanied by chromosomopathies. The origin of this state is highly variable:[45,38] in 52% is caused by cardiopathy, sometimes is associated with nephropathy, placental and cord anomalies,

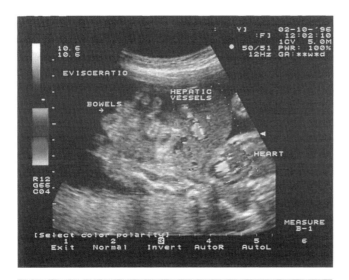

FIGURE 26-18 Huge abdominal wall defect shows and extrusion of an important portion of the intraabdominal structures paralleled with an outlet of the vessels emerging from the defect.

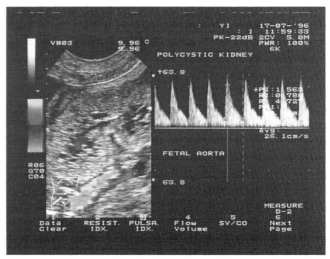

FIGURE 26-20 The same patient as in Figure 26-19. Fetal aorta blood flow demonstrates an initial decrease. Blood flow alterations of the fetal aorta and renal artery are proportional to the status of the fetus and stage of oligohydramnios.

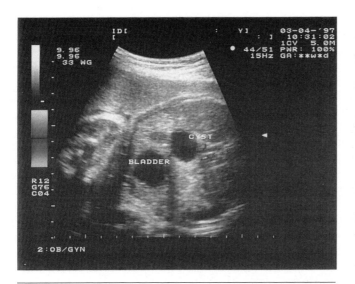

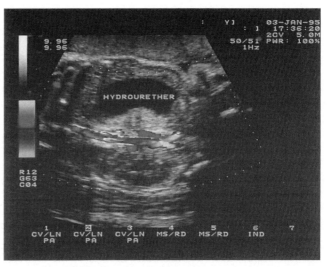

FIGURE 26-21 Color Doppler may be helpful in differentiation of the abdominal cystic structures and fetal bladder. Small cystic structure filled with anechoic fluid is visualized above the bladder. Pericystic vessels are depicted using color Doppler imaging.

sacrococcygeal teratomas, and so on. In severe cases complicated by anemia, hypopoteinemia, and cardiac insufficiency color Doppler measurements show significant alterations (Figs. 26-25, 26-26).

Doppler features of some vascular hepatic tumors such as cavernous hemangiomas[46] or hemangioendotheliomas [47,48,49] were reported as well. Sacrococcygeal teratomas are highly vascularized tumors characterized with numerous arteriovenous shunts, polyhydramnios, hypertrophic placenta, and congestive cardiac insufficiency.[50,51,52] Therefore, color Doppler seems to be useful in detection and follow-up of the hemodynamic changes in pregnancies complicated by sacrococcygeal teratoma.

FIGURE 26-23 Obstructive uropathy at 27 weeks' gestation. Color signals are easily obtained from the fetal aorta.

This method allows us to study the kinetic patterns of different fluids, such as amniotic fluid or fetal urine. Abnormal movements of these fluids may lead an ultrasonographer to definition of some anomalies that are difficult to be detected such as cleft lip and palate, pharyngeal anomalies, and so on.

COLOR DOPPLER IN DIAGNOSIS OF INDIRECT SIGNS OF CHROMOSOMAL DEFECTS

A single umbilical artery is commonly associated with chromosomal defects, perinatal complications, intrauterine growth retardation, and existence of fetal malformations. Since the

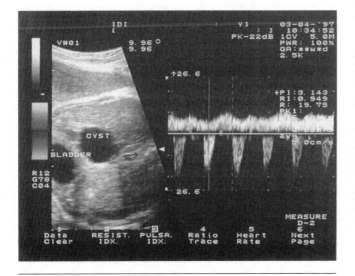

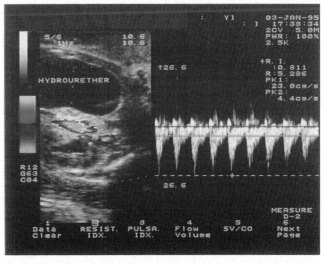

FIGURE 26-22 Unilocular abdominal cyst at 19 weeks' gestation demonstrates increased vascular resistance (RI = 0.95) in the supplying artery.

FIGURE 26-24 The same patient as in Figure 26-23. Blood flow signals obtained from the fetal aorta demonstrate continuous diastolic blood flow and RI of 0.81.

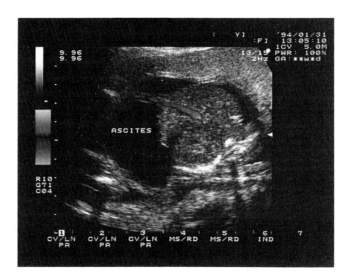

FIGURE 26-25 Generalized edema at 27 weeks' gestation. Hepatic vessels, ductus venosus and umbilical vein are depicted using color flow mapping.

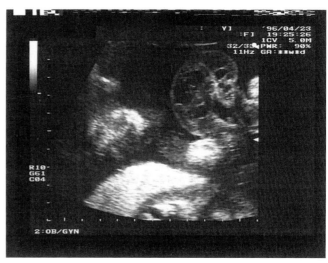

FIGURE 26-27 Conventional ultrasound examination of the umbilical cord at 22 weeks' gestation. Note cystic-like appearance at the free loop of the umbilical cord.

incidence of this sign is around 1% in singleton pregnancies, and 4.6% in twin gestations, one should be aware of the importance of the early and safe detection of this entity by color and pulsed Doppler.[31]

Pseudocysts of the umbilical cord display focal degeneration of the Wharton's jelly without involving embryonic vestigial structures of the omphalomesenteric or alantoid canals. Since these structures are associated with trisomies 18 and 13, their visualization by color Doppler indicates further cytogenetic evaluation.

Cord angiomyxomas are vascular tumors in a close contact with one or more umbilical vessels from which they arise (Figs.

26-27, 26-28). Due to infiltration of the cord by the angiomatous tissue and progressive shortening of the cord, a cesarean section is recommended.

Shortening of the length of the umbilical cord is associated with several chromosomal defects and congenital malformations.[53] Color Doppler allows precise measurement of the umbilical cord, and exact "tracing" from the placenta insertion to the fetal insertion (Fig. 26-29).

Increased resistance of the umbilical artery blood flow, without simultaneous alteration of the uterine flow is a warning signal, commonly described in patients with chromosomal defects and perinatal complications.[54] Umbilical vein pulsations indicate alterations in cardiac function (Fig. 26-30). They are

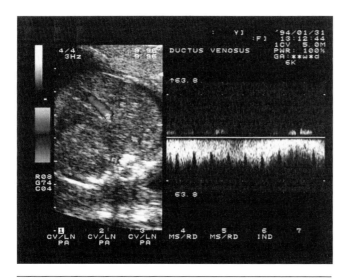

FIGURE 26-26 Color coded blood flow in ductus venosus (blue). Ductus venosus, which macroscopically resembles a continuation of the intra-abdominal part of the umbilical vein, has a typical blood flow velocity waveform (right).

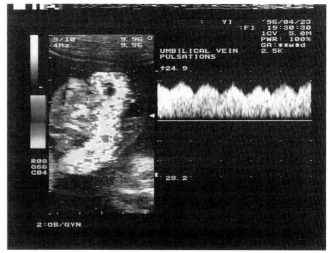

FIGURE 26-28 Color flow image of the same umbilical cord as in Figure 26-27 shows an abnormal vascular pattern suggestive of cord angioma.

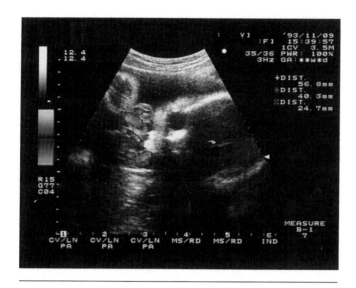

FIGURE 26-29 Color flow image of a shortened umbilical cord coiled around the fetal neck.

associated with severe growth retardation, end-diastolic velocities in the umbilical artery and abnormal fetal heart rates.

Color Doppler does not improve the imaging of the markers of aneuploidy such as nuchal translucency, intestinal hyperechogenicity, or visualization of the pyelectasis.

However, the use of color Doppler may significantly improve the identification of the heart defects. Because between 16 and 20% of fetuses with congenital heart defects are carriers of chromosomal anomalies[55,56] and between 50 and 52% of the chromosomal defects indicate complex heart defects, there is an obvious need for early and proper recognition of heart defects.

The results of ultrasound examinations in the study carried out by DeVore and Alfi[55] are clearly very different depending

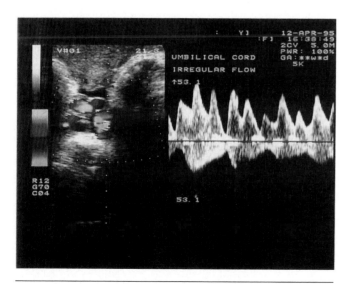

FIGURE 26-30 Irregular pulsations obtained from the umbilical artery indicated a cesarean section.

on whether conventional echography is done in real time or whether color Doppler is added. In the first case only 12% of trisomy 21 cases would have been suspected, the percentage increased to 47% using color Doppler ($p < 0.05$ and R = 6.1). The differences are even more significant if all chromosomal abnormalities are grouped together: 7% sensitivity in real time as compared to 43% with color Doppler ($p < 0.004$ and R = 9.7).

Carrera[31] clearly stated that in pregnant women aged 35 or over, echographic examination using color Doppler considerably alters the thoretical risk of trisomy 21. If we accept that the potential risk of this trisomy is 1 in 270 at the age of 35 and 1 in 134 for any chromosomal anomaly, these indices are only reached at age 42 if a color Doppler examination is performed to exclude anomalies. Beyond that age, the risk of trisomy 21 or any other anomaly increases as it usually does beyond the age of 35. Therefore, if the color Doppler study is normal, no cytogenetic study needs to be carried out until after the age of 42.

CONCLUSIONS

Since the introduction of diagnostic ultrasound to obstetrics, there has been a dramatic increase in the quantity and quality of fetal malformation information that can be obtained. Color Doppler imaging has opened new fields in the investigation of the physiology and pathophysiology of pregnancy. Apart from investigations during the first trimester of pregnancy,[57–59] analysis of the early cerebral flow,[60,61] fetomaternal circulation in patients with threatened abortions[62] and studies on intervillous circulation[63] our group conducted a prospective study on fetuses with congenital defects. Part of these results are demonstrated and illustrated in this chapter indicating that color Doppler provides information that can contribute to the improved diagnosis of structural abnormalities of the fetus.

References

1. Rottem S, Bronshtein M, Thaler I, et al. First trimester transvaginal sonography diagnosis of fetal anomalies. *Lancet.* 1989;1: 444–445.

2. Benacerraf BR. First-trimester diagnosis of fetal abnormalities. A report of three cases. *J Reprod Med.* 1988;33:777–780.

3. Goldstein RD, Filly RA, Cullen PW. Sonography of anencephaly: pitfalls in early diagnosis. *J Clin Ultrasound.* 1989;17:397–402.

4. Johnson A, Losure TA, Neiner S. Early diagnosis of fetal anencephaly. *J Clin Ultrasound* 1989;13:503–505.

5. Bonilla-Musoles F, Ballester MJ, Raga F. Transvaginal color Doppler in early embryonic malformations. In: Kurjak A, ed. *An Atlas of Transvaginal Color Doppler: The Current State of the Art*, pp. 105–123, (London-Casterton-New York: Parthenon; 1994.

6. Gustavii B, Edvall H. First trimester diagnosis of cystic nuchal hygroma. *Acta Obstet Gynecol Scand.* 1984;63:377–378.

7. Van Salen-Sprock MM, Van Vugt JMG, Van der Harten HJ, et al. Cephalocele and cystic hygroma: diagnosis and differentiation in the first trimester of pregnancy with transvaginal sonography: report of two cases. *Ultrasound Obstet Gynecol.* 1992;2:289–292.

8. Bronshtein M, Rotterm S, Yoffe N, et al. First-semester and early second-trimester diagnosis of nuchal cystic hygroma by transvaginal sonography: diverse prognosis of the septated from the non septated lesion. *Am J Obstet Gynecol.* 1989;161:78–84.

9. Mostello DJ, Bofinger MK, Siddigi TA. Spontaneous resolution of fetal cystic hygroma and hydrops in Turner syndrome. *Obstet Gynecol.* 1989;73:862–865.

10. Rodis JF, Vintzileos AM, Campbell WA, et al. Spontaneous resolution of fetal cystic hygroma in Down syndrome. *Obstet Gynecol.* 1988;71:976–977.

11. Rahmani MR, Fong KW, Connor TP. The varied sonographic appearance of cystic hygromas in utero. *J Ultrasound Med.* 1986;5:165–168.

12. Fisk N, Vaugghan J, Smidt M, et al. Transvaginal ultrasound recognition of nuchal edema in the first-trimester diagnosis of achondrogenesis. *J Clin Ultrasound.* 1991;19:586–590.

13. Ville Y, Lalondrelle C, Doumerc S, et al. First trimester diagnosis of nuchal anomalies: significance and fetal outcome. *Ultrasound Obstet Gynecol.* 1992;2:314–316.

14. Cullen MT, Gabrielli S, Green JJ, et al. Diagnosis and significance of cystic hygroma in the first trimester. *Prenat Diagn.* 1990;10:643–651.

15. Nicolaides KH, Azar G, Byrne D, et al. Fetal nuchal translucency: ultrasound screening for chromosomal defects in first trimester of pregnancy. *Br Med J.* 1992;304:867–869.

16. Schulman LP, Emerson DS, Myers CM, et al. Longitudinal evaluation of 11 fetuses with cystic hygromata detected in the first trimester. *Am J Obstet Gynecol.* 1991;164:351–352.

17. Podobnik M, Singer Z, Podobnik-Sarkanji S, et al. First-trimester diagnosis of cystic hygromata by transvaginal sonography. *Ultrasound Obstet Gynecol.* 1992;2:124–125.

18. Van Zalen-Spock MM, Van Vugt JMG, Gein HP. First trimester diagnosis of cystic hygroma, course and outcome. *Am J Obstet Gynecol.* 1992;167:94–98.

19. Rebarber A, Mohon R. Prenatal diagnosis of cystic adenomatoid malformation of one fetus in a twin pregnancy: an unusual presentation. *J Ultrasound Med.* 1992;11:305–308.

20. Shulman LP, Emerson DS, Felker RE, et al. High frequency of cytogenetic abnormalities in fetuses with cystic hygroma diagnosed in the first trimester. *Obstet Gynecol.* 1992;80:80–82.

21. Reuss A, Pijpers L, Van Swaij E, et al. First-trimester diagnosis of recurrence of cystic hygroma using a vaginal ultrasound transducer. *Eur J Obstet Gynecol Reprod Biol.* 1987;26:271–273.

22. Cullen MT, Gabrielli S, Green JJ. Diagnosis of significance of cystic hygroma in the first trimester. *Prenat Diagn.* 1990;10:643–651.

23. Johnson W, Berry JM, Einzig S, et al. Doppler findings in nonimmune hydrops fetalis and cerebral arteriovenous malformation. *Am Heart J.* 1988;115:1138–1140.

24. Hirsch JH, Cyr D, Eberhardt H, et al. Ultrasonographic diagnosis of an aneurysm of the vein of Galen *in utero* by duplex scanning. *J Ultrasound Med.* 1983;2:231–233.

25. Rizzo G, Arduini D, Colosimo C, et al. Abnormal fetal cerebral blood flow velocity waveforms as a sign of an aneurysm of the vein of Galen. *Fetal Ther.* 1987;2:70–75.

26. Hata T, Hata K, Senoh D. Antenatal Doppler color flow mapping of arteriovenous malformation of the vein of Galen. *J Cardiovasc Ultrasonogr.* 1988;7:301–303.

27. Bonilla-Musoles F, Simon C, Sampaio M, et al. Transvaginal ultrasound in the first trimester of pregnancy. *Revista Obstet Gynecol.* 1989;1:247–251.

28. Bronshtein M, Ben-Shlomo I. Choroid plexus dysmorphism detected by transvaginal sonography: the earliest sign of fetal hydrocephalus. *J Clin Ultrasound.* 1991;19:547–553.

29. Rotmensch S, Luo JS, Nores JA, et al. Bilateral choroid plexus cyst in trisomy 21. *Am J Obstet Gynecol.* 1992;166:591–592.

30. Jaffe R, Warsof SR, Kurjak A, et al. Color Doppler in congenital anomalies. In: Kurjak A, Kupesic S, (eds.). *An Atlas of Transvaginal Color Doppler.* New York, London: Parthenon 2000;65–72.

31. Carrera JM, Devesa R, Torrents M, et al. Color Doppler in prenatal diagnosis. In: Chervenak FA, Kurjak A, (eds). *Current Perspectives on the Fetus as a Patient.* New York-London: Parthenon; 1996: 39–48.

32. De Vore GR. The use of color Doppler imaging to examine the fetal heart. Normal and pathologic anatomy. In: Jaffe R, ed. *Color Doppler Imaging in Obstetrics and Gynecology.* 1992:121–154.

33. Mortera C, Carrera JM, Torrents M. Doppler pulsado codificado en color. Mapa Doppler color de la circulacion fetal. In: Carrera JM, ed. *Doppler en Obstetricia.* Barcelona: Salvat-Masson; 1992: 185–198.

34. Copel JA, Morotti R, Hobbins JC, et al. The antenatal diagnosis of congenital heart disease using fetal echocardiography; is color flow mapping necessary? *Obstet Gynecol.* 1991;78:1–8.

35. Cyr DR, Mack LA, Schoenecker SA. Bowel migration in the normal fetus: US detection. *Radiology.* 1986;161:119–123.

36. Schmidt W, Yarkoni S, Crelin ES, et al. Sonographic visualization of physiologic anterior abdominal wall hernia in the first trimester. *Obstet Gynecol.* 1987;69:911–915.

37. Timor-Tritsch IE, Warren WB, Peisner DB, et al. First-trimester midgut hemiation: a high frequency transvaginal sonographic study. *Am J Obstet Gynecol.* 1989;161:831–833.

38. Merz E. *Ultrasound in Gynecology and Obstetrics.* Stuttgart: Thieme Verlag; 1991.

39. Bronshtein M, Kushnir O, Ben-Rafael Z, et al. Transvaginal sonographic measurement of fetal kidneys in the first trimester of pregnancy. *J Clin Ultrasound.* 1990;18:299–301.

40. Jaffe R, Warsof SR. *Color Doppler Imaging in Obstetrics and Gynecology.* New York: McGraw-Hill; 1992.

41. Campbell S, Vyas S. Color flow mapping in measurement of flow velocity in fetal renal arteries. Presented at the *First International Meeting, Fetal and Neonatal Color Flow Mapping,* Dubrovnik, Croatia. 1988.

42. Hecker K, Spernol R, Szalay S. Doppler blood flow velocity waveforms in the fetal renal artery. *Arch Gynecol Obstet.* 1989;246: 133–137.

43. Kaminopetros P, Dukes EH, Nicolaides KH. Fetal renal artery blood velocimetry in multicystic kidney disease. *Ultrasound Obstet Gynecol.* 1991;1:410–412.

44. Zimmer EZ, Bronshtein M. Fetal intra-abdominal cysts detected in the first and early second trimester by transvaginal sonography. *J Clin Ultrasound.* 1991;19:564–567.

45. Bonilla-Musoles F. *Diagnostico Prenatal de las Malformaciones Fetales.* Barcelona: Jims; 1983.

46. Rizzo G, Arduini D. Prenatal diagnosis of an intraabdominal ectasia of the umbilical vein with color Doppler ultrasonography. *Ultrasound Obstet Gynecol.* 1992;2:55–57.

47. Diakoumakis EE, Weinberg B, Seife B, et al. Infantile hemangioendothelioma of the liver. *J Clin Ultrasound.* 1986;14:137–139.

48. Nakamoto SK, Dreilinger A, Dattel B. The sonographic appearance of hepatic hemangioma in-utero. *J Ultrasound Med.* 1983;2: 239–241.

49. Platt LD, De Vore GR, Brenner P, et al. Antenatal diagnosis of a fetal liver mass. *J Ultrasound Med.* 1983;2:521–522.

50. Gergely RZ, Eden R, Schifrin BS, et al. Antenatal diagnosis of congenital sacral teratoma. *J Reprod Med.* 1989;24:229–231.

51. Kohler HG. Sacrococcygeal teratoma and nonimmunological hydrops fetalis. *Br Med J.* 1976;2:422–424.

52. Alter DN, Reed KL, Marx GR, et al. Prenatal diagnosis of congestive heart failure in a fetus with a sacrococcygeal teratoma. *Obstet Gynecol.* 1988;71:978–981.

53. Szabo J, Gellen J, Szemere G. Nuchal edema as an ultrasonic sign of trisomy 21 during the first trimester of pregnancy. *Orv Hetil.* 1992;133:3167–3168.

54. Carrera JM, Mortera C. Estudio Doppler de los Defectos Congeni-
tos. Presented at *I Congreso Mundial de Obstetricia y Ginecologia.*
January, London; 1991.

55. DeVore GR, Alfi O. The use of color Doppler ultrasound to identify fetuses at increased risk for trisomy 21: an alternative for high-
risk patients who decline genetic amniocentesis. *Obstet Gynecol.*
1995;85:378–386.

56. Allan LD, Sharland GK, Chita SK, et al. Chromosomal anomalies in
fetal congenital heart disease. *Ultrasound Obstet Gynecol.* 1991;1:
8–11.

57. Kupesic S. The first three weeks assessed by transvaginal color
Doppler. *J Perinat Med.* 1996;24:301–317.

58. Kurjak A, Zudenigo D, Predanic M, et al. Recent advances in the
Doppler study of early fetomaternal circulation. *J Perinat Med.*
1994;22:419–423.

59. Kurjak A, Zalud I, Predanic M, et al. Transvaginal color and pulsed
Doppler study of uterine blood flow in the first and early second
trimester of pregnancy: normal vs. abnormal. *J Ultrasound Med.*
1994;13:43–47.

60. Kurjak A, Schulman H, Predanic M, et al. Fetal choroid plexus vascularization assessed by color and pulsed Doppler. *J Ultrasound Med.*
1994;13:841–844.

61. Kupesic S, Kurjak A, Babic MM. New data on early cerebral circulation. *Prenatal Neonatal Med.* 1997;2:48–55.

62. Kurjak A, Schulman H, Zudenigo D, et al. Subchorionic hematomas
in early pregnancy: clinical outcome and blood flow patterns. *J Matern
Fetal Med.* 1996;5:41–44.

63. Kurjak A, Kupesic S. Doppler assessment of the intervillous blood
flow in normal and abnormal early pregnancy. *Obstet Gynecol.*
1997;89:252–256.

DOPPLER AND FETAL ABNORMALITIES IN THE SECOND TRIMESTER

Brian Trudinger / Jill Ablett

Doppler ultrasound is widely used to study blood flow. Two distinct approaches are in use. Blood flow can be imaged to display vascular architecture. Either the frequencies of the Doppler frequency shift signals arising from the ultrasound beam striking a moving column of blood in a blood vessel or the power of the signals (with a Doppler frequency shift) created by the motion can be displayed. In the former, color flow mapping, blood flow is displayed with color coding of velocity and direction of the flow. In the latter there is no directional information. In the second approach the Doppler frequency shift signals from blood flow are displayed on a time base to create a flow velocity waveform. Velocity of flow is proportional to the frequency shift. The waveform shape is influenced by a wide variety of hemodynamic factors including the upstream pump, downstream resistance, vessel branching and local lesions, and properties of the contained blood. Volume blood flow can be calculated from an assessment of velocity and vessel area.

In pregnancy Doppler ultrasound has been widely used to study blood flow. The fact that much of the pioneering work and initial clinical applications using Doppler ultrasound in clinical practice have been focussed on obstetrics is explained by the noninvasive nature of ultrasound studies. This is an essential requirement for pregnancy. In the presence of a fetal anomaly, Doppler studies may provide diagnostic information through an effect on blood flow, imaging characterization of the particular abnormality, or adjunctive information as a result of the effects of the anomaly on cardiac output, fetal growth, and development or placental function.

In this review the information provided by Doppler ultrasound studies in the presence of fetal abnormality will be discussed. The use of Doppler will be divided into the 2 groups outlined above: Doppler flow velocity waveform studies and imaging studies of vascular anatomy.

DOPPLER FLOW VELOCITY WAVEFORM STUDY WITH FETAL ABNORMALITY

UMBILICAL PLACENTAL FLOW VELOCITY WAVEFORMS

Flow velocity waveform (FVW) study by Doppler ultrasound within the gravid uterus includes studies of the umbilical artery and the umbilical placental circulation and studies of the intrafetal vessels. The study of flow velocity waveforms from the umbilical artery provides valuable information about the umbilical placental circulation. Normally the resistance in this vascular bed decreases with advancing gestation as the placenta grows and blood flow increases.[1] The various indices of resistance (the systolic diastolic ratio, the pulsatility index and the resistance index) are measured to quantify the changing waveform shape as end diastolic flow velocities increase relative to the systolic peak velocity of the maximum velocity envelope

of the flow velocity waveform. Mathematical modeling from a computer model of the placenta suggests that these indices may be thought of as a measure of the number of small arterial channels in the placenta.[2] Experimental evidence of this comes from studies in fetal lambs in which the umbilical circulation was embolized with microspheres.[3] In the circumstance of fetal growth restriction these indices are high. This finding has been correlated with an obliteration and loss of small muscular arteries and arterioles from the umbilical placental villous tree.[4]

Major fetal anomaly may be associated with the "high resistance" pattern of reduced, absent, or even reversed diastolic flow velocities in the umbilical artery flow velocity waveform. As stated previously this finding signals a reduced number of small arterial/arteriolar channels in the resistance vessels of the umbilical villous vascular tree. There are 2 explanations for this which are associated with characteristic disturbances in the patterns of fetal growth.[5] Low growth potential in association with the fetal anomaly may lead to a small fetus and placenta. With advancing gestation the fetus and placenta continue to grow but do not achieve normal size and so are small when compared to normal standards. The index of resistance although high will decrease with gestation because the vascular bed (number of channels) is continuing to increase. Alternatively the fetal anomaly may be associated with an obliterative vascular disease in the umbilical placental circulation which is a feature of "placental insufficiency" growth restriction. In this case the number of vascular channels will decrease with advancing gestation and so the index of resistance will increase. It is interesting to speculate that the abnormal conceptus may have a lower threshold or greater propensity for this process to occur. Activation of platelet and endothelial cells, thrombosis and obliteration of placental microcirculation are all part of this process. In a report of 96 fetuses from pregnancy considered at high fetal risk with an extremely abnormal umbilical artery, Doppler study major fetal anomaly was present in 9 cases (10%).[6]

Fetal aneuploidy has been associated with a high-resistance umbilical artery Doppler study. This diagnosis should be sought in the antenatal period for a fetus presenting with profound intrauterine growth restriction or if any "soft sign" abnormality is present in a small fetus. Umbilical artery Doppler may be regarded as another soft sign. It is another aid in management when relevant to the clinical presentation. Although Trisomy 21 is the most frequent karyotype anomaly recognized the number of cases of fetal triploidy is noteworthy. Trisomy 18 fetuses may not be recognized until late in pregnancy when they present as a profoundly "growth restricted" fetus with a high-resistance Doppler study.

The results of published studies of umbilical artery Doppler in association with fetal abnormality are tabulated in Table 27-1. The first study listed, from the writers institution, involved patients in whom an umbilical Doppler study had been performed and major fetal anomaly was evident at birth. All

TABLE 27-1 | ASSOCIATIONS WITH THE ANTENATAL FINDING OF ABSENT END DIASTOLIC FLOW RELOCATION IN THE UMBILICAL ARTERY DOPPLER WAVEFORM

Author	Referral Reason Study Group	Total Cases	Chromosomal Abnormality Present		Major Structural Abnormality Present	
			Umbilical Artery Doppler		Umbilical Artery Doppler	
			Normal	Abnormal	Normal	Abnormal
Trudinger et al. 1991[7]	"major anom."	88	6	16 (73%)	37	29 (52%)
Wenstrom et al. 1991[6]	"high risk"	450 cases 22 with AEDV	N/A	4	16	6 (27%)
Rochelson et al. 1987[9]	AEDF	95	N/A	12 (12.6%)	N/A	N/A
Rizzo et al. 1993[10]	AEDF	192	N/A	16 (8.3%)	N/A	25 (13.0%)
Snijders et al. 1993[11]	IUGR	458	63	26 (5.7%)	167	N/A
Farine et al. 1993[12]	AEDF	916	N/A	50	N/A	65

patients were initially referred because of concerns about the pregnancy and fetal welfare. All patients had routine detailed anatomical studies and umbilical artery Doppler studies. There was no statistically significant difference between those structurally abnormal fetuses with normal or abnormal Doppler studies. However, there was a significant difference in those karyotypically abnormal fetuses with abnormal Doppler studies, compared to normal studies ($p = 0.02$). In this series, 4 of the 5 cases of Trisomy 18 had SD ratios above the 95th percentile, and although the Trisomy 21 cases were distributed between both groups, 8 of these 11 cases had abnormal umbilical artery Doppler studies. Interestingly, all of the perinatal losses in this group with Trisomy 21 had abnormal Doppler studies. In total, there were 5 perinatal deaths in this group ($n = 88$). The overall losses were similar in groups with normal and abnormal Doppler studies.[7]

In the study from Wenstrom et al. the 450 patients were again referred for suspected pregnancy complications.[8] All had detailed ultrasound examination including Doppler studies. Twenty-two fetuses between 20–36 weeks gestation were found to have absent or reversed end-diastolic flow in the umbilical artery Doppler. Of these, 18 underwent karyotyping and 4 were found to be abnormal (22%). Of these the 2 had a Trisomy 18 and resulted in intrauterine fetal death. A fetus with the chromosomal inversion had other serious structural abnormalities and the pregnancy was terminated. The fourth case with a mosaic Trisomy 21 survived. Thus 22% of those with AEDF or reversed flow in the umbilical artery Doppler study had an abnormal karyotype. Six of the 22 with congenital malformations were also noted to have an abnormal umbilical Doppler study (27%).

Two other groups studied the incidence of chromosomal abnormalities in fetuses with AEDF after 20 weeks gestation. The incidences found were 12.6% and 8.3% respectively.[9,10] The second study also noted a significantly earlier gestational age at diagnosis of AEDF in chromosomally abnormal fetuses than those with a normal karyotype (26.7 ± 3.2 weeks vs. 30.1 ± 2.8 weeks, $p < 0.001$). In addition they found that 13% of fetuses with AEDV had associated structural abnormalities. With regard to fetal demise associated with abnormal Doppler studies and aneuploidy it is noted in Rochelson's paper that the 3 fetuses with Trisomy 18 did not survive, but no other follow-up data is reported.[9] Similarly no follow-up data is reported in the paper by Rizzo et al.[10]

The final study from Snijders et al. included patients who were referred for IUGR only. An abdominal circumference less than the 5th percentile for gestational age and no other apparent abnormalities were the entry criteria for the 458 patients who were between 17 and 40 weeks gestation (mean 29).[11] Detailed assessment was performed and Doppler studies of both umbilical and uterine arteries were performed, together with routine karyotyping. There were 89 fetuses with abnormal karyotypes from this group, and again these were detected more frequently in those referred in the second trimester. Fetal malformations were present in 40% of those with abnormal karyotypes compared to 2% with no abnormalities detected ($p < 0.001$). They noted that the incidence of chromosomal abnormalities in the group with normal umbilical and uterine Doppler studies was significantly higher than those where both vessel waveforms were abnormal (44% vs. 8%, $p < 0.001$). This can be interpreted to mean that if the fetus is small and every other fetal welfare study is normal then one should have a high index of suspicion of the possibility of karyotype abnormality. By using only AEDF in the umbilical artery Doppler rather than the uterine Doppler measurements the detection rate was lifted to 32% of the karyotypically abnormal fetuses. Only 6% of these fetuses with IUGR and abnormal karyotype survived the neonatal period, though the majority elected to terminate the pregnancy. By comparison 63% of those fetuses with IUGR and a normal karyotype survived into infancy.

The study report of Farine et al.[12] is a compilation of published and unpublished data and clearly confirms the association of karyotype abnormality and high resistance umbilical artery Doppler study.

There is contradictory evidence on the possible association between abnormal umbilical artery Doppler measurements in the first trimester and aneuploidy. Martinez et al. reported that the umbilical artery Doppler was raised above the 95th percentile in 55% of their 9 cases of Trisomy 21 and this was not always associated with an increased nuchal translucency measurement.[13] In contrast Jauniaux et al.[14] and Brown et al.[15] reported no significant association between the umbilical artery Doppler studies of fetuses with normal and abnormal karyotypes.

The ductus venosus is a unique shunt in the fetal circulation carrying well-oxygenated blood from the umbilical vein through the liver to the right atrium. That blood passes then across the foramen ovale to the left heart and upper body. It appears to be a most useful vessel in assessing disturbed cardiac function.[16] Abnormal patterns probably arise from a high central venous pressure, the result of altered ventricular contractility. It is possible to assess the ductus venosus flow from 11 weeks onward. A study examining ductal flow at 11–14 weeks in fetuses with increased nuchal translucency reported absent or reversed flow during atrial contraction in 57 of 63 (90.5%) chromosomally abnormal fetuses and in only 13 of 423 (3.1%) chromosomally normal fetuses.[17]

FETAL ANEMIA

Study of intrafetal flow velocity waveforms may indicate the presence of fetal anemia. Recent attention has focussed on measurement of peak velocity of the middle cerebral artery flow velocity waveform envelope.[18] Peak velocity correlates with volume blood flow. If the fetus is anemic then blood flow to the brain will increase to ensure oxygen delivery. This is a very plausible explanation for the increase in peak velocity which correlates with the degree of fetal anemia. From a normal range of middle cerebral artery peak velocities plotted against gestational age action values for gestation have been defined for use in rhesus isoimmunization. However this information has the potential for much wider applications. Hydrops fetalis may be of nonimmune origin. Assuming normal cardiac function and control then the same abnormal middle cerebral artery flow velocity waveform pattern will be present when the hydrops is due to fetal anemia of nonimmune origin. Causes of fetal anemia include parvovirus infection, a variety of metabolic errors causing anemia, and the thalassemia group of disorders. Assessment of cerebral artery Doppler is a useful tool to check for anemia in an otherwise unexplained case of hydrops and may reduce the need for invasive fetal testing. Before hydrops is apparent dilatation of the cardiac chambers may be seen.

FETAL CARDIAC ANOMALY, ARRHYTHMIA

It is not the scope of this chapter to describe the Doppler findings of congenital heart disease. Color flow is useful for defining cardiac chambers and great vessels both arterial and venous. Flow velocity waveforms may be used to index volume flow across valves and orifices. Failure of the heart to maintain an adequate output will lead to a high venous pressure.[19]

Characteristic patterns in the flow velocity waveforms recorded from the central fetal vein results. Reversal of flow at the time of atrial contraction (a wave) and during ventricular uptake when the atrial/ventricular valves are closed but tricuspid regurgitation may occur in association with dilatation of the heart. Pulsation in the umbilical vein in the cord may also be seen.[20]

DOPPLER STUDIES OF VASCULAR ANATOMY

Doppler may be used to demonstrate blood flow in fetal vessels. Color Doppler imaging can be simply used to demonstrate the presence or absence of vessels or their situation. Power Doppler imaging is quicker and simpler but does not give velocity or directional information. Study of vascular architecture has diagnostic applications in the workup of fetal developmental anomalies.

TUMORS

The precise diagnosis of fetal tumors imaged in utero can be difficult. The use of color Doppler imaging techniques may assist in the determination of the origins of a mass seen in utero.

Teratoma

Teratomas are the most common of the congenital tumors. They may contain cells derived from all 3 germ layers. The most common sites are the sacrococcygeal region (1 in 40,000 births), the neck, mediastinum, and intracranial areas. These tumors present as a mass, with cystic or solid areas and are typically well vascularized. They may grow to a diameter of 30 cm and show divergent differentiation. Malignant elements are rare in utero but may develop thereafter. Their large blood supply may cause hydrops from high output cardiac failure and arteriovenous shunting from within the tumor. The associated placentomegaly may produce the "mirror syndrome" in the mother, with the manifestations of severe preeclampsia.[21]

The vascularity may be demonstrated using color Doppler imaging techniques. This helps in diagnosis. A cervical teratoma is readily distinguished from a cystic hygroma. The cervical teratoma may also contain calcifications and solid areas, and be associated with hydrops. A sacrococcygeal teratoma may appear in a similar location to a meningomyelocele and again the vascularity of this mass should aid the identification.

The prediction of fetal hydrops and poor outcome was best done by studying vascularity and morphology of a tumor rather than size. Rate of growth is associated with local compression effects and also the development of hydrops. Fetuses with hydrops tended to have tumors that were mainly solid and highly vascularized. There was no significant difference in the incidence of polyhydramnios between fetuses with poor or good outcomes.[22,23]

Tumors of Vascular Origin

Hepatic Hemangioma

Liver tumors are uncommon, representing only 6–8% of all fetal tumors. Hemangiomas can be diagnosed using color Doppler imaging. Arteriovenous shunting and an enlarged artery arising from the aorta supplying the mass may be seen. This may produce cardiac failure and may result in fetal hydrops.[24]

Neuroblastoma

Neuroblastoma arises from the tissue of the neural crest. It is the most common congenital malignant tumor. It may have a cystic or solid appearance and color Doppler may illustrate its highly vascular nature, with pulsatile flow.[21,25] It may be associated with placental metastases. The most common location is the fetal abdomen, with the majority being located in the adrenal medulla.

Renal Tumors

Fetal renal tumors comprise only 5% of all congenital tumors. Mesoblastic nephroma is most common and appears as a non-capsulated mass compressing the renal parenchyma. It has no characteristic vascular pattern. A Wilm's tumor has a more vascular appearance.

Central Nervous System Tumors

Prenatal diagnosis of intracranial tumors is limited, as they are extremely rare. Teratomas are the most common intracranial tumor, and are identified by the hyperechoic multicystic mass with demonstrable vascularity, which may distort the intracranial architecture.[26] Prenatal diagnosis of intracranial vascular malformations have also been reported using color Doppler imaging techniques.[27]

DEVELOPMENTAL ANOMALIES

Bronchopulmonary sequestration is a rare foregut malformation where a mass of lung tissue loses its connection to the rest of the bronchial tree early in development. The circulatory supply to this tissue is usually derived directly from the aorta, suggesting the abnormality occurred early in development. The sequestered lobe may be situated in the fetal thorax or less commonly in the abdomen. This abnormality may be associated in up to 60% of cases with other foregut malformations such as diaphragmatic hernia, tracheoesophageal fistula, or cardiac defects. Bronchopulmonary sequestration can be seen as a unilateral solid or cystic mass in the thorax or abdomen and is difficult to distinguish from a CCAM. However, Doppler imaging techniques may help to identify the blood supply to the sequestered lobe, directly from the aorta. CCAM however, shows no increased vascularity patterns. The distinction between a fetal neuroblastoma and a subdiaphragmatic pulmonary sequestration may be difficult as both are similar in appearance and highly vascular. Curtis et al. in 1997 published an algorhythm following a literature review of this topic.[28] Subdiaphragmatic bronchopulmonary sequestration was more likely to be hyperechoic, be diagnosed in the second trimester, and situated on the left side. The neuroblastoma was mostly identified in the third trimester, the lesion was predominantly cystic and more often right sided.

The anomalous blood supply can rarely cause cardiac failure, manifest as hydrops, and slow polyhydramnios.

ORGAN IDENTIFICATION

The renal arteries can be easily demonstrated branching from the aorta using color Doppler imaging. The failure of development of a single kidney may be seen by the absence of the ipsilateral renal artery. The presence of renal arteries demonstrated by color Doppler techniques will help differentiate between premature rupture of the fetal membranes and renal agenesis in the second trimester fetus with anhydramnios.

CHORIOANGIOMA OF THE PLACENTA

Hemangioma of the placenta has been reported in up to 1% of all placentae. Most tumors are small, single and of no clinical significance. Chorioangiomas larger than 5cm may cause polyhydramnios. Arterio venous shunting may cause fetal hydrops. These tumors may be demonstrated with color Doppler imaging.[21]

References

1. Trudinger BJ, Giles WB, Cook CM, et al. Fetal umbilical artery flow velocity waveforms and placental resistance: clinical significance. *Br J Obstet Gynaecol.* 1985;92:23–30.
2. Thompson RS, Trudinger BJ. Doppler waveform pulsatility index and resistance, pressure and flow in the umbilical placental circulation: an investigation using a mathematical model. *Ultrasound Med Biol.* 1990;16:449–458.
3. Trudinger BJ, Stevens D, Connelly A, et al. Umbilical artery flow velocity waveforms and placental resistance: the effects of embolization of the umbilical circulation. *Am J Obstet Gynecol.* 1987;157:1443–1449.
4. Giles WB, Trudinger BJ, Baird P. Fetal umbilical artery flow velocity waveforms and placental resistance: pathological correlation. *Br J Obstet Gynaecol.* 1985;92:31–38.
5. Trudinger BJ, Cook CM. Umbilical and uterine artery flow velocity waveforms in pregnancy associated with major fetal abnormality. *Br J Obstet Gynaecol.* 1985;92:666–670.
6. Trudinger BJ, Cook CM, Giles WB, et al. Fetal umbilical artery velocity waveforms and subsequent neonatal outcome. *Br J Obstet Gynaecol.* 1991;98:378–384.
7. Trudinger BJ. Doppler ultrasound studies and fetal abnormality. In: *Antenatal Diagnosis of Fetal Abnormalities.* Drife JO, Donnai D, eds. London, England: Springer-Velag; 1991:113–125.
8. Wenstrom KD, Weiner CP, Williamson RA. Diverse maternal and fetal pathology associated with absent diastolic flow in the umbilical artery of high risk fetus. *Obstet Gynecol.* 1991;77:374–378.
9. Rochelson B. The clinical significance of absent end diastolic velocity in the umbilical artery waveform. *Clin Obstet Gynecol.* 1989;32:692–702.
10. Rizzo G, Pietropolli A, Copponi A, et al. Chromosome abnormalities in fetuses with absent end diastolic velocity in umbilical artery: analysis of risk factors for an abnormal karyotype. *Am J Obstet Gynecol.* 1994;171:827–831.

11. Snijders RJ, Sherrod C, Gosden CM, et al. Fetal growth retardation: associated malformations and chromosomal abnormalities. *Am J Obstet Gynecol*. 1993;168:547–555.

12. Farine D, Kelly EN, Ryan G, et al. In: *Doppler Ultrasound in Obstetrics and Gynecology*. Copel J, Reed KL, eds. New York, NY: Raven Press, Ltd; 1995:187–197.

13. Martinez JM, Borrell A, Antonin E, et al. Combining nuchal translucency and umbilical Doppler velocimetry for detecting fetal trisomies in the first trimester of pregnancy. *Br J Obstet Gynaecol*. 1997;104:11–14.

14. Jauniaux E, Garrill P, Khun P, et al. Fetal heart rate and umbilicoplacental Doppler flow velocity waveforms in early pregnancies with a chromosomal abnormality and/or an increased nuchal translucency thickness. *Hum Reprod*. 1996;11:435–439.

15. Brown R, Di Luzio L, Gomes C, et al. The umbilical artery pulsatility index in the first trimester: is there an association with increased nuchal translucency or chromosomal abnormality? *Ultrasound Obstet Gynecol*. 1998;12:244–247.

16. Kiserud T. In a different vein: the ductus venous could yield much valuable information. *Ultrasound Obstet Gynecol*. 1997;9:369–372.

17. Matias A, Gomes C, Flack N, et al. Screening for chromosomal abnormalities at 11–14 weeks: the role of ductus venous blood flow. *Ultrasound Obstet Gynecol*. 1998;12:380–384.

18. Mari G, Deter RL, Carpenter RL, et al. Collaborative Group for Doppler Assessment of Blood velocity in Anaemic Fetuses. Noninvasive diagnosis by Doppler ultrasonography of fetal anemia due to maternal red cell alloimmunization. *N Engl J Med*. 2000;342:9–14.

19. Mori A, Trudinger B, Mori R, et al. The fetal central venous pressure waveform in normal pregnancy and umbilical placental insufficiency. *Am J Obstet Gynecol*. 1995;172:51–57.

20. Reed KL, Anderson CF. Changes in umbilical venous velocities with physiological perturbations. *Am J Obstet Gynecol*. 2000;182:835–838.

21. Goldstein I. *Fetal Neoplasm in Medicine of the Fetus and Mother*. Reece EA, Hobbins JC, eds. 2nd ed. Lippincott-Raven; 1999:643–666.

22. Brace V, Grant SR, Brackley KJ, et al. Prenatal diagnosis and outcome in sacrococcygeal tumors: a review of cases between 1992 and 1998. *Prenat Diagn*. 2000;20:51–55.

23. Westerburg B, Feldstein VA, Sandberg PL, et al. Sonographic prognostic factors in fetuses with sacrococcygeal teratoma. *J Pediatr Surg*. 2000;35:322–326.

24. Meirowitz NB, Guzman ER, Underberg-Davies SJ, et al. Hepatic hemangioendothelioma: prenatal sonographic findings and evolution of the lesion. *J Clin Ultrasound*. 2000;28:258–263.

25. Heling KS, Chaoui R, Hartung J, et al. Prenatal diagnosis of congenital neuroblastoma: analysis of 4 cases and review of the literature. *Fetal Diagn Ther*. 1999;14:47–52.

26. Sherer DM, Onyeije CI. Prenatal ultrasonographic diagnosis of fetal intracranial tumors: a review. *Am J Perinatol*. 1998;15:319–328.

27. Yuval Y, Lerner A, Lipitz S, et al. Prenatal diagnosis of Vein of Galen aneurismal malformation: report of two cases with proposal for prognostic indices. *Prenat Diagn*. 1997;17:972–977.

28. Curtis MR, Mooney DP, Vaccaro TJ, et al. Prenatal ultrasound characterization of the suprarenal mass: distinction between neuroblastoma and subdiaphragmatic extralobar pulmonary sequestration. *J Ultrasound Med*. 1997;16:75–83.

ULTRASOUND IN MULTIPLE GESTATION

Yaron Zalel / Zvi Leibovitz

INTRODUCTION

Although twin pregnancies account for approximately 1–2% of all births, they are associated with 11% of all perinatal mortality.[1] This perinatal mortality is 4–6 times higher than in singletons.[2,3] Stillbirths account for one third of perinatal deaths and two thirds are due to complications of prematurity. The incidence of major malformations in monochorionic twins is 2.3% vs. 1% in singletons and that of minor malformations is 4.1% vs. 2.5% in singletons.[4] Since the highest mortality rate is associated with monoamniotic pregnancies, the most important step toward management of multiple gestations is the precise determination of zygocity (the number of zygotes that produced the multifetal pregnancy) chorionicity (the number of placentas) and amnionicity (the number of amniotic sacs), as described in Table 28-1. It is also important to determine at an early stage the precise number of fetuses, since this number correlates with the risk of prematurity and its complications. The usual length of gestation in a singleton pregnancy (39 weeks) is reduced to 35 weeks in twins, 33 weeks in triplets, and 29 weeks gestation in quadruplets. Recognizing the number of fetuses, chorionicity, and amnionicity as early as possible in pregnancy, may reduce the expected risks and complications (Table 28-2). The aim of this chapter is to describe the important role of ultrasonography in determining zygocity, chorionicity, and amnionicity.

The most common mechanism of twinning (two thirds of cases) is fertilization of several oocytes in 1 menstrual cycle, resulting in genetically different individuals (nonidentical, dizygotic or fraternal twins). The incidence of dizygotic twins varies widely in different populations (from 0.18% in Japan to 5.7% in Nigeria) and has a hereditary tendency. It also varies with maternal age, parity, genetic factors, and obviously—the use of assisted reproductive techniques. Inter-twin circulatory complications are rare, since every zygote develops its own chorion, placenta, and amniotic cavity. In one third of cases, however, the mechanism of twinning is early embryonic splitting of a single zygote (ie, monozygotic). The frequency of monozygotic twinning is relatively constant across populations, occurring at a rate of 1 in 250 births and is independent of maternal age, race, or parity.[5,7]

The type and outcome of monozygotic twinning depends on the time when the zygote undergoes splitting and the degree of differentiation of the chorion and amnion, as described in Table 28-3. The chorion differentiates at day 4 after fertilization and the amnion at day 8. Therefore, splitting before day 3 post-fertilization (prior to the formation of the inner-cell mass at the 2–8 cells stage) results in dichorionic-diamniotic twinning with 2 separate chorions, amnions, and placentas (one third of cases). Splitting on days 4–7 post-fertilization (the early blastocyst stage after the formation of the inner-cell mass) results in development of a single placenta with 2 amniotic cavities (monochorionic-diamniotic). If separation occurs > day 8 post-fertilization (after the embryonic disk and the amnion have already formed) a monochorionic-monoamniotic pregnancy results. Splitting beyond day 13 results in conjoined twins.[8,9]

ULTRASONOGRAPHY

As much as 9.5–12% of natural conceptions are identified as multiple gestations by early first trimester trans-vaginal sonography (TVS).[10,11] Evaluation of chorionicity can be performed by TVS as early as 5 weeks gestation, when separate sacs can clearly be visualized.[12] However, chorionicity and amnionicity are optimally determined at 8–10 weeks. The unique findings in each type of twins are described in the following sections.

DICHORIONIC TWINS

Dichorionic twins are easy to recognize during the first trimester by the demonstration of a thick membrane or "septum" between the 2 embryos (Fig. 28-1). Since the inter-twin membrane in composed of a layer of chorion between 2 layers of amnion, the membrane is thick, especially when seen during 6–9 weeks of gestation. Some authors tried to count the number of membranes to determine chorionicity, but this is not useful as a single marker. The implantation of 2 zygotes will result in 2 separate gestational sacs without a sharing of chorion or amnion. This leads to the insertion of the placenta between the 2 gestational sacs creating the "twin-peak sign" or the "lambda sign."[13,14] Later on, dichorionic twins may be identified by the demonstration of separated placentas or discordant sex. When the twins are of different sexes, most likely that the fetuses are dichorionic.

According to the Birmingham twin survey,[4] 65% of twins have the same sex, among whom 28% are monozygotic and 37% are dizygotic. Thus, discordant sexes virtually exclude monochorionicity. Sonographic follow-up of dichorionic diamniotic twins is demonstrated in Figure 28-3.

MONOCHORIONIC TWINS

The perinatal mortality rate for monozygotic twins is approximately 3 times higher than that of dizygotic twins.[15] The complications associated with monochorionic gestation are twin-to-twin transfusion syndrome (TTTS) in 10–15% of monochorionic gestations, accounting for 17% of the perinatal mortality in multiple pregnancies.[16] Another complication occurs with demise of one co-twin with subsequent damage in the survivor, occurring in as much as 50% of the cases.[17]

In monoamniotic twins there is up to 60% perinatal mortality mainly due to cord entanglement.[18] These complications mandate the early identification of this condition. In addition, monochorionic twins may rarely manifest in unique complications such as conjoined twins and acardiac twin.

| TABLE 28-1 | DIFFERENT TYPES AND FREQUENCIES OF TWIN GESTATIONS ACCORDING TO ZYGOCITY, CHORIONICITY, AND AMNIONICITY |

| | *Chorionicity* | | | |
| | *Monochorionic* | | *Dichorionic* | |
Zygocity	*Monoamniotic*	*Diamniotic*	*Fused[a] Placentas*	*Separate Placentas*
Monozygotic (4/1000)	1%	65%	25%	10%
Dizygotic (8/1000)	—	—	40%	60%

Adapted from reference 6.
[a] Secondary fusion.

MONOCHORIONIC-DIAMNIOTIC TWINS

All monochorionic twins are monozygotic. Monochorionic twinning occurs in two thirds of monozygotic twins.[19] The fetuses share the same chorion and can either share the same amnion (monochorionic-monoamniotic twins) or each have a separate amnion (monochorionic-diamniotic). In monochorionic-diamniotic twins, the preimplantation embryo splits after 4–8 days after fertilization, when the chorion has already differentiated and cannot split. In early pregnancy the 2 embryos are separated by a very thin membrane (Fig. 28-4). Since the chorion is shared, the growing placenta can not infiltrate between the gestational sacs. As a result, the insertion of the dividing membranes to the placenta is in a T-shape. Furthermore, since the dividing membrane is composed of only 2 layers of amnion, it is very thin. It is so thin, that in many instances it cannot be visualized and the pregnancy is misdiagnosed as monoamniotic until later in pregnancy, when the dividing membrane becomes more visible. Moreover, in many instances the monochorionic pregnancy is diagnosed in early pregnancy as a singleton pregnancy when the membrane is barely visible and the other fetus is unnoticed. The sonographic follow-up of monochorionic twins is shown in Fig. 28-5.

The first sonographic clue to a monochorionic gestation is the presence of 2 separate embryo-yolk sac complexes in a single chorionic sac. Later in the pregnancy, it is common to encounter sonographic evidence of TTTS, the severity of which is determined by degree of polyhydramnios and edema in the "recipient," and oligohydramnios in the "donor," leading to a condition of "stuck twin." (Fig. 28-6)

MONOCHORIONIC-MONOAMNIOTIC TWINS

Monoamniotic twins account for 1% of all twin gestations and result from splitting between 7–13 days after fertilization.[8,9] Both fetuses lie in the same gestational sac and share the same chorion and amnion. Monochorionic-monoamniotic pregnancies are often misdiagnosed as singleton gestations on early scans performed at 5–7 weeks. Thus, the diagnosis of monoamniotic twins should not be done before 8 weeks gestation, when the inter-twin membrane should be clearly visible. Further sonographic signs of monochorionic-monoamniotic twinning include a single placenta; the absence of an inter-twin dividing membrane; the presence of a single yolk sacs (in most cases); concordant gender and later in pregnancy cord entanglement (Fig. 28-8). Although monoamniotic twinning is usually associated with a single yolk sac, some cases demonstrate 2 yolk sacs, resulting from a relatively early splitting.

Later in pregnancy, diagnosis of chorionicity is based on the structure of the placenta, the thickness of the inter-twin membrane and the shape of its insertion to the placenta, as described in Table 28-4. One must bear in mind, however, the pitfalls associated with the sonographic markers of chorionicity and amnionicity: While sex discordance implies dizygocity, there are reported cases of monozygotic pregnancies with discordant sex due to anaphase lag in monozygotic twins resulting in a normal 46,XY male and a 45,X Turner syndrome female. Another pitfall is the visualization of what appears to be 2 placentas. While separate placentas imply a dichorionic pregnancy, a succenturiate (accessory) placenta may mimic 2 placentas in a monochorionic pregnancy. Conversely,

| TABLE 28-2 | THE FREQUENCY AND ASSOCIATED MORTALITY RATES IN MONOZYGOTIC TWIN GESTATIONS ACCORDING TO CHORIONICITY AND AMNIONICITY |

Type	*Frequency*	*Mortality*
Dichorionic-diamniotic	30%	9%
Monochorionic-diamniotic	68%	25%
Monochorionic-monoamniotic	1–2%	5–60%

Adapted from reference 5.

| TABLE 28-3 | THE TYPE OF MONOZYGOTIC TWINNING ACCORDING TO THE TIME OF SPLITTING |

Type of Twinning	*Time of Embryo Splitting (Days Post Fertilization)*
Dichorionic-diamniotic	1–3
Monochorionic-diamniotic	4–7
Monochorionic-monoamniotic	8–10
Conjoined	13–15

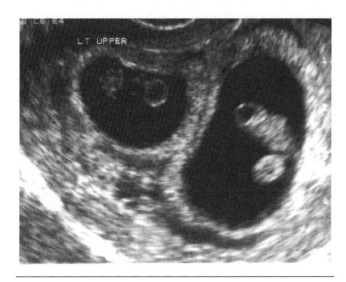

FIGURE 28-1 Dichorionic twins. Note the thick septum between sacs.

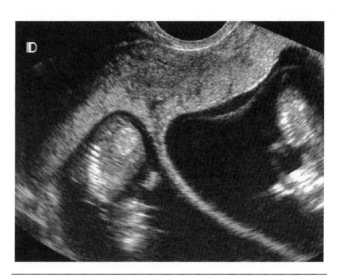

FIGURE 28-2 Lambda or twin-peak sign.

secondary fusion of the placentas occurs in 40% of dizygotic and 25% of monozygotic twins, giving the impression of a single placenta, which may not necessarily be the case. Finally, in a monochorionic pregnancy with TTTS, the "stuck" twin has oligohydramnios bringing the inter-twin membrane in direct contact with its body. This lack of a visible membrane may lead to a misdiagnosis of a monoamniotic pregnancy.

Sepulveda[14] introduced the "Lambda sign." It is applied to the placental edge of the dividing membrane, it is best done at 10–14 weeks' gestation and it has approximately 100% ac-

curacy if it is done correctly. A word of caution, the correct site for evaluating the sign is the attachment to the placenta. In addition, it is important to use a perpendicular plane of insonation, since a wrong plane may lead to a misdiagnosis of inter-twin membrane while there is only a membrane folding.

CONJOINED TWINS

Division of the embryonic disk 13 days or more after fertilization is usually incomplete and results in conjoined twins.[20] All conjoined twins are monozygotic and share the same chorion and amnion. Conjoined twins are a rare anomaly with

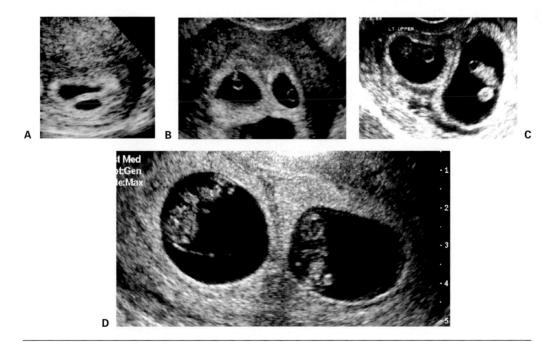

FIGURE 28-3 Natural history of diochorionic-diamniotic twin gestation (**A**) 4 weeks and 4 days; (**B**) 5 weeks and 4 days; (**C**) 7 weeks and 3 days; (**D**) 9 weeks and 2 days.

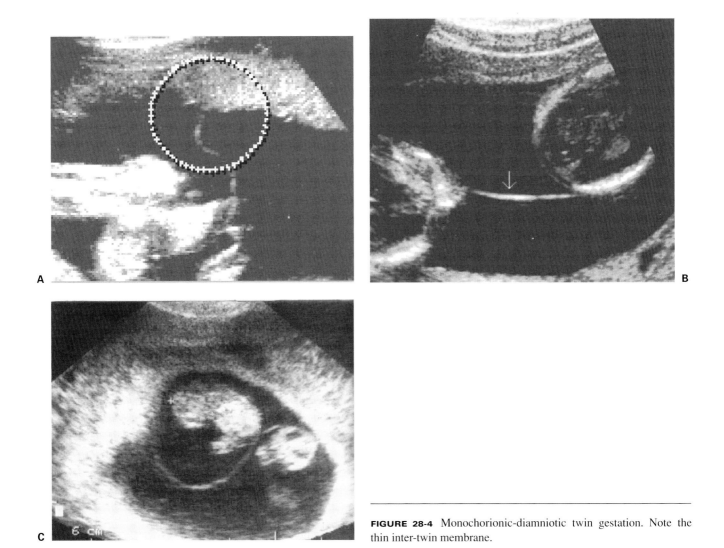

FIGURE 28-4 Monochorionic-diamniotic twin gestation. Note the thin inter-twin membrane.

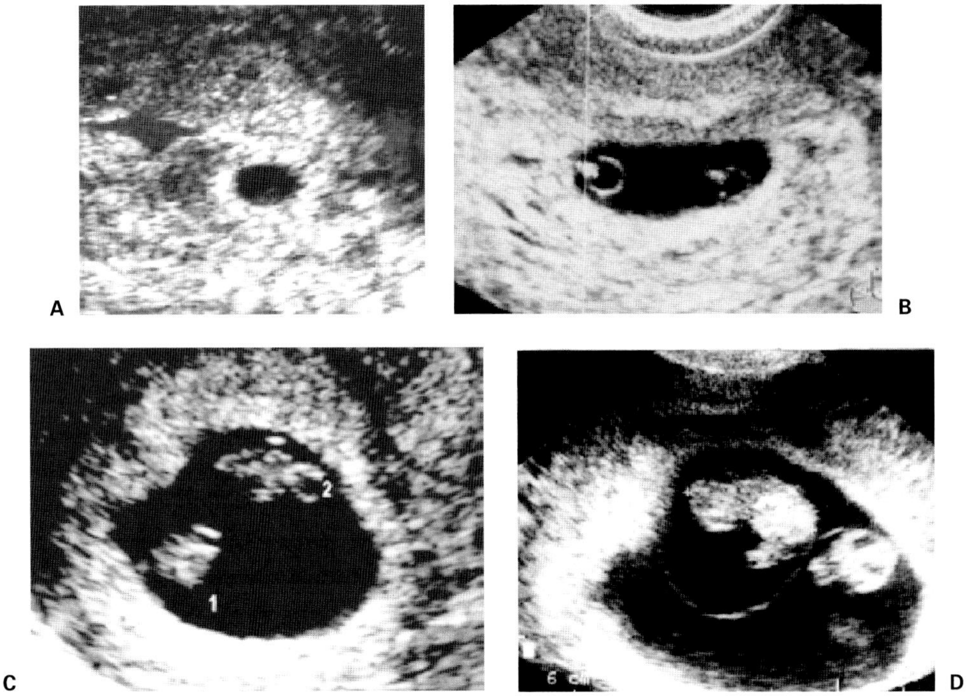

FIGURE 28-5 Natural history of monochorionic-diamniotic twin gestation: (**A**) 4 weeks + 3 days; (**B**) 5 weeks + 2 days; (**C**) 6 weeks + 3 days; (**D**) 9 weeks.

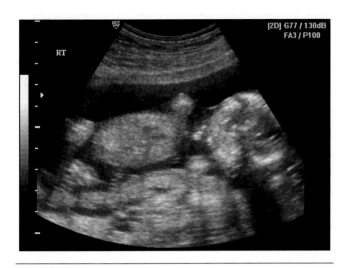

FIGURE 28-6 Monochorionic twins with twin-to-twin transfusion syndrome (TTTS). Note the polyhydramnios in the receipient (upper) and oligohydramnios in the donor (lower) stuck twin.

an estimated frequency of 1 in 50,000–100,000 pregnancies.[21] The nomenclature is based on the site of fusion followed by the suffix *pagus*, the Greek term for "fastened." The most common form is thoraco-omphalopagus—fusion of the thorax and abdomen. These fusions tend to be limited to 1 region and are usually anterior. A side-by-side fusion is more extensive and the term is based on the parts that are separated (Di-cephalic, for example).

Sonographically, conjoined twins should be suspected in a monoamniotic twin gestation in which the fetuses lie in close proximity to each other or when they both move together in tandem. The heart is sometimes shared and there may be a single umbilical cord with more than 3 vessels. Multiple malformations are the rule and polyhydramnios is common. The diagnosis however, should be done with caution: The inter-twin membrane in monochorionic diamniotic twins is sometimes very thin and invisible, especially in TTTS with stuck twins, 1 of the fetuses could be so malformed that the pregnancy could be misdiagnosed as a singleton pregnancy. Finally, discordant presentation does not exclude conjoined twins, on the contrary—it is more common in omphalo-pagus twins. Figure 28-9 describes a thoracopagus (fusion at the thoracic region) at 14 weeks gestation.

THE TWIN REVERSE ARTERIAL PERFUSION (TRAP) SEQUENCE

The twin reverse arterial perfusion (TRAP) sequence is a rare complication of monochorionic multifetal pregnancies, and affects approximately 1% of monochorionic twins—a prevalence of 1 in 35,000 pregnancies.[22,23] A constant feature of the TRAP sequence is artery-to-artery anastomosis, leading to reversed blood perfusion from the donor pump to the acardiac twin. However, the pathogenesis and the initial insult of the TRAP sequence are controversial issues. The phenotype of the acardiac twin is classified according to the mode of development and growth. The TRAP sequence leads mainly to the *acardius acephalus* phenotype (no cranial or thoracic structures and usually malformed upper extremities). However, *acardius anceps* (some cranial structures), and *acardius amorphous* (the most malformed

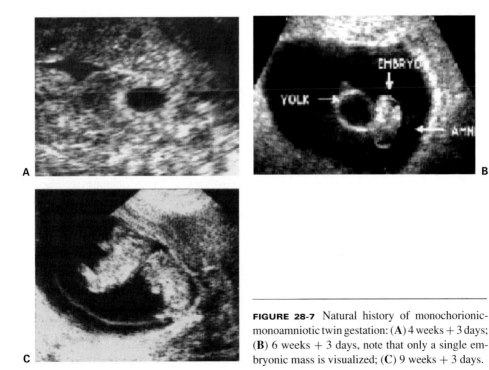

FIGURE 28-7 Natural history of monochorionic-monoamniotic twin gestation: (**A**) 4 weeks + 3 days; (**B**) 6 weeks + 3 days, note that only a single embryonic mass is visualized; (**C**) 9 weeks + 3 days.

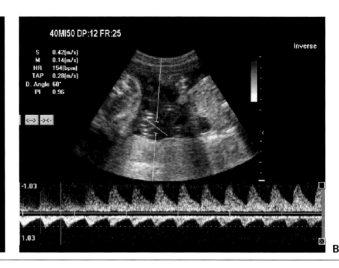

FIGURE 28-8 Cord entanglement in monoamniotic twins at 25 weeks' gestation. (**A**) Color Doppler demonstrating cord entanglement (courtesy of Dr. Israel Shapiro). (**B**) Simultaneous spectral Doppler tracing demonstrating two different heart rates in adjacent umbilical cord loops, "gallop sign."

structure) phenotypes were also described. The rarest phenotype is *acardius acormus* that exhibits cranial elements but no body structure. The diagnosis of TRAP sequence is already available in the first trimester.[24]

HIGHER-ORDER MULTIFETAL PREGNANCIES

Higher order multifetal pregnancies often present a diagnostic challenge. In Western countries, most cases of triploidy are the result of assisted reproductive technologies (ARTs), and are therefore most commonly, trizygotic. However, there are numerous reports of different types of chorionicity in triplet pregnancies, even following ARTs. Such pregnancies may be trichorionic, dichorionic, or monochorionic. Sepulveda et al.[25] suggested using ultrasonographic assessment of the ipsilon zone (the junction of the 3 interfetal membranes) to determine chorionicity in triplet pregnancies. They studied the thickness of the component membranes in the ipsilon zone in 28 triplet pregnancies and detected 22 trichorionic, 5 dichorionic, and 1 monochorionic, and found the assessment correct in all but 1 trichorionic pregnancy, which was misclassified as dichorionic. The issue of chorionicity is particularly important to de-

termine prior to performing multifetal pregnancy reduction (MFPR), in order to avoid reduction of a fetus that shares a chorion with a nonreduced one. In addition, evaluating fetal size prior to MFPR facilitates the choice of fetus for reduction, which would be the smallest one or the one with the largest nuchal translucency. Also, the degree of size discordance in multifetal pregnancy may predict overall outcome.[26]

SUMMARY

In this chapter we illustrated the sonographic findings in twin gestations. As shown, the perinatal mortality rate is proportionally directed to the different types of twinning, with monochorionic (and particularly monoamniotic) twins carrying the highest risk. It is therefore of utmost importance to recognize the type of multi-fetal pregnancy as early as possible, including determination of chorionicity based on the presence and form of the septum between the fetuses. This diagnosis is possible as early as 5 weeks of gestation. Also important is the sonographic follow-up, in the first trimester and later on during gestation in order to detect the complications of twinning and to try to prevent them.

TABLE 28-4	LATE DIAGNOSIS OF TWINNING		
	Dichorionic-Diamniotic	*Monochorionic-Diamniotic*	*Monochorionic-Monoamniotic*
Placentas	Separate	Fused	Fused
Septal insertion	Y-sign	T-sign	
Septal thickness	Thick, layered	Thin, no layers	No septum #

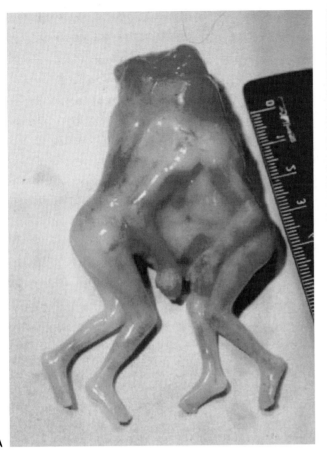

A

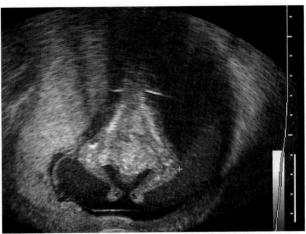

B

FIGURE 28-9 Conjoined twins.

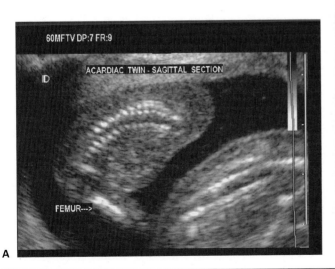

A

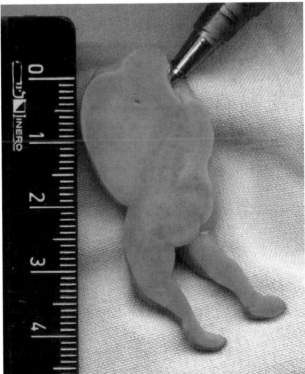

B

FIGURE 28-10 Acardiac twins. Pre- and post-natal illustration of two cases of acardiac twins (Courtesy of Dr. Israel Shapiro). Note the edematous acardiac fetuses which developed from the lower chest downwards.

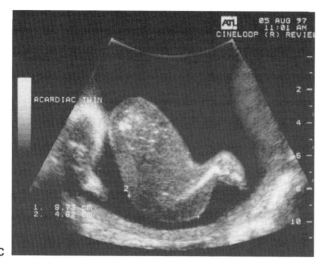

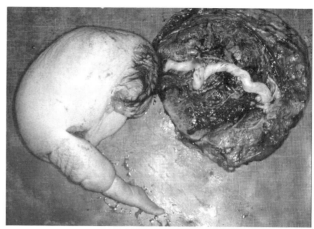

FIGURE 28-10 (*Continued*).

References

1. Hrubec Z, Robinette CD. The study of human twins in medical research. *N Engl J Med.* 1984;310:345.
2. Ghai V, Vidyasagar D. Morbidity and mortality factors in twins. An epidemiologic approach. *Clin Perinatol.* 1988;15:123.
3. Sebire NJ, Nicolaides KH. Screening for fetal abnormalities in multiple pregnancies. *Baillieres Clin Obstet Gynaecol.* 1998;12:19–36.
4. Cameron AH. The Birmingham twin survey. *Proc R Soc Med.* 1968;61:229–234.
5. Benirschke K, Kim CK. Multiple pregnancy. *N Engl J Med.* 1973;288:1276.
6. Thompson MW, et al. *Thompson and Thompson Genetics in Medicine.* 5th ed. Philadelphia: WB Saunders; 1991.
7. Moore KL, Persaud TV. The placenta and fetal membranes in the developing human. In: *Clinical Oriented Embryology.* 5th ed. Philadelphia: WB Saunders; 1993.
8. Baldwin VJ. *Pathology of Multiple Pregnancies.* New York: Springer-Verlag; 1994.
9. Rumack CM, Wilson SR, Charboneau JW, eds. *Diagnostic Ultrasound.* St Louis, MO: Mosby Year Book; 1991;745–758.
10. Bateman BG, Nunley WC Jr., Kolp LA, et al. Vaginal sonography findings and hCG dynamics of early intrauterine and tubal pregnancies. *Obstet Gynecol.* 1990;75:421–427.
11. Boklage CE. Survival probability of human conceptions from fertilization to term. *Int J Fertil.* 1990;35:75–94.
12. Monteagudo A, Timor-Tritsch IE, Sharma S. Early and simple determination of chorionic and amniotic type in multi-fetal gestations in the first fourteen weeks by high-frequency transvaginal ultrasonography. *Am J Obstet Gynecol.* 1994;170:824–829.
13. Finberg HJ. The "twin-peak" sign: reliable evidence of dichorionic twinning. *J Ultrasound Med.* 1992;11:571–577.
14. Sepulveda W, Sebire NJ, Nicolaides KH. The lambda sign in twin pregnancies. *Ultrasound Obstet Gynecol.* 1996;8:429.
15. Naeye RL, Tafari N, Judge D. Twins: causes of perinatal deaths in 12 United States cities and one African city. *Am J Obstet Gynecol.* 1978;131:267.
16. Pietrantoni M, Stewart DL, Ssemakula N, et al. Mortality conference: twin-to-twin transfusion. *J Pediatr.* 1998;132:1071–1076.
17. Liu S, Benirschke K, Scioscia AL, et al. Intrauterine death in multiple gestation. *Acta Genet Med Gemellol (Roma).* 1992;41: 5–26.
18. Colburn DW, Pasquale SA. Monoamniotic twin pregnancy. *J Reprod Med.* 1982;27:165–168.
19. Benirschke K. The biology of the twinning process: how placentation influences outcome. *Semin Perinatol.* 1995;193:42–50.
20. Rudolf AJ, Michaels JP, Nichols BL. Obstetric management of conjoined twins. *Birth Defects.* 1967;3:28.
21. Edmonds LD, Layde PM. Conjoined twins in the United States, 1970–1977. *Teratology.* 1982;25:301.
22. James WH. A note on the epidemiology of acardiac monster. *Teratology.* 1977;16:211–216.
23. Napolitani FD, Schreiber I. The acardiac monster: a review of the world literature and presentation of 2 cases. *Am J Obstet Gynecol.* 1960;80:582.
24. Shalev E, Zalel Y, Ben-Ami M, et al. First trimester ultrasonic diagnosis of twin reversed arterial perfusion sequence. *Prenat Diagn.* 1992;12:219–222.
25. Sepulveda W, Sebire NJ, Odibo A, et al. Prenatal determination of chorionicity in triplet pregnancy by ultrasonographic examination of the ipsilon zone. *Obstet Gynecol.* 1996;88:855–858.
26. Carreno CA, Yaron Y, Feldman B, et al. First trimester embryo size discordance: a predictor of premature birth following multi-fetal pregnancy reduction. *Fertil Steril.* 2001;75:391–393.

CHAPTER 29

THREE-DIMENSIONAL ULTRASOUND IN PRENATAL DIAGNOSIS

Donna D. Johnson / Dolores H. Pretorius

Ultrasound is one of the most important technological advances introduced into modern obstetrics. Its use has revolutionized the prenatal detection of fetal structural anomalies, growth aberrations, and multiple gestations. The advantages of real-time ultrasound include its moderate cost, biosafety for the fetus and mother, the ability to observe in utero behavior, and the ability to do a fetal structural evaluation and obtain biometry noninvasively.[1] The disadvantage of conventional sonography is that acquisition of many fetal images are required to enable the physician interpreting the scan to mentally recreate an impression of a 3-dimensional (3D) structure. Visualization of curved structures and complex anatomical deformities is challenging with conventional technology to the most experienced physician.

Recently, 3D ultrasound has been introduced into clinical medicine.[2-5] The clinical impact of this new technology is broad and very promising in perinatal medicine. An overview of 3D imaging is warranted to understand the potential benefits of 3D ultrasound over existing technology. Although the specific details may vary between machines, the basic concepts are the same. Volume data may be obtained with commercially available 2-dimensional (2D) or annular array transducers. The volume data contain continual 2D images approximately a millimeter apart across an arc of 60–90 degrees. The amount of volume data obtained is dependent on the sweeping arc used, the duration of the acquisition, and the number of acquired images per second. The volume data are stored in a computer memory system. The images in the volume data are displayed in 3 different arbitrary planes, which are perpendicular to each other. These images are referred to as planar images. Using an interactive display, the 3 planar images can be rotated to a standard orientation for ease of interpretation. This feature allows volume data to be collected with ease from any fetal position. For example, the fetal face is oriented so that the images in the three planes correspond to the frontal, sagittal, and axial planes, respectively. Each plane contains many images and each image may be seen by simply scrolling through the desired plane with the interactive display. In addition, the images may be magnified without the need to rescan the patient.

Inexpensive, powerful microprocessors and the development of parellel processors has allowed 3D scanning in real time. In the past, a 3D rendered image was computer generated from a subvolume of the planar images. However, now the fetus may be scanned with real time 3D imaging. The images obtained may be stored as a 3D image or the 3D image plus the planar images. Being able to generate 3D images in real time has drastically reduced the time and complexity of generating a three dimensional image to be viewed with the planar images. In the past computing time for the rendered image varied, depending on the size of the image generated, but could be less than 10 seconds with simple structures like the fetal face to as long as a few minutes with more complicated structures such as the fetal skeletal survey.[2-4,6] Today these images can be displayed in real time.

Viewing fetal structures with 3D images has several significant advantages. First, the 3D rendered image allows the physician to view complex structures in a single image (Fig. 29-1). The physician does not depend on mental reconstruction of the image to define the defect so they may be more confident in the diagnosis. Second, the 3D rendered image may serve as a reference so the exact location on the planar image is well defined. Third, the volume data can be reviewed and processed many times after the ultrasonographic examination is complete. This feature enables the physician to teach residents and sonographers without the patient's presence. The volume can be reviewed millimeter by millimeter in any plane which is more effective than viewing a videotape from 2D sonography. In addition, the volume data can easily be reviewed with other colleagues to obtain second opinions. Fourth, the 2D image is an image that most families can comprehend. Unlike the abstract images obtained with conventional technology, 3D ultrasound provides a realistic presentation, especially of the fetal face. This allows the family to view the normal as well as any abnormal features of their infant with more ease.[7-9]

Never before have we been able to capture such real images of the fetus in utero. Although the medical profession and more importantly the expectant parents may be spellbound by 3D technology, its application and its usefulness in prenatal diagnosis must be studied with scientific rigor. Early investigators showed that 3D ultrasound was clearly applicable in prenatal diagnosis.[2-3,10,11] More recently, articles have been published to demonstrate some of the advantages of 3D ultrasound while others have suggested benefits that are not yet proven.

In one of the largest studies published thus far, Merz et al. examined 242 normal fetuses and 216 fetuses with anomalies with both 2D and 3D ultrasound. Using only the display of the 3 planar images simultaneously, they found diagnostic gain with 3D ultrasound in 46% of the cases. Construction of a 3D rendered image provided more information in 64% of the cases. The highest yield in diagnostic gain (72%) resulted when the 3D image was displayed together with the planar images.[12] This display often improves our ability to evaluate the fetus because fetal structures can be seen in planes that cannot be obtained with traditional ultrasound.

In a similar study, Merz et al. studied 204 fetuses with anomalies. They found 3D ultrasound was advantageous over 2D ultrasound in diagnosing and defining the extent of congenital malformations in 62% of their population. Three-dimensional ultrasound provides the same information in 36% of the cases and was disadvantageous in 2%.[13] Dyson et al. has published similar findings in 63 fetuses with 103 malformations. Three-dimensional ultrasound provided additional diagnostic information in 51% of the anomalies, equivalent to conventional technology in 45% and disadvantageous in 4% of the malformations.[14] In these 2 studies, 3D ultrasound was

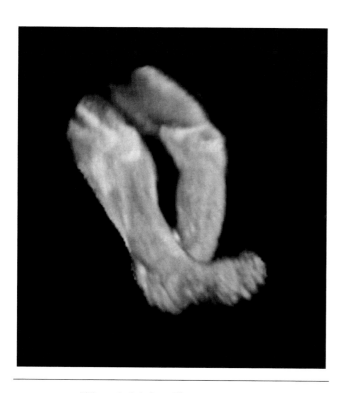

FIGURE 29-1 Bilateral club feet. The varus angulation was present in both ankles. On 3D render view, the position of the feet is more clearly seen. The club foot is seen in the front foot. 3DUS can provide understandable image to patient.

disadvantageous in cases of cardiac defects due to motion artifacts that occurred during volume data acquisition and in complex anomalies with gross disruption where localization of normal landmarks was difficult.

With the addition of spatio-temperol image correlation (STIC), the problems created by motion artifact from cardiac movement should be overcome. This technique allows for temporal resolution which corresponds to a B-mode frame rate. The cardiac volumes are displayed as a single real-time cardiac cycle in a cine loop. The examiner may play the cine loop in slow motion or view static images for a detailed view of specific phases of the cardiac cycle. Each of the planar images can be moved and rotated while maintaining the synchronized cardiac loop.[15] Viñals et al. studied the feasibility and capability of the STIC technology. A general obstetrician collected an acquisition from 100 fetuses with gestational range of 18–37 weeks. A complete cardiac exam was collected in 94% of the fetuses. The only disadvantage of the technology was Doppler velocimetry was not possible however it is available now.[16]

Physicians often have difficulty in correctly identifying facial anomalies and results of studies from several centers confirm a poor detection rate.[17,18] Curvature of the face and inability to obtain views necessary to see all of the facial features limit our diagnostic capabilities. Three-dimensional ultrasound may eliminate some of these obstacles. Pretorius and Nelson studied the face of 27 fetuses and satisfactory surface

rendered 3D images of the fetal face were obtained in 24 fetuses. The lack of a fluid-skin interface was the critical factor limiting visualization in the remaining 3 fetuses. Scanning after 19 weeks produced a higher quality, 3D rendered image of the face.[19] These results have been confirmed by Merz et al. in an additional 125 patients.[20]

In another study, Pretorius et al. examined the fetal lips on both 2D and 3D ultrasound. In 63 fetuses, the presence of a normal lip was confirmed in 92% with 3D sonography compared with only 76% with 2D sonography. Three-dimensional ultrasound showed the greatest diagnostic advantage in the subgroup of fetuses younger than 24 weeks.[21] Although the resolution of the rendered image was difficult to interpret alone in the younger fetuses, it was important as a reference guide for determining the exact location of the lips in the planar images.

Although identification of a paranasal echogenic mass on 2D imaging can assist in the identification of a bilateral cleft palate, the diagnosis of a cleft palate is often very difficult. Johnson et al. examined 31 fetuses with a cleft lip to determine if 3D ultrasound improved the detection of palate involvement (Fig. 29-2). The involvement of the palate was more clearly delineated in more fetuses than with conventional sonography.[22] Lee et al. reported on 7 fetuses with facial cleft abnormalities and added that 3D ultrasound was helpful in identifying the premaxillary protrusion from bilateral cleft lip and palate that was not appreciated on multiplanar images (Fig. 29-2).[23]

Abnormal profiles or dysmorphic faces can be detected by 3D sonography and even related to specific syndromes in some cases. Merz et al. studied 125 fetal facial profiles with 2D and 3D sonography. They found that the facial profile shown in the 2D image represented the true mid-sagittal profile in only 70% of cases. In the remaining 30%, the profile deviated from a true mid-sagittal section by up to 20. Comparison of the surface-rendered profile views provided striking images of the abnormal profiles that may provide additional information to the physician.[20] Profile images are technically much easier to obtain and review with volume imaging than conventional imaging.

Micrognathia can be diagnosed more easily with 3D ultrasound than 2D ultrasound because the profile can be accurately obtained from the volume. Lee et al. examined 9 cases of micrognathia with 3D ultrasound and reported the following advantages: (1) the true mid-sagittal plane was obtained, (2) surface rendering images were helpful in consulting with physicians and counselling patients, (3) improved assessment for facial dysmorphology, particularly for associated cleft lip and palate.[24] Rotten et al. reported on a quantitative method of examining the face for micrognathia and retrognathia which included measurement of the inferior facial angle (normal being greater than 49 degrees).[25] This work is very encouraging.

Lee et al. reported a rendered image of a fetus with Trisomy 13 that clearly demonstrated the absence of normal facial features and a midline single orbit located above a proboscis.[26] Pretorius and Nelson demonstrated a fetus with hypotelorism and a cleft lip on a single rendered image.[19] Van Wymersch

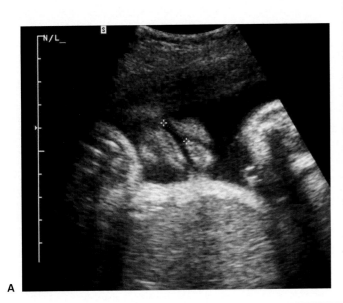

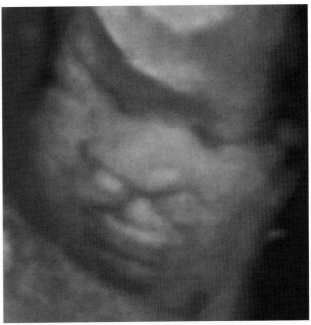

FIGURE 29-2 Unilateral large cleft lip and palate at 34 weeks. (**A**) 2D image in frontal plane shows a cleft in the upper lip marked by the calipers (+). (**B**) A large defect in upper lip and deviated nostril are seen on 4D surface rendering image. On real time 4DUS, the tongue is protruded through the defect for a moment.

et al. established a prenatal diagnosis of Fryns Syndrome using 3D imaging.[27]

Conventional sonography has been of little use in identifying abnormal sutures and fontanelles. Often our evaluation is limited to identifying "overlapping" sutures seen in fetal demise or abnormal cranial contours such as a cloverleaf skull seen in a thanatophoric dwarf. Pretorius and Nelson examined 8 normal volunteer pregnant women with 3D sonography and found that cranial sutures and fontanelles were easily identifiable in all fetuses. The sutures most commonly identified included the coronal, lambdoidal, and squamosal. The fontanelles most often identified included the anterior, posterior, mastoid, and sphenoid.[28] Merz et al. has recently demonstrated delayed ossification of the fetal calvarium in a 20-week fetus affected by achondroplasia.[20] Besides cranial sutures the fetal ear[29] and developing dentention can be addressed.[31] So, 3D sonography offers the potential to identify cranial lesions currently not seen with 2D sonography.

Spinal anomalies, such as neural tube defects, scoliosis, and hemivertebrae (Fig. 29-3) are common congenital defects. Accurate diagnosis of spinal defects requires an appreciation of normal anatomy as well as artifacts produced by the transducer, such as pseudodysmorphism.[31] The recognition of associated sonographic abnormalities in the fetal skull and cerebellum has enhanced the antenatal detection of neural tube defects.[32] However, localization of the neural tube defect is often difficult with conventional sonography.[33] Johnson et al. studied a small group of 9 fetuses with neural tube defects. The spinal defects were examined on both 2D and 3D sonography. Using 3D ultrasound, they localized the neural tube defect on average 2

vertebral bodies higher on 3D ultrasound. In the cases in which the exact location of the lesion was known, the level of vertebral body involvement was determined more accurately with 3D imaging. In addition, they were able to localize one lesion that could not be defined on conventional equipment.[34] Mueller et al. also looked at a small number of patients with neural tube defects and found 3D ultrasound was helpful in delineating the exact anatomic level of the defect. They reported that the increased confidence of the precise lesion location improved patient counseling.[35] Lee et al. also reported similar findings in a study of 9 fetuses with spina bifida.[36] In all 3 of these studies, the 3D rendered image was beneficial in defining both normal anatomy (Figs. 29-5, 29-6) as well as spinal pathology (Fig. 29-7).[34–36] After key landmarks such as the twelfth thoracic vertebral body were identified on the 3D rendered image, the lesion could be localized in the coronal, sagittal, and transverse view without concern for fetal motion that is encountered in real-time scanning.

Three-dimensional ultrasound may be useful in diagnosing and studying other central nervous system abnormalities. Blaas et al. examined 3 first trimester fetuses at 7–11 weeks gestation and found that at 7 weeks, the rhombencephali as well as both hemispheres and their connection to the third ventricle were readily identifiable. They followed the development of brain cavities and demonstrated the dominant size of the hemispheres by 11 weeks. They predicted 3D ultrasound would enhance detection of early developmental central nervous system abnormalities.[37] Benoit et al. also reported on neurosonography in the first trimester and emphasized the development of the ventricular system and the fact that lucencies should

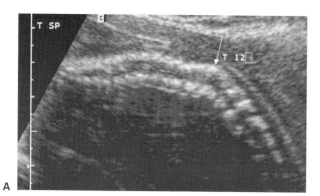

A

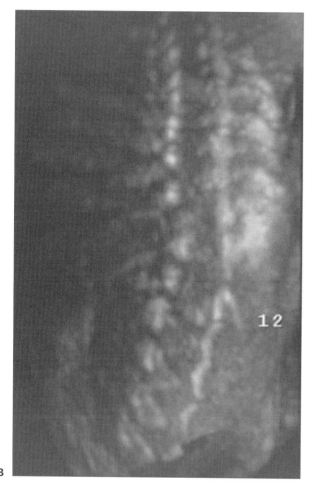

B

FIGURE 29-3 Hemivertebrae. Scoliosis of the lower thoracic spine in a 31 weeks' gestational age fetus. (**A**) 2D image shows scoliosis of lower lumbar spine (T 12 = 12th thoracic vertebra level). (**B**) 3D rendered image of scoliosis at the 10th and 12th thoracic vertebrae levels.

be seen in the brain as early as 8 weeks.[38] In older fetuses, Mueller et al. examined 4 fetuses with hydrocephalus. The 3 planar views allowed them to clarify intracranial anatomy especially in cases that fetal position limited the information obtained from the 2D scan[35] (Fig. 29-4). Examination of the fetal central nervous system by Hamper et al. also demonstrated

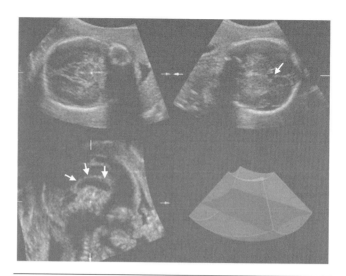

FIGURE 29-4 Multiplanar display of the midline structures of the brain. Upper left image is axial, upper right image is coronal and lower left image is sagittal. The septum pellucidum (arrows) is best seen on the sagittal plane in the lower left image however it is also seen on the coronal image in the upper right image.

that 3D ultrasound reduced reverberation artifacts in the fetal head.[11]

Screening ultrasound with conventional technology for urogenital malformations is accurate for simple renal anomalies, such as hydronephrosis, with detection rates greater than 95% reported.[17] However, detecting and defining more complex urogenital anomalies such as a horseshoe kidney and ambiguous genitalia is much less reliable. In this organ system, 3D ultrasound may provide additional diagnostic information

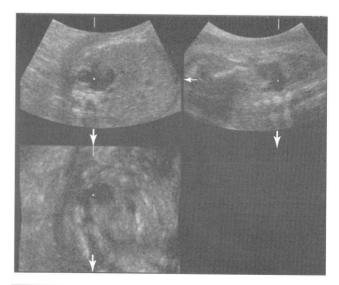

FIGURE 29-5 Unilateral hydronephrosis. The pelvis and ureter could be followed using the cursor dot to the bladder. The cursor dot is positioned within the dilated renal pelvis in all three planes: upper left is axial, upper right is coronal and lower left is sagittal.

especially in the more complex anomalies. Merz and his colleagues examined 51 cases of urogenital malformations including: hydronephrosis, Potter syndrome, Wilm tumor, Prune Belly syndrome, and hydrocele. Three-dimensional ultrasound was advantageous in 43% of the malformations. Two-dimensional and three-dimensional ultrasound provided the same information in 57% of the cases.[13] Other case reports have suggested detailed benefits to 3D ultrasound in urogenital malformations. Steiner and his colleagues were able to differentiate a fetal abdominal retroperitoneal cystic structure from dilated ureters. They used a feature known as a flight path on the 3D ultrasound, which allows the sonographer to mark a tortuous structure so the marked structure can be evaluated in consecutive axial plane images in the volume data (Fig. 29-5). The authors were able to demonstrate prenatally that a retroperitoneal cystic structure was not connected to the renal structures.[8] In another case, Lee et al. were able to define a complex malformation of the external genitalia in a 27-week-old male fetus. On 2D ultrasound, 2 echogenic areas consistent with enlarged female labia were seen in the region of the genitalia. Yet, the karyotype was consistent with a male fetus. Despite proper fetal position, a scrotum and penis could not be simultaneously imaged with conventional technology. Three-dimensional surface rendered image of the external genitalia revealed a bipartite scrotum. The accuracy and resolution of the 3D surface rendered image was striking when compared to the photographs of the infant taken after delivery.[39]

Evaluation of the fetal extremities is useful in patients at risk for a chromosome anomaly, limb reduction defects, neural tube defects, neuromuscular disorders, and skeletal dysplasia as these fetuses are at risk for abnormal hand posture, club feet, rocker bottom feet, and abnormal bones in the limb.[40–42] While some limb anomalies are associated with specific abnormalities, others are isolated birth defects. The detection rate of limb abnormalities with current technology is difficult to ascertain since limbs were only recently added to the guidelines adopted by the A.I.U.M. and the American College of Obstetrics and Gynecology.[1,43] In a study of the upper extremity, Budorick et al. examined 31 normal and 12 abnormal upper extremities with both 2D and 3D ultrasound. The 2 technologies were similar in determining if the upper extremity was normal or abnormal. However, 3D ultrasound provided additional information in both normal and abnormal hands. With the newer technology, the volume data could be rotated such that the hands could be evaluated in planes not possible with conventional technology. In the surface rendered image, the relationship of the thumb and fingers could be routinely evaluated on the same image, and the digits counted easily. A loosely curled fist with normal digits could be readily distinguished from a clenched fist with overlapping digits. In the abnormal upper extremities, most wrists were found to be severely flexed which was easily demostrated with 3D ultrasound. The 3D image improved the physician's understanding of the precise relationship of the wrist, hand, and digits of the upper extremity.[44]

In another study, Ulm and co-workers examined the fetal upper extremity of 70 low-risk patients from 10 to 32 weeks.

They were able to evaluate all of the digits in 74% of cases with 3D ultrasound but only 53% with 2D ultrasound. Optimal visualization was achieved between 20 and 23 weeks. In this subgroup, all fingers were visualized in 100% of the fetuses with 3D technology. The time required to visualize all of the digits on the upper extremity was less with the newer technology because the authors did not have to wait for the fetus to optimally position the upper extremity and hand.[45]

In a similar study of the lower extremity, Budorick et al. studied 36 high-risk fetuses. As expected, 3D ultrasound provided 3 planes (coronal, sagittal, and axial) to view the lower extremity with 1 volume acquisition. Normal features of the distal lower extremity were demonstrated more frequently with 3D ultrasound than 2D ultrasound in the coronal view. In the sagittal view, normal features were equally demonstrated with both technologies. Abnormal features were seen equally as well as in the coronal and sagittal views with both modalities. The advantage of 3D imaging of the lower extremity was the ability to view the distal lower extremity during rotation of the surface rendered image (Fig. 29-1). As in the upper extremity, the anatomical relationship of the lower leg and foot could be more clearly defined in the 3D image. In addition, in this image the digits of the lower extremity could be counted without spending extra time to obtain a specific view of the foot in real-time.[46]

Favre and his colleagues studied limb circumferences obtained by 3D ultrasound to predict fetal birthweight. Using a formulae that incorporated thigh and arm circumference, this group was able to predict fetal birthweight more accurately than traditional formulae. The most accurate results were obtained for macrosomic fetuses. Three-dimensional ultrasound was advantageous because reproducible limb circumference measurements could be obtained. The midpoint of the extremity on the sagittal view was determined while simultaneously displaying the transverse view in the same location. With conventional sonography, the circumference of the limbs were very difficult to standardize. They concluded that the use of 3D ultrasound could facilitate a more accurate prediction of fetal weight.[47]

One of the most promising applications of 3D ultrasound in obstetrics is volume measurements. In vitro studies of various shaped balloons by Riccabona et al. have demonstrated greater accuracy of 3D ultrasound volume measurements compared to conventional 2D ultrasound volume calculations. Three-dimensional volume measurements revealed a mean absolute error of $6.4 \pm 4.4\%$ which was more accurate than 2D volume calculations with a mean absolute error of $12.6 \pm 8.7\%$. For irregularly shaped objects, conventional sonography was even more inaccurate than 3D technology.[48] These results were also confirmed in vivo by studying adult bladder volumes.[49] Their work has also been confirmed by Brunner et al. Follicular cyst volumes were measured with 3D ultrasound prior to transvaginal needle-guided aspiration. A good correlation was seen between the sonographic volumes and the amount of fluid obtained.[50]

The volume of the gestational sac has been investigated as a possible predictor of pregnancy outcome by Steiner and co-workers. They evaluated 38 pregnancies between 5 and 11 weeks gestation, of which 31 had a normal outcome and 7 had complications. Complications included blighted ovum or embryonic demise. Their results revealed gestational sac volume correlated well to gestational age. In addition, 3D volume measurements of the gestational sac were highly accurate between different observers. Most of the abnormal outcomes had a gestational sac volume greater than two standard deviations below the mean.[51]

Precise lung volume measurements may be able to more accurately predict fetal outcome in conditions associated with pulmonary hypoplasia such as congenital diaphragmatic hernia and oligohydramnios. Measuring total fetal lung volume in utero is difficult with existing technology. However, measuring fetal pulmonary volume in utero with 3D ultrasound is promising. D'Arcy et al. measured fetal lung volumes in 20 healthy women with a singleton pregnancy between 24 and 36 weeks of gestation. They found that total lung volume increased exponentially with gestational age. Right lung volume measured consistently greater than left lung volume.[52] Lee et al. reported similar findings in 78 fetuses from 14 weeks of gestation to term.[53] Both studies suggested that 3D volume measurements accurately reflect fetal lung volume.[52,53] The reliability of this new technology in predicting abnormal lung volumes has not been studied yet.

As with 2D ultrasound, artifacts can be confused with an anomaly on 3D images. Pretorius et al. reported a false-positive cleft lip on a 3D surface rendered image of a fetal face. In this 36-week fetus, the upper lip appeared normal with conventional technology and was normal at birth. Upon reviewing the volume data, the umbilical cord was lying adjacent to the upper lip simulating a cleft.[21] Riccabona et al. reported narrowing of the thoracic spine in a 3D rendered image, yet the infant was normal at birth. Pseudo-narrowing was created by reduced echogenicity of the ossification center in the lateral arch and higher echo intensity of the ossification of the central vertebral body.[54] Both of these artifacts could have been detected by viewing the 3D rendered image simultaneously with the 3 planar images.

Three-dimensional ultrasound also has limitations. First, motion artifacts are produced in the volume data when the fetus moves. Fetal motion is readily seen during data collection and the scan can be repeated quickly. Second, the size of the scanned volume is limited. This is usually not a problem in the first half of gestation but can limit the amount of a fetal structure, such as the spine, that can be seen in a single 3D rendered image later in gestation. Third, 3D images containing many planar images and a large degree of rotation may be time consuming to construct. As technology advances, the time will likely decrease. Finally, the physician must be knowledgeable in 3D device handling. Inadequate selection of postprocessing modalities may cause suboptimal display of the 3D image. Although general guidelines are available, postprocessing features are learned by trial and error. However, the volume data may be manipulated as often as you desire without the need to rescan the patient.

Unfortunately, 3D does not immediately change a less skilled sonography into an excellent one. Where there is an optical barrier, no ultrasound information is obtained regardless of whether 2D or 3D ultrasound is used. Unfavorable scanning conditions, such as oligohydramnios, severe maternal obesity, and absence of tissue borderlines cause the same problems in both scanning modalities. In short, both scanning techniques are dependent on the same physical principles.

In summary, 3D ultrasound offers some distinct advantages over existing technology. This technology has undergone rapid advances in recent years and continues to progress quickly. Unquestionably, 3D ultrasound is gaining increasing importance in prenatal diagnosis and will likely become an integral part of it in the near future.

References

1. Ultrasound in Pregnancy. *ACOG Technical Bulletin.* 1993;187.
2. Baba K, Satoh K, Sakamoto S, et al. Development of an ultrasonic system for three-dimensional reconstruction of the fetus. *J Perinat Med.* 1989;17:19–24.
3. Kuo HC, Chang FM, Wu CH, et al. The primary application of three-dimensional ultrasonography in obstetrics. *Am J Obstet Gynecol.* 1992;166:880–886.
4. Kirbach D, Whittingham. 3D ultrasound—the Kretztechnik-Voluson approach. *Eur J Ultrasound.* 1994;1:85–89.
5. Pretorius DH, Nelson TR, Jaffe JS. 3D sonographic analysis based on color flow Doppler and gray scale image data: a preliminary report. *J Ultrasound Med.* 1992;11:225–232.
6. Riccabona M, Pretorius DH, Nelson TR, et al. Three-dimensional ultrasound: display modalities in obstetrics. *J Clin Ultrasound.* 1997;25:157–167.
7. Rankin RN, Fenster A, Downey DB, et al. Three-dimensional sonographic reconstruction: techniques and diagnostic applications. *AJR Am J Roentgenol.* 1993;161:695–702.
8. Steiner H, Staudach A, Spitzer D, et al. Three-dimensional ultrasound in obstetrics and gynecology: technique, possibilities and limitations. *Hum Reprod.* 1994;9:1773–1778.
9. Pretorius DH, Nelson TR. Three-dimensional ultrasound imaging in patient diagnosis and management: the future. *Ultrasound Obstet Gynecol.* 1995;5:219–221.
10. Nelson TR, Pretorius DH. Three-dimensional ultrasound of fetal surface features. *Ultrasound Obstet Gynecol.* 1992;2:166–174.
11. Hamper UM, Trapanotto V, Sheth S, et al. Three-dimensional ultrasound: preliminary clinical experience. *Radiology.* 1994;191:397–401.
12. Merz E, Bahlmann F, Weber G, et al. Three-dimensional ultrasound in prenatal diagnosis. *J Perinat Med.* 1995;23:213–222.
13. Merz E, Bahlmann F, Weber G. Volume scanning in the evaluation of fetal malformations: a new dimension in prenatal diagnosis. *Ultrasound Obstet Gynecol.* 1995;5:222–227.
14. Dyson R, Pretorius DH, Budorick NE, et al. Three-dimensional ultrasound in evaluation of fetal anomalies. *Ultrasound Obstet Gynecol.* 2000;16:321–328.
15. DeVore GR, Falkensammer P, Sklansky MS, et al. Spatio-temporol image correlation (STIC): new technology for evaluation of the fetal heart. *Ultrasound Obstet Gynecol.* 2003;22:380–387.

16. Vinals F, Poblete P, Giuliano A. Spatio-temperol image correlation (STIC): a new tool for the screening of congenital heart defects. *Ultrasound Obstet Gynecol.* 2003;22:380–387.

17. Crane JP, LeFevre ML, Winborn RC, et al. A randomized trial of prenatal ultrasonographic screening: impact on detection, management and outcome of anomalous fetuses. *Am J Obstet Gynecol.* 1994;171:392–399.

18. Chitty LS, Hunt GH, Moore J, et al. Effectiveness of routine ultrasonography in detecting fetal structural abnormalities in a low risk population. *BMJ.* 1991;303:1165–1169.

19. Pretorius DH, Nelson TR. Fetal face visualization using three-dimensional ultrasonography. *J Ultrasound Med.* 1995;14:349–356.

20. Merz E, Weber G, Bahlmann F, et al. Application of transvaginal and abdominal three-dimensional ultrasound for detection or exclusion of malformations of the fetal face. *Ultrasound Obstet Gynecol.* 1997;9:237–243.

21. Pretorius DH, House M, Nelson TR, et al. Evaluation of normal and abnormal lips in fetuses: comparison between three- and two-dimensional sonography. *AJR Am J Roentgenol.* 1995;165:1233–1237.

22. Johnson DD, Pretorius DH, Budorick NE, et al. Three-dimensional ultrasound of the fetal lip and primary palate: three-dimensional versus two-dimensional ultrasound. *Radiology.* 2000;217:236–239.

23. Lee W, Kirk JS, Shaheen KW, et al. Fetal cleft lip and palate detection by three-dimensional ultrasonography. *Ultrasound Obstet Gynecol.* 2000;16:314–320.

24. Lee W, McNie B, Chaiworapongsa T, et al. Three-dimensional ultrasonographic presentation of micrognathia. *J Ultrasound Med.* 2002;21:775–781.

25. Rotten K, Levaillant JM, Martinez H, et al. The fetal mandible: a 2D and 3D sonographic approach to the diagnosis of retrognathia and micrognathia. *Ultrasound Obstet Gynecol.* 2002;19:122–130.

26. Lee A, Deutinger J, Bernaschek G. Three-dimensional ultrasound: abnormalities of the fetal face in surface and volume rendering mode. *Br J Obstet Gynaecol.* 1995;102:302–306.

27. van Wymersch D, Favre R, Gasser B. Use of three-dimensional ultrasound to establish the prenatal diagnosis of Fryns syndrome. *Fetal Diagn Ther.* 1996;11:335–340.

28. Pretorius DH, Nelson TR. Prenatal visualization of cranial sutures and fontanelles with three-dimensional ultrasonography. *J Ultrasound Med.* 1994;13:871–876.

29. Shih JC, Shyu MK, Lee CN, et al. Antenatal depiction of the fetal ear with three-dimensional ultrasonography. *Obstet Gynecol.* 1998;91:500–505.

30. Ulm MR, Kratochwil A, Ulm B, et al. Three-dimensional ultrasound evaluation of fetal tooth germs. *Ultrasound Obstet Gynecol.* 1998;12:240–243.

31. Dennis MA, Drose JA, Pretorius DH, et al. Normal fetal sacrum simulating spina bifida: pseudo dysraphism. *Radiology.* 1985;155:751–754.

32. van den Hof MC, Nicolaides K, Campbell J, et al. Evaluation of the lemon and banana signs in one hundred thirty fetuses with open spina bifida. *Am J Obstet Gynecol.* 1990;162:322–327.

33. Kollias SS, Goldstein RB, Cogen PH, et al. Prenatally detected myelomeningoceles: sonographic accuracy in estimation of the spina level. *Radiology.* 1992;185:109–112.

34. Johnson DD, Pretorius DH, Riccabona M, et al. Three-dimensional ultrasound of the fetal spine. *Obstet Gynecol.* 1997;89:434–438.

35. Mueller GM, Weiner CP, Yankowitz J. Three-dimensional ultrasound in the evaluation of fetal head and spine anomalies. *Obstet Gynecol.* 1996;88:372–378.

36. Lee W, Chaiworapongsa T, Romero R, et al. A diagnostic approach for the evaluation of spina bifida by three-dimensional ultrasonography. *J Ultrasound Med.* 2002;21:619–626.

37. Blaas HG, Eik-Nes SH, Kiserud T, et al. Three-dimensional imaging of the brain cavities in human embryos. *Ultrasound Obstet Gynecol.* 1995;5:228–232.

38. Benoit B, Hafner T, Kurjak A. Three-dimensional neurosonography in the first trimester of pregnancy. *Ultrasound Rev Obstet Gynecol.* 2001;1:128–137.

39. Lee A, Deutinger J, Bernaschek G. "Voluvision:" three-dimensional ultrasonography of fetal malformations. *Am J Obstet Gynecol.* 1994;170:1312–1314.

40. Benacerraf BR, Frigoletto FD, Greene MF. Abnormal facial features and extremities in human trisomy. *Radiology.* 1986;159:243–246.

41. Bromley B, Benacerraf BR. Abnormalities of the hands and feet in the fetus: sonographic findings. *AJR Am J Roentgenol.* 1995;165:1239–1243.

42. Benacerraf BR. Antenatal sonographic diagnosis of congenital clubfoot: a possible indication for amniocentesis. *J Clin Ultrasound.* 1986;14:703–706.

43. Laurel, MD. Standards for the performance of the antepartum obstetrical ultrasound examination. *American Institute of Ultrasound in Medicine.* 1994.

44. Budorick NE, Pretorius DH, Johnson DD, et al. Three-dimensional ultrasound examination of the fetal hands: normal and abnormal. *Ultrasound Obstet Gynecol.* 1998;12:1–8.

45. Ploeckinger-Ulm B, Ulm MR, Lee A, et al. Antenatal depiction of fetal digits with three-dimensional ultrasonography. *Am J Obstet Gynecol.* 1996;175:571–574.

46. Budorick NE, Pretorius DH, Johnson DD, et al. Three-dimensional ultrasonography of the fetal distal lower extremity: normal and abnormal. *J Ultrasound Med.* 1998;17:649–660.

47. Favre R, Bader AM, Nisand G. Prospective study on fetal weight estimation using limb circumferences obtained by three-dimensional ultrasound. *Ultrasound Obstet Gynecol.* 1995;6:140–144.

48. Riccabona M, Nelson TR, Pretorius DH. Three-dimensional ultrasound: accuracy of distance and volume measurements. *Ultrasound Obstet Gynecol.* 1996;7:429–434.

49. Riccabona M, Nelson TR, Pretorius D, et al. In vivo three-dimensional sonographic measurement of organ volume: validation in the urinary bladder. *J Ultrasound Med.* 1996;15:627–632.

50. Brunner M, Obruca A, Bauer P, et al. Clinical application of volume estimation based on three-dimensional ultrasonography. *Ultrasound Obstet Gynecol.* 1995;6:358–361.

51. Steiner H, Gregg AR, Bogner G, et al. First trimester three-dimensional ultrasound volumetry of the gestational sac. *Arch Gynecol Obstet.* 1994;255:165–170.

52. D'Arcy TJ, Hughes SW, Chiu WSC, et al. Estimation of fetal lung volume using enhanced 3D ultrasound: a new method and first result. *Br J Obstet Gynaecol.* 1996;103:1015–1020.

53. Lee A, Kratochwil A, Stumpflen I, et al. Fetal lung volume determination by three-dimensional ultrasound. *Am J Obstet Gynecol.* 1996;175:588–592.

54. Riccabona M, Johnson DD, Pretorius DH, et al. Three-dimensional ultrasound: display modalities in the fetal spine and thorax. *Eur J Radiol.* 1996;22:141–145.

THREE-DIMENSIONAL FETAL NEUROSCAN

Ilan E. Timor-Tritsch / Ana Monteagudo

In one of our earlier publications we said that, there is no other part in the fetal body that undergoes as much change in a short time until delivery occurs than the central nervous system (CNS). Other fetal organs or organ systems reach their final sonographic appearance early in gestation. The only change that takes place in these systems is that they increase in volume and in size.[1]

For those who engage in scanning the CNS, ultrasound knowledge and understanding of the developmental changes of the brain that occur during fetal life is of utmost importance. Since we would like to detect fetal malformations as early as possible, we have to be aware of the developmental changes in the fetal CNS which are a function of gestational age. An important ingredient to achieve a clinical and meaningful sonographic diagnosis of the developing fetal brain is to use high-frequency ultrasound transducers. These produce sonographic pictures of high quality. Examining these high quality sonographic pictures enable us to detect subtle changes and pathologies in the fetal brain. Our and other worker's approach has always been that high-frequency probes can be used throughout the pregnancy to obtain high-quality and high-resolution images of the fetal brain.[2-13]

Before we engage in the discussion of the three-dimensional (3D) technique of the fetal neurosonography the basic technique of the transvaginal approach to scan the fetal brain has to be addressed.

THE TECHNIQUE OF TRANSVAGINAL FETAL NEUROSCAN

Two kinds of ultrasound probes can be utilized for fetal neuroscan: transabdominal and transvaginal ultrasound probes. The former employs lower frequencies as opposed to the transvaginal probes, which are built to emit higher frequencies to accomplish the examination. Preferentially, during the first half of the pregnancy, high-frequency transvaginal probes should be used. The reason for this is that the fetal skull in early pregnancy is relatively thin and sound waves penetrate easily to image the brain. Logically, this is also the reason that high-frequency transvaginal probes should be the "first line" choice regardless of fetal position. If the fetus is in vertex presentation it is possible to continue and employ TVS scanning anytime in pregnancy. However, if the fetal head is above the pelvis—transverse or breech presentation—transabdominal probes are usually used. Maybe one has to repeat the fact that TVS utilizes probes which operate at frequency 5–10 MHz while TAS probes utilizes frequencies of 3–5 and up to 7 MHz. This is true regardless of two-dimensional (2D) or 3D scanning. As pregnancy progresses, the fetal skull thickens/increases; therefore, ways to circumvent this obstacle have to be found. Scanning through the relatively large and open anterior and posterior or fontanelle is one of the solutions.

Transvaginal transfontanelle scanning generates clinically diagnostic pictures. The planes obtained by the transfontanelle scanning window are: the median and paramedian (or oblique) sections in the traditional sagittal direction and by turning the transducer 90°: several coronal sections. The advantage of transvaginal transfontanelle fetal neuroscan is that we can use identical and comparable planes and sections to those obtained by the neonatal transfontanelle neuroscan. If suspicion of a fetal brain malformation arises, showing the pictures to the pediatric neurologists they will have a clear understanding of the location, identity, and extent of the lesion.

Using transabdominal scanning, the images are generated through the bones and will result in a relatively less detailed picture of the fetal brain, mainly in the axial plane (Fig. 30-1). However, using the transvaginal transfontanelle approach we can obtain the diagnostically important sagittal as well as the coronal planes. 3D volume scan of the fetal brain, as it will be pointed out later, will circumvent some of the problems mentioned here.

The technique of transvaginal fetal neuroscan is simple. The technique of acquiring the images is similar in the 2D and 3D scanning methods. The probe is prepared as usual for transvaginal scanning. The patient is placed in the position advancing the probe slowly into the vagina. The patient's bladder should be as empty as possible to enable the probe to come closer to the fetal head. The tip or the footprint of the transvaginal probe has to be maneuvered to "sit" opposite the anterior fontanelle. This can be obtained by tilting the vaginal probe until the best images obtained, while the abdominally placed second hand of the operator is stabilizing the fetal head in the desired position for the clearest ultrasound picture (Fig. 30-2). We emphasize that, if a reasonably strong suspicion of a malformation is entertained and the fetus is in the breech presentation, one should strongly consider performing an external version to turn the fetus into the more desirable vertex presentation. This can quite easily be obtained in the late first or early second trimester or sometimes even later under the safeguards of performing the external version.

We use an end-firing transvaginal transducer type, which will enable symmetrical pictures on both sides of the scanning axis. Using a non-end firing, out-of-axis vaginal probe may become very cumbersome to use, since the probe has to constantly be twisted and tilted into the right position and the operator will be confused by the position of the probe and the exact location of certain structures in the brain.

SCANNING PLANES EMPLOYED BY 2D SCANNING

Using transvaginal fetal neuroscan it is virtually impossible to obtain the "classical" planes since the footprint of the probe touches the anterior fontanelle and it is fanned from anterior and posterior in the sagittal planes, and from side to side in the coronal planes. This by no means represents the "classical" sagittal and coronal planes which should be parallel to each

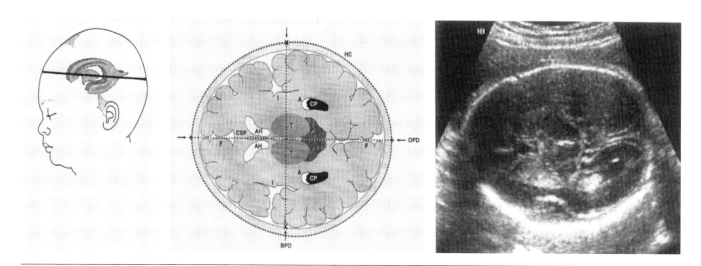

FIGURE 30-1 Axial section of the fetal head at the level shown on the head icon. Note that the hemisphere close to the ultrasound probe (upper) is less clear than the one far from the foot print of the ultrasound probe (lower).

other. Using transfontanelle scanning these newly "created" planes radiate from a common point: the anterior fontanelle or several other points along the sagittal suture (Fig. 30-3). These points are used as the window to the fetal brain. However, as mentioned previously, these planes are identical to those obtained by the neonatal transfontanelle imaging of the fetal brain. Exploiting these similarities between the neonatal and fetal scanning planes and sections will present a practical advantage, when prenatal and neonatal brain images have to be compared and a certain pathology discussed. Toward a better understanding of these planes a new nomenclature

was proposed.[14] To define each of these newly proposed sections a number of landmarks and anatomic structures were defined. The clustering and the combination of these landmark structures present in each plane enables a precise identification of each plane. The following landmarks and anatomic structures were considered when defining the above mentioned planes: orbits, meningeal folds, different parts of the ventricles and their connections, interhemispheric foramina, the choroid plexus and the tela choroidea, midbrain structures as the corpus callosum, head of the caudate nucleus, the thalamus, the cavum septi pellucidi, cerebellum with its hemispheres, and the vermis, among others.

The coronal planes are depicted in Fig. 30-4 and are subdivided into three groups: the frontal, the middle, and the occipital group. (a) The frontal group contains two sections. The Frontal-1 which we also called the "steer head

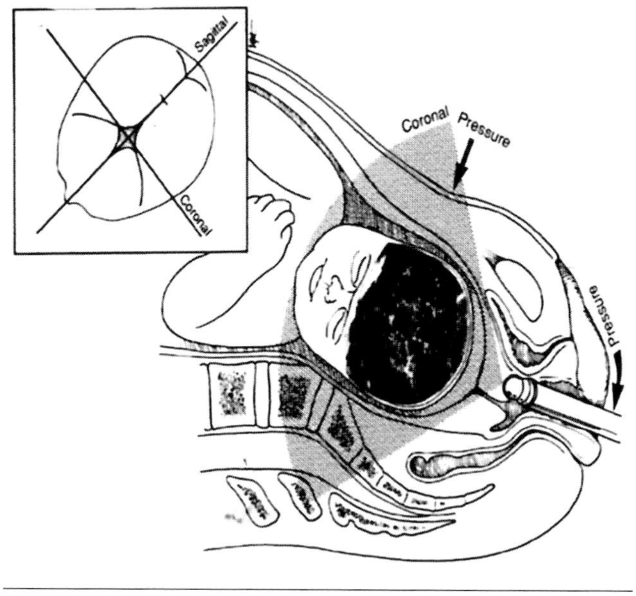

FIGURE 30-2 Schematic drawing depicting the technique of transvaginal sonography during the second and third trimesters. Inset: The relationship of the anterior fontanelle to the transvaginal transducer is demonstrated.

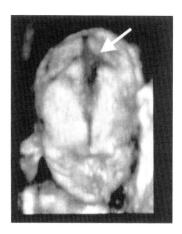

FIGURE 30-3 On this 3D rendering of a fetal skull the location of the anterior fontanelle and the open sagittal suture (arrow) are clearly seen.

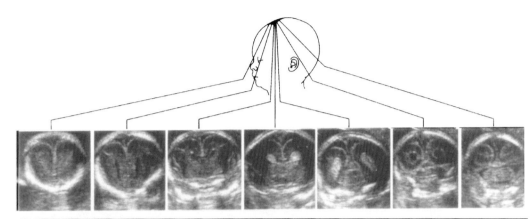

Anatomical Structures		FRONTAL 1	FRONTAL 2	MID-CORONAL 1	MID-CORONAL 2	MID-CORONAL 3	OCCIPITAL 1	OCCIPITAL 2
Skull			Orbit					
Ventricles & Connections	Lateral	Only at < 16w	Ant. horn	Body	Body / Choroid plexus	Atrium	Post. horn	
	Intravent. foramen				With choroid plexus			
	Third				(Virtual space) Tela choroidea			
Cavum septi pellucidi				Cavum septi pellucidi				
Midbrain	Corp. callosum			Genu	Trunk	Splenium		
	Head of caudate nucl.			Caudate nucleus				
	Thalamus				Thalamus			
Cerebellum	Hemisphere						Hemispheres	
	Vermis							Vermis
	4th Ventr.						4th Ventricle (at times)	
Meninges	Falx	F	A		L		X	
	Tentorium						Tentorium	
Cisterna magna								Cist. magna

FIGURE 30-4 This figure summarizes the brain structures imaged on each of the consecutive frontal, midcoronal and occipital sections (From Timor-Tritsch et al., by permission).

configuration" since it features the orbit and some facial structures. The tip of the anterior horn is seen only before the sixteenth postmenstrual week on this section. (b) The Frontal-2 section depicts the orbits, the tip of the anterior horns as well as the falx.

The middle group has three sections: (a) Midcoronal-1 in which the lateral ventricles, the body of the lateral ventricles choroid corpus callosum and the head of the caudate nucleus are seen. (b) Midcoronal-2 contains the lateral ventricles, choroid plexus, and the third ventricle as well as the cross section of the corpus callosum. (c) Midcoronal-3 section contains the lateral ventricles with the choroid plexuses and the thalami.

The occipital group has two sections (a) Occipital-1, on which the cross section of the posterior horns, cerebellar hemispheres, and the vermis are seen (b) Occipital-2 where the structures are: the cerebellar hemispheres, the vermis, the tentorium, and the cisterna magna.

The sagittal planes are depicted in Fig. 30-5 these are subdivided into the following groups:

The Median plane (previously termed "mid-sagittal"). The structures seen on this plane are: the entire corpus callosum (prior to the eighteenth or twentieth week only parts of this structure can be seen). The cavum septi pellucidi and cavum vergae, the head of the caudate nucleus, the thalamus, midbrain structures such as the corpora quadrigemina, the vermis, the cisterna magna, and the fourth ventricle.

The right and left Oblique-1 sections were previously termed parasagittal sections. These contain the anterior horns, the atria, and the posterior horns of the lateral ventricles. On this section, the inferior horns should not be visible, since they are lateral to this plane.

The right and left Oblique-2 these contain mostly brain tissue with a horizontally oriented gaping lateral sulcus in the shape of the letter V turned 90 degrees on its side. The upper arm of the V is the lower edge of the parietal lobe and is called

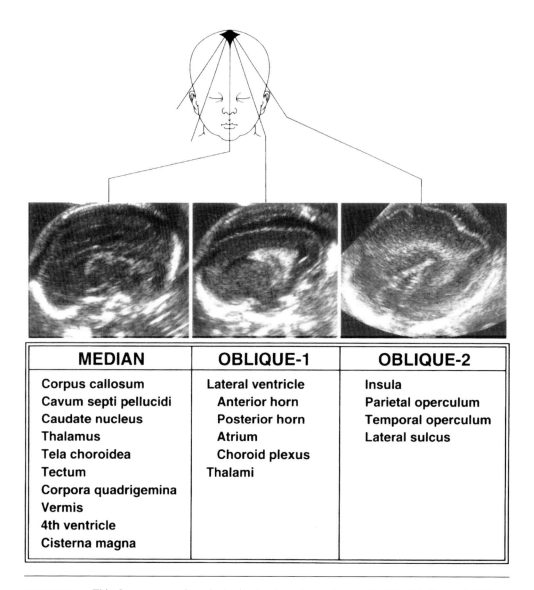

MEDIAN	OBLIQUE-1	OBLIQUE-2
Corpus callosum	Lateral ventricle	Insula
Cavum septi pellucidi	Anterior horn	Parietal operculum
Caudate nucleus	Posterior horn	Temporal operculum
Thalamus	Atrium	Lateral sulcus
Tela choroidea	Choroid plexus	
Tectum	Thalami	
Corpora quadrigemina		
Vermis		
4th ventricle		
Cisterna magna		

FIGURE 30-5 This figure summarizes the brain structures imaged on each of the Median and Oblique sections (From Timor-Tritsch et al., by permission).

parietal operculum. The lower arm is formed by the upper edge of the temporal lobe and is called temporal operculum. These 2 structures enclose the insula. As term approaches the insulae are progressively covered by the 2 closing opercula.

The logic behind the introduction of this systematic method of fetal neuroscan transvaginal sonography helped us to better define the normal and abnormal fetal brain. As stated previously, it emulates neonatal neuroscan, therefore creates a common ground with the pediatric neurologist and neurosurgeon. Even after the introduction of the 3D fetal neuroscan the above mentioned systematic 2D fetal neuroscan will and probably should be used as a first line scanning modality of the fetal CNS.

DESCRIPTION OF VARIOUS BRAIN STRUCTURES

The ventricular system consists of 2 symmetrically positioned C-shaped lateral ventricles, which connects to the third ven-

tricle, in the midline, through the 2 interventricular foramina (Monroe). The CNS fluid produced by the choroid plexuses drains from the lateral ventricles through their openings into the third ventricle and then through the aqueduct into the fourth ventricle. In continuation, through the median and lateral aperture, the fluid reaches the cerebellopeduncular cistern or cisterna magna. From there it is dispersed throughout the surface of the hemispheres where it is absorbed by special structures of the arachnoid membranes.

The 3 horns of the lateral ventricles, easily seen by 2D or 3D transvaginal sonography are—as previously mentioned— anterior, posterior, and inferior horns. These are sometimes called in the literature as frontal, occipital, and temporal horns respectively. All 3 horns are relatively large at 12–14 weeks however the posterior horn is gradually increasing its size toward term. Classically the size of the lateral ventricle is measured on an axial section. If the width of the lateral ventricle is measured above 10 mm it should be suspicious for true ventriculomegaly.[15] If only the posterior horn dilates it is called colpocephaly, which is a very sensitive indicator of certain brain anomalies (e.g., agenesis of the corpus callosum). Using the transvaginal imaging it is easy to measure various aspects of the lateral ventricles.[7,16–17] Pertinent nomograms were published on this subject.[18] The anterior horn is relatively large in the late first and early second trimesters (Fig. 30-6). This should not be misdiagnosed as ventricular dilatation. It becomes progressively narrower and it is slit-like at term. The inferior horn extends laterally and low into the temporal lobe. The size of this horn remains relatively stationary while the rest of the brain is growing. Later after 24 weeks it is hard to detect the inferior horn. Therefore if on an Oblique-1 section, using 2D ultrasound, or on the 3-horn view obtained by the 3D transvaginal fetal neuroscan this horn can be distinctly seen, ventriculomegaly should be seriously suspected.[19]

The third ventricle is rarely imaged and any measurement above 5 mm using the Midcoronal-2 section should indeed subject the CNS to a detailed fetal neuroscan and to examine the lateral ventricle system.

The fourth ventricle is usually seen on the median plane as a sonolucent triangle at the level of the cerebellum. It can also be seen on a horizontal or tilted axial section at the level of the cerebellum. Its connection to the cisterna magna in late first and early second trimester can be clearly identified. This connection is quite wide and should not trigger a suspicion of vermian pathology.

Choroid plexuses are found in the lateral ventricles, as well as in the third and fourth ventricles. The choroid plexuses of the lateral ventricles are best evaluated using the Midcoronal-3 and/or the left and right Oblique-1 planes. They appear as cottonlike structures with irregular borders. They are richly supplied by capillaries if they become thin or dangling this is a sensitive marker of lateral ventriculomegaly. At times cystic structures within the choroid plexus can be detected. An ongoing controversy exists as to the importance of this cystic structure to serve as markers of chromosomal anomalies of the fetus.

THE CORPUS CALLOSUM AND MIDBRAIN STRUCTURES

The best plane to study the midbrain is the median plane. Some of the most important structures seen on this plane that should be scrutinized are the corpus callosum, the cavum septi pellucidi, and the pericallosal artery. The corpus callosum starts to form at around 12 weeks and it completes its development around 20–22 weeks.[20] It is a C-shaped structure that extends from the beak (rostrum), the knee (genu), the body (corpus), and the tail (splenium). Below it one can find the cavum septi pellucidi and above it the pericallosal artery. The posterior compartment of the cavum septi pellucidi is called cavum vergae (Fig. 30-7A). The cava are not part of the ventricular system because they do not communicate with them. The cavum vergae diminishes in size and almost disappears close to term. Above the corpus callosum, the pericallosal artery runs in the pericallosal sulcus. Color or power Doppler interrogation of the medical hemisphere on the median plane can image this important landmark (Fig. 30-7B). On this median plane one can study the medial part of the thalami, caudate nuclei, the fourth ventricle, and the medulla. The median plane should be included in every detailed fetal neuroscan.

THE POSTERIOR FOSSA

The posterior coronal sections such as the Midcoronal-3, Occipital-1, and -2 provide a good view of the posterior fossa. At times in order to complete the examination and reveal subtle anatomic features it is advantageous to use a posteriorly tilted axial (Fig. 30-8) or even a sagittal plane. If possible the tip of the transducer should be slid over the sagittal suture closer to the posterior fontanelle. If this procedure is possible, a surprisingly clear image of the posterior fossa can be obtained. If only a more anterior position of the foot print of the probe

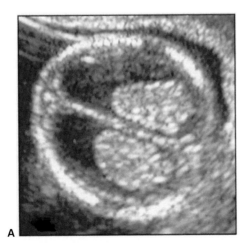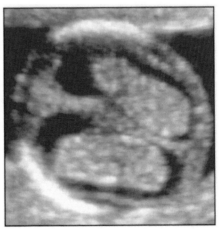

FIGURE 30-6 The relatively large size of the anterior horn on axial sections: (**A**) at 10 postmenstrual weeks; (**B**) at 14 postmenstrual weeks.

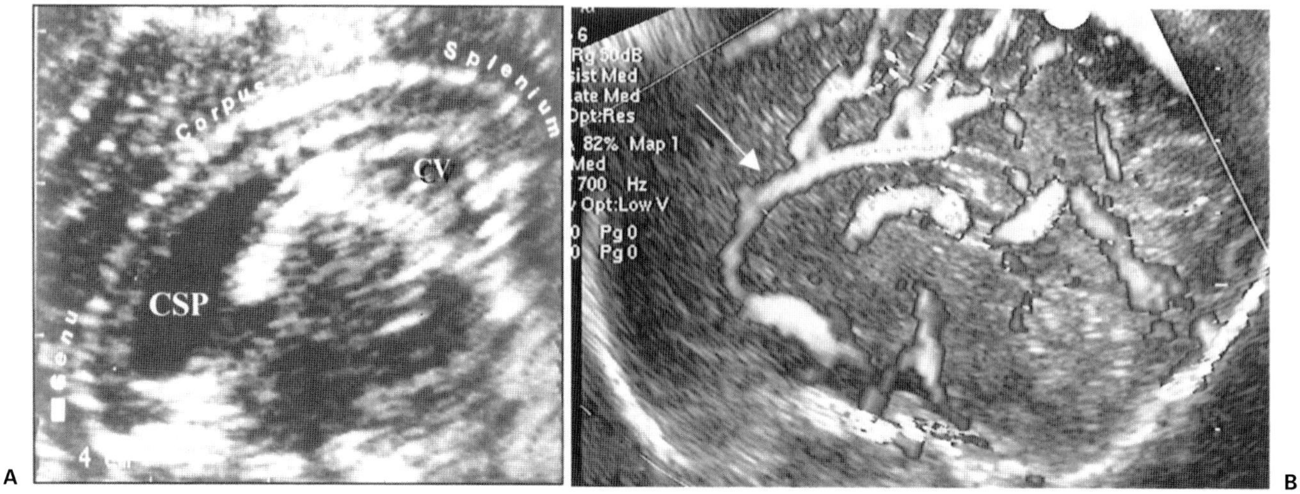

FIGURE 30-7 Median sections of the fetal brain: (**A**) The knee, body, and splenum of the corpus callosum below which the cavum septi pellucidi (CSP) and vergae (CV) are seen. (**B**) The pericallosal artery (arrow) above the corpus callosum (Power Doppler examination).

is possible, the posterior fossa may not always be viewed in a sufficient manner. At 14–16 post menstrual weeks the vermis is still incompletely formed (Fig. 30-9) and one can see the communication between the cisterna magna and the fourth ventricle through the open median aperture (Magendie). On the Occipital-2 section, at times, it is possible to detect the fluid filled cisterns above the lateral aspects of the cerebellum (cisterna ambiens) and below the cerebellum itself. When the scanning the posterior fossa one should be aware of the fine linear echoes generated by the arachnoid or some vessels crossing the arachnoid. These are sometimes visualized in the cerebello-peduncular cisterna (cisterna magna). These are normal and should not be confused with pathology. The vermis is particularly hyperechoic and it should be easy to recognize it by transvaginal transfontanelle fetal neuroscan.

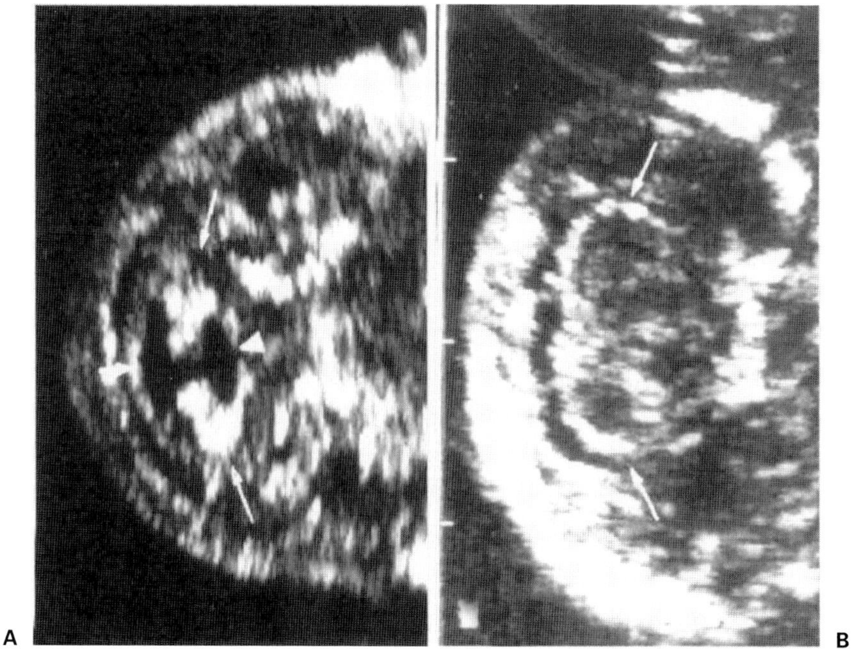

The cerebral cortex: since ultrasonography is only able to depict flat surfaces it is clear that the lateral and superior convex surfaces of the hemispheres can not be imaged using these standard planes. The only flat surface of the hemisphere lending itself to sonographic scrutiny is the medial surface of the cerebral hemispheres. This can be best scanned using the Median section, which will image the major sulci and gyri along the falx cerebri. One can also use a cross section of the brain such as the Midcoronal-1, 2, and 3 in order to get some insight into the sulci and gyri along the medial surface of the brain. The image of the singulate gyri and singulate sucli as well as 1 of 2 gyri and sulci in branching can be seen adequately on such coronal sections.

The cerebral hemispheres are still smooth around the twenty second post week. At around the twenty-fourth post menstrual week the singulate sulci and gyrus can be detected. The biggest increase of the number and the depth of the sulci takes place between twenty-eighth and thirtieth postmenstrual weeks. After the twenty-eighth

FIGURE 30-8 The posterior fossa at 16 postmenstrual weeks. (**A**) A low axial section showing the tonsils of the cerebellum (arrows) and the connection of the cisterna magna to the fourth ventricle (arrowhead). (**B**) A higher axial section in the same fetus shows the normal cerebellum (arrows).

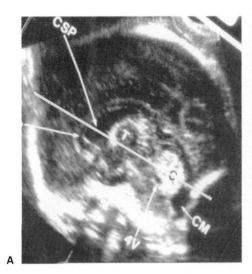 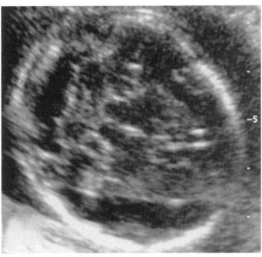

FIGURE 30-9 Tilted axial section of the brain. (**A**) The white line indicates the plane at which the image on (**B**) was generated. (CSP-cavum septi pellucidi, T-thalamus, CM-cisterna magna, 4V-fourth ventricle, C-cerebellar vermis).

postmenstrual week typically, the above mentioned, 2 or 3 sections of the fetal brain can be looked at to study the brain surface. Lack of some of the landmark structures detectable using transvaginal technique may raise suspicion regarding developmental problems of the brain surface.[21]

THREE-DIMENSIONAL FETAL NEUROSCAN

Three-dimensional fetal neuroscan is an additional imaging tool to enable better understanding of the fetal brain and better localize some of the hard-to-detect pathologies. The possibility of acquiring a volume of the fetal brain and simultaneously displaying the traditional and classical coronal sagittal and axial planes is a significant development in achieving a better definition of the brain anatomy and its possible pathologies. After obtaining a volume scan of the fetal brain it is easy to scroll or navigate within the volume and scrutinize the sagittal plane from "ear-to-ear" the axial planes from the base of the skull to the top of the head and in the coronal plane from the orbit back to the occipital areas. The 3 planes are at right angles to each other, therefore they are referred to as the multiplanar orthogonal display (Figs. 30-10, 30-11). At this time several ultrasound machines make this kind of volume acquisition possible and the ability to scroll within the volume is thus available. It is also possible to create any other desired plane by rotating the volume to a different position. Transabdominal and transvaginal transducers can be used to acquire fetal brain volume data.[19,22]

The subarachnoid space is most evident on sagittal sections. This space extends from anterior to posterior on the outer surface of the hemispheres and in the second trimester appears quite wide (Fig. 30-11), however as pregnancy advances this space narrows.

The technique of 3D ultrasound is uniform for almost all transducers and ultrasound machines. The reason of interest is selected and fit into the x and y planes in order to include all the important structures. The volume is then acquired using a free hand or a motor-driven, advanced acquisition technique. After the volume is obtained the 3 classical planes: the coronal sagittal and the axial planes are displayed on the monitor. Minor adjustments to correct tilts and undesired head positions can then be achieved. Using the Medison/GE 3D US machine we usually display the coronal plane in the upper left box of the image, the sagittal plane in the upper right box and the axial plane in the lower right box. However any other display that better serves the sonologist is possible. Some ultrasound machines can display a continuous series of consecutive sections much like the images that are displayed in MRI and CAT scans. An example of enabling a combination of the planes is to look at the lateral ventricles using the three horn view.[19–22]

It should be stressed that the planes and sections obtained by the previously described transvaginal-transfontanelle fetal neuroscan differ only slightly from the ones imaged by the 3D technique. The main differences between 2D and 3D fetal neuroscan are described in the following sections.

By 2D transfontanelle fetal neuroscan it is very rare to obtain axial sections. This reconstructed plane is readily available using the 3D technique. In 2D transfontanelle fetal sagittal coronal planes are radiating from the footprint of the probe that is placed adjacent to the fontanelle while 3D enables an imaging in which the scanning planes are always parallel to each other.

Using the 2D technique in the everyday practice the sonologist and/or the sonographer usually recreates 3D images in his or her brain. Using 3D ultrasound, first a volume is created in the memory bank of the machine, then the various sections are generated and available on the monitor. The intersection of the three planes is displayed on the screen as a "marker dot."

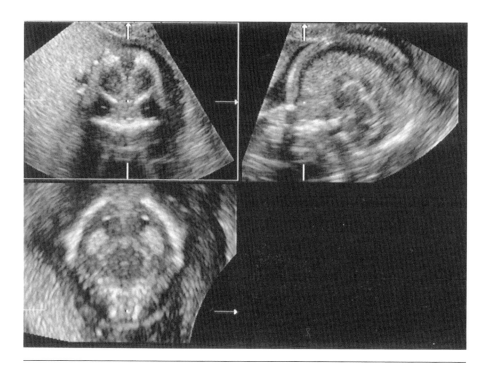

FIGURE 30-10 The orthogonal display. Once the volume is acquired and stored in a Cartesian system, it is displayed on the monitor. Using the agreed upon positioning controls, the following is the basic orientation of the cranium and the brain. Box A (upper left) contains all coronal views. In this picture Box B is the active box and it is bordered by a square around it. Fetal right is on the left of the picture. Box B (upper right) contains the sagittal planes, in this case the median plane is seen. The coronal view in the active Box A is generated using the plane across the white arrow under Box B. The fetus faces the left. Box C (lower left) contains the axial (horizontal) views. This view is generated using the plane across the horizontal dotted line in Box A.

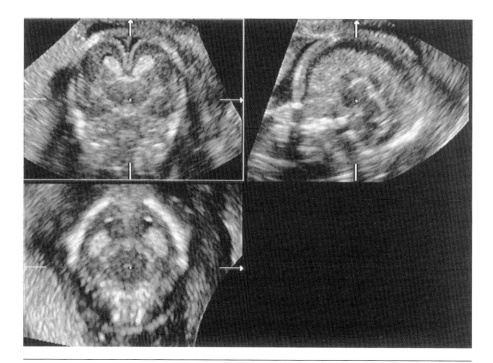

FIGURE 30-11 Same 3D display as in Figure 30-10. This time the active Box A (upper left) displays a Midcoronal plane.

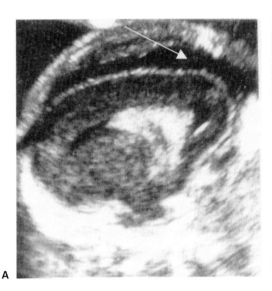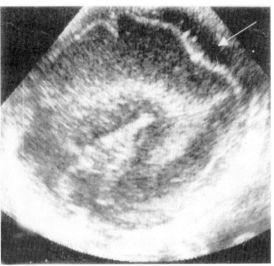

FIGURE 30-12 The subarachnoid space. (**A**) On this Oblique-1 section the wide open (but normal) subarachnoid space is shown (arrow). This is also a good example of the 3 horn view. (**B**) On the Oblique-2 section the same wide space is shown (arrow).

The position of this dot enables the observer to pinpoint the pathology on all 3 planes at the same time (Fig. 30-12).

Using 3D imaging the pathology can easily be conveyed to the radiologist, MRI specialist, who also uses similar parallel (to each other) sections of any scanned body part. There are numerous advantages of the 3D fetal scanning, among them: (1) scrolling in any direction is possible, (2) any plane can be generated by tilting the brain into any desired direction, (3) the observer can scrutinize the brain simultaneously in coronal sagittal and axial planes, (4) the volume can be stored for future reference and evaluation, (5) patient education counseling is easy, (6) the volume can be sent to experts over networks and using a special software program the volume can be looked at in all desired planes as if it would be on the monitor of the acquiring machine, and (7) color Doppler can be used.

There are few limitations of ultrasound of the fetal brain.[1] Fetal movements, for instance, create artifacts. However newer 3D ultrasound machines enable increasingly faster acquisition times which help in acquiring a quick volume between 2 periods of fetal movement. The biggest limitations of the technique are that the equipment is not widespread, operators are still inexperienced about scanning techniques, but more importantly few are familiar with transfontanelle fetal neuroscan.

We are confident that the 3D fetal neuroscan will be progressively widespread as the imaging modality to maximize visual information on brain anatomy or pathology.

FETAL BRAIN PATHOLOGY SEEN BY 2D AND 3D TRANSVAGINAL FETAL NEUROSCAN

To diagnose and define anomalies of the CNS, the sonographer has to be familiar with the developmental stages of the fetal brain. Many structures that appear to be pathological are indeed normal milestones in the development of the brain (examples of this can be found by looking at the corpus callosum, the surface of the brain with its sulci gyri the relatively late closure of the foramen Magendie (median aperture) and finally the form and shape of the lateral ventricles. We cannot emphasize enough that the fetal brain is the only organ that undergoes large anatomic changes throughout gestation. As far as the different fetal brain pathologies are concerned, it is impossible to list all of them here and at the same time to present illustrative examples of them. The reader is referred to the classical textbooks.[23–24]

SELECTED FETAL NEUROPATHOLOGY USING 2D AND 3D TRANSVAGINAL TRANSFONTANELLE SCANNING

If any part of the fetal brain deviates from its normal sonographic appearance one is dealing with CNS malformations. These may be a result of pathologic development or they may be acquired during gestation (e.g., infection). Regardless of the cause they are called congenital brain anomalies. To properly diagnoses such anomalies the sonographer or the sonologist has to be familiar with the developmental stages of the fetal brain. We cannot stress enough that some structures may be normal early in pregnancy, however, if they are found later they may represent pathological development. As stated previously, the fetal brain is the only organ that undergoes tremendous anatomic changes throughout gestation.

Following this, some of the anomalies detectable by both the 2D and 3D transvaginal sonography will be presented. As stated previously, the images obtained by the 2 techniques are

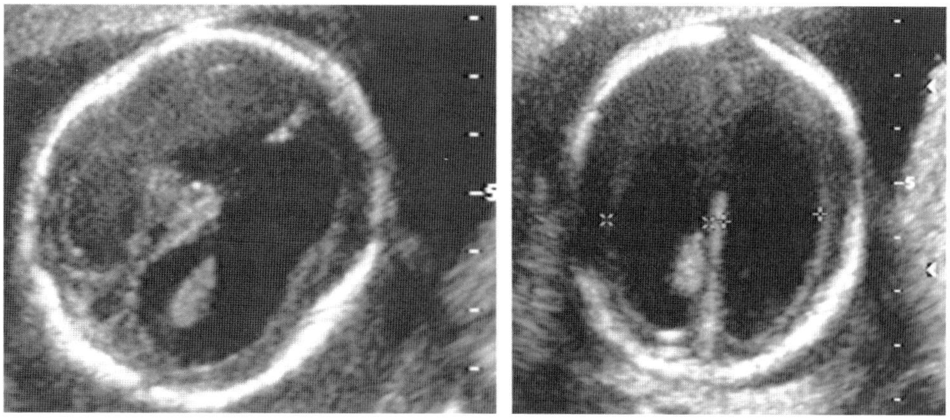

FIGURE 30-13   Axial sections of a fetal brain with aqueductal stenosis at 21 postmenstrual weeks. With the degree of the hydrocephaly, the thin cortical and white matter and the dangling choroid plexus are seen.

similar in appearance. To define a certain plane or section we may use the nomenclature developed by the 2D transvaginal transfontanelle technique (e.g., Mid-coronal 1–3 or Oblique 1 and 2). By scrolling through a stored brain volume one can generate almost identical planes. The important aspect of both techniques is that the brain is thoroughly scanned at short intervals. It is beyond the scope of this chapter to list all the fetal CNS anomalies; however, the images presented here will enable the reader to understand the principle of the scanning methods and their advantages.

VENTRICULOMEGALY AND HYDROCEPHALY

Ventriculomegaly and hydrocephaly are sometimes used interchangeably. Ventriculomegaly is an increase in size of the lateral ventricles with normal CNS fluid pressure and without an increase in head size, while hydrocephaly is more than ventriculomegaly, since there is an increase in the pressure of the CFS fluid, causing increasing fetal head size with thinning of the brain tissue. Hydrocephaly is divided into noncommunicating and communicating types. Ventriculomegaly and hydrocephaly are relatively simple to detect, as there are relatively large fluid-filled spaces, which can be detected easily even by transabdominal fetal neuroscan (Fig. 30-13).

There are several ways to assess the size of the ventricles subjectively or qualitatively using transvaginal sonography: (a) relying on *indirect signs* such as the thickness of the cortical mantle, detection of the inferior horn (which, as mentioned previously should normally not be seen on an Oblique-1 section!), or the shape and the mobility of the choroid plexus on any coronal section (Fig. 30-14) if these structures are thin and dangling it signifies ventricular dilatation; (b) the *gestalt approach*, defined as relying on the observers experience in judging the appearance of the ventricular system; (c) looking at the third ventricle on the Mid-coronal-1 or -2 sections. Anytime this ventricle is seen (usually it is slitlike!) attention to the entire ventricular system should be given.

The 3 horn views are instrumental sections that provide valuable information about the extent of this pathology.[19] They are evident on the Oblique-1 sections if 2D scans are used. Using the 3D volume they are achieved by tilting the coronal sections to the left and to the right and then passing the sagittal plane through the lateral ventricles. Figures 30-15 and 30-16 depict a fetus with agenesis of the corpus callosum also demonstrates the left and right 3 horn views. The objective assessment of ventricular size is based on the published measurements of different parts of the lateral and the third ventricles or their ratios. These measurements are based upon TAS[15,25] or transvaginal sonography.[18]

Transvaginal sonographic evaluation of the ventricular system seems to be of high specificity in detecting mild ventriculomegaly as well as asymmetric ventriculomegaly. However, the most important prognostic factors in the outcome of prenatally detected hydrocephaly are: associated chromosomal anomalies, the amount of residual brain tissue around the ventricles, and the presence or absence of any other anomaly.

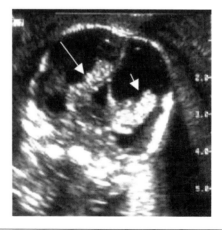

FIGURE 30-14   Coronal section of the same brain shown on Fig. 30-13. The arrows point to the dangling choroid plexuses.

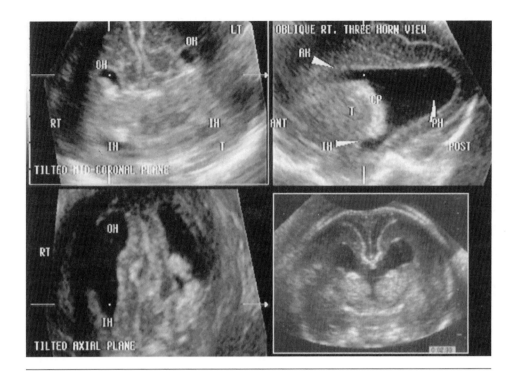

FIGURE 30-15 Agenesis of the corpus callosum. Upper right box: coronal section; upper right box: sagittal section; lower left box: axial section. All the indirect signs are present: wide lateral ventricles, colpocephaly and dilatation of the inferior horn (in the right three horn view), teardrop-shaped lateral ventricles on the axial section. In the inset: a coronal section showing the upward displaced third ventricle.

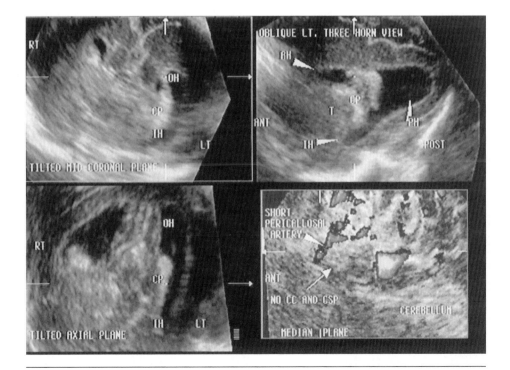

FIGURE 30-16 The same brain scanned as in Fig. 30-15. The upper left box shows the coronal plane titled to the left. The upper left right box contains the sagittal view of the left three horn view with the obvious colpocephaly. The inset: color Doppler reveals only the short pericallosal artery, no corpus callosum, and no cavum septi pellucidi.

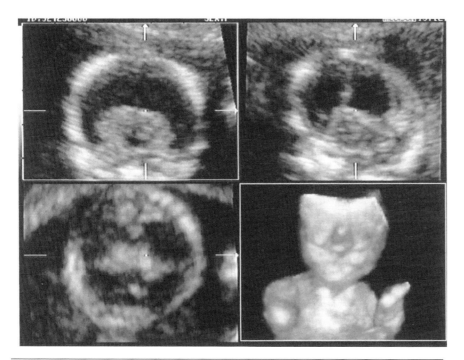

FIGURE 30-17 3D images of lobar holoprosencephaly at 16 postmenstrual weeks. Coronal(upper left), sagittal (upper right), and axial (lower left) are shown. The inset shows the rendering of the face with proboscis and cyclops.

HOLOPROSENCEPHALY

At birth its incidence is about 1 per 1,600 births, however, in the late first and early second trimester this anomaly will be seen more frequently.

Two of the more frequent forms: alobar (Fig. 30-17) and semilobar types are relatively easily diagnosed. Absence of the interhemispheric fissure (total or partial), nondisjunction of the thalami, no corpus callosum and cavum septi pellucidi, and several facial anomalies (cyclops, proboscis, median clefts, etc.) are the most frequent, but not the only features (Fig. 30-17 inset and Fig. 30-18).

The lobar type has more subtle features. At times the only sign are seen around corpus callosum, cavum septi pellucidi, and the third ventricle. The box-shaped cavity in the midbrain, below the corpus callosum without the 2 lateral walls of the septum pellucidum give rise to the suggestion of lobar holoprosencephaly and its closest differential diagnosis: septo-optic displasia.[26] The final diagnosis usually is made only after birth.

Several types of alobar holoprosencephaly were described (pancake, ball, and cup types) however the most important sonographic feature of all the above types is the presence of the primitive single telencephalic ventricle. Figure 30-19 depicts a ball type holoprosencephaly. Chromosomal aneuploidies are almost always the case and the prognosis is universally dismal.

NEURAL TUBE DEFECTS (NTDs)

Since the incidence of the NTDs in most of the world is 2–3 per 1,000 births it is important to recognize them at the earliest possible stage. Figure 30-17 illustrates a fetus with anencephaly. It is possible to detect the exencephaly-anencephaly sequence as early as 9–10 weeks by carefully scanning the fetal head. The head shape in the coronal, sagittal as well as in the axial plane are pathognomonic and are part of the diagnosis at these gestational ages

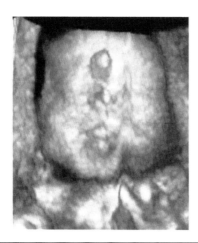

FIGURE 30-18 The face of the fetus shown in Fig. 30-17.

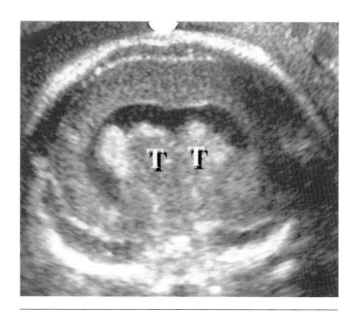

FIGURE 30-19 Ball type alobar holoprosencephaly using a Midcoronal-2 section (T-thalamus).

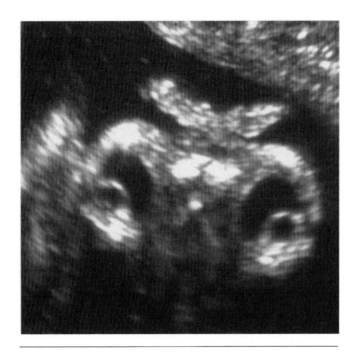

FIGURE 30-20 Coronal image of the orbits and some dangling, degenerating brain tissue above them of an anencephalic fetus at 14 postmenstrual weeks.

(Fig. 30-20). Bronshtein et al.[27] believes that the anencephaly results from the rubbing off of exposing brain tissue, by observing the progressively diminishing amount of brain tissue in cases of exencephaly and by detecting free-floating neural cells. It is therefore felt that the exposed brain tissue is disintegrating and diminishing as gestation progresses.[27–28]

AGENESIS OF THE CORPUS CALLOSUM (ACC)

Transvaginal sonography seems to us indispensable to make or rule out this diagnosis in a reliable and straightforward manner. The indirect diagnostic features of ACC such as the teardrop-shaped lateral ventricles on the axial section; the widely displaced upward pointing anterior horns, the upward displaced third ventricle connecting with the interhemispheric fissure on coronal sections can be seen using transabdominal sonography (Figs. 30-15, 30-16). However, these are indirect signs. The direct observation of the presence or absence (or partial absence) of the corpus callosum is the most reliable way to arrive at the correct diagnosis and is possible only by using the median plane. Transvaginal sonography may be the only means to provide this plane. Since the corpus callosum develops parallel to the development of the pericallosal artery and the cavum septi pellucidi, it is important to track and localize all 3 structures at the same time using the median plane (Fig. 30-16, inset).

Our impression during the last 5 or 6 years was that many sonologists and sonographers using only transabdominal sonography diagnose and report the associated and more obvious hydrocephaly and miss the real diagnosis (ie, ACC or partial ACC).

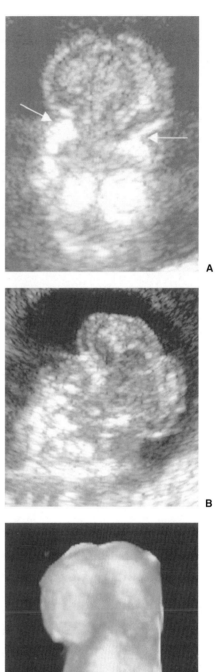
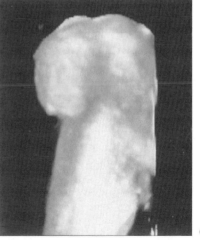

FIGURE 30-21 Exencephaly in a fetus at 13 postmenstrual weeks. (**A**) Coronal image. Brain tissue bulges out between the skull bones (arrows). (**B**) Sagittal image. (**C**) 3D rendering of the coverless brain tissue.

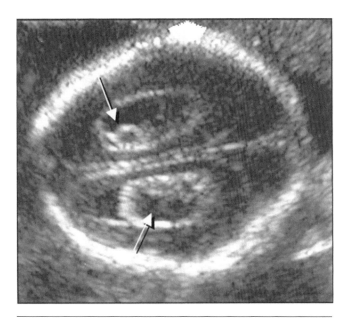

FIGURE 30-22 Choroid plexus cysts (arrows).

CHOROID PLEXUS CYST (CPC)

Choroid plexus cysts (CPCs) are fluid-filled cystic lesions within the choroid plexus and have a approximate incidence of 1% of all pregnancies. They are usually benign and disappear about the twenty-fourth postmenstrual week. An ongoing debate is reflected in the literature as to whether they are indeed markers of chromosomal anomalies. They can be detected as early as week 11–12 of gestation. Figure 30-22 depicts bilateral cysts on an axial section. Table 30-1 provides a compilation based on the literature[26–30] in which, of 55,

218 patients scanned, there were 764 (1.4%) choroid plexus cysts. Of these 674 (88%) were isolated. Of the isolated cases 5 (0.74%) had chromosomal aneuploidy whereas there was a group of 90 patients with additional sonographic abnormalities. In this group there were 20 fetuses (22%) with chromosomal aneuploidies.[29–33] We conclude, therefore, that karyotyping for CPC should be offered to women carrying a fetus with other associated anomalies, and abnormal biochemical test result or women over age 35.

ARACHNOID CYSTS

These are CSF-filled spaces that do not connect to the ventricles or the cava. They are space-occupying lesions with all the effects of such lesions; however, they are histologically benign. They appear as sonolucent, thin-walled structures. The left-sided lesions are most common; 10% of which are located in the quadrigeminal cistern (Fig. 30-23). Five to ten percent are in the posterior fossa and about 10% of arachnoid cysts are in potentially dangerous areas (e.g., the suprasellar cistern). By exerting pressure on the flow of the CSF they may cause bilateral hydrocephaly (e.g., pressure on the interventricular foramen). If they are located on the convexity of the brain, the outcome is usually good.

PORENCEPHALIC CYST

This lesion is a result of degenerating brain tissue following a severe insult to the brain caused by hemorrhage, ischemia, or a vessel obliteration (Fig. 30-24). These lesions are not symmetrical and present with a variety of apolarances from hyerechoic areas (clots) and irregular, bizarre-shaped sonolucences. Their prognosis is dependent on the size of the lesion but tends to be uniformly poor.

TABLE 30-1 | ISOLATED CHOROID PLEXUS CYST(S) (CPC) AND CHROMOSOMAL ANEUPLOIDY

Author/Year	Total Number of Patients Scanned	Number of CPC	Incidence (percent)	Isolated CPC	Isolated with Chromosomal Aneuploidy (percent)	Additional Sonographic Abnormalities	Chromosomal Aneuploidy in Patient with Additional Sonographic Findings (percent)
Geary 1997 (29)	13,690	84	0.6	78	0	6	3 Trisomy 18
Sohn 1997 (30)	4,326	41	0.94	40[d]	0	1[e]	1 Trisomy 18
Reinsch 1997 (31)	16,059	301	1.8	263	0	38[a]	3 (2 trisomy 18; 1 trisomy 21)
Morcos 1998 (32)	7,617	210	2.8	181	1 (Trisomy 21)[b]	29	1 (trisomy 18)[b]
Sullivan 1999 (33)	13,526	128	0.95	112[c]	4 (3 trisomy 18;1 unbalanced translocation)[c]	16	12 (9 trisomy 18; 1 trisomy 21; 1 balanced translocation; 1 chromosomal inversion)
Total	55,218	764	1.4	674 (88%)	5 (0.74%)	90 (12%)	20 (22%)

[a] In addition to the CPC other risk factors included: other sonographic abnormalities, AMA, past obstetrical, and family history.
[b] Patient reported to be at least 35 years of age.
[c] This group included 1 patient age 38 years who had trisomy 18; 6 patients with abnormal MSAFP; and 16 patients with abnormal triple screens.
[d] Only 38 had amniocentesis.
[e] 2 fetuses lost to follow up.

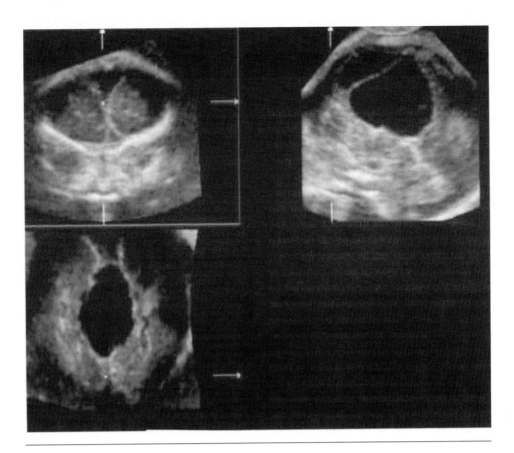

FIGURE 30-23 Arachnoid cyst of the quadrigeminal plate clearly shown in Box B (upper right) on the sagittal plane.

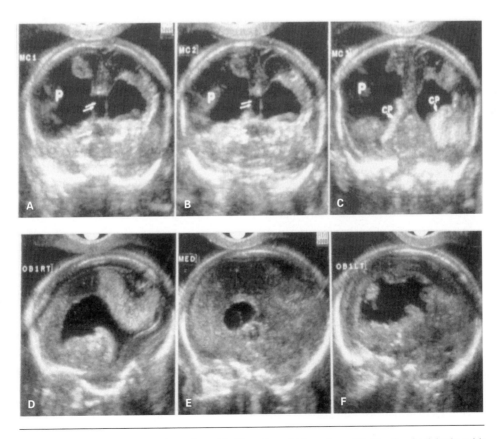

FIGURE 30-24 Several coronal sections (**A–C**) and sagittal sections (**D–F**) of a fetal brain with porencephaly.

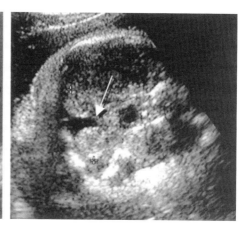

FIGURE 30-25 Dandy-Walker Variant on the left axial section shows a slightly enlarged cisterna magna (arrow) on the right the arrow points to the site of the absent vermis.

LESIONS OF THE POSTERIOR FOSSA

The most frequent pathology of the posterior fossa is Dandy-Walker malformation (DWM). The full-blown picture of DWM is relatively easy to diagnose. It is frequently associated with hydrocephaly. If only part of the vermis is missing and the cisterna magna is not excessively large the diagnosis is Dandy-Walker variant (Fig. 30-25). As mentioned previously, this diagnosis should not be finalized before the expected time of completion of the vermian development.

Hypoplasia of the cerebellum is a relatively rare diagnosis (Fig. 30-26). It may be familial or X linked.

ANEURYSM OF THE VEIN OF GALEN

Rarely seen, however, if the proper diagnostic tools (color or Doppler flow studies) are not employed, the aneurysm of the vein of Galen diagnosis can be missed. It is diagnosed on the basis of a sonolucent, elongated midline structure posterior to the corpus callosum and above the cerebellum (Fig. 30-27). It is usually evident on a second trimester fetal neuroscan.

INTRACRANIAL HEMORRHAGE

Intracranial hemorrhage rarely occurs in utero; however, if it occurs it is caused by hypoxemia, congenital vascular anomalies, clotting defects, drugs, thrombosis of the umbilical cord or its entanglement, and other anomalies.

One can detect fresh clots by their hyperechoic appearance within the parenchyma or in the ventricles. Sites of longstanding clots may disintegrate and become porencephalic cysts.

The neurodevelopmental long-term outcome of fetuses diagnosed with intracranial hemorrhages is related to the severity and the location of the hemorrhage.

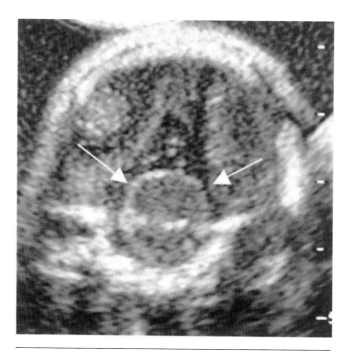

FIGURE 30-26 Cerebellar hypoplasia. The arrows point to the small fused cerebellar hemispheres.

SUMMARY AND KEY POINTS

- Fetal neuroscan, using transvaginal sonography in particular can detect the overwhelming majority of structural anomalies of the CNS. Its strength is that it can detect the anomalies developing early in gestation.
- It is important to stress that knowledge of the "developmental timetable" of the fetal brain is essential for proper assessment of the normal and abnormal fetal CNS. In addition, it is necessary that high-resolution ultrasound machines are operated only by skillfully trained sonographers and sonologists.
- Three-dimensional fetal neuroscan is a promising tool that undoubtedly will be of pivotal importance in the future.

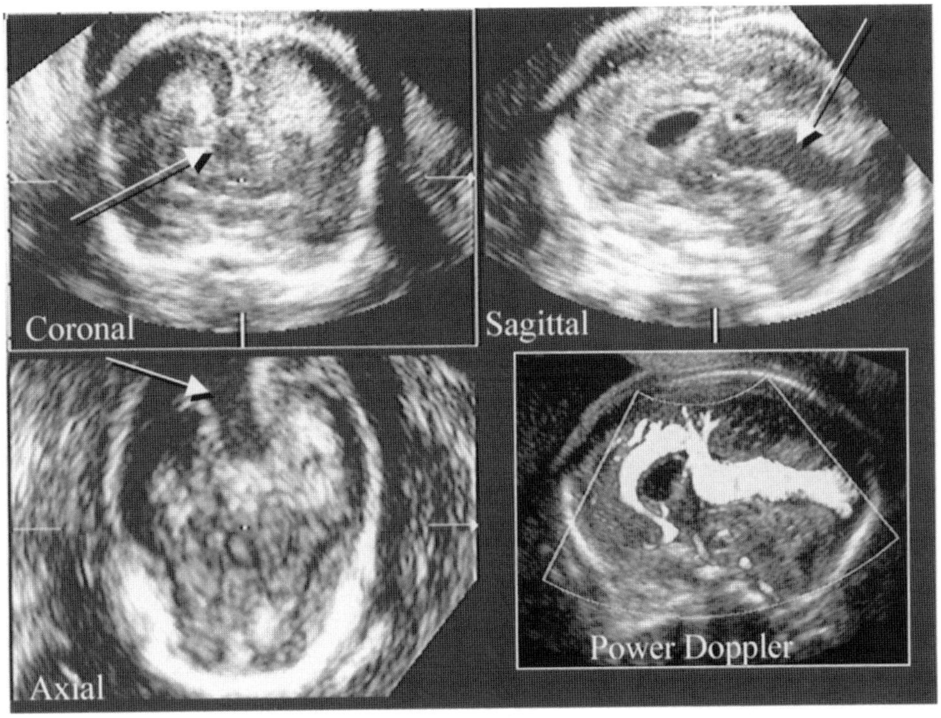

FIGURE 30-27 Aneurysm of the vein of Galen. The arrow points to the dilated vein on the coronal (upper left), sagittal (upper right), and the axial (lower left) planes. The inset: Power color flow of the dilated vein of Galen.

References

1. Monteagudo A. Fetal neurosonography: should it be routine? Should it be detailed? (editorial) *Ultrasound Obstet Gynecol.* 1998;12 (1): 1–5.

2. Timor-Tritsch IE, Farine D, Rosen MG. A close look at early embryonic development with the high-frequency transvaginal transducer. *Am J Obstet Gynecol.* 1988;159:676–681.

3. Timor-Tritsch IE, Monteagudo A, Warren WB. Transvaginal ultrasonographic definition of the central nervous system in the first and early second trimesters. *Am J Obstet Gynecol.* 1991;164:747–753.

4. Kushnir U, Shalev J, Bronshtein M, et al. Fetal intracranial anatomy in the first trimester of pregnancy: transvaginal ultrasonographic evaluation. *Neuroradiology.* 1989;31:222–225.

5. Timor-Tritsch IE, Blumenfeld Z, Rottem S. Sonoembryology. In: Timor-Tritsch IE, Rottem S, eds. *Transvaginal sonography,* 2nd ed. New York: Chapman & Hall, 1991:241.

6. Monteagudo A, Timor-Tritsch IE, Reuss ML, et al. Transvaginal sonography of the second and third trimester fetal brain. In: Timor-Tritsch IE, Rottem S, eds. *Transvaginal sonography,* 2nd ed. New York: Chapman & Hall, 1991:393–425.

7. Monteagudo A, Timor-Tritsch IE, Moomjy M. In utero detection of ventriculomegaly during the second and third trimesters by transvaginal sonography. *Ultrasound Obstet Gynecol.* 1994;4:193–198.

8. Achiron R, Achiron A. Transvaginal ultrasonic assessment of the early fetal brain. *Ultrasound Obstet Gynecol.* 1991;1:336–344.

9. Blaas HG, Eik-Nes SH, Kiserud T, et al. Early development of the hindbrain: a longitudinal ultrasound study from 7 to 12 weeks of gestation. *Ultrasound Obstet Gynecol.* 1995;5:151–160.

10. Blaas HG, Eik-Nes SH, Kiserud T, et al. Three-dimensional imaging of the brain cavities in human embryos. *Ultrasound Obstet Gynecol.* 1995;5:228–232.

11. Blaas HG, Eik-Nes SH, Kiserud T, et al. Early development of the forebrain and midbrain: a longitudinal ultrasound study from 7 to 12 postmenstrual weeks of gestation. *Ultrasound Obstet Gynecol.* 1994;4:183–192.

12. Timor-Tritsch IE, Greenebaum E, Monteagudo A, et al. The exencephaly-anencephaly sequence: proof by ultrasound imaging and amniotic fluid cytology. *Matern Fet Med.* 1996;5:182–185.

13. Warren WB, Timor-Tritsch IE, Peisner DB, et al. Dating the early pregnancy by sequential appearance of embryonic structures. *Am J Obstet Gynecol.* 1989;161:747–753.

14. Timor-Tritsch IE, Monteagudo A. Transvaginal fetal neurosonography: standardization of the planes and sections by anatomic landmarks. *Ultrasound Obstet Gynecol.* 1996. *Am J Obstet Gynecol.* 8:42–47.

15. Cardoza ID, Goldstein RB, Filly RA. Exclusion of fetal ventriculomegaly with a single measurement of the width of the lateral ventricular atrium. *Radiology.* 1988;169:711–714.

16. Monteagudo A, Timor-Tritsch IE, Moomjy M. In utero detection of ventriculomegaly during the second and third trimesters by transvaginal sonography. *Ultrasound Obstet Gynecol.* 1994;4:193–198.

17. Monteagudo A, Reuss ML, Timor-Tritsch IE. Imaging the fetal brain in the second and third trimesters using transvaginal sonography. *Obstet Gynecol.* 1991;77:27–32.

18. Monteagudo A, Timor-Tritsch IE, Moomjy M. Nomograms of the fetal lateral ventricles using transvaginal sonography. *J Ultrasound Med.* 1993;5:265–269.

19. Timor-Tritsch IE, Monteagudo A, Mayberry P. 3D ultrasound evaluation of the fetal brain: the three horn view. *Ultrasound Obstet Gynecol.* 2000;16:302–306.

20. Malinger G, Zakut H. The corpus callosum: normal fetal development as shown by transvaginal sonography. *AJR*. 1993;161:1041–1043.

21. Monteagudo A, Timor-Tritsch IE. Development of fetal gyri, sulci and fissures: a transvaginal sonographic study. *Ultrasound Obstet Gynecol*. 1997;9:222–228.

22. Timor-Tritsch IE, Monteagudo A, Mayberry P. Three dimensional transvaginal neurosonography of the fetal brain: navigating in the volume scan. *Ultrasound Obstet Gynecol*. 2000;16:307–313.

23. Timor-Tritsch IE, Monteagudo A, Cohen H. Ultrasound of the prenatal and neonatal brain. 2nd ed. New York: McGraw Hill; 2001.

24. Chervenak FA, Kurjak A, Comstock CH. Ultrasound and the fetal brain. Parthenon; 1995.

25. Pretorius DH, Drose JA, Manco-Johnson ML. Fetal lateral ventricular ratio determination during the second-trimester. *J Ultrasound Med*. 1986;5:121–124.

26. Pilu G, Perolo A, David C. Midline anomalies of the brain. In: Timor-Tritsch IE, Monteagudo A, Cohen HL, eds. Ultrasonography of the prenatal and neonatal brain. Stamford, CT: Appleton & Lange; 1996:241–258.

27. Bronshtein M, Ornoy A. Acrania: anencephaly results from secondary degeneration of a closed neural tube: Two cases in the same family. *J Clin Ultrasound*. 1991;19:230–234.

28. Greenebaum E, Mansakhani MM, Heller DS, et al. Open neural tube defects: immunocytochemical demonstration of neuroepithelial cells in amniotic fluid. *Diagn Cytopathol*. 1997;16(2):143–144.

29. Geary M, Patel S, Lamont R. Isolated choroid plexus cysts and association with fetal aneuploidy in an unselected population. *Ultrasound Obstet Gynecol*. 1997;10:171–173.

30. Sohn C, Gast AS, Krapfl E. Isolated fetal choroid plexus cysts: Not an indication for genetic diagnosis? *Fetal Diagn Ther*. 1997;12:255–259.

31. Reinsch RC. Choroid plexus cysts-Association with trisomy: Prospective review of 16,059 patients. *Am J Obstet Gynecol*. 1997;176:1381–1383.

32. Morcos CL, Platt LD, Carlson DE, et al. The isolated choroid plexus cyst [see comments]. *Obstet Gynecol*. 1998;92:232–236.

33. Sullivan A, Giudice T, Vavelidis F, et al. Choroid plexus cysts: Is biochemical testing a valuable adjunct to targeted ultrasonography? *Am J Obstet Gynecol*. 1999;181:260–265.

CHAPTER 31

COMPUTER AND ULTRASOUND

Sean C. Blackwell / Ivan Zador / Ryan Blackwell

PAST AND PRESENT

Computerized perinatal database systems have been integral parts of clinical and research programs at academic obstetrics/gynecology departments since the 1970s.[1] These relational databases optimally link all obstetrical data with both short- and long-term neonatal outcomes. They are episodic and longitudinal databases designed to enhance clinical care and expedite epidemiological research.[2] In particular, the ability to develop large perinatal datasets has facilitated the study of infrequent, but critically important pregnancy complications.[3,4]

At Wayne State University/Hutzel Hospital, we have been using POPRAS (Problem Oriented Perinatal Risk Assessment System) forms for perinatal risk assessment since 1985.[5] Demographic and antenatal data are recorded at prenatal care sites and then sent to Hutzel Hospital for direct entry by trained technicians who batch enter data after checks for completeness and internal consistency. The perinatal database is used to generate summaries of antepartum information and delivery outcomes, ultrasound reports, and service statistics. It supports immediate availability of ultrasound reports and other key clinical information at multiple sites where care is provided. It has captured extensive obstetrical and neonatal outcome data for over 100,000 consecutive births. Currently, the perinatal database is a single relational database in the Microsoft Access format and is easily converted into one of many different statistical programs including SPSS, SAS, and Epistat, thus accessible to faculty and fellows for research purposes.

Data elements specific to prenatal genetics included in our perinatal database include family history of genetic conditions, prior history of pregnancies complicated by structural anomalies/chromosomal abnormalities, second trimester serum screening results (MSAFP, beta HCG, and unconjugated estriol), targeted ultrasound examination findings (major structural anomalies as well as "soft" markers for aneuploidy), and invasive genetic testing results (CVS, amniocentesis, and fetal blood sampling).

TECHNOLOGY ISSUES

Because of the significant labor costs associated with this type of "off-line" data entry, the feasibility of financially supporting a team of specific perinatal data entry personnel is a limiting factor for many departments. Even with database systems for which patient information is inputted directly into a computerized medical record by physicians, nurses, or other health care team members (e.g., ultrasound technicians) the initial and maintenance hardware and network costs may also be prohibitive. For these reasons, there is much interest in the development and application of an electronic medical record (EMR) that may run over the Internet.

There are several potential advantages and disadvantages to this approach (Table 31-1). First, if the perinatal EMR is maintained through an Application Service Provider (ASP), there is limited computer and network infrastructure costs. As long as there is access to high-speed Internet connections, which are available at relatively low costs at most health care sites, standard desktop computers can readily be used. Since the EMR application is administrated and maintained over the Internet at the server level, there is a low burden on the local client computer, which further decreases the departmental burden on in-house information technology support. The second advantage is immediate and widespread access to data from different health care sites. Although a patient may have antenatal encounters at her prenatal care clinic or an off-site ultrasound unit, this data may be inputted into the same database that ultimately contains all inpatient data, thus providing a potentially more seamless integration of antenatal outpatient and inpatient data. Furthermore, if the same EMR is used within a medical center but at different hospitals, there is the potential for more uniform data collection, more consistent data definitions, and subsequently improved clinical care. This may be increased further if disease specific clinical pathways are part of the EMR as well as quality assurance program.

There are currently few entirely web-based perinatal database systems in clinical use. Concerns over the stability and reliability of Internet access coupled with unknown security risks are major reasons for this hesitation. Although high-speed Internet access is relatively easy and inexpensive to obtain, the unknown risk of system downtime due to virus or denial of service attacks still plague potential users. Furthermore, security and privacy of sensitive patient data is another issue. The potential for unauthorized remote access by "hackers" to patient information such as genetic testing or HIV results remains of concern. Despite use of security measures such as username and password protection, role-based security, IP address restriction, and data encryption, administrators and risk managers remain wary. Anticipated governmental guidelines for the electronic transmission of patient information are a further potential burden that affects initiation of an Internet-based system. This is due to the fear of an inability to be compliant with these regulations and the potential punitive action from the government.[6]

FUTURE

Regardless of the technology employed, there are several promising avenues for further development of reproductive genetics-based EMRs for both clinical and research application. In the following section, we will briefly describe 2 examples that are in development at Wayne State University/Hutzel Hospital.

TABLE 31-1	POTENTIAL ADVANTAGES AND DISADVANTAGES OF AN INTERNET-BASED PERINATAL DATABASE	
Advantages	*Disadvantages*
Limited computer and network costs	Unknown future down time of Internet
Immediate and widespread access	Security of system or data from "hackers," denial of service attacks, or viruses.
More standardized collection of data across health care system	Unknown effect of future governmental regulations
Lower in-house IT costs	

There is significant interest in the combined use of biochemical and ultrasound markers in the first trimester for the detection of aneuploidy. Results from several large multicenter trials suggest that research in this area will continue and clinical practice has already changed with widespread use of nuchal translucency measurements. In order to continue to prospectively collect useful research data, as well integrate the available clinical information, we are developing within our Perinatal EMR an "Integrated" First Trimester Genetic Screening Module. This module combines maternal demographic and clinical data, maternal biochemical markers, first trimester ultrasound markers, and results of invasive genetic tests (see Fig. 31-1). It will display in one combined report: maternal age, maternal serum free beta-HCG and PAPP-A levels, ultrasound images of nuchal translucency measurement, ductus venosus waveform, and fetal profile for identification of the nasal bone. It will also provide risk assessment based on these individual markers or in combination, as well as normative and/or adjusted values. For both quality-control pur-

poses, a digital image of each ultrasound marker will be part of the report. Finally, it will have the ability for easy expansion and incorporation of new "tests" as they are developed.

Integration and dissemination of this information to genetic counselors, reproductive geneticists, maternal-fetal medicine specialists, and sonographers will continue to promote collaboration between these disciplines and improved patient care. As more data is collected from ongoing clinical trials and clinical strategies are evaluated, this "Integrated" Genetic module will serve as a computer-based clinical support system that provides a specific patient risk that is based on ethnicity, maternal age, serum screening tests, and ultrasound markers.

Another module within our Perinatal EMR that is relevant to reproductive genetics is our Multi-disciplinary Dysmorphology Database. This web-based database combines data input from maternal-fetal medicine, prenatal imaging, reproductive and pediatric genetics, pediatric dysmorphology, and perinatal pathology (Fig. 31-2). For each case clinical information and cytogenetic results are linked with prenatal images from 2D ultrasound, 3D/4D ultrasound, and ultrafast fetal MRI. Finally, perinatal pathologists contribute autopsy data including photographs of gross pathology, results of other postmortem imaging studies (radiography, dye studies, MRI), and histology findings. All cases are electronically archived and users with permission are able to search cases by ultrasound and/or cytogenetic findings, by diagnosis, and finally by key word(s). Interesting or difficult cases are presented at a monthly Dysmorphology Conference. This interdisciplinary approach has been successful at other institutions.[7]

In summary, regardless of the manner in which data is collected as part of a perinatal database, a good system must have 3 basic features. It must link information from all obstetrical encounters; antepartum and delivery information must be linked to all other clinical information, such as data from

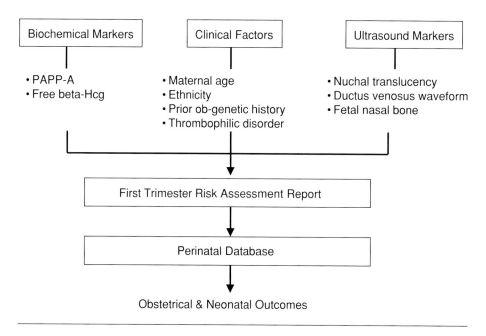

FIGURE 31-1 Diagram of components of an Integrated First Trimester Genetic Screening Electronic Medical Record.

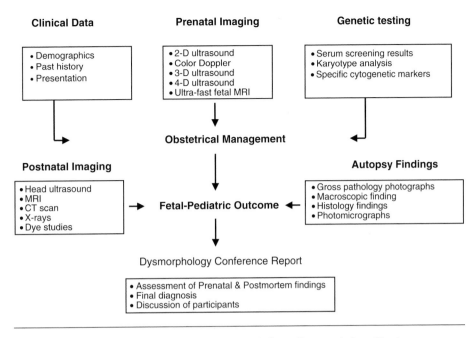

FIGURE 31-2 Diagram of components of Multi-disciplinary Dysmorphology Database.

prenatal ultrasound and genetic testing. Second, obstetrical conditions and outcomes must be actively linked to neonatal data; the disconnection of these data elements threatens the utility of having a perinatal database. Finally, data must be able to be retrieved from the database, not merely collected, in order to be useful for research and vital statistics reporting.

References

1. Rosen MG, Sokol RJ, Chik L. Use of computers in the labor and delivery suite: an overview. *Am J Obstet Gynecol.* 1978;132:589–594.

2. Chik L, Sokol J, Kooi R, et al. A perinatal database management system. *Methods Inf Med.* 1981;20:133–141.

3. Smith RS, Bottoms SF. Ultrasonographic prediction of neonatal survival in extremely low-birth-weight infants. *Am J Obstet Gynecol.* 1993;169:490–493.

4. Sorokin Y, Blackwell S, Reinke T, et al. Demographic and intrapartum characteristics of term pregnancies with early-onset neonatal seizures. *J Perinatol.* 2001;21:90–92.

5. Sokol RJ, Chik L. Perinatal computing: an overview. *Acta Obstet Gynecol Scand Suppl.* 1982;109:7–10.

6. The buzz on HIPAA: how HIPAA will affect the electronic transmission of health information. *Health Devices.* 2000;12:472–476.

7. Tennstedt C, Hufnagl P, Korner H, et al. Fetal autopsy: the most important contribution of pathology in a center for perinatal medicine. *Fetal Diagn Ther.* 2001;16:384–393.

FETAL AGE DETERMINATION AND GROWTH ASSESSMENT: THEIR ROLES IN PRENATAL DIAGNOSIS

Russell L. Deter

IS FETAL AGE DETERMINATION AND GROWTH ASSESSMENT IMPORTANT TO PRENATAL DIAGNOSIS?

The concept of prenatal diagnosis is usually associated with the detection of biochemical, structural, or chromosome abnormalities of the fetus. Fetal age determination and growth assessment may not be commonly considered a part of the procedures needed to identify such abnormalities but on closer inspection, they can be shown to be important or essential to many of the prenatal diagnostic methods currently in use. The most obvious examples are the hormone and biochemical assays used to screen patients for various chromosomal and structural abnormalities.[1] The reference ranges for most hormones and biochemical markers change with fetal age so determining whether a given value is abnormal requires an accurate fetal age estimate. Similarly, the risk for several chromosome abnormalities is fetal age dependent[2] and therefore cannot be determined accurately without knowing the fetal age. With respect to structural anomalies, many evolve over time and thus the likelihood of detection depends on the age of the fetus.[3] Finally, the incidence of postnatal problems resulting from such abnormalities has been shown to be dependent on both the magnitude of the lesion and the fetal age at which it is detected in a number of instances.[4,5] For these reasons determining the fetal age is an integral part of any prenatal diagnostic procedure if it has not been done for other reasons.[6,7]

With respect to growth assessment, a number of studies have shown that size abnormalities frequently occur in the late first trimester, second trimester, and third trimester in fetuses with chromosome abnormalities[8–11] and that different types of size abnormalities are associated with different chromosome abnormalities.[12–15] This suggests that growth assessments could play an important role in helping to identify fetuses who are at risk for such chromosomal problems. Benacerraf et al.[16] have proposed a scoring system for use in ultrasound screening for Trisomy 21 that includes evaluation of both the femur and humerus diaphysis lengths. Many structural anomalies are detected by making measurements on specific anatomic structures and comparing these measurements to their appropriate reference ranges. An example of this is the use of measurements of the atrium of the ventricular system of the brain to detect hydrocephalus and other brain abnormalities.[17] The seriousness of the anatomical abnormality has frequently been shown to be related to the magnitude of the deviation from normal and the degree of change occurring over time.[4,5] Structural anomalies are frequently associated with impaired fetal growth[18,19] although excessive growth occurs in some cases (eg, the head in hydrocephalus and the trunk in ascites, bowel obstruction and urethral obstruction). For these reasons, growth assessments can frequently contribute significantly to the prenatal diagnosis of fetal abnormalities, their subsequent obstetrical management, and patient counseling.

FETAL AGE DETERMINATION

DEFINITION OF FETAL AGE

Currently, the age of the fetus is most commonly called the gestational age. A survey of medical dictionaries, textbooks, and monographs from the 1950s and 1960s suggests that this terminology came into use around 1960, perhaps in conjunction with efforts to standardize definitions of viability, prematurity, and maturity.[20] However, this author has not been able to find the document that first formally defines gestational age as being determined from the first day of the last menstrual period. In discussing fetal age, use of the term gestational age introduces considerable confusion, which is getting worse with the wider use of assisted reproduction techniques, and is in fact biologically incorrect. Fetal development obviously starts with fertilization so the most biologically appropriate way to determine the age of the fetus is from the date of conception (this can now be done for pregnancies resulting from in vitro fertilization). Such fetal age estimates can logically be called conceptual age estimates. As the date of conception is not known in most pregnancies, conceptual age cannot be used except in a small number of cases at present. The more general way of determining fetal age is of course based on the first day of the last menstrual period (LMP), a point in time *before* there is even a fertilized zygote! To indicate that the fetal age was derived from the LMP, these fetal age estimates should be called menstrual age estimates. Since gestation does not begin until after fertilization, gestational age is actually synonymous with conceptual age, not menstrual age as its current definition indicates. In fact, there is no real need for the term gestational age since conceptual age and menstrual age provide a much more explicit and biologically correct indication of the basis for determining the age of the fetus. Since the time interval between the first day of the last menstrual period and ovulation is approximately 2 weeks,[21] it is reasonable to add 2 weeks to the conceptual age estimate to obtain a menstrual age estimate. In the following discussion of fetal age determination, only the terms menstrual age and conceptual age will be used.

DETERMINATION OF FETAL AGE FUNCTIONS

Although the age of the fetus is most commonly determined from the LMP, anatomical measurements made with ultrasound can also be utilized for this purpose. This requires specification of a fetal age function for each of the anatomical parameters used. A fetal age function is a mathematical equation that defines the relationship between the fetal age (usually

TABLE 32-1	REGRESSION EQUATIONS FOR DETERMINING FETAL AGE
Mean Gestational Sac Diameter [mGSD]: [Ref 35]	$MA = -2.67091 + 0.80396\ (mGSD) - 0.01342\ (mGSD^2)$
Maximal Straight Line Length [MSLL]: [Ref 42]	$Log_e\ (MA) = 1.684969 + 0.315646\ (MSLL) - 0.049306\ (MSLL^2) + 0.004057\ (MSLL^3) - 0.000120456\ (MSLL^4)$
Biparietal Diameter [BPD]:	
[Ref 33]	$MA = 9.54 + 1.482\ (BPD) + 0.1676\ (BPD^2)$
[Ref 27]	$Log_e\ (MA) = 1.985 + 0.04557\ (BPD) - 0.0061838\ (BPD \times log_e\ \{BPD\})$
Head Circumference [HC]:	
[Ref 33]	$MA = 8.96 + 0.540\ (HC) + 0.0003\ (HC^3)$
[Ref 27]	$Log_e\ (MA) = 1.848 + 0.01061\ (HC) - 0.000030321\ (HC^2) + 0.43498 \times 10^{-7}\ (HC^3)$
Abdominal Circumference [AC]: [Ref 33]	$MA = 8.14 + 0.753\ (AC) + 0.0036\ (AC^2)$
Femur Diaphysis Length [FDL]: [Ref 32]	$Log_e\ (MA) = 2.353301 + 0.231815\ (FDL) - 0.007804\ (FDL^2)$
[Ref 27]	$Log_e\ (MA) = 2.306 + 0.034375\ (FDL) - 0.0037254\ (FDL \times log_e\ \{FDL\})$

Menstrual age in weeks, anatomical parameters in centimeters.

the menstrual age), the dependent variable, and the anatomical measurement, the independent variable (Table 32-1). Fetal age functions are used to determine the expected menstrual age associated with a particular value of the anatomical parameter and are derived by regression analysis from known values for menstrual age-anatomical measurement pairs. Their validity depends on the accuracy of the menstrual age and anatomical measurement data, the absence of growth abnormalities in the fetuses from which such data were obtained, the representativeness of the sample used in the regression analysis and the appropriateness of the mathematical model chosen as the fetal age function. The latter should meet the criteria discussed previously for fetal size models.[22] The widely used fetal age functions of Hadlock et al.[23–26] and more recently those of Altman and Chitty,[27] satisfy these requirements except that the information on the growth status of the fetuses studied was rather limited.

Using a sample better controlled for growth abnormalities, Chervenak et al.[28] showed that the second trimester age estimates provided by the functions of Hadlock et al. and others were in good agreement with age estimates determined from the date of conception in IVF pregnancies. Similar results were found by Mull et al.[29] using less precise methods. Wennerholm et al.[30] and Tunon et al.[31] also report good agreement between first and second trimester age estimates derived from ultrasound measurements, using other fetal age functions, and those determined from dates of conceptions in IVF pregnancies. These investigations indicate that currently used dating methods based on ultrasound measurement of anatomical parameters provide accurate age estimates in the early part of pregnancy.

However, because of variability in fetal growth patterns, every fetus with a given value for a specific anatomical measurement does not have the same age. Therefore, it is important to specify both the expected menstrual age and the variability associated with that value. The variability determines the magnitude of the age error that one could be making if the *expected* menstrual age is taken as the *actual* fetal age, as is usually done. Determining this variability is another aspect of regression analysis as one is evaluating the pattern of menstrual age variability around the regression line given by the fetal age function. If this variability is found to be uniform as a function of the value of the anatomical measurement, the standard error of the estimate obtained in the course of the regression analysis can be used as the variability measure for *all* expected menstrual age values obtained using the fetal age function. However, if this variability changes as a function of the value of the anatomical measurement, as is usually the case, the change in variability must be defined. This may require transformation of the original data[32] and use of a variety of mathematical techniques that can vary with the anatomical parameter studied. Satisfactory evaluation of menstrual age variability has been carried out in only some cases.[32] The variability data given for most of the fetal age functions published by Hadlock et al.[23–26,33] are based on dividing the available data into fetal age-based subgroups and determining the differences between the actual and estimated ages in each age interval. This procedure does not use the entire data set to determine variability parameters, thus reducing the effective sample size, and assumes that the variability within each age interval is constant, an assumption shown to be incorrect for BPD, HC, Head Profile Area (HA), Transverse Cerebellar Diameter (TCD), and FDL.[27,32] As a result, the variabilities in age estimation given by Hadlock et al. are not optimal but in many cases they have been the best available. Altman and Chitty[27] have re-examined this issue using a larger sample and more rigorous statistical methods. New measures of age estimate variability were provided but all dating parameters were not studied and no data on age estimate variability after 36 weeks were given.

MEASUREMENTS USED TO ESTIMATE FETAL AGE

First Trimester

Fertilization and Ovulation: As can be seen in Table 32-2, fetal age determination is most accurate in the first trimester. The ideal fetal age parameter is the time of fertilization, which can now be determined for pregnancies resulting from in vitro

TABLE 32-2 | **VARIABILITY ASSOCIATED WITH FETAL AGE ESTIMATES**

Age Estimation Parameter	Subgroup Variability[a]						
	2–3 wks[b]	6–12 wks	12–18 wks	18–24 wks	24–30 wks	30–36 wks	36–42 wks
Ovulation	0.2	—	—	—	—	—	—
Fertilization	0.1	—	—	—	—	—	—
Mean Gestational Sac Diameter	—	+/−1.8	—	—	—	—	—
Maximal Straight Line Length	—	+/−0.6 to +/−1.2	+/−1.2 to +/−1.7	—	—	—	—
Biparietal Diameter (BPD)							
[Ref 33]	—	—	+/−1.2	+/−1.7	+/−2.2	+/−3.1	+/−3.2
[Ref 27]	—	—	+/−1.0 to +/−1.4	+/−1.4 to +/−2.1	+/−2.3 to +/−3.0	+/−3.0 to +/−3.9	—
Head Circumference (HC)							
[Ref 33]	—	—	+/−1.2	+/−1.5	+/−2.1	+/−3.0	+/−2.7
[Ref 27]	—	—	+/−1.1 to +/−1.3	+/−1.1 to +/−1.6	+/−1.7 to +/−2.6	+/−2.6 to +/−4.1	—
Abdominal Circumference (AC)	—	—	+/−1.7	+/−2.1	+/−2.2	+/−3.0	+/−3.0
Femur Diaphysis Length (FDL)							
[Ref 32]	—	—	+/−1.3 to +/−1.9	+/−1.9 to +/−2.5	+/−2.5 to +/−3.1	+/−3.1 to +/−3.6	+/−3.6 to +/−4.2
BPD, HC, AC, FDL	—	—	+/−1.1	+/−1.4	+/−1.8	+/−2.4	+/−2.3

[a] Variability given as +/− 2 SD where indicated.
[b] Subgroup age ranges given as menstrual age.

fertilization within 1 day.[21] However, this procedure is invasive and expensive so is not likely to be widely used. Because of the limited time (mean: 0.7 [99% range: +/−3.2] days) that is available for oocyte fertilization after ovulation,[21] the day of fertilization can be approximated from the day of ovulation. Ovulation can be determined from the LH surge[21] and by ultrasound.[34] Such estimates have an error of approximately 2 days.

Gestational Sac: From the first few days of gestation until approximately 3 weeks, conceptual age (CA) (5 weeks, menstrual age (MA)), it is not possible to determine fetal age with current technology. However, beginning at 5 weeks, MA, fetal age can be estimated from the mean gestational sac diameter (mGSD) measured by ultrasound.[35] This is possible until approximately 10 weeks, MA, with the accuracy of the age estimate being +/−1.8 weeks. This significant variability is due to the fact that gestational sacs do not have simple shapes and vary in their growth. Therefore, considerable differences in the mGSD can be expected even in pregnancies of the same age.

Longest Longitudinal Dimension and Crown-Rump Length: Beginning at 5.7 weeks, MA, and continuing until 18 weeks, MA, fetal age can be determined from the "length" of the fetus[36] as measured by ultrasound. This measurement was originally called the crown-rump length (CRL),[37] follow-

ing the practice of embryologists. However, as pointed out by Goldstein,[38] the measurement usually made is actually the longest longitudinal dimension (LLD) of the fetal pole. Prior to 8 weeks, MA, the head and trunk cannot be separately identified with conventional ultrasound methods and thus this measurement is frequently the "neck-rump length" because of the extreme curvature of these early embryos.[37] The effect of curvature on this measurement was recognized by Goldstein[38] and Wisser et al.,[39] the latter defining both a "crown-rump length" and a "greatest embryonic length" but using the latter measurement for fetal age determinations. However, the most anatomically correct measurement of embryo or fetal length would be along the long axis of the maximal longitudinal section of the embryo or fetus (maximal axial length {MAL}[40]) as illustrated in Fig. 32-1. If the fetus is not curved, this measurement is the same as the true crown-rump length measurement or the longest longitudinal dimension. However, in the presence of curvature these measurements can be different (see Fig. 32-1). Such curvature problems have been found with current technology between 8 and 13 weeks, MA, and the differences have ranged from –2% to –25% for the CRL and 0% to –14% for the LLD using the MAL as reference.[40] With the application of new technologies to first trimester pregnancies, such as the catheter containing an ultrasound transducer,[41] this problem may become significantly more important.

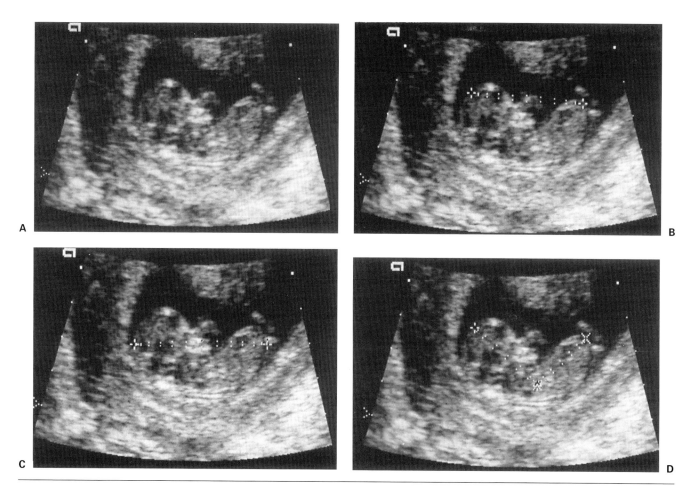

FIGURE 32-1 First trimester measurements of fetal length. This figure illustrates measurement problems caused by fetuses who are in a curved lie (**A**). The conventional measurement made on such fetuses is the maximal straight line length (MSLL) as shown in (**B**). This measurement is usually called the crown-rump length (CRL) but as shown in (**C**), the actual CRL measurement is quite different. The most appropriate measurement from the anatomical point of view would be along the long axis of the fetal profile (**D**), which we call the maximal axial length (MAL). The double broken lines in subfigures B–D were added to emphasize the anatomical locations of the measurements, not for measurement purposes themselves. CRL = 3.2 cm; MSLL = 3.7 cm; MAL = 4.4 cm. Data from reference 40, with permission.

Such imaging systems will permit the use of much higher ultrasound frequencies and produce very high-resolution images. In such images the marked curvature of early embryos could be visualized and it will be essential to use the most appropriate measuring procedure for determining the length of the embryo.

To determine fetal age from any of these measurements of fetal length requires the use of a fetal age function such as that given in Table 32-1. However, it is important to know which measuring procedure was employed as almost all measurements of fetal length are called crown-rump length measurements even if different measuring procedures were used. A given fetal age estimate is only valid if the measurement entered into the fetal age function is the same as that used to derive the function. Also, most fetal age functions using fetal length measurements are not valid beyond 12–13 weeks, MA, because data collection stopped at that point. The function of Hadlock et al.[42] is an exception. The errors associated with age estimates based on fetal length have been shown to increase progressively with menstrual age, being around +/−0.5 weeks at 6 weeks, MA, rising to +/−1.0 weeks at 13 weeks, MA, and finally reaching +/−1.4 weeks by 18 weeks, MA.[42] After 14 weeks, MA, other anatomical measurements are usually used to estimate age because they are easier to make and can provide a more detailed assessment of fetal size.

Second and Third Trimesters

Fetal age determination in the second and third trimesters is very similar to that in the first trimester except that different anatomical parameters are used. Fetal age functions (Table 32-1) are required and the errors in age estimates increase progressively toward term (Table 32-2). There are 4 primary anatomical measurements used for fetal age estimates, namely the biparietal diameter (BPD),[23] the head circumference (HC),[24] the abdominal circumference (AC)[25] and the femur diaphysis length (FDL).[26,32] The latter is also called the "femur length" but as shown by Mahoney et al. in 1985, the femur diaphysis is actually being measured.[43] The anatomically correct designation for this measurement was introduced by Deter et al. in 1987.[44] As can be seen in Table 32-2, the errors associated with individual age estimates are significantly greater than those in the first trimester except in the first half of the second trimester. However, the actual magnitudes of these errors are well defined only for FDL[32] and partially well defined for BPD, HC, HA, and TCD,[27] as indicated earlier. Despite this problem, it is clear that age estimation in the third trimester needs to be improved over what can be obtained using individual measurements. Hadlock et al.[33] found that a reduction in age estimation errors of approximately 16–23%, depending on when in pregnancy the age estimates were obtained, could be obtained by averaging the age estimates determined from the BPD, HC, AC, and FDL. This is probably due to the fact that technical errors and growth variations are not in the same direction for all age parameters and thus tend to cancel each other. This average age estimate, called the *composite menstrual age*, provides the best ultrasound estimate of fetal age in the second and third trimesters. It should be noted, however, that ultrasound age estimates are affected by significant technical problems, growth abnormalities and structural anomalies involving 1 or more of the anatomical parameters included in the calculation of the composite menstrual age.[33] If there is evidence that any of these anatomical parameters are affected by 1 or more of these problems, it should be omitted from the calculation of the composite menstrual age.

Growth Abnormality-Insensitive Measurement for Estimating Fetal Age

Although most growth retardation is due to utero-placental insufficiency or maternal disease, it is well known that chromosome abnormalities[13] and structural anomalies[19] are associated with growth abnormalities. As most anatomical parameters used to estimate fetal age are also important in monitoring fetal growth,[45] they can be affected by growth abnormalities and thus may give erroneous age estimates. For that reason there has been considerable interest in identifying parameters for estimating fetal age that are *not* sensitive to growth abnormalities. In the first trimester, those parameters used to determine the date of ovulation or conception are obviously such parameters but are not generally available. mGSD measurements are not known to be affected by fetal growth abnormalities but this cannot be tested directly and the high variability associated with age estimates based on this measurement limit its usefulness. Fetal length has been shown to be affected by Trisomy 18 and triploidy (at least after 12 weeks, MA, for the latter) but not other chromosome abnormalities.[8,9] Decreased fetal length growth has been reported in diabetic pregnancies[46] but this has not been confirmed in a more recent study.[47] However, there were reduced first trimester fetal lengths in diabetic pregnancies where subsequent structural anomalies were found.[46] Similarly, fetuses with anencephaly may have reduced lengths between 12 and 14 weeks, MA, but not before.[48] In twins, decreased length has been seen in fetuses with structural anomalies.[18] Thus it appears that first trimester length measurements can provide accurate age estimates even

if later growth abnormalities occur but only under certain circumstances.

In the second and third trimesters the only anatomic parameter receiving significant attention as a growth abnormality-insensitive parameter has been the transverse cerebellar diameter (TCD).[49–56] There has been considerable controversy concerning the insensitivity of this parameter to growth abnormalities with a number of authors finding it insensitive[50,52,54,56] while others have reported that it is sensitive.[49,51,53,57] The type of growth abnormality being studied may explain this discrepancy. If one evaluates fetuses with early onset of symmetric growth retardation, cerebellar growth *is* affected but in those fetuses with later asymmetric growth retardation or macrosomia, cerebellar growth *is not* affected.[49] The conclusion concerning asymmetrically growth-retarded fetuses has been questioned by Hill et al.[51] This controversy may also be partially a result of measurement error, which could be resolved by the use of 3-dimensional ultrasound.[58] Currently, it appears that the TCD may be an effective parameter for determining fetal age in some cases where growth abnormalities are present but not in others.

CHOOSING THE APPROPRIATE AGE ESTIMATE

From the foregoing discussion, it should be obvious that the best fetal age estimate would be that determined from the date of conception when known, with the date of ovulation being a close second. Age estimates based on these parameters have an accuracy unmatched by those based on any other parameter. Except before the sixth week, MA, when they cannot be measured, first trimester fetal length measurements provide age estimates, when appropriate, that are superior to those based on the LMP or subsequent ultrasound measurements because these age estimates have a maximum error of around 1 week or less. Therefore, the first trimester is the optimal time in pregnancy to determine the fetal age.

In the second and third trimesters it has been common practice to base the age of the fetus on the LMP unless the menstrual history was questionable or the ultrasound studies indicated that the ultrasound age estimates were not consistent with that derived from the LMP, in the absence of growth abnormalities. As reviewed by Geirsson[59] and Gardosi,[60] there is considerable evidence suggesting that this reliance on LMP age estimates is not warranted. Geirsson has shown that even in patients with normal, well-documented last menstrual periods, whose cycles were regular and 28 days in length, fetal age discrepancies of 3–4 weeks can be found when age estimates based on the LMP were compared to those based on late first trimester or early second ultrasound studies.[61] Mongelli et al.[62] found that second trimester ultrasound age estimates were better predictors of the duration of pregnancy than the LMP. Both Geirsson[59] and Mongelli et al.[62] recommend fetal age determinations by ultrasound in the first or early second trimester for all pregnancies. This is quite possible in Europe and Canada where routine ultrasound examinations in the second trimester are common practice but ultrasound examinations in all pregnancies is not the standard of care in the United States. Moreover,

A

MENSTRUAL AGE DETERMINATION

		Values	Predicted Values	±	2 SD	Use in Composite
FETAL MEASURMENTS						
Crown Rump Length	CRL :	cm		±	wks	N
Head	BPD :	4.7 cm	20.2	±	1.7 wks	Y
"	FOD :	5.9 cm				
"	HSA :	4.8 cm				
"	HLA :	6.1 cm				
"	HC :	17.2 cm	19.7	±	1.5 wks	Y
Abdomen	ASA :	4.4 cm				
"	ALA :	4.6 cm				
"	AC :	14.1 cm	19.2	±	2.1 wks	Y
Thigh	FDL :	3.1 cm	20.0	±	2.1 wks	Y
"	THC :	cm				
Cephalic Index	HSA/HLA :	0.79	0.78	±	0.04	

| MENSTRUAL AGE LMP: | 21.4 wks | Others: | 21.4 wks | Estimated Date of | |
| Composite: | 19.8 wks | Selected: | 21.4 wks | Delivery | 24 JUN 1995 |

B

FETAL GROWTH EVALUATION   x = Value   o = Beyond Graph

Expected Range

Selected MA:	21.4 wks	Low »————■————« High
MEASURMENTS HC:	17.2 cm*	x »————■————«
AC:	14.1 cm*	x»————■——«
FDL:	3.1 cm*	x »————■————«
THC:	cm	

RATIOS	HC/AC:	1.22	»————■——x————«
	FDL/HC:	0.18	
	FDL/AC:	0.22	

GROWTH RATES	HC:	1.0 cm/wk*	x »————■———«
	AC:	0.9 cm/wk*	x »————■——«
	FDL:	0.3 cm/wk	»————x——■————«

| WEIGHT | Estimated: | 298g ± | 44g | 16th Percentile |

FIGURE 32-2 Fetal age determination and growth assessment report forms. This figure illustrates the report forms generated by the Obstetrical Ultrasound Assessment software (Fetal Assessment International, Houston, Texas) to summarize the information used in determining fetal age (**A**) and assessing the growth status of the fetus (**B**). In this particular patient, the last menstrual period was normal, the menstrual cycle was regular and the ultrasound age estimates in a previous scan were consistent with the LMP age. For these reasons the LMP age was chosen as the fetal age and used to specify the normal ranges for HC, AC and FDL and their growth rates. The ultrasound age estimates in this examination were close to that based on the LMP, the composite menstrual age being within 1.6 weeks of the LMP age. However, all 3 anatomic parameters were below the lower limit of their respective normal ranges as were the growth rates for HC and AC. These results demonstrate that fetal age determination and fetal growth assessment are *not* the same thing.

most current ultrasound scanning protocols used in Europe and Canada do not directly address the possibility of growth abnormalities affecting ultrasound age estimates. Evaluation of this possibility would require an ultrasound examination in the first trimester (as is done in Germany) or 2 second trimester scans to evaluate growth rates.[45] Even without growth abnormalities, there is still the problem of the normal, genetically small, or large fetus. These fetuses could have anatomical measurements in the second trimester that would result in erroneous ultrasound age estimates. Growth rates may or may not be helpful in separating such fetuses for those with true growth abnormalities, depending on the timing of the scans. Therefore it is possible that the age of fetuses with unusual growth

patterns in the second trimester would be more reliably determined from the LMP if there were no abnormalities in the menstrual history.

Although the most reliable fetal age estimates are obtained in the first or early second trimester, it is frequently necessary to determine fetal age in the late second or third trimester. This is considerably more difficult than earlier in pregnancy because growth problems are more likely and the variation associated with age estimates is greater (Table 32-2). Frequently this results in a lack of correspondence between age estimates based on the LMP and those derived from ultrasound measurements, some of the latter may agree with the LMP age estimate and some may not. Our approach to this problem (Fig. 32-2), based on making fetal age assessments in more than 85,000 scans over the last 16 years, begins with a validity assessment of the LMP. As LMP age estimates in patients with "perfect" menstrual histories have differed significantly from those based on ultrasound,[61] the LMP age estimate is provisionally set aside in patients with *any* menstrual history abnormality. Age estimation based on the ultrasound findings is given priority, at least up to 30 weeks, MA. If the ultrasound age estimates do not differ by more than the errors associated with their estimation (Table 32-2) and there are no findings associated with growth abnormalities (ie, anatomical asymmetry, amniotic fluid abnormalities, abnormal physiologic parameters, risk factors, etc.), the composite menstrual age is accepted as the fetal age. If there are major discrepancies in the ultrasound age estimates or a growth abnormality is possible, the composite menstrual age is accepted provisionally as the fetal age and the patient rescanned in 3 weeks. Based primarily on a growth rate analysis (Fig. 32-2), a decision is made as to whether there is a growth problem. If no growth problem is found, the composite menstrual age determined in the first scan is considered the fetal age and all subsequent fetal ages determined from that age. If a growth abnormality is found, it may have been present at the time of the first scan, thus affecting the age determined from the ultrasound measurements. At this point a clinical decision has to be made as to what is the best estimate of the fetal age.

If there is no reason to question the reliability of the LMP age estimate, we consider all age estimates in determining the fetal age. When 2 or more of the 4 ultrasound age estimates differ from the LMP age estimate by less than the errors associated with the ultrasound age estimation process (Table 32-2), the LMP age estimate is taken as the fetal age. If the differences are greater that these errors for 3 or more ultrasound age estimates, the composite menstrual age is provisionally chosen as the fetal age, at least until 36 weeks, MA. If a growth abnormality is possible, based on the assessment described previously, the patient is rescanned in 3 weeks and a growth evaluation carried out. If no growth abnormality is found, the composite menstrual age is taken as the fetal age. For those fetuses with growth problems, the LMP age estimate is considered the fetal age.

In patients being scanned for the first time after 36 weeks, MA, there is a real problem because of the large errors associated with the ultrasound age estimates (Table 32-2), the possibility of growth problems and the proximity to delivery. For those fetuses with reliable LMP age estimates, it is reasonable to consider the LMP age estimate to be the fetal age regardless of whether or not the ultrasound age estimates are consistent with this age estimate. However, when there is evidence that the LMP age estimate is not reliable, one is faced with a situation in which all age estimates may be unreliable. In these late scans, the growth status of the fetus cannot be evaluated. There is evidence of growth cessation after 38 weeks, MA, even in normal fetuses,[63–65] so a sufficient interval between scans to determine growth rates reliably is not available. Again, a clinical decision as to which age estimate should be used is required.

SOME COMMON MISCONCEPTIONS CONCERNING FETAL GROWTH ASSESSMENT

Before considering how the growth of the fetus should be evaluated, there are several commonly held concepts that cause confusion and make it difficult to think clearly about growth assessment procedures. The following is a brief discussion of these ideas that hopefully will make the subsequent discussion of growth assessment more understandable.

EVALUATING THE SIZE OF A FETUS IS *NOT* THE SAME AS EVALUATING ITS GROWTH

For many years investigators interested in fetal growth have been collecting measurements of various anatomical structures at specific time points in pregnancy and using these data pairs to construct "growth curves." However, as pointed out by Altman,[66] such curves are not growth curves but rather "size curves." Growth is defined biologically as a change in size over time.[67] Therefore growth can only be evaluated by determining growth rates, which requires at least 2 measurements of size. Standards for the growth rates of a number of anatomic parameters are now available.[45,68] A given size is the result of growth rates some time in the past and may or may not indicate the way in which the fetus is growing at the time of the examination. Serial evaluation of growth rates is required to follow growth over any length of time during pregnancy.

DETERMINING THE AGE OF THE FETUS IS *NOT* THE SAME AS EVALUATING ITS GROWTH

It is common practice to evaluate fetal growth (actually fetal size) by determining the magnitude of the discrepancy between the expected fetal age and the fetal age determined by ultrasound. This procedure has no logical, mathematical, or scientific foundation whatsoever and it has not been justified by any empirical study. Its continued use in clinical obstetrics is a direct result of a lack of understanding of the basic mathematical ideas underlying both fetal age determination and growth assessment. This situation has arisen from the fact that both age determination and size assessment utilize the same anatomical measurement—menstrual age pairs.[23–26;32] However, whether one is determining fetal age or evaluating fetal size depends on what is defined as being unknown (the dependent variable) and what is defined as being known (the independent variable). This results in 2 types of plots of the original anatomical measurement-menstrual age pairs, the dating curve for fetal age determination and the size curve for evaluating fetal size (Figs. 32-3, 32-4). Regression analysis is used to determine the expected curves relating the dependent variable to the independent variable (solid line in both plots), which are the same except for orientation. This results in expected anatomical measurement—menstrual age pairs that

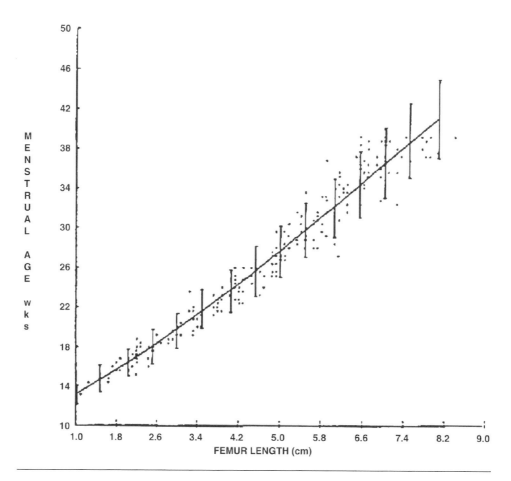

FIGURE 32-3   Age curve used in determining fetal age. This figure is an example of a data plot obtained in a cross-sectional study used to specify fetal age estimates from the femur diaphysis length. The dependent variable is the menstrual age (MA) and the independent variable is the femur diaphysis length (FDL). The function relating MA to FDL obtained by regression analysis, is given in Table 32-1 and was used to determine the expected menstrual ages at different values of the FDL (solid line). The vertical lines represent the normal ranges (+/−2 SD) in weeks for different FDL values. Data from reference 32, with permission.

are the same for both types of curves but the variability around these expected curves is not the same. For the dating curve the variability is in menstrual weeks (as it should be) while that for the size curve is in centimeters (as it should be). Usually the variability around the expected curve is affected by whether one is working with a dating curve or a size curve and different mathematical methods are frequently needed to define the normal variability associated with these 2 types of curves. This results in different reference ranges for the age estimate and the size of the anatomical measurement. As shown in Figure 32-2, an erroneous classification of fetal size can occur if it is based on whether there is agreement between ultrasound age estimates and the LMP age. This procedure provides no direct information on growth. The logical way to deal with this situation is to focus first on determining the best fetal age estimate then, using that age estimate, to define the appropriate reference ranges for classifying the anatomical measurements.

GROWTH AND SIZE PARAMETERS REFLECT LONG-TERM PROCESSES, NOT SHORT-TERM PROCESSES

The anatomical changes being used to monitor fetal growth usually occur only over a period of weeks, not days, hours, or even minutes as is the case with physiologic parameters. Current ultrasound methods for making anatomical measurements have intra- and inter-observer errors[69] and there are significant differences between prenatal and postnatal measurements even when the interval between these measurements is quite short.[70] This is particularly true for parameters such as weight that are *not* measured directly.[45] To be detected, anatomic changes due to growth must be larger than such errors and even in normally growing fetuses, this occurs only over a period of several weeks. We have found that determining reliable growth rates usually requires an interval between scans of approximately 3 weeks for most parameters. If significant growth retardation is present, an even longer interval may be needed.

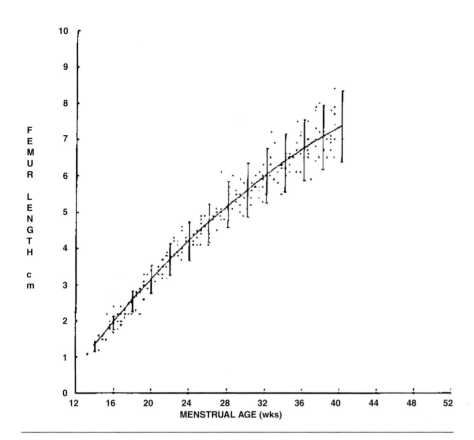

FIGURE 32-4 Size curve used in assessing fetal size. This figure is an example of a data plot obtained in the same cross-sectional study described in Figure 32-3 to assess fetal size at different menstrual ages. The dependent variable is the femur diaphysis length (FLD) and the independent variable is the menstrual age (MA). The function relating FDL to MA obtained by regression analysis is $FDL = -3.8929 + 0.42062(MA) - 0.0034513(MA^2)$. This function was used to determine the expected FDL values at different menstrual ages (solid line). The vertical lines represent the normal ranges ($+/-2$ SD) in centimeters at different menstrual ages. Data from reference 32, with permission.

Because of this characteristic, growth assessment can best be used to evaluate processes that have been going on over a considerable length of time. It is likely that such assessments will be useful for long-term predictions of subsequent pathology rather than short-term predictions.

FETAL GROWTH ASSESSMENT

SELECTION OF ANATOMIC PARAMETERS

In evaluating the growth of any fetus, it is first necessary to decide which anatomical parameters will be measured. There are parameters reflecting the general growth of the fetus (weight, length, soft tissue mass, etc.) and those giving information about major components of the fetal body (head, trunk, long bones, etc.). In addition there are various organs that can be measured,[71] which may be of use in detecting and following the progression of specific congenital anomalies or disease

processes. In general volume measurements would be most appropriate because the structures studied are 3-dimensional (3D), volume measurements are not sensitive to shape changes and a direct relationship to mass can be obtained if the density is known. Although longitudinal studies of volume growth parameters have been carried out[72] and the recent development of 3D ultrasound scanners have made volume measurements much simpler,[73] the use of volume parameters in fetal growth assessments is still under investigation. Although normal ranges for a number of volume parameters are now available, their use in growth assessment has been limited. At present, based on the most widely available technology, attention is primarily focused on measurements of length, either directly or in the form of diameters or circumferences, measured on 2-dimensional sections of anatomical structures at specific locations.[45]

Prenatal Parameters

For general growth assessment, the parameters available depend on the age of the fetus and quality of the ultrasound scanner being used. Prior to 5 weeks, MA, no fetal structure can be seen while between 5 and 6 weeks only the yolk sac can be measured.[35] From 6 to 18 weeks, MA, the length of the fetus can be measured[42] although this measurement is not well standardized as discussed above (Fig. 32-1). Between 9 and 14 weeks, MA, measurements of the head circumference (HC) and abdominal circumference (AC) have been made.[74] However, whether such measurements are comparable to those made after 14 weeks is difficult to determine because the anatomical landmarks used for plane selection are not as well defined. The quality of the image used for these measurements may also be important since the anatomical detail needed for plane selection is difficult to visualize without a high-quality image.

In the second and third trimesters, a set of parameters can be used to evaluate fetal growth that we have called the Prenatal Growth Profile (Table 32-3).[45] This set of parameters was chosen because the individual components have been found to be abnormal in neonates with growth problems[75] and they reflect the growth of most major components of the fetus. Other measures of trunk size, such as the chest circumference,[76] could have been used but because of the size of the liver and its central role in energy balance,[77] the AC was considered

TABLE 32-3	PRENATAL GROWTH PROFILE	
Variable	**Measured Anatomical Parameter**
Weight	Estimated Weight
Length	Femur Diaphysis Length
Head size	Head Circumference
Trunk size	Abdominal Circumference
Soft tissue mass	Thigh Circumference
Body proportionality	HC/AC, HC/FDL, AC/FDL

more useful. Similarly, other long bone measurements could probably be used to monitor skeletal growth but the FDL has been shown to be strongly related to the Crown-Heel Length (CHL)[78–80] and has proven effective in detecting skeletal dysplasias.[81] The use of the thigh circumference (ThC) to monitor soft tissue mass is more problematical. Although quite well defined prenatally[45] and important in the postnatal detection of IUGR[82] and Macrosomia,[125] its high normal variability, most likely due to the lack of leg position control but also other factors,[83] has made it relatively insensitive to prenatal changes in soft tissue readily detected with the same parameter postnatally.[82,84,125] This is a significant problem since postnatal studies strongly indicate that a decrease in soft tissue is the earliest stage of IUGR[84] and it is likely that this will be the case for Macrosomia due to diabetes. Several other measures of soft tissue have been proposed[85–88] but they have not been completely evaluated. It is also possible that more than 1 measure may be needed to accurately evaluate this widely distributed anatomical structure.[89]

Postnatal Parameters

Although Prenatal Diagnosis focuses primarily on events before birth, postnatal evaluations are also very important for confirming or not confirming observations and interpretations made prenatally. The situation is similar for growth assessment so appropriate evaluations of the neonatal growth status should be made. For this purpose, a Neonatal Growth Profile (Table 32-4) has been proposed for many of the same reasons given for the Prenatal Growth Profile.[45] As can be seen, these 2 profiles are quite similar except that weight (WT) and length (CHL) can be measured directly at birth instead of being estimated or inferred from other measurements as is the case

TABLE 32-4	NEONATAL GROWTH PROFILE	
Variable	**Measured Anatomical Parameter**
Weight	Weight
Length	Crown-Heel Length
Head size	Head Circumference
Trunk size	Abdominal Circumference
Soft tissue mass	Thigh Circumference
Body proportionality	HC/AC, WT/CHL, WT/CHL³

prenatally.[45,90] However, it should be kept in mind that even direct measurements such as HC and AC are not the same prenatally and postnatally even when made close together in time.[70]

Parameter Sets vs. Single Parameters

Instead of using sets of parameters such as those mentioned above, many clinicians follow the growth of the fetus, or evaluate the growth status of the neonate, with only a single anatomic parameter, in a majority of cases the estimated fetal weight or the birth weight. This is because of clinical practice developed many decades before ultrasound was available, the simplicity of this approach and the considerable clinical experience in relating weight to patient management. However, detailed studies of fetuses at risk for both IUGR and Macrosomia have revealed that all fetuses with growth problems do not manifest these problems in the same way (Fig. 32-5) and the use of single parameters (including weight) results in significant misclassification of the growth status of individuals, both in the third trimester[91] and at birth[82,125] (Table 32-5). Neonates with birth weights below the 2.5th percentile have been found to have no abnormal estimated weight measurements in the third trimester, even when using individualized estimated weight standards.[92] As can be seen in Figure 32-5, other parameters will often indicate that a growth abnormality is present even when this is not seen with the estimated weight. As the purpose of growth assessment is to detect pathological processes that manifest themselves as growth problems or to predict subsequent fetal compromise correctly and early, detection of who has a growth problem and who does not is essential. This requires the use of a set of anatomical measurements that can accurately characterize the growth status of all individuals.

Other Anatomical Measurements

Although there are a large number of specific anatomical measurements that can be made on different parts of the body, particularly with respect to individual organs,[71] relatively few have been widely used to detect different types of abnormalities. Exceptions to this are measurements of the diameter of the atrium of the brain,[17] the anterior-posterior diameter of the renal pelvis,[5] width of the nuchal translucency,[93] and various dimensions of the heart.[94] The thoracic circumference measurement has been suggested for fetuses at risk for pulmonary hyperplasia[76] while femur diaphysis length/abdominal circumference[95] and femur diaphysis length/foot length[96] have been used in the detection of skeletal dysplasias. Measurements of the orbits and lens (to detect eye abnormalities),[97] the alveolar ridge (to detect cleft palate),[98] the jaw (to detect micrognathia),[99] and sternum (to help in the diagnosis of various genetic disorders)[100] have been proposed. However, these more specific aspects of growth assessment should be explored further to determine which are effective and which are not. With the advent of 3-dimensional ultrasound scanners, evaluation of structures with complex shapes (e.g., the liver) have become much easier since volume growth parameters can be

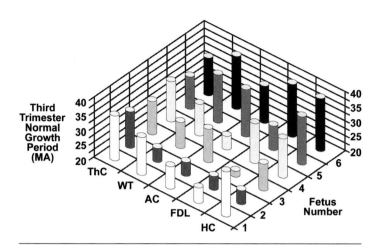

FIGURE 32-5 Variability in the manifestation of IUGR in the third trimester. This figure gives examples of the variability in affected anatomical parameters and age of onset seen in fetuses found to be IUGR at birth based on their mNGAS$_{51}$ values. Growth of a given parameter was considered to be abnormal when its %Dev value was below its normal range. In certain individuals the growth of some parameters was never abnormal, including that of EWT and AC. Data from reference 126, with permission.

used. Even though the scanning volume of current instruments is still rather small, it is sufficient for organs and other structures of the size usually found in the fetus.[73] Several volume parameters have been suggested as detectors of various abnormalities but this remains to be verified.

SIZE ASSESSMENT

At the time of the first ultrasound examination in any patient, a single set of fetal measurements is obtained and must be evaluated. The conventional procedure is to determine the age of the fetus and then compare each measurement to its age specific reference range as given by an appropriate 'growth' curve. The measurements are classified as 'within the normal range,' 'above the normal range,' or 'below the normal range,' and based on these classifications, the growth of the fetus is considered normal or showing evidence of a 'growth problem' of some type. A new set of second and third trimester standards for this purpose has recently been published by Chitty et al.[101–103]

In critically evaluating this procedure, several comments need to be made. The first concerns the importance of fetal age. A large number of both cross-sectional and longitudinal studies have shown that both the average size and the range of normal variability increase with the age of the fetus for almost all fetal measurements (Fig. 32-4 is an example) except for some ratios.[104] Therefore it is essential that fetal age be known before growth assessment is carried out (as discussed in detail in the previous section, fetal age determination is *not* the same as fetal growth assessment!).

Secondly, the so-called growth curves are not in fact growth curves but rather size curves, as pointed out by Altman[66] and discussed above. For that reason they are related to growth in the past but exactly when in the past cannot be determined. The relevancy of the size classifications to current growth status is not known.

Thirdly, the age-specific "reference ranges" against which the measurements will be compared are determined from population samples using regression analysis and must be defined properly.[22] This first requires a population sample with demographic characteristics similar to the patient under study or evidence that any differences in such characteristics do not affect normal variability. Next an appropriate definition of the "reference range" must be used. A definition of +/−2 SD includes 95% of the measurements from what would be considered normal fetuses and is appropriate if the distribution of measurements is symmetrical. The 2.5th percentile and the 97.5th percentile give a similar range for asymmetric distributions and can also be used for symmetric distributions. Some investigators have defined the reference range as the 5th and 95th percentiles or the 10th and 90th percentiles. These definitions reduce the range to 90% and 80% of reference values, respectively. Since use of such definitions of the reference range increases the number of measurements considered abnormal, their use needs to be justified before they are accepted. Finally, the method giving the actual values of the reference range at different times in pregnancy must be valid for the data being used.

Since the data available at any given time point are usually small, variability measures (e.g., standard deviation) based on such data are subject to significant sampling error and

TABLE 32-5 | EFFECTIVENESS OF SINGLE ANATOMICAL PARAMETERS IN SEPARATING IUGR, NORMAL AND MACROSOMIC NEONATES

| Growth Status[a] | N | Abnormal GPRI Values[b] | | | | | Abnormal Measurements[c] | | | | | SGA % | LGA % |
		WT %	CHL %	HC %	AC %	ThC %	WT %	CHL %	HC %	AC %	ThC %		
Normal	52	5.8	3.8	7.7	11.6	11.6	0.0	5.8	3.8	7.7	3.8	0.0	0.0
IUGR	22	77.3	27.3	40.9	50.0	77.3	27.3	36.4	18.2	13.6	50.0	45.5	0.0
Macrosomia	22	78.3	13.0	21.7	69.6	43.5	21.7	7.0	7.0	17.4	13.0	0.0	60.9

Data from reference 125.

[a]Growth status determined from m$_3$NGAS$_{51}$ values: IUGR<182.5%, Normal-182.5% to 210.0%, Macrosomia >210% (reference 125).

[b]GPRI values compared to normal ranges given in references 90,113.

[c]Measurements < −2 SD below age-specific mean considered abnormal using normal ranges given in reference 124.

are not reliable. Use of the entire sample studied is necessary to obtain reliable measurements of variability at all time points. This can be done by transforming the original data to eliminate the dependence of the variability on the fetal age or by fitting a function to the variability data and using that function to specify the reference range at all time points.[105] Use of the standard error of the estimate to calculate the reference range is only valid if the variability is *not* a function of fetal age,[22] a rare situation for fetal size parameters.

Customized size standards: Classifications utilizing traditional size curves do *not* correct for differences in growth potential so genetically small or large normal fetuses cannot be separated from those with IUGR or Macrosomia. Some fetuses with normal measurements may in fact be IUGR or Macrosomic if one were to compare their actual measurements to those expected from their growth potential rather than to the *population* reference range.[82,106,125] As a result, misclassifications can occur and deciding who has a growth problem and who does not becomes increasingly difficult. Individualized Growth Assessment[45,126] deals with this problem quite well since it provides the ultimate in customized size and growth standards (each fetus is its own control). However, because it involves mathematical modeling and requires 2 scans before 26 weeks to define an individual's growth potential, this procedure has not been widely accepted. Rather, efforts have been made to customize population size curves to provide a more appropriate normal range. In the simpler procedures, the size is compared to an age-specific mean value at the time of the first scan[107] or the birth measurement is compared to an optimal value, determined by regression analysis from data on birth age and a specific set of demographic variables.[108] In the former, differences from mean values are expressed as a percent of the mean value, which is assumed to be constant until delivery. In the latter case actual measurements are expressed as a percent of the optimal value. The normal range is based on specific percentile values derived from a reference sample and thus contains the high inter-individual variability due to differences in growth potential (as do all reference ranges defined in this way). A more complex procedure[109] also uses regression analysis and a specific reference sample to determine the relationship between birth weight and a set of variables, which includes birth age and certain demographic characteristics. A function is derived which allows calculation of the optimal birth weight for any specific neonate. It is then assumed that the actual weight growth curve for the fetus being studied has the same shape as the expected estimated weight growth curve (e.g., the 50th percentile line) determined in the cross-sectional study by Hadlock et al.[110] One then chooses the particular percentile line of the Hadlock estimated weight growth curve that would result in the optimal weight at 40 weeks, MA. This curve gives the expected fetal weight at any given time point. The normal range is considered to be plus or minus this expected value times $1.28 \times$ (S.D. / mean weight at 40 weeks for the reference sample) (10th and 90th percentiles). The previously described methods have only been applied to weight and can adjust the normal range only for variables that can be identified and measured or classified.

The methods of Wilcox et al.[108] and Gardosi et al.[109] assume that the regression models give the optimal predicted weight even though in the only instance for which it was reported, just 28% of the weight variance was accounted for by the model.[108] Gardosi et al.[109] and Santonja-Lucas et al.[107] assume that actual individual growth curves parallel the percentile lines determined in cross-sectional studies of population samples and that fetuses follow their percentile lines if growth is normal. Actual longitudinal studies of weight growth curves[112] do *not* support such assumptions and there is only 1 appropriately done investigation which has attempted to test them by trying to predict birth weight.[107] In this study the error in weight prediction at birth was twice as high assuming fetuses follow percentile lines as has been found using IGA methods that make *no* such assumptions.[113] At the present time there is *no* direct scientific evidence which justifies assuming that actual individual growth curves are parallel to the percentile lines of population size curves or that normally growing fetuses stay on their percentile lines throughout pregnancy. These concepts are factoids not facts!

The appropriate statistical approach to the problem of customizing the normal range is 2-level statistical modeling that has recently been used by Pang et al.[127] with several fetal growth parameters. This method, utilizing longitudinal studies of fetal growth, characterizes the growth of normal fetuses in the first level and the effect of identifiable variables affecting this growth in the second level. Any given expected value is adjusted for the values of factors affecting growth in that individual. An age-dependent variance function provides the appropriate SD value for any given time point. This procedure requires none of the assumptions utilized by the methods previously described but does give normal ranges that include the biological variability of the reference sample and only adjusts for identifiable and measurable variables.

Royston[111] has introduced a similar customization procedure that specifies the reference range at a subsequent time point based on the size of the measurement at the current time point and the time interval between scans. This dependence of the subsequent reference range on current size implies that the growth rate is size dependent, as has also been shown for growth rates based on the Rossavik growth model (Table 32-6). Since size is an indirect measure of growth potential (determined by both known and unknown causes), this approach can adjust the normal range for variables that are not known or cannot be measured. The Royston method is derived from longitudinal studies of fetal growth and has been applied to the BPD, HC, AC, FDL, and EWT. However, a special computer program is required for its implementation because of the mathematical complexity involved. It should also be noted that the Royston method does not eliminate the biological variability of the reference sample.

GROWTH ASSESSMENT

Growth Rates

To actually evaluate growth, as opposed to size, it is necessary to determine the change in size over time. To make such

| TABLE 32-6 | MATHEMATICAL FUNCTIONS USED IN INDIVIDUALIZED GROWTH ASSESSMENT |

A. Rossavik Growth Model

$P = c\,(t)^{k+s(t)}$ P: anatomical parameter   t: MA minus start point

Growth rate $= dP/dt = P\,[s + k/t + s\log_e(t)]$

B. Percent Deviation (%Dev)

%Dev = (actual measurement − expected measurement)/(expected measurement) × 100

C. Pathological Percent Deviation ($\%Dev_p$)

$\%Dev = \%Dev_p + \%Dev_r$

$\%Dev_p = \%Dev - \%Dev_r$ $\%Dev_r$: upper or lower limit of normal range for %Dev provides an estimate of $\%Dev_r$

$\%Dev_p$: values less than $\%Dev_r$ set equal to zero

D. Prenatal Growth Assessment Score ($PGAS_{at}$)

$$PGAS_{at} = \sum_{i=1}^{a}\sum_{j=1}^{t}(\%Dev_{Pij})/(N_T)$$

a: number of anatomical parameters studied

t: number of time points studied

N_T: total number of deviations studied

E. Percent Difference at Birth (%Diff)

(%Diff) = (predicted measurement − actual measurement)/(actual measurement) × 100

F. Growth Potential Realization Index (GPRI)

GPRI = (actual measurement at birth)/(predicted measurement at birth) × 100 [Predicted measurements are corrected for systematic prediction errors when indicated]

G. Neonatal Growth Assessment Score (NGAS)

$$NGAS_4 = \sqrt{(GPRI_{ThC}-100)^2 + (GPRI_{WT}-100)^2 + (GPRI_{AC}-100)^2 + (GPRI_{HC}-100)^2}$$

H. Modified Neonatal Growth Assessment Score (mNGAS)

$m_1NGAS_{51} = 0.685\,(GPRI_{ThC}) + 0.600\,(GPRI_{WT})$
$\quad + 0.349\,(GPRI_{AC}) + 0.169\,(GPRI_{CHL}) + 0.142\,(GPRI_{HC})$

$m_2NGAS_{51} = 0.700\,(GPRI_{WT}) + 0.556\,(GPRI_{ThC})$
$\quad + 0.401\,(GPRI_{AC}) + 0.156\,(GPRI_{CHL}) + 0.129\,(GPRI_{HC})$

$m_3NGAS_{51} = 0.660\,(GPRI_{WT}) + 0.602\,(GPRI_{ThC})$
$\quad + 0.394\,(GPRI_{AC}) + 0.159\,(GPRI_{CHL}) + 0.146\,(GPRI_{HC})$

an assessment, one obviously needs anatomical measurements from at least 2 ultrasound examinations. With this information the average growth rate for the interval between scans can be calculated by simply dividing the difference in the anatomic measurements by the difference in menstrual ages. This interval growth assessment can be carried out at 3–4 weeks intervals using serial scans in those patients with significant risk for growth problems.[45] Although it may be desirable to reduce this interval to 2 weeks in some cases, we have found that this often results in growth rates that are difficult to interpret, probably because the change in size due to growth is not large compared to the measurement errors. Mongelli et al.[114] found that the use of scan intervals of less than 3 weeks increased the rate of false positives in the detection of growth restriction based on AC growth rates. The noncontinuous fetal growth seen by Bernstein et al. in normal fetuses[115] led these authors to conclude that the absence of growth for less than 3 weeks could not be considered abnormal.

The principal problem in using growth rate measurements is finding an appropriate growth rate standard against which to compare a given measurement. This is because the data needed for such standards comes from longitudinal studies of fetal growth while determining the age-specific reference ranges requires that the statistical analysis be carried out on data which are completely independent,[68] unless special conditional probability techniques are used.[111] To assure independence, only 1 entity per fetus can be included in the analysis. If one growth rate measurement per fetus were used, in a sample where the number of fetuses and the time intervals were large enough and appropriately distributed throughout pregnancy, reference ranges could be determined by regression analysis as has been done for individual anatomical measurements.[22] This is relatively easy if growth is linear (or linear over a defined time interval)[40] but is much more difficult if growth is curvilinear as is often the case.[112] As one might imagine, obtaining the needed sample is extremely difficult and such a sample has not been used in previous growth rate studies.[68,116] What has generally been done is to carry out serial ultrasound studies over most of pregnancy then use multiple growth rate measurements from each fetus in the statistical analysis. As has been pointed out previously in the statistical literature,[117] measurements from the same individual are correlated and thus are not independent. Therefore reference ranges determined from such data sets are biased (usually underestimated).

To deal with these sampling problems, Deter and Harrist introduced a new method for determining growth rate standards based on the Rossavik growth model.[68] This model, introduced in 1984,[118] has been shown to fit longitudinal data sets of 1-, 2- and 3-dimensional parameters with a very high degree of accuracy (R^2: 97–99%).[45] There are only 3 coefficients in this model (Table 32-6), one of which (k) is a constant specified by the anatomical measurement being studied.[45] Thus virtually all the information in the entire longitudinal growth curve of any specific parameter in a given fetus is captured by the two other Rossavik model coefficients (c,s). The procedure of Deter and Harrist takes advantage of these characteristics of Rossavik models by carrying out all variability analyses on the coefficients c and s. Thus, the entire longitudinal growth curve becomes the entity whose variability is being evaluated. As there is only one such curve for each fetus for a given parameter, data independence is assured. This procedure also takes into account differences in measurement error, time point distributions, and fitting errors. To obtain growth rate standards, data from fetuses with normal growth outcomes were used to define the Rossavik growth models for 40 extreme growth curves (specified by the values for c and s). Instantaneous growth rates at specified time points were then determined using these models (see equation in Table 32-6). The limits of the reference range at any given time were defined as the highest and lowest values obtained at that time.[68] Depending on the shape of these growth curves, which is not limited in any way, different growth curves contributed the extreme values at different times. This approach has provided reference ranges at weekly intervals for the growth rates of 1-, 2-, and 3-dimensional parameters throughout pregnancy.[45,68]

Individualized Growth Assessment

Although serial growth rate assessments can be made throughout pregnancy to monitor fetal growth, such assessments do not correct for differences in growth potential. Thus, as with size curves (see previous section), determination of fetal growth status is difficult because the significant inherent variability of even normally growing fetuses is still present in the growth rate standards described above and misclassification occurs. This problem can be circumvented by use of individual growth curve standards which utilizes each fetus as its own control.[119] Such standards can be specified from the data obtained in two ultrasound examinations during the second trimester, separated by 4–8 weeks,[120,121] provided there is no evidence of abnormal growth during this period (this criterion has been satisfied even in fetuses which later were considered to be either IUGR[91] or Macrosomic[122] at birth). The slopes of the second trimester growth curves are determined from the ultrasound data and used to specify a Rossavik growth model for each anatomical parameter in each fetus. Expected growth trajectories, and birth characteristics if growth continues to be normal, can be obtained using these growth models.[45] Comparisons of actual measurements to expected ones in fetuses with normal growth outcomes at birth have shown that HC, AC, and FDL growth can be predicted with an accuracy of 5–10% in singletons, twins and triplets. Similar data for ThC and EWT are 15–18%.[113] WT, CHL, HC, AC, and ThC at birth can be predicted with random errors of 5–10% for singletons, twins, and triplets.[113] This high level of accuracy in predicting third trimester growth and birth characteristics has permitted the definition of new measures of fetal growth and growth status at birth that are independent of differences in growth potential (Table 32-6).[63,82,125,126] The use of these measures has provided new insights into the development of IUGR and Macrosomia in both fetuses and neonates.[82,84,91,92,122,123,125,126]

USE OF SIZE AND GROWTH ASSESSMENTS

First Examination

As indicated above, the data available after the first ultrasound examination does not permit a direct evaluation of growth but only size, and only if the age of the fetus is well known. However, since size is a result of growth in the past, it can be used with other information to provide a preliminary assessment of the growth status of the fetus. If abnormal size measurements are associated with appropriate risk factors (e.g., abnormally small fetus in patient with severe pregnancy-induced hypertension) or other abnormal ultrasound findings (e.g., abnormally large fetus and polyhydramnios), one might suspect that a growth problem is present and order a repeat scan to see if a growth problem is actually present. In this regard, ratios of anatomic parameters (e.g., HC/AC, AC/FDL, HC/FDL) can be helpful as fetal asymmetry can occur at different stages of both IUGR and Macrosomia.[91,92,122] Some of these ratios (e.g., AC/FDL, HC/FDL) have the useful characteristic of being constant, at least after 20 weeks, MA, so an accurate age estimate is not needed. However, it should be noted that growth pathology can exist in the presence of normal ratios (e.g., 'symmetrical' growth retardation) and abnormal ratios occur in fetuses with normal growth.[67] Because of the latter, we do not consider an abnormal ratio to be significant unless 1 of the 2 components of the ratio is outside its age-specific reference range.

If there are no risk factors or other abnormal findings associated with abnormal size measurements, one must consider the possibility that the growth of the fetus is normal and the fetus is small or large because of the set points of its genetic growth controllers. Since this situation cannot be determined directly, this diagnosis can only be made indirectly by searching for previously unknown pathologic conditions (to exclude other causes) or by obtaining historical information (e.g., small or large babies at term in previous pregnancies) consistent with this condition. Obviously a repeat scan is indicated to see if the growth rates are abnormal.

If all anatomic measurements are within their age-specific normal ranges but risk factors or other abnormal findings are present, a growth abnormality should still be considered. However, it is known that normally growing fetuses can be found in mothers with significant risk factors.[82] This is because the correct interpretation of a size measurement is not possible unless one knows what the measurement should have been, something that can only be known using Individualized Growth Assessment (IGA) methods.[45,126] Using conventional growth assessment procedures, normal anatomical measurements have been found in both fetuses and neonates who are IUGR or Macrosomic by IGA methods.[82,91,92,122,123,125] However, having all measurements of the Prenatal or Neonatal Growth Profiles within their reference size ranges in a fetus or neonate with a growth problem would be very unusual but possible (e.g., 'symmetric' IUGR), depending on how well the age of the fetus of neonate was known. Given these possibilities, a repeat scan to evaluate growth rates is quite reasonable.

Finally, if all anatomic measurements are within their age-specific reference ranges and there are no risk factors or other abnormal findings, it is reasonable, at least on a probabilistic basis, to conclude that the growth status at the time of the scan was normal. However, this situation can change later in pregnancy and numerous studies of low birth weight neonates have indicated that only approximately 50% of the decrease in weight can be attributed to known causes. Therefore subsequent clinical developments or indirect evidence of growth problems (e.g., abnormal fundal height measurements) justify a repeat scan to evaluate the amount of growth since the last scan.

Second Examination

With 2 ultrasound examinations, one has 2 sets of anatomical measurements and ratios which can be evaluated as described above and also compared to see if they indicate persistence of any abnormalities found in the first scan. However, in addition, one can now calculate average growth rates, as indicated above, and make an actual evaluation of growth, at least for the interval between the scans. To do this, appropriate reference ranges for average growth rates must be constructed from the data on the age-specific reference ranges for instantaneous growth rates.[68] This involves determining the ages with instantaneous growth rate values that are closest to the actual ages at each end of the interval. The 2 lower limit values are then averaged, followed by an averaging of the 2 upper limit values, to obtain estimated upper and lower normal limits of the average growth rate reference range. If all of the measured average growth rates are within their reference range limits, one has presumptive evidence that growth is normal. However, it should be kept in mind that these reference ranges are population growth standards and not individual growth standards. Thus such assessments are subject to the same problems described above for other population standards, namely they do not correct for differences in growth potential.

If average growth rates are abnormal, particularly if present in conjunction with abnormal size measurements, asymmetry, significant risk factors, or other abnormal findings associated with growth problems, a growth problem is likely. However, in the absence of other confirmatory evidence, abnormal average growth rates at the time of the second scan do not necessarily indicate abnormal growth although multiple abnormal average growth rates are more worrisome. A normal but genetically small or large fetus would be expected to have abnormal average growth rates sometime in pregnancy, most likely in the second trimester, since having anatomical measurements outside their reference ranges implies average growth rates outside their reference ranges. Exactly when the growth of such fetuses is below or above reference range values remains to be defined. Another possibility results from an aspect of fetal growth patterns that has not been previously described. Our longitudinal studies of fetuses with normal growth outcomes, using 2–3 week intervals between scans, suggest that normal early growth is not truly linear (more sinusoidal) although linear models fit the growth of many anatomical parameters quite well.[112] We have found periodicities in the growth patterns that are similar for different parameters in the same fetus but different in different fetuses (Deter, unpublished). If the measurement times correspond to the peak (first scan) and the trough (second scan) of such periodicities, one obtains an abnormally low average growth rate while the converse occurs if the relationship of the times of measurement to the growth period is reversed. This can result in abnormal average growth rates for a specific time interval even in fetuses whose overall growth during pregnancy is normal. Regardless of whether the abnormal average growth rates indicate abnormal growth, repeat scanning is indicated to determine if the growth abnormality is persistent and progressive, the hallmarks of true pathological processes.

Subsequent Examinations

Serial assessments of average growth rates can be used to resolve the issues described in the previous section. Normal, genetically small or large normal fetuses will not show progression of their growth rate abnormality and it is our impression that these growth rates fall within their reference ranges

later in pregnancy although this has not been documented by a scientific study. Growth rate abnormalities due to the timing of the scans relative to the growth period will show an alternating pattern, the abnormality (or location within the reference range) being first in 1 direction for a given interval then in the opposite direction for the subsequent interval. This oscillation seems to dampen as pregnancy progresses. For true growth rate abnormalities, persistence in one direction as well as progression is usually seen if there are no effective changes in management. When the cause of the growth abnormality can be identified and either eliminated or its effect reduced, subsequent average growth rates will go back into the reference range or may show compensatory growth acceleration or deceleration for some period of time. This ability of interval growth rates to reflect the changing growth pattern of the fetus over time makes these measurements very useful for managing patients with growth abnormalities.

Individualized Growth Assessment

As indicated previously, using serial average growth rate assessment to follow changing fetal growth patterns utilizes growth rate standards that contain inter-fetus variability and do not correct for differences in growth potential. Thus such assessments lack sensitivity and result in misclassifications as has been pointed out for size assessments using standards with similar characteristics. The use of Individualized Growth Assessment (IGA)[126] corrects for these problems, except for the second trimester time interval used for model specification, as was indicated for size assessment, since each fetus is its own control. Growth during the model specification interval, a period when growth is assumed to be normal, is characterized by the coefficient c and must be evaluated using population standards.[113] If found to be abnormal, additional information is needed to determine if this finding indicates a growth problem starting in the first trimester (eg, chromosome abnormality) or a low or high set point for the genetic growth controllers (at present we know of no way to distinguish between these two possibilities using growth parameters). The former would be a violation of the basic assumption of IGA so this method should not be used while the latter would indicate a normal variant and use of IGA methods is justified. Once the validity of using IGA methods is established, one then has an individualized standard for growth rate assessment. The expected growth rate is given by the difference in the expected anatomical measurements at the 2 time points defining the growth interval divided by that time interval. The range of normal variation (due to measurement and modeling errors, not biological differences between fetuses) is given by using the upper and lower limits of the expected value at the second time point, together with the expected value at the first time point, in two separate growth rate calculations. The measured growth rate between the 2 time points can be compared to this individualized normal range. Alternatively, one can calculate the Percent Deviation[126] ([Observed – Predicted/Predicted] × 100) at a given time point. In a recent publication[126] it has been shown mathematically that the Percent Deviation is proportional to the difference between the expected growth rate and the observed growth rate in the third trimester. Thus, Percent Deviations (see Table 32-6) and their normal ranges[113] can be used in place of growth rates in serial growth assessments as they give equivalent information and are simpler to follow.

As shown in Table 32-6, percent deviations represent a comparison of the actual anatomical measurement to its expected value and thus are individualized growth assessment parameters. They differ from zero due to random measurement and fitting errors as well as pathologic processes[91] but not the normal biological variability between fetuses as each fetus is its own control. The variability found in fetuses with normal growth outcomes[92] is a measure of former types of errors so Percent Deviations outside their reference ranges indicate the presence of pathology. Because different fetuses manifest their growth abnormalities in significantly different ways (Fig. 32-5), it has been found necessary to combine information from 5 parameters (EWT, HC, AC, ThC, FDL) of the Prenatal Growth Profile in order to optimize detection of IUGR in the third trimester.[91] As indicated in Table 32-6, the pathological components of the percent deviations for these 5 parameters over any specified number of time points can be summed and divided by the number of time points studied to give an average pathological percent deviation, called the Prenatal Growth Assessment Score (PGAS$_{At}$). The PGAS$_{At}$ stays above its normal limit of –0.4%[92] if growth is normal but becomes progressively more negative in fetuses with IUGR (Fig. 32-6). Abnormal PGAS$_{At}$ values have been found, on average, at 31

(+/–3.7) weeks, MA, 5.4 (+/–2.5) weeks before delivery.[91,92] The PGAS$_{At}$ has been very effective in identifying normally growing and IUGR fetuses in the third trimester except when the growth abnormality was limited to a decrease in soft tissue deposition,[92] the earliest stage of growth retardation as indicated by studies of neonatal growth status.[84] This is probably because the parameters most sensitive to changes in soft tissue, EWT and ThC, have high normal variability.[113] Better methods for the detection of soft tissue abnormalities are needed to improve the early detection of IUGR. Third trimester detection of Macrosomia using these methods has not been extensively investigated.[126]

In the neonate, the evaluation of birth characteristics can be made on an individualized basis using Growth Potential Realization Index (Table 32-6) values for WT, CHL, HC, AC, and ThC.[113] However, heterogeneity in the expression of growth abnormalities seen in fetuses is also found in neonates.[84,125] Therefore use of a set of parameters instead of a single parameter optimizes the detection of IUGR[82] and Macrosomia.[125] At the present time, the modified Neonatal Growth Assessment Score (mNGAS) (Table 32-6) provides the most comprehensive means for identifying IUGR[82] and Macrosomic neonates.[125] A boundary value of 181.7% for the m$_1$NGAS$_{51}$ separated IUGR and Normal neonates with an accuracy of 97.3%. Normal and Macrosomic neonates were separated with an accuracy of 97.3% using a boundary value of 207.5% for the m$_2$NGAS$_{51}$. Boundary values of 182.5% and 210% for the m$_3$NGAS$_{51}$ separated IUGR, Normal and Macrosomia neonates with an accuracy of 96.9%.[125] This single composite measure of growth outcome is much more effective than any single anatomical parameter in separating IUGR, Normal, and Macrosomic neonates, regardless of whether corrections for differences in growth potential are made in the latter.[125]

It is hoped that this chapter on fetal age determination and growth assessment will help the clinician use these powerful tools to more accurately diagnose a wide range of prenatal conditions.

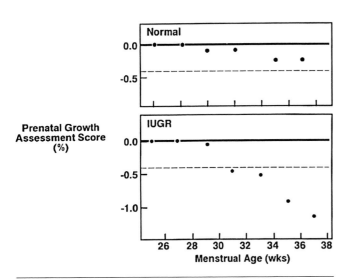

FIGURE 32-6 Change in PGAS$_{At}$ values during the third trimester in fetuses that were normal or IUGR at birth. This figure gives the PGAS$_{At}$ values at sequential time points in the third trimester for a fetus with a normal growth outcome at birth (upper panel) and one considered to have IUGR (lower panel), based on their NGAS$_4$ values. The PGAS$_{At}$ values in the normally growing fetus stay above the lower boundary of the normal range (broken line) while those for the IUGR fetus are initially above this boundary but go below it at approximately 31 weeks, MA, and become progressively more negative. Data from reference 91, with permission.

References

1. Kuller JA, Chescheir NC, Cefalo RC. *Prenatal Diagnosis and Reproductive Genetics*. St. Louis, MO: Mosby; 1996:78–95.

2. Snijders RJ, Sebire NJ, Nicolaides KH. Maternal age and gestational age-specific risk for chromosomal defects. *Fetal Diagn Ther*. 1995;10:356–367.

3. Romero R, Pilu G, Jeanty P, et al. *Prenatal Diagnosis of Congenital Anomalies*. Norwalk, VA: Appleton & Lange; 1988.

4. Chervenak FA, Isaacson GC, Campbell S. Anomalies of the cranium and its contents. In: Chervenak FA, Isaacson GC, Campbell S eds. *Ultrasound in Obstetrics and Gynecology*. Boston, MA: Little, Brown and Company: 1993:825–852.

5. Wickstrom E, Maizels M, Sabbagha RE, et al. Isolated fetal pyelectasis: assessment of risk for postnatal uropathy and Down syndrome. *Ultrasound Obstet Gynecol*. 1996;8:236–240.

6. Phillips OP, Shulman LP. Abnormal maternal serum screening results and ultrasonography: elevated MSAFP (part I). *The Female Patient.* 1999;24(2):15–26.

7. Phillips OP, Shulman LP. Abnormal maternal serum screening results and ultrasonography: screen-positive for chromosome abnormalities: (part II). *The Female Patient.* 1999;24:15–23.

8. Kuhn P, Brizot ML, Pandya PP, et al. Crown-rump length in chromosomally abnormal fetuses at 10 to 13 weeks' gestation. *Am J Obstet Gynecol.* 1995;172:32–34.

9. Jauniaux EP, Brown RM, Snijders RJ, et al. Early prenatal diagnosis of triploidy. *Am J Obstet Gynecol.* 1997;176:550–554.

10. Ranzini AC, Guzman ER, Ananth CV, et al. Sonographic identification of fetuses with Down syndrome in the third trimester: a matched control study. *Obstet Gynecol.* 1999;93:702–706.

11. Bahado-Singh RO, Oz AU, Gomez K, et al. Combined ultrasound biometry, serum markers and age for Down syndrome risk estimation. *Ultrasound Obstet Gynecol.* 2000;15:199–204.

12. Benacerraf BR. The second trimester fetus with Down syndrome: detection using sonographic features. *Ultrasound Obstet Gynecol.* 1996;7:147.

13. Lin CC, Evans MI. Intrinsic causes of fetal growth retardation: the genetic component. In: Lin CC, Evans MI, eds. *Intrauterine Growth Retardation: Pathophysiology and Clinical Management.* New York, NY: McGraw Hill; 1984:68–80.

14. Johnson MP, Barr Jr M, Qureshi F, et al. Symmetrical intrauterine growth retardation is not symmetrical: organ-specific gravimetric deficits in midtrimester and neonatal trisomy 18. *Fetal Diagn Ther.* 1989;4:110–119.

15. Snijders RJ, Sherrod C, Gosden CM, et al. Fetal growth retardation: associated malformations and chromosomal abnormalities. *Am J Obstet Gynecol.* 1993;168:547–555.

16. Benacerraf BR, Nadel A, Bromley B. Identification of second trimester fetuses with autosomal trisomy by use of a sonographic scoring index. *Radiology.* 1994;193:135–140.

17. Cardoza JD, Goldstein RB, Filly RA. Exclusion of ventriculomegaly with a single measurement: the width of the lateral ventricular atrium. *Radiology.* 1988;169:711–714.

18. Weisman A, Achiron R, Lipitz S, et al. The first trimester growth-discordant twin: an ominous prenatal finding. *Obstet Gynecol.* 1994;84:110–114.

19. Khoury MJ, Erickson JD, Cordero JF, et al. Congenital malformations and intrauterine growth retardation: a population study. *Pediatrics.* 1988;82:83–90.

20. Reid DE. Fetal Growth and Physiology. Reid DE, ed. In: *A Textbook of Obstetrics.* Philadelphia, PA: WB Saunders Company; 1962:88–129.

21. Buster JE, Sauer MV. Endocrinology of conception. In: Brody SA, Ueland K, eds. *Endocrine Disorders in Pregnancy.* Norwalk, VA: Appleton & Lange; 1989:39–63.

22. Deter RL. Evaluation of quantitative obstetrical ultrasound studies. In: Deter RL, Harrist RB, Birnholz JC, Hadlock FP, eds. *Quantitative Obstetrical Ultrasonography.* New York, NY: John Wiley & Sons; 1986:15–30.

23. Hadlock TP, Deter RL, Harrist RB, et al. Fetal biparietal diameter: a critical reevaluation of the relation to menstrual age by means of real time ultrasound. *J Ultrasound Med.* 1982;1:97–104.

24. Hadlock FP, Deter RL, Harriest RB, et al. Fetal head circumference: relation to menstrual age. *AJR Am J Roentgenol.* 1982;138:649–653.

25. Hadlock FP, Deter RL, Harriest RB, et al. Fetal abdominal circumference as a predictor of menstrual age. *AJR Am J Roentgenol.* 1982;139:367–370.

26. Hadlock FP, Harriest RB, Deter RL, et al. Femur length as a predictor of menstrual age: sonographically measured. *AJR Am J Roentgenol.* 1982;138:875–878.

27. Altman DG, Chitty LS. New charts for ultrasound dating of pregnancy. *Ultrasound Obstet Gynecol.* 1997;10:174–191.

28. Chervenak FK, Skupski DW, Romero R, et al. How accurate is fetal biometry in the assessment of fetal age? *Am J Obstet Gynecol.* 1998;178:678–687.

29. Mul T, Mongelli M, Gardosi J. A comparative analysis of second trimester ultrasound dating formulae in pregnancies conceived with artificial reproductive techniques. *Ultrasound Obstet Gynecol.* 1996;8:397–402.

30. Wennerholm UB, Bergh C, Hagberg H, et al. Gestational age in pregnancies after in vitro fertilization: comparison between ultrasound measurements and actual age. *Ultrasound Obstet Gynecol.* 1998;12:170–174.

31. Tunon K, Eik-Nes SH, Grottum P, et al. Gestational age in pregnancies conceived after in vitro fertilization: a comparison between age assessed from oocyte retrieval, crown-rump length and biparietal diameter. *Ultrasound Obstet Gynecol.* 2000;15:41–46.

32. Warda A, Deter RL, Rossavik IK, et al. Fetal femur length: a critical re-evaluation of the relationship to menstrual age. *Obstet Gynecol.* 1985;66:69–75.

33. Hadlock FP, Deter RL, Harrist RB, et al. Estimating fetal age: computer assisted analysis of multiple fetal growth parameters. *Radiology.* 1984;152:497–502.

34. Ritchie WG. Ultrasound in the evaluation of normal and induced ovulation. In: Wallach EE, Kempers RD, eds. *Modern Trends in Infertility and Conception Control.* Vol 4. Chicago: Year Book Medical Publishers, Inc; 1988:167–181.

35. Grisolia G, Milano V, Pilu G, et al. Biometry of early pregnancy with transvaginal sonography. *Ultrasound Obstet Gynecol.* 1993;3:403–411.

36. Robinson HP. Sonar measurement of fetal crown-rump length as means of assessing maturity in first trimester of pregnancy. *BMJ.* 1973;4:28–31.

37. O'Rahilly R, Muller F. *Developmental Stages in Human Embryos.* Washington, D.C.: Carnegie Institution of Washington; 1987.

38. Goldstein SR. Embryonic ultrasonographic measurements: crown-rump length revisited. *Am J Obstet Gynecol.* 1991;165:497–501.

39. Wisser J, Dirschedl P, Krone S. Estimation of gestational age by transvaginal sonographic measurement of greatest embryonic length in dated human embryos. *Ultrasound Obstet Gynecol.* 1994;4:457–462.

40. Deter RL, Buster JE, Casson PR, et al. Individual growth patterns in the first trimester: evidence for difference in embryonic and fetal growth rates. *Ultrasound Obstet Gynecol.* 1999;13:90–98.

41. Fujiwaki R, Hata TP, Hata KP, et al. Intrauterine ultrasonographic assessments of embryonic development. *Am J Obstet Gynecol.* 1995;173:1770–1774.

42. Hadlock FP, Shah YP, Kanon OJ, et al. Fetal crown-rump length: reevaluation of relation to menstrual age (5–18 weeks) with high-resolution real-time ultrasound. *Radiology.* 1992;182:501–505.

43. Mahony BS, Filly RA. High-resolution sonographic assessment of the fetal extremities. *J Ultrasound Med.* 1984;3:489–498.

44. Deter RL, Rossavik IK, Hill RM, et al. Longitudinal studies of femur growth in normal fetuses. *J Clin Ultrasound.* 1987;15:299–305.

45. Deter RL, Harrist RB. Assessment of normal fetal growth. Chervenal FA, Isaacson G, Campbell S, eds. In: *Ultrasonography in Obstetrics and Gynecology.* Boston, MA: Little, Brown and Co; 1993:361–386.

46. Pedersen JF, Molsted-Pedersen L. Early fetal growth delay detected by ultrasound marks increased risk of congenital malformation in diabetic pregnancy. *BMJ.* 1981;283:269–271.

47. Steel JM, Wu PS, Johnstone FD, et al. Does early growth delay occur in diabetic pregnancy? *Br J Obstet Gynaecol.* 1995;102:224–227.

48. Johnson SP, Sebire NJ, Snijders RJ, et al. Ultrasound screening for anencephaly at 10–14 weeks of gestation. *Ultrasound Obstet Gynecol.* 1997;9:14–16.

49. Campbell WA, Vintzileos AM, Rodis JF, et al. Use of the transverse cerebellar diameter/abdominal circumference ratio in pregnancies at risk for intrauterine growth retardation. *J Clin Ultrasound.* 1994;22:497–502.

50. Hill LM, Guzick D, Fries J, et al. The transverse cerebellar diameter in estimating gestational age in the large for gestational age fetus. *Obstet Gynecol.* 1990;75:981–985.

51. Hill LM, Guzick D, Rivello D, et al. The transverse cerebellar diameter cannot be used to assess gestational age in the small for gestational age fetus. *Obstet Gynecol.* 1990;75:329–333.

52. Lee W, Barton S, Comstock CH, et al. Transverse cerebellar diameter: a useful predictor of gestational age for fetuses with asymmetric growth retardation. *Am J Obstet Gynecol.* 1991;165:1044–1050.

53. Capponi A, Rizzo G, Pietropolli A, et al. Transverse cerebellar diameter in small-for-gestational-age fetuses: pregnancy dating is possible only when growth retardation is secondary to urteroplacental insufficiency. *Ultrasound Obstet Gynecol.* 1994;4:104–108.

54. Goldstein I, Reece EA. Cerebellar growth in normal and growth-restricted fetuses of multiple gestations. *Am J Obstet Gynecology.* 1995;173:1343–1348.

55. Goldstein I, Reece EA, Pilu G, et al. Cerebellar measurements with ultrasonography in the evaluation of fetal growth and development. *Am J Obstet Gynecol.* 1987;156:1065–1068.

56. Reece EA, Goldstein I, Pilu G, et al. Fetal cerebellar growth unaffected by intrauterine growth retardation: a new parameter for prenatal diagnosis. *Am J Obstet Gynecol.* 1987;157:632–637.

57. Vinkesteijn AS, Mulder PG, Wladimiroff JW. Fetal transverse cerebellar diameter measurements in normal and reduced fetal growth. *Ultrasound Obstet Gynecol.* 2000;15:47–51.

58. Chang CH, Chang FM, Yu CH, et al. Three-dimensional ultrasound in the assessment of fetal cerebellar transverse and antero-posterior diameters. *Ultrasound Med Biol.* 2000;26:175–182.

59. Geirsson RT. Ultrasound instead of last menstrual period as the basis of gestational age assignment. *Ultrasound Obstet Gynecol.* 1991;1:212–219.

60. Gardosi J. The menstrual history: old limitations, new prospects. *Ultrasound Obstet Gynecol.* 1999;13:84–85.

61. Geirsson RT, Busby-Earle RM. Certain dates may not provide a reliable estimate of gestational age. *Brit J Obstet Gynaecol.* 1991;98:108–109.

62. Mongelli M, Wilcox M, Gardosi J. Estimating the date of confinement: ultrasonographic biometry versus certain menstrual dates. *Am J Obstet Gyencol.* 1996;174:278–281.

63. Deter RL, Hill RM, Tennyson LM. Predicting the birth characteristics of normal fetuses 14 weeks before delivery. *J Clin Ultrasound.* 1989;17:89–93.

64. Kurniawan YS, Deter RL, Visser GH, et al. Prediction of the neonatal crown-heel length from femur diaphysis length measurements. *J Clin Ultrasound.* 1994;22:245–252.

65. Kurniawan YS, Deter RL, Visser GH. Predicting head circumference at birth: a study in a Dutch population using the Rossavik growth model. *Ultrasound Obstet Gynecol.* 1995;5:123–128.

66. Altman DG, Hytten FE. Assessment of fetal size and fetal growth. In: Chalmers I, Enkin M, Keirse MJ, eds. *Effective Care in Pregnancy and Childbirth.* Vol 411. Oxford, England: Oxford University Press; 1987.

67. Deter RL, Harrist RB, Hadlock FP, et al. The use of ultrasound in the assessment of normal fetal growth: a review. *J Clin Ultrasound.* 1981;9:481–493.

68. Deter RL, Harrist RB. Growth standards for anatomic measurements and growth rates derived from longitudinal studies of normal fetal growth. *J Clin Ultrasound.* 1992;20:381–388.

69. Simon NV, Deter RL, Kofinas AD, et al. Effect of measurement variability on Rossavik growth model specification and prediction of growth outcome at birth. *J Clin Ultrasound.* 1992;20:239–246.

70. Deter RL, Hadlock FP, Harrist RB, et al. Fetal head and abdominal circumference: Evaluation of measurement errors (part I). *J Clin Ultrasound.* 1982;10:357–363.

71. Hata T, Deter RL. A review of fetal organ measurements obtained with ultrasound: normal growth. *J Clin Ultrasound.* 1992;20:155–174.

72. Deter RL, Harrist RB, Hadlock FP, et al. Longitudinal studies of fetal growth using volume parameters determined with ultrasound. *J Clin Ultrasound.* 1984;12:313–324.

73. Riccabona M, Nelson TR, Pretorius DH. Three-dimensional ultrasound: accuracy of distance and volume measurements. *Ultrasound Obstet Gynecol.* 1996;7:429–434.

74. Lasser DM, Peisner DB, Vollebergh J, et al. First trimester fetal biometry using transvaginal sonography. *Ultrasound Obstet Gynecol.* 1993;3:104–108.

75. Deter RL, Hadlock FP, Harrist RB. Evaluation of normal fetal growth and the detection of intrauterine growth retardation. In: Callen W, ed. *Ultrasonography in Obstetrics and Gynecology.* 1983:113–140.

76. Fong K, Ohlsson A, Zalev A. Fetal thoracic circumference: a prospective cross-sectional study with real-time ultrasound. *Am J Obstet Gyencol.* 1988;158:1154–1160.

77. Polin RA, Fox WW. *Fetal and Neonatal Physiology.* Philadelphia, PA: WB Saunders Company; 1992.

78. Hadlock FP, Deter RL, Roecker E, et al. Relation of fetal femur length to neonatal crown-heel length. *J Ultrasound Med.* 1984;3:1–3.

79. Ventzileos AM, Campbell WA, Neckles S, et al. The ultrasound femur length as a predictor of fetal length. *Obstet Gynecol.* 1984;64:779–782.

80. Lim JM, Hong AG, Raman S, et al. Relationship between fetal femur diaphysis length and neonatal crown-heel length: the effect of race. *Ultrasound Obstet Gynecol.* 2000;15:131–137.

81. Goncalves L, Jeanty P. Fetal biometry of skeletal dysplasias: a multicentric study. *J Ultrasound Med.* 1994;13:977–986.

82. Deter RL, Nazar R, Milner LL. Modified neonatal growth assessment score: a multivariate approach to the detection of intrauterine growth retardation in the neonate. *Ultasound Obstet Gynecol.* 1995;6:400–410.

83. Deter RL, Rossavik IK, Cortissoz C, et al. Longitudinal studies of thigh circumference growth in normal fetuses. *J Clin Ultrasound.* 1987;15:388–393.

84. Xu B, Deter RL, Milner LL, et al. Evaluation of twin growth status at birth using individualized growth assessment: comparison with conventional methods. *J Clin Ultrasound.* 1995;22:277–286.

85. Abramowicz JS, Sherer DM, Bar-Tov EP, et al. The cheek-to-cheek diameter in the ultrasonographic assessment of fetal growth. *Am J Obstet Gynecol.* 1991;165:846–852.

86. Abramowicz JS, Sherer DM, Woods JR. Ultrasonographic measurement of cheek-to-cheek diameter in fetal growth disturbances. *Am J Obstet Gynecol.* 1993;169:405–408.

87. Sood AK, Yancey M, Richards D. Prediction of fetal macrosomia using humeral soft tissue thickness. *Obstet Gynecol.* 1995;85:937–940.

88. Gardeil F, Greene R, Stuart B, et al. Subcutaneous fat in the fetal abdomen as a predictor of growth restriction. *Obstet Gyencol.* 1999;94:209–212.

89. Fiorotto ML, Cochran WJ, Klish WJ. Fat-free mass and total body water of infants estimated from total body electrical conductivity measurements. *Pediatr Res.* 1987;22:417–421.

90. Milner LL, Deter RL, Hill RB, et al. Prediction of crown-heel length in normal singletons, twins and triplets using individualized growth assessment. *J Clin Ultrasound.* 1994;22:253–256.

91. Deter RL, Stefos T, Harrist RB, et al. Detection of intrauterine growth retardation in twins using individual growth assessment: evaluation of third trimester growth and prediction of growth outcome at birth (part II). *J Clin Ultrasound.* 1992;20:579–586.

92. Deter RL, Xu B, Milner LL. Prenatal prediction of neonatal growth status in twins using individualized growth assessment. *J Clin Ultrasound.* 1996;24:53–60.

93. Pandya PP, Brizot ML, Kuhn P, et al. First trimester fetal nuchal translucency thickness and risk for trisomies. *Obstet Gynecol.* 1994;84:420–423.

94. deVore GR. Fetal Echocardiography. Chernvenak FA, Isaccson GC, Campbell S, eds. In: *Ultrasound in Obstetrics and Gynecology.* Boston, MA: Little, Brown and Company, 1993:199–219.

95. Ramus RM, Martin LB, Twickler MD. Ultrasonographic prediction of fetal outcome in suspected skeletal dysplasias with use of the femur length-to-abdominal circumference ratio. *Am J Obstet Gynecol.* 1998;179:1348–1352.

96. Campbell J, Henderson A, Campbell S. The fetal femur/foot length ratio: a new parameter to assess dysplastic limb reduction. *Obstet Gyencol.* 1988;72:181–184.

97. Goldstein I, Tamir A, Zimmer EZ, et al. Growth of the fetal orbit and lens in normal pregnancies. *Ultrasound Obstet Gynecol.* 1998;12:175–179.

98. Goldstein I, Jakobi P, Tamir A, et al. Nomogram of the fetal alveolar ridge: a possible screening tool for the detection of primary cleft palate. *Ultrasound Obstet Gynecol.* 1999;14:333–337.

99. Paladini D, Morra T, Teodoro A, et al. Objective diagnosis of micrognathia in the fetus: the jaw index. *Obstet Gynecol.* 1999;93:382–386.

100. Zalel Y, Lipitz S, Soriano D, et al. The development of the fetal sternum: a cross-sectional sonographic study. *Ultrasound Obstet Gynecol.* 1999;13:187–190.

101. Chitty LS, Altman DG, Henderson A, et al. Charts of fetal size: head measurement (part II). *Br J Obstet Gynaecol.* 1994;101:35–43.

102. Chitty LS, Altman DG, Henderson A, et al. Charts of fetal size: abdominal measurements (part III). *Br J Obstet Gynaecol.* 1994;101:125–131.

103. Chitty LS, Altman DG, Henderson A, et al. Charts of fetal size: femur length (part IV). *Br J Obstet Gynaecol.* 1994;101:132–135.

104. Deter RL. Evaluation of normal growth. In: Deter RL, Harriest JC, Birnholz RB, Hadlock FP, eds. *Quantitative Obstetrical Ultrasonography.* New York, NY: John Wiley and Sons; 1986:65–112.

105. Altman DG, Chitty LS. Charts of fetal size: methodology (part I). *Br J Obstet Gynaecol.* 1994;101:29–34.

106. Ariyuki Y, Hata RP, Kitao MP. Evaluation of perinatal outcome using individualized growth assessment: comparison with conventional methods. *Pediatrics.* 1995;96:36–42.

107. Santonja-Lucas JJ, Armero CP, Martinez-Gonzalez LM. Long-term prediction of birth weight. *J Ultrasound Med.* 1993;12:431–436.

108. Wilcox MA, Johnson IR, Maynard PV, et al. The individualized birth weight ratio: a more logical outcome measure of pregnancy than birth weight alone. *Br J Obstet Gynaecol.* 1993;100:342–347.

109. Gardosi J, Mongelli M, Wilcox M, et al. An adjustable fetal weight standard. *Ultrasound Obstet Gynecol.* 1995;6:168–174.

110. Hadlock FP, Harrist RB, Martinez-Poyer J. In utero analysis of fetal growth: a sonographic weight standard. *Radiology.* 1991;181:129–133.

111. Royston P. Calculation of unconditional and conditional reference intervals for fetal size and growth from longitudinal measurements. *Stat Med.* 1995;14:1417–1436.

112. Deter RL, Harrist RB, Hadlock FP, et al. Longitudinal studies of fetal growth with the use of dynamic image ultrasonography. *Am J Obstet Gynecol.* 1982;143:545–554.

113. Hata T, Deter RL, Hill RM, et al. Individual growth curve standards in triplets: prediction of third trimester growth and birth characteristics. *Obstet Gynecol.* 1991;78:379–384.

114. Mongelli M, Sverker EK, Tambyrajia R. Screening for fetal growth restriction: a mathematical model of the effect of time interval and ultrasound error. *Obstet Gynecol.* 1998;92:908–912.

115. Bernstein IM, Blake K, Wall B, et al. Evidence that normal fetal growth can be non-continuous. *J Matern Fetal Med.* 1995;4:197–201.

116. Owen P, Donnet ML, Ogston SA, et al. Standards for ultrasound fetal growth velocity. *Brit J Obstet Gynaecol.* 1996;103:60–69.

117. Elston RC, Grizzle JE. Estimation of time-response curves and their confidence bands. *Biometrics.* 1962;18:148–159.

118. Rossavik IK, Deter RL. Mathematical modeling of fetal growth: basic principles (part I). *J Clin Ultrasound.* 1984;12:529–533.

119. Deter RL, Rossavik IK, Harrist RB, et al. Mathematical modeling of fetal growth: development of individual growth curve standards. *Obstet Gynecol.* 1986;68:156–161.

120. Deter RL, Rossavik IK. A simplified method for determining individual growth curve standards. *Obstet Gynecol.* 1987;70:801–805.

121. Stefos T, Deter RL, Simon NV. Effect of timing of initial scan and interval between scans on Rossavik growth model specification. *J Clin Ultrasound.* 1989;17:319–326.

122. Simon NV, Deter RL, Grow DR, et al. Detection of macrosomia using the individual growth curve assessment method. *Obstet Gynecol.* 1991;77:793–797.

123. Simon NV, Deter RL, Kofinas AD, et al. Small-for-menstrual-age infants: different subgroups detected with individualized fetal growth assessment. *J Clin Ultrasound.* 1994;22:3–10.

124. Usher R, McLean F. Intrauterine growth of live born Caucasian infants at sea level: standards obtained from measurements in 7 dimensions of infants born between 25 and 44 weeks of gestation. *J Pediatr.* 1969;74:901–910.

125. Deter RL, Spence LR. Identification of marcosomic, normal and intrauterine growth retarded neonates using the modified neonatal growth assessment score. *Fetal Diagn Ther.* 2004;19:58–67.

126. Deter RL. Individualized growth assessment: evaluation of growth using each fetus as its own control. *Semin Perinatol.* 2004;28:23–32.

127. Pang MW, Leung TN, Sahota DS, et al. Customizing fetal biometric charts. *Ultrasound Obstet Gynecol.* 2003;22:271–276.

ULTRASOUND EVALUATION OF THE PLACENTA

Byron Calhoun

The placenta is a remarkable organ that serves as the interface between a mother and her fetus. It accomplishes a wide range of endocrine, exocrine, and respiratory functions including transportation of nutrients and oxygen to the fetus and transportation of metabolic waste and carbon dioxide from the fetus. Such diverse characteristics have made the placenta the focus of much study. As ultrasound technology has advanced, a large volume of information has been gathered on physiologic and pathologic conditions of the placenta and future investigations are certain to reveal information that will enhance provider's ability to provide care to pregnant women.

EMBRYOLOGY OF THE PLACENTA

The maternal contribution to the placenta is called the decidua (L. deciduus, meaning a falling off) and is derived from the endometrium. The fetal component develops from the chorionic sac. The 3 distinct layers of the decidua are the decidua basalis, decidua capsularis, and decidua parietalis (vera). The decidua basalis forms the deepest layer and is adjacent to the uterine myometrium. The decidua capsularis is the superficial layer immediately adjacent to the chorion of the conceptus. The decidua parietalis makes up the middle layer of the deciduas and is the most prominent portion of the decidua.

Blastocyst implantation occurs 5–6 days after fertilization. The outer cell layer is formed by the trophoblast cell mass that differentiates into cytotrophoblast and syncitiotrophoblast. By day 7–12 syncitiotrophoblast erode into the endometrial glands and blood vessels. Lacunae are formed that eventually become the intervillous space.

Beginning around the eighth embryonic week, chorionic villi associated with the decidua capsularis are compressed and degenerate to form the chorion levae. The villi associated with the decidua basalis undergo hypertrophy, hyperplasia, and develop a complex branching pattern. The proliferative portion of the chorionic sac is known as the chorion frondosum. The placenta increases in thickness as the stem villi continue to branch. The villi from the chorion frondosum project into the intervillous space and specialized stem villi anchor the chorion frondosum to the decidua basalis through the cytotrophoblastic shell. At maturity, the placenta accounts for 15–30% of the decidual thickness. Maternal arteries and veins pass into the intervillous space through gaps in the cytotrophoblastic shell. Branch villi that arise from the stem villi provide a large surface area for transfer of material between fetal and maternal circulations across the placental membrane.[1]

During sonographic evaluation, the placenta may appear as a thickening in the hyperechoic rim around the gestational sac around 10 weeks gestation. Intervillous blood flow is not typically demonstrated until 12–13 weeks gestation using Doppler sonography. A 1–2 centimeter hypoechoic area just deep to the placenta referred to as the "retroplacental complex" is typically seen sonographically by 14–15 weeks gestation. Decidua, myometrium, and uterine vessels form this complex. By the third trimester, the placenta is highly vascular and a plethora of intraplacental and retroplacental vessels can be identified.

PLACENTA LOCATION AND ATTACHMENT

Sonographic evaluation of the placenta begins with defining the location of the placenta and the extent of its margins. The placental attachment site has significant clinical implications, particularly if the placental site is adjacent to the cervical os. Transabdominal ultrasonography is often adequate in evaluating placental location; however, placentas located in the lower uterine segment may falsely appear to cover the cervical os when the patient's bladder is over distended or a focal contraction occurs in the lower uterine segment. To avoid some of the pitfalls of transabdominal imaging, many sonographers recommend transvaginal ultrasonography for all patients with placentas that appear to be low-lying or covering the cervical os.

Smith et al. used transvaginal sonography to evaluate placental location on 168 patients who were noted to have placenta covering or within 2 centimeters of cervical os on transabdominal ultrasound at 15 weeks or greater. One hundred thirty-one cases were analyzed. In 65 cases, transvaginal and transabdominal sonography both demonstrated good visualization of the cervical os and placental edge. Visualization by transabdominal sonography was suboptimal in 66 cases, and transvaginal ultrasound changed the diagnosis in 26% of the cases.[2]

Some sonographers have also espoused translabial sonography in evaluation of the low-lying placenta. Dawson et al. demonstrated the utility of this technique in 40 patients with suspected placenta previa. Translabial imaging was superior to transabdominal imaging in correctly diagnosing and excluding placenta previa.[3]

Diagnosis of placenta previa during the second trimester is certainly important clinically; however, the patient is not certainly destined to have placenta previa at the time of delivery. Due to the discordant growth of myometrial cells in the upper and lower uterus, the placenta appears to "migrate" away from the cervical os as pregnancy progresses. Page et al. retrospectively evaluated the outcomes of 732 patients cared for at the British Military Hospital, Munster. Seventy-nine of the patients were diagnosed with "low-lying" placenta by sonography at 15–20 weeks gestation. None of these patients developed placenta previa and pregnancy outcomes were similar to patients without low-lying placenta in the second trimester.[4]

Zelop et al. evaluated the outcomes of 925 patients who were diagnosed with placenta previa during second trimester sonography. Forty-three (4.6%) of the 925 patients had placenta previa at the time of delivery. Over half (22/43) had no vaginal bleeding prior to delivery. Review of the second trimester studies demonstrated a good correlation between degree of placental symmetry with respect to the internal cervical os. Placentas that asymmetrically covered the internal cervical os were less likely to persist as a previa. Symmetry of the placenta over the cervical os at the time of the second trimester ultrasound study had a sensitivity of 49% and a specificity of 93% for predicting a placenta previa at birth.[5]

In addition to clearly defining location and extent of the placenta, one should evaluate the placental attachment site. A retroplacental complex and fairly distinct placental margins are typically noted sonographically. Abnormalities of this region should cause concern for potential placenta accreta. Patients at particularly high risk for placenta accreta are those with a prior history of uterine surgery and a placenta previa. Color Doppler imaging is a useful adjunct to transabdominal and transvaginal sonography in the evaluation of possible placenta accreta.[6,7]

Chou et al. evaluated the efficacy of transabdominal color Doppler sonography in diagnosing placenta accreta associated with placenta previa. Diffuse intraparenchymal placental lacunar flow, focal intraparenchymal placental lacunar flow, bladder-uterine serosa interphase hypervascularity, prominent subplacental venous complex, and loss of subplacental Doppler vascular signals were used as criteria. Sixteen of 80 patients evaluated had sonographic findings consistent with placenta accreta using these criteria, and 14 of the 16 had pathologic confirmation of placenta accreta. Two false-positives were related to bladder varicosities that were mistaken for interphase hypervascularity. The sensitivity of color Doppler in diagnosing placenta accreta in the setting of placenta previa was 82.45 (14/17). The specificity was 96.8% (61/63), positive predictive value 87.5% (14/16), and negative predictive value 95.3% (61/64).[7]

Finberg et al. prospectively evaluated 34 patients with placenta previa and prior Cesarean delivery using the following criteria: (1) Loss of normal hypoechoic retroplacental myometrial zone, (2) Thinning or disruption of the hyperechoic uterine serosa-bladder interface, and (3) Presence of a focal exophytic mass. Using these criteria 14 of 18 patients with positive sonographic findings had an accreta and 1 of 16 patients with negative sonographic findings had an accreta. In addition to the criteria used in the study, the presence of numerous intraplacental vascular lacunae appeared to be correlated with placenta accreta.[8]

Levine et al. also demonstrated the usefulness of transvaginal ultrasound with power Doppler sonography in evaluation of patients with possible placenta accreta at increased risk due to previous uterine surgery. Magnetic resonance imaging was superior to ultrasound in evaluation of possible posterior placenta accreta.[9]

Most cases of placenta previa that are diagnosed antenatally are in patients with placenta previa and prior uterine surgery. There is at least 1 case in the literature, however, of antenatal diagnosis of placenta accreta in a low-risk primiparous patient by gray scale imaging.[10]

PLACENTA SIZE AND SHAPE

The placenta is normally discoid to ovoid in shape although its symmetry can demonstrate marked variation. Average placental thickness is roughly equal to the number of weeks gestation converted to millimeters $+/-10$ mm. At term, the placenta is generally less than 40 mm. Placenta thickness >40 mm is often associated with maternal diabetes, hydrops, and perinatal infection.

Elchalal et al. followed 561 normal pregnancies to determine the correlation between placental thickness and perinatal morbidity and mortality. Patients with placental thickness over the 90th percentile were designated as the study group and those with placental thickness between 10–90% were used as controls. Perinatal mortality was significantly higher in the group with placental thickening (6.82% vs. 0.66%, $p = 0.037$). There were also a significantly higher number of neonates with birth weight >4,000 grams (20.45% vs. 5.3%, $p = 0.001$). Interestingly, there were also more neonates with birth weight <2,500 grams in the thickened placenta group (15.9% vs. 7.3%, $p = 0.03$). Fetal anomalies were identified in 9.1% of the study group and 3.97% of the controls; however, this difference did not reach statistical significance.[11] The study does demonstrate an association between placental thickness and perinatal risk.

Jauniaux et al. completed a prospective cross-sectional study of 210 normal pregnancies to evaluate the incidence of placental abnormalities by ultrasonography and to determine the usefulness of measuring placental size. The group completed measurements of placental thickness, circumference, and volume in addition to morphologic evaluation. They identified an association between abnormal placental development, placenta morphology, and abnormal fetal growth and pregnancy-related hypertension. They concluded that ultrasound evaluation of placental thickness, placental morphology, uterine Doppler analysis, and maternal serum alpha-fetoprotein may provide efficient screening for subsequent abnormal fetal growth or pregnancy related hypertension.[12]

With modern ultrasound resolution many abnormalities of placental architecture such as accessory lobes, circumvallate and velamentous cord insertion can be diagnosed antenatally. Color and pulse wave Doppler can be particularly useful in evaluation of the cord-placenta junction and in identification of vascular connections between succenturiate lobes or bilobate placentas. These diagnoses are important clinically when the vessels are near the cervical os creating a vasa previa. Additionally, abnormal cord insertion may be associated with intrauterine growth restriction.

The complete circumference of the placenta should be evaluated. Careful inspection can reveal a circumvallate placenta.

This is a condition of extrachorial placentation characterized by a thickened, "rolled" appearing periphery due to the amnion folding in on itself and maintaining only a loose association with peripheral chorion. The placental rim in this condition is often associated with infarction or hemorrhage. Antepartum diagnosis is useful clinically because complete circumvallation has been associated with major fetal malformations, intrauterine growth restriction, abruptio placenta, pre-eclampsia, and perinatal death.[13]

PLACENTAL LESIONS

Placental abruption is the most common cause of significant vaginal bleeding in the third trimester of pregnancy and it is still one of the leading causes of perinatal mortality. The incidence of placental abruption is around 1 in 200 pregnancies[14,15] and the incidence of placental abruption significant enough to result in fetal demise is around 1 in 1,550.[16] Preeclampsia is associated with a 3-fold increase incidence in abruption, and the incidence rises 4-fold in patients with chronic hypertension.[17] Smoking cigarettes, cocaine use, and advanced maternal age are also associated with increased risk. The diagnosis of placental abruption is typically made clinically by vaginal bleeding, acute abdominal pain, and uterine tenderness. Uterine contractions and nonreassuring fetal heart tones are also common.

Attempts to verify clinical suspicion and diagnose placental abruption sonographically have proven less than favorable. The sonographic appearance of a placental abruption depends on the age of the hemorrhage to a great extent. In the early phase of an abruption (up to 48 hours) the lesion is frequently hyperechoic. Over the next 3–7 days its appearance becomes more isoechoic and by 1–2 weeks it becomes progressively hypoechoic.[18]

Subchorionic lucencies are frequently noted by sonography of the placenta. Katz et al. evaluated the outcomes of 40 patients who had subchorionic placental lucencies identified at a perinatal diagnostic referral center. They concluded that this ultrasound finding was not associated with increased risk of adverse pregnancy outcome and was not associated with an increased incidence of fetal anomalies.[19] Lesions located near the decidual surface have the highest likelihood of having clinical significance. Conditions that have such an appearance include retroplacental hematomas, maternal floor infarctions, and perivillous fibrin depositions. If the lesion affects 30–40% of the placental site there is likely an increased risk of perinatal complications including intrauterine growth restriction and preterm labor.

Placental calcifications are commonly seen during sonographic evaluation of the placenta as pregnancy progresses and represent the normal "aging" of the placenta. Historically, attempts were made to associate the calcifications with fetal lung maturity; however, no consistent relationship could be established.[20] Premature calcification of the placenta has been noted in patients who smoke.[21] Other sonographers report accelerated calcifications in patients with thrombotic disorders treated with heparin or aspirin.[22]

The most common benign tumor of the placenta is a chorangioma. The incidence of grossly apparent chorangioma is 1 in 1,194.[23] Microchorangioma may be as frequent as 1%, but the clinical importance of these microscopic lesions is likely minimal and these lesions would not be visible sonographically. Chorangioma are typically well circumscribed, predominantly hypoechoic and may vary in size from microscopic to several centimeters in diameter. Doppler imaging techniques are useful in the evaluation of suspected chorangioma since this is a vascular lesion with prominent flow differentiating it from a hematoma or fibrin collection that would have no flow.

Prapas et al. retrospectively reviewed all cases referred to Yale for suspicion of chorangioma over a $9^1/_2$-year period. They confirmed the utility of color flow mapping and pulsed Doppler examination.[24] Their findings were also consistent with prior studies indicating an increased risk of polyhydramnios, preterm labor, and intrauterine growth restriction.

Chorangioma over 4 cm in maximum diameter or multiple smaller chorangioma have been associated with adverse perinatal outcomes including intrauterine growth restriction, polyhydramnios, massive fetomaternal hemorrhage, disseminated intravascular coagulopathy, platelet sequestration, and neonatal hypoalbuminemia.[23] Frequent ultrasound evaluation every 2–3 weeks is warranted in these patients to observe for rapid growth of the tumor or adverse fetal effects.

Metastatic tumors of maternal and fetal origin have been identified in the placenta. Fortunately, they are exceedingly rare.

MULTIPLE GESTATIONS

Evaluation of the placenta(s) can be helpful in multiple gestations as one attempts to determine the chorionicity of the pregnancy. Determination of chorionicity is clinically useful to help rule in or exclude potential pathologic processes such as twin-twin transfusion syndrome or karyotype abnormalities. In monozygotic twins when zygotic division occurs prior to trophoblastic differentiation (day 4 following fertilization) each embryo will have its own amnion and chorion. If zygotic division occurs on days 4–7, the embryos will each have its own amnion, but share a single chorion. Zygotic division after day 7 results in a shared amnion and shared chorion. Identification of 2 separate placentas confirms a diamnionic, dichorionic gestation. Occasionally, there will be fusion of placentas and it is not possible to determine chorionicity by placenta evaluation alone. In this setting, further evaluation of membranes is useful. Dichorionic diamnionic gestations will have a more prominent membrane prior to 26 weeks and will form a "peak sign" at its junction with the placenta. Monochorionic diamnionic gestations will have a thin, wispy membrane and intersect perpendicularly with the placenta.

ULTRASOUND EVALUATION OF AMNIOTIC FLUID

Amniotic fluid is a complex physiologic substance that provides the essential environmental factors required for fetal growth and development. The aqueous environment provides protection from physical trauma by dampening the impact of external forces while at the same time providing an atmosphere that facilitates fetal development by allowing for relatively unrestricted fetal movement. Adequate amniotic fluid volume also protects the umbilical cord from compression by the fetus and is a fundamental requirement for normal fetal lung development. Immunologic properties of amniotic fluid help maintain a sterile environment while nutritional components and growth factors in amniotic fluid are likely an important supplement to transplacentally acquired nutrients.

Abnormalities of amniotic fluid volume may result from a number of maternal and fetal disorders ranging from maternal diabetes mellitus to preterm premature rupture of membranes to fetal renal agenesis. Additionally, an abnormal amniotic fluid volume is associated with increased neonatal morbidity and mortality.[25,26]

PHYSIOLOGY OF AMNIOTIC FLUID

Amniotic fluid volume and composition are dynamic throughout pregnancy. The balance between production and resorption determines amniotic fluid volume. Volume increases at a rate of 10 milliliters per week at 8 weeks gestation and increases to a rate of 60 milliliters per week by 21 weeks gestation. After mid-pregnancy, the rate of production relative to resorption decreases and amniotic fluid volume plateaus around 33 weeks gestation.[27] At term, a typical amniotic fluid volume is roughly 700–800 milliliters although there is wide variation in physiologic fluid volumes. Generally, less than 500 milliliters is considered low (oligohydramnios) and greater than 2,500 milliliters is considered excessive (hydramnios).

During the first few weeks of gestation, amniotic fluid is derived predominantly as a transudate of maternal plasma across the amnion and chorion. By 12–14 weeks gestation the amniotic fluid is largely fetal in origin and is derived by diffusion through fetal skin and fetal urine production. After mid-pregnancy, fetal skin is keratinized and amniotic fluid is composed predominantly of fetal urine. The fetal lungs also excrete significant volumes of fluid each day, contributing to the total volume. Fetal swallowing is the major mechanism of amniotic fluid resorption. Although transmembranous absorption does occur, this phenomenon is not as well understood.

USE OF ULTRASOUND IN AMNIOTIC FLUID ASSESSMENT

Sonography is an invaluable tool in the evaluation of amniotic fluid. Real-time ultrasonography has allowed for precise needle localization during amniocentesis and cordocentesis. Investigation of amniotic fluid composition and amniocyte evaluation has revolutionized antenatal diagnosis and offer great promise in the area of fetal therapy. Ultrasound directed sampling of amniotic fluid is routinely employed in evaluation of suspected fetal gene or karyotype abnormality, nonimmune hydrops, possible chorioamnionitis, and determination of fetal lung maturity.

Sonography has also demonstrated utility in the evaluation of suspected amniotic fluid volumes. It has long been recognized that abnormally high or abnormally low amniotic fluid volume is associated with maternal and fetal complication leading to increased perinatal morbidity and mortality. Historically, quantitative assessment of amniotic fluid volume was only possible by directly measuring the amount of amniotic fluid removed from the uterus at the time of hysterotomy or pregnancy termination. In the 1960s, techniques were standardized to quantify amniotic fluid volume using an indicator dilution technique.[28] Although the indicator dilution technique has demonstrated reliability, it requires an amniocentesis and its associated risk of infection, rupture of membranes and initiation of labor. A noninvasive substitute has been pursued.

Subjective sonographic assessment of amniotic fluid volume has demonstrated clinical utility,[29,30] however, it requires an experienced sonographer and does not provide nominal data that can be compared to subsequent evaluations to demonstrate improvement or worsening of a volume disturbance. As ultrasound equipment has improved, several semiquantitative methods of evaluating amniotic fluid volume have been investigated and put into clinical practice. Three semiquantitative methods have been described and adopted.

Manning et al. included an amniotic fluid assessment in their description of the biophysical profile in 1980. In their original work, oligohydramnios was diagnosed when no amniotic fluid pocket measuring at least 1 cm in the vertical plane could be identified.[31] Chamberlain and Manning expanded the investigation of amniotic fluid measurement in 1984 and noted an association between an abnormality in the maximum vertical pocket and adverse perinatal outcome. Patients who had a sonographically determined maximum vertical pocket of amniotic fluid less than 2 centimeters or more than 8 centimeters had a higher incidence of intrauterine growth restriction, perinatal mortality, and major congenital anomalies. Determination of maximum vertical pocket has a low negative predictive value for perinatal morbidity, however.[26]

One disadvantage to the maximum vertical pocket assessment is that only 1 area of the uterus is evaluated and it may not be a good representation of the entire intrauterine environment. To overcome this characteristic, Phelan and colleagues described the amniotic fluid index in 1987. In the initial description of this technique, the sonographer divided the abdomen into 4 quadrants around the umbilicus.[32] Moore and Cayle described a similar technique in 1990 dividing the uterus into quadrants with a midline sagittal plane and a tranverse plane halfway up the uterine fundus.[33] With both techniques the ultrasound transducer is held in the longitudinal plane and the largest vertical pocket is determined in each quadrant. The 4 measurements are then summed. Oligohydramnios is defined as an amniotic fluid index of less than 5 centimeters and hydramnios is defined as an amniotic fluid index of greater than 24 centimeters. An amniotic fluid index between 5 and 8 centimeters is considered borderline. Since amniotic fluid volume is dynamic throughout pregnancy, some authors prefer to define oligohydramnios as less than the 5th percentile for gestational age and hydramnios as an amniotic fluid index greater than the 95th percentile. Moore and Cayle have published normative data for amniotic fluid index from 16–42 weeks gestation.[33] Porter and colleagues have published normative data for amniotic fluid index in twin gestations.[34]

Magann and colleagues described a 2-diameter pocket measurement.[35] To obtain this measurement, the sonographer identifies the maximum vertical pocket and multiplies the vertical measurement by the horizontal measurement of the same pocket. Oligohydramnios is defined as a 2-diameter pocket measurement of less than 15 centimeters square, and values greater than 50 centimeters square represent hydramnios.

Magann compared ultrasound assessment of amniotic fluid volume to quantitative assessment using indicator dilution testing with sodium aminohipurate. The 2-diameter pocket correctly identified 75% of the cases of oligohydramnios and 67% of the cases of hydramnios. The 2-diameter pocket measurement was slightly better than amniotic fluid index measurement that correctly classified 65% of the cases of oligohydramnios and maximum vertical pocket measurement that identified 63%. Magann concluded that the 2-diameter pocket technique is an acceptable semiquantitative measurement of amniotic fluid volume.[35]

Subsequent work by the group has demonstrated less favorable accuracy of the semiquantitative techniques. One hundred seventy-nine patients had dye-dilution measurement of amniotic fluid volume following sonographic estimation by amniotic fluid index and maximum vertical pocket. Amniotic fluid index less than 5 centimeters had a sensitivity of 10% and specificity of 96% in correctly identifying oligohydramnios. Maximum vertical pocket of less than 2 cm has a sensitivity and specificity of 5% and 98%. Neither technique was reliable in identifying true amniotic fluid volumes and neither technique was superior for identifying truly abnormal amniotic fluid volumes.[36]

Dildy and colleagues also compared ultrasound assessment of amniotic fluid with indicator dilution techniques and concluded that sonographic assessment is adequate for diagnosing amniotic fluid volume abnormalities; however, ultrasound techniques do not accurately measure actual amniotic fluid volume. Amniotic fluid index correctly identified oligo-

hydramnios in 67% of the cases, and hydramnios in 60% of the cases.[37]

Advances in techniques to assess amniotic fluid volumes sonographically beg the question as to whether or not such measurements can predict unsatisfactory outcomes. Phelan studied 330 patients undergoing antepartum fetal testing and noted a correlation between oligohydramnios and fetal heart rate tracing abnormalities including nonreactivity and variable decelerations. Adverse fetal outcomes were also associated with an amniotic fluid index of less than 5 centimeters. He concluded that the amniotic fluid index is a useful tool to assess amniotic fluid volume and can predict an increased risk for perinatal morbidity.[37]

Magann and colleagues prospectively enrolled 1,001 high-risk patients undergoing antenatal testing and followed the patients to determine subsequent pregnancy outcome. No difference was noted in the outcomes of patients with an amniotic fluid index less than 5 centimeters or a 2-diameter pocket measurement of less than 15 centimeters square compared to controls. Outcome variables studied included nonreactive nonstress test, meconium-stained amniotic fluid, cesarean delivery for fetal distress, low Apgar scores, and cord pH less than 7.10. The group concluded that current ultrasound techniques are poor predictors of adverse perinatal outcome.[38]

Chauchan and colleagues performed a meta-analysis of studies on the risk of cesarean delivery for fetal distress, 5-minute Apgar score less than 7, and umbilical artery pH less than 7.00 in patients with an amniotic fluid index less than 5 centimeters compared to patients with an amniotic fluid index greater than 5 centimeters. The analysis included 18 studies and 10,551 patients. The results demonstrate an increased risk of cesarean delivery for fetal distress and increased risk of low Apgar score at 5 minutes in patients who have an amniotic fluid index less than 5 centimeters. They also determined that more than 23,000 patients would be necessary to demonstrate a 1.5 times increased risk of umbilical artery pH less than 7.00 in patients with a low amniotic fluid index.[39]

Three-dimensional ultrasonography is gaining support in the clinical setting and may demonstrate utility in the assessment of amniotic fluid volume in the future. Three-dimensional methods for determination of amniotic fluid have been described,[40] but further investigation is required to determine its role in the management of patients.

In summary, sonographic techniques described to date do not accurately measure amniotic fluid; however, semiquantitative sonographic assessment of amniotic is clinically useful and establishes an objective measurement that can be followed over time.

References

1. Moore KL, Persaud TV, Shiota K. *Color Atlas of Clinical Embryology.* 2nd ed. Philadelphia, PA: WB Saunders; 2000.

2. Smith RS, Lauria MR, Comstock CH, et al. Transvaginal ultrasonography for all placentas that appear to be low-lying or over the internal cervical os. *Ultrasound Obstet Gynecol*. 1997;9:22–24.

3. Dawson WB, Dumas MD, Romano WM, et al. Translabial ultrasonography and placenta previa: does measurement of the os-placenta distance predict outcome? *J Ultrasound Med*. 1996;15:441–446.

4. Page IJ, Wolstenhulme S. Does the ultrasound diagnosis of low-lying placenta in early pregnancy warrant a repeat scan? *J R Army Med Corps*. 1991;137:84–87.

5. Zelop CC, Bromley B, Frigoletto Jr FD, et al. Second trimester sonographically diagnosed placenta previa: prediction of persistent previa at birth. *Int J Gynaecol Obstet*. 1994;44:207–210.

6. Timor-Tritsch IE, Monteagudo A. Diagnosis of placenta previa by transvaginal sonography. *Ann Med*. 1993;25:279–283.

7. Chou MM, Ho ES, Lee YH. Prenatal diagnosis of placenta previa-accreta by transabdominal color Doppler ultrasound. *Ultrasound Obstet Gynecol*. 2000;15:28–35.

8. Finberg HJ, Williams JW. Placenta accreta: prospective sonographic diagnosis in patients with placenta previa and prior cesarean section. *J Ultrasound Med*. 1992;11:333–343.

9. Levine D, Hulka CA, Ludmir J, et al. Placenta accreta: evaluation with color Doppler US, power Doppler US and MR imaging. *Radiology*. 1997;205:773–776.

10. Jauniaux E, Toplis PJ, Nicolaides KH. Sonographic diagnosis of a non-previa placenta accreta. *Ultrasound Obstet Gynecol*. 1996;7: 58–60.

11. Elchalal U, Ezra Y, Levi Y, et al. Sonographically thick placenta: a marker for increased perinatal risk—a prospective cross-sectional study. *Placenta*. 2000;21:268–272.

12. Jauniaux E, Ramsay B, Campbell S. Ultrasonographic investigation of placental morphologic characteristics and size during the second trimester of pregnancy. *Am J Obstet Gynecol*. 1994;170(1 Pt 1):130–137.

13. Lewis SH, Benirschke K. Overview of placental pathology and justification for examination of the placenta. In: Lewis SH, Perrin E. (eds.) *Pathology of the Placenta*. 2nd ed. Philadelphia, PA: Churchill-Livingstone; 1999.

14. Karegard M, Gennser G. Incidence and recurrence rate of abruptio placentae in Sweden. *Obstet Gynecol*. 1986;67:523–528.

15. Ananth CV, Smulian JC, Vintzileos AM. Incidence of placental abruption in relation to cigarette smoking and hypertensive disorders during pregnancy: a meta-analysis of observational studies. *Obstet Gynecol*. 1999;93:622–628.

16. Cunningham FG, Gant NF, Leveno KJ, et al. *Williams Obstetrics*. 21st ed. New York, NY: McGraw-Hill; 2001.

17. Ananth CV, Berkowitz GS, Savitz DA, et al. Placental abruption and adverse perinatal outcomes. *JAMA*. 1999;282:1646–1651.

18. Nyberg DA, Cyr DR, Mack LA, et al. Sonographic spectrum of placental abruption. *AJR Am J Roentgenol*. 1987;148:161–164.

19. Katz VL, Blanchard GF, Watson WJ, et al. The clinical implications of subchorionic placental lucencies. *Am J Obstet Gynecol*. 1991; 164(1 Pt 1):99–100.

20. Vosmar MB, Jongsma HW, van Dongen PW. The value of ultrasonic placental grading: no correlation with intrauterine growth retardation or with maternal smoking. *J Perinat Med*. 1989;17:137–143.

21. Pinette. *Obstet Gynecol*. 1989.

22. Harris RD, Alexander RD. Ultrasound of the placenta and umbilical cord. In: Callen PW, ed. *Ultrasonography in Obstetrics and Gynecology*. 4th ed. Philadelphia, PA; WB Saunders; 2000.

23. Shanklin DR. Chorangiomas and other tumors. In: Lewis SH, Perrin E, eds. *Pathology of the Placenta*. 2nd ed. Philadelphia, PA: Churchill-Livingstone; 1999.

24. Prapas N, Liang RI, Hunter D, et al. Color Doppler imaging of placental masses: differential diagnosis and fetal outcome. *Ultrasound Obstet Gynecol*. 2000;16:559–563.

25. Chamberlain PF, Manning FA, Morrison I, et al. Ultrasound evaluation of amniotic fluid volume: the relationship of marginal and decreased amniotic fluid volumes to perinatal outcome (part I). *Am J Obstet Gynecol*. 1984;150:245–249.

26. Chamberlain PF, Manning FA, Morrison I, et al. Ultrasound evaluation of amniotic fluid volume: the relationship of increased amniotic fluid volume to perinatal outcome (part II). *Am J Obstet Gynecol*. 1984;150:250–254.

27. Brace RA, Wolf EJ. Normal amniotic fluid volume changes throughout pregnancy. *Am J Obstet Gynecol*. 1989;161:382–388.

28. Charles D, Jacoby HE, Burgess F. Amniotic fluid volumes in the second half of pregnancy. *Am J Obstet Gynecol*. 1965;93:1042–1047.

29. Goldstein RB, Filly RA. Sonographic estimation of amniotic fluid volume: subjective assessment versus pocket measurements. *J Ultrasound Med*. 1988;7:363–369.

30. Hallak M, Kirshon B, O'Brian-Smith E, et al. Subjective ultrasonographic assessment of amniotic fluid depth: comparison with the amniotic fluid index. *Fetal Diagn Ther*. 1993;8:256–260.

31. Manning FA, Platt LD, Sipos L. Antepartum fetal evaluation: development of a fetal biophysical profile. *Am J Obstet Gynecol*. 1980; 136:787–795.

32. Phelan JP, Smith CV, Broussard P, et al. Amniotic fluid volume assessment with the four-quadrant technique at 36–42 weeks' gestation. *J Reprod Med*. 1987;32:540–542.

33. Moore TR, Cayle JE. The amniotic fluid index in normal human pregnancy. *Am J Obstet Gynecol*. 1990;162:1168–1173.

34. Porter TF, Dildy GA, Blanchard JR, et al. Normal values for amniotic fluid index during uncomplicated twin pregnancy. *Obstet Gynecol*. 1996;87(5 pt 1):699–702.

35. Magann EF, Nolan TE, Hess LW, et al. Measurement of amniotic fluid volume: accuracy of ultrasonography techniques. *Am J Obstet Gynecol*. 1992;167:1533–1537.

36. Magann EF, Chauhan SP, Barrilleaux PS, et al. Amniotic fluid index and single deepest pocket: weak indicators of abnormal amniotic volumes. *Obstet Gynecol*. 2000;96(5 pt 1):737–740.

37. Dildy GA, Lira N, Moise KJ, et al. Amniotic fluid volume assessment: comparison of ultrasonographic estimates versus direct measurements with a dye-dilution technique in human pregnancy. *Am J Obstet Gynecol*. 1992;167(4 pt 1):986–994.

38. Phelan JP. Antepartum fetal assessment—newer techniques. *Semin Perinatol*. 1988;12:57–65.

39. Magann EF, Chauhan SP, Kinsella MJ, et al. Antenatal testing among 1001 patients at high risk: the role of ultrasonographic estimate of amniotic fluid volume. *Am J Obstet Gynecol*. 1999;180(6 pt 1):1330–1336.

40. Chauhan SP, Sanderson M, Hendrix NW, et al. Perinatal outcome and amniotic fluid index in the antepartum and intrapartum periods: a meta-analysis. *Am J Obstet Gynecol*. 1999;181:1473–1478.

41. Grover J, Mentakis EA, Ross MG. Three-dimensional method for determination of amniotic fluid volume in intrauterine pocket. *Obstet Gynecol*. 1997;90:1007–1010.

SECTION III

Procedures

AMNIOCENTESIS

Arie Drugan / Mark I. Evans

INTRODUCTION

The diagnosis of genetic disorders in samples of amniotic fluid and cells was introduced in the early 1960s. The first diagnoses of fetal chromosome anomalies performed on amniocytes[1,2] were shortly followed by the development of enzymatic assays for prenatal diagnosis of metabolic disorders (eg, galactosemia).[3] The diagnostic accuracy and the relatively low risk of fetal or maternal compromise associated with amniocentesis established it as the basic procedure in modern prenatal diagnosis.[4] Amniocentesis is considered frequently the "gold standard" to which other methods for prenatal diagnosis are compared.

The most common indication for amniocentesis is evaluation of fetal karyotype by cytogenetic analysis of amniotic fluid cells.[5] Amniocytes are removed from amniotic fluid by centrifugation and are placed in appropriate culture conditions to grow in monolayers. The dividing cells are arrested in metaphase, harvested, and placed in hypotonic saline, which allows better spreading of the chromosomes during slide preparation. After fixation, the chromosome spreads are stained for analysis. Modification of cell culture techniques[6,7] allow karyotype results to be available in 2 weeks or less, as opposed to 4 weeks or longer when traditional methodologies were employed. Some laboratories use fluorescence in situ hybridization (FISH) with probes for chromosomes 13, 18, 21, X, and Y, diagnosing most cases of potentially viable trisomies within 24 hours from sampling.[8] FISH is applied to uncultured amniocytes, obviating the possibility of culture failure, a complication that affects about 1 in 700 amniotic fluid samplings in midtrimester, but is apparently more common in aneuploid gestations.[9] The use of FISH to diagnose numerical chromosome anomalies is very reliable and efficient in patients that need rapid results.[10] It must be emphasized, however, that FISH is still an adjunct to standard cytogenetics since the commercially available probes will not identify some cases of mosaicism, translocations, or marker chromosomes, which are observed only with probes constructed and directed to the specific aberration. In addition, FISH analysis can be used to identify microdeletions that cannot be diagnosed with standard cytogenetics, as in the Di George, Angelman, Prader Willi, or Smith Magenis syndromes.[11]

INDICATIONS FOR PRENATAL DIAGNOSIS BY AMNIOCENTESIS

The most common indication for prenatal cytogenetic studies is advanced maternal age. The association of maternal age over 35 years with an increased risk of chromosomally abnormal conceptions is well documented.[12,13] It is considered standard of care to offer prenatal diagnosis to all women who are 35 years of age or more at delivery.[13] Almost all chromosomal abnormalities increase in incidence with advanced maternal age, but the most common is Trisomy 21, which affects approximately 50% of all aneuploid live births.

Other indications for genetic amniocentesis are summarized in Table 34-1. A previous aneuploid offspring born to a woman younger than 30 years of age confers a 1% risk of recurrence in future pregnancies, like the risk of chromosome anomalies observed in a 38 year old.[14] A balanced structural rearrangement of parental chromosomes (translocation or inversion) is encountered in 2–4% of couples investigated for repeated spontaneous abortions and is associated with an increased risk of unbalanced offspring, which may be as high as 15%.[15] Recurrent pregnancy loss in itself may be associated with an increased risk of chromosomally abnormal conceptions, even if the parents have normal karyotypes[13,16] and, in our opinion, prenatal diagnosis should be considered in these cases.

Chromosome anomalies are detected in 30–35% of amnioceteses performed for ultrasound diagnosis of major fetal malformations.[17,18] Some minor isolated ultrasound findings (ie, fetal choroid plexus cysts, nuchal edema, nonseptated cervical cystic hygroma, or pyelectasis) observed in pregnancies of women younger than 35 years may confer a risk of aneuploidy between 1–4%[19–24] and amniocentesis should be considered in these cases. In women older than 35 years, ultrasound can be used to modify genetic risks at counseling, since the diagnosis of ultrasound markers for aneuploidy in these patients significantly increase the risk of a chromosomal abnormality in pregnancy.[20,22,25] On the other hand, a normal ultrasound study may reduce the risk of aneuploidy in these patients to one fifth of the age-related risk.[22,26]

Biochemical screening of specific markers in maternal serum is increasingly employed to detect additional pregnancies in the low-risk population that need fetal karyotype evaluation. Low levels of alpha-fetoprotein (AFP) and unconjugated estriol and high levels of HCG in maternal serum are associated with increased risk of a chromosomally abnormal pregnancy. Amniocentesis should be offered when the combined risk of serum biochemical markers and maternal age equals or is higher than the risk of aneuploidy in the gestation of 35 year olds. Such would occur in about 6–8% of gestations.[27] When amniocentesis is performed according to these criteria, the prevalence of chromosome anomalies diagnosed is 2%.[28] Only half of the anomalies diagnosed are Trisomy 21. Other chromosome aberrations associated with abnormal maternal serum screening include triploidy, trisomy 13, and trisomy 18, unbalanced translocations and sex chromosome anomalies.[29] In amnioceteses performed for "maternal anxiety" in women without serum screening, the rate of chromosome anomalies was apparently similar to that observed when the procedure was indicated for low alpha-fetoprotein in maternal serum.[30] The judicious use of additional biochemical markers in maternal serum, in the first and second trimesters, may increase the accuracy of risk assessment and may target the invasive

TABLE 34-1	INDICATIONS FOR AMNIOCENTESIS AND RISK OF A POSITIVE RESULT	
Indications		*Risk of Anomaly*
A. Increased risk for chromosome anomalies		
1. Advanced maternal age		> 0.5%
2. Previous aneuploid offspring		1%
3. Parental balanced structural rearrangement		
a: reciprocal translocations		12–15%
b: Robertsonian translocations		1–3%
c: Inversions		6%
4. Maternal abnormal serum screening		2%
5. Ultrasound diagnosis of anomalies		
a: major malformations[a]		25–30%
b: minor anomalies[b]		1–3%
B. Previous offspring with NTD		3%
C. Parents carriers of Mendelian traits		25–50%

[a]Omphalocele, duodenal atresia, atrio-ventricular septal defects, horseshoe kidneys, septated cystic hygroma.
[b]Fetal pyelectasis, nuchal edema, choroid plexus cyst, nonseptated cystic hygroma.

procedures to those that need it most.[31] In combination with nuchal translucency screening, 6 biochemical markers in maternal serum will detect 85–94% of affected pregnancies without changing the designed 5% false positive rate.[32]

Elevated levels of maternal serum AFP (higher than 2.5 MOM) are observed in approximately 4% of screened pregnancies. After excluding wrong dates or multiple gestations, half of these cases will remain without a benign explanation for the abnormal result. In these, the risk for fetal anomalies is 5–10% and amniocentesis for AFP, acetyl cholinesterase (AChE), and karyotype as well as meticulous ultrasound examination of the fetus for exclusion of fetal malformation are recommended.[33] Neural tube defects (NTD), abdominal wall defects (ie, omphalocele or gastroschisis), sacrococcygeal teratoma, Meckel's Syndrome, congenital skin defects, esophageal atresia, and fetal demise have all been reported in association with elevated AFP in amniotic fluid.[33] Although the need for fetal karyotyping in pregnancies complicated by elevated AFP in maternal serum has been questioned recently,[34] it is our belief that fetal karyotype should be evaluated in these cases, even when a NTD is diagnosed on ultrasonography. Aneuploidy (mostly trisomy 18) is observed in as many as 7% of these pregnancies and will affect prognosis of the malformed fetus as well as recurrence risks and recommendations for future gestations.[35]

Prenatal diagnosis of inborn errors of metabolism can be made by analysis of precursor levels in cell-free amniotic fluid,[36] or, more commonly, by enzymatic assays of cultured amniocytes.[37] Hormonal changes in pregnancy may modify the expression of specific enzymes in amniotic fluid or amniocytes, causing an increase in the rate of false-positive or false-negative results.[38,39] Increasing utilization of molecular diagnosis for single gene disorders, through the use of restriction fragment length polymorphisms (RFLPs) and oligonucleotide gene probes combined with polymerase chain (PCR) amplification of specific DNA segments, should reduce the rate of false results to a minimum.[40,41] Since diagnosis of these disorders is expensive and laborious, it should be offered only when couples are at substantial risk (25–50%) for an affected child. Such would be the situation if the couple already had a child affected by an autosomal or X-linked recessive disorder, if 1 of the parents is affected by an autosomal or X-linked dominant disorder or when carrier testing reveals that both parents carry a recessive trait. Some traits are more common in specific ethnic groups—sickle cell anemia in blacks, α-thalassemia in Southeast Asian populations, β-thalassemia in couples of Mediterranean origin, and Tay Sachs, Cystic Fibrosis, and Gaucher in Ashkenazi Jews. Carrier testing should be offered routinely to these patients.[42]

TECHNICAL ASPECTS OF AMNIOCENTESIS

Amniocentesis should be performed by an obstetrician trained and experienced in the procedure. It should be preceded by genetic counseling,[43,44] in which the family pedigree and genetic risk are evaluated and the advantages and risks of the procedure are explained. A detailed ultrasound examination should assess gestational age, amniotic fluid volume, and fetal and placental location and should exclude gross fetal malformations.[44] Patient's blood type and antibody status should be known prior to amniocentesis and Rh-negative women with negative antibody screening should receive Rh immuno-prophylaxis after the procedure. In Rh-negative patients, the risk of Rh isosensitization is probably slightly increased by transplacental passage of the needle.[45] Though several studies documented that pregnancy outcome is not worsened by transplacental amniocentesis[46,47] and the rate of amniotic fluid leakage may actually be reduced with the transplacental approach,[47] the selected needle path should avoid, if possible, the placenta in Rh-negative patients. However, if necessary, we do not hesitate to go through the placenta to reach a pocket of amniotic fluid that is free of fetal parts.

Our technique is to use ultrasound to locate a suitable pocket of fluid that is devoid of fetus and of cord. It is important that the ultrasound transducer be held perpendicular to the ground and not at an angle, such that the ultrasound image clearly represents the true relationships and distances below the transducer. Once a suitable pocket of fluid has been selected, the transducer should be turned 90° to get a transverse view and confirm relationships and distances. Often, a minor correction side to side may be necessary. If there is a narrow pocket, an oblique approach may be preferable, providing more distance through the pocket. The operator can angle the ultrasound transducer to delineate such an approach. The use of

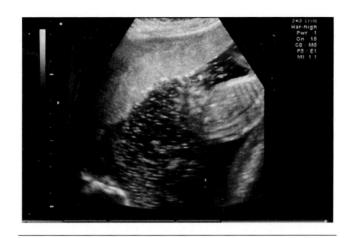

FIGURE 34-1 After aspiration of fluid from first sac, a small amount of fluid is pushed back into cavity stirring up debris creating "bubbles" that allow operator to distinguish between the sacs.

local anesthetics is not necessary, as it may be more uncomfortable to the patient than the actual amniocentesis. The optimal spot for needle insertion is in the upper fundal region. Procedures done near the bladder tend to be more uncomfortable and are associated with a higher incidence of amniotic fluid leaks. Leakage of amniotic fluid after amniocentesis performed in a high fundal pocket is rare.

After sterile preparation of the skin, abdominal layers are penetrated to the amniotic cavity with a 20- or 22-gauge, 3.5-inch long, spinal needle. The needle, held in 1 hand with the finger on top of the stylet, should be inserted smoothly, in a single motion, into the pocket of amniotic fluid. The experienced operator should be able to feel the needle entering the amniotic cavity by a sudden change in tissue resistance. Real-time ultrasonographic guidance during amniocentesis is, however, strongly advocated, since it may reduce the frequency of multiple needle insertions, of bloody taps, and of failure to obtain amniotic fluid.[48-50] The incidence of fetal trauma and fetal loss from amniocentesis[51] are apparently lowered by continuous ultrasonic visualization of the needle tip, which may also help to identify technical difficulties, such as membrane tenting during the procedure.[52] In the latter situation, rotating the needle while inserting it, or using a stylet that is longer than the needle to pierce the membranes,[53] may help.

When the needle tip, seen on ultrasound (Fig. 34-1) as a bright spot, is placed satisfactorily into a pocket of amniotic fluid, the stylet is removed and a 5 ml syringe is attached. The first 2–5 ml of fluid are aspirated and discarded, in order to minimize the risk of contamination from maternal cells drawn by the needle in its pathway. Twenty to 30 ml of amniotic fluid are then gently aspirated into syringes, transferred to sterile tubes and transported at room temperature to the laboratory for processing.

Patients are released after a brief period of observation and ultrasound documentation of fetal viability. Following amniocentesis, we recommend to postpone sexual activity and strenuous exercise for 2–3 days. Patients are also instructed to report

immediately signs of infection, vaginal bleeding, leakage of amniotic fluid, and regular uterine contractions.

INTERPRETATION OF RESULTS

The karyotype obtained in amniocytes reflects the accurate fetal status in over 99% of cases. However, false negative results of amniocentesis have been reported.[54] One or more hypermodal cells are observed in 2–3% of karyotypes analyzed.[55] Most of these cases are caused by extra embryonic nondisjunction (pseudomosaicism) and are associated with a normal phenotype.[56] True fetal mosaicism is considered when hypermodal cells are identified in at least 2 colonies in the same culture flask (as encountered in 0.7% of amniotic cells cultures) or in multiple flasks (observed in 0.2% of cultures).[56-58] Even in these cases, however, mosaicism in cultured amniocytes will not always represent *true* fetal mosaicism. Fetal blood karyotypes evaluated after the diagnosis of chromosomal mosaicism in amniotic cell cultures were normal in 15 of 16 mosaic autosomal trisomy cases and in all 8 cases of mosaic sex chromosome trisomy diagnosed by amniocentesis.[59] Mosaicism for chromosome structural rearrangements was confirmed in fetal blood from 5 of 11 cases with mosaic translocation or inversion and in 4 of 6 cases of de novo supernumerary marker chromosome mosaicism. Although a normal blood karyotype may not exclude cases of true fetal mosaicism confined to specific fetal tissues,[56] follow up of mosaicism in cultured amniocytes with fetal blood sampling should help to avoid termination of pregnancy of some normal fetuses.

Balanced translocations or inversions diagnosed at amniocentesis may be inherited or de novo, implying that evaluation of parental karyotypes is frequently needed. If the balanced structural rearrangement is inherited from 1 of the parents, they may be reassured that the phenotype of the offspring will also be normal. If, however, the abnormality occurred for the first time (de novo) in that specific conception, the risk of major fetal malformations and of mental retardation is probably around 8–10%.[60]

Brown or green tinged amniotic fluid is aspirated in 1–6% of midtrimester amniocenteses and may be associated with an increased risk (5–9%) of perinatal mortality and pregnancy loss.[61,62] Analysis of discolored fluid samples indicates that in most cases the discoloring pigment is hemoglobin. Vaginal bleeding prior to amniocentesis seems to predispose for presence of discolored amniotic fluid.

Alpha-fetoprotein concentration in amniotic fluid is routinely evaluated in most laboratories, irrespective of indication for sampling, although the usefulness of this measurement has been questioned recently.[63,64] An alpha-fetoprotein level in amniotic fluid higher than 2.5 MoM for gestational age is an indication to check for acetylcholine esterase (AChE). The combination of elevated AFP and positive AChE in amniotic fluid is by far more accurate than AFP alone for prenatal diagnosis of NTD and the false positive rate is only 1:300 or less.[65,66] Traditionally, amniotic fluid AChE was considered a bimodal test, with either positive or negative result. However, with sensitive laboratory techniques, a faint but true band can sometimes be detected in the specific AChE position on gel electrophoresis. This "inconclusive" result is more common in amniotic fluid samples of early gestational age (before 15 weeks of gestation), at which time it is only seldom associated with fetal malformations. Later in pregnancy, an "inconclusive" AChE band is relatively rare (<2%), but fetal anomalies are observed in more than half of such cases.[67,68]

SPECIAL CONDITIONS FOR AMNIOCENTESIS

MULTIPLE GESTATIONS

Twinning occurs once in every 87 pregnancies of white North American women and its frequency may increase with advancing parity and maternal age. Infertility treatments are offered to about 10% of women and carry also a substantial risk of multiples—25–50% of twins to 5–7% of triplets. Thus, about 1.2–2.4% of patients presenting for prenatal diagnosis will carry multiple fetuses.[69] Only one third of multiple gestations are monozygotic, the twin fetuses having identical karyotypes, but identification of chorionicity by ultrasound is troublesome. Thus, in most cases separate sampling of amniotic fluid from both sacs is necessary to assess correctly the karyotype of each fetus. In general, the chance that at least 1 twin has an abnormal karyotype should be quoted as almost twice the age-related risk[70] and the danger of pregnancy loss related to amniocentesis should probably be increased accordingly.[71,72] When the anatomic relationship of the sacs and the chorioamniotic membrane between them is clearly discernible, it is generally easy to sample separately both sacs, with continuous ultrasound guidance. Using a curvilinear or linear array ultrasound transducer, the first needle can be left in situ while introducing another amniocentesis needle into the second sac, so that both needles are observed on ultrasound in the same plane simultaneously, with the chorioamniotic membrane between them.[73] A technique by which a single needle is progressively advanced under ultrasound guidance from the first to the second sac has also been promoted.[74,75]

When the relationship between the sacs is not evident, injection of a dye-like Indigo Carmine or Congo red into the first sac after aspiration of amniotic fluid may be a helpful marker. After injection of dye into the first amniotic cavity, aspiration of clear fluid proves that the current sample is from the second sac. Dye can also be used to prove that a multiple pregnancy is monoamniotic, if no membrane is visible on ultrasound. The use of dyes in pregnancy should be approached, however, cautiously. Exposure to methylene blue as a dye marker for genetic amniocentesis in twins has been repeatedly associated with jejunal atresia.[76,77] Cases of fetal death after exposure to

methylene blue have also been reported.[78] A membrane free maternal hemoglobin hemolysate appears to be a useful inert and safe biologic dye for this purpose.[79]

In singleton pregnancies, abnormally elevated amniotic fluid AFP indicates the need to test for AChE in amniotic fluid. An abnormally elevated amniotic fluid AFP and a positive AChE is associated in most cases with fetal malformations or with fetal death. Transfer of these materials across the membranes may confuse clinical interpretation of amniotic fluid AFP and AChE results in twin pregnancies. Discordant amniotic fluid AFP results are more common in dizygotic twins, perhaps due to the bichorionic biamniotic membrane between the sacs. AChE diffuses readily across the membranes and cannot be used to determine which twin is abnormal.[80]

"EARLY" AMNIOCENTESIS

Improved ultrasound technology, increasing experience with ultrasound-guided needle manipulation and patient preference for more private, earlier genetic diagnosis have motivated a shift from second trimester amniocentesis toward earlier procedures—CVS and "early" amniocentesis. Early amniocentesis refers to procedures performed before 15 weeks' gestation (most commonly between 12–14 gestational weeks). The approach technique is somewhat different from that used at midtrimester, for 2 reasons. First, ultrasound guidance is essential as the size of the fluid pocket is much smaller and requires greater experience to access safely. Second, if one pushes the needle slowly into the pocket, there is a much higher likelihood of tenting the fetal membranes, which did not adhere yet to the uterine wall. We use a 22-gauge needle, which is inserted to the myometrium. After fetal position is verified, the needle is advanced in a single, swift thrust into the pocket of fluid. Sometimes, rotating the needle may also help to overcome tenting of the membranes. One ml of amniotic fluid per every week of gestation is aspirated into a syringe, transferred into sterile tubes and sent to the laboratory for processing.

Increasing experience with this procedure shows it to be comparable to mid trimester amniocentesis in terms of sampling success or accurate cytogenetic diagnosis but to provide earlier counseling, testing, and availability of results.[81–86] Our experience with over 500 such procedures also suggests that "early" amniocentesis is safe and reliable, with amniotic fluid samples obtained in all cases. However, because of slower growth in culture of cells obtained from early amniotic fluid, the latency period between procedure and results is 3–4 weeks, about 1 week longer than after midtrimester amniocentesis.[87] The use of filtration techniques to increase the yield of amniocytes obtained in a relatively low volume of fluid aspirated may help to overcome this difficulty.[88,89] Early amniocentesis results are available 4–6 weeks before standard amniocentesis and 1–3 weeks after CVS,[86] presenting an attractive method for prenatal diagnosis in the early second trimester, despite a somewhat higher rate of immediate post procedure complications.[90–92]

An advantage of early amniocentesis is the ability to measure AFP and AChE in amniotic fluid. Alpha-fetoprotein peaks in amniotic fluid at 12–13 weeks gestation and then gradually decline, following the trend of AFP in fetal blood.[93,94] In amniotic fluid obtained from pregnancies at 10–15 weeks of gestation, elevated AFP has been found in association with fetal structural anomalies and low AFP values were observed in some of the pregnancies that were aneuploid, as reported for pregnancies of later gestational age.[93,94] A faint, "inconclusive," AChE band was frequently observed on gel electrophoresis of "early" amniotic fluid samples—this seems, however, to be less commonly associated with fetal anomalies than when this finding appears in amniotic fluid samples obtained later on in gestation.[67] Thus, until larger databases are accumulated, results of AFP and AChE in "early" amniocentesis specimens should be interpreted with extreme caution.

SAFETY AND COMPLICATIONS OF AMNIOCENTESIS

Amniocentesis is a relatively safe procedure, with almost nonexistent severe sequelae. The frequency of severe chorioamnionitis following amniocentesis is about 0.1%; however, maternal septicemia with pulmonary edema, renal failure, and DIC has been reported occasionally.[95] Leakage of amniotic fluid is a relatively frequent complication, experienced by 1–2% of patients after amniocentesis, but is of minor clinical significance and usually resolves within 48–72 hours.[96] Although rare, persistent and significant amniotic fluid leakage may however lead to oligohydramnion and may result in fetal pressure deformities and pulmonary hypoplasia.[97] In experienced hands, the overall procedure related pregnancy loss is 0.2–0.5% above the spontaneous pregnancy loss rate at 16 weeks gestation, the latter being estimated at 2–3%.[98,99] Pregnancy loss rates seem to be associated with number of failed attempts (needle insertions) at the same session and with vaginal bleeding following amniocentesis, but not with gestational age at the time of amniocentesis, the volume of fluid removed or whether the procedure is repeated following a failed attempt at a previous date. Advanced maternal age (over 40), episodes of vaginal bleeding earlier in pregnancy and a history of multiple previous losses may also increase the risk of complications from amniocentesis.[99] Pregnancy loss related to early amniocentesis is somewhat higher than at midtrimester, about 0.7–0.8%,[84–86] comparable to that observed at CVS.[91,100] Apparently, the rate of complications associated with amniocentesis is directly related to the experience of the operator.[101]

Fetal injury by the amniocentesis needle should be very rare with ultrasound-guided procedures. Traumatization of the fetus by the amniocentesis needle has, however, been reported.[102–104] Another rare complication believed to be associated with amniocentesis, the amniotic band syndrome, has been reported only a few times and other causes are suggested now as its etiology.[105]

It has been suggested that removal of amniotic fluid at amniocentesis, especially when performed early in gestation, may affect fetal lung development. Lung function tests performed after birth to babies subjected to amniocentesis apparently demonstrated lower dynamic compliance and higher resistance compared to controls.[106] Other studies could not document an effect on neonatal lung function tests but noted a significantly higher incidence of respiratory distress and admissions to special care units for neonates subjected to chorionic villus sampling (CVS) in the first trimester.[107] Apparently, both amniocentesis and CVS performed in the first trimester may impair antenatal lung growth.[108] However, recent population-based studies on long-term outcomes after amniocentesis[109,110] could not document any long-term adverse effects on children born after this procedure.

In summary, amniocentesis is a relatively safe, well-established, and widely utilized procedure for prenatal diagnosis and most practicing obstetricians are familiar with it. However, failure to offer prenatal diagnosis to couples whose increased genetic risk had not been recognized or complications occurring to patients during procedures a physician does not do very commonly are areas of potential liability which bring us to question whether amniocentesis should be a routine, office procedure. Thus, although amniocentesis was labeled by CREOG as a procedure that should be learned by residents, in many large cities most private practitioners do not perform it but rather refer their patients to genetic centers with vast experience, where many of these procedures are performed daily. Nevertheless, a practicing obstetrician who is well experienced with amniocentesis and has the backup of a genetic center for counseling, would certainly not be considered below the standard of care if performing his own amniocenteses for prenatal diagnosis.

References

1. Jacobson CB, Barter RH. Intrauterine diagnosis and management of genetic defects. *Am J Obstet Gynecol.* 1967;99:795.
2. Valenti C, Schutta EJ, Kehaty T. Prenatal diagnosis of Down syndrome. *Lancet.* 1968;2:220.
3. Nadler HL. Antenatal detection of hereditary disorders. *Pediatrics.* 1968;42:912.
4. Nadler HL, Gerbie AB. Role of amniocentesis in the intrauterine detection of genetic disorders. *N Engl J Med.* 1970;282:596.
5. Evans MI, Schulman JD. Prenatal diagnosis: invasive techniques and alpha-fetoprotein screening. In: Avery GB, ed. *Neonatal Pathophysiology and Management of the Newborn.* 3rd ed. Philadelphia, PA: Lippincott Harper; 1986.
6. Freshney RI. *Culture of Animal Cells: A Manual of Basic Techniques.* New York, NY: Allan R Liss, Inc; 1983.
7. Cheung SW, Crane JP, Johnson A, et al. A simple method to prepare metaphase chromosomes from amniotic fluid cell cultures. *Prenat Diagn.* 1987;7:383.

8. D'Alton ME, Malone FD, Chelmow D, et al. Defining the role of fluorescence in situ hybridization on uncultured amniocytes for prenatal diagnosis of aneuploidies. *Am J Obstet Gynecol.* 1997;176:769–774.

9. Reid R, Sepuvelda W, Kyle PM, et al. Amniotic fluid culture failure: clinical significance and association with aneuploidy. *Obstet Gynecol.* 1996;87:588–592.

10. Evans MI, Henry GP, Miller WA, et al. International collaborative assessment of 146,000 prenatal karyotypes: expected limitations if only chromosome specific probes and fluorescent in situ hybridization are used. *Hum Reprod.* 2000;15:228–230.

11. Ligon AH, Beaudet AL, Sheffer LG. Simultaneous multilocus FISH analysis for detection of microdeletions in the diagnostic evaluation of developmental delay and mental retardation. *Am J Hum Genet.* 1997;61:51.

12. Hook EB, Cross PK, Schreimachers DM. Chromosomal abnormality rates at amniocentesis and in live born infants. *JAMA.* 1983;249:2034–2038.

13. ACOG Practice Bulletin. Clinical management guidelines for Obstetricians–Gynecologists: prenatal diagnosis of fetal chromosome abnormalities. *Obstet Gynecol.* 2001;97(5 Pt 1):1–12.

14. Stene J, Stene K, Mikkelsen M. Risk for chromosome abnormality at amniocentesis following a child with a non-inherited chromosome aberration. *Prenat Diagn.* 1984;4 Suppl 1:81.

15. Boue A, Gallano P. A collaborative study of the segregation of inherited chromosome structural rearrangements in 1356 prenatal diagnoses. *Prenat Diagn.* 1984;4 Suppl 1:45.

16. Drugan A, Koppitch FC, Williams JC, et al. Prenatal diagnosis following recurrent early pregnancy loss. *Obstet Gynecol.* 1990;75:381–384.

17. Platt LD, DeVore GR, Lopez E, et al. Role of amniocentesis in ultrasound detected fetal malformations. *Obstet Gynecol.* 1986;68:153.

18. Williamson RA, Weiner CP, Patil S, et al. Abnormal pregnancy sonogram: selective indication for fetal karyotype. *Obstet Gynecol.* 1987;69:15.

19. Drugan A, Reichler A, Bronshtein M, et al. Abnormal biochemical serum screening versus second trimester ultrasound-detected minor anomalies as predictors of aneuploidy in low risk patients. *Fetal Diagn Ther.* 1996;115:301.

20. Drugan A, Johnson MP, Evans MI. Ultrasound screening for fetal chromosome anomalies. *Am J Med Genetics.* 2000;90:98–107.

21. Wickstrom EA, Thangavelu M, Parilla BV, et al. A prospective study of the association between isolated fetal pyelectasis and chromosomal abnormality. *Obstet Gynecol.* 1996;88:379–382.

22. Vintzileos AM, Egan JF. Adjusting the risk for trisomy 21 on the basis of second trimester ultrasonography. *Am J Obstet Gynecol.* 1995;172:837–844.

23. Kupferminc MJ, Tamura RK, Sabbagha RE, et al. Isolated choroid plexus cyst(s): an indication for amniocentesis. *Am J Obstet Gynecol.* 1994;171:1068–1071.

24. Corteville JE, Dicke JM, Crane JP. Fetal pyelectasis and Down syndrome: is genetic amniocentesis warranted? *Obstet Gynecol.* 1992;79:770–772.

25. Drugan A, Johnson MP, Reichler A, et al. Second trimester minor ultrasound anomalies: impact on the risk of aneuploidy associated with advanced maternal age. *Obstet Gynecol.* 1996;88:203–206.

26. Yeo L, Vintzileos AM. The use of genetic sonography to reduce the need for amniocentesis in women at high risk for Down syndrome. *Semin Perinatol.* 2003;27:152–159.

27. Kellner LH, Weiss RR, Weiner Z, et al. The advantages of using triple-marker screening for chromosomal abnormalities. *Am J Obstet Gynecol.* 1995;172:831–836.

28. Phillips OP, Elias S, Schulman LP, et al. Maternal serum screening for fetal Down syndrome in women less than 35 years of age using alpha-fetoprotein, HCG and unconjugated estriol: a prospective 2 year study. *Obstet Gynecol.* 1992;80:353–358.

29. Drugan A, O'Brien JE, Gambino RB, et al. Prenatal biochemical screening. In: Evans MI, Johnson MP, eds. *Prenatal Diagnosis in the 90's.* J Reprod Med Symposium, 1992.

30. Kaffe S, Hsu LY. Maternal serum alpha-fetoprotein screening and fetal chromosome anomalies: is lowering maternal age for amniocentesis preferable? *Am J Med Genet.* 1992;42:801–806.

31. Benn PA, Ying J, Beazoglou T, et al. Estimates for the sensitivity and false positive rates for second trimester serum screening for Down syndrome and trisomy 18 with adjustment for cross identification and double positive results. *Prenat Diagn.* 2001;21:46–51.

32. Wald NJ, Watt HC, Hackshaw AK. Integrated screening for Down syndrome on the basis of tests performed during the first and second trimesters. *N Engl J Med.* 1999;341:461–467.

33. Drugan A, Dvorin E, O'Brien JE, et al. Alpha-fetoprotein screening. *Curr Opin Obstet Gynecol.* 1991;3:230–234.

34. Gonzalez D, Barrett T, Apuzzio J. Is routine fetal karyotyping necessary for patients undergoing amniocentesis for elevated maternal serum alpha-fetoprotein. *J Matern Fetal Med.* 2001;10:376–379.

35. Hume RF, Drugan A, Reichler A, et al. Aneuploidy among prenatally detected neural tube defects. *Am J Med Genet.* 1996;61:171–173.

36. Warsoff SL, Larsen JW, Kent SG, et al. Prenatal diagnosis of congenital adrenal hyperplasia. *Obstet Gynecol.* 1980;55:751.

37. Arnon J, Ornoi A, Bach G. Cultured amniotic fluid cells for prenatal diagnosis of lysosomal storage disease: a methodological study. *Prenat Diagn.* 1986;6:351–361.

38. Wiederschain GY, Rosenfeld EL, Brusilowski AI, et al. Alpha L-fucosidase and other glycosidases in human placenta, fetus, liver and amniotic fluid at various stages of gestation. *Clin Chim Acta.* 1971;35:99–107.

39. Hultberg B, Sjoblad S, Gustavii B. Acid hydrolases in amniotic fluid and chorionic villi at various stages of pregnancy. *Clin Chim Acta.* 1974;53:221–227.

40. Weatherall DJ, Old JM, Their SL, et al. Prenatal diagnosis of the common hemoglobin disorders. *J Med Genet.* 1985;22:422–430.

41. Butler WJ, McDonough PG. The new genetics-molecular technology and reproductive biology. *Fertil Steril.* 1989;51:375–386.

42. ACOG technology assessment. Genetics and molecular diagnostic testing. *Int J Gynaecol Obstet.* 2002;79:67–85.

43. Cohn GM, Gould M, Miller RC, et al. The importance of genetic counseling before amniocentesis. *J Perinatol.* 1996;16:352–357.

44. Evans MI, Hume RF, Johnson MP, et al. Integration of genetics and ultrasonography in prenatal diagnosis: just looking is not enough. *Am J Obstet Gynecol.* 1996;174:1925–1931.

45. Murray JC, Karp LE, Williamson RA, et al. Rh isoimmunization as related to amniocentesis. *Am J Hum Genet.* 1983;16:527.

46. Bravo RR, Shulman LP, Phillips OP, et al. Transplacental needle passage in early amniocentesis and pregnancy loss. *Obstet Gynecol.* 1995;86:437–440.

47. Giorlandino C, Mobili L, Bilancioni E, et al. Transplacental amniocentesis: is it really a higher risk procedure? *Prenat Diagn.* 1994;14:803–806.

48. Benaceraff BR, Frigoletto FD. Amniocentesis under continuous ultrasound guidance: a series of 232 cases. *Obstet Gynecol.* 1983;62:760.

49. McDicken WN, Anderson T, MacKenzie WE, et al. Ultrasonic identification of needle tips at amniocentesis. *Lancet.* 1984;2:198.

50. Romero R, Jeanty P, Reece EA, et al. Sonographically monitored amniocentesis to decrease intraoperative complications. *Obstet Gynecol.* 1985;64:426.

51. Williamson RA, Varner MW, Grant SS. Reduction in amniocentesis risks using real time needle guide puncture. *Obstet Gynecol.* 1985;65:751.

52. Platt LD, DeVore GR, Gimowsky ML. Failed amniocentesis: the role of membrane tenting. *Am J Obstet Gynecol.* 1982;144:479–480.

53. Dombrowsky MP, Isada NB, Johnson MP, et al. Modified stylet technique for tenting of amniotic membranes. *Obstet Gynecol.* 1996;87:455–456.

54. Fraser S, Drew JH, Fraser C. False negative cytogenetic results following amniocentesis. *Aust N Z J Obstet Gynaecol.* 1996;36:149–151.

55. Simpson JL. Amniocentesis: what it can tell you and what it can't. *Contemp Obstet Gynecol.* 1988;31:31–36.

56. Hsu YF, Kaffe S, Perlis ET. Trisomy 20 mosaicism in prenatal diagnosis: a review and update. *Prenat Diagn.* 1987;7:581–596.

57. Worton RG, Stern RA. A Canadian collaborative study of mosaicism in amniotic fluid cell cultures. *Prenat Diagn.* 1984;4:131–144.

58. Hsu LY, Yu MT, Richkind KE, et al. Incidence and significance of chromosome mosaicism involving an autosomal structural abnormality diagnosed prenatally through amniocentesis: a collaborative study. *Prenat Diagn.* 1996;16:1–28.

59. Gosden C, Nikolaides KH, Rodeck CH. Fetal blood sampling in the investigation of chromosome mosaicism in amniotic fluid cell culture. *Lancet.* 1988;1:613–616.

60. Warburton D. Outcome of cases of de novo structural rearrangements diagnosed at amniocentesis. *Prenat Diagn.* 1984;4:69–80.

61. Allen R. The significance of meconium in midtrimester genetic amniocentesis. *Am J Obstet Gynecol.* 1985;152:413–417.

62. Zorn EM, Hanson FW, Greve IC, et al. Analysis of the significance of discolored amniotic fluid at midtrimester amniocentesis. *Am J Obstet Gynecol.* 1986;154:1234–1240.

63. Shields LE, Uhrich SB, Komarniski CA, et al. Amniotic fluid alpha-fetoprotein determination at the time of genetic amniocentesis: has it outlived its usefulness? *J Ultrasound Med.* 1996;15:735–739.

64. Silver RK, Leeth EA, Check IJ. A reappraisal of amniotic fluid alpha-fetoprotein measurement at the time of genetic amniocentesis and midtrimester ultrasonography. *J Ultrasound Med.* 2001;20:631–637.

65. Wald JN, Cuckle HS: Amniotic fluid acetyl cholinesterase electrophoresis as a secondary test in the diagnosis of anencephaly and spina bifida in early pregnancy: report of the collaborative acetyl cholinesterase study. *Lancet.* 1981;2:321–324.

66. Crandall BF, Matsumoto M. Routine amniotic fluid alpha-fetoprotein assay: experience with 40,000 pregnancies. *Am J Med Genet.* 1986;24:143.

67. Drugan A, Syner FN, Belski-Gold RL, et al. Amniotic fluid acetyl cholinesterase: implications of an inconclusive result. *Am J Obstet Gynecol.* 1988;159:469–474.

68. Brown CL, Colden KA, Hume RF, et al. Faint and positive amniotic fluid acetyl cholinesterase with a normal sonogram. *Am J Obstet Gynecol.* 1996;175:1000–1003.

69. Jewell SE, Yip R. Increasing trends in plural births in the United States. *Obstet Gynecol.* 1995;85:229–232.

70. Meyers C, Adam R, Dungan J, et al. Aneuploidy in twin gestations: when is maternal age advanced? *Obstet Gynecol.* 1997;89:248–251.

71. Kidd SA, Lancaster PA, Anderson JC, et al. A cohort study of pregnancy outcome after amniocentesis in twin pregnancy. *Paediatr Perinat Epidemiol.* 1997;11:200–213.

72. Yukobowich E, Anteby EY, Cohen SM, et al. Risk of fetal loss in twin pregnancies undergoing second trimester amniocentesis. *Obstet Gynecol.* 2001;98:876–877.

73. Bahado-Singh R, Schmitt R, Hobbins JC. New technique for genetic amniocentesis in twins. *Obstet Gynecol.* 1992;79:304–307.

74. van Vugt JMG, Niewwint A, van Geijn HP. Single needle insertion: an alternative technique for early second trimester genetic twin amniocentesis. *Fetal Diagn Ther.* 1995;10:178.

75. Sebire NJ, Noble PL, Odibo A, et al. Single uterine entry for genetic amniocentesis in twin pregnancies. *Ultrasound Obstet Gynecol.* 1996;7:26–31.

76. van der Pol JS, Wolf H, Boer K, et al. Jejunal atresia related to the use of methylene blue in genetic amniocentesis in twins. *Br J Obstet Gynecol.* 1992;99:141–143.

77. Gluer S. Intestinal atresia following intra-amniotic use of dyes. *Eur J Pediatr Surg.* 1995;5:240–242.

78. Kidd SA, Lancaster PA, Anderson JC, et al. Fetal death after exposure to methylene blue dye during mid-trimester amniocentesis in twin pregnancy. *Prenat Diagn.* 1996;16:39–47.

79. Beekhuis JR, de Bruijn HW, van Lith JM, et al. Second trimester amniocentesis in twin pregnancies: maternal hemoglobin as a dye marker to differentiate biamniotic twins. *Br J Obstet Gynecol.* 1992;99:126–127.

80. Drugan A, Sokol RJ, Syner FN, et al. Clinical implications of amniotic fluid AFP in twin pregnancies. *J Reprod Med.* 1989;34:977–981.

81. Assel BG, Lewis SM, Dickerman LH, et al. Single operator comparison of early and mid-second trimester amniocentesis. *Obstet Gynecol.* 1992;79:940–944.

82. Diaz Vega M, de la Cueva P, Leal C, et al. Early amniocentesis at 10–12 weeks' gestation. *Prenat Diagn.* 1996;16:307–312.

83. Henry GP, Miller WA. Early amniocentesis. *J Reprod Med.* 1992; 37:305–402.

84. Hanson FW, Tennant F, Hune S, et al. Early amniocentesis: outcome, risks and technical problems at less than 12.8 weeks. *Am J Obstet Gynecol.* 1992;166:1707–1711.

85. Johnson JM, Wilson RD, Winsor EJ, et al. The early amniocentesis study: a randomized clinical trial of early amniocentesis versus midtrimester amniocentesis. *Fetal Diagn Ther.* 1996;11:85–93.

86. Crandall BF, Kulch P, Tabsh K. Risk assessment of amniocentesis between 11 to 15 weeks: comparison to later amniocentesis controls. *Prenat Diagn.* 1994;14:913–919.

87. Evans MI, Koppitch FC, Nemmitz B, et al. Early genetic amniocentesis and chorionic villus sampling. *J Reprod Med.* 1988;33:450–452.

88. Sundberg K, Bang J, Brocks V, et al. Early sonographically guided amniocenteses with filtration technique: follow up on 249 procedures. *J Ultrasound Med.* 195;14:585–590.

89. Farran I, Sanchez MA, Mediano C, et al. Early amniocentesis with the filtration technique: neonatal outcome in 123 singleton pregnancies. *Prenat Diagn.* 2002;22:859–863.

90. Brumfield CG, Lin S, Conner W, et al. Pregancy outcome following genetic amniocentesis at 11–14 versus 16–19 weeks' gestation. *Obstet Gynecol.* 1996;88:114–118.

91. Nicolaides KH, Brizot ML, Patel F, et al. Comparison of chorion villus sampling and early amniocentesis for karyotyping in 1942 singleton pregnancies. *Fetal Diagn Ther.* 1996;11:9–15.

92. Alfirevic Z. Early amniocentesis versus transabdominal chorionic villus sampling for prenatal diagnosis. (Cochrane Review) In: The Cochrane Library, Issue 2, 2000. Oxford, England: Update Software.

93. Drugan A, Syner FN, Greb A, et al. Amniotic fluid alpha fetoprotein and acetyl cholinesterase in early genetic amniocentesis. *Obstet Gynecol.* 1988;72:33–35.

94. Jorgensen FS, Sundberg K, Loft AG, et al. Alpha-fetoprotein and acetyl cholinesterase activity in first and early second trimester amniotic fluid. *Prenat Diagn.* 1995;15:621–625.

95. Hamoda H, Chamberlain PF: Clostridium welchii infection following amniocentesis: a case report and review of the literature. *Prenat Diagn.* 2002;22:783–785.

96. Borgida AF, Mills AA, Feldman DM, et al. Outcome of pregnancies complicated by ruptured membranes after genetic amniocentesis. *Am J Obstet Gynecol.* 2000;183:937–939.

97. Nimrod C, Varela-Gittings F, Machin G, et al: The effect of very prolonged membrane rupture on fetal development. *Am J Obstet Gynecol.* 1984;148:540–543.

98. Antsaklis A, Papaantoniou N, Xygakis A, et al. Genetic amniocentesis in women 20–34 years old: associated risks. *Prenat Diagn.* 2000;20:247–250.

99. Papantoniou NE, Daskalakis GJ, Tziotis JG, et al. Risk factors predisposing to fetal loss following a second trimester amniocentesis. *Br J Obstet Gynaecol.* 2001;108:1053–1056.

100. Alfirevic Z, Sundberg K, Brigham S. Amniocentesis and chorionic villus sampling for prenatal diagnosis. (Cochrane Review) In: The Cochrane Library, Issue 3, 2003. Oxford, England: Update Software.

101. Anandakumar C, Wong YC, Annapoorna V, et al. Amniocentesis and its complications. *Aust N Z J Obstet Gynecol.* 1992;32:97–99.

102. Ledbetter DJ, Hall DG. Traumatic arteriovenous fistula: a complication of amniocentesis. *J Pediatr Surg.* 1992;27:720–721.

103. Eller KM, Kuller JA. Porencephaly secondary to fetal trauma during amniocentesis. *Obstet Gynecol.* 1995;85:865–867.

104. Squier M, Chamberlain P, Zaiwalla Z, et al. Five cases of brain injury following amniocentesis in midterm pregnancy. *Dev Med Child Neurol.* 2000;42:554–560.

105. Lockwood C, Ghidini A, Romero R, et al. Amniotic band syndrome: reevaluation of its pathogenesis. *Am J Obstet Gynecol.* 1989;160:1030–1033.

106. Milner AD, Hoskins EW, Hopkin IE. The effect of midtrimester amniocentesis on lung function in the neonatal period. *Eur J Pediatr.* 1992;151:458–460.

107. Thompson PJ, Greenough A, Nikolaides KH. Lung volume measured by functional residual capacity in infants following first trimester amniocentesis or chorionic villus sampling. *Br J Obstet Gynecol.* 1992;99:479–482.

108. Yuksel B, Greenough A, Naik S, et al. Perinatal lung function and invasive antenatal procedures. *Thorax.* 1997;52:181–184.

109. Baird PA, Yee IM, Sadovnick AD. Population-based study on long-term outcomes after amniocentesis. *Lancet.* 1994;344:1134–1136.

110. Finegan JA, Sitarenios G, Bolan PL, et al. Children whose mothers had second trimester amniocentesis: follow up at school age. *Br J Obstet Gynecol.* 1996;103:214–218.

CHAPTER 35

EARLY AMNIOCENTESIS: RISK ASSESSMENT

R. Douglas Wilson

INTRODUCTION

Invasive prenatal diagnosis has been available since the 1950s and 1960s with initial studies allowing fetal sex determination followed by complete karyotype analysis.[1,2,3] Aneuploidy is present in approximately 6–11% of all stillbirths and neonatal deaths while chromosome defects compatible with life but resulting in significant morbidity is present in 0.65% of newborns. Genetic amniocentesis was initially evaluated in the mid 1970s and became the gold standard for invasive prenatal diagnosis in the 1980s. Earlier prenatal diagnosis was considered a definite advantage and techniques such as chorionic villus sampling (CVS) were evaluated and introduced in the mid 1980s. Earlier prenatal diagnosis had the advantage for patient with abnormal results, the option for an earlier and safer termination of pregnancy with the possible reduced social and physiological trauma.[4,5,6] In situations where couples had genetic risks as high as 25%, CVS had a distinctive advantage with earlier diagnosis.[7] There were several disadvantages with CVS identified, which included the absence of alphafetoprotein (AFP) testing, placental mosaicism, and increased incidence of maternal cell contamination.[4,6,8] The risks of limb reduction vascular disruption sequence and facial abnormalities associated with CVS are related to gestational ages of less than 9 weeks at the time of the procedure.[4] Early amniocentesis (EA) was considered as an early prenatal diagnosis technique option due to the concerns related to CVS and the wide spread use of amniocentesis at 15–16 weeks gave false reassurance that amniocentesis could be used safely at an earlier gestational age. The ultrasound-guided amniocentesis technique was moved down in gestational age with procedures being undertaken in the 11–14 gestation weeks. Early observational studies were not able to identify the risks of the procedure and it was only after 3 randomized trials were completed that the true risks of the procedure were identified.[9,10,11] These early amniocentesis risks included higher total pregnancy loss, a significant increase incidence of musculoskeletal foot deformity, a significant increased culture failure rate, and an increased post amniocentesis rate of leakage compared with the gold standard mid-trimester amniocentesis. The early amniocentesis window considered in these randomized trials were 11 weeks and 0 days to 13 weeks and 6 days. The specific risk of EA in a gestational window of 14 weeks 0 days to 14 weeks 6 days has not been clearly defined.

Three recent reviews[12,13,14] evaluated EA and CVS. Meta analysis (3 studies) concluded that EA is associated with a greater risk of spontaneous miscarriage and neonatal talipes compared to transabdominal CVS.[12] All invasive procedures should be performed under continuous ultrasound guidance by experienced operators. Mid-trimester amniocentesis remains the safest invasive procedure as both CVS and EA can induce fetal structural defects and should be abandoned as routine invasive tests.[13]

DEFINITION

Early amniocentesis is defined as a first trimester procedure performed before 14 weeks of gestation (from 11 + 0 to 13 + 6).[4,5] Some series have included procedures as early as 9 + 0 weeks. Traditional amniocentesis is usually performed after 15 + 0 weeks of gestation; invasive procedures between 14 + 0 and 14 + 6 are usually considered early and have been included in some series (Table 35-1).

EMBRYOLOGY

As implantation of the blastocyst progresses, a small cavity called the primordium of the amniotic cavity appears in the inner cell mass at around 7–8 days postfertilization.[51] Amnioblasts separate from the epiblast and form a thin membrane called the amnion, which encloses the amniotic cavity. The epiblast, 1 of the 2 layers of the embryonic disk, forms the floor of the amniotic cavity. The other layer of the embryonic disk, the hypoblast, forms the roof of the exocoelomic cavity and is continuous with the thin exocoelomic membrane.[49] This membrane and its cavity become the primary yolk sac. The embryonic disk lies then between the amniotic cavity and primary yolk sac.

The extraembryonic coelom is formed by the fusion of isolated spaces within the extraembryonic forms, the primary yolk sac decreases in size and a smaller secondary yolk sac forms. The extraembryonic mesoderm and the 2 layers of trophoblast constitute the chorion. The chorion forms the wall of the chorionic sac (gestational sac) within which the embryo and its amniotic and yolk sacs are suspended by the connecting stalk (future umbilical cord). By development day 13 (postfertilization), the future amniotic cavity is approximately one third the size of the secondary yolk sac. The amniotic cavity has surrounded the embryo as well as the connecting stalk by day 28 (postfertilization). At 10 weeks of gestation, the embryo is still connected to the yolk sac by the vitelline duct. The yolk sac is located between the 2 gestational sac membranes (amnio, chorion). By the end of the twelfth postfertilization week (fourteenth week of gestation), the amnion is usually in direct contact with the chorion, obliterating the chorionic cavity.[4,51,52] The yolk sac has shrunk and disappeared.

The physiology and the anatomy of the fetal membranes differ at 16 weeks of gestation compared with the late first

TABLE 35-1 | RANDOMIZED, PARTIALLY RANDOMIZED, AND OBSERVATIONAL STUDIES ON EARLY AMNIOCENTESIS

		Gestational Age						Needle Size	Leakage Amniotic Fluid %	Sampling Failure Rate (Lab Failure)%	Loss Rates	
	No.	<11	11	12	13	14	15				Overall%	Postamnio%
Randomized studies												
EATA[11] (2004)	1,820	—	I–161	–I	1216	501	—	22	9.7	0.5 (0.2)	2.6	0.3
CEMAT[10] (1998)	1,916	43	885	998	119	21	34	22	4.6	1.7	7.6	2.6
Sundberg[9] (1997)	581	—	157	372	52	—	—	20	2.4	0.1	5.4	2.6
Johnson[15] (1996)	344	—	I–334–	–I	—	—	—	22	2.1	0.6	7.8	2.4
Partially randomized studies												
Nagel[16]	130	—	—	I–	130	—	I	22	—	1.5	6.2	—
Cederholm[17] (1997)	147	—	I–	—	147	–I	—	20	7.5	6.8	6.8	4
Nicolaides[18] (1996)	840	I 537	I–	303–	I	—	—	20			2	7	4.9
Observational studies (1994–2001)												
Collins[19] (1999)	1,207	—	—	I	1207	I	—	—	3.2	—	3.9	2.2
Daniel[20] (1998)	279	I–33–	I	74	78	94	181	22	1.4	—	2.2	
Jorgensen[21] (1998)	1,678	—	I–	—	1,678–	I	—	22	1.3	0.9 (0.9)	3	1.5
Eiben[22] (1997)	3,277	—	I–	640–I	I 2636	I	—	22	1.1	0.3	—	2
Brumfield[23] (1996)	413	—	63	139	112	—	—	22	2.9	—	—	2.2
Diaz Vega[24] (1996)	181	3	86	92	—	—	—	22	1.6	1.6 (5.5)	2.1	0.5
Shulman[25] (1994)	250	3	8	25	84	130	—	22	0.1		3.8	2.4
Crandall[7] (1994)	693	—	16	116	258	303	—		<1			0.2
Eiben[26] (1994)	1,554	—	5	153	520	876	—	20	0			0.3
(1987–1993)[6,27–50]	11,982	57	381	I–	10450	-I	1,094	20/22	1.6	3.3	4.1	2.6

trimester (11 + 0 to 13 + 6 weeks of gestation).[53] The amniotic membranes have 5 layers of amnion and 3 layers of chorion.[51] At gestational ages of 14–15 weeks, the amnion has not completely expanded to become adjacent and occluding the extraembryonic coelom.[54]

BACKGROUND POPULATIONS FOR COMPARING BENEFITS AND RISKS OF INVASIVE PRENATAL DIAGNOSIS

The mid-trimester amniocentesis population is important to establish the background pregnancy risks if no procedures are undertaken as well as the risks of mid-trimester amniocentesis done after 15 + 0 weeks of pregnancy. The determination of the background rate of pregnancy loss with no invasive prenatal diagnosis is necessary as a variety of factors can affect the incidence. Spontaneous miscarriage rate decreases with increasing gestational age, 15–20% of recognized pregnancies result in a spontaneous pregnancy loss before 20 weeks gestation.[32] In pregnancies with normal ultrasound before 14 weeks gestation, the total spontaneous abortion rate is 2.7%, with 1.5% occurring before 16 weeks gestation.[55] Other background overall loss rates have been reported from 2.1–3.2% in ultrasound observed populations.[56–58] Advanced maternal age increases the risk of pregnancy loss to as high as 14% in women of 40 years of age.[56] Higher background loss rates

are inherent with starting evaluation in earlier gestational age coupled with longer observation time. The specific etiology causing the pregnancy loss whether it is a fetal anomaly, aneuploidy, or placental factors can lead to a higher background pregnancy loss rate.[5]

Recent publications and reviews continue to look at post amniocentesis loss rates.[59–61] There has been a change in the primary indications for genetic amniocentesis over the last 2 decades. Initially genetic amniocentesis was used mainly for women of advanced maternal age but with the introduction of fetal screening techniques such as maternal serum triple screen and ultrasound, these indications have significantly added to the need for diagnostic amniocentesis. A collaborative study on 11,000 prenatal genetic amniocentesis showed that maternal serum abnormality was the indication for 45% of the procedures. In the group with an abnormal ultrasound indication, 6.5% had a chromosomal abnormality. From their total population, 2.5% were detected to have a chromosomal abnormality.[59] Consideration of the gestational age specific pregnancy outcome indicated in a review of 2,924 amniocenteses that the total miscarriage rate was 1% after early amniocentesis (11 + 0 to 14 + 6 weeks), 1.2% after traditional mid-trimester amniocentesis (15 + 0 to 18 + 6) and 3.1% for amniocentesis performed after 18 + 6 weeks gestation. The cumulative miscarriage risks increased from 0.03% 1 week after the procedure to plateau at 1.1% 5 weeks after the procedure. The preterm and stillbirth rates following amniocentesis were similar for the early and traditional mid-term amniocentesis but was significantly higher when the amniocentesis was performed after 19 weeks gestation.[60]

As women become more knowledgeable about genetic screening and invasive prenatal diagnosis, other aspects must be considered with regard to their counseling and decisions. Fewer United States patients at risk for Down syndrome in 1998 than in 1995 requested amniocentesis both before and after genetic counseling and ultrasound examination. Risk factors identified for this population were advanced maternal age, abnormal serum triple screen, or ultrasound abnormalities.[62] Women undergoing counseling for amniocentesis identified the main source of information had been their doctors or midwives. The majority of women (65%) made the decision with their partner. The women's concerns were focused mainly about fetal injury, miscarriage, and waiting for the results. The amniocentesis test did not have a major physiological impact on the women in general but a substantial minority reacted with anxiety and distress.[63,64]

The frequency of chromosomal abnormalities at amniocentesis showed the overall rate is 1.8% in a 20-year follow-up study. Within this group, 21% of all abnormalities were structural rearrangements (including markers) and less than half of all abnormalities were Trisomy 21. The advanced maternal age specific risk of aneuploidy in the second trimester is 1.24%. Recurrence risks for aneuploidy is 1.29% but is higher (4.84%) for women greater than or equal to 35 years of age. For couples, with a balanced translocation in 1 parent, the overall risk is 10.2% for an unbalanced translocation and 37.3% for a balanced translocation in the fetus.[65] The cytogenetic trend over the last decade showed overall increases for both amniocentesis and CVS. CVS made up 18% of the total samples in 1997 compared with 7.4% in 1988. Reporting times and culture success rates have improved with the overall reporting time falling from 20.2 to 13.8 days for amniotic fluid specimens and 21.3 to 14.5 for CVS specimens.[66]

AMNIOTIC FLUID SAMPLING AND RESULTS

TECHNIQUE

The EA technique is similar to amniocentesis performed at later gestational ages.[67] A spinal needle (length 9 or 14 cm) is inserted through the maternal abdomen wall and uterine wall into a pocket of amniotic fluid within the amniotic sac. Continuous ultrasonographic guidance is necessary to visualize the needle tip throughout and enhance success and safety. The amniotic fluid is aspirated usually into a 10–20 mL syringe[67] or through a filtration system.[9] A 22-gauge needle is most often used (Table 35-1) and approximately 1 mL of amniotic fluid per week of gestation is aspirated. Recent laboratory techniques allow smaller volumes of amniotic fluid to be aspirated, because higher post procedural fetal loss rates have been associated with larger extracted volumes at earlier gestational ages.[43]

"Tenting" of the amniotic membrane may occur in front of the spinal needle preventing access to the amniotic cavity and

the amniotic fluid.[5] This has been reported in up to 5% of the amniocentesis.[44] The approach, unique to the EA technique, may require the use of a more vigorous movement of the needle through the amnion membrane, in an amniotic fluid area, clear of the fetus.

The sampling failure rate associated with EA reported has ranged between 0.2% and 2.7% (Table 35-1). The Canadian Early and Mid-trimester Amniocentesis Trial (CEMAT),[10] through a secondary analysis focusing on procedural/technical variables, showed that failed or unsuccessful procedures (not attempted or not completed) were significantly more common with the EA technique than the traditional mid-trimester amniocentesis (1.6 vs. 0.4; $P < 0.01$).[68] This technical difficulty did not directly correlate with an increased fetal loss rate. Tenting of the amnion was significantly associated with increased procedure failure rate for early procedures (12.5% vs. 1.4%) as well as for mid-trimester procedures (3% vs. 0.2%).[66] The number of needle insertions has been a concern in early procedures. Series report between 89% to 100% success with the first EA attempt,[40,41,43,50] but the chance of more than 1 needle insertion being required to obtain sufficient amniotic fluid was found to be twice as high among EA patients (5.4% vs. 2.1%; $P < .01$).[68] However, no direct correlation with an increased fetal loss rate was apparent with the requirement of 2 or more insertions.

Other technical aspects involve the site of needle insertion and the placental localization. Although avoiding the placental continues to be part of the recommended technique for amniocentesis, no specific complications have been associated with the transplacental approach.[6,50,69,70] Even if more amniotic fluid specimens stained by maternal blood are obtained, these are not associated with a decreased amniocyte culture success rate.[71] Moreover, when the placental membranes are in close apposition, less amniotic tenting occurs[71] and the relative risk for post procedure amniotic fluid leakage is significantly reduced (1.8% vs. 3.5%; relative risk 1.9).[68] Patients with a transplacental early amniocentesis had significantly lower incidence of late procedure-related antenatal complications such as preterm labor and preterm rupture of membranes.[72] Thus, it appears that transplacental needle insertion should not be avoided when performing an EA.[72]

A syringe adapter is reported to facilitate aspiration at amniocentesis by permitting aspiration by barrel advancement rather than withdrawal.[71] Other technique variations, such as the use of local anesthesia or light pressure effleurage, do not affect the pain experience during amniocentesis.[74,75]

ACCURACY OF AMNIOTIC FLUID RESULTS

Numerous studies have showed that EA is reliable for early routine prenatal cytogenetic analysis.[4] The success rate of amniocytes culture and karyotyping increased with duration of pregnancy from gestational week $11 + 0$.[72] Rooney et al.[45] and Rebello et al.[76] reported sufficient material for cytogenetic analysis as early as 12 weeks of gestation. The small, but increasing viable cells number added to the dramatic rise in the total cell count result in a stable concentration of cells from 8–18 weeks of gestation.[77] However, the earlier the sample is taken, the fewer the number of viable cells are able to be plated and divide.[29,31] The rate of successful amniocyte cultures reported in recent series ranged from 97% to 100%.[21,22,26,36,40–42] In the CEMAT[10] trial, 2.38% of EA and 0.25% of mid-trimester amniocentesis resulted in culture failures (P < 0.001).[78] Consequently due to the culture failure, more repeat amniocentesis were required in the EA patients to obtain a cytogenetic result.[78] There were also a higher number of analyses obtained from less than standard number of cells in the EA group. This had no clinical implication, however, because no results were reported by the cytogenesis as inadequate.

The majority of series found a slightly longer average time in culture for the earlier gestations compared with traditional amniocentesis.[20,29,41,50,79] This slightly longer duration of time required for karyotype results for EA does not have clinical importance. In the harvest of cells was longer for EA (9.4 ± 2.7 days vs. 8.2 ± 2.4 days).[78]

In contrast with CVS, early amniocentesis has the advantage of a low rate of maternal cell contamination.[5] Few EA reports have encountered this cytogenetic interpretive challenge. Penso et al.[6] and Sundberg et al.[9] report a rate of 0.25%. The extended experience of the filtered EA (12.5 weeks) technique has shown a lower culture failure rate compared to CVS (11.0 weeks) and other EA reports. The chromosome preparations were considered high quality with low risk of ambiguous results.[80] The estimated frequency of maternal cell contamination in the CEMAT trial was not statistically increased in the EA (0.7%) compared with mid-trimester amniocentesis.[78] It is useful to remember that even if the proportion of maternal cells is increased in a bloody amniotic fluid specimen, the absence of visible blood does not eliminate the possibility of maternal cells in the amniotic fluid specimen.[78]

The measurement of AFP in amniotic fluid is an established method of diagnosis of neural tube defect in the second trimester. The adjunction of this measurement with EA had been assessed in few studies. The normal levels of amniotic fluid AFP in the first trimester were recently established. Levels from 11 weeks of gestation have been described by Brumfield et al.,[81] Drugan et al.,[82] and Crandall et al.;[83] they show a similar pattern to those in fetal serum, with levels rising to 13 weeks of gestation and then falling. Wathen et al.[84] showed high levels of AFP in amniotic fluid at 8 weeks, which fall rapidly up to 10 weeks after which there is a small rise.

The determination of the presence of acetylcholinesterase AChE in amniotic fluid by gel electrophoresis is a useful test in the prenatal diagnosis of open neural tube defect or fetal ventral wall defect.[85] It is useful to identify false-positive rate amniotic fluid AFP elevation.[46] Acetylcholinesterase is believed to be fetal in origin.[86] The main source is the neural tube and the level should decrease gradually after its closure at 6 weeks of gestation.[86] In Campbell's study, all samples at 8 weeks of gestation and less were positive and all samples after 12 weeks were negative.[86] There is progressive decreasing of amniotic fluid AChE between 9 and 11 gestational weeks.[86] Therefore, amniotic fluid AChE cannot be used to diagnose neural tube defects before 12 weeks of gestation.[86] Durgan et al.[82] found inconclusive results of amniotic fluid AChE up until 14 weeks of gestation. After 93 AChE determinations performed on amniotic fluid samples from 11–14 weeks of gestation (5 false-positive results), Burton et al.[85] concluded that positive results should be interpreted cautiously in EA samples.

Molecular technologies can be used for rapid determination of zygosity and common aneuploidies from amniotic fluid cells using quantitative fluorescent polymerize chain reaction following genetic amniocentesis (second trimester) in multiple pregnancies.[87] This technology could be used in the first trimester as small amniotic fluid specimens of 5 cc are required but further studies are required to confirm this consideration.

COMPLICATIONS

POST-PROCEDURE LOSS RATE

Fetal losses associated with mid-trimester standard amniocentesis were evaluated by randomized studies and are estimated at 1% (0.7% to 1.7%) (Table 35-2). The mid-trimester procedure was randomly allocated to procedure versus no procedure

TABLE 35-2	RANDOMIZED OR RECENT COHORT STUDIES WITH MID-TRIMESTER AMNIOCENTESIS GROUP TO ESTIMATE MID-TRIMESTER POST-PROCEDURE LOSS RATE			
Study		*Mid-trimester Amniocentesis*	*Compared With No.*	*Post-Mid-trimester Amnio Fetal Loss Rate*
CEMAT[10] (1998)	(R)	1,775	Early amnio (1,916)	0.8% (2.6% for EA)
Canadian Trial[8] (1992)	(R)	1,200	CVS (1,191)	0.7% (1.1% for CVS)
Tabor[88] (1986)	(R)	2,302	No procedure (2,304)	1.7% (0.7% for control)
Collins[19] (1998)	(C)	1,747	Early amnio (1207)	1.1% (2.5 for EA)
Reid[89] (1999)	(C)	3,953	No control group	0.7%
Horger[90] (2001)	(C)	4,600	No control group	0.95%

R—randomized; C—cohort.

in 1 study,[88] versus transabdominal CVS in another study,[8] and versus EA in the last study.[10]

Any other invasive technique for prenatal diagnosis should be compared with this mid-trimester amniocentesis because it remains the gold standard with respect to diagnostic reliability and the low complication rate.[22] However, different background biological factors do not allow the comparison of 2 invasive procedures performed at different gestational ages. Spontaneous miscarriage rates decrease with increasing gestational age. Fifteen to twenty percent of recognized pregnancies result in spontaneous pregnancy loss before 20 weeks of gestation.[32] In pregnancies with normal ultrasounds before 14 weeks of gestation, the total spontaneous abortion rate is 2.7%, with 1.5% occurring before 16 weeks gestation.[55] Lippman et al.[91] reported in a CVS population a total loss rate of 10 in 7% between gestational week 10 and 16, with a decrease to 3.9% between 12 and 16 weeks of gestation. Other background overall loss rates have been reported from 2.1–3.2% in ultrasound observed population.[56–58] Gilmore and Mcnay[56] reported a loss rate of up to 13.6% with advance maternal age (40 years old). Saltvedt and Almstran[92] concluded that EA (13 weeks) was followed by an increased fetal loss rate that could not be explained solely by a higher risk of spontaneous abortion at that gestational age. Thus, higher background loss rates are inherent to starting evaluation at an earlier gestational age coupled with a longer observation time.[5] Moreover, the specific etiology that causes a pregnancy to be at increased risk for fetal anomaly or aneuploidy could also lead to a higher background pregnancy loss rate.[5]

History of spontaneous or induced abortion and bleeding in the current pregnancy was associated with a substantial rise of fetal loss following amniocentesis (2.1%) and in the nonprocedure control group (1.5%) for women aged 20–34 years. The background loss rate in a population with no predisposing factors was 0.03%.[93]

The overall pregnancy loss rates and postprocedure fetal loss rates organized in randomized, partially randomized, or observational studies are summarized in the Table 35-1. Since 1987, various sized observational studies on EA have been published in the English literature reporting rates of procedure-related fetal loss from 1.4–8.1% (Table 35-1). The largest of these series was published by Eiben et al.;[22] the total fetal loss rate was 2% after 3,277 EA procedures from 10 + 4 weeks to 13 + 6 weeks compared with 1.4% in the nonrandomized control group of standard amniocentesis (14 + 0 weeks to 19 + 6 weeks). Penso et al.[6] observed a post amniocentesis loss of 2.3% which is comparable with contemporary publications. They concluded that EA is an appropriate technique for early diagnosis but is associated with an increased fetal loss rate.[6] The increased pregnancy loss was also observed by Hanson et al.[32] in a series of amniocentesis performed before 12.8 weeks (3.4%). However, postprocedural fetal loss rates are difficult to compare, because there is a gestational age bias. In an observational study, Assel et al.[31] compared EA with mid-trimester amniocentesis and found a significant increased post procedure fetal loss rate (1.8% vs. 0.4%) but discloses again

the gestational age bias. On the other hand, when EA was compared with CVS, it was reported to be associated with a higher total pregnancy loss rate (3.8% vs. 2%).[25] Brumfield et al.[23] reported an observational study that showed an increased fetal loss rate after EA compared with traditional amniocentesis (2.2% vs. 0.2%). Similar results were published by Daniel et al.[20] Although EA became more available, most authors concluded on the need for randomized trials with adequate power to evaluate safety and accuracy before providing routine EA procedures.

A prospective partially randomized study by Nicolaides et al.[18,94] disclosed a significant increased risk of spontaneous loss with EA (10–13 weeks of gestation) compared with CVS. The final report presented the results of 840 EA (278 randomized) and showed a higher rate of fetal loss after EA compared with CVS (4.9% vs. 2.1%), which was significant for pregnancies at 10–11 weeks but not significant for the 12–13 weeks gestation period. Cederholm et al.[17] reported a partially randomized prospective trial comparing EA and transabdominal CVS; all procedures were performed at 10–13 weeks of gestation, with a fetal loss rate 4 times higher in the EA group (6.8% vs. 1.7%). A fully randomized trial comparing EA and CVS reported on 581 EA and 579 CVS.[9] In this article, the amniocentesis technique involved a filter system (Sterivex DV, Millipore, Denmark) that filtered 25 mL of amniotic fluid to actually retrieve only a 1-mL specimen through a 20-gauge needle. This technique makes comparison with other studies using the standard amniocentesis technique more difficult. The results showed that EA (filter technique) is associated with a postprocedure abortion rate similar to CVS; however, the size of this study population reduced the strength of this conclusion.[9] The CEMAT study compared EA between 11 + 0 and 12 + 6 weeks with standard amniocentesis (15 + 0 to 16 + 6). This multi center randomized trial reporting on 1,916 EA procedures showed an increased total pregnancy loss (preprocedure and postprocedure losses including intrauterine and neonatal deaths) with the EA procedure (7.6% vs. 5.9; p = .012).[10]

EA between 13 + 0 to 14 + 0 weeks of gestation has not been adequately assessed; however, the results concerning EA at 11 + 0 to 12 + 6 weeks should be part of the preprocedure counseling, if the invasive prenatal diagnosis is considered to allow appropriate informed consent.

A recent randomized trial evaluated the safety and accuracy of amniocentesis and transabdominal chorionic villus sampling (CVS) performed at 11–14 weeks of gestation.[11] There were 3775 women randomized into two groups (1914 to CVS; 1861 to amniocentesis). The primary outcome measure of a composite of fetal loss plus preterm delivery before 28 weeks of gestation in cytogenetically normal fetuses was similar for both groups (2.1% for CVS vs. 2.3% for amniocentesis, p = NS). Spontaneous pregnancy losses before 20 weeks and procedure-related indicated termination appeared increased in the amniocentesis groups (RR 1.74.95%, CI 0.94, 3.22, p = .07). There was a 4.65 fold increase in the rate of talipes equinovarus after early amniocentesis (95% CI 1.01, 21.5, p = 0.17). The study concluded that amniocentesis at 13 weeks carries a significantly increased risk of talipes equinovarus compared with CVS and a possible increase in early, unintended pregnancy loss.

POSTPROCEDURE AMNIOTIC FLUID LEAKAGE

Besides fetal loss, additional complications have been reported as being directly related to an invasive prenatal diagnosis procedure. Leakage of amniotic fluid after the amniocentesis procedure is concerning because of the risk for infection, miscarriage, preterm labor/delivery, and fetal neonatal complications. The reported incidence varies from 0–4.6% (Table 35-1). Penso et al.[6] reported 40% fetal loss after leakage of amniotic fluid in 407 EA procedures. A similar rate of fetal loss after 936 EA procedures at less than 12.8 weeks was also reported by Hansen et al.[32] Brumfield et al.[23] reported a 2.9% incidence of leakage and this was found to be significantly higher compared with 0.2% in the cohort control group of mid-trimester amniocentesis. This post procedural complication contributed to a 22% fetal loss rate. Cederholm et al.[17] described the highest rate of postprocedure leakage (7.5%) in a partially randomized series of 147 EA procedures compared with 174 transabdominal CVS (7.5% vs. 1.1%). The CEMAT study reported an increased rate of fluid leakage that was statistically significant before 22 weeks of gestation when EA were compared with standard amniocentesis (3.5% vs. 1.7%).[10]

A review paper evaluated thirteen recent studies of amniotic fluid leakage following amniocentesis. There were 17,136 amniocentesis and 280 cases of amniotic fluid leakage for an incidence of 1.6%. Factors such as gestational age of less than 15 weeks and avoiding the placenta were found to increase the risk. Conservative management with bed rest was found to be useful in allowing the leakage site to seal. Amnio patch technique was also considered.[95]

MUSCULOSKELETAL

The smaller amounts of amniotic fluid and the gestational age dependant extraembryonic coelome separating the amnion and the chorion membranes are a major concern, if prenatal diagnosis is required in fetuses at less than 15 gestational weeks.[53] The total volume of amniotic fluid is limited to 30–50 mL at around 12 gestational weeks.[63] The vulnerability of the fetal lungs and extremities after removal of up to 50% of the amniotic volume and the effects on the fetus if the amniotic membrane collapses are known.[53] Many reports have suggested an association between EA and congenital abnormalities (Table 35-3). The lower limb extremity appears to have increased susceptibility with temporary disturbances from a diminution in intraamniotic volume.[22] A randomized study of second trimester amniocentesis has shown that the incidence of talipes (0.8%) was not significantly different from controls that did not have invasive testing.[88] Penso et al.[6] 2.2% of orthopedic postural deformity including 4 club feet, 1 hyperextended knee, 1 scoliosis, 1 congenital dislocation of the hip, and 1 of the knee. Three pregnancies (38%) had leakage of amniotic fluid.[6] Nevin

| TABLE 35-3 | EARLY AMNIOCENTESIS: ASSOCIATED MUSCULOSKELETAL AND RESPIRATORY COMPLICATIONS | | | | | |

Randomized Studies	No.	Needle Size	Volume AF(mL)	Complications Leakage AF %	Musculoskeletal %	Respiratory %
EATA[11] (2004)	1,820	22	12–14	9.7	1.5	0.4
CEMAT[10] (1998)	1,916	22	11	4.6	1.3	—
Sunberg[9] (1997)	518	20	25 filtered	2.4	2.4	0.9
Johnson[15] (1996)	344	22	11	2.1	1.2	2
Partially randomized studies						
Nagel[16] (1998)	130	22	11	—	3.1	—
Cederholm[17] (1997)	147	20	10	7.5	0	—
Nicolaides[18] (1996)	840	20	11	—	1.6	—
Observational studies						
Yoon[96] (2001)	980	22	11–12	—	1.1	—
Tharmaratnam[97] (1998)	412	22	7		1.6	2.7
Eiben[22] (1997)	3,277	22	3–6	1.1	0.4	—
Henry[30] (1992)	1,805	22	11–17	1.7	0.5	—
Hanson[32] (1992)	879	22	12–15	1.1	<0.4	—
Hackett[36] (1991)	106	20	10–18	1	2.0	—
Nevin[42] (1990)	222	20	2–17	—	0.5	—
Penson[6] (1990)	407	22	12–15	2.6	2.2	6.1

AF—amniotic fluid.

et al.[42] described a single case of bilateral talipes equinovarus (0.5%) in their 222 EA procedures. Hackett et al.[36] identified 4 congenital anomalies from their series of 62 EA procedures; 2 were positional talipes. Eiben et al.[22] reported an incidence of 0.4% of hip dislocation and talipes. Sundberg et al.[9] reported a higher rate of talipes equinovarus after filtered EA compared with CVS in a randomized trial but the number of EA procedures were not sufficient to allow definitive conclusion.[22] The 2 congenital anomalies mentioned in the Cederholm and Axelsson[17] study did not involve the musculoskeletal system (large hemangioma on the trunk, cleft palate). Nicolaides' partially randomized trial showed a higher incidence of talipes equinovarus in the EA group (1.66%) than in the CVS group (0.48%), but this difference was not statistically significant.[18] The partially randomized trial of Nagel et al.[16] comparing EA and transabdominal CVS had to be terminated early because of an unintended increased fetal loss rate and substantially more frequent incidence of talipes [3.1% (0.8–7.7%)]. The CEMAT[10] trial showed a significant increased rate of a foot anomaly (1.3% vs. 0.1%; $p = 001$) for EA from 11 + 0 week to 12 + 0.

EATA[11] study found a 4.65 fold increase in talips with amniocentesis during week 13 of pregnancy. Yoon et al.[96] reviewed a non randomized cohort following EA and found a 1.1% incidence of talips. Tharmaratnam et al.[97] reported a rate of fixed flexion deformities of 1.6%. Their conclusion was that there is a positive association with the amount of amniotic fluid removed and the rate of musculoskeletal deformities.[97]

An orthopedic review group hypothesized that the foot deformities are secondary to decreased fetal movement during a key phase in foot and ankle development.[98]

Even before the evaluation of EA, there have been concerns of possible lung complications related to traditional amniocentesis.[67] Some suboptimal lung growth and development have been demonstrated in a monkey model.[98] Milner et al.[99] compared immediate neonatal lung function tests in 39 full-term babies that had had an amniocentesis in the second trimester with 43 unexposed babies. Their results showed a significantly lower dynamic compliance of the lungs and an increased resistance in the group exposed to amniocentesis.[99] The incidence of respiratory difficulties in newborns after EA varies from 1%[30] to 6.1%.[6] Calhoun et al.[101] reported on a prospective controlled pilot study evaluating short-term complications of EA versus mid-trimester amniocentesis. They identified a clinically but not significant difference in pulmonary complications between the EA group and the standard group.[101] Tharmaratnam et al.[97] reported a series of 404 EA procedures; the incidence of respiratory problems at birth was 2.7% after removing only 7 mL of amniotic fluid. These results for lung complications were comparable with other studies.[97] Recently, Greenough et al.[102] evaluated the impact of EA and CVS on respiratory morbidity in very young children. The functional residual capacity was higher as well as the number of chest-related hospital admissions for the EA group compared with the control group.[102] They concluded that first trimester procedures are associated with increased respiratory morbidity in children within their first year of life.[102]

OTHER POSSIBLE FINDINGS FOLLOWING AMNIOCENTESIS

Evidence of bacterial and viral organisms present in the amniotic fluid at the time of second trimester amniocentesis has been reported.[103,104] In 22 consecutive asymptomatic women with intact membranes at mid gestation, 3 (13.6%) specimens found chlamydia trachomatis (2) and corynebacterium group (1).[104] Preexisting intrauterine viral infections were identified in 8% of post amniocentesis losses within 30 days of procedure and 15% of matched controls without pregnancy loss. Adenovirus was present in both groups while cytomegalovirus was found in only the control group. The conclusion was that the presence of virus in second trimester amniotic fluid is not significantly associated with elevated IL-6 levels or with early post amniocentesis pregnancy loss.[103] These infection studies have not been evaluated in the first trimester.

Reports of amniocentesis fetal needle trauma at second trimester are rare with the use of continuous ultrasound guidance.[105,106] These risks may be present in first trimester as well.

A secondary analysis[107] of the EATA Trial[11] identified an observation that focal disruption of the placenta at 13–14 weeks may increase the risk of hypertension/preeclampsia. These findings provide support for the theory that disturbances in early placentation lead subsequently to maternal hypertension.[107]

CONCLUSION

Over the years, many observational studies and partially randomized and randomized trials had shown that early amniocentesis can be performed effectively. The results are generally compared with a mid-trimester amniocentesis at a comparable time. This technique, attractive because of a shorter learning curve, the availability, the low rate of maternal-cell contamination, and the early gestational timing, has been performed widely in many centers. During this last decade, more and more articles have started to raise questions about the safety of the EA procedure. The increased rate of post procedure fetal loss was often explained by many authors to be due to the early timing of the procedure compared with the standard amniocentesis. Recently, multicenter randomized trials (CEMAT[10]; EATA[11]) comparing EA and mid-trimester amniocentesis and late chorionic villus sampling reported statistically and clinically significant results. The CEMAT[10] study showed the EA group to have a total pregnancy loss to be significantly higher, a significant increased incidence of musculoskeletal foot deformities, an increased culture failure rate, and an increased post-amniocentesis rate of leakage when compared with standard mid-trimester amniocentesis. The EATA[11] study showed an increased risk of talips with amniocentesis at 13 weeks gestation and possible increased pregnancy loss. These results should certainly be part of any pre-procedure counseling when EA procedure is considered. There is still the need to evaluate early amniocentesis between 14 + 0 to 14 + 6 weeks.

References

1. Riis P, Fuchs F. Antenatal determination of foetal sex in the prevention of hereditary diseases. *Lancet*. 2:180–12.
2. Steele MW, Berg WR. Chromosome analysis of human amniotic fluid cells. *Lancet*. 1966;1:383–35.
3. Jacobson CS, Barter RH. Intrauterine diagnosis and management of genetic defects. *Am J Obstet Gynecol*. 1967;99:795–807.
4. Wilson RD. Early amniocentesis: a clinical review. *Prenat Diagn*. 1995;15:1259–12.
5. Penso CA, Frigoletto FD. Early amniocentesis. *Semin Perinatol*. 1990;14:465–40.
6. Penso CA, Sanstrom MM, Garber MF, et al. Early amniocentesis: report of 407 cases with neonatal follow-up. *Obstet Gynecol*. 1990;76:1032–1016.
7. Crandall BF, Kulch P, Tabsh K. Risk assessment of amniocentesis between 11 and 15 weeks: compared to later amniocentesis controls. *Prenat Diagn*. 1994;14:913–919.
8. Canadian Multicentre Randomized Clinical Trial of Chorionic villus Sampling and Amniocentesis. Final report. *Prenat Diagn*. 1992;12:3876–4476.
9. Sundberg K, Bang J, Smidt-Jensen S, et al. Randomized study of risk of fetal loss related to early amniocentesis versus chorionic villus sampling. *Lancet*. 1997;350:697–703.
10. The Canadian Early and Mid-trimester Amniocentesis Trial (CEMAT) Group. Randomized trial to assess safety and fetal outcome of early and mid-trimester amniocentesis. *Lancet*. 1998;351:242–247.
11. Philip J, Silver RK, Wilson RD, et al. Late first trimester invasive prenatal diagnosis results of an international randomized trial. *Obstet Gynecol*. 2004;103:1164–1173.
12. Alfirevic Z. Early amniocentesis versus transabdominal chorion villus sampling for prenatal diagnosis. (Cochrane Review) In: The Cochrane Database of Systemic Reviews, The Cochrane Library, The Cochrane Collaboration, 2003.
13. Jauniaux E, Pahal GS, Rodeck CH. What invasive procedure to use in early pregnancy? [Review] *Best Practice and Research in Clinical Obstetrics and Gynecol*. 2000;14(4):651–662.
14. Nanal R, Kyle P, Soothill PW. A classification of pregnancy losses after invasive prenatal diagnostic procedures: an approach to allow comparison of units with a different case mix. *Prenat Diagn*. 2003;23:488–492.
15. Johnson J, Wilson RD, Windsor E, et al. The early amniocentesis study: a randomized clinical trial of early amniocentesis versus mid-trimester amniocentesis. *Fetal Diagn Ther*. 1996;11:85–93.
16. Nagel HT, Vandenbussche FP, Keirse MJ, et al. Amniocentesis before 14 completed weeks as an alternative to transabdominal chorionic villus sampling: a controlled trial with infant follow-up. *Prenat Diagn*. 1998;18:465–475.
17. Cederholm M, Axelsson O. A prospective comparative study on transabdominal chorionic villus sampling and amniocentesis performed at 10–13 weeks' gestation. *Prenat Diagn*. 1997;17:411–417.
18. Nicolaides K, de Lourdes Brizot M, Patel F, et al. Comparison of chorion villus sampling and early amniocentesis for karyotyping in 1,492 singleton pregnancies. *Fetal Diagn Ther*. 1996;11:9–15.
19. Collins VR, Webley C, Sheffield LJ, et al. Fetal outcome and maternal morbidity after early amniocentesis. *Prenat Diagn*. 1998;18:767–772.
20. Daniel A, HG A, Kuah KB, et al. A study of early amniocentesis for prenatal cytogenetic diagnosis. *Prenat Diagn*. 1998;18:21–28.
21. Jorgensen C, Andolf E. Amniocentesis before the 15th gestational week in single and twin gestations: complications and quality of genetic analysis. *Acta Obstet Gynecol Scand*. 1998;77:151–154.
22. Eiben B, Hammons W, Nanson S, et al. On the complication risk of early amniocentesis versus standard amniocentesis. *Fetal Diagn Ther*. 1997;12:140–144.
23. Brumfield CG, Lin S, Conner W, et al. Pregnancy outcome following genetic amniocentesis at 11–14 versus 16–19 weeks gestation. *Obstet Gynecol*. 1996;88:114–118.
24. Diaz Vega M, de la Cueva, Leal C, et al. Early amniocentesis at 10–12 weeks gestation. *Prenat Diagn*. 16:307–312.
25. Shulman LP, Elias S, Phillips OP, et al. Amniocentesis performed at 14 weeks' gestation or earlier: comparison with first trimester transabdominal chorionic villus sampling. *Obstet Gynecol*. 83:543–548.
26. Eiben B, Goebel R, Hansen S, et al. Early amniocentesis: a cytogenetic evaluation of over 1,500 cases. *Prenat Diagn*. 1994;14:497–501.
27. Eiben B, Goebel R, Rutt G, et al. Early amniocentesis between the 12th–14th week of pregnancy: clinical experiences with 1100 cases. *Geburtshilfe Frauenhelkd*. 1993;53:538–554.
28. Kerber S, Held KR. Early genetic amniocentesis: 4 years experience. *Prenat Diagn*. 1993;12:21–27.
29. Djalali M, Barbi G, Kennerknecht L, et al. Introduction of early amniocentesis to routine prenatal diagnosis. *Prenat Diagn*. 1992;12:661–669.
30. Henry GP, Miller WA. Early amniocentesis. *J Reprod Med*. 37:396–402.
31. Assel BG, Lewis SM, Dickerman LH, et al. Single operator comparison of early and mid-second trimester amniocentesis. *Obstet Gynecol*. 1992;79:940–944.
32. Hanson FW, Tennant F, Hune S, et al. Early amniocentesis: outcome, risks, and technical problems at ≤12.8 weeks. *Am J Obstet Gynecol*. 166:1707–1711.
33. Sato M, Witt D. Early amniocentesis: prospective follow-up of 604 cases. *Am J Hum Genet*. 1991;49:230.
34. Shulman LP, Elias S, Simpson JL. Early amniocentesis: complications in initial 150 cases compared to complications in initial 150 cases of transabdominal chorionic villus sampling. *Am J Hum Genet*. 1991;49:231.
35. Nevin J, Nevin NC, Dorman JC, et al. Early amniocentesis: clinical and cytogenetic evaluation of 500 cases. *Am J Hum Genet*. 1991;49:226.
36. Hackett GA, Smith JH, Rebello MT, et al. Early amniocentesis at 11–14 weeks' gestation for the diagnosis of fetal chromosomal abnormality: a clinical evaluation. *Prenat Diagn*. 1991;11:311–315.
37. Klapp J, Nicolaides KH, Hager HD, et al. Examinations in regards to early amniocentesis. *Geburtshilfe Frauenheilkd*. 1990;50:443–446.
38. Lindner C, Huneke B, Masson D, et al. Early amniocentesis for prenatal diagnosis. *Geburshilfe Frauenheilkd*. 1990;50:954–958.
39. Thayer B, Braddock B, Spitzer K, et al. Clinical and laboratory experience with early amniocentesis. *Birth Defects Original Article Series*. 1990;26:58–63.
40. Stripparo L, Buscaglia M, Longatti L, et al. Genetic amniocentesis: 505 cases performed before the sixteenth week of gestation. *Prenat Diagn*. 1990;10:359–364.
41. Elejalde BR, de Elejalde MM, Acuna JA, et al. Prospective study of amniocentesis performed between weeks 9 and 16 of gestation:

its feasibility, risks, complications and use in early genetic prenatal diagnosis. *Am J Med Genet*. 1990;35:188–196.

42. Nevin J, Nevin N, Dornan J, et al. Early amniocentesis: experience of 222 consecutive patients. *Prenat Diagn*. 1990;1:79–83.

43. Hanson F, Happ R, Tennant F, et al. Ultrasonography guided early amniocentesis in singleton pregnancies. *Am J Obstet Gynecol*. 1990;162:1376–1383.

44. Evans MI, Drugan A, Kopitch III FC, et al. Genetic diagnosis in the first trimester: the norm for the 1990's. *Am J Obstet Gynecol*. 1989;160:1332–1336.

45. Rooney DE, MacLachlan N, Smith J, et al. Early amniocentesis: a cytogenetic evaluation. *Br Med J*. 1989;299:25.

46. Benacerraf BR, Greene MF, Saltzman DH, et al. Early amniocentesis for prenatal cytogenetic evaluation. *Radiology*. 1988;169:709–710.

47. Johnson A, Godmilow L. Genetic amniocentesis at 14 weeks or less. *Clin Obstet Gynecol*. 1988;31:345–351.

48. Godmilow L, Weiner S, Dunn L. Genetic amniocentesis performed between 12 and 14 weeks gestation. *Am J Hum Genet*. 1987;41:818.

49. Miller W, Davies R, Thayer B, et al. Success, safety and accuracy of early amniocentesis. *Am J Hum Genet*. 1987;41:835.

50. Hanson FW, Zorn Em, Tennant FR, et al. Amniocentesis before 15 weeks' gestation: outcome, risks and technical problems. *Am J Obstet Gynecol*. 1987;156:1524–1531.

51. Moore KL, Persaud TVN. *The Developing Human*. 6th ed. Philadelphia, PA: WB Saunders; 1998:40–55.

52. Wilson RD. An evaluation of early amniocentesis. *J Soc Obstet Gynaecol*. 1996;18:773–785.

53. Smidt-Jensen S, Sundberg K. Early amniocentesis. *Curr Opin Obstet Gynecol*. 1995;7:117–121.

54. Sundberg K, Jorgensen FS, Tabor A, et al. Experience with early amniocentesis. *J Perinatol Med*. 1995;23:149–158.

55. Liu DTY, Jesvons B, Preston C, et al. A prospective study of spontaneous miscarriage in ultrasonically normal pregnancies and relevance to chorion villus sampling. *Prenat Diagn*. 1987;7:223–227.

56. Gilmore DH, Mcnay MB. Spontaneous fetal loss rate in early pregnancy. *Lancet*. 1985;I:107.

57. Wilson RD, Kendrick E, Wittmann BK, et al. Risk of spontaneous abortions in ultrasonically normal pregnancies. *Lancet*. 1984;II:920–921.

58. National Institute of Child Health and Human Development. National registry for amniocentesis for prenatal diagnosis: safety and accuracy. *JAMA*. 1976;236:1471–1476.

59. Yang YH, Ju KS, Kim SB, et al. The Korean collaborative study of 11,00 prenatal genetic amniocentesis. *Yonsei Med*. 1999;40:460–466.

60. Roper EC, Konje JC, DeChazal RC, et al. Genetic amniocentesis: gestation-specific pregnancy outcome and comparison of outcome following early and traditional amniocentesis. *Prenat Diagn*. 19:803–807.

61. American College of Obstetricians and Gynecologists Committee on Practice Bulletins-Obstetrics. ACOG Practice Bulletin. Clinical Management Guidelines for Obstetricians-Gynecologist: prenatal diagnosis of fetal chromosomal abnormalities. *Obstet & Gynecol*. 2001;97(5 pt 1):suppl 1–12.

62. Kucun CC, Harrigan JT, Canterino JC, et al. Changing trends in patient decisions concerning genetic amniocentesis. *Am J Obstet Gynecol*. 2000;182:10118–10120.

63. Cederholm M, Axelsson O, Sjoden PO. Women's knowledge, concerns and psychological reactions before undergoing an invasive procedure for prenatal karyotyping. *Ultra Obstet Gynecol*. 1999;14:267–272.

64. Cedarholm M, Sjoden PO, Axelsson O. Psychological distress before and prenatal invasive karyotyping. *Acta Obstet Gynecol Scand*. 2001;80:539–545.

65. Caron L, Tihy F, Dallaire L. Frequencies of chromosomal abnormalities at amniocentesis: over 20 years of cytogenetic analyses in one laboratory. *Am J Med Genet*. 1999;82:149–154.

66. Waters JJ, Waters KS. Trends in cytogenetic prenatal diagnosis in the UK: results from UKNEQAS external audit, 1987–1998. *Prenatal Diagn*. 1999;19:1023–1026.

67. Wilson RD, Johnson J, Windrim R, et al. The early amniocentesis study: a randomized clinical trial of early amniocentesis and mid-trimester amniocentesis. *Fetal Diagn Ther*. 1997;12:97–101.

68. Johnson JM, Wilson RD, Singer J, et al. Technical factors in early amniocentesis predict adverse outcome: results of the Canadian Early (EA) vs Mid-trimester (MA) Amniocentesis trial. *Prenat Diagn*. 1999;19:732–738.

69. Creasy RK, Resnik R. *Maternal-Fetal Medicine*. 4th ed. Philadelphia, PA: WB Saunders; 1999;56–57.

70. Bravo RR, Shulman LP, Philips OP, et al. Transplacental needle passage in early amniocentesis and pregnancy loss. *Obstet Gynecol*. 1995;86:437–440.

71. Tharmaratnam S, Sadek S, Steele EK, et al. Transplacental early amniocentesis and pregnancy outcome. *Br J Obstet Gynaecol*. 1998;105:228–230.

72. Jorgensen FS, Band J, Lind AM, et al. Genetic amniocentesis at 7–14 weeks. *Prenat Diagn*. 1992;12:277–283.

73. Robinson JN, Loeffler HH, Norwitz ER. A syringe adapter to facilitate aspiration at amniocentesis. *Obstet Gynecol*. 2000;96(1):138–140.

74. van Schoubroeck D, Verhaeghe J. Does local anesthesia at mid-trimester amniocentesis decrease pain experience? a randomized trial in 220 patients. *Ultrasound Obstet Gynecol*. 2000;16:536–538.

75. Fischer RL, Bianculli KW, Sehdex H, et al. Does light pressure effleurage reduced pain and anxiety associated with genetic amniocentesis? a randomized clinical trial. *J Matern Fetal Med*. 2000;9:294–297.

76. Rebello MT, Gray CTH, Rooney DE, et al. Cytogenetic studies of amniotic fluid taken before the 15th week of pregnancy for earlier prenatal diagnosis: a report of 114 consecutive cases. *Prenat Diagn*. 11:35–40.

77. Byrne D, Azar G, Nicolaides K. Why cell culture is successful after early amniocentesis. *Fetal Diagn Ther*. 1991;6:84–86.

78. Winsor EJ, Tomkins DJ, Dalousek D, et al. Cytogenetic aspects of the Canadian Early Med-Trimester Amniocentesis fluid trial (CEMAT). *Prenat Diagn*. 1999;19:620–627.

79. Lockwood DH, Neu RL. Cytogenetic analysis of 1375 amniotic fluid specimens from pregnancies with gestational age less than 14 weeks. *Prenat Diagn*. 1993;13:801–805.

80. Sundberg K, Lundsteen C, Philip J. Comparison cell cultures, chromosome quality and karyotypes obtained after chorionic villus sampling and early amniocentesis with filter technique. *Prenat Diagn*. 1999;19:12–16.

81. Brumfield CG, Cloud GA, Davis RO, et al. The relationship between maternal serum and amniotic fluid alphafetoprotein in women undergoing early amniocentesis. *Am J Obstet Gynecol*. 1990;163:903–906.

82. Drugan A, Syner FN, Greb A, et al. Amniocentesis fluid alphafetoprotein and acetylcholinesterase in early genetic amniocentesis. *Obstet Gynecol*. 1988;72:35–38.

83. Crandall BF, Hanson FW, Tennant F, et al. Alpha-fetoprotein levels in amniotic fluid between 11 and 15 weeks. *Am J Obstet Gynecol*. 1989;160:1204–1206.

84. Wathen NC, Peter LC, Campbell DJ, et al. Early amniocentesis: Alphafetoprotein levels in amniotic fluid, extraembryonic coelomic fluid and maternal serum between 8 and 13 weeks. *Br J Obstet Gynecol*. 1991;98:866–870.

85. Burton BK, Lewis HN, Pettenati MJ. False-positive acetylcholinesterase with early amniocentesis. *Obstet Gynecol*. 1989;74:607–610.

86. Campbell J, Cass P, Warhen N, et al. First-trimester amniotic fluid and extraembryonic coelomic fluid acetylcholinesterase electrophoresis. *Prenat Diagn*. 1992;12:609–612.

87. Chen CP, Chern SR, Wang W. Rapid determination of zygosity and common aneuploidies from amniotic fluid cells using quantitative fluorescent polymerase chain reaction following genetic amniocentesis in multiple pregnancies. *Hum Reprod.* 2000;15:929–934.

88. Tabor A, Philip J, Madsen M, et al. Randomized controlled trial of genetic amniocentesis in 4,606 low risk women. *Lancet.* 1986;I:1287–1293.

89. Reid KP, Gurrin LC, Dickinson JE, et al. Pregnancy loss rates following second trimester genetic amniocentesis. *Aust N Z J Obstet Gynecol.* 1999;39:281–285.

90. Horger EO, Finch H, Vincent VA. A single physician's experience with four thousand six hundred genetic amniocenteses. *Am J Obstet Gynecol.* 2001;185:279–288.

91. Lippman A, Vekemans MJ, Perry TB. Fetal mortality at the time of chorionic villi sampling. *Hum Genet.* 1984;68:337–338.

92. Saltvedt S, Almstrom H. Fetal loss rate after second trimester amniocentesis at different gestational age. *Act Obstet Gynecol Scand.* 1999;78:10–14.

93. Antsaklis A, Papantoiou N, Xygakis A, et al. Genetic amniocentesis in women 20–34 years old: associates risks. *Prenat Diagn.* 2000;29:247–250.

94. Nicolaides K, deLourdes Brizot M, Patel F, et al. Comparison of chorionic villous sampling and amniocentesis for fetal karyotyping at 10–13 weeks' gestation. *Lancet.* 1994;344:435–439.

95. Abboud P, Zejli A, Mansour G, et al. Amniotic fluid leakage and premature rupture of membranes after amniocentesis: a review of the literature. *J Gynecol Obstet Biol Reprod.* 2000;29:741–745.

96. Yoon G, Chernos J, Sibbald B, et al. Association Between Amniocentesis and Congenital Foot Anomalies (abstract). Department of Medical Genetics, Department of Obstetrics and Gynecology, Alberta Congenital Anomalies Surveillance System (ACASS), University of Calgary.

97. Tharmaratnam S, Sadex S, Steele EK, et al. Early amniocentesis: effect of removing a reduced volume of amniotic fluid on pregnancy outcome. *Prenat Diagn.* 1998;18:773–778.

98. Tredwell SJ, Wilson RD, Wilmink MA, et al. Review of the effect of early amniocentesis on foot deformity in the neonate. *J Pediatr Orthop.* 2001;21:636–641.

99. Hislop A, Fairweather DV. Amniocentesis and lung growth: an animal experiment with clinical implications. *Lancet.* 1982:II:1271–1272.

100. Milner AD, Hoskyns EW, Hopkin IE. The effects of mid-trimester amniocentesis on lung function in the neonatal period. *Eur J Pediatr.* 1992;151:458–460.

101. Calhoun BC, Brehm W, Bombard AT. Early genetic amniocentesis and its relationship to respiratory difficulties in pediatric patients: a report of findings in patients and matched controls 3–5 years postprocedure. *Prenat Diagn.* 1994;14:209–212.

102. Greenough A, Yuksel B, Maik S, et al. First trimester invasive procedures: effects on symptom status and lung volume in very young children. *Pediatr Pulmonol.* 1997;22:415–422.

103. Wenstrom KD, Andrews WW, Bowles NE, et al. Intrauterine viral infection at the time of second trimester genetic amniocentesis. *Obstet Gynecol.* 1998;92:420–422.

104. Mandar R, Livukene K, Ehrenberg A, et al. Amniotic fluid microflora in asymptomatic women at mid-gestation. *Scand J Infect Dis.* 2001;33(1):60–62.

105. Cambiaghi S, Restano L, Cavalli R, et al. Skin dimpling as a consequence of amniocentesis. *J Am Acad Dermatol.* 1998;39(5 pt 2):888–890.

106. Squier M, Chamberlain P, Zaiwalla Z, et al. Five cases of brain injury following amniocentesis in mid-term pregnancy. *Dev Med Child Neurol.* 2000;42:554–560.

107. Silver RK, Wilson RD, Philip J, et al. Late first trimester placental disruption and subsequent gestational hypertension/preeclampsia. *Obstet Gynecol.* 2005;105:587–592.

CHAPTER 36

CHORIONIC VILLUS SAMPLING

Mark I. Evans / Guy Rosner / Yuval Yaron / Ronald J. Wapner

Since the development of amniocentesis more than 30 years ago, there has been a constant desire to move prenatal diagnosis to as early in gestation as possible.[1] In the mid-1980s, the combination of increasingly sophisticated ultrasound and laboratory cytogenetic advances made first trimester sampling of chorionic villi possible. Two decades of experience have now shown that chorionic villus sampling (CVS), in experienced hands, is both safe and effective (Fig. 36-1). Despite allegations in the early 1990s of increased risk of birth defects[2,3] now clearly disproved at the usual gestational ages by objective data (although still disputed by some), CVS gained rapid acceptance, then decline, and now re-acceptance in prenatal diagnosis in the hands of experienced operators.

In the 1980s, several US and European centers began performing CVS for the purpose of prenatal diagnosis in the clinical setting. Multiple single institutions and collaborative papers documented its accuracy and safety. Following the 1990 FDA approval of the Trophocan[TM] catheter (Concord/Portex; Keene, New Hampshire) for use in transcervical CVS, an increasing number of US physicians began offering the procedure. To obtain privileges to perform CVS, some states enacted legislation requiring the performance of 50 CVS procedures in pregnancies in which the patient has already chosen first trimester abortion.[1] This practice has not always been feasible because of the controversies already surrounding elective abortion, or because of the increased medical costs if this experience were acquired in a hospital setting. Other states and hospitals had no guidelines at all, which resulted in physicians performing the procedure without guidance and experience of trained operators.

INDICATIONS

The most common indications for CVS are advanced maternal age, and a biochemical or molecularly diagnosable genetic disorder abnormalities. Over the last decade, nuchal translucency (NT) measurement in the first trimester has become a routine in many centers worldwide (see Chapter 23). Increased NT in the first trimester has been shown to be a prognostic marker of fetal aneuploidy as well as structural anomalies.[4] The risk for fetal trisomy increases with NT, and that NT of 3, 4, 5, and >6 mm are associated with a 4-fold, 21-fold, 26-fold, and 41-fold increase, respectively, in the maternal age-related risks for trisomies 21, 18, and 13.[5] Over the last few years, combined first trimester screening has been employed, using first trimester NT and maternal serum pregnancy associated plasma protein A (PAPP-A) and free $\tilde{\beta}$-hCG.[6-8] This combined screening strategy is estimated to achieve a DS detection rate of 80–85% for a 5% false positive rate.[9] The test may be performed at 11–13 weeks of gestation, and screen positive patients may be offered CVS. Other general indications have been reviewed elsewhere and will not be repeated here.

With the exception of those patients whose primary risk is for a neural tube defect, any patient considered a candidate for amniocentesis could be offered CVS if they are seen in the first trimester. CVS has the advantage of earlier diagnosis, allowing earlier intervention when mandated guaranteeing privacy in reproductive choices. While we used to check routinely at 9–10 weeks, we generally attempt to schedule patients interested in CVS to be seen at 11–12 weeks gestational age in order to obtain translucency measurements at the same time. If an abnormality is found, they may choose to terminate by the safer, easier, quicker, and cheaper suction method rather than techniques used in the second trimester, which are more expensive, have higher complication rates, and are without privacy as often many of the pregnant status of the patient becomes obvious.

MULTIPLE GESTATIONS

CVS can be performed in the setting of multiple gestations if separate, discrete placentas are clearly identified. Twins are the most common multiple gestation even in the era of assisted reproductive technologies (ARTs). We commonly perform CVS in higher order multiples prior to fetal reduction, but usually sample only the 2 or 3 fetuses likely to be kept. Placental and fetal locations must be meticulously noted in order to avoid the issues of mis-identification and of sampling 1 twin twice, and the other not at all (Fig. 36-2). Operators performing transcervical/transcervical CVS may run the risk of cross-contamination of samples. With twins, a transabdominal/transcervical CVS or transabdominal/transabdominal dual CVS procedure can commonly be performed to minimize cytogenetic contamination.

In the setting of a "vanishing twin," which may occur in up to 3% of pregnancies,[10] studies suggest an increased risk of aneuploidy in the remaining placental tissue of the "vanished twin".[11] Therefore, care must be taken during sampling if only the remaining twin is being evaluated.

PROCEDURE

After counseling, the next step is the ultrasound evaluation. First, fetal viability is confirmed. About 7% of patients are discovered to have a blighted ovum or an embryonic/fetal demise.[12] Fetal size discrepancies should also be noted. Of significant concern is the smaller-than-expected fetus, even in the first trimester. We have found that such fetuses are at increased risk for aneuploidy,[13,14] and that such cases merit CVS to shorten the time to diagnosis.

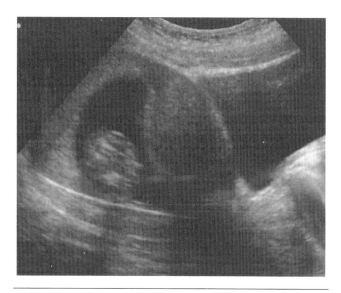

FIGURE 36-1 CVS ultrasound—transcervical.

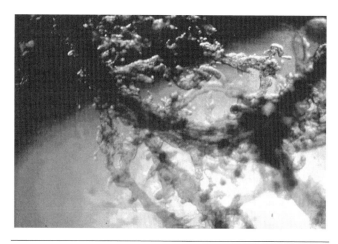

FIGURE 36-3 Villi in dish.

Appropriate dating of the pregnancy is of particular importance in some cases of prenatal diagnosis by DNA studies. Some disorders such as fragile X syndrome or other diseases diagnosed by Southern blot may require larger amounts of tissue (20–40 mg), compared to PCR-based diagnosis (Fig. 36-3). If the indication for CVS is such that requires large amounts of tissue, we prefer to schedule the patient at 11–12 weeks gestation because the placental mass is generally larger, and multiple passes may be necessary to obtain sufficient material for DNA extraction and analysis.

Placental evaluation is of utmost importance in properly assessing patients for transcervical CVS. In general, placental location determines whether the approach will be transcervical or transabdominal. For most cases, this decision will be straightforward. If the placenta is low-lying and posterior, a transcervical approach is appropriate. Such cases are easier to perform and may be attempted by novices under guidance.

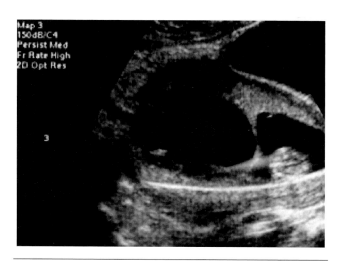

FIGURE 36-2 Twin CVS ultrasound.

If the placenta is anterior and fundal, an abdominal approach is usually indicated. The placenta can sometimes be maneuvered into a vertical configuration by judicious manipulation of bladder volume. There is wide variation among operators in the percentage of cases done cervically versus abdominally. In general, it is easier for less experienced physicians to do transabdominally because of their prior amniocentesis experience. However, most patients prefer an experience akin to a pap smear rather than a needle. It is critical that operators be able to perform both methods.

Other factors must be considered before attempting CVS. At times the patient gives a history of genital herpes simplex or a recent group B streptococcus (GBS) infection. Such cases should be individualized, and the small or theoretical risk of introducing an infection into the fetal-placental tissues should be discussed with the patient. Transabdominal CVS (TA-CVS) or amniocentesis are usually offered when a significant risk of active GBS is present as data are in favor that uterine infection in such cases might occur almost entirely after transcervical aspiration.[15,16] Additionally, because of the possibility of GBS septic abortion after transcervical CVS procedure (TC-CVS) in known GBS carriers, prophylactic antibiotic therapy may be advocated prior to TC-CVS in such selected cases. Silverman et al.[16] have showed, however, that CVS was associated with a low rate of post CVS bacteremia (4.1% after TC-CVS compared to none after TA-CVS). Additionally, although catheter tips used for TC-CVS yielded positive cultures in as much as 16.3% of procedures, the actual rate of bacteremia was much lower. Baumann et al. compared cervical bacterial carrier status in women performing TC-CVS and TA-CVS and its implications on pregnancy outcome.[17] They reported an increased incidence of miscarriages in the TC-CVS group where bacteria/yeast or mycoplasma were found in cervical cultures. In comparison, none of the miscarriages after TA-CVS was associated with bacterial- or fungal-positive cervical cultures other than mycoplasma. The authors concluded that regarding TA-CVS positive cervical mycoplasma culture might be associated with late miscarriage (greater than 2 weeks post procedure). The choice of whether to perform TA-CVS or TC-CVS should be made according to the experienced operator's judgment, based on the previously described conditions and in accordance with the patient's bacterial/fungal cervical carrier status.

SAFETY

Over the past 2 decades, multiple reports from individual centers have demonstrated the safety and low rates of pregnancy loss following CVS.[18–23] In experienced centers, the total rate of miscarriage from the time of CVS until 28 weeks' gestation is approximately 2–3%.[23,24,25] However, adjustments for the relatively high background loss at this gestational age are necessary to determine procedure-related pregnancy loss.

In the late 1980s and early 1990s most data regarding the safety of either transabdominal or transcervical CVS procedures was reported by 3 collaborative groups. The Canadian Collaborative CVS-Amniocentesis Clinical Trial Group reported a prospective, randomized trial comparing CVS to second trimester amniocentesis.[26] There were 7.6% fetal losses (defined as spontaneous abortions, induced abortions, and late losses) in the CVS group, and 7.0% in the amniocentesis group. The difference of 0.6% for CVS over amniocentesis was not statistically significant, however, the overall loss was relatively high.

The first American Collaborative Report was a prospective, nonrandomized trial of over 2,200 women who chose either TC-CVS or second trimester amniocentesis.[27] Patients in both groups were recruited in the first trimester of pregnancy. As in the Canadian study, advanced maternal age was the primary indication for prenatal diagnosis. When the loss rates were adjusted for slight group differences in maternal and gestational ages, an excess pregnancy loss rate of 0.8% referable to CVS over amniocentesis was calculated, which again was neither clinically nor statistically significant.

A prospective, randomized collaborative comparison of over 3,200 pregnancies sponsored by the European MRC Working Party on the Evaluation of CVS demonstrated a 4.6% greater pregnancy loss rate following CVS when compared with amniocentesis (95%; CI 1.6–7.5%).[28] However, there were major flaws with this study. Operator experience, or lack therefore would likely explain this difference. The US trial included 7 centers and the Canadian trial included 11 centers, whereas the European trial included 31. There were, on average, 325 cases per center in the United States study, 106 in the Canadian study, but only 52 in the European trial. While no significant change in pregnancy loss rate was demonstrated during the course of the European trial, the learning curve for both transcervical and transabdominal CVS probably exceeds 400 or more cases.[29,30] Operators having performed fewer than 100 cases may have 2–3 times the postprocedure loss rate of operators who have performed more than 1,000 procedures.[31]

Nicolaides et al., compared the pregnancy outcome following prenatal diagnosis procedure between CVS and early amniocentesis, done at 10 and 13 weeks' gestation, and found that the spontaneous loss rate was significantly higher after early amniocentesis (5.3%) than after CVS (2.3%).[32]

In a more recent work on the safety of TA-CVS, Brun et al. reported of their experience in 10,741 CVSs during 1990–1999.[23] The rate of fetal loss at <28 weeks was 1.64% in all pregnancies and 1.92% when CVS was performed before 13 weeks. The authors explain their low fetal loss rate by the fact that CVS was done at a higher median gestational age (15 weeks) and in contrast to other studies, not done exclusively during the first trimester. In concordance with other studies, advanced maternal age appeared to be the single factor significantly associated with fetal loss.

Several randomized trials have compared the transcervical and transabdominal approaches.[24,30,33,34] In the United States collaborative CVS Project, no difference was found in the postprocedure pregnancy loss rates between the 2 approaches (TC-CVS 2.5%, TA-CVS 2.3%).[24] Equally important was that the overall post-CVS loss rate in the study (2.5%) was 0.8% lower than that in the initial US study, which compared CVS to second trimester amniocentesis. Because 0.8% was the quantitative difference in loss rates between amniocentesis and CVS in the original study, this finding suggests that when centers become equivalently experienced, amniocentesis and CVS may have the same risk of pregnancy loss. Smidt-Jensen also found no difference in pregnancy loss between TA-CVS and second trimester amniocentesis, but he showed an increased risk for TC-CVS, the procedure for which their center was least experienced. In a retrospective review of their experience with over 9,000 CVS procedures, Church has shown that in their center, transcervical CVS has a slightly greater risk of pregnancy loss than transabdominal sampling.[35] Recently, an international randomized trial of late first trimester invasive prenatal diagnosis to assess the safety and accuracy of amniocentesis and TA-CVS performed at 11–14 weeks was reported.[36] No difference in fetal loss or preterm delivery was observed for both procedures (2.3% and 2.1%, respectively). However, a 4-fold increase in the rate of talipes equinovarus was observed in cases where early amniocentesis was the technique used. The authors concluded that amniocentesis at, or before,13 weeks carries an increase risk for this specific limb defect and an additional increase in early, unintended pregnancy loss. In another study, Alfirevic et al.[37] have analyzed 14 randomized studies from the Cochrane Pregnancy and Childbirth Group Trials Registry and from the Cochrane Central Registry and Control Trials, in order to assess the safety and accuracy of the various invasive procedures employed for early prenatal diagnosis. Based on their results they concluded that early amniocentesis is not a safe alternative to second trimester amniocentesis because of increased pregnancy loss (relative risk 1.29), and higher rates of talipes equinovarus (relative risk 6.43). According to their results, TC-CVS appeared to carry a significant higher rate of pregnancy loss and spontaneous miscarriage (relative risk 1.4 and 1.5, respectively) in comparison to second trimester amniocentesis. Notably, the absolute percentages reported in that study were higher than those reported by others (ie, fetal loss after transcervical CVS 14.5%).

In conclusion, for first trimester diagnosis, either TA-CVS or TC-CVS are the preferred method of choice, while early amniocentesis carries a significant risk for fetal loss and fetal malformations. It appears safe to speculate that fetal loss rates between transcervical and transabdominal sampling will be similar in most centers once equivalent expertise is gained with either approach. We believe utilization of both methods is necessary to have the most complete, practical, and safe approach to first trimester diagnosis.

RISK OF FETAL ABNORMALITIES FOLLOWING CVS

In the first half of the 1990s it was suggested that CVS may be associated with specific fetal malformations, particularly limb reduction defects (LRDs). Today, based on the published data, it appears safe to state that there is no increased risk for LRDs or any other birth defect when CVS is performed at >70 days of gestation from LMP.[38–41] Nonetheless, the subject will be reviewed in greater detail.

The first suggestion of an increased risk for fetal abnormalities following CVS was reported by Firth et al.[2] In a series of 539 CVS-exposed pregnancies, there were 5 infants with severe limb abnormalities in a cohort of 289 pregnancies sampled by TA-CVS at 55–66 days gestation. Four of these infants had the unusual and very rare oromandibular-limb hypogenesis syndrome, and the fifth had a terminal transverse LRD. Based on the estimation that oromandibular-limb hypogenesis syndrome occurs in 1 per 175,000 live births,[42] and LRDs occurs in 1 per 1690 births,[43] the occurrence of these abnormalities in more than 1% of CVS-sampled cases raised a high level of suspicion of a causative association. Subsequently, other groups have reported the occurrence of LRDs and oromandibular hypogenesis in following CVS.[44–49] Currently, an abundant data has accumulated concerning with the possibility and statistics of fetal abnormalities following a CVS procedure.[39–41] In 1992, a case-control study using the Italian Multi-Center Birth Defects Registry, reported an odds ratio of 11.3 (95%; CI 5.6–21.3) for transverse limb abnormalities following first trimester CVS.[44]). When stratified by gestational age at sampling, pregnancies sampled prior to 70 days had a 19.7% increased risk of transverse limb reduction defects, while patients sampled later did not demonstrate a significantly increased risk. Other case-control studies, however, have not seen any association of CVS with LRDs.[39,40]

Currently, there are ample data suggesting an increased risk for fetal malformations when CVS is done at an earlier gestation age (i.e., prior to 70 days of gestation).[2,3,46] Brambati et al. reported a of 1.6% incidence of severe LRDs in a group of patients sampled at 6 and 7 weeks gestation.[46] This

rate decreased to 0.1% at 8–9 weeks. In a report of the Taiwan CVS experience, Hsieh reported 29 cases of limb reduction defects following CVS from September 1990 until June 1992; 4 cases had oromandibular limb hypogenesis syndrome.[47] However, there were 2 remarkable aspects of this report. First, although the gestational age at sampling was not known with certainty in all cases, most were performed at <63 days. Secondly, the cases with LRDs were performed by inexperienced community-based operators, whereas no defects were seen in cases performed at major medical centers. These data support the assumption that early gestational sampling and excessive placental trauma may be etiologic in the reported clusters of post-CVS LRDs. In contrast, Wapner and Evans have shown that in very experienced centers, CVS can be safely and reliably performed even in very early gestation.[38] In a study they conducted CVS was performed at less than 8 weeks' gestation in a population of Orthodox Jews who by their religion are permitted abortion only before 40 days post conception. Of the 82 cases of early CVS, there was only a single case of severe LRDs, a rate of 1.6% (Fig. 36-4).

The question whether CVS sampling after 10 weeks has the potential of causing more subtle defects, such as shortening of the distal phalanx or nail hypoplasia was a major concern debated thoroughly in the literature.[48,50] Presently, as the overall incidence of limb reduction defects after CVS is estimated to be 1 in 1881 (ranging from 5.2–5.7 per 10,000), compared with 1 in 1642 (ranging from 4.8–5.97 per 10,000) in the general population[41,50] there are no data to substantiate this concern. As noted, in most experienced centers performing CVS after 10 weeks, no increase in limb defects of any type was observed.[39,41,49,50] Based on the WHO CVS Registry Data (216,381 cases) published in 1999,[50] it was concluded that CVS does not carry an increased risk for fetal loss or birth defects. Furthermore, no difference in the incidence of LRDs was found in the WHO report even when data regarding LRDs and other birth defects in nonviable fetuses and terminated pregnancies was also included. Therefore, as the possibility of fetal malformations occurring after CVS seems negligible after 70 days of gestation, it is speculated that the few reported

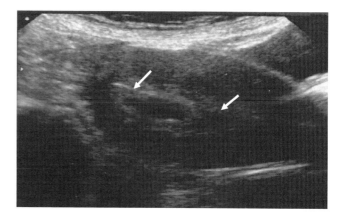

FIGURE 36-4 Posterior early CVS.

clusters are either statistical flukes or related to center-specific practices.

Mechanisms by which CVS could potentially lead to fetal malformations continue to be disputed. Placental thrombosis with subsequent fetal embolization has been raised as a potential etiology, but is unlikely because fetal clotting factors appear to be insufficient at this early gestational age. Inadvertent entry into the extra embryonic coelom with resulting amniotic bands has also been raised as a potential mechanism. This appears unlikely as well, because actual bands have not been observed. Additionally, many of these cases of oromandibular-limb hypogenesis syndrome had internal CNS anomalies that cannot be accounted for by fetal entanglement or compression.

Uterine or placental vascular disruption appears to be the most plausible mechanism at present.[42,51] According to this hypothesis, CVS causes injury, vasospasm, or compression of the uterine vessels, which subsequently results in under-perfusion of the fetal peripheral circulation. Following the initial insult, there may be subsequent rupture of the thin-walled vessels of the damaged distal embryonic circulation, leading to further hypoxia, necrosis, and eventually re-absorption of preexisting structures. Theoretically, an overly traumatic CVS technique could lead to significant uterine or placental disruption with secondary fetal hypovolemia, vasospasm, and peripheral shut down, especially in very early gestation. A similar mechanism leading to limb defects has been demonstrated in animal models following uterine vascular clamping, maternal exposure to cocaine and to the prostanglandin E1 analogue misoprostol, or even simple uterine palpation.[49,52,53] A variation of this hypothesis implicates fetal hemorrhage rather than vasospasm as the etiology of fetal hypo-perfusion. Because the fetal and maternal circulations are contiguous, a significant fetal bleed will result in a fetal-to-maternal hemorrhage detectable as an increase in the maternal serum alpha fetoprotein (AFP) level. Smidt-Jensen et al. found that spontaneous fetal loss occurs more frequently among women whose serum AFP increased substantially after TA-CVS,[54] suggesting that severe fetal hemorrhage may result in fetal death, whereas lesser degrees of hemorrhage may allow the pregnancy to continue, but result in a transient episode of fetal hypo-perfusion. Brent[55] suggested that as a consequence of CVS, bleeding from the chorion might deprive the embryo a portion of its blood supply during a critical period (50–70 days post conception) and therefore could lead to birth defects.

As an increased incidence of fetal hemangiomas in conjunction with fetal oromandibular and limb disruption has been reported to occur when CVS was performed prior to 9 weeks of gestation,[25,56] plausible mechanisms of fetal hypo-perfusion secondary to placental bleeding has been suggested. Quintero et al.[57] added additional information by using transabdominal embryoscopic visualization of the first-trimester embryo. In their study, Quintero et al. demonstrated the occurrence of fetal facial, head, and thoracic echymotic lesions following traumatically induced detachment of the placenta with sub-chorionic hematoma formation, while no changes in fetal heart rate were seen. Although these lesions consistently appeared following

significant physical trauma to the placental site, it was speculated that these findings were unlikely to be produced by the passage of a standard CVS catheter.

A different hypothesis concerning mechanisms of fetal malformations following CVS was postulated by Van der Zee et al.[58] who studied the possibility of maternal-embryonic transfusion following CVS as a cause of immunogenic stimulation and a local antibody-mediated reaction. The authors have demonstrated that in experimental animals, maternal-embryonic transfusion after CVS can lead to an antibody-mediated reaction with vascular disruption at the level of the "end arteries," causing increased apoptotic cell death. When an increased apoptotic cell death occurs early in pregnancy, birth defects in general, and limb defects in particular is predicted to be more extensive than later in pregnancy.

Any theory of CVS-induced limb defects must consider the varying stages of fetal sensitivity and should demonstrate a correlation between the severity of the defects and the gestational age at sampling. As was shown by Firth et al.[3] and by others[25,46,47,55,56] it appears that sampling prior to 9 weeks' gestation may induce LRDs, but rates are not increased following CVS performed after 70 days of gestation, compared to the baseline risk and provided that the procedure is performed in an experienced center by a trained operator. Patients should be informed, however, of the theoretical risk to the fetus, and in particular LRDs and feta anomalies documented when CVS is performed prior to 10 weeks of gestation.

COMPLICATIONS OF CHORIONIC VILLUS SAMPLING

BLEEDING

Vaginal bleeding is less common after TA-CVS, but is seen in as many as 7–10% of patients sampled transcervically. Minimal spotting is more common and may occur in almost one third of women sampled by the transcervical route.[27,28] In most cases, the bleeding is self-limited and the pregnancy outcome is excellent.

INFECTION

Since the initial development of TC-CVS, there has been concern that TC-CVS would introduce vaginal flora into the uterus. This possibility was confirmed by cultures that isolated bacteria from up to 30% of catheters used for CVS.[59–64] In clinical practice, however, the incidence of post-CVS chorioamnionitis is low.[26,27,60,65] In a recently published United States study of over 2,000 cases of TC-CVS, infection was suspected as a possible etiology of pregnancy loss in only 0.3% of cases.[27] Infection following TA-CVS also occurs and has been demonstrated, at least in some cases, to be secondary to bowel flora introduced by inadvertent puncture by the sampling needle.

RUPTURE OF MEMBRANES

Gross rupture of the membranes days to weeks after the procedure is acknowledged as a possible post-CVS complication. Rupture can result from either mechanical or chemical injury to the chorion, allowing exposure of the amnion to subsequent damage or infection. One group reported a 0.3% incidence of delayed rupture of the membranes following CVS,[65] a rate confirmed by Brambati et al.[66,67] Unexplained midtrimester oligohydramnios has also been suggested as being a rare complication of TC-CVS which occurs from delayed chorio-amnion rupture and slow leakage of amniotic fluid.[68]

ELEVATED MSAFP AND Rh SENSITIZATION

An acute rise in MSAFP after CVS has been consistently reported, implying a detectable degree of fetal-maternal bleeding.[69-72] The elevation is transient, occurs more frequently after TA-CVS, and appears to depend on the quantity of tissue aspirated.[72] In Rh negative women, this otherwise negligible bleeding accrues special importance because Rh-positive cells in volumes as low as 0.1 mL have been shown to cause Rh sensitization.[73] Because all women with even a single pass of a catheter or needle show detectable rises in MSAFP, it seems prudent that all Rh-negative, nonsensitized women undergoing CVS receive Rho (D) immunoglobulin following the procedure. Further support to the feto-maternal cell trafficking comes from another study showing fetal erythroblasts to be proportionally elevated in the maternal blood, correlated directly to the period post CVS so that the closer the time to the procedure the higher the percentage of fetal erythroblasts detected.[74]

Implications of trends in MSAFP and beta hCG levels following CVS were demonstrated to be predictive of adverse pregnancy outcome.[75] In this study, patients who miscarry had a greater rise in MSAFP and a greater decrease in maternal serum beta hCG levels following CVS (compared to control subjects with normal pregnancy outcome) implying that pre- and post-CVS MSAFP and beta hCG levels might assist in prediction of an increased risk for subsequent miscarriage.

PERINATAL COMPLICATIONS

No increases in preterm labor, premature rupture of the membranes, small-for-gestational age infants, maternal morbidity, or other obstetric complications have occurred in sampled patients.[76] Although the Canadian Collaborative Study showed an increased prenatal mortality in CVS sampled patients, with the greatest imbalance being beyond 28 weeks, no obvious recurrent event was identified.[26] To date, CVS is not considered to harbor additional prenatal complication as long as the procedure is performed by an experienced operator and after 10 weeks' gestation.

LONG-TERM INFANT DEVELOPMENT

Long-term infant follow up has been performed by Chinese investigators who evaluated 53 children from their initial placental biopsy experience of the 1970s. All were reported in good health, with normal development and school performance.[77] Schaap et al.[78] obtained long-term follow-up data after CVS and amniocentesis and found no significant differences for neonatal and pediatric morbidity. Based on their data the authors concluded that TC-CVS performed around 10 weeks' gestation is not associated with an increased frequency of congenital malformations compared with second trimester amniocentesis.

ACCURACY OF CVS CYTOGENETIC RESULTS

A major concern with all prenatal diagnostic procedures is the possibility of discordance between the prenatal cytogenetic diagnosis and the actual fetal karyotype. With CVS, these discrepancies can occur from either maternal tissue contamination or from true biologic differences between the extra embryonic tissue (ie, placenta) and the fetus. Fortunately, genetic evaluation of chorionic villi provides a high degree of success and accuracy, particularly in regard to the diagnosis of common trisomies.[79,80] The United States Collaborative Study revealed a 99.7% rate of successful cytogenetic diagnosis, with 1.1% of the patients requiring a second diagnostic test, such as amniocentesis or fetal blood analysis, to further interpret the results.[79] In most cases, the additional testing was required to delineate the clinical significance of mosaicism or other ambiguous results (76%), although laboratory failure (21%) and maternal cell contamination (3%) may also require repeated testing. Clinical errors or misinterpretation are rare, however, and the need for repeat testing continues to decrease, as more knowledge about the characteristics of chorionic villi is obtained. Indeed, recent studies[23,36] have demonstrated that CVS is associated with a low rate of maternal cell contamination or chromosomal abnormalities confined to the placenta, as will be described in the following section.

MATERNAL CELL CONTAMINATION (MCC)

Contamination of samples with a significant amount of maternal decidual tissue may lead to diagnostic errors, underlining the importance of preventing this occurrence. Generally, decidual contamination in CVS is almost always due to a small sample size, making appropriate tissue selection difficult. In experienced centers, in which adequate quantities of tissue are available, this problem has become increasingly rare, with MCC occurring in less than 1% of CVS procedures. In recent years there has been much progress in the molecular techniques suitable for detection of MCC, allowing more accurate results in cases of molecular diagnoses, where MCC may jeopardize the validity of the test.

In order to separate maternal tissue from the sample, the chorionic "fronds" are distinguished from the maternal decidua under the microscope, making decidual removal by careful dissection possible. Various molecular techniques have been applied to detect MCC when it occurs. Most are based on the assessment of specific polymorphic loci in the human genome. Batanian et al.[81] reported a simple, rapid, and sensitive method for detection of MCC in prenatal tissue, using the highly polymorphic markers such as variable number of tandem repeats (VNTRs) or microsatellites (stretches of DNA consisting of repeating units of 2–4 nucleotides) that are fluorescently or radioactively labeled. The appropriate genetic locus must be determined by simultaneous screening of the parents in order to distinguish informative from noninformative markers.

CONFINED PLACENTAL MOSAICISM

True discrepancies between the karyotype of the villus and the actual fetal karyotype can occur, leading to either false-positive or false-negative clinical results. Although initially there was concern that this might invalidate CVS as a prenatal diagnostic tool, subsequent investigations have led not only to a clearer understanding of the clinical interpretation of villus tissue results, but also revealed new information about the etiology of pregnancy loss, possible causes of intrauterine growth retardation (IUGR), and the biologic mechanisms for uniparental disomy and associated clinical syndromes.

Mosaicism occurs in about 1–2% of all CVSs[80,82–84] but is confirmed in the fetus in only 10% to 40% of these cases. In contrast, amniocentesis mosaicism is observed in only 0.1–0.3% of cultures but when found, it is confirmed in the fetus in ~70% of cases.[85–87] These feto-placental discrepancies are known to occur because the chorionic villi consist of a combination of extra embryonic tissue of different sources that become separated and distinct from those of the embryo in early developmental stages. Specifically, at the 32- to 64-celled blastocyst, only 3–4 blastomeres differentiate into the inner cell mass (ICM), which forms the embryo, mesenchymal core of the chorionic villi, the amnion, yolk sac, and chorion, whereas the rest of the cells become the precursors of the extra embryonic tissues.[88]

A chromosomal aberration that does not involve the fetal cell lineage will produce a confined placental mosaicism (CPM), in which the trophoblast and perhaps the extra embryonic mesoderm may demonstrate aneuploid cells, but the fetus is euploid. Several mechanisms may apply in pregnancies where CVS mosaicism or nonmosaic feto-placental discrepancies are detected: One possible explanation may be a lineage-specific, nondisjunction. Another is selection for or against a particular aneuploidy in certain cell lineages.[89] This may be the result of postzygotic, mitotic nondisjunction or anaphase lag in conceptuses originally diploid or through mitotic loss of a supernumerary chromosome in subsequent divisions in initially trisomic conceptions. The probability of mosaic or non-mosaic trisomy in the fetus itself depends on the placental lineages in which the trisomic cell line was found. CVS culture represents the villus mesenchymal core and therefore reflects the chromosomal constitution of the fetus proper to a greater extent than the direct preparation, which represent the chorionic ectoderm, farther removed from the fetus. Thus, if a mosaic chromosomal aberration is detected on both direct preparation and long-term culture, it is more likely to represent a true mosaicism of the fetus.[84] Nevertheless, it is advised that in all gestations involving mosaic trisomic villus mesenchyme (with or without evidence of trisomy in direct cytotrophoblast examination) to further examine the fetal karyotype by amniocentesis and perform a thorough fetal ultrasound scan to rule out fetal malformations.

Another adverse outcome that may be associated with CPM is that of uniparental disomy (UPD). In UPD, both chromosome of a given pair are inherited from a single parent, rather than 1 from each. UPD results when the original trisomic embryo is "rescued" by the loss of the 1 extra chromosome. Because in the trisomic embryos 2 of chromosomes come from 1 parent and 1 from the other, there is a theoretical 1 in 3 chance that the 2 remaining chromosomes originate from the same parent, leading to UPD. This may have clinical consequences if the chromosome involved harbors imprinted genes whose expression vary according to the parent-of-origin or if the 2 remaining chromosomes carry a mutant recessive gene, creating a homozygous state. In general, UPD has been reported for almost every chromosomal pair, although clinical consequences have been observed mainly in cases involving specific chromosomes (ie chromosomes 2, 6, 7, 10, 11, 14, 15, 16, 20) and depending on the parent of origin.[90] For instance, despite a relative high frequency of CPM for Trisomy 2 and Trisomy 7, maternal UPD(2) and maternal UPD(7) have only been reported rarely.[91–93]

The most common CPM involving chromosome 15 is encountered in 27/100,000 samples.[94] This is associated with risk for UPD(15) which may lead to well-recognized clinical syndromes. This is due to the fact that chromosome 15 is known to carry genes that are subject to both paternal and maternal imprinting. Maternal UPD(15), resulting from the relatively more common maternally derived Trisomy 15, causes the Prader-Willi syndrome. In contrast, paternal UPD(15) caused by rescue of the less common paternal Trisomy 15, results in the less frequent Angelman syndrome.

In rare cases, CPM for Trisomy 15 offers the important clue that UPD may be present in the "chromosomally normal" fetus, which may be at risk of having Prader Willi/Angelman syndrome.[95,96] For this reason, cases in which CVS reveals Trisomy 15 (either complete or mosaic) should be evaluated for UPD if the amniotic fluid demonstrates an apparently euploid fetus.[94,97,98]

SUMMARY

As a result of the Human Genome Project, we have witnessed constant progress in prenatal diagnosis of genetic disorders in families at risk. In addition, over the last decade first trimester aneuploidy screening using nuchal translucency, PAPP-A and free beta hCG has become routine in many centers worldwide. These have significantly increased the need for early prenatal diagnosis. Due to the association between early amniocentesis and increased fetal malformations and fetal loss, this procedure is no longer recommended for first trimester diagnosis. At the time of writing, the use of fetal cells from maternal blood for genetic diagnosis remains largely experimental, making CVS the earliest technique for prenatal diagnosis in the clinical setting. CVS has proved to be a relatively safe procedure with approximately 2–3% fetal loss in experienced centers. Based on published data regarding the possibility of fetal anomalies post CVS, it seems that there is no increased risk for limb reduction defects (LRDs) or any other birth defect when CVS is done at >70 days of gestation. Evidence from multiple studies demonstrates the high accuracy of this technique, with a low rate of both maternal cell contamination or chromosomal abnormalities confined to the placenta. Technically, CVS can be performed transabdominally or transcervically. The choice between TA-CVS or TC-CVS should be made according to the experienced operator's judgment, based on the experience gained in the particular route. A very recent review by us shows that there is no significant difference in risk between CVS and midtrimester amniocentesis.[99] In experienced hands, CVS can be offered to virtually any patient who would be offerred a genetic amniocentesis.

References

1. Evans MI, Johnson MP. Chorionic villous sampling. In: Evans MI, ed. *Reproductive Risks and Prenatal Diagnosis.* Norwalk, CT: Appleton & Lange. 1992;175–184.

2. Firth HV, Boyd P, Chamberlain P, et al. Severe limb abnormalities after chorion villus sampling at 56–66 days' gestation. *Lancet.* 1991;337:726.

3. Firth HV, Boyd PA, Chamberlain PF, et al. Analysis of limb reduction defects in babies exposed to chorionic villus sampling. *Lancet.* 1994;343:1069–1071.

4. Nicolaides KH, Brizot ML, Snijders RJ. Fetal nuchal translucency: ultrasound screening for fetal trisomy in the first trimester of pregnancy. *Br J Obstet Gynaecol.* 1994;101:782–786.

5. Pandya PP, Brizot ML, Kuhn P, et al. First-trimester fetal nuchal translucency thickness and risk for trisomies. *Obstet Gynecol.* 1994;84:420–423.

6. Wald NJ, Hackshaw AK. Combining ultrasound and biochemistry in first-trimester screening for Down syndrome. *Prenat Diagn.* 1997; 17:821–829.

7. Wald NJ, Kennard A, Hackshaw AK. First trimester serum screening for Down syndrome. *Prenat Diagn.* 1995;15:1227–1240.

8. Nicolaides KH, Sebire NJ, Snijders RJ. Down syndrome screening with nuchal translucency. *Lancet.* 1997;349:438.

9. Wald NJ, Watt HC, Hackshaw AK. Integrated screening for Down syndrome on the basis of tests performed during the first and second trimesters. *N Engl J Med.* 1999;341:461–467.

10. Landy HL, Weiner S, Carson SL. The "vanishing twin": ultrasonographic assessment of fetal disappearance in the first trimester. *Am J Obstet Gynecol.* 1986;155:14.

11. Rudnicki M, Vejerslev LO, Junge J. The vanishing twin: morphologic and cytogenetic evaluation of an ultrasonographic phenomenon. *Gynecol Obstet Invest.* 1991;31:141–145.

12. Johnson MP, Drugan A, Koppitch FC, et al. Postmortem CVS is a better method for cytogenetic evaluation of early fetal loss than culture of abortus material. *Am J Obstet Gynecol.* 1990;163:1505–1510.

13. Drugan A, Johnson MP, Isada NB, et al. The smaller than expected first trimester fetus is at increased risk for chromosome anomalies. *Am J Obstet Gynecol.* 1992;167:1525–1528.

14. Sorokin Y, Johnson MP, Uhlmann WR, et al. Postmortem chorionic villus sampling: correlation of cytogenetic and ultrasound findings. *Am J Med Gen.* 1991;39:314–316.

15. Brambati B, Lanzani A, Tului L. Transabdominal and transcervical chorionic villus sampling: efficiency and risk evaluation of 2,411 cases. *Am J Med Genet.* 1990;35:160–164.

16. Silverman NS, Sullivan MW, Jungkind DL, et al. Incidence of bacteremia associated with chorionic villus sampling. *Obstet Gynecol.* 1994;84:1021–1024.

17. Baumann P, Jovanovic V, Gellert G, et al. Risk of miscarriage after transcervical and transabdominal CVS in relation to bacterial colonization of the cervix. *Prenat Diagn.* 1991;11:551–557.

18. Clark BA, Bissonnette J, Olson SB, et al. Pregnancy loss in a small chorionic villus sampling series. *Am J Obstet Gynecol.* 1989;161:301.

19. Green JE, Dorfman A, Jones SL, et al. Chorionic villus sampling: experience with an initial 940 cases. *Obstet Gynecol.* 1988;71:208.

20. Gustavii B, Claesson V, Kristoffersson U, et al. Risk of miscarriage after chorionic biopsy is probably not higher than after amniocentesis. *Lakartidningen.* 1989;86:4221.

21. Jahoda MG, Pijpers L, Reuss A, et al. Evaluation of transcervical chorionic villus sampling with a completed follow-up of 1550 consecutive pregnancies. *Prenat Diagn.* 1989;9:621.

22. Young SR, Shipley CF, Wade RV, et al. Single-center comparison of results of 1000 prenatal diagnoses with chorionic villus sampling and 1000 diagnoses with amniocentesis. *Am J Obstet Gynecol.* 1991;165:255.

23. Brun JL, Mangione R, Gangbo F, et al. Feasibility, accuracy and safety of chorionic villus sampling: a report of 10741 cases. *Prenat Diagn.* 2003;23:295–301.

24. Jackson LG, Zachary JM, et al. Randomized comparison of transcervical and transabdominal chorionic villus sampling. *N Engl J Med.* 1992;327:594–598.

25. Brambati B, Tului L, Cislaghi C, et al. First 10,000 chorionic villus samplings performed on singleton pregnancies by a single operator. *Prenat Diagn.* 1998;18:255–266.

26. Canadian Collaborative CVS–Amniocentesis Clinical Trial Group. Multicentre randomized clinical trial of chorionic villus sampling and amniocentesis. *Lancet.* 1989;1:1.

27. Rhoads GG, Jackson LG, Schlesselman SE, et al. The safety and efficacy of chorionic villus sampling for early prenatal diagnosis of cytogenetic abnormalities. *N Engl J Med.* 1989;320:609.

28. MRC Working Party on the Evaluation of Chorionic Villus Sampling and the Medical Research Council European Trial of Chorionic Villus Sampling. *Lancet.* 1991;337:1491.

29. Saura R, Gauthier B, Taine L, et al. Operator experiences and fetal loss rate in transabdominal CVS. *Prenat Diagn.* 1994;14:70.

30. Wapner RI, Barr MA, Heeger S, et al. Chorionic villus sampling: a 10-year, over 13,000 consecutive case experience [abstract]. American College of Medical Genetics First Annual Meeting; 1994 March; Orlando, FL.

31. Brambati B, Lanzani A, Tului L: Transabdominal and transcervical chorionic villus sampling: efficacy and risk evaluation of 2411 cases. *Am J Hum Genet.* 1990;35:160.

32. Nicolaides KH, deLourdes-Brigit M, Patel F, et al. Comparison of chorionic villus sampling and amniocentesis for fetal karyotyping at 10–13 weeks gestation. *Lancet.* 1994;344:435–439.

33. Brambati B, Terzian E, Tognoni G. Randomized clinical trial of transabdominal versus transcervical chorionic villus sampling methods. *Prenat Diagn.* 1991;11:285.

34. Smidt-Jensen S, Permin M, Philip J. Sampling success and risk by transabdominal chorionic villus sampling, transcervical chorionic villus sampling and amniocentesis: a randomized study. *Ultrasound Obstet Gynecol.* 1991;1:86.

35. Church JT, Goldberg JD, Wohifered NM, et al. Comparison of transcervical and transabdominal chorionic villus sampling loss rates in nine thousand cases from a single center. *Am J Obstet Gynecol.* 1995;173:1277.

36. Philip J, Silver RK, Wilson RD, et al. for the NICHD EATA Trial Group. Late first-trimester invasive prenatal diagnosis: results of an international randomized trial. *Obstet Gynecol*. 2004;103:1164–1173.

37. Alfirevic Z, Sundberg K, Brigham S. Amniocentesis and chorionic villus sampling for prenatal diagnosis. (Cochrane Review) In: *Cochrane Library*, Issue 3, 2003. Oxford: Update Software.

38. Wapner RJ, Evans MI, Davis DO, et al. Procedural risks versus theology: chorionic villus sampling for orthodox Jews at less than 8 weeks' gestation. *Am J Obstet Gynecol*. 2002;186:1133–1136.

39. Wapner R, Jackson L, Evans MI, et al. Limb reduction defects are not increased following first-trimester chorionic villus sampling. Proceedings of the 16th annual meeting of the society of perinatal obstetricians; 1996 Feb; Kona, Hawaii. Kona: The Society: 1996.

40. Froster UG, Jackson L. Limb defects and chorionic villus sampling: results from an international registry, 1992–94. *Lancet*. 1996; 347:489–494.

41. Kuliev A, Jackson L, Froster U, et al. Chorionic villus sampling safety. Report of World Health Organization/EURO meeting in association with the Seventh International Conference on Early Prenatal Diagnosis of Genetic Diseases, Tel-Aviv, Israel, May 21, 1994. *Am J Obstet Gynecol*. 1996;174:807–811.

42. Hoyme F, Jones KL, Van Allen MI, et al. Vascular pathogenesis of transverse limb reduction defects. *J Pediatr*. 1982;101:839.

43. Foster-Iskenius U, Baird P. Limb reduction defects in over 1,000,000 consecutive live births. *Teratology*. 1989;39:127.

44. Mastroiacovo P, Botto LD, Cavalcanti DP. Limb anomalies following chorionic villus sampling: a registry based case control study. *Am J Med Genet*. 1992;44:856–863.

45. Dolk H, Bertrend F, Lechat MF, and the EUROCAT Working Group. Chorionic villus sampling and limb abnormalities. *Lancet*. 1992;339:876.

46. Brambati B, Simoni G, Traui M. Genetic diagnosis by chorionic villus sampling before 8 gestational weeks: efficiency, reliability and risks on 317 completed pregnancies. *Prenat Diagn*. 1992;12:784–789.

47. Hsieh FJ, Shvu MK, Sheu BC, et al. Limb defects after chorionic villus sampling. *Obstet Gynecol*. 1995;85:84.

48. Burton BK, Schultz CJ, Burd LI. Spectrum of limb disruption defects associated with chorionic villus sampling. *Pediatrics*. 1993;91: 989–993.

49. Brent RL. Relationship between uterine vascular clamping, vascular disruption syndrome and cocaine teratology. *Teratology*. 1990;41:757.

50. WHO/PAHO consultation on CVS. Evaluation of chorionic villus sampling safety. *Prenat Diagn*. 1999;19:97–99.

51. Golden CM, Ryan LM, Holmes LB. Chorionic villus sampling: a distinctive teratogenic effect on fingers? *Birth Defects Res Part A Clin Mol Teratol*. 2003;67:557–562.

52. Webster W, Brown-Woodman T. Cocaine as a cause of congenital malformations of vascular origin: experimental evidence in the rat. *Teratology*. 1990;41:689.

53. Gonzalez CH, Marques-Dias MJ, Kim CA, et al. Congenital abnormalities in Brazilian children associated with misoprostol misuse in first trimester of pregnancy. *Lancet*. 1998;351:1624–1627.

54. Smidt-Jensen S, Philip J, Zachary J, et al. Implications of maternal serum alphafetoprotein elevation caused by transabdominal and transcervical CVS. *Prenat Diagn*. 1994;14:35–46.

55. Brent RL. What is the relationship between birth defects and pregnancy bleeding?: new perspectives provided by the NICHD workshop dealing with the association of chorionic villous sampling and the occurrence of limb reduction defects. *Teratology*. 1993;48:93–95.

56. Greenough A, Naik S, Yuksel B, et al. First-trimester invasive procedures and congenital abnormalities. *Acta Paediatr*. 1997;86:1220–1223.

57. Quintero R, Romero R, Mahoney M, et al. Fetal hemorrhagic lesions after chorionic villus sampling. *Lancet*. 1992;339:193.

58. van der Zee DC, Bax KM, Vermeij-Keers C. Maternoembryonic transfusion and congenital malformations. *Prenat Diagn*. 1997;17:59–69.

59. Brambati B, Matarrelli M, Varotto F. Septic complications after chorionic villus sampling. *Lancet*. 1987;1:1212.

60. Brambati B, Varotti F. Infection and chorionic villus sampling. *Lancet*. 1985;2:609.

61. Garden AS, Reid G, Benzie RJ. Chorionic villus sampling. *Lancet* 1985;1:1270.

62. McFadven IR, Taylor-Robinson D, Furr PM, et al. Infection and chorionic villus sampling. *Lancet*. 1985;2:610.

63. Scialli AR, Neugebauer DL, Fabro SE. Microbiology of the endocervix in patients undergoing chorionic villus sampling. In: Fracearo M, Simoni G, Brambati B, eds. *First-trimester Fetal Diagnosis*. New York, NY: Springer-Verlag; 1985:69–73.

64. Wass D, Bennett MJ. Infection and chorionic villus sampling. *Lancet*. 1985;2:338.

65. Hogge WA, Schonberg SA, Golbus MS. Chorionic villus sampling: experience of the first 1000 cases. *Am J Obstet Gynecol*. 1986;154:1249.

66. Brambati B, Oldrini A, Ferrazzi E, et al. Chorionic villus sampling: an analysis of the obstetric experience of 1000 cases. *Prenat Diagn*. 1987;7:157–169.

67. Brambati B, Tului L, Cislaghi C, et al. First 10,000 chorionic villus samplings performed on singleton pregnancies by a single operator. *Prenat Diagn*. 1998;18:255–266.

68. Cheng EY, Luth DA, Hickok D, et al. Transcervical chorionic villus sampling and midtrimester oligohydramnios. *Am J Obstet Gynecol*. 1991;165:1063.

69. Blakemore K, Baumgarten A, Schoenfeld-Dimaio M, et al. Rise in maternal serum alpha-fetoprotein concentration after chorionic villus sampling. *Lancet*. 1985;2:339.

70. Brambati B, Guercilena S, Bonacchi I, et al. Fetomatemal transfusion after chorionic villus sampling: clinical implications. *Hum Reprod*. 1986;1:37–40.

71. Shulman LP, Mevers CM, Simpson JL, et al. Fetomatemal transfusion depends on amount of chorionic villi aspirated but not on method of chorionic villus sampling. *Am J Obstet Gynecol*. 1990;162: 1185.

72. Brezinka C, Hagenaars AM, Wladimiroff JW, et al. Fetal ductus venosus flow velocity waveforms and maternal serum AFP before and after first-trimester transabdominal chorionic villus sampling. *Prenat Diagn*. 1995;15:699–703.

73. Zipursky A, Israels LG. The pathogenesis and prevention of Rh immunization. *CMAJ*. 1967;97:1245–1257.

74. Al-Mufti R, Hambley H, Farzaneh F, et al. Distribution of fetal erythroblasts in maternal blood after chorionic villous sampling. *BJOG*. 2003;110:33–38.

75. Barkai G, Reichman B, Ries L, et al. The association between alpha-fetoprotein and beta hCG levels prior to and following chorionic villus sampling in cases that spontaneously miscarried. *Prenat Diagn*. 1994;14:793–798.

76. Williams J, Medearis AL, Bear MD, et al. Chorionic villus sampling is associated with normal fetal growth. *Am J Obstet Gynecol*. 1987;157:708.

77. Angue H, Bingru Z, Hong W. Long-term follow-up results after aspiration of chorionic villi during early pregnancy. In: Fraccaro M, Simoni G, Brambati B, eds. *First-Trimester Fetal Diagnosis*. New York, NY: Springer-Verlag; 1985:1.

78. Schaap AH, van der Pol HG, Boer K, et al. Long-term follow-up of infants after transcervical chorionic villus sampling and after amniocentesis to compare congenital abnormalities and health status. *Prenat Diagn*. 2002;22:598–604.

79. Ledbetter DH, Martin AO, Verlinsky Y, et al. Cytogenetic results of chorionic villus sampling: high success rate and diagnostic accuracy in the United States collaborative study. *Am J Obstet Gynecol*. 1990;162:495.

80. Mikkelsen M, Avme S. Chromosomal findings in chorionic villi. In: Vogel F, Sperling K, eds. *Human Genetics*. Berlin, Germany; Springer-Verlag; 1987:597.

81. Batanian JR, Ledbetter DH, Fenwick RG. A simple VNTR-PCR method for detecting maternal cell contamination in prenatal diagnosis. *Genet Test*. 1998;2:347–350.

82. Ledbetter DH, Zachary JL, Simpson MS, et al. Cytogenetic results from the US collaborative study on CVS. *Prenat Diagn*. 1992;12:317.

83. Vejerslev LO, Mikkelsen M. The European collaborative study on mosaicism: data from 1986–1987. *Prenat Diagn*. 1989;9:575–579.

84. Hahnemann JM, Vejerslev LO. European collaborative research on mosaicism in CVS (EUCROMIC) fetal and extrafetal cell lineages in 192 gestations with CVS mosaicism involving single autosomal trisomy. *Am J Hum Genet*. 1997;60:917–927.

85. Breed AS, Mantingh A, Vosters R, et al. Follow-up and pregnancy outcome after a diagnosis of mosaicism in CVS. *Prenat Diagn*. 1991;11:577.

86. Bui TH, Iselius L, Linsten J. European collaborative study on prenatal diagnosis: mosaicism, pseudomosaicism and single abnormal cells in amniotic fluid cell cultures. *Prenat Diagn*. 1984;4:145.

87. Hsu LY, Perlis TE. United States survey on chromosome mosaicism and pseudomosaicism in prenatal diagnosis. *Prenat Diagn*. 1984;4:97.

88. Markert C, Petters R. Manufactured hexaparenteral mice show that adults are derived from three embryonic cells. *Science*. 1978;202:56.

89. Wolsenholme J. Confined placental mosaicism for trisomies 2. 3, 7, 8, 9, 16, and 22: their incidence, likely origins and mechanisms for cell lineage compartmentalization. *Prenat Diagn*. 1996;16:511–524.

90. Kotzot D. Abnormal phenotypes in uniparental disomy (UPD): fundamental aspects and a critical review with bibliography of UPD other than 15. *Am J Med Genet*. 1999;82:265–274.

91. Harrison K, Eisenger K, Anyane-Yeboa K, et al. Maternal uniparental disomy of chromosome 2 in a baby with trisomy 2 mosaicism in amniotic fluid culture. *Am J Med Genet*. 1995;58:147–51.

92. Webb AL, Sturgiss S, Warwicker P, et al. Maternal uniparental disomy for chromosome 2 in association with confined placental mosaicism for trisomy 2 and severe intrauterine growth retardation. *Prenat Diagn*. 1996;16:958–962.

93. Langolis S, Yong SL, Wilson RD, et al. Prenatal and postnatal growth failure associated with maternal heterodisomy for chromosome 7. *J Med Genet*. 1995;32:871–875.

94. European Collaborative Research on Mosaicism in CVS (EUCROMIC). Trisomy 15 CPM: probable origins, pregnancy outcome and risk of fetal UPD. *Prenat Diagn*. 1998;18:35–44.

95. Cassidy SB, Lai LW, Erickson RP, et al. Trisomy 15 with loss of the paternal 15 as a cause of Prader-Willi syndrome due to maternal disomy. *Am J Hum Genet*. 1992;51:701.

96. Purvis-Smith SG, Saville T, Manass S, et al. Uniparental disomy 15 resulting from "correction" of an initial trisomy 15. *Am J Hum Genet*. 1992;50:1348.

97. Kalousek DK, Langlois S, Barrett I, et al. Uniparental disomy for chromosome 16 in humans. *Am J Hum Genet*. 1993;52:8.

98. Post JG, Nijhuis JG. Trisomy 16 confined to the placenta. *Prenat Diagn*. 1992;12:1001.

99. Evans MI, Wapner JS: Invasive prenatal diagnostic procedures 2005. *Prenat Diagn*. 2005;29:215–218.

CORDOCENTESIS

Carl P. Weiner

CORDOCENTESIS

Fetal blood sampling was first performed in the 1960s using a fetoscope to identify the targeted vessel. Fetoscopy was cumbersome and risky—the procedure-related loss rate exceeded 5%. Fortunately, the development of high-resolution ultrasound made it possible to clearly image the umbilical cord. Spurred by the need for an accurate method to diagnose fetal toxoplasmosis, the first intentional percutaneous umbilical blood sampling under ultrasound guidance (cordocentesis) was performed by Fernand Daffos in 1980s.[1] The procedure rapidly gained favor with demonstration of its safety[2-4] directly leading to the development of fetal medicine. A wide range of gestationally appropriate norms[5-13] permit new insight into fetal pathophysiology. And while some early indications for cordocentesis have been replaced by less invasive techniques, the information gained allows the practice of fetal medicine based on direct knowledge of the pathophysiology rather than "educated" guesses.

METHODS

Cordocentesis can be performed as early as 12 weeks gestation, though it is technically more difficult prior to 20 weeks and the loss rate much higher prior to 16 weeks gestation.

There are 2 methods for cordocentesis: freehand and using a fixed needle guide. Regardless of technique, the preferred location for cord puncture is the placental origin where it is relatively fixed. The first few centimeters of the fetal origin of the umbilical cord is innervated. Its puncture causes pain and should be avoided. The umbilical vein rather than the artery is the preferred target because of its lower association with complications discussed subsequently. Like all percutaneous procedures, a "no touch" philosophy is essential. If you do not touch the shaft of the needle that enters the patient, you cannot contaminate it.

The technique described by Daffos uses a 20-gauge spinal needle 8–12 centimeters long.[1] The needle course is tracked by imaging the tip and shaft with a high-resolution ultrasound transducer held either in the opposite hand of the operator or by their assistant. This is a matter of operator preference. Since the needle is not fixed, the tip can move several centimeters in all axes should either the site of insertion be suboptimal or the fetus move during the procedure. Once punctured, the operator secures the needle while the assistant aspirates a series of 1 ml syringes. It is a fairly common mistake to use a single, large syringe to eliminate the need to change syringes. Aspiration with a syringe much larger than a milliliter can generate enough negative pressure to collapse the umbilical vein leading to the erroneous conclusion that the position has been lost.

Pre-heparinization of the syringe is unnecessary unless a fetal blood gas is needed. The sample is immediately placed into a specimen container prepared with the required preservative. The freehand technique remains the most popular method for cordocentesis no doubt because of the flexibility it allows the operator.

Cordocentesis may also be performed using a fixed needle guide which is attached to the base of the ultrasound transducer. Typically, the transducer is held by the operator's assistant. The predicted course of the needle, which can travel only in the vertical plane is displayed on the ultrasound screen. This allows the operator to select in advance a precise target for puncture. Deviation from the predicted path occurs only when there is an abrupt change in the relationship between the puncture site in the maternal abdominal wall and the uterus as the needle traverses between the 2. The most common causes are abrupt patient movement and failure of the assistant to hold the transducer head flat against the maternal abdomen. Because lateral movement of the needle is neither desired nor possible, a smaller gauge needle such as a 22 or 25 is typically used. It is important to line up the cord longitudinally rather than in cross section. I prefer to target the "easiest" location for a direct approach rather than confine myself to the placental cord origin. In fact, a free loop is my target more than 50% of the time. The preferred puncture is on the near side of the bend in the loop. Placental puncture should be avoided if possible when the indication for the blood sample is alloimmunization (RBC or platelet) just as the informed practitioner would do with amniocentesis.

Many practitioners use local anesthesia and prophylactic antibiotics. The former is unnecessary for diagnostic procedures if a 22-gauge needle is used, but may be beneficial with the freehand technique because of the larger needle caliper and movement outside the vertical axis. A local anesthetic placed subcutaneously is useful independent of technique when the procedure is lengthy (e.g., intravascular transfusion). Prophylactic antibiotics are not indicated for either cordocentesis or intravascular transfusion. There is no evidence they reduce the already low risk of amnionitis. In my experience, amnionitis complicates less than 1 in 800 diagnostic procedures when the "no touch" philosophy is rigorously adhered to and a needle guide is used.

Fetal movement can either prevent a successful puncture or shorten the available access time regardless of the technique used. Fetal movement while the needle is intraluminal is likely to increase the risk of trauma to the cord. Many operators administer a neuromuscular antagonist to eliminate fetal movement. I routinely use pancuronium: 0.3 mg/kg when performing a mid loop puncture. The pancuronium may be given either intramuscular into the fetal buttock, or preferably, intravenously as soon as the vein is punctured. The effect is evident within seconds when given intravascularly. Recent study suggests vercurnium may provide some advantage over pancuronium. Its shorter duration of action is an advantage for diagnostic procedures since it is associated with a more rapid return of fetal movement and heart rate variability.[14]

INDICATIONS AND APPLICATIONS FOR CORDOCENTESIS

The indications for cordocentesis are dictated by the risk of a significant complication. Risk does vary by indication (see the following section). Typical indications for cordocentesis are listed in Table 37-1.

The Doppler resistance index of several fetal vessels correlates with the fetal acid base status.[15,16] As such, its use has been advocated when the fetus is presumed small. However, cordocentesis is not indicated to determine the acid base status of a fetus whose umbilical artery Doppler resistance index is normal in the absence of labor. Assuming the mother is well ventilated and the vessel punctured is correctly identified, the blood gases are less likely to be abnormal than the chance of a fetal loss. In over 1,200 procedures, we have yet to identify a fetus with abnormal blood gases and a normal Doppler resistance index in the absence of either hydrops or fetal sepsis (unpublished).

More provocative and potentially clinically relevant is the application for cordocentesis in the preterm growth restricted fetus who has an elevated Doppler resistance index but still has diastolic flow present if in the umbilical artery solely to measure the acid base status. With these Doppler measurements, the range of fetal blood gases is wide encompassing normal to acidemia. Recent study of children who as growth restricted fetuses had undergone cordocentesis suggests that it is the acidemia not the hypoxemia alone which is associated with compromised neurodevelopment.[17] Should these exciting findings be confirmed, proof that a preterm fetus was hypoxic but not acidemic would allow the delay of delivery at least until there is time to complete a course of maternal corticosteroids to enhance postnatal lung function.

TABLE 37-1	**INDICATIONS FOR CORDOCENTESIS**
Indication	**%[a]**
Rapid karyotype	50.7
Hemolytic disease	33.7
Severe, early onset growth restriction	21.7
Congenital infection	16.9
Miscellaneous	4.2
Nonimmune hydrops fetalis	
Stuck twin syndrome	
Fetal drug therapy	
Maternal TSiG	
Alloimmune thrombocytopenia	

[a]Percentages taken from reference 16. Some patients had more than 1 indication.

Cordocentesis is not indicated solely for fetal blood typing in most instances of maternal RBC alloimmunization. This can now be accomplished by the application of PCR to either trophoblast or amniocytes obtained early second trimester when the risk of exacerbating sensitization is lower.

Immune thrombocytopenia (ITP) is not an indication for cordocentesis (it is indicated for alloimmune thrombocytopenia (ATP)).[8] The pro-cordocentesis argument is based on the assumed risk to the fetus of intracranial hemorrhage during labor. While the argument is logical, it is not supported by the aggregate experience of the last 2 decades. There is no more than 1 fetal loss documented in the literature secondary to an intrapartum fetal hemorrhage.[18] Most losses attributed to ITP have either been associated with a maternal connective tissue disorder or where associated with a neonatal bleed. In almost all other instances of a reported loss, either the cause of death or the timing of death is either not stated or not known. ITP is the most common autoimmune disorder of reproductive age women; if true, there should be no controversy that thrombocytopenia secondary to ITP posed a significant fetal risk during labor. Yet, the loss rate from cordocentesis in the best hands for a "low risk" fetus is 0.2%.[19] In addition, there is no direct or indirect evidence that cesarean section for the indication of autoimmune thrombocytopenia improves neonatal outcome. In short, the use of cordocentesis to obtain a fetal platelet count in a woman with ITP adds more risk than benefit.

Preliminary reports suggest that cordocentesis for the diagnosis of fetal toxoplasmosis has been supplanted the application of PCR to samples of amniotic fluid, though this remains controversial. Though a fetal blood sample had been thought central to the diagnosis of fetal infection for all viruses other than CMV, this indication too will likely be supplanted by the application of PCR to amniotic fluid samples.

Not yet widely accepted but a likely valid indication for cordocentesis is presence of maternal thyroid stimulating antibody (TSiG) or active maternal Graves disease.[20,21] Emerging evidence suggests that even mild degrees of thyroid dysfunction impairs long-term neurodevelopment.[22–24] While there is a relationship between the degree of maternal and fetal thyroid suppression with such agents as propylthiouracil, it is not uncommon to find the fetus is significantly over- or under-treated despite the mother being euthyroid. In the instance of fetal hyperthyroidism, the maternal PTU dose is increased and the woman given thyroxine replacement.[20] In the instance of fetal hypothyroidism, the fetus can be given thyroxine intra-amniotically on a weekly basis.[25] Women with a history of Graves disease who have undergone thyroid ablation should be screened for the presence of TSiG. The fetus is at minimal risk if the TSiG study is negative.

The performance of cordocentesis is essential for a complete evaluation of nonimmune hydrops since it allows the separation of cardiac from noncardiac etiologies.[10,26] The UVP is a surrogate for the central venous pressure. Recent studies of human fetuses[27] indicate that is very similar to the right-sided heart pressure. An elevated umbilical venous pressure (UVP) is consistent with myocardial dysfunction whether caused by anemia (eg, parvovirus infection, hemolytic disease), or my-ocarditis, or obstructed cardiac return (thoracic mass effect). I am unaware of any medical or surgical treatment for noncar-diac hydrops. Successful treatment of cardiogenic hydrops is associated with normalization of the UVP before the hydrops resolves.[26] The UVP also predicts which fetus with a hydro-thorax and hydrops whose hydrops will be cured by place-ment of a thoraco-amniotic shunt. Hydrops that is responsive to shunting is caused by a shift of the mediastinum which then obstructs cardiac return. If the UVP is neither elevated nor normalizes after draining the chest, a shunt will not help. The underlying problem lies elsewhere.

MAJOR COMPLICATIONS AND RISK FACTORS FOR CORDOCENTESIS

The principle major complications of cordocentesis are listed in Table 37-2. They include all those complications associ-ated with amniocentesis plus fetal bradycardia, umbilical cord laceration, and thrombosis. Risk factors for cordocentesis are noted in Table 37-3.

Umbilical cord laceration and thrombosis are seen prin-cipally with freehand procedures and have not been reported when a needle guide was used.[19] Though bleeding from the umbilical puncture site is common, prolonged bleeding with sequelae is uncommon. Application of a "no touch" technique and the use of disposable needles for a single puncture will minimize the risk of amnionitis. Bradycardia is the major com-plication of cordocentesis. Virtually all emergency cesarean deliveries and most perinatal losses are associated with a fetal bradycardia (Table 37-4). A method to block its development is greatly needed. Umbilical artery puncture and hypoxia are the major risk factors for bradycardia. In the absence of pro-found anemia or myocardial failure, fetal hypoxia is associ-ated with an elevated umbilical artery resistance index and it can be used as a risk marker. The incidence of bradycardia with absent and/or reversed diastolic flow approaches 25%. Umbilical artery puncture increases the risk of fetal bradycar-dia 5–10 fold.[3,19,28] The presence of either oligohydramnios or a 2-vessel cord increases the risk of arterial puncture in my experience. I have seen during bradycardic episodes that

TABLE 37-2 | COMPLICATIONS OF CORDOCENTESIS

1. Bradycardia or asystole
2. Premature rupture of membranes
3. Premature labor
4. Umbilical hemorrhage
5. Placental hemorrhage
6. Chorioamnionitis
7. Umbilical thrombosis
8. Fetal to maternal hemorrhage

TABLE 37-3 | RISK FACTORS FOR CORDOCENTESIS

1. Umbilical artery puncture (associated with bradycardia)
2. Fetal hypoxemia (associated with bradycardia)
3. Technique—freehand versus needle guide
4. Gestational age—prior to 20 weeks, both techniques
5. Number of punctures (freehand technique only)
6. Duration of procedure (freehand technique only)
7. Experience (freehand technique only, presumably be-cause of #4, 5)

the Doppler resistance index is elevated in only 1 of the um-bilical arteries suggesting the vasospasm is localized. I have also demonstrated that pancuronium reduces the incidence of bradycardia in appropriately grown but not growth restricted fetuses.[28] It is likely that some episodes of bradycardia result when the fetus tugs on its cord causing needle trauma and irritation of the underlying vascular smooth muscle. The asso-ciation of bradycardia with umbilical vein puncture may reflect disruption of the adjacent umbilical artery smooth muscle as the tip traverses the cord. There is no known treatment for fe-tal bradycardia in response to a cordocentesis. Based on direct observation, I believe that vigorous fetal stimulation is bene-ficial since the heart will slow again if the manual stimulation is stopped too early. I have, on occasion administered a vari-ety of chronotropes (e.g., atropine) and bicarbonate as part of a fetal resuscitation. I am unconvinced they have predictable value.

Even when performed at a mid loop, the fetus does "re-act" to the cordocentesis. Umbilical artery resistance typically declines after either a diagnostic procedure or a fetal intravas-cular transfusion.[29] As a rule, the higher the "normal" base-line resistance index, the greater the decline. The decrease is the result of prostacyclin release from the vascular endo-thelium.[30,31]

Endothelial adaptation to hypoxia also explains why hy-poxemia is a risk factor for bradycardia.[28] Rizzo demonstrated that umbilical vein puncture released a potent vasoconstrictor, endothelin, in growth restricted but not appropriately grown fetuses.[32] Bradycardic fetuses released more endothelin. It is reasonable to speculate that the release of a large amount of endothelin causes focal vasocontriction at or near the puncture site. Future studies of growth restricted fetuses might test an ET antagonist as prophylaxis against bradycardia.

Both techniques for cordocentesis have a learning curve. Based on considerable experience with both, I believe the learning curve is shorter when a needle guide is used. However, use of a needle guide requires a trained assistant with steady hands. Until recently, it was generally accepted that the tech-nique selected was a matter of operator preference and had no impact on outcome.

I have long believed that the "advantage" of the freehand technique, flexibility, also poses a risk to the fetus based on indirect evidence. Analogous to a lever, a small movement at the hub of the needle amplifies the distance the tip moves.

| TABLE 37-4 | FREQUENCY OF MAJOR COMPLICATIONS OF CORDOCENTESIS WHEN A NEEDLE GUIDE IS USED | | | |

Final Diagnosis	GA (Weeks) at Cordocentesis	Percent Emergency Delivery[a]	Percent Death Within 2 Weeks[b]
RBC alloimmunization	28 ± 4	0.2	0.2
Uteroplacental dysfunction	32 ± 4	5.0	0.9
Chromosome abnormality	29 ± 6	7.7	9.9
All others	28 ± 6	0.3	0.2

[a]Weiner, unpublished.

[b]From Weiner and Okamura.[19] Fetuses with a chromosome abnormality delivered by cesarean section were delivered before the karyotype was completed.

For example, a freehand cordocentesis produces a significantly greater incremental increase in the MSAFP than does amniocentesis after controlling for placental puncture.[33] In contrast, the change in MSAFP when a needle guide is used is similar to amniocentesis.[34] Further, the association between fetal thrombocytopenia and bleeding from the umbilical puncture site after a freehand cordocentesis is high enough to have prompted 1 investigator to suggest prophylactic platelet transfusion of all fetuses at risk.[35] In contrast, there is no relationship between the fetal platelet count and bleeding from the puncture site when a needle guide is used.[36] The latter may also be explained by the use of the thinner gauge needle which is another potential advantage of the needle guide. Second trimester amniocentesis studies report lower loss rates when thinner needles are used.[37] Not surprising, there are also reports which suggest that an amniocentesis performed with a needle guide is safer than 1 performed freehand.[38]

Comparisons of loss rates sustained by groups using the freehand and needle guide techniques are difficult since it is hard to separate procedure related losses from those secondary to the natural progression of disease. No single center has adequate volume for a randomized trial and up to now there is no interest in a multicenter trial. Recently, I combined my experience with diagnostic cordocentesis with that of Professor Okamura from Tokohu University in Sendai Japan.[19] Our 2 sites shared only the use of a fixed needle guide and a long experience involving many operators ($n = 25$) with varying levels of experience.

In this study, 1,260 diagnostic cordocenteses were performed at a mean gestational age of 29 weeks. The umbilical vein (confirmed by the blood pressure reading) was punctured in 90% demonstrating the desired vessel can be targeted. We defined a procedure-related loss as any loss within 2 weeks of the procedure except that resulting from elective pregnancy termination. Overall, there were 12 losses (0.9%) (Table 37-4). Ghidini et al. reviewed the experience of the world's largest centers.[39] All cordocenteses were performed freehand except those from the University of Iowa where a needle guide was used. Therefore, the Iowa contribution was deleted from the following analyses.

The overall loss rate with the freehand method was 7.2% (96/1,328).[39] This rate was significantly higher than the overall loss rate when a needle guide was used (0.9%, 12/1,260; $p < 0.00001$). To exclude the contribution of the underlying pathology to the loss rate, Ghidini subdivided the procedures into high and low risk with the latter excluding chromosomal abnormalities, nonimmune hydrops, intrauterine growth restriction, and fetal infection. Such exclusions virtually eliminate all abnormal fetuses who might be at risk for a loss *unrelated* to the procedure. The perinatal loss rate for these low risk procedures using the freehand technique was 3% (20/660). This rate is 15 times the needle guide rate (0.2%, 2/1021; $p < 000001$) which *includes* fetuses with either infection, hydrops, or structural malformations.

It might be argued that the Ghidini review included many centers early in their learning curve and that a single center would provide a more suitable comparison. That opportunity came when Donner et al. reported 759 diagnostic cordocenteses *with a known outcome* using the freehand technique.[40] Acknowledging several limitations (final diagnoses were not necessarily reported and 87% (34/39) of their perinatal losses were excluded as being unrelated to the procedure), their stated loss rate was 0.8% including 94 therapeutic terminations in the denominator. Subtracting the terminations from their total yields a loss of 1.1% (7/665). Of these pregnancies, 160 were sampled because of severe early onset growth restriction. We can estimate their low-risk group if we exclude the growth restricted fetuses and assume that all fetuses with chromosomal abnormalities were either in the growth restriction group, therapeutic termination group, or the 1 fetus with trisomy 18 noted in the paper. This leaves a low-risk group of 504 in which there were 6 fetal/neonatal losses (1.2%). This rate is significantly higher than that achieved with a needle guide ($p = 0.03$).

I do not believe the needle guide is a panacea. But while a few skilled operators might duplicate the results obtained with a needle guide, the majority of practitioners perform only a few cordocenteses per year and would benefit from use of the guide.

References

1. Daffos F, Capella-Pavlovsky M, Forestier F. A new procedure for fetal blood sampling in utero: preliminary results of fifty-three cases. *Am J Obstet Gynecol*. 1983;146:985–987.
2. Weiner, CP. Cordocentesis for diagnostic indications—two years experience. *Obstet Gynecol*. 1987;70:664–668.

3. Daffos F. Access to the other patient [review]. *Semin Perinatol.* 1989;13:252–259.

4. Maxwell DJ, Johnson P, Hurley P, et al. Fetal blood sampling and pregnancy loss in relation to indication. *Br J Obstet Gynaecol.* 1991;98:892–897.

5. Soothill PW, Lestas AN, Nicolaides KH, et al. 2, 3-Diphosphoglycerate in normal, anemic and transfused human fetuses. *Clin Sci.* 1988;74:527–530.

6. Economides DL, Nicolaides KH, Linton EA, et al. Plasma cortisol and adrenocorticotropin in appropriate and small for gestational age fetuses. *Fetal Ther.* 1988;3:158–164.

7. Forestier F, Daffos F, Catherine N, et al. Developmental hematopoiesis in normal human fetal blood. *Blood.* 1991;77:2360–2363.

8. Andreux JP, Renard M, Daffos F, et al. Erythropoietic progenitor cells in human fetal blood. *Nouvelle Revue Francaise d Hematologie.* 1991;33:223–226.

9. Nicolaides KH, Rodeck CH, Mibashan RS, et al. Have Liley charts outlived their usefulness? *Am J Obstet Gynecol.* 1986;155:90–94.

10. Weiner CP, Heilskov J, Pelzer GD, et al. Normal values for human umbilical venous and amniotic fluid pressures and their alteration by fetal disease. *Am J Obstet Gynecol.* 1989;161:714–717.

11. Weiner CP, Sipes SL, Wenstrom KD. The effect of gestation upon normal fetal laboratory parameters and venous pressure. *Obstet Gynecol.* 1992;79:713–718.

12. Weiner CP, Williamson RA, Wenstrom KD, et al. Management of fetal hemolytic disease by cordocentesis: prediction of fetal anemia (part I). *Am J Obstet Gynecol.* 1991;165:546–553.

13. Thorpe-Beeston JG, Nicolaides KH, Felton CV, et al. Maturation of the secretion of thyroid hormone and thyroid-stimulating hormone in the fetus [see comments]. *N Engl J Med.* 1991;324:532–536.

14. Mouw RJ, Hermans J, Brandenburg HC, et al. Effects of pancuronium or atracurium on the anemic fetus during and directly after intrauterine transfusion (IUT): a double blind randomized study. *Am J Obstet Gynecol.* 1997;176(suppl):S18.

15. Weiner, CP. The relationship between the umbilical artery systolic: diastolic ratio and umbilical blood gas measurements in specimens obtained by cordocentesis. *Am J Obstet Gynecol.* 1990;162:1198–1202.

16. Hecher K, Snijders R, Campbell S, et al. Fetal venous, intracardiac, and arterial blood flow measurements in intrauterine growth retardation: relationship with fetal blood gases. *Am J Obstet Gynecol.* 1995;173:10–15.

17. Soothill PW, Ajayi RA, Campbell S, et al. Fetal oxygenation at cordocentesis, maternal smoking and childhood neurodevelopment. *Eur J Obstet Gynecol Reprod Biol.* 1995;59:21–24.

18. Weiner CP. Why fuss over diagnosing fetal thrombocytopenia secondary to ITP? *Contemp Obstet Gynecol.* 1995;40:45–50.

19. Weiner CP, Okamura K. Diagnostic fetal blood sampling—technique related losses. *Fetal Diagn Ther.* 1996;11:169–175.

20. Wenstrom KD, Weiner CP, Williamson RA, et al. Prenatal diagnosis of fetal hyperthyroidism using funipuncture. *Obstet Gynecol.* 1990;75:1–5.

21. Yankowitz J, Weiner CP. Medical Fetal Therapy. *Clin Obstet Gynaecol.* 1995;9:553–570.

22. Salerno M, Di Maio S, Militerni R, et al. Prognostic factors in the intellectual development at 7 years of age in children with congenital hypothyroidism. *J Endocrinol Invest.* 1995;18:774–779.

23. Kooistra L, van der Meere JJ, Vulsma T, et al. Sustained attention problems in children with early treated congenital hypothyroidism. *Acta Paediatrica* 1996;85:425–429.

24. Weber G, Siragusa V, Rondanini GF, et al. Neurophysiologic studies and cognitive function in congenital hypothyroid children. *Pediatr Res.* 1995;37:736–740.

25. Van Loon AJ, Derksen JT, Bos AF, et al. In utero diagnosis and treatment of fetal goitrous hypothyroidism, caused by maternal use of propylthiouracil. *Prenat Diagn.* 1995;15:599–604.

26. Weiner CP. Umbilical venous pressure measurement in the evaluation of nonimmune hydrops. *Am J Obstet Gynecol.* 1993;168:817–823.

27. Weiner Z, Efrat Z, Zimmer EZ, et al. Direct measurement of central venous pressure in human fetuses. *Am J Obstet Gynecol.* 1997;176 (suppl):S19.

28. Weiner CP, Wenstrom KD, Sipes SL, et al. Risk factors for cordocentesis and fetal intravascular transfusions. *Am J Obstet Gynecol.* 1991;165:1020–1023.

29. Weiner CP, Anderson T. The acute effect of cordocentesis with or without fetal curarization and of intravascular transfusion upon umbilical artery waveform indices. *Obstet Gynecol.* 1989;73:219–224.

30. Weiner CP, Robillard JE. Effect of acute intravascular volume expansion upon human fetal prostaglandin concentrations. *Am J Obstet Gynecol.* 1989;161:1494–1497.

31. Capponi A, Rizzo G, Pasquini L, et al. Indomethacin modifies the fetal hemodynamic response induced by cordocentesis. *Am J Obstet Gynecol.* 1997;176 (suppl):S19.

32. Rizzo G, Capponi A, Rinaldo D, et al. Release of vasoactive agents during cordocentesis: differences between normally grown and growth-restricted fetuses. *Am J Obstet Gynecol.* 1996;175:563–570.

33. Nicolini U, Kochenour NK, Greco P, et al. Consequences of fetomaternal hemorrhage after intrauterine transfusion. *BMJ.* 1988;297:1379–1381.

34. Weiner CP, Grant SS, Hudson J, et al. Effect of diagnostic and therapeutic cordocentesis upon maternal serum alpha fetoprotein concentration. *Am J Obstet Gynecol.* 1989;161:706–708.

35. Paidas MJ, Lynch L, Lockwood CJ, et al. Alloimmune thrombocytopenia: fetal and neonatal losses related to fetal blood sampling. *Am J Obstet Gynecol.* 1995;172:475–479.

36. Weiner CP. Fetal blood sampling and fetal thrombocytopenia. *Fetal Diagn Ther.* 1995;10:173–177.

37. Tabor A, Philip J, Bang J, et al. Needle size and risk of miscarriage after amniocentesis [letter]. *Lancet.* 1988;1:183–184.

38. Weiner CP, Williamson RA, Varner MW, et al. Safety of second trimester amniocentesis [letter]. *Lancet.* 1986;2:226.

39. Ghidini A, Sepulveda W, Lockwood CJ, et al. Complications of fetal blood sampling. *Am J Obstet Gynecol.* 1993;168:1339–1344.

40. Donner C, Simon P, Karioun A, et al. Experience of a single team of operators in 891 diagnostic funipunctures. *Obstet Gynecol.* 1994;84:827–831.

TISSUE BIOPSIES

Mark I. Evans / Wolfgang Holzgreve / Eric L. Krivchenia / Eric P. Hoffman

Over 2 decades, there has been a dramatic shift away from the need for tissue-specific diagnoses to those that can be accomplished by DNA methodologies. However, there are many disorders for which only a tissue-specific histological or immuno-histochemical examination of the tissue will provide accurate prenatal diagnosis.[1] A classic example is ornithine trans-cabamylase deficiency which previously required a fetal liver biopsy, but now can be done at DNA level from amniotic fluid, chorionic villi, or fetal blood.[2] There are still numerous inborn errors of metabolism and other genetic disorders in which a tissue-specific sample is necessary. For example, several liver specific enzymes such as glycogen storage diseases require tissue biopsy. In other disorders such as Duchenne Muscular Dystrophy (DMD), the isolation of the dystrophin gene in the late 1980s allowed for the vast majority of patients at risk for DMD to have the diagnosis in the first trimester through CVS and subsequent DNA analysis.[3] However, not all cases of DMD are informative. When there is only 1 affected family member, and there are no other data to definitively discern whether a pregnant woman is a carrier, molecular diagnosis can be particularly problematic.

Prenatal diagnostic techniques have centered on 2 major areas, the first of which has been visualization of fetal structure and function. Over the decades, these techniques have included X-ray, amniography, direct visualization by fetoscopy, and ultrasound.[4] The second major approach to prenatal diagnosis has been through the laboratory study of fetal tissue. After 3 decades of use, the most utilized clinical technique remains amniocentesis. Chorionic villus sampling (CVS) and cordocentesis have emerged as additional techniques for obtaining fetal material. The combination of cytogenetic, biochemical, and molecular analyses in conjunction with highly detailed ultrasound examination has enabled the prenatal diagnosis of multiple fetal diseases and anatomic defects.

There has been a movement over the past decade away from needing specific tissue material for diagnosis. The major advantage of molecular diagnosis is that it allows, in general, for the use of any fetal tissue to look at DNA structure and expected function rather than at enzymatic reactions which are tissue-limited to their actual site of action.[5] However, in some cases, the availability of DNA diagnoses has increased both the possibilities for diagnosis, but also developed the need for fetal tissue-specific biopsies for previously undiagnosable cases for which molecular approaches do not work.

FETAL SKIN BIOPSY

Only a few of the serious dermatologic disorders are associated with chromosomal abnormalities or enzyme defects that can be detected in amniotic fluid or chorionic villi.[6] Furthermore, in the majority of serious cutaneous abnormalities, ultrasonic visualization is useless. Actual visualization of the skin and histology are the only ways to make such diagnoses. Examples of conditions for which prenatal diagnosis requires study of the fetal skin include:

- harlequin ichthyosis
- Sjögren-Larsson syndrome
- epidermolytic hyperkeratosis
- epidermolysis bullosa dystrophica
- epidermolysis bullosa lethalis
- oculocutaneous albinism
- congenital ichthyosiform ertheraderma
- congenital bullous epidermolysis[6–11] (Fig. 38-1)

Fetal skin biopsies have been obtained in 1 of 2 ways: Either under direct visualization via fetoscopy or under ultrasound guidance.[12]

FETOSCOPY

For fetoscopy, the site of entry of the fetoscope is chosen to allow easy access to biopsy sites such as the back, thighs, or scalp.[13–15] From 1970–1990, fetal skin biopsies have been obtained by fetoscopic methods which carried a 2–5% risk of miscarriage. The newer fiberoptic scopes simplify the procedure and have lowered the risks. The skin is prepared as for any invasive fetal procedure. Lidocaine 1% is injected subcutaneously into the maternal skin for anesthesia. A no. 15 scalpel blade is used to nick the skin and, if the patient is thin, down to the fascia. Then, under ultrasound guidance, the trocar of the fetoscope—which can be as simple as a 16- or 18-gauge needle—is inserted into the amniotic sac. If the procedure is being performed under direct visualization, the fetoscope is directed to the biopsy site. A significant advantage of direct visualization is that the specimen can be obtained at the site of obvious pathology. Though ultrasound-guided "blind" biopsy has gained popularity because the quality of fiber optics had previously been so poor, recent advances of fiber optic scopes have changed the equation back in favor of direct visualization. Fetoscopic techniques are described more fully in Chapter 41.

ULTRASOUND-GUIDED BIOPSIES

Recently, a modified approach to obtaining percutaneous ultrasound-guided fetal skin biopsies has been developed using a fine needle system.[16] The maternal skin is anesthetized with 1% Xylocaine. A good site is fetal buttock and outer thigh. Traditionally, an 18-gauge, 16-cm-long needle with trocar is inserted into the abdominal wall through the uterine cavity. Then, the sharp point of the trocar is withdrawn to avoid trauma. The tip of the needle is guided until it is about 1 cm away from the biopsy site. A 20-cm-long, 20-gauge biopsy forceps is inserted until it touches the fetal scalp, and a biopsy is obtained. The biopsy may be repeated to ensure that adequate material is obtained.

Alternatively, we have recently begun using the core biopsy needle/gun as for muscle biopsies. Here, the major issue is

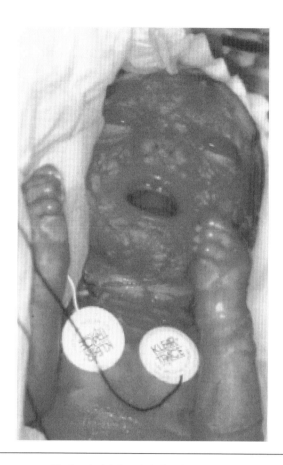

FIGURE 38-1 Harlequin ichthyosis baby shortly before death.

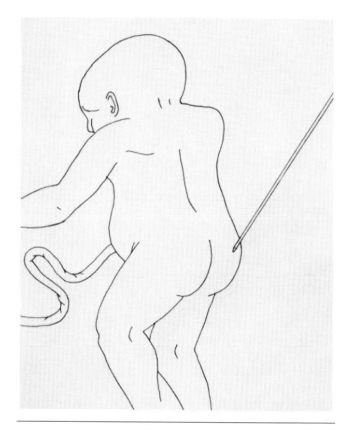

FIGURE 38-2 Skin biopsy: biopsy needle hovering over buttock.

making sure that the core starts external to the skin so that as the core is excised it includes the entire skin thickness (Figs. 38-2, 38-3, and 38-4).

One potential concern applicable to all skin biopsies is scarring from the procedure. However, recent evidence, predominantly secondary to fetal surgical experience, suggests that fetal skin heals by a different mechanism than it does postnatally. The process of regeneration is to reorganize properly, and fetal incisions therefore tend to heal without scar.[17]

Methods of diagnosis include histology and biochemical studies. For example, in harlequin ichthyosis, there is premature hyperkeratosis, most marked around the hair follicles and sweat ducts.[13] Sjögren-Larsson syndrome is diagnosed by finding of hyperkeratosis with increased keratohyaline.[18] In epidermolysis bullosa dystrophica, a cleavage plane below the basal lamina, and focal collagenolysis of the upper dermis, appears below the dermal/epidermal junction in unseparated regions.[19]

Significant advances in the biochemical examination of pathological fetal skin have been made over the past 5 years concurrent with our understanding of the ontogeny of structural proteins of normal fetal skin.[11,20] Biochemical studies have the advantages of allowing diagnoses earlier in gestation before direct visualization would be possible. The biochemical analyses of skin may also be applicable for genetic diagnosis using amniocytes and amniotic fluid. For example, prenatal diagnosis of several ichthyoses and other genetic disorders of

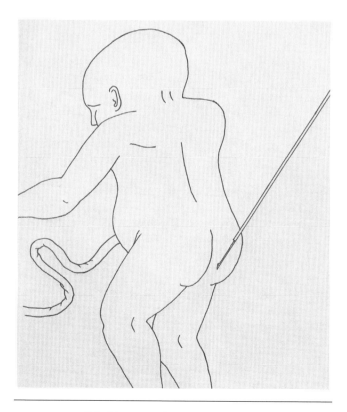

FIGURE 38-3 Skin biopsy: coring element extended through skin thickness.

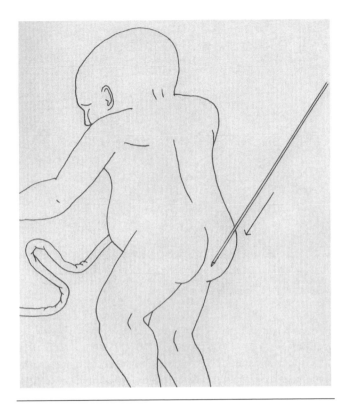

FIGURE 38-4 Skin biopsy: coring gun barrel shot forward obtaining specimen.

which ichthyosis is a component, has been performed using amniotic fluid obtained between 14 and 16 weeks gestation.

Such studies have concluded, for example, that harlequin ichthyosis is not 1 disorder, but a genetically heterogeneous group of disorders with altered glomerular granules, intercellular lipids, and variation in expression and/or processing of structural protein markers of normal epidermal keratinization.

As with all invasive procedures, risks include rupture of membranes, bleeding, infection, and miscarriage. Improvement in the fiber optic technologies have allowed decreasing size and time to complete procedures, and therefore increasing safety.

FETAL LIVER BIOPSY

The liver has hundreds of metabolic functions. For a large number of these enzymatic reactions, enzyme activity can be documented in many different tissues including amniotic fluid and chorionic villi.[21] Though it was necessary to learn that there were different normal activity values in different tissues,[22,23] the diagnoses of conditions such as the mucopolysaccharidoses and Tay Sachs disease (among countless others) have been routine for a number of years. Unfortunately, enzyme activity is strictly limited to the liver for certain disorders.

Fetal liver biopsies have been used successfully for the prenatal diagnosis of:

- ornithine transcarbamylase deficiency [24–28]
- Von Gierke's disease
- carbamyl phosphate synthetase deficiency
- primary hyperoxaluria type 1

The technique for fetal liver biopsy is similar to that for skin except that a needle or coring biopsy instrument is inserted into the upper right quadrant of the fetal abdomen. If a needle is used, a syringe is attached to create suction, and the needle is then removed, taking a careful specimen with it.[14] It is important for all of these biopsy techniques to have a dissecting microscopy readily available to ensure that an adequate specimen has been obtained. Likewise, the coring biopsy gun can be used.

Multiple enzymes, in addition to the 1 of interest, must be tested to eliminate the possibility that a low level of activity is a function of a poor specimen rather than disease. Otherwise, the enzymatic procedures are similar to those well known for pediatric specimens.

FETAL MUSCLE BIOPSY

After nearly 3 decades of research in the United States and millions of dollars in funding from highly publicized charitable campaigns, the gene for the muscle protein dystrophin, whose absence causes Duchenne muscular dystrophy (DMD), was finally isolated in 1987.[3] This gene encompasses more than 2 1/2 million base pairs of the X chromosome and is by far the largest gene ever described.[29] Analyses of children with DMD have revealed that multiple molecular defects can produce the clinical picture of DMD.[30]

Many of the children with DMD have sizable deletions of the gene. In about 45% of patients, however, no deletion is detectable. Attempts to diagnose DMD prenatally had been futile for nearly 20 years. It was hoped, for example, that muscle proteins could be demonstrable in fetal blood, as it is known that elevated levels of creatine phosphokinase (CPK) are often elevated in carriers of DMD as well as significantly elevated in patients with DMD. Unfortunately, these levels do not begin to rise until at least the very end of pregnancy, making it impractical for prenatal diagnosis.

With the isolation of the DMD gene, the majority of fetal cases could be diagnosed by the molecular analysis of the gene, either through detection of deletion mutations or by linkage analysis. Thus, the majority of cases of DMD are currently diagnosed from tissue specimens obtained via chorionic villus sampling. However, there are a number of situations in which a deletion mutation is not found and DNA molecular diagnosis will not work. These can be divided into 4 different categories:

- Those with only prior family member affected, and it cannot be determined whether the single affected family member inherited an abnormal X chromosome from his mother, or was a spontaneous mutation himself.

- Those for which analysis of polymorphisms proves uninformative (ie, fails to reveal any differences between 2 maternal X chromosomes).
- Those for which there has been a crossover in meiosis between maternal X chromosomes such that it cannot be determined whether or not the DMD gene mutation was inherited.
- Those for which there is an X-autosomal translocation in a male or even female fetus. Such female DMD cases are possible because an X-autosomal translocation break can be in the DMD region,[31] and these translocations will usually not be inactivated because Barr bodies are intact X chromosomes.

For example, a 41-year-old, gravida 3, para 2 woman came for prenatal diagnosis at 11 weeks gestation by CVS for advanced maternal age. On family history, however, it was first revealed that she had a 19-year-old son from a previous marriage, who had classic DMD. No other family members were affected. CVS was obtained demonstrating abnormal male karyotype. DNA analysis was performed on the fetus, the mother and the son with DMD which showed that the fetus had inherited the same X chromosome as his affected half-brother. By Bayesian analysis, it was determined that the chance that the fetus was affected was the same risk as that the mother was a carrier, which was felt to be about 30% in this case. Typically, patients in this circumstance have been advised to consider termination of pregnancy followed by postmortem analysis for dystrophin. If dystrophin was absent, then the fetus was affected by DMD and the mother was a carrier. Therefore, future fetuses would be at risk. If dystrophin were present, it could be concluded that the deceased brother was affected with DMD due to a spontaneous mutation, and that there was little risk to future pregnancies. A muscle biopsy specimen showed the presence of dystrophin was documented both by Western blotting and by immunofluorescence of muscle tissue.[32] The pregnancy continued successfully, and the child was born without symptoms or scarring.

Under ultrasound guidance, a site of entry for the biopsy is chosen, the maternal abdomen anesthetized, and a small nick made in the skin to ease entry. For 10 years we used a Perry Kidney biopsy gun, but recently we have switched to a Temno core biopsy needle system that is thinner but gets a cleaner, larger layer core biopsy specimen (Fig. 38-5). The biopsy device is inserted into the uterine cavity and into the fetal buttock in a downward and outward direction (Fig. 38-6). The coring guide is extended and then the trigger pulled, creating a core biopsy. It is important to carefully pick the fetal entry site attempting to avoid likely sites of bleeding, nerve location, or the fetal testes. By definition, however, the procedure is somewhat crude, and some complications will inevitably eventually occur. Collaborative data to this point are encouraging about patient safety, and the procedure should

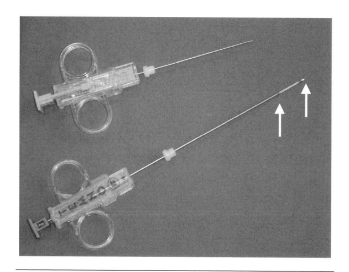

FIGURE 38-5 Temno biopsy needle.

be used when indicated, and only performed by experienced operators.[33,34]

Care must continue to be exerted in the performance of the procedure, as sampling has the potential for damage to fetal nerves and vascular supply. In our experience, there were no scars or nerve damage, and all liveborns were correctly diagnosed. No specific nerve studies have been done postnatally as none seemed to be indicated. In a collaborative report from 1994, 2 of 12 cases aborted, both secondary to ruptured membranes which is a risk with any invasive procedure. With experience, the procedure has been performed faster and safer, with losses predicted to be about 1–3%, consistent with comparable invasive procedures. In our experience, we have not seen losses in over 30 cases (unpublished). However, fetal muscle biopsy

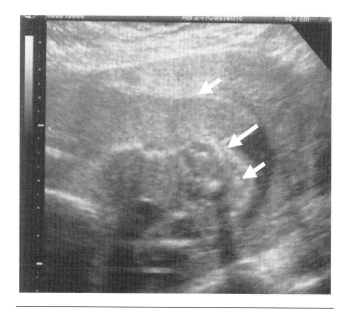

FIGURE 38-6 Ultrasound showing coring biopsy needle extending through fetal gluteal muscle. Arrows show path of needle.

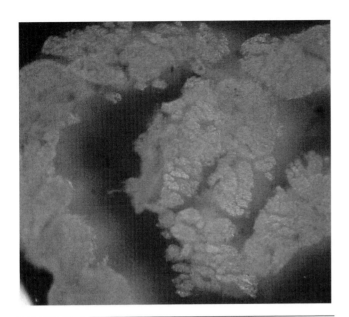

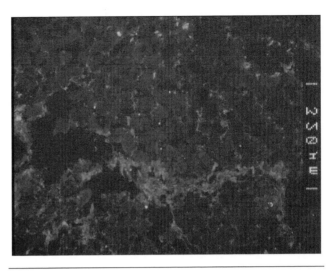

FIGURE 38-9 Immunohistochemical staining of Duchenne Muscle showing lack of uptake of stain.

FIGURE 38-7 Fetal muscle biopsy specimen.

procedures should clearly be seen as a last resort following inability to obtain a diagnosis by less invasive techniques.

The dystrophin protein is present only in muscle. Assays for the dystropin protein are immunoblotting and immunofluorescence, though the former requires a relatively large amount of muscle tissue (50 mg). Immunofluorescence is accurate with as few as 6 muscle cells.[31] It is important to use multiple antibodies directed against different regions of the very large dystrophin protein, and to include control antibodies which demonstrate the presence of fetal muscle cells in the biopsy, which is usually predominantly epidermal tissue (Fig. 38-7). Additional tissue controls of known normal and known affected fetal muscle should be carried out in parallel. Our experience suggests that the incubation of serial cryostat sections with

anti-dystrophin antibodies 60kD (amnio-terminal region) and d10 (carboxyl-terminal region), and a myosin heavy chain antibody (F59), allows the accurate differentiation of Duchenne dystrophy from normal (Fig. 38-9).

The high incidence of DMD and the frequent difficulties encountered in arriving at unambiguous molecular genetic predictions suggest that fetal muscle biopsy will become a standard procedure for the in utero diagnosis of DMD. As progress is made in the molecular pathology of other neuromuscular conditions, it is conceivable that this methodology could be extended to the diagnosis of other muscle diseases.

OTHER ORGANS

It is easy to imagine the desirability of having a fetal tissue biopsy of a tumor or mediastinal mass.[12] Kidney biopsies may be useful to document the degree and type of renal dysplasia associated with an obstructive uropathy. Currently, however, most of these other indications would not seem strong enough to outweigh the risk of obtaining the fetal tissue.

A major risk in performing a biopsy of a tumor or a mediastinal mass would be uncontrollable bleeding. As visualization techniques and instrumentation improve, however, the balance of the equation might certainly change, and one should be very hesitant to be dogmatic about the desirability of any particular procedure.

CONCLUSIONS

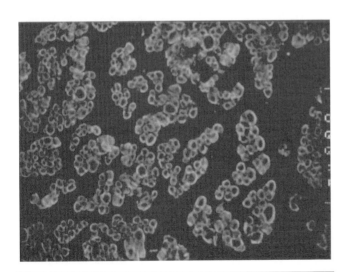

FIGURE 38-8 Immunohistochemical staining of normal fetal muscle showing normal staining pattern.

Though most prenatal diagnoses can be made either by visualization or the obtaining of either amniotic fluid or blood, other rare disorders require a specific tissue such as skin, liver, or muscle. Fetal tissue biopsy may be performed either fetoscopically or under sonographic guidance. The risks of pregnancy wastage are relatively high. Thus, these biopsies should be performed only when the yield exceeds that risk. Because of their rarity and the complexity involved in the analyses of the specimens, these procedures should be performed only in specialized referral units.

References

1. Evans MI, Greb A, Kinkel LM, et al. In utero fetal muscle biopsy for the diagnosis of Duchenne muscular dystrophy. *Am J Obstet Gynecol.* 1991;165:728–732.
2. Brusilow SW, Horwick AL. Urea Cycle Enzymes. In: Scriver CR, Beaudet AL, Sly WS, Valle D, eds. *The Metabolic and Molecular Bases of Inherited Disease.* 7th ed. New York, NY: McGraw-Hill Publishing Co; 1995:1187–1200.
3. Hoffman EP, Brown RH, Kunkel LM. Dystrophin: the protein product of the Duchenne muscular dystrophy locus. *Cell.* 1987;51:919–928.
4. Charrow J, Nadler HL, Evans MI. Prenatal diagnosis. In: Emery AE, Rimoin DL, eds. *Principles and Practice of Medical Genetics.* 2nd ed. New York: Churchill Livingstone;1991:1959–1994.
5. Caskey CT, Rossiter BJ. Molecular genetics. In: Evans MI ed. *Reproductive Risks and Prenatal Diagnosis.* Norwalk, CT: Appleton & Lange;1992:265–277.
6. Epstein E. Diagnosis of metabolic diseases that affect the skin using cultured amniotic fluid cells. *Semin Dermatol.* 1984;3:167–171.
7. Nazzaro V. Sviluppo normale della cute umana fetale. *Giornale Italiano di Dermatologia E Venereologia.* 1989;124:421–427.
8. Dale BA, Holbrook KA, Fleckman P, et al. Heterogeneity in harlequin ichthyosis, an inborn error of epidermal keratinization: variable morphology and structural protein expression and the defect in lamellar granules. *J Invest Dermatol.* 1990;94:618.
9. Holbrook KA, Dale BA, Williams ML, et al. The expression of congenital ichthyosiform erythroderma in second trimester fetuses of the same family: morphologic and biochemical studies. *J Invest Dermatol.* 1988;91:521–531.
10. Nazzaro V, Nicolini U, DeLuca L, et al. Prenatal diagnosis of junctional epidermolysis bullosa associated with pyloric atresia. *J Med Genet.* 1990;27:244–248.
11. Dale BA, Perry TB, Holbrook KA, et al. Biochemical examination of fetal skin biopsy specimens obtained by fetoscopy: use of the method for analysis of keratins and filaggrin. *Prenat Diagn.* 1986;6:37–44.
12. Rodeck CH, Nicolaides KH. Fetal tissue biopsy: techniques and indications. *Fetal Ther.* 1986;1:46–58.
13. Elias J, Mazur M, Sabbagha R, et al. Prenatal diagnosis of harlequin ichthyosis. *Clin Genet.* 1980;17:275–279.
14. Hobbins JC, Mahoney MJ. In utero diagnosis of hemoglobinopathies: technique for obtaining fetal blood. *N Engl J Med.* 1974;290:1065–1067.
15. Bang J. Intrauterine needle diagnosis. In: Holm K, ed. *Interventional Ultrasound.* Munksgaard, Elsevier, Copenhagen: 1985;122–128.
16. Buckshee K, Parveen S, Mittal S, et al. Percutaneous ultrasound guided fetal skin biopsy: a new approach. *Int J Gynaecol Obstet.* 1991;34:267–270.
17. Adzick NS, Longaker MT. *Fetal Wound Healing.* New York: Elsevier Science Inc; 1992:53–70.
18. Kusseff BG, Matsouka LY, Stenn KS, et al. Prenatal diagnosis of Sjogren-Larsson syndrome. *J Pediatr.* 1982;101:998–1001.
19. Ant N, Lambrect L, Jovanovic V, et al. Prenatal diagnosis of epidermolysis bullosa dystrophic hallopean siemens with electron microscopy of fetal skin. *Lancet.* 1981;2:1677–1679.
20. Moll, R, Moll I, Wiest W. Changes in the pattern of cytokeratin polypeptides epidermis and hair follicles during skin development in human fetuses. *Differentiation.* 1983;23:170–178.
21. Ben-Yoseph Y. Biochemical genetics. In: Evans MI, ed. *Reproductive Risks and Prenatal Diagnosis.* Norwalk, CT: Appleton & Lange; 1992:251–265.
22. Evans MI, Moore C, Kolodny E, et al. Lyosomal enzymes in chorionic villi, cultured amniocytes and cultured skin fibroblasts. *Clin Chem Acta.* 1986;157:109–113.
23. Ben-Yoseph Y, Evans MI, Bottoms SF, et al. Lyosomal enzyme activities in fresh and frozen chorionic villi and in cultured trophoblasts. *Clin Chem Acta.* 1986;161:307–313.
24. Rodeck CH, Patrick AD, Pemberg ME, et al. Fetal liver biopsy for prenatal diagnosis of ornithine carbamoyl transferase deficiency. *Lancet.* 1982;1:297–299.
25. Holzgreve W, Golbus MS. Prenatal diagnosis of ornithine transcarbamylase deficiency utilizing fetal liver biopsy. *Am J Hum Genet.* 1984;36:320–328.
26. Danpure CJ, Jennings PR, Penketh RJ, et al. Fetal liver alanine: glyoxylate aminotransferase and the prenatal diagnosis of primary hyperoxaluria type I. *Prenat Diagn.* 1989;9:271–291.
27. Golbus MS, Simpson TJ, Koresawa M, et al. The prenatal determination of glucose-6-phosphatase activity by fetal liver biopsy. *Prenat Diagn.* 1988;8:401–404.
28. Piceni Sereni L, Bachmann C, Pfister U, et al. Prenatal diagnosis of carbamoylphosphate synthetase deficiency by fetal liver biopsy. *Prenat Diagn.* 1988;8:307–309.
29. Hoffman EP, Fishbeck KH, Brown RH, et al. Dystrophin characterization in muscle biopsies from Duchenne and Becker muscular dystrophy patients. *N Engl J Med.* 1988;318:1363–368.
30. Hoffman EP. Genotype/phenotype correlations in Duchenne/Becker muscular dystrophy. In: Partridge TA, ed. *Molecular and Cell Biology of Muscular Dystrophy.* London, England: Chapman and Hall; 1993:57–63.
31. Evans MI, Farrell SA, Greb A, et al. In utero fetal muscle biopsy for the diagnosis of Duchenne muscular dystrophy in a female fetus "suddenly at risk". *Am J Med Genet.* 1003;46:309–312.
32. Kuller JA, Hoffman EP, Fries MJ, et al. Prenatal diagnosis of Duchenne muscular dystrophy by fetal muscle biopsy. *Hum Genet.* 1992;90:34–40.
33. Evans MI, Hoffman EP, Cadrin C, et al. Fetal muscle biopsy: collaborative experience with varied indications. *Obstet Gynecol.* 1994;84:913–917.
34. Evans MI, Quintero RA, King M, et al. Endoscopically assisted, ultrasound guided fetal muscle biopsy. *Fetal Diagn Ther.* 1995;10:168–173.

CHAPTER 39

FETAL SKIN SAMPLING AND PRENATAL DIAGNOSIS OF GENODERMATOSES

Anthony R. Gregg / Sherman Elias

BACKGROUND

In the past, the accurate prenatal diagnosis of serious inherited skin disorders (genodermatoses) relied exclusively on the procedure of fetal skin biopsy. This was first described in 1980 and 1981.[1,2] At that time, the fetal skin biopsy required fetoscopy, which had its beginnings in the early 1970s.[3] Fetoscopy allows direct visualization of the fetus through a variably sized (0.7–6.8 mm) endoscope.[4] During the 1980s and early 1990s real-time ultrasound technology advanced significantly. Thus, skill in performing fetoscopy is no longer a prerequisite to fetal skin biopsy procedures.

The laboratory diagnostic approach to genodermatoses, like the technique of fetal skin biopsy, has also evolved since the earliest reports of successful prenatal diagnosis of genodermatoses.[5] Establishing a diagnosis once relied on clinical history and confirmed diagnosis in the proband combined with histologic assessment of the fetal skin. In some cases these requirements could not be met and prenatal diagnosis was not possible. Molecular genetics based testing is currently available for many genodermatoses.[6] This approach to establishing the diagnosis may eliminate the need for an exact clinical diagnosis in the proband, may allow for greater accuracy in establishing diagnoses, and may provide a more rapid turn-around time from sample collection to diagnosis. Importantly, this approach to the diagnosis of genodermatoses is less invasive. Furthermore, fetal cells obtained by chorionic villus sampling (CVS) or amniocentesis can provide the DNA needed for establishing a diagnosis rapidly, and is far less invasive than fetal skin sampling.

Many of the specific proteins that are integral to the proper structure and function of the skin have been identified. In many cases their chromosomal location and gene structure have been identified (Table 39-1). Further, we are rapidly expanding our understanding of the exact mutations responsible for these disorders. As our understanding of the genetic basis of genodermatoses expands, it is anticipated that the demand for fetal skin biopsy as a clinical service for prenatal diagnosis will become virtually nonexistent. Rather physicians trained in the procedure of CVS or amniocentesis will be capable of acquiring specimens for diagnosis. In the meantime, however, fetal skin sampling may still be needed for some cases in which the molecular diagnosis is not possible.

Although rapid advances in fetal imaging technology and molecular diagnostics have made prenatal diagnosis of genodermatoses easier, the low prevalence of these disorders (Table 39-2) and rapid acquisition of molecular data relating to these disorders establishes the need to manage at-risk families in specialized centers. Certainly the importance of proper genetics counseling should not be dismissed due to ease of sample collection. Genetic counseling services are an important means of providing accurate information to families, physicians, and laboratory personnel.

TECHNIQUE

Fetal skin biopsy is a procedure performed most often between 17 and 20 weeks gestation.[9] Prior to proceeding with the procedure the ability to establish a diagnosis using fetal skin for histologic or immunohistologic studies should have been established. Furthermore, the diagnosis should be performed using this invasive technique only when a molecular-based diagnosis is not possible using cells obtained by CVS or amniocentesis. After obtaining the patient's informed consent, an ultrasound examination is performed. This examination seeks to determine or confirm the gestational age of the fetus. Immunohistologic assessment of the fetal skin is dependent on gestational age. Many proteins assayed by immunostaining are not expressed prior to 12 weeks gestation; therefore, establishing the gestational age of the fetus is of paramount importance.[5] The initial ultrasound also allows screening for fetal malformations, which might preclude further testing. This approach will also allow early diagnosis of multiple gestation and localization of the placenta and umbilical cord.

Using ultrasound the safest approach to the fetal skin over the back, thorax, or buttocks is established. It is prudent to avoid the placenta, umbilical cord, head, neck, and genitalia whenever possible. Once a suitable entry site is selected, the skin is prepared with an antiseptic, and the abdomen sterily draped. Due to the need for a larger bore needle in this procedure as compared to amniocentesis and the slightly greater procedure time, the patient may be sedated with an appropriate agent such as diazepam (10 mg intravenous). This may cross the placenta thereby reducing fetal movement during the procedure. The maternal skin is anesthetized over the chosen entry site (1% lidocaine hydrochloride, subcutaneous). A stab wound in the skin is made at the entry site using a no. 11 scalpel blade. This allows easy entry of a 14-gauge Angiocath (Desert Medical, Sandy, UT) past the skin, subcutaneous tissue, uterine smooth muscle, and into the amniotic cavity. The stylet is withdrawn and amniotic fluid specimens are obtained via a syringe attached to the Angiocath. Amniotic fluid is sent for cytogenetic analysis, acetylcholinesterase, and alpha Feto-protein studies. Depending on the genodermatosis being investigated, amniotic fluid may be used to complement the diagnosis made by histology or immunohistochemistry (ie, presence or absence of small macrophages in amniotic fluid). After the syringe is removed, biopsy forceps, Storaz 27071Z (Karl Storz Endoscopy America, Culver City, CA) are passed through the catheter into the

| TABLE 39-1 | GENODERMATOSES AND THE PROTEINS IMPLICATED IN THE CLINICAL CONDITION. THE CHROMOSOMAL LOCATION FOR EACH GENE THAT ENCODES THE LISTED PROTEIN IS KNOWN. FOR NEARLY, EVERY GENODERMATOSIS LISTED ONE OR MORE GENE MUTATIONS HAVE BEEN DESCRIBED. NEW MUTATIONS ARE BEING CATALOGUED AT A VERY RAPID RATE | | |

Genodermatosis	Protein	Chromosome[7]
Lamellar ichthyosis	Loracrin	1q21-q22
	Profilaggrin	1q21-q22
	Involucrin	1q21-q22
	Cornifin	1q21-q22
	Trichohyalin	1q21.3
	Transglutaminase I	14q11
Epidermolysis hyperkeratosis	Desmoglein I	18q21-q22
Palmar plantar keratosis	Keratin 1	12q13
	Keratin 10	17q21-q22
	Desmocollin 1	18
Darier's disease	Desmoglein III	18q12.1-q12.2
	Desmoglein II	18q12.1-q12.2
Epidermolysis bullosa simplex	Keratin 5	12q13
	Keratin 14	17q12-q21
	BPAG 1	6p12-p11
Junctional epidermolysis bullosa	BPAG 2	10q24.3
	α6 integrins	2
	β4 integrins	17q11-qter
	Laminin 5	10q24.3
Dystrophic epidermolysis bullosa	Type VII Collagen	3p21.3

amniotic cavity and against the fetal skin (Fig. 39-1). Multiple biopsies are taken (2–5) depending on the focal nature of the genodermatosis. Furthermore, it should be kept in mind that false positive histology may result from traumatic injury to the tissue during the biopsy procedure.[5] Skin biopsy specimens (1 × 1 mm) are placed into the appropriate transport container with fixative or media as needed for the planned studies.

Upon completing the sampling procedure, the Angiocath is removed from the maternal abdomen and pressure is applied for about 5 minutes. Afterward maternal vital signs are monitored for a period of about 1 hour. Women at risk for Rh immunization should receive Rh immunoglobulin (300 μg) after the procedure.

SAFETY

The safety of fetal skin biopsy procedures will vary depending on operator experience and whether or not the biopsies are obtained under ultrasound guidance or by direct visualization using fetoscopy. Fetal skin biopsy obtained by fetoscopy has been studied more extensively than ultrasound-guided skin biopsy techniques. The general risks associated with fetoscopy are described in detail in Chapter 41. The risks from fetoscopy for fetal loss and perinatal loss is related to the invasive fetal procedure performed. For fetal skin biopsy a risk of fetal loss after fetoscopy was reported as 16%. Perinatal loss was determined to be 4.8%.[10] Overall fetoscopy may be associated with a 10% increase in preterm delivery.[11] The safety of ultrasound directed fetal skin biopsy has been reported once.[9] Among 17 reported cases, 5 were found to be affected and terminated. The remaining 12 cases continued uneventfully

| TABLE 39-2 | THE INCIDENCE OF SELECTED GENODERMATOSES AND THEIR INHERITANCE PATTERNS | | |

Genodermatoses	Incidence[8]	Inheritance
Lamellar ichthyosis	<1:300,000	A_R
Epidermolysis hyperkeratosis	Rare U.S. (3,000)	A_D
Palmar plantar keratosis	1:200 N. Sweden	A_D
	1:40,000 N. Ireland	
Darier's disease	1:55,000–1:100,000	A_D
Epidermolysis bullosa simplex	50,000 U.S.	A_D (A_R)
Junctional epidermolysis bullosa	Rare	A_R
Dystrophic epidermolysis bullosa	6,500	A_D
	10,000	A_R

A_R—autosomal recessive; A_D—autosomal dominant, A_D—(A_R)—autosomal dominant with autosomal recessive less common mode of inheritance.

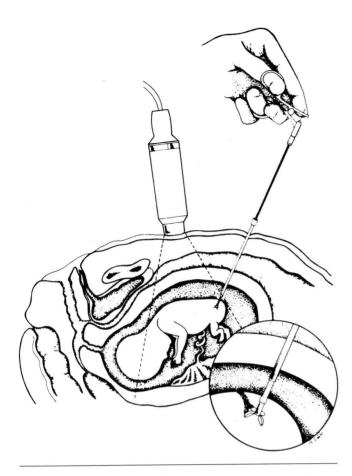

FIGURE 39-1 Fetal skin sampling with ultrasound guidance. Reproduced with permission.

to term with no cases of preterm labor, or preterm rupture of the fetal membranes. There were no serious functional or cosmetic injuries reported. Skin blemishes thought to be attributable to fetal skin biopsy were noted in 25% of term infants. The limited safety data available for the ultrasound guided approach makes it impossible to properly draw conclusions as to its safety over fetoscopy. However, use of a smaller gauge instrument and smaller biopsy forceps suggests greater safety with the ultrasound-guided approach.

SUMMARY

Advances in ultrasound technology and molecular diagnostics have dramatically altered the approach to the prenatal diagnosis of genodermatoses. An ultrasound-guided approach to fetal skin biopsy rather than fetoscopy may be safer when fetal skin is required to establish the diagnosis of a genodermatosis antenatally.

References

1. Elias S, Esterly NB. Prenatal diagnosis of hereditary skin disorders. *Clin Obstet Gynecol.* 1981;24:1069–1087.
2. Elias S, Mazur M, Shabbagha R, et al. Prenatal diagnosis of harlequin ichthyosis. *Clin Genet.* 1980;17:275–280.
3. Hobbins JC, Mahoney MJ, Goldstein LA. New methods of intrauterine evaluation by the combined use of fetoscopy and ultrasound. *Am J Obstet Gynecol.* 1974;118:1069–1072.
4. Montemagno R, Soothill P. In: *Fetal Therapy Invasive and Transplacental.* Fisk NM, Moise KJ, eds. New York: Cambridge University Press; 1997;9–26.
5. Holbrook K, Christiano A, Elias S, et al. Prenatal diagnosis of inherited EB: Ultrastructural, antigenic, and molecular approaches. In: *Epidermolysis Bullosa: Epidemiologic, and Laboratory Advances, and the Findings of the National Epidermolysis Bullosa Registry.* Fine J-D, Bauer EA, McGuire J, Moshell A, eds. Baltimore: Johns Hopkins University Press.
6. Sybert VP. In: *Genetic Skin Disorders.* New York: Oxford University press; 1997.
7. Online Mendelian Inheritance in Man, OMIM (TM). Center for Medical Genetics. Johns Hopkins University (Baltimore, MD) and National Center for Biotechnology Information, National Library of Medicine (Bethesda, MD), 1997. Available *http://www.ncbi.nlm.nih.gov/omim/*
8. Spitz JL. In: *Genodermatoses a Full-Color Clinical Guide to Genetic Skin Disorders.* Baltimore: Williams and Wilkins; 1996.
9. Elias S, Emerson DS, Simpson JL, et al. Ultrasound-guided fetal skin sampling for prenatal diagnosis of genodermatoses. *Obstet Gynecol.* 1994;83:337–341.
10. Special Report: The status of fetoscopy and fetal tissue sampling. *Prenat Diag.* 1984;4:79–81.
11. Hobbins JC. Doing fetoscopy. *Contemp Obstet Gynecol.* 1985;25:31–35.

OPERATIVE FETOSCOPY

Jan Deprest / Dominique van Schoubroeck / Gerard Barki / Eduardo Gratacos

INTRODUCTION

Fetoscopy is the direct fetal visualization through endoscopy, which was introduced in the 1970s to solve some uncommon first and second trimester diagnostic problems.[1] In addition to the demonstration of some external pathognomic malformations, fetoscopy was used to obtain or transfuse fetal blood or to guide fetal biopsies. It however never became widely implemented because of the required skills and special instruments but mostly because of its invasiveness. The overall abortion rate was 4%, being more frequent for specific procedures such as skin biopsy (16%).[2] This number should be seen in proportion to the diameter of the instrumentation used at that time: rod lens telescopes had a minimal diameter of 3 mm for sufficient illumination and image resolution. As high-resolution ultrasound (US) made its introduction in fetal medicine, fetoscopy became redundant. Today we witness a revival of fetoscopy, thanks to rapid advances in video endoscopy in general, and fiberoptic endoscopic technology in particular. Fiber endoscopes with a high number of pixels offer excellent image quality at a very small diameter, making intrauterine operative interventions possible.[3,4] By the year 2000, clinical interventions involve mainly procedures on the placenta, umbilical cord, and fetal membranes. In other words these are interventions on the fetal adnexae, also called "obstetrical endoscopy."[5] But as time goes by and skills increase, the field of operative fetoscopy extends towards interventions on the fetus itself: endoscopic fetal surgery has become a clinical reality.[6] In this chapter, we first introduce the reader to instrumental requirements for and surgical aspects of fetoscopy, as successful fetoscopy depends highly on technical details. Thereafter some of the main clinical applications are discussed.

INSTRUMENTATION AND TECHNIQUES

ENDOSCOPES

Basic requirements are the same as for any endoscopic procedure, such as a good quality light fountain and a video camera. We use a Xenon light source, and a 1 or 3 chip digital camera. Fetoscopic images are projected on a video screen together with the US images. A special "Twin" video system (Karl Storz, Tuttlingen, Germany) mixes both types of images at variable magnification according to the surgeon's needs. Alternatively, 2 screens can be used. The *endoscopes* are completely different from their hysteroscopic or laparoscopic counterparts and specially developed for this purpose. There has been a considerable innovation in this field, thanks to an investment of the European Commission with its "Biomed 2 Programme" referred to as the "Eurofoetus project."[7] The European manufacturer *Karl Storz Endoskope* received funds

to develop an entire line of purpose designed instruments with a group of clinicians. This kind of funding is designed for instrumentation that would otherwise never make its way to the market. Fetoscopes typically come in diameters of 1.0–2.3 mm, and the most modern generation has deported eyepieces rather than standard fixed eyecaps. This reduces weight during the operation and facilitates precise movements, because the camera and eyepiece rest far away from the insertion site. This makes manipulation very similar to other needle-based invasive procedures in fetal medicine. Image and light transmission can be either through fiber-optic bundles or through a conventional rod lens system. Fiberscopes of 1.0–2.0 mm form the core of our instrumentation, they have a wide opening angle (60°) and come in different lengths depending on the gestational age they will be used for. We have a 1.0 mm diameter, 20 cm long endoscope for early gestation, a 1.2 mm endoscope of 30 cm for early second trimester (both 10,000 pixels) and a 2.0 mm endoscope with 50,000 pixels, offering excellent quality and therefore preferred for most procedures above 20 weeks. Fiberscopes have the advantage that they are semiflexible and can thus be curved to a certain extent. All these scopes have a 0° angle of view or look straight ahead. At present we experiment with 12–30° rod lens fetoscopes of 2.0 mm (length: 26.5 cm). These are for instance used to work on an anteriorly located placenta or in case the target of the fetoscopy lays out of the axis of the endoscope (Fig. 40-1). In the absence of such scopes, we have been using successfully curved fiber endoscopes to overcome the limitation of a 0° angle of view. Earlier experience with steerable (flexible) endoscopes was not very convincing in terms of light transmission and resolution when used for laser coagulation on an anteriorly located placenta.[8–10]

SHEATHS, TROCARS, AND CANNULAS

The scopes are used within a *sheath*, which protects the semi-flexible fiber or fragile rod lens endoscope. Its form and diameter are dependant on the purpose of the procedure. For straightforward fetal visualisation a round sheath or needle can be used fitting tightly around the endoscope and allowing minimal flow of infusion fluid. For instance an 18 G needle is large enough to house the embryofetoscope. If instruments are needed and the same single entry port is to be used, the sheath needs to be larger. For the most common procedure such as photocoagulation, a laser fiber is inserted through the upper part of an oval shaped sheath. As the upper part of the sheath is narrower the laser fiber is kept in a stable position. Most sheaths have luer lock connections for irrigation fluid through luer lock fittings.

The sheath can be introduced into the amniotic cavity either directly or through a cannula. For direct introduction, sheaths come with an accompanying *trocar* (this is a sharpened obturator). The combination of sheath and cannula is directly stabbed through the skin abdominal and uterine wall. As in operative

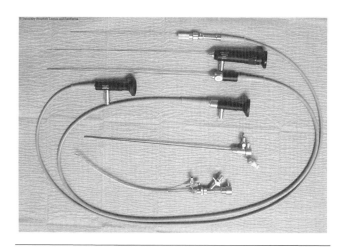

FIGURE 40-1 Overview of our fiber-optic endoscopes. 1.0, 1.2, and 2.0 mm 0° fiber scope with deported eyepiece. Straight and curved sheaths are shown at the bottom of the image.

laparoscopy, it may be necessary to change instruments or endoscopes during the procedure. Therefore we feel more comfortable to work with formal *cannulas*—ports that stay during the entire procedure, and through which instruments and scopes can be introduced. This allows easy instrument changes and in theory reduces the risk for membrane dislodgement, as the cannula does not move much in relation to the membranes during the procedure. The diameter of the cannula is determined according to the largest instrument to be used during the operation. At present we have a wide range of thin-walled, semiflexible cannulas commercially available in any diameter between 4 and 15 Fr (1.6–5 mm; Performa, Cook, Belgium). They can be inserted either with the *Seldinger* technique,[11] which gradually expands the myometrial and membrane stab wound up to the desired diameter, or *directly* with purpose-designed pyramidal trocars (Karl Storz; Fig. 40-2). Cannulas have a silicone seal at the rear end of the port house, allowing the introduction of irregularly shaped instruments of different diameters, without fluid leak. Ideally we would prefer to use

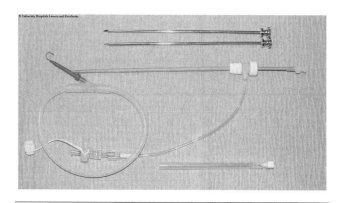

FIGURE 40-2 A set of a 9.0 and 10 Fr trocar and a thin walled Teflon cannula. Alternatively the trocar can be introduced using the Seldinger technique, for which the depicted needle and guide wire is used.

the type of cannulas we used in experimental fetal surgical procedures: these are balloon-tipped which in its turn prevents membrane dislodgement.[12] A commercial and approved product is however not available yet.

DISTENSION MEDIUM AND INSTRUMENTS

Although fetoscopy can be performed in a natural amniotic fluid environment, the use of a distension medium can improve visualisation or create more working space. When blood, debris, particles, or other substances hamper proper visualisation it is used to exchange the fluid present in the amniotic cavity. This is not so uncommon: it occurs in around 5% of cases of fetoscopic vessel coagulation for FFTS.[13] One can use warmed Hartmann's solution; during longer operations a blood warmer or a special amnio-irrigator is used to keep its temperature at 38°C.[13] Care should be taken to avoid a rise in intra-amniotic pressure by (intermittent) drainage.[14,15] Gas distension is now being reconsidered, particularly for complex procedures. We recently conducted a randomised experimental trial demonstrating that working in gas conditions cuts operation time by more than half and improves surgical accuracy when clipping a trachea.[16] The use of CO_2 for that purpose is discouraged, as it causes variable degrees of fetal acidosis, which can not be corrected by maternal hyperventilation.[13,17] N_2O is the suggested alternative.[16]

The choice of instruments depends on the purpose of the procedure. For most obstetrical interventions, a laser with appropriate coagulation abilities is needed. We use either a Nd:YAG laser (minimal power requirements 60–100 W) or diode laser (30–60 W) (Dornier Medilas, Germany) with fibres of 400–600 μm. Recently Quintero described the use of larger fibres with side-firing capabilities, which are used to coagulate anteriorly located placentas, but require a second introduction port as they are too large to work through the working channel.[10] Miniaturized forceps, scissors, and others can be inserted through an operative sheath, or more easily through an additional port. The length of these instruments should be sufficient, and their diameter not too small to resist bending. The use of bipolar forceps will be addressed further.

CLINICAL APPLICATIONS

DIAGNOSTIC EMBRYOSCOPY AND FETOSCOPY IN THE FIRST TRIMESTER

Embryoscopy is the introduction of an endoscope in the exocoelomic space, by penetration of the chorion and looking through contact with the amnion. Optimally this should be done at 9 weeks gestation and, by definition, before 12 weeks, at which stage the chorion fuses with the amnion. This can be done transvaginally or transabdominally. Later in gestation the fetus should be visualised within the amniotic cavity, which is done transabdominally. Embryoscopy is likely to remain confined to the early investigation in a few families at high risk of recurrence of genetic conditions showing pathognomic external fetal abnormalities. With the increasing use of early fetal anomaly scans at 10–14 weeks, patients may be anxious to rule out as early as possible abnormal US findings found at that time, rather than waiting until US has sufficient diagnostic capability. Several congenital malformations have been diagnosed in the first trimester, but embryo-fetoscopy has its physical restrictions.[18,19] Fetoscopic visualization of the fetal anatomy is by definition only partial, as the needlescope looks only straight forward (0° angle) and at a restricted opening angle. The needle must therefore be directed toward the fetal part most likely to be affected. For further details, and a list of conditions diagnosed by embryo-fetoscopy, we refer to the specialised literature.[19]

"OBSTETRICAL ENDOSCOPY": FETOSCOPIC SURGERY ON THE PLACENTA, CORD AND MEMBRANES

Apart from case reports on ligation of the major vessels in a placental chorioangioma and section of amniotic membranes or webs,[20,21] laser coagulation of the chorionic plate vessels and cord obliteration account for the majority of present obstetrical indications for operative fetoscopy.

ND:YAG LASER COAGULATION OF CHORIONIC PLATE VESSELS FOR FETO-FETAL TRANSFUSION SYNDROME

Pathophysiology

Monochorionic (MC) twins represent 75% of monozygous twins, and have a 3- to 10-fold increased perinatal morbidity and mortality in comparison to dichorionic twins. This is thought to be related mostly to the presence of vascular anastomoses between the 2 (or more) fetal circulations. Anastomoses exist in virtually all monochorionic placentas and feto-fetal transfusion is a balanced phenomenon. In about 6–35% of MC twins, a chronic imbalance in the net flow of blood across these communications occurs, resulting in pathologic interfetal transfusion, usually referred to as "feto-fetal transfusion syndrome" (FFTS). This chronic imbalanced transfusion across vascular communications is the consequence of a certain type of angioarchitecture in the MC placenta of these twins.[22,23] FFTS seems related to the presence of 1 (or few) arterio-venous (A-V) anastomoses in combination with a paucity (or absence) of arterio-arterious (A-A) rather than veno-venous (V-V) anastomoses, which normally compensate for the hemodynamic effects of A-V communications.[24,25] Probably oversimplifying the pathophysiology one can think of the situation as follows. The "donor" provides a net transfusion and suffers therefore from hypovolemia and eventually hypoxia. It may suffer from growth retardation, which probably is more related to the proportion of the placenta it has recruited earlier on, but also to the angioarchitecture. Due to hypovolemia, it develops oligo-uria and oligohydramnios, showing as a fetus being stuck in its membranes. The recipient becomes hypervolemic, compensates with polyuria—leading to polyhydramnios—and will develop circularly overload and congestive cardiac failure.

When occurring before 28 weeks of gestation, FFTS is associated with more than 80% fetal or perinatal loss.[9] FFTS covers a wide spectrum, and may be progressive, a concept that is reflected in a proposed staging of the disease. Whether this is clinically relevant and has any impact on therapy is under investigation.[26] For a more detailed review on pathophysiologic considerations we refer to the literature.[25,27]

Main problems associated to FFTS are preterm labour and premature birth, PPROM and its associated morbidity and mortality, mainly all as a consequence of extreme polyhydramnios. Intra Uterine Fetal Death (IUFD) is another complication, and unfortunately enough does not arrest the transfusion process nor improve the prognosis for the remainder. On the contrary, at that time the survivor acutely exsanguinates in the circulation of the dying fetus, with a high risk of severe neurological damage.[28,29] Therapy consisted for years in serial amnioreductions. Potential mechanisms explaining the rationale and benefits of this therapy are detailed in the previously mentioned reviews but are out of the scope of this chapter. Despite improving fetal survival rate (usually around 60%), significant neurological morbidity is reported in 20% of survivors or more.[9,24,30,31] Amniodrainage does not interfere with the vascular basis of the condition neither does it prevent the risk of neurological damage in case of IUFD of 1 fetus. Intentionally puncturing the intertwin septum ("septostomy") with or without amnioreduction has been suggested to have beneficial effects but not much data today is available to support this technique, and the pathophysiologic rationale behind it must still be proven.[32] Selective feticide is another option but usually only contemplated in case of end-stage disease. Adapted techniques will be dealt with in a separate section.

Fetoscopic laser coagulation of chorionic plate vessels is considered as a cause-oriented approach to severe midgestational FFTS. It intervenes at the level of the pathophysiological basis of the disease, namely by obliterating anastomosing vessels. To avoid an ongoing confusion, we remind the reader that an arterio-venous anastomosis is not a real 'anatomical' anastomosis, but actually a shared cotyledon, fed by an artery from 1 fetus, and drained by a vein from the other. The afferent and efferent branches of this shared cotyledon run over the placental surface and plunge into the chorionic plate close to each other and anastomose at the villous capillary level of that "shared" cotyledon (Fig. 40-3).[33] The anastomotic process thus occurs deeply in the placenta but the feeding vessels run on the surface of the placenta. Provided that the "vascular" hypothesis is correct and that anastomosing vessels can be identified in utero, their occlusion will result in arresting the abnormal inter-twin blood transfer. It has been demonstrated in experimental conditions and by placental perfusion studies that the obliteration of the superficially located feeding vessels indeed eliminates the deeply located circulation or the "shared" cotyledon.[34,35] Julian De Lia should be credited for introducing the clinical technique[36,37] but the procedure became more widely implemented in Europe, after Ville and Nicolaides reported a modified percutaneous technique.[38]

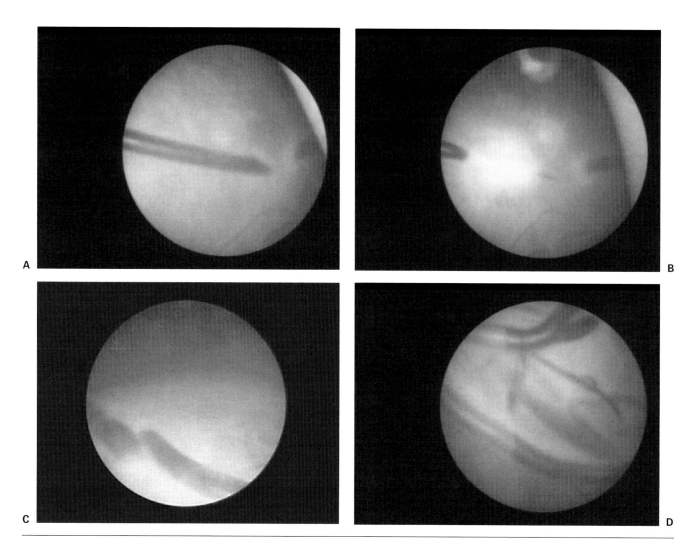

FIGURE 40-3 Fetoscopic appearance of anastomosing vessels on a monochorionic placenta. (**A**) Artery to vein anastomosis prior to and (**B**) after coagulation; (**C**) artery-to-artery anastomosis; (**D**) superficial chorionic plate vessels crossing the intertwin membrane.

Operative Technique

In Europe, laser coagulation is usually performed by percutaneous approach and under local or loco-regional anaesthesia. The need for general anesthesia is therefore questionable. A cannula or fetoscopic sheath is inserted under US guidance into the polyhydramniotic sac. According to gestational age different diameter fetoscopes and 400–600 μm laser fibers are used. The laser tip is directed as close as possible to a 90° angle toward the target vessels and with a nontouch technique vessels are photocoagulated. We ablate sections of approximately 1 cm and confirm obliteration always at the end of the procedure. During surgery amnioinfusion may improve visualisation or clear the fiber from debris. The procedure is completed by amniodrainage till normal amniotic fluid pockets are seen on US.

There are 2 important technical aspects for the surgeon doing this procedure. The first issue is the entry point into the amniotic sac. Obviously the port should be inserted in an area free of placenta. When the placenta is anterior, 2 problems

arise when using straight fetoscopes and laser fibers. It may (1) be difficult to avoid inserting the trocar through the lateral edge of the placenta, as the polyhydramnios stretches the placenta sometimes that much that one underestimates its size. (2) An anterior trocar insertion makes it by definition difficult to achieve a close to 90° angle with the target area with the instruments, reducing the possibility for appropriate fetoscopic inspection and effective coagulation. Different modifications can reduce this problem. We proposed a transfundal technique (Figs. 40-4, 40-5, 40-6),[39] either by percutaneous approach, or in exceptional cases by a mini-laparotomy. An alternative solution is the use of a 12 or 30° fetoscope and a device that inclines the laser fiber towards the placenta. However this new instrument requires a cannula of 4.3 mm. Alternatively a double puncture technique was proposed[40] that combines a 30° fetoscope through 1 port and a side-firing laser fiber through a second insertion, ending up with 2 stab wounds.

Another issue of debate and misunderstanding is the selection of vessels at the time of fetoscopic inspection of the

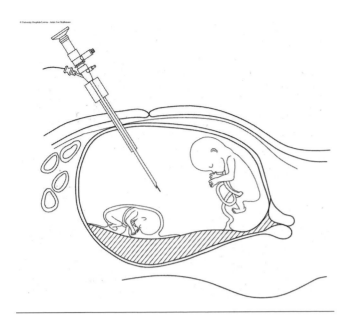

FIGURE 40-4 Schematic drawing of fetoscopic Nd:YAG laser coagulation of chorionic plate vessels, in case of a posterior placenta. The trocar is inserted percutaneously. (Drawing: Luc Brullemans, artist KU Leuven).

chorionic plate. Ideally one should strive to be consequent with the pathophysiology and obliterate anastomoses selectively at the exact site they can be seen on the placenta. De Lia called this Fetoscopic Laser Occlusion of the Chorioangiopagus vessels (FLOC).[41] The placenta is inspected along the vascular equator, not necessarily bearing any relationship to the membranous equator (Fig. 40-3). By definition some part of the placenta is covered by membranes of the stuck twin, or may

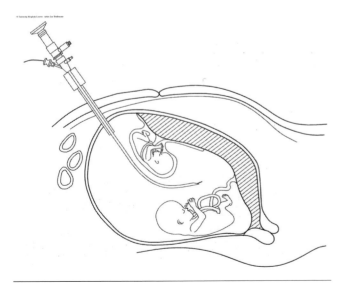

FIGURE 40-5 Schematic drawing of fetoscopic Nd:YAG laser coagulation of chorionic plate vessels in case of an anterior placenta. A percutaneous trocar insertion has been used; the curved endoscope overcomes this shortcoming. (Drawing: Luc Brullemans, artist KU Leuven).

be rendered inaccessible by a fetus, and therefore excluded for fetoscopic inspection. This means not all vessels can be inspected. In a more pragmatic approach, Ville et al.[38] described the surgical division of the vascular territory by coagulating all vessels crossing the intertwin membrane. The latter is certainly overtreating, but reproducible and faster because of its readily identifiable landmarks. However in reality most surgeons we know are as selective as possible and use a mix of selective and less-selective coagulation, including:

(1) follow all vessels connecting the 2 cords (mapping of the placenta)

(2) identifying and coagulating all clearly anastomosing vessels and

(3) if it cannot be excluded that a certain vessel is connected to the other fetus because part of it is out of reach of the scope, it will be coagulated at the level where it crosses the membrane or close to the fetus with the largest part of the placenta.

We are at present not agreeable with a technique leaving open certain types of anastomoses believed to be protective, as one cannot predict the effect of it based on intra-operative findings. It would also leave the fetal circulations connected which inevitably poses the one fetus at risk in case of IUFD of the other one. We have even seen a few exceptional failures, where seemingly there was persisting of transfusion and one case with sudden reversed transfusion, because of incomplete ablation of anastomoses. These were found at second look intervention and successfully treated at second intervention. As with any surgical intervention, there are and will ever be technical (and human) limitations, such as improper visualisation by blood or stained fluid, feto-placental position, next to an inherent risk of PPROM (>5%) with this invasive procedure. In addition the consequences of unequal placental sharing are not solved with this operation. These limitations will by definition also limit the results or explain therapeutic failures.

Results

Fetal survival has been consistently around 55–68%, with a risk for neurologic sequellae in survivors of about 5% (Table 40-1).[30,37,38,41–43] The comparable outcomes confirm that the technique is reproducible in different but experienced hands. Hecher[44] indeed demonstrated a clear effect on results of the learning curve, an argument against scattering of experience over too many centres with occasional exposure to cases. Particularly the number of double survivors increases with experience, which in its turn may also relate to a more accurate selection of vessels coagulated. Results appear to be better than those reported for amniodrainage, at least in respect to the occurrence of neurologic damage. Both a retrospective compilation of amniodrainage series published until 1997[9] and a recently reported prospective multicentre study on amniodrainages[45] yielded a 60% survival rate with about 19% risk for neurological impairment. In a recent German prospective (but not randomized) comparative study of laser versus amniodrainage, the results of laser (n = 73) at 1 institution

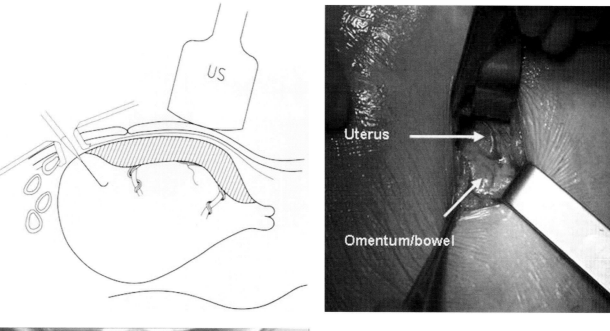

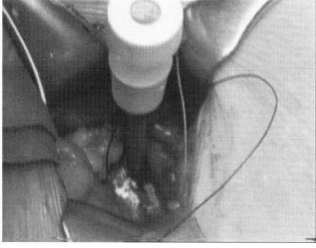

FIGURE 40-6 In exceptional situations, this may require a mini-laparotomy, to introduce the trocar safely through the fundus or toward the posterior side of the uterus. Reprinted, with permission, from Parthenon Publishers (Deprest 1998a). Insert: outside view of a mini-laparotomy and trocar insertion.

were prospectively compared with those of amniodrainage ($n = 43$) at another, using the same restrictive criteria.[30] The survival rate and neurological morbidity for the laser group were 61% and 6% respectively, and those of amniodrainage 51% and 19% (Table 40-2). This study probably represents the best available comparison at present, but still has the drawback of not being a randomized study.

The procedure-associated risk of single IUFD is around 20–25%; it is usually the donor and occurs early after the procedure. This may be due to several reasons. Not infrequently there is a degree of unequal placental sharing, which after separation of the fetal circulations and infarctization of the coagulated cotyledons, may reach a critical level. Due to limitations of fetoscopic vessel identification some vessels not involved in the pathological transfusion process may end up being coag-

ulated, which may further reduce the placental mass. The fact that only 1 fetus dies, without double fetal death, and with a low neurological morbidity, such as in drained patients, underscores that the 2 fetal circulations are indeed separated. Double IUFD is complicating up to 30% of amnioreductions.[30,46] Amnio drainage does not interfere with the anastomoses, so at the time of single IUFD the remaining fetus can exsanguinate into the other and die shortly after, a phenomenon prevented by appropriate coagulation.

Because at present it is unknown which is the best therapy to offer, a randomized trial was designed by the EUROFOETUS group. Although the initiative is supported by European funds, participation is open to all centers throughout the world via a website on the internet (www.eurofoetus.org). Inclusion criteria for the study are (1) diagnosis of FFTS

TABLE 40-1 FETOSCOPIC Nd:YAG LASER COAGULATION FOR FFTS; GROUPED BY REPORTS INCLUDING INITIAL EXPERIENCE AND REPORTS FOR WHICH THE LEARNING CURVE WAS EXCLUDED

Author, Year	Number of Cases	Fetal Survival	Survival of at Least 1 Fetus	Neurologic Morbidity
Series including first cases				
De Lia et al. 1990[36]	31	53%	69%	4%
Ville et al. 1995[38]	45	53%	71%	2%
Ville et al. 1998[42]	132	55%	73%	5%
After the learning curve				
Hecher et al. 1999[30]	69	61%	79%	6%
De Lia et al. 1999[41]	100	69%	82%	4.3%
Hecher et al. 2000[44]	127[a]	68%	81%	N/A

[a]Paper includes 200 cases, last 127 are given in 2000 series; first cases are included in earlier study (1999).

established at less than 25 weeks of gestation, (2) confirmed monochorionicity and (3) polyhydramnios/oligohydramnios sequence as defined by well described US criteria, varying with gestational age (Table 40-3).

The randomization and the use of strict inclusion criteria aim at evaluating only severe and pre-viable cases of FFTS overcoming the limited comparability of most available data in the literature. The international scientific world has always been criticizing the fact that both therapies are supported by their proponents on emotional rather than scientific arguments, and the answer can only come from a well conducted RCT. Despite that, still the majority of cases are treated according to the patient's (or physician's) preference. Data from those cases are also considered to be of value: they can be entered via the same website into a so-called observational study on FFTS, provided they meet the same criteria as in the trial (Table 40-3). Again, both initiatives are not limited to Europe, but open to all fetal medicine units worldwide (consult

http://www.eurofoetus.org). A large pool of data may become an important source of information particularly for certain subanalyses or uncommon complications.

FETOSCOPIC CORD OBLITERATION

MC twinning may be complicated by a number of rare conditions, such as Twin Reversed Arterial Perfusion Sequence (TRAP), or discordant structural and/or genetic anomalies, for which they are at higher risk than singletons.[47] Selective feticide may then be contemplated but the conventional techniques of intracardiac potassium chloride injection used in *multichorionic* pregnancies cannot be used, as the product by definition can reach the other fetus via the ever present anastomoses in a MC placenta. Patent intertwin vessels may be the source of acute feto-fetal haemorrhage after IUFD of one MC twin. This may lead to hypovolemic shock in the survivor, causing either central nervous system damage or IUFD of the survivor. Accordingly, methods strive to arrest both arterial and venous flow in the cord of the target fetus completely and permanently.[11]

INDICATIONS FOR SELECTIVE TERMINATION IN MC TWINS

Twin Reversed Arterial Perfusion Sequence (TRAP)

TRAP is an uncommon condition (1% of MZ pregnancies) where a parasitic relationship exists between a pump and acardiac twin, the latter surviving only on blood provided by the pump twin. Deoxygenated blood flows from an umbilical artery of the pump twin in a reversed direction into the umbilical artery of the acardiac fetus. This arterio-arterial anastomosis can usually be visualised by Doppler examination. The umbilical vein of the parasitic fetus returns blood into the placenta and so back to the pump twin. The acardiac usually is grossly abnormal, with failure of development of the upper part of the body. The condition places the pump twin at risk for high output cardiac failure and hydrops, potentially leading to IUFD and/or to polyhydramnios and its complications.[48] According to Healey, TRAP-sequence is complicated by polyhydramnios in 51% of cases and by preterm labour in 75%.[49] Congestive heart failure occurs in 28% and intrauterine demise of the pump twin in 25%. Perinatal mortality is estimated to be about 30%. The proportional size of the acardiac to the pump

TABLE 40-2 PROSPECTIVE, COMPARATIVE STUDY OF FFTS PATIENTS, TREATED WITH FETOSCOPIC LASER COAGULATION OR SERIAL AMNIODRAINAGE[30]

	Laser (n = 73)	Serial Amniodrainage (n = 43)	P-value
GA at diagnosis[a]	20.7 (17–25)	20.4 (17.6–25)	0.438
Fluid drained (mL)	2500 (650–7,500)	1990 (350–3,000)	<0.001
GA at delivery[a]	33.7 (25–40)	30.7 (28–37)	0.438
Survival (%)	61 %	51 %	0.239
% 2 survivors	42 %	42 %	1.0
% 1 survivor	37 %	19 %	0.058
% no survivors	21 %	40 %	0.033
Neonatal deaths	6 %	14 %	0.221
Neurologic morbidity[b]	6 %	18 %	0.030
Birthweight (gram)			
Donor	1750 g	1145 g	0.034
Recipient	2000 g	1560 g	0.076

Modified from reference 30.

[a]GA = gestational age.

[b]Defined as periventricular leukomalacia, grade III and IV intraventricular hemorrhage, parenchymal defects and microcephaly.

TABLE 40-3	CRITERIA FOR EUROFOETUS TRIAL FOR TREATMENT OF SEVERE FFTS PRIOR TO 26 + 0 WEEKS	

Inclusion Diagnostic Criteria	*Exclusion Criteria*

1. Twin pregnancy known to be monochorionic on a first trimester scan and/or a single placental mass and concordant sex on the second trimester scan.
2. Polyhydramnios in 1 sac with a deepest vertical pool of amniotic fluid of at least
  • 8 cm at less than 20 weeks' gestation,
  • 10 cm at more than 20 weeks.
  The polyhydramnios should be related to polyuria with a distended fetal bladder during most of the examination period.
3. Oligohydramnios (stuck twin) in the other sac with a deepest vertical pool of amniotic fluid of at most 2.0 cm. The oligohydramnios should be likely related to fetal oliguria with a collapsed bladder during most of the examination period.
	1. Major fetal anomaly.
	2. Ruptured membranes.
	3. Maternal condition mandating delivery.
	4. Previous amniodrainage or other invasive therapy for the same condition.
	5. Multiple pregnancies of higher order than 2.
	6. Will also be excluded post factum:
	  – Lack of confirmation of chorionicity after delivery.
	  – Late diagnosis of major fetal anomaly.

Consult *www.eurofoetus.org.*

twin seems to be a predictive factor. A twin weight ratio of above 50% (acardiac/pump twin) has a 71% predictive value for preterm delivery and a 45% predictive value for the death of the pump twin.[50] Although some pregnancies complicated by acardiac twinning will progress uneventfully into the viable period, allowing treatment by timed delivery; we recommend a more active approach. These pregnancies are followed up by ultrasound for subtle signs of cardiac failure in the pump, i.e. reversed atrial flow in the ductus venosus, pulsatile flow in the umbilical vein or tricuspid regurgitation. Whether it is wise to wait until terminal cardiac failure develops or not, is uncertain. Particularly early in gestation the above-mentioned criteria may not apply as we have seen several pregnancies resulting in IUFD without previously worrying hemodynamic alterations.

Discordant Congenital or Acquired Anomalies in MC Twins

Some FFTS patients may present with irreversible damage, such as cerebral ventriculomegaly or hydrocephalus or have severe cardiac failure with impending IUFD. Another group are MC twins discordant for severe congenital anomalies. Structural abnormalities are more common in MC twins, including anencephaly, sirenomelia, neural tube defects and holoprosencephaly.[51,52] In only about 15% of cases both twins are affected by the anomaly (concordant), while in the majority of cases only 1 twin is affected (discordant).[53] In such case, the expected results of selective feticide must be weighed against the risk of spontaneous IUFD, and the invasiveness and risks of the procedure.

TECHNIQUES FOR CORD OCCLUSION IN MONOCHORIONIC TWINS

Fetoscopy definitely plays a role in selective feticide in MC twins: fetoscopic cord ligation was the first multiple entry endoscopic in utero operation ever done in human pregnancy.[54] However technology is evolving very fast, and a number of procedures has been suggested as competing alternatives, that

do not necessarily require fetoscopy. At present it is unclear which technique is the most effective and puts the co-twin at the lowest risk. Umbilical cord embolization is merely a historical technique. Denbow recently discouraged embolization because of incomplete vessel occlusion and an overall success rate of only 33%.[55]

- Laser coagulation: A simple and straightforward procedure is laser coagulation of the umbilical cord with instruments described in the previous section. This procedure has been done as early as 16 weeks using a double-needle loaded with 1.0 mm fetoscope and a 400 μm laser fiber.[56] The cord root of the target fetus is visualized and the vessels are coagulated using a "no touch" technique (Fig. 40-7). Limitation for this technique is mainly the size of the vessels

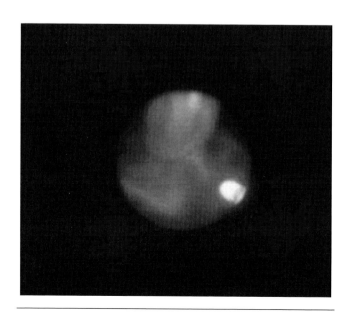

FIGURE 40-7 Nd:YAG laser coagulation of cord vessels. A 400 μm fiber is used.

TABLE 40-4 **FETOSCOPIC CORD LIGATIONS**

Author, Year	Number of Cases	Failure of Ligation	IUFD	PPROM =<32 Weeks[b]	PPROM >32 Weeks[b]	Amnionleakage	Neonatal Survival
McCurdy 1993[54]	1	0	1	—	—	—	0/1
Willcourt 1996[59]	1	0	0	0/1	0/1	0	1/1
Lémery 1994[60]	2	0	0	NA	NA	0	2/2
Quintero 1996b[61]	14[a]	2	3	3/14	1/14	1	8/14
Deprest 1996[62]	4	0	0	2/4	0/4	1	3/4
Crombleholme 1996[63]	1	0	0	1/1	0/1	0	1/1
Totals	23	2/23	4/21	6/17	2/17	2/17	15/23

Modified from Deprest 1998a.
IUFD = in utero fetal death; NA = not available.
[a] 13 pregnancies, of which 1 was a quadruplet pregnancy, with 2 cord ligations.
[b] Calculation only for the successfully performed procedures with in utero surviving co-twin.

to be coagulated, with exceptional success as late as 24 weeks.[57] As a rule of thumb failure of laser coagulation of the cord is possible till 20–22 weeks onward and one should have a alternative available.[58]

- Fetoscopic cord ligation: Surgical ligation of the umbilical cord causes immediate, complete, and permanent interruption of both arterial and venous flow in the umbilical cord, irrespective of its diameter. It is therefore in theory the most attractive technique, and it became clinically acceptable since it was feasible by endoscopy. One or 2 ports are being inserted as described above and with a nonabsorbable suture 1 or more extra-corporeal knots are slipped in. Quintero advocates to make several knots with section of the cord in between, to prevent later IUFD by cord entanglement. The procedure yielded over 70% survivors. We have however abandoned fetoscopic cord ligation because (1) the procedure is associated with an unacceptably high risk for PPROM (>30%) and (2) it remains very technically difficult and cumbersome (Table 40-4).[11]

- Bipolar coagulation: Today less complex and as efficient alternatives are available. We recently described occlusion of the umbilical cord using bipolar coagulation forceps.[64] The procedure can be carried out using only US guidance and through a single port. It requires only readily available and inexpensive instrumentation. Occasionally we use fetoscopic guidance, although not essential, significantly reducing the operation time and perhaps the risk for unintentional collateral damage (Figure 40-8). Because it requires an ancillary port, which may increase the access-related complications, we only do so when the procedure is difficult. We always try to work completely within the sac of the target fetus, but this is not always possible. Amnioinfusion can be helpful to improve accessibility to the target sac. Even when entering the sac of the fetus to survive, the cord can be grasped and coagulated through the intertwin membranes. Key instrument is a small diameter bipolar coagulation forceps. We initially used a disposable 3.0 mm forceps (Everest Medical, Minneapolis, Minnesota, USA) but now have a 2.3 and a 3.0 mm reusable instrument (Karl Storz). In our initial series of 10 cases, 2 patients had PPROM and underwent

termination. The other 8 patients delivered at a mean gestational age of 35 weeks—more than 15 weeks after the procedure. Nicolini et al.[65] confirmed the feasibility and similar efficacy of this procedure. One out of the 17 cases treated was complicated by fatal cord perforation, and the survival rate was 81% (13/16 survivors; 1 patient had TOP because of an abnormality diagnosed later). Of interest is that bipolar cord coagulation can be done even late in pregnancy—beyond 28 weeks.[66]

- Monopolar coagulation: Another minimally invasive alternative is the use of monopolar needles, as described by Rodeck et al. and Holmes et al.[67,68] Under US guidance a needle is inserted towards the cord or fetal aorta. Their published experience includes so far 11 cases of TRAP sequence. Three procedures failed at first attempt (27%), but in 2 re-intervention was successful. Total survival rate was 72% (8/11). Undoubtedly somewhat biased by our own views, and perhaps also due to the limited experience, we fear that vessel diameter may be a limitation: 2 procedures at 24 weeks failed or complicated by IUFD. The procedure also has a high failure risk in normal or hyperdynamic circulatory conditions: it has not been successfully applied in case of FFTS. These limitations were suggested by our experimental work, where ineffectiveness and vessel perforation was shown in typical fetal hemodynamic conditions at higher vessel diameters.[69]

There is at present no objective way to evaluate which is the optimal method of selective feticide in MC pregnancies. Given the rarity of the indications, it is unlikely that this judgement will soon (or ever?) be possible. Based on the data presented in the previous section, and our own experience we suggest that the simplest procedure, if possible with the fewest ports, is likely to have the best chance for success and fewest complications. Accordingly we apply today the following clinical algorithm (Fig. 40-9). Prior to about 21 weeks, we try Nd:YAG laser coagulation first. If unsuccessful, or for pregnancy beyond 21 weeks, we proceed with bipolar cord coagulation. We do not hesitate to put a needle scope if the conditions are difficult. Of interest is that cord coagulation can be done even late in

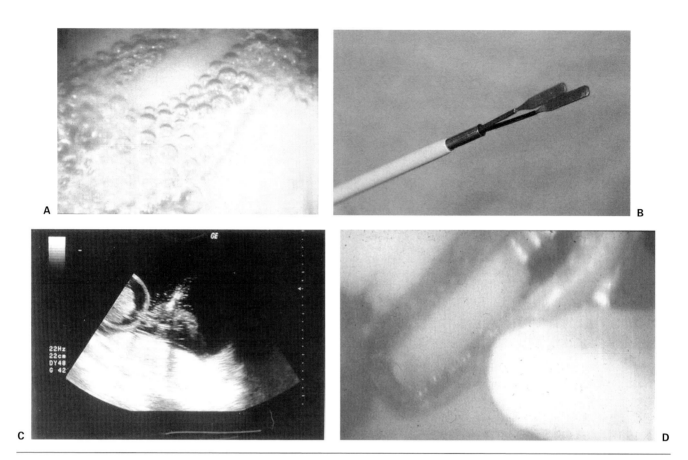

FIGURE 40-8 (**A**) Technique of fetoscopic cord bipolar coagulation, using a 3.0 mm bipolar forceps; (**B**) smaller instruments are now available, like this 7.0 Fr (2.3 mm) bipolar forceps, which can be manipulated under ultrasound control; (**C**) local heat production is visible as steam bubbles; (**D**) view of coagulated cord.

pregnancy—beyond 28 weeks.[66] Sono-endoscopic cord ligation is reserved as a (theoretical) backup.

AMNIOTIC BAND SYNDROME (ABSd)

ABSd refers to amputation of fingers and/or limbs, and a wide spectrum of associated trunk and craniofacial anomalies. Two theories have been proposed to explain the pathogenesis. One is based on a developmental anomaly of the embryonic germinal disc[70] where the amniotic band would be a by-product rather than the cause of fetal anomalies. The second theory claims that the primary problem is rupture of the amniotic membrane and its detachment from the chorion.[71] In that scenario, the fetus would exit the amniotic cavity, and the outer amnion and naked chorion produce mesodermic fibrous strings which entangle and entrap different fetal organs like a "guillotine" leading to constriction and amputation. This theory became widely accepted, despite the small number of cases and inconsistent findings.[72] Moerman[73] proposed to reconcile both theories, and accepts that both entities exist and are just of different origin. Whatever the cause, today the condition can be diagnosed in utero and progressive constriction of the lower limbs from 21 weeks onward has been well documented making the case of fetal intervention.[74] In utero release of amniotic bands in humans was therefore only a logical step pioneered by Quintero et al.[21] He lysed amniotic bands in 2 cases at 22 and 23 weeks. The procedure restored adequate blood flow distal to the obstruction and the extremity could be preserved. In both cases, only minimal to mild limb dysfunction was present at birth.

COMPLICATIONS OF FETOSCOPIC SURGERY

Most of these are related to the access method to the amniotic cavity. The most relevant side effect of operative fetoscopy is the high risk of (Preterm) Prelabor Rupture of the Membranes

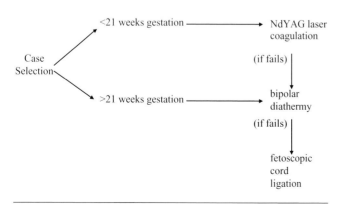

FIGURE 40-9 Suggested clinical flow chart of techniques for cord occlusion.

(PPROM). Since this event is related to the invasiveness of the procedure, and thus has other causes than spontaneous PPROM, we called it "iatrogenic" PPROM (iPPROM).[43,75] The exact incidence of iPPROM is difficult to define, given the limited and underreported experience with operative fetoscopy. In the pooled series of 17 successful cord ligations with surviving pump twin, there was frank rupture of the membranes in 8 cases (47%) and in an additional 2 patients there was temporary amniotic fluid leakage prior to 32 weeks.[11] This remained as high even when considering only the series of 1 single surgeon. For a much more common procedure such as laser photocoagulation of chorionic plate vessels, Ville reported an iPPROM rate of 10%[42] and Hecher quoted a total fetal loss rate of 12%, part of them related to iPPROM. We speculated that the number of ports used is a risk factor for iPPROM but other factors, such as operating time, complexity of the procedure, diameter of the port, previous invasive procedure, uterine bleeding, premature labor, and the need for excessive amnioinfusion may also be risk determinants.

iPPROM will remain an inevitable complication and the search for an effective therapy for this complication has been going on. Some innovative techniques to seal traumatic membrane defect have been proposed. Quintero reported the use of a cryo-precipitate plug (amniopatch). Platelets seem to adhere to the extracellular matrix of the membrane defect and the procedure is clinically most effective in case of iPPROM.[76] We use the amniopatch at present as a first step in case of postoperative iPPROM. However we would in theory prefer a preventive measure—prophylactic sealing the membrane defect at the end of the procedure. We have been proposing the insertion of a collagen plug based on our experimental models.[5,77,78] Detailed experimentation in a primate model is ongoing at the time of writing this chapter and we wait for results prior to using it in clinical procedures. It is also hoped that any knowledge on the dynamics of fetal membrane wound healing may ultimately be beneficial for patients with spontaneous PPROM. Disruption of the fetal membranes leading to amniotic bands is also a potential risk; we have seen it in a case of fetoscopic cord ligation,[62] and also once after laser for FFTS (Fig. 40-10).

The exact nature and incidence of other, less frequent complications are less clear. One of these is inherently haemorrhage from the trocar insertion site, but this risk may be reduced significantly by using US guidance and smaller diameter instruments. When the bleeding is intra-amniotic it hampers fetoscopic view and the procedure may have to be discontinued. Severe bleeding may prompt the need for transfusion.[35,42] Just as with serial amnioreductions, chorioamnionitis, and abruptio placentae are possible. Amniotic fluid embolism leading to maternal death has been reported in one case.[79] If one considers the number of fetoscopies done over the last 20 years, this seems to be an extremely rare event. However, fatal amniotic fluid embolism is a potential complication of any invasive procedure, and an underlying condition such as polyhydramnios may be a co-risk factor. In addition, one has to take into account this event can occur after apparently simple procedures such as diagnostic amniocentesis[80] or amnioinfusion.[81]

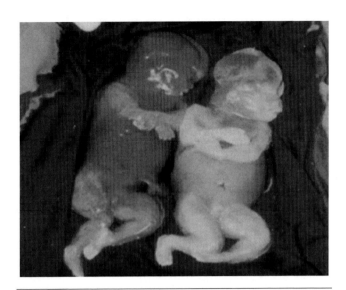

FIGURE 40-10 View of an amniotic band a few weeks after laser coagulation. The band caused a cord accident and fetal death. (Courtesy of Dr. H. Brandenburg, Rotterdam, the Netherlands).

There are some other complications that may be observed, but that are probably more related to the underlying fetal condition. Maternal "hydrops" associated to severe hydrops fetoplacentalis has been described once by Ville, and we have seen this once following a laser procedure for FFTS.[19,82] In another case however this was mildly present prior to the operation, but resolved completely after the laser procedure.[83] This suggests that this condition is probably more an epiphenomenon of the primary condition rather than from the invasive procedure. The same should be said about a patient in the series by Ville,[42] who died of complicated preeclampsia weeks after the procedure.

These serious complications demonstrate uncommon but inherent risks to this procedure. Patients should be counselled accordingly and monitored closely for any of these complications. Theoretically all known side effects of invasive in utero procedures might eventually be expected, including bowel perforation, sepsis, and eventually maternal death. This is 1 of the reasons driving the set up of a registry of fetoscopic procedures, irrespective of their indication.[84] We have done so with support of the European Commission and data can be entered via the internet. Just as for the studies regarding FFTS, the registry is open to all centers worldwide (http://www.eurofoetus.org). Maternal safety is the primary objective, but registration of large numbers may help to learn about fetal safety and outcome.

ACKNOWLEDGMENT

Work supported by the Biomed Programme of the European Commission (EUROFOETUS, BMH4 CT972383, cofinanced by the Flemish Government COF 98/012). E.G. was a recipient of a research fellowship of the European Commission. The members of the Eurofoetus group (Y. Ville, G. Barki, T. H. Bui,

K. Hecher, U. Nicolini) are acknowledged for their efforts to set up the Eurofoetus project.

References

1. Dumez Y, Mandelbort L, Dommergues M. Embryoscopy in continuing pregnancies. Proceedings of the annual meeting of the International Fetal Medicine Society; May 1992; Evian, France.
2. International Fetoscopy Group. The status of fetoscopy and fetal tissue sampling. *Prenat Diagn*. 1984;4:79–81.
3. Luks F, Deprest J. Endoscopic fetal surgery a new alternative? *Eur J Obstet Gynecol Reprod Biol*. 1993;52:1–3.
4. Quintero RA, Abuhamad A, Hobbins JC, et al. Transabdominal thin gauge cmbryofetoscopy: A technique for early prenatal diagnosis and its use in the diagnosis of a case of Meckel-Gruber Syndrome. *Am J Obstet Gynecol*. 1993;168:1552–1557.
5. Deprest JA, Gratacos E. Obstetrical Endoscopy. *Curr Opinion Obstet Gynecol*. 1999;11:195–203.
6. Harrison MR, Mychaliska GB, Albanese CT, et al. Correction of congenital diaphragmatic hernia in utero IX: fetuses with poor prognosis (liver herniation and low lung-to-head ratio) can be saved by fetoscopic temporary tracheal occlusion. *J Pediatr Surg*. 1998;33:1017–1022.
7. Eurofetus. Endoscopic feto-placental surgery: from animal experimentation to early human experimentation. Program funded by the European Commission, within the Biomed 2 Program. 1997:2382.
8. Luks FI, Deprest JA, Marcus M, et al. Carbon dioxide pneumoamnios causes acidosis in the fetal lamb. *Fetal Diagn Ther*. 1994;9:101–104.
9. Ville Y. Monochorionic twin pregnancies: "les liasons dangereuses." *US Obstet Gynecol*. 1997;10:82–85.
10. Quintero RA, Bornick PW, Allen MH, et al. Selective photocoagulation of communicating vessels in severe twin-twin transfusion syndrome in women with an anterior placenta. *Obstet Gynecol*. 2001;97:477–481.
11. Deprest JA, Evrard VA, Van Ballaer PP, et al. Experience with fetoscopic cord ligation. *Eur J Obstet Gynaecol Reprod Biol*. 1998;81:157–164.
12. Luks FI, Deprest JA, Gilchrist BF, et al. Access techniques in endoscopic fetal surgery. *Eur J Pediatr Surg*. 1997;7:131–134.
13. Gratacos E, Wu J, Devlieger R, et al. Nitrous oxide amniodistention reduces operation time as compared to fluid amniodistention while inducing no changes in fetal acid-base status in a sheep model for endoscopic surgery. *Am J Obstet Gynecol*. 2002;186:538–543.
14. Fisk NM, Ronderos-Dumit D, Soliani A, et al. Diagnostic and therapeutic transabdominal amnio-infusion in oligohydramnios. *Obstet Gynecol*. 1991;78:270–278.
15. Evrard V, Deprest J, Luks F, et al. Amnio-infusion with Hartmann's solution: a safe distension medium for endoscopic fetal surgery in the ovine model. *Fetal Diagn Ther*. 1997;12:188–192.
16. Gratacos E, Wu J, Devlieger R, et al. Effects of amniodistention with carbon dioxide on fetal acid-base status during fetoscopic surgery in a sheep model. *Surg Endosc*. 2001;15:368–372.
17. Luks FI, Deprest JA, Vandenberghe K, et al. Fetoscopy-guided fetal endoscopy in a sheep model. *J Am Coll Surg*. 1994;178:609–612.
18. Ville Y, Hyett JA, Vandenbussche F, et al. Endoscopic laser coagulation of umbilical cord vessels in twin reversed arterial perfusion sequence. *US Obstet Gynecol*. 1994;4:396–398.
19. Ville Y, Van Peborgh P, Gagnon A, et al. Traitement chirurgical du syndrome transfuseur-transfusé: coagulation des anastomoses par un laser Nd:YAG sous contrôle écho-endoscopique. *J Gynecol Obstet Biol Reprod*. 1997;26:175–181.
20. Quintero RA, Reich H, Romero R, et al. In utero endoscopic devascularization of a large chorioangioma. *Ultrasound Obstet Gynecol*. 1996;8:48–52.
21. Quintero RA, Morales WJ, Kalter CS, et al. In utero lysis of amniotic bands. *US Obstet Gynecol*. 1997;10:316–320.
22. Bajoria R, Wigglesworth J, Fisk N. Angioarchitecture of monochorionic placentas in relation to the twin-twin transfusion syndrome. *Am J Obstet Gynecol*. 1995;172:856–863.
23. Machin G, Still K, Lalani T. Correlations of placental vascular anatomy and clinical outcomes in 69 monochorionic twin pregnancies. *Am J Med Genet*. 1996;61:229–236.
24. Denbow ML, Cox P, Taylor M, et al. Placental angioarchitecture in monochorionic twin pregnancies: relationship to fetal growth, fetofetal transfusion syndrome and pregnancy outcome. *Am J Obstet Gynecol*. 2000;182:417–426.
25. van Gemert M, Umur A, Tijssen J, et al. Twin-twin transfusion syndrome: etiology, severity and rational treatment. *Curr Opinion Obstet Gynaecol*. 2001;2:193–206.
26. Quintero RA, Morales WJ, Allen MH, et al. Staging of twin-twin transfusion syndrome. 1999;19:550–555.
27. Fisk NM, Taylor M. The fetus with twin-twin transfusion syndrome. In: Harrison M, Evans MI, Adzick N, Holzgreve W, eds. *The Unborn Patient*. Philadelphia, PA: WB Saunders; 2001:341–356.
28. Fusi L, McParland P, Fisk NM, et al. Acute twin-twin transfusion: a possible mechanism for brain-damaged surviors after intrauterine death of a monochorionic twin. *Obstet Gynecol*. 1991;78:517–520.
29. Nicolini U, Pisoni MP, Cele E, et al. Fetal blood sampling immediately before and within 24 hours of death in MC twin pregnancies complicated by single in utero fetal death. *Am J Obstet Gynecol*. 1998;179:800–803.
30. Hecher K, Plath H, Bregenzer T, et al. Endoscopic laser surgery versus serial amniocenteses in the treatment of severe twin-twin transfusion syndrome. *Am J Obstet Gynecol*. 1999;180:717–724.
31. Deprest J. Endoscopic Feto-Placental Surgery: From animal experience to early clinical applications. Leuven University Press, *Acta Biomedica Lovaniensia*. 1999;199:1–179.
32. Hubinont C, Bernard P, Pirot N, et al. Twin-to-twin transfusion syndrome: treatment by amnio drainage septostomy. *Eur J Obstet Gynecol Repr Biol*. 2000;92:141–144.
33. De Lia JE, Cruikshank DP. Feticide versus laser surgery for twin-twin transfusion syndrome [letter]. *Am J Obstet Gynecol*. 1994;170:1480–1481.
34. Dumitrascu-Branisteanu I, Deprest J, Evrard V, et al. Time-related cotyledonary effects of laser coagulation of superficial chorionic vessels in an ovine model. *Prenat Diagn*. 1999;19:205–210.
35. Van Peborgh P, Rambaud C, Ville Y. Effect of laser coagulation on placental vessels: histological aspects. *Fetal Diagn Ther*. 1997;12:32–35.
36. De Lia JE, Cruikshank DP, Keye WR. Fetoscopic neodymium: YAG laser occlusion of placental vessels in severe twin-twin transfusion syndrome. *Obstet Gynecol*. 1990;75:1046–1053.
37. De Lia JE, Kuhlmann RS, Harstad TW, et al. Fetoscopic laser ablation of placental vessels in severe previable twin-twin transfusion syndrome. *Am J Obstet Gynecol*. 1994;172:1202–1211.
38. Ville Y, Hyett J, Hecher K, et al. Preliminary experience with endoscopic laser surgery for severe twin-twin transfusion syndrome. *N Engl J Med*. 1995;332:224–227.
39. Deprest J, Van Schoubroeck D, Van Ballaer P, et al. Alternative access for fetoscopic Nd:YAG laser in TTS with anterior placenta. *Ultrasound Obstet Gynecol*. 1998;12:347–352.
40. Quintero RA, Bornick PW, Allen MH, et al. Selective laser photocoagulation of communicating vessels in severe twin-twin transfusion syndrome in women with an anterior placenta. *Obstet Gynecol*. 2001;97(3):477–481.

41. De Lia JE, Kuhlmann RS, Lopez KP. Treating previable twin-twin transfusion syndrome with fetoscopic laser surgery: outcomes following the learning curve. *J Perinat Med.* 1999;27:61–67.

42. Ville Y, Hecher K, Gagnon A, et al. Endoscopic laser coagulation in the management of severe twin transfusion syndrome. *Brit J Obstet Gynecol.* 1998;105:446–453.

43. Deprest JA. *Endoscopic Feto-Placental Surgery: from Animal Experience to Early Clinical Applications* [dissertation]. Acta Biomedica Lovaniensia. Leuven University Press; 1999;Vol 199:1–179.

44. Hecher K, Diehl W, Zikulnig L, et al. Endoscopic laser coagulation of placental anastomoses in 200 pregnancies with severe mid-trimester twin-to-twin transfusion syndrome. *Eur J Obstet Gynaecol Reprod Biol.* 2000;92:135–140.

45. Mari G. Amnioreduction in twin-twin transfusion syndrome—a multicenter registry, evaluation of 579 procedures [abstract]. *Am J Obstet Gynecol.* 1998;177 suppl:S28.

46. Mari G, Roberts A, Detti L, et al. Perinatal morbidity and mortality rates in severe twin-twin transfusion syndrome: Results of the International Amnioreduct Registry. *Am J Obstet Gynecol.* 2001;186:708–715.

47. MacGillivray I. Epidemiology of twin pregnancy. *Semin Perinatol.* 1984;10:4.

48. Gilliam DL, CH Hendricks. Holoacardius: review of the literature and case report. *Obstet Gynecol.* 1953;2:647–653.

49. Healey MG. Acardia: predictive risk factors for the co-twin's survival. *Teratology.* 1994;50:205.

50. Moore TR, Gale S, Bernischke K. Perinatal outcome of forty-nine pregnancies complicated by acardiac twinning. *Am J Obstet Gynecol.* 1990;163:907–912.

51. Adams D, Chevernak F. Multifetal pregnancies: epidemiology, clinical characteristics and management. In: E. Reece, et al., eds. *Medicine of the Fetus and Mother.* Philadelphia, PA: JB Lippincott; 1992:269.

52. Evans M, et al. Efficacy of second trimester selective termination for fetal abnormalities: International collaborative experience amongst the world's largest centers. *Am J Obstet Gynecol.* 1994;171:90.

53. Onyskowova A, Dolezal A, Jedlica V. The frequency and the character of malformations in multiple births. *Acta Univ Carol Med.* 1970;16:333.

54. McCurdy CM, Childers JM, Seeds JW. Ligation of the umbilical cord of an acardiac-acephalus twin with an endoscopic intrauterine technique. *Obstet Gynecol.* 1993;82:708–711.

55. Denbow ML, Overton TG, Duncan KR, et al. High failure rate of umbilical vessel occlusion by ultrasound guided injection of absolute alcohol or enbucrilate gel. *Prenat Diagn.* 1999;19:527–532.

56. Hecher K, Hackeloër BJ, Ville Y. Umbilical cord coagulation by operative microendoscopy at 16 weeks gestation in an acardiac twin. *Ultrasound Obstet Gynecol.* 1997;10:130.

57. Arias F, Sunderji S, Gimpelson R, et al. Treatment of acardiac twinning. *Obstet Gynecol.* 1998;91:818.

58. Challis D, Gratacos E, Deprest J. Selective termination in monochrorionic twins. *J Perinat Med.* 1999;27:327–338.

59. Willcourt RJ, Naughton MJ, Knutzen VK. Ligation of an umbilical cord of an acardiac fetus: laparoscopic technique. *J Am Assoc Gynecol Laparosc.* 1995;2:319–321.

60. Lemery DJ, Vanlieferinghen P, Gasq M, et al. Umbilical cord ligation under US guidance. *Obstet Gynecol.* 1994;4:399–401.

61. Quintero Romero R, Reich H, et al. In utero percutaneous umbilical cord ligation in the management of complicated monochorionic multiple gestations. *Ultrasound Obstet Gynecol.* 1996;8:16–22.

62. Deprest J, Evrard V, Van Schoubroeck D, et al. Fetoscopic cord ligation. *Lancet.* 1996;348:890–891.

63. Crombleholme TM, Robertson F, Marx G, et al. Fetoscopic cord ligation to prevent neurological injury in monozygous twins. *Lancet.* 1996;348:191.

64. Deprest J, Audibert F, Van Schoubroeck D, et al. Bipolar cord coagulation of the umbilical cord in complicated monochorionic twin pregnancy. *Am J Obstet Gynecol.* 2000;182:340–345.

65. Nicolini U, Poblete A, Boschetto C, et al. Complicated monochorionic twin pregnancies: experience with bipolar cord coagulation. *Am J Obstet Gynecol.* 2000;185:703–707.

66. Vandenbussche FP, Deprest JA, Klumper FJ, et al. Foetale therapie bij monochoriale meerlingzwangerschappen gecompliceerd door een acardiacus. *Ned Tijdsch Geneesk.* 2003;931–936.

67. Rodeck C, Deans A, Jauniaux E. Thermocoagulation for the early treatment of pregnancy with an acardiac twin. *New Engl J Med.* 1998;339:1293–1294.

68. Holmes A, Jauniaux E, Rodeck C. Monopolar thermocoagulation in acardiac twinning. *Brit J Obstet Gynecol.* 2001;108:1000–1002.

69. Perales A, Bonati F, Rheinwald M, et al. Monopolar an dinterstitial laser coagulation for umbilical cord occlusion: an experimental study. In: *A Journey from Gamete to Newborn* [abstract book]. Leuven;2000:19.

70. Streeter GL. Focal deficiencies in fetal tissues and their relation to intrauterine amputation. *Contrib Embryol.* 1930;22:1.

71. Torpin R. Amniochorionic mesoblastic fibrous strings and amniotic bands: associated constricting fetal anomalies or fetal death. *Am J Obstet Gynecol.* 1965;91:65–75.

72. Bronshtein M, Zimmer EZ. Do amniotic bands amputate fetal organs? *Ultrasound Obstet Gynecol.* 1997;10:309–311.

73. Moerman P, Fryns JP, Vandenberghe K, et al. Constrictive amniotic bands, amniotic adhesions, and limb-body wall complex: discrete disruption sequences with pathogenetic overlap. *Am J Med Genet.* 1992;42:470–479.

74. Tadmor O, Kreisberg G, Achiron R, et al. Limb amputation in amniotic band syndrome: serial ultrasonographic and Doppler observations. *Ultrasound Obstet Gynecol.* 1997;10:312–315.

75. Gratacos E, Wu J, Yesildaglar N, et al. Successful sealing of fetoscopic access sites with collagen plugs in the rabbit model. *Am J Obstet Gynecol.* 2000;182:142–146.

76. Quintero RA, Morlaes WJ, Bornick AM, et al. Treatment of iatrogenic previable premature rupture of the membranes with intra-amniotic injection of platelets and cryoprecipitate (amniopatch): preliminary experience. *Am J Obstet Gynecol.* 1999;1812:744–749.

77. Deprest J, Papadopulos NA, Dumitrascu I, et al. Closure techniques for fetoscopic access sites in the midgestational rabbit model. *Human Reprod.* 1999;14:1730–1734.

78. Luks FI, Deprest JA, Peers KH, et al. Gelatin sponge plug to seal fetoscopy port sites: technique in ovine and primate models. *Am J Obstet Gynecol.* 1999;181:995–996.

79. Quintero RA. Personal communication at the Meeting of International Fetal Medicine and Surgery Society; 2000; Nantucket Island, MA.

80. Hasaart TH, Essed GG. Amniotic fluid embolism after transabdominal amniocentesis. *Eur J Obstet Gynecol Reprod Biol.* 1983;16:25–30.

81. Maher JE, Wenstrom KD, Hauth JC, et al. Amniotic fluid embolism after saline amnioinfusion: two cases and review of the literature. *Obstet Gynecol.* 1994;83:951–954.

82. Demeyere T, Van Schoubroeck D, Deprest J, et al. Maternal hydrops after laser surgery in twin-to-twin transfusion syndrome. *Fet Diagn Ther.* 1998;17suppl:S124.

83. Claerhout F, Deprest J, Van Schoubroeck D, et al. In utero recovery of fetal hydrops and maternal hydrops in twin-twin transfusion syndrome. *Fet Diagn Ther.* 1998;17suppl:S125.

84. Gratacós E, Deprest J. Current experience with fetoscopy and the Eurofoetus registry for fetoscopic procedures. *Europ J Obstet Gynecol Reprod Biol.* 2000;92:151–160.

SECTION
IV

Laboratory Diagnostics

CYTOGENETICS AND MOLECULAR CYTOGENETICS

Alan E. Donnenfeld / Allen N. Lamb

Since the development of amniocentesis in the late 1960s, testing for aneuploidy has become a routine component of obstetric care. New prenatal diagnosis techniques have been developed that permit the analysis of numerous embryonic tissues. These include traditional amniocentesis, early amniocentesis (<14 weeks), transabdominal and transcervical chorionic villus sampling (CVS), fetal blood sampling, fetal skin biopsy, analysis of fetal urine, and testing of fetal cystic hygroma fluid. These clinical procedures are described in other chapters. Over the past decade, the laboratory evaluation of samples derived from these tissues has expanded dramatically. For decades, traditional cytogenetic analysis had been the exclusive test for chromosome abnormalities. Current methodologies include interphase fluorescence in situ hybridization (FISH) for common aneuploidies involving chromosomes 13, 18, 21, X, and Y, as well as other molecular cytogenetic tests. These molecular cytogenetic tests permit evaluation and further characterization of more subtle abnormalities, including microdeletions, marker chromosomes, translocations, deletions, inversions, and subtelomeric deletions. DNA-based tests can be used to search for uniparental disomy (UPD).

AMNIOTIC FLUID

Amniocentesis is the most common procedure performed for prenatal diagnosis. Most laboratories performing cytogenetic studies handle large numbers of samples so that appropriate specimen handling and labeling is critical. The sample volume and gross appearance (clear, bloody, brown, etc.) are recorded. The sample, often in 2 tubes, is centrifuged and most of the amniotic fluid is removed and saved. A small volume of tissue culture medium is added (usually .5 mL), and the cell pellet is resuspended. Highly supplemented tissue culture medium optimized for the growth of amniocytes is commonly utilized. Two of the most commonly used medias in the United States are Amniomax (GIBCO, Carlsbad, CA) and Chang (Irvine Scientific, Santa Ana, CA).

There are 2 culture methods for amniocytes: in situ and flask. Most laboratories now use the in situ method. The resuspended cells are placed on the surface of a coverslip in a small culture dish, cells are allowed to attach overnight, and then the coverslip is flooded with more medium on the second day. The cells attach and grow on coverslips as individual colonies and the sample can be harvested without subculturing. Four cultures are generally established for amniocytes, 2 from each original sample tube. Both A-side cultures and both B-side cultures (representing the 2 original sample tubes) are split between 2 incubators.

Cytogenetic analysis is performed on metaphase spreads found in the in situ colonies, which usually results in a faster turnaround time (TAT) than the flask method. The specific advantage is that subculturing, with subsequent slide making, is avoided. TAT with the in situ method is in the 6- to 10-day range for most patient cultures. Small-volume and bloody samples are often at the upper end of the TAT range or longer. Early amniocentesis may take up to 1½ days longer than the average 16-week amniocentesis sample because there are fewer cells.[1]

The culture medium is removed from cultures selected for harvest. The cells are then exposed to a hypotonic solution to help separate the chromosomes. The hypotonic treatment is followed by fixation steps with Carnoy's fixative (3:1, methanol:acetic acid). The chromosomes are spread in a temperature- and humidity-controlled environment, and the coverslips are allowed to dry. The coverslips are then placed in a dilute trypsin solution to induce banding, stained, and mounted on a slide. Most laboratories use a trypsin G-band technique to analyze chromosomes, with an average banding resolution of between 400–500 bands per haploid genome.

CHROMOSOME ANALYSIS

Requirements and guidelines for chromosome analysis for all sample types are available from the College of American Pathologists (CAP) at www.cap.org/toolbox/index.htm (Checklists, Cytogenetics) and the American College of Medical Genetics (ACMG) at www.acmg.net (educational materials, Standards and Guidelines for Clinical Genetics Laboratories, 2002 edition).

For amniotic fluid cell culture, the recommended CAP standard is 15 cells from 15 colonies from 2 independent cultures. The ACMG Guidelines state that if 15 colonies are not available, 10–15 cells from at least 10 colonies are acceptable. Neither CAP nor ACMG provide recommendations on what to do or report if fewer than 10 cells are available.

The number of cells studied affects the ability to detect mosaicism, which is the presence of 2 or more cell lines with different karyotypes in at least 2 independent cultures. To be considered a cell line, there must be at least 2 cells with the same karyotype for trisomies or structural rearrangements, or 3 cells monosomic for the same chromosome. The routine analysis of 15 cells from 15 colonies excludes 19% mosaicism at the 95% confidence level, and 9–6 cells excludes from 29–41% mosaicism.[2] As the ability to detect mosaicism decreases with 6–9 cells, and is not possible to exclude with 5 cells or less, some laboratories include a statement about this reduced ability on the final report.

Cytogenetic laboratories commonly have several layers of review of the karyotypes, which may include (1) 2 technologists reading the case at the scope and each doing a band-by-band analysis of all chromosomes in at least 2 cells, (2) another person cutting out chromosomes and karyotyping 2–3 cells, either from electronic computer images or from photographic paper, (3) a supervisor or senior technologist review, and (4) a director review. Following a band-by-band analysis, the director must also review the clinical indication and any other clinical information and decide whether additional chromosome analysis or other studies must be performed prior to signing out the case.

Biochemical evaluation of amniotic fluid from early amniocentesis specimens can be problematic. There is a significant rate of false positive acetylcholinesterase (AChE) results from specimens less than 13 weeks gestation. In 1 study involving 476 early amniocentesis procedures, a 10.6% rate of positive AChE results was identified compared to a 2.5% rate in routine amniocentesis specimens. This difference was statistically significant.[3] This may result in difficulty determining the risk of a neural tube defect in these early pregnancies. For instance, if the amniotic fluid alpha-fetoprotein (AFP) level is elevated, it is not possible to determine if a subsequent positive AChE is a true- or false-positive result. In addition, because of the reduced sample volume obtained, a slight increase in cell culture growth failure has been observed in most studies.

CHORIONIC VILLUS SAMPLING

For a CVS procedure, a small sample of chorionic villi is obtained. Amniotic fluid is not withdrawn. As such, biochemical analysis of amniotic fluid, including assaying amniotic fluid AFP, is not possible. For this reason, evaluation for neural tube defects through CVS is not possible.

The primary advantage of CVS is earlier results. This is especially important to couples at extremely high risk for a genetic abnormality or those who have had a genetic abnormality in a previous pregnancy and find it unbearable to wait until the mid second trimester for amniocentesis. Transcervical CVS was initially introduced in the mid 1970s. The technique involves the introduction of a flexible catheter with a metal stylet through the cervix. After the catheter is properly placed within the placenta, the metal stylet is withdrawn and a 20-cc syringe filled with 5 cc of sterile aspiration medium is attached. Aspiration medium consists of modified Eagle's medium or other medium, L-glutamine, and penicillin–streptomycin. No fetal bovine serum (FBS) is used to avoid generating bubbles that may interfere with the aspiration. Aspiration of villi is performed as the catheter is withdrawn. The sample is then placed in transport medium, which is the aspiration medium with 15% FBS added, and sent to the laboratory for analysis.

Excluding confined placental mosaicism (a finding in approximately 1% of CVS samples), the genetic makeup of the placenta is identical to that of the fetus. For this reason, chorionic villi may be utilized to determine the chromosomal, enzymatic, or molecular genetic status of the fetus. As such, the indications for CVS are similar to those for amniocentesis. The only exceptions are that CVS cannot test for neural tube defects and CVS is unreliable as a test for fragile X syndrome because inaccurate DNA methylation patterns in chorionic villi compared to the fetus are frequently observed.

As noted, confined placental mosaicism is encountered in approximately 1% of CVS specimens. In these situations, amniocentesis should be offered. Although a normal amniocentesis result does not eliminate the possibility of true mosaicism in the fetus, it does substantially reduce the chance that true mosaicism exists. Only approximately 10–20% of mosaicism identified on CVS is confirmed on amniocentesis.[4] If confined placental mosaicism is identified, there is an association with poor perinatal outcome, including an increased risk of pregnancy loss, fetal growth restriction, and stillbirth.[5]

LABORATORY METHODOLOGY

Villi are composed of trophoblastic cells that consist of an outer cytotrophoblastic layer and an inner mesenchymal core. The cytotrophoblastic layer contains spontaneously dividing cells and is used for direct chromosome preparations. For short-term culture, the mesenchymal core cells are broken up by enzyme digestion and set up in culture.

When a chorionic villus sample is received in the laboratory, it is placed in a sterile tissue culture dish and examined under a dissecting microscope. The volume and quality of the sample are determined; maternal decidua are separated from the villi and discarded. If a direct preparation is requested, the sample is split. Ideally, there are 10–15 mg available for the direct preparation and 15–20 mg for the culture. Today, laboratories either do both the direct preparation and the culture or only the culture. Direct preparations are not used any longer as a standalone test because of potential false-positive and -negative results. In addition, the poor banding quality and morphology as compared to those obtained from the short-term cultures make it more difficult to detect small rearrangements. Direct and cultured preparations may yield different cytogenetic results; they are derived from different cell layers. When this occurs, or when mosaicism is found in the culture, a follow-up amniocentesis is often needed to clarify the results.

For direct preparations, villi are placed in aspiration or culture medium and treated with a hypotonic solution and several changes of Carnoy's fixative. The fixative is removed and a solution of 1:1 acetic acid:water is added and gently mixed. A small amount of this suspension is added to a warm slide on hotplate. The slide is allowed to dry, which results in the spreading of any spontaneous dividing cells. Banding and staining are the same as for amniocytes.

For CVS cultures, cleaned villi are rinsed and incubated in aspiration media to wash off the FBS from the transport medium (which is inhibitory to digestive enzymes). The sample is then placed in a dish containing 10× trypsin-EDTA and incubated at 37°C. The sample is next transferred to a centrifuge tube and pelleted. The trypsin solution is aspirated off and the cell pellet is resuspended in a solution with collagenase and incubated at 37°C. The sample is centrifuged, the solution aspirated off, and the cells are resuspended in a supplemented tissue culture medium such as Amniomax or Chang (see discussion under amniocyte cell culture). For the in situ method, resuspended cells are placed on the surface of a coverslip in a small culture dish, cells are allowed to attach overnight, and then the coverslip is flooded with more medium on the second day. Banding and staining is as described for amniocytes. The TAT averages 5–7 days, but may take longer if a small volume or poor quality of villi is received.

Five cells are usually examined from the direct preparation and 20 cells from the culture. As cells are disassociated and in large numbers, growth is not in obvious colonies as it is with amniocytes.

PRENATAL DIAGNOSIS FROM CYSTIC HYGROMA FLUID AND FETAL URINE

CYSTIC HYGROMA FLUID

Cystic hygromas are congenital malformations of the lymphatic system appearing as septated or nonseptated fluid-filled cavities, usually involving the neck. They are often associated with a chromosome abnormality, most commonly 45,X, trisomy 21, or trisomy 18, in descending order of frequency. They may also be associated with several different Mendelian syndromes.[6]

Obtaining fluid from a cystic hygroma for prenatal diagnostic studies has been suggested as an easier procedure than obtaining amniotic fluid in cases involving large posterior nuchal cystic hygromas associated with oligohydramnios. The largest series of cytogenetic and FISH analysis from cystic hygroma fluid involved 83 cystic hygroma specimens; all 83 samples were evaluated by traditional cytogenetics and 23 also evaluated by FISH for chromosomes 13, 18, 21, X, and Y.[7] When >5 mL of fluid was submitted to the laboratory, the success rate for cytogenetic analysis was 76%. If the sample was <5 mL, cytogenetic analysis was successful in only 9%. FISH on cystic hygroma specimens was successful for 78% of the samples submitted, including several where cell culture failed. The optimal approach was to perform both traditional cytogenetic analysis and FISH. Using this combined approach, a successful result was obtained in 90% of cases when >5 mL of fluid was submitted for analysis. The mean TAT was 8.2 days (range, 4–17 days). Results were available in <12 days in 91% of cases. There was a 91% aneuploidy rate identified, with 45,X occurring in 86% of the samples.

FETAL URINE

The sonographic appearance of a fetus with bladder outlet obstruction is characterized by a large, distended bladder, oligohydramnios, and hydronephrosis. An investigation involving the chromosome analysis of 75 fetal urine specimens from fetuses with bladder outlet obstruction, including 31 evaluated by interphase FISH, was recently reported.[8] Traditional cytogenetic analysis was successful on 95% of samples and FISH was informative on 65% of specimens. The combination of traditional cytogenetic analysis and FISH yielded a 96% chromosome analysis diagnostic success rate. The mean TAT was 8 days (range, 5–14) for traditional cytogenetic analysis and

1.6 days (range, 1.0–4.0) for FISH. Chromosome abnormalities were detected in 8%. The authors concluded that traditional cytogenetic analysis achieved a high success rate (95%) and was superior to FISH for chromosome evaluation of fetal urine. However, the rapid TAT achieved with FISH allowed for expeditious clinical management of bladder outlet obstruction and placement of a vesicoamniotic shunt, when applicable, approximately 6 days sooner than would be possible if waiting for traditional cytogenetic results to become available. For this reason, FISH is warranted in the management of fetal bladder outlet obstruction. It is apparent that the optimal approach for health care providers submitting fetal urine for prenatal diagnosis of chromosome abnormalities should be to request both traditional cytogenetic studies and a FISH evaluation for the most common aneuploidies involving chromosomes 13, 18, 21, X, and Y.

LABORATORY METHODOLOGY

The culturing of cystic hygroma fluid and fetal urine is the same as for amniotic fluid cells. For cystic hygroma fluid, some labs may also set up a phytohemagluttanin (PHA)-stimulated culture in an attempt to stimulate any fetal white cells that may be in the fluid. Chromosome analysis is the same as for amniocytes.

FETAL BLOOD SAMPLING

Gaining direct access to the fetal circulation was considered an impossibility (and far too risky to attempt) until Daffos et al.[9] published their series of 606 fetal blood sampling procedures in 1985.

LABORATORY METHODOLOGY

Standard PHA-stimulated blood culture techniques are used for fetal blood samples (AGT Manual). To ensure that fetal and not maternal blood has been cultured and analyzed, a distinguishing test should be performed (CAP requirement), preferably at the time of sampling. Twenty metaphase cells are examined.

FETAL SKIN BIOPSY

A fetal skin biopsy for chromosome analysis is rarely performed. More commonly, a skin biopsy may be considered for the prenatal diagnosis of a heritable, severe congenital skin disorder such as epidermolysis bullosa. However, some investigators have encouraged the use of a fetal skin biopsy to evaluate mosaicism identified either on amniocentesis or fetal blood sampling. Once obtained, the cells can be separated by collagenase and placed on coverslips, in flasks, or both. At least 21 instances in which an abnormal cell line was observed on a fetal skin biopsy, but not in fetal blood peripheral lymphocytes, have been reported.[10] Thus, to clarify the prenatal cytogenetic status of a fetus following the diagnosis of mosaicism on amniocentesis, fetal skin biopsy should be considered. The ectodermally derived cells from fetal skin may be more reflective of the true fetal chromosome status than mesodermally derived tissue such as blood lymphocytes. Fetal skin biopsy appears to be a relatively safe procedure. In the largest series reported of 54 such procedures, no fetal complications were encountered and no pregnancy losses occurred.[11]

CYTOGENETIC RESULTS AND ISSUES COMMON TO ALL PRENATAL SAMPLE TYPES

The majority (80%) of clinically significant chromosome abnormalities are trisomies involving chromosomes 21, 18, and 13, aneuploidies involving the sex chromosomes, or mosaicism involving these chromosomes. Most of the remaining 20% of the chromosome abnormalities involve unbalanced translocations or deletions (Figs. 41-1, 41-2), either de novo or inherited, other rare mosaic trisomies, and marker chromosomes. If the chromosome abnormality can be defined based on G-bands or with the use of FISH, prognostic information may be provided to the parents after a search of the literature for similar cases.

A number of prenatal cytogenetic findings require the study of parental blood chromosomes to help define the significance of a finding in the fetal karyotype. These include balanced translocations, unbalanced translocations (Fig. 41-3), inversions, marker chromosomes, and potential variant chromosomes.

If a rearrangement appears to be a balanced translocation or inversion, studying the parents to see if this rearrangement has been "tested" in a phenotypically normal person often provides useful prognostic information. If the rearrangement is de novo, more general risks may be provided based on the literature.[12]

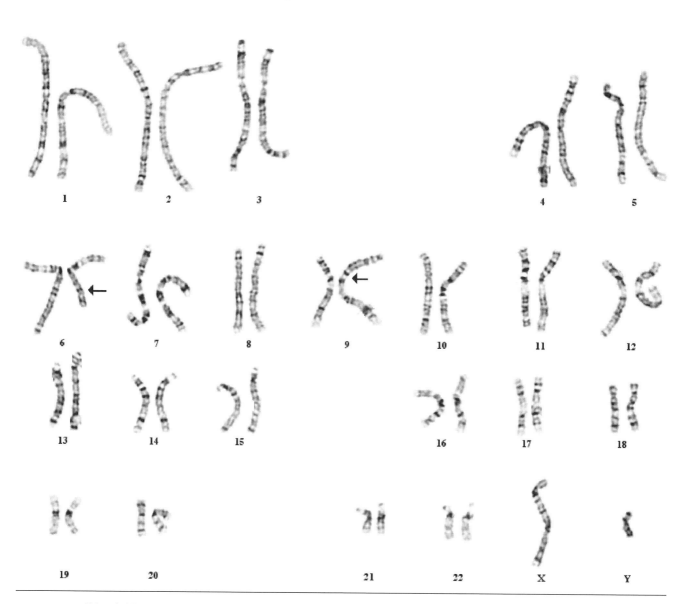

FIGURE 41-1 G-banded karyotype revealing a balanced reciprocal translocation between chromosomes 6 and 9.

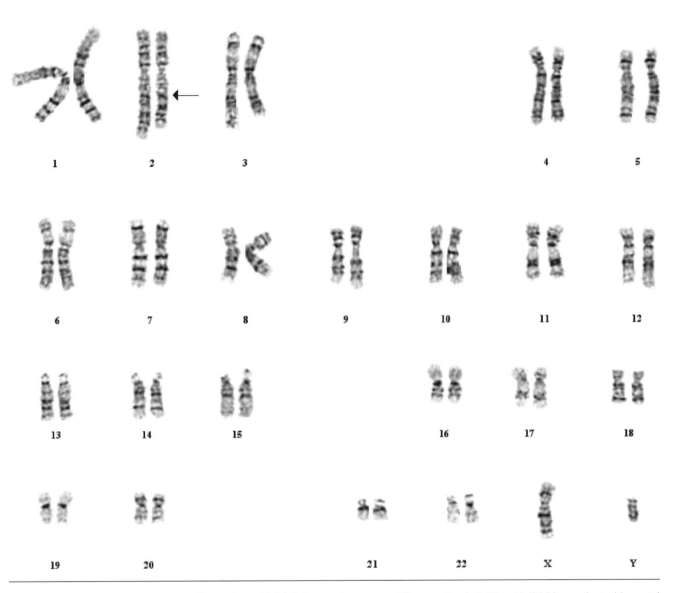

FIGURE 41-2 G-banded karyotype revealing an interstitial deletion on chromosome 2 between bands 2q23 and 2q24.2 in a patient with mental retardation.

Because parental blood chromosomes are often of a better quality and higher banding resolution, it is possible that what was thought to be an unbalanced rearrangement in the fetus turns out to be balanced. This may occur as parental studies are usually performed at a higher banding resolution. This may lead to discovery of both derivative chromosomes from a parental balanced translocation. A reexamination of the fetal karyotype may show that what was originally thought to be an apparently unbalanced translocation is actually an inherited balanced translocation. Therefore, caution should always be used until parental studies are completed before making pregnancy management decisions. Routine FISH on obvious abnormalities may also uncover balanced rearrangements (see below).

Marker chromosomes provide a challenge if inherited or de novo, requiring both FISH and C-bands, and are discussed further under Molecular Techniques.

Parental studies are also useful for determining if the presence of additional material around the centromeres of any of the chromosomes, or in the short arm regions of acrocentric chromosomes (chromosomes 13, 14, 15, 21, and 22), is clinically significant or represents a normal variant chromosome. C-banding and/or FISH can also be useful in resolving the clinical significance of this category of chromosome variations.

The finding of a 45,X karyotype without abnormal ultrasound findings requires a cautious approach to rule out mosaicism with a normal cell line with 2 sex chromosomes (X or Y), or mosaicism with a cell line that contains an abnormal X or Y chromosome. A discussion with the clinician of the ultrasound findings can be helpful, especially if male genitalia are observed. This cautious approach has uncovered additional cell lines when more cells are examined (with the second sex chromosome X or Y derived) and/or when FISH

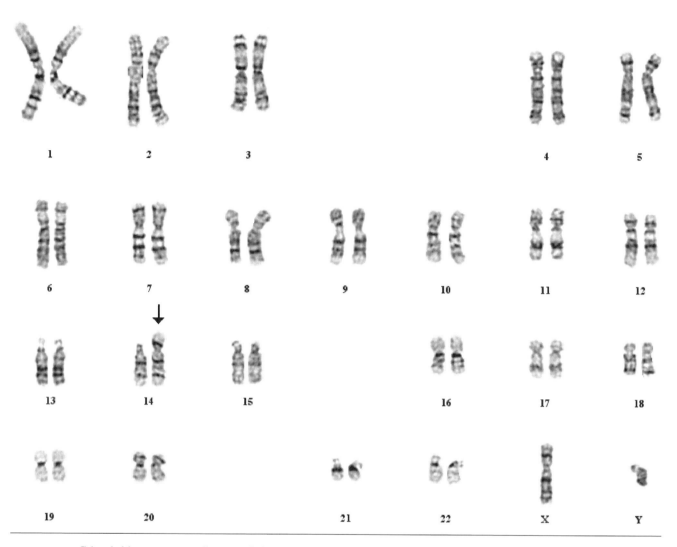

FIGURE 41-3 G-banded karyotype revealing an unbalanced Robertsonian translocation involving chromosomes 14 and 21 in a child with Down syndrome.

is included. Depending on the ultrasound results, FISH using *SRY* and/or the Y centromere and *Yqh* probes, and the X centromeric probe may be necessary. Some rare 45,X cases may have the testis determining-gene, *SRY*, translocated to the short arm of an acrocentric chromosome where it may not be distinguishable from a normal acrocentric short arm variant. In cases of a 46,XX karyotype and male genitalia, *SRY* is frequently translocated to the tip of the X chromosome short arm (see the section on Prenatal Diagnosis From Cystic Hygroma Fluid).

Carriers of Robertsonian translocations that involve chromosomes 14 and/or 15 are at risk of having offspring with UPD. UPD is the inheritance of a chromosome pair from only 1 parent, with no contribution from the other. This is a concern if genes are *imprinted*, which refers to the expression of certain genes only on the paternal homolog and others only on the maternal homolog. The best known examples of imprinted diseases in humans are Prader-Willi syndrome (PWS) and Angelman syndrome (AS). Paternal and

maternal UPD for chromosome 14 has been reported to be associated with an abnormal phenotype (reviewed in Shaffer et al.[13] and Drugan et al.[3]). Therefore, in both inherited and de novo cases involving Robertsonian translocations with chromosomes 14 and/or 15, UPD needs to be ruled out. The risk of UPD is approximately 0.5% for Robertsonian translocations involving nonhomologous chromosomes, and as high as 66% if isochromosomes of 14 or 15 are seen in a fetus.[14]

MOLECULAR CYTOGENETICS

Molecular techniques have complemented and improved the diagnostic capabilities of prenatal and postnatal chromosome analysis over the past 12 years. The major molecular cytogenetic technique is FISH, where fluorescently tagged DNA probes are hybridized to metaphase spreads or interphase cells from all tissue types.

GUIDELINES FOR FISH STUDIES

Requirements and guidelines for FISH analysis for all sample types are available from the CAP at www.cap.org/toolbox/index.htm (Checklists, Cytogenetics) and in more detail from the ACMG at www.acmg.net (educational materials, Standards and Guidelines for Clinical Genetics Laboratories, 2002 edition). The guidelines ensure rigorous quality control and validation of probes, both commercially prepared and "homebrew." Probes not cleared or approved by the Food and Drug Administration (FDA) are considered to be analyte-specific reagents (ASRs). The following disclaimer must be included on any test report using ASRs: "This test was developed and its performance characteristics determined by [laboratory name] as required by the CLIA '88 regulations. It has not been cleared or approved for specific uses by the U.S. Food and Drug Administration." ACMG suggests that the following clarifying language may follow the above disclaimer: "The FDA has determined that such clearance or approval is not necessary. This test is used for clinical purposes. It should not be regarded as investigational or for research." A laboratory must test and validate all of its probes on a lot-by-lot basis. For interphase use, databases should be made to establish confidence intervals for interpreting results.

TYPES OF FISH PROBES AND CLINICAL STUDIES

The main categories of FISH probes include locus-specific probes, painting probes, and repetitive sequence probes. Locus-specific probes can be from any unique locus on a chromosome, such as those used to detect microdeletions (Table 41-1), specific subtelomeric regions, and other unique regions of various chromosomes. A FISH laboratory likes to have probes covering as many different regions of all the chromosomes as possible. This allows many structural rearrangements to be further investigated, although it is often fortuitous if a probe happens to be located in a region so that it provides useful information. This used to also be true of the regions at the ends of the chromosomes until the development of chromosome-specific subtelomeric probes. Now suspected or unexpected rearrangements at the chromosome ends can be verified or discovered.

Subtelomeric Probes

A subtelomeric check of all the chromosome ends is indicated in postnatal cases with indications of mental retardation or developmental delay and dysmorphic features (mild or severe). This has uncovered many cryptic or subtle rearrangements, approximately half of which may be present in a balanced form in 1 of the parents (reviewed in Berend et al.[14] and de Vries et al.[15]). Although many parents wish to pursue the perfect child and want to eliminate as many uncertainties for their fetus

TABLE 41-1 | DISORDERS ASSOCIATED WITH MICRODELETIONS DIAGNOSABLE BY MOLECULAR CYTOGENETIC TECHNOLOGY

Syndrome	Microdeletion	Features
DiGeorge/VCFS	22q11.2	Thymus hypoplasia, abnormal facies, moderate mental retardation, hypoplastic parathyroid glands, cardiac malformations
Angelman	15q11.2(mat)	Severe mental retardation, seizures, ataxia, hyperactivity, absence of speech, inappropriate laughter
Prader-Willi	15q11.2(pat)	Hypotonia in infancy, hyperphagia, obesity, developmental delay, hypogonadism
Cri-du-Chat	5p15.2	Cat cry in infancy, mental retardation, microcephaly, round face, hypotonia, hypertelorism
Kallman	Xp22.3	Anosmia and hypogonadism
Miller-Dieker	17p13.3	Type I lissencephaly; agyria; high, narrow, wrinkled forehead; wide, flat lip; micrognathia
Smith-Magenis	17p11.2	Mental retardation, brachycephaly, brachydactyly, sleep disorders, failure to thrive, hypotonia, self-destructive behavior as an adult
Steroid sulfatase deficiency	Xp22.3	X-linked ichthyosis
Williams	7q11.23	Mental retardation, elfin facies, supravalvular aortic stenosis and/or other cardiac defects, gregarious personality, infantile hypercalcemia, stellate iris
Wolf-Hirschhorn	4p16.3	Severe growth and mental retardation, cleft lip and palate, microcephaly, hypertelorism, hypospadias, cryptorchidism

VCFS—velocardiofacial syndrome.

as possible, a subtelomeric check of all the chromosome ends in a prenatal study is not a practical or feasible approach with current labor-intensive FISH methodologies. If family history leads to a suspicion of a subtle rearrangement, it is more appropriate to study the affected child, if possible. If this is not possible, a study of the parental chromosomes is the next choice. If a rearrangement is found, then FISH studies on fetal chromosomes can be performed with the specific probes involved.

Microdeletion Syndromes

For the microdeletion syndromes listed in Table 41-1, most are based on a previous child with, or a family history of, a specific syndrome. The 1 major exception is the 22q11.2 deletion seen in DiGeorge/velocardiofacial syndrome (DGS/VCFS). The ultrasound finding of a congenital heart defect increases the risk that the fetus has DGS/VCFS. Certain cardiac defects, most specifically tetralogy of Fallot and conotruncal anomalies, may be signs of DGS/VCFS syndrome.[17] The risk of DiGeorge syndrome in the presence of a prenatally diagnosed congenital heart defect is approximately 5%. The risk is higher when the specific defect is identified as tetralogy of Fallot or truncus arteriosus. In addition, the presence of excess nuchal translucency, an ultrasound finding identifiable in the late first trimester, has been identified as a risk factor for DiGeorge syndrome.[18] The prevalence of DGS/VCFS has been estimated to be 1 in 3000. This is a higher frequency than many conditions that are studied prenatally.

Painting Probes

Whole chromosome painting probes, which hybridize to the entire length of a specific chromosome, are most often used for broader questions, such as "Is the extra material on a chromosome from another chromosome or a duplication of material from the same chromosome?" Almost every lab has been surprised investigating what was thought to be a simple deletion or unbalanced rearrangement, only to use a painting probe and see a small amount of the painting probe on another chromosome. A focused reexamination of the G-banded chromosomes usually reveals the balanced rearrangement.

Centromeric Probes

Centromeric probes are the most common and useful chromosome-specific repetitive probes. These can be used as control probes to mark a specific centromeric region in relation to a locus-specific probe, to investigate centromeric variants, or to identify marker chromosomes.

MARKER CHROMOSOMES

Marker chromosomes can be difficult and frustrating to deal with for the laboratory, the clinician, and the patient. A marker chromosome may be present in a mosaic or nonmosaic state, vary in size, or may be satellited or nonsatellited. As with most any unusual cytogenetic observation in fetal cells, parental chromosomes should be studied when a marker chromosome is found. FISH technology now allows the chromosome origin (but not usually the gene content) of a marker chromosome to

be identified. Centromeric probes and painting probes (either as individual painting probes or as multicolor painting probes) can now be used to identify almost all marker chromosomes. This information, however, does not always change the quality of information presented to patients. Further detailed characterization of the marker with probes adjacent to the centromere is not currently readily available to determine if markers derived from the same chromosome contain the same genes. In addition, the level and distribution of abnormal cells in a mosaic state may also make comparisons difficult. The number of characterized published cases is limited but growing.[19] Other than for chromosomes 15, 22, and the X chromosome, no consistent genotype/phenotype correlations have been found that can provide prognostic information. Therefore, C-band characterization and the pre-FISH era risks of 11–15% risk for serious congenital anomalies[12] are often the most useful information that can be provided.

Chromosome 15–Derived Markers

Markers derived from chromosome 15 represent an opportunity to provide the patient with specific prognostic information. The majority of these markers are bisatellited and are also referred to as inverted duplicated 15 markers (inv dup[15]) or psu dic (15;15) markers. If these markers have the PWS/AS region present (easily shown by FISH studies), then the marker is associated with a well-characterized abnormal phenotype distinct from PWS or AS.[20,21] If the PWS/AS region is missing, a normal phenotype is often, but not always, observed.[21] The exception is when the marker is associated with PWS or AS owing to UPD (2 copies of chromosome 15 inherited from 1 parent).[20] If detected prenatally, there appears to be a 10% risk of UPD for chromosome 15.[22]

X Chromosome–Derived Markers

An X chromosome–derived marker can also provide the patient with specific prognostic information (reviewed in Leppig and Disteche[23] and Willard[24]). The determination of the presence or absence of the XIST gene can help predict the phenotype in prenatal cases of 45,X/46,r(X). If a small ring X chromosome lacks the XIST gene that is associated with X inactivation and there are genes present on the marker, then genes that are usually inactivated will be active and associated with an abnormal phenotype that includes mental retardation. If there are no genes present on the small r(X) chromosome, then Turner syndrome is expected. Also, if the marker is larger and contains a functional XIST gene, then this r(X) marker is inactivated and also results in a Turner syndrome phenotype.

PRENATAL INTERPHASE FISH

Prenatal interphase FISH is the rapid assessment of aneuploidy status in uncultured interphase cells from amniotic fluid, CVS, fetal blood, fetal urine, and cystic hygroma fluid. This technique is designed to detect aneuploidies of chromosomes 13, 18, 21, X, and Y. Experience has demonstrated the reliability and usefulness of prenatal interphase FISH for providing rapid, useful information to the clinician and patient (see review in

Miny et al.[25] and Schwartz[26]). Issues such as the presence of maternal blood in the sample, either grossly visible or only noticeable after centrifugation of the sample, still prevent results from being obtained on 2–5% of amniotic fluid samples. These samples are either not analyzed or called uninformative if male fetal cells are not observed.

NEW MOLECULAR DEVELOPMENTS

Because many of the FISH approaches discussed are labor intensive and costly, development of new, more cost-effective technologies is a desired goal. Another goal for new technology is the development of more powerful and routine analysis of the genome at a resolution higher than that attained with traditional G-banded chromosome analysis and with some of the FISH probes.

A recent successful molecular technique for the replacement of prenatal interphase FISH that is becoming widespread in Europe is QF–PCR[27,28] (reviewed in Miny et al.[25]). This quantitative approach uses polymorphic DNA markers (STRs) for the common trisomies and sex chromosome aneuploidies.

Microarrays (DNA chips) with genomic clones are being developed and hold promise for providing a replacement for FISH for microdeletion syndromes and subtelomere analysis, and potentially as a high-resolution banding technique, providing a more detailed reading of the complete genome than current G-banding.[29]

SUMMARY

Over the past 10 years, prenatal chromosome diagnosis has rapidly changed; both sampling methodologies and molecular techniques complement chromosome analysis. This review summarizes current techniques and their risks used by the clinician, and selected aspects of cytogenetic and molecular techniques used by the laboratories. Within the next 3–5 years, DNA techniques are expected to complement, and potentially replace, aspects of current cytogenetic and FISH techniques, and provide more detailed information on the genetic status of the fetus.

References

1. Lockwood DH, Neu RL. Cytogenetic analysis of 1375 amniotic fluid specimens from pregnancies with gestational age less than 14 weeks. *Prenat Diagn*. 1993;13:801–805.

2. Hook EB. Exclusion of chromosomal mosaicism: tables of 90%, 95% and 99% confidence limits and comments on use. *Am J Hum Genet*. 1977;29:94–97.

3. Drugan A, Syner FN, Greb A, et al. Amniotic fluid alpha-fetoprotein and acetylcholinesterase in early genetic amniocentesis. *Obstet Gynecol*. 1988;72:35–38.

4. Goldberg JD, Wohlferd MM. Incidence and outcome of chromosomal mosaicism found at the time of chorionic villus sampling. *Am J Obstet Gynecol*. 1997;176:1349–1353.

5. Johnson A, Wapner R, Davis GH, et al. Mosaicism in chorionic villus sampling: an association with poor perinatal outcome. *Obstet Gynecol*. 1990;75:573–576.

6. Descamps P, Jourdain O, Paillet C, et al. Etiology, prognosis and management of fetal cystic hygroma: 25 new cases and literature review. *Eur J Obstet Gynecol Reprod Biol*. 1997;71:3–10.

7. Donnenfeld AE, Lockwood D, Lamb AN. Prenatal diagnosis from cystic hygroma fluid: the value of fluorescence in situ hybridization. *Am J Obstet Gynecol*. 2001;185:1004–1008.

8. Donnenfeld AE, Lockwood D, Custer T, et al. Prenatal diagnosis from fetal urine in bladder outlet obstruction: success rates for traditional cytogenetic evaluation and interphase fluorescence in situ hybridization. *Genet Med*. 2002;4:444–447.

9. Daffos F, Capella-Pavlovsky M, Forestier F. Fetal blood sampling during pregnancy with use of a needle guided by ultrasound. A study of 606 consecutive cases. *Am J Obstet Gynecol*. 1985;153:655–659.

10. Berghella V, Wapner RJ, Yang-Feng T, et al. Prenatal confirmation of true fetal trisomy 22 mosaicism by fetal skin biopsy following normal fetal blood sampling. *Prenat Diagn*. 1998;18:384–389.

11. Nicolini U, Rodeck CH. Fetal blood and tissue sampling. In: Brock DJH, Rodeck CH, Ferguson-Smith MA, eds. *Prenatal Diagnosis and Screening*. London, England: Churchill Livingstone; 1992:39–51.

12. Warburton D. De novo balanced chromosome rearrangements and extra marker chromosomes identified at prenatal diagnosis: clinical significance and distribution of breakpoints. *Am J Hum Genet*. 1991;49: 995–1013.

13. Shaffer LG, Agan N, Goldberg JD, et al: American College of Medical Genetics Statement on Diagnostic Testing for Uniparental disomy. *Genet Med*. 2001;3:206–211.

14. Berend SA, Horwitz J, McCaskill C, et al. Identification of uniparental disomy following prenatal detection of Robertsonian translocations and isochromosomes. *Am J Hum Genet*. 2000;66:1787–1793.

15. de Vries BBA, White SM, Knight SLJ, et al. Clinical studies of submicroscopic subtelomeric rearrangements: a checklist. *J Med Genet*. 2001;38:145–150.

16. Knight S, Flint J. Perfect endings: a review of subtelomeric probes and their use in clinical diagnosis. *J Med Genet*. 2000;37:401–409.

17. Driscoll DA. Prenatal diagnosis of the 22q11.2 deletion syndrome. *Genet Med*. 2001;3:14–18.

18. Lazanakis MS, Rodgers K, Economides DL. Increased nuchal translucency and CATCH 22. *Prenat Diagn*. 1998;18:507–510.

19. Crolla JA. FISH and molecular studies of autosomal supernumerary marker chromosomes excluding those derived from chromosome 15. II. Review of the literature. *Am J Med Genet*. 1998;75:367–381.

20. Engel E, Antonarakis SE. *Genomic Imprinting and Uniparental Disomy in Medicine*. New York, NY: Wiley-Liss; 2002.

21. Webb T. Inv dup(15) supernumerary marker chromosomes. *J Med Genet*. 1994;31:585–594.

22. Christian SL, Mills P, Das S, et al. High risk of uniparental disomy associated with amniotic fluid containing de novo small supernumerary marker chromosomes [abstract]. *Am J Hum Genet Suppl*. 63:A11. 1998;Abstract 54.

23. Leppig KA, Disteche. Ring X and other structural X chromosome abnormalities: X inactivation and phenotype. *Semin Reprod Med*. 2001;19:147–157.

24. Willard HF. The sex chromosomes and X chromosome inactivation. In Scriver CR, Beaudet AL, Sly WS, Valle D, eds. *The Metabolic*

and Molecular Bases of Inherited Diseases. 8th ed. New York, NY: McGraw-Hill; 2001:1191–1211.

25. Miny P, Tercani S, Holzgreve W. Developments in laboratory techniques for prenatal diagnosis. *Curr Opin Obstet Gynecol.* 2002;14: 161–168.

26. Schwartz S. Molecular cytogenetics and prenatal diagnosis. In: Milunsky A, ed. *Genetic Disorders and the Fetus.* 4th ed. Baltimore, Md: The Johns Hopkins University Press; 1998:286–313.

27. Adinolfi M, Sherlock J. Prenatal detection of chromosome disorders by QF-PCR. *Lancet.* 2001;358:1030–1031.

28. Mann K, Fox SP, Abbs SJ, et al. Development and implementation of a new aneuploidy diagnostic service within the UK National Health Service and implications for the future of prenatal diagnosis. *Lancet.* 2001;358:1057–1061.

29. Antonarakis SE. BACing up the promises. *Nat Genet.* 2001;27:230–232.

BIOCHEMICAL GENETICS

Yoav Ben-Yoseph

Biochemical tests for diagnosis of inherited metabolic disorders consist of identification of abnormal metabolites or abnormal levels of metabolites that reflect the metabolic block or alteration, and ultimately identification, quantitation and characterization of the defective or deficient gene product that is responsible for the metabolic block or alteration.[1,2] The disorders covered here are monogenic disorders that are caused by single mutant genes. Such disorders are caused by mutant genes that produce no protein, produce small quantity of protein, or produce abnormal protein whose functional activity is altered. The 1 gene–1 enzyme concept has been extended to cover RNA as the final gene product and to cover proteins that are not enzymes as well as complex proteins composed of nonidentical polypeptide chains. Posttranslational cleavage to generate multiple peptides, alternative splicing, and alternative promoter sequences contribute complexities to the concept. Additional intricacies are introduced as mutations in transcription factors, gain-of-function mutations, somatic mutations, unstable mutations, and imprinting of genes.

When the underlying biochemical defect is known and is expressed in obtainable specimens of fetal tissue (chorionic villi and fetal liver biopsy) or cells (trophoblasts, amniotic fluid cells, fetal erythrocytes, and leukocytes), prenatal diagnosis is ultimately based on analysis of the enzyme or other protein primarily involved. In other cases, the test is based on measurement of secondary biochemical events such as elevation or absence of a particular metabolite(s) or protein(s) in cell-free amniotic fluid or in fetal plasma or serum.

The purpose of this chapter is to describe some of the considerations used in prenatal diagnosis of monogenic diseases, and to delineate the principles of the biochemical methodology. The various points are illustrated by examples of representative diseases and assay systems.

Mode of inheritance and family studies are important issues in prenatal diagnosis of monogenic disorders, especially for interpretation of the test results. Specific points of consideration relating mostly to autosomal recessive disorders include genotype assignments among relatives of an index case, fetal contribution to maternal serum enzyme levels during pregnancy, problems with pseudodeficiencies, and carrier detection screening programs. Other points addressed are distinction between affected heterozygotes and homozygotes in autosomal-dominant diseases, identification of heterozygous females in X-linked diseases and non-Mendelian inheritance.

Fetal samples of various types and origins serve as diagnostic material for prenatal evaluations. Specific points discussed include availability of the respective normal control samples, maternal contamination, distribution of various enzymes and isozymes in different cells and tissue types, direct versus cultured specimens, cell morphology and cell culture conditions, amniotic fluid metabolites, fetal blood sampling and fetal liver biopsy, and handling of processed and unprocessed tissue and fluid specimens.

Biochemically analyzable materials include gene products such as enzymes, receptors, transporters, activators, peptide hormones, immunoglobulins, collagens, coagulation factors and transcription factors, and metabolites such as amino acids, organic acids, and vitamins. In describing the methodologic principles, the emphasis is on enzymes which are the most commonly analyzed gene products. Topics addressed are enzyme preparations, assay conditions, controls and blanks, substrates and cofactors, separation and detection methods, and nonenzymatic defects.

MODE OF INHERITANCE AND FAMILY STUDIES

Definitive diagnosis of an inherited metabolic disorder must be based on clear-cut distinction between the values of affected and unaffected fetuses. In the case of an autosomal-recessive disease, the assay employed should ideally discriminate between homozygous affected, heterozygous unaffected, and homozygous normal fetuses. Because variability owing to different genomic backgrounds does exist among family members, testing of leukocytes or cultured skin fibroblasts from the parents, the index case and unaffected siblings can provide valuable information on the respective values of different genotypes within a particular family. In addition to the benefit in interpretation of the results of the prenatal evaluation, it may prove to be a reliable means for identification of carriers among members of the extended family. Valuable information concerning the fetus can be obtained in some cases by determination of maternal serum enzyme activities during pregnancy. For example, the normal increase in serum hexosaminidase A during pregnancy appears to be of fetal origin and unchanged levels in pregnancies at risk for Tay-Sachs disease may indicate an affected fetus.[3,4]

Low levels of enzymatic activity in apparently healthy individuals (pseudodeficiency) make prenatal diagnosis a more difficult task. Deficiency of galactocerebrosidase activity toward galactosylceramide and deficiency of arylsulfatase A activity toward both p-nitrocatechol sulfate (artificial substrate) and cerebroside sulfate (natural substrate) have been described in unaffected members of families with Krabbe disease[5] and metachromatic leukodystrophy,[6] respectively. Prenatal diagnosis cannot be made in such families on tissue or cell extracts, but is possible by loading tests that are based on growing intact cells in culture in the presence of the appropriate substrate or its precursor.[7] Alternatively, mutations causing pseudodeficiency may be identified by molecular methods.[8]

Screening for carriers is usually limited to populations at high risk for a diagnosable disease. Carrier detection for Tay-Sachs disease is routinely offered to all individuals of Ashkenazi Jewish descent, in whom the combined frequency for 2 common Mutations In the α-chain gene of hexosaminidases is 1 in 30.[9,10] The ultimate benefit of carrier detection programs is the identification of couples at risk prior to having an affected child. In 1995–1996 (International Tay-Sachs Disease Quality Control and Data Collection Center), 61,017 young adults were screened by 102 centers worldwide to determine their Tay-Sachs disease carrier status and 60 at-risk couples (both partners heterozygotes) were identified.

Assays for detection of autosomal-dominant diseases such as some of the porphyrias[11,12] are usually capable of identifying affected homozygotes but fail sometimes to differentiate conclusively affected heterozygotes from unaffected fetuses. In genetic disorders, there is potential for overlap between the normal and heterozygous ranges for enzyme activities. This is caused in part by variability in assay conditions, but mainly by the wide variation found for almost any activity in the normal population. Consequently, the demonstration of reduced enzyme activities comparable with heterozygous forms of autosomal dominant porphyrias usually is not considered an indication for termination of pregnancy. On the other hand, deficient enzyme activities consistent with homozygous forms of dominant porphyrias are often considered for termination of pregnancy because of their more severe clinical course.

X-linked disorders present some specific difficulties in heterozygote detection. Recessive and dominant inheritance refer only to expression of the gene in females and this is often highly variable owing to random X inactivation.[13] This has led to some arbitrary and inconsistent assignments. Ornithine carbamoyltransferase deficiency often has been described as X-linked dominant, whereas Fabry disease often has been described as X-linked recessive. Phenotypic abnormalities occur in some heterozygotes for either disorder. Because there is no clear convention, it may be best to consider such disorders as simply X-linked without a dominant or recessive designation. The recessive or dominant descriptors are more useful for X-linked disorders where, respectively, heterozygotes are quite consistently asymptomatic as in X-linked recessive Hunter disease or are quite consistently symptomatic in a manner similar to hemizygous males as in X-linked dominant hypophosphatemic rickets. Depending on the proportions of active mutant and normal X chromosomes in the tissues involved in the pathogenesis of the disease, a female heterozygous for Fabry disease, for example, may be clinically normal through her life or she may develop mild or severe manifestations of the disease with increasing age.[14]

Biochemical methods are seldom completely accurate in identifying X-linked carriers because of the randomness of the X inactivation that sometimes may lead to a normal biochemical result. As the variable clinical manifestation, enzyme activities measured also vary depending on the ratio between active mutant and active normal X chromosomes in the specimen analyzed. Hence, activity levels may not correlate with clinical expression. Accuracy can be increased to some extent by sampling relatively clonal cell sources such as hair roots and cloned skin fibroblasts or by testing related metabolites under induced conditions such as orotic aciduria in carriers of ornithine carbamoyltransferase deficiency.[15] Molecular methods can circumvent the problems of biochemical analysis of the gene product in some families, particularly when the mutation can be detected directly. Males, on the other hand, have only 1 X chromosome and they are either hemizygote affected with deficient enzyme activity or hemizygote normal with activity within the normal range.

Some X-linked disorders are lethal in utero in males and severely or completely impair reproduction in females. Such disorders occur in females primarily or exclusively as sporadic events owing to new mutations. Obviously, in such disorders mode of inheritance is not an issue. Microphthalmia with linear skin defects syndrome[16] and Rett[17] syndrome are probably such disorders. Some genes on the X chromosome fall in the pseudoautosomal region and have a homologous copy on the Y chromosome. For pseudoautosomal genes, modes of inheritance are indistinguishable from those of autosomal genes, as the term implies.

There are also some monogenic disorders with non-Mendelian inheritance. Mutations in mitochondrial DNA are inherited maternally because oocytes carry multiple copies of the mitochondrial genome and none are transferred by the sperm. Females pass the trait to all offspring and males do not transmit the trait. The situation is complicated because there are multiple copies of mitochondrial genome per cell, and the copies can be heterogeneous; some carry a mutation and others do not. This may lead to phenotypic variation among family members with the same mutation, to tissue-specific variation, and to variation with age of the individual. Another example of non-Mendelian mode is the inheritance of 2 copies of a whole chromosome or a portion of a chromosome from 1 parent and no copy from the other parent. Although this phenomenon of uniparental disomy is relatively rare, it can contribute to the occurrence of the well-known clinical disorders, Prader-Willi and Angelman syndromes. The significance of uniparental disomy is in large part related to the phenomenon of imprinting whereby the maternal copy of a gene and the paternal copy of a gene may be differentially expressed.

GENETIC HETEROGENEITY

Genetic heterogeneity may result from the existence of different mutations at a single locus (allelic heterogeneity) or from mutations at different genetic loci (nonallelic heterogeneity). A clinically similar bleeding disorder can be caused by mutations at either of 2 loci on the X chromosome, 1 leading to a deficiency of factor VIII (classical hemophilia or hemophilia A) and the other causing a deficiency of factor IX (Christmas disease or hemophilia B).[18] Hereditary methemoglobinemia, which was once regarded as a homogeneous clinical entity, is the result of 10 different mutations occurring at 3 distinct gene loci: 2 at the locus coding for the α-chain of hemoglobin, 3 at the locus coding for the β-chain of hemoglobin, and 5 at the NADH-cytochrome b$_5$ reductase locus.[19] Most inherited diseases, when analyzed thoroughly, are found to be genetically heterogeneous. The extent of allelic heterogeneity is especially high as being demonstrated by molecular techniques. Sickle cell anemia that results from a single mutation at a single locus is 1 of the rare exceptions. This disorder, however, has a quite varied expression due to different genetic backgrounds.

In most diseases there is a classic phenotype in which no functional gene product is produced. Many different alleles that encode no functional gene product cause this severe phenotype. There are also milder expressions arising from mutations that do not totally eliminate the functional gene product. The occurrence of compound heterozygotes contributes to the complexity of the clinical and biochemical spectra. Description of Hurler-Scheie compound heterozygotes among mucopolysaccharidosis I patients was first based on the existence of intermediate phenotypes between the "classical" Hurler syndrome and the mild Scheie syndrome. At the mild end of the spectrum are those mutant alleles that encode a product that has substantial activity and leads to a nearly normal clinical phenotype or to one that is normal under most environmental conditions. This spectrum extends into biochemical variation usually not associated with a clinical effect.

Hartnup disorder and mild forms of hyperphenylalaninemia and methylmalonic acidemia are examples of these "benign" phenotypes that are still subject to acute symptoms if stressed. The amount of functional gene product required to prevent clinical symptoms depends on other genetic factors and on exogenous factors such as diet and catabolic events. An individual with benign methylmalonic acidemia must be considered to be at greater risk than other individuals in the face of major catabolic episodes, so that the benign designation in such cases is merely conditional. The individual with Hartnup disorder is at some risk for a pellagra complication. This type of genetic heterogeneity forms 1 part of the border between monogenic disorders and multifactorial diseases.

FETAL SAMPLES

The use of direct and cultured fetal specimens for prenatal evaluation of metabolic disorders requires the availability of the respective normal control preparations. This applies to readily obtainable specimens such as chorionic villus tissue, cultured trophoblasts, cultured amniotic fluid cells, and amniotic fluid supernatant, as well as to those obtained by more invasive procedures such as fetal blood sampling and fetal liver biopsy. Except for trophoblasts and amniotic fluid cells that can be maintained in culture, availability of fresh controls is often a problem, and in most instances one has to resort to frozen controls, which may have lost some activity. There are also other potential pitfalls specific for each of these tissue, cell, and fluid types.

In the case of chorionic villus sampling, it is crucial to obtain samples that are of fetal origin and in which maternal cells are either completely absent or extremely rare. The quantity of tissue obtained is usually limited and may be insufficient for a thorough analysis. The use of frozen controls may affect adversely the interpretation of the results (false-negative diagnoses) especially when the enzyme in question is very labile such as sialidase (sialidosis) or when the normal activity levels in chorionic villi are extremely low as described for α-iduronidase (mucopolysaccharidosis I or Hurler, Scheie, or Hurler/Scheie syndrome).[20,21] Specific problems may be encountered because of different distribution of enzymes and isozymes. The presence of high levels of arylsulfatase C activity in chorionic villi hampers the differential detection of arylsulfatases A (metachromatic leukodystrophy) and B (mucopolysaccharidosis VI or Maroteaux-Lamy syndrome), and therefore precautions must be taken to avoid false-negative diagnoses. This can be accomplished by separating the arylsulfatase isozymes using electrophoresis or chromatography.[22]

For most first trimester prenatal tests, the recommended practice is to utilize the chorionic villi results for preliminary evaluation and to use cultured trophoblasts for confirmation of the diagnosis. Nonketotic hyperglycinemia is an exception. The feasibility of prenatal diagnosis of this disease by chorionic villus sampling has been supported by demonstration of the presence of the glycine cleavage system in placenta obtained by abortion at 12 weeks of gestation.[23] The evaluation in this case must rely exclusively on the results obtained in chorionic villi because the glycine cleavage system is not expressed in amniotic fluid cells or trophoblasts. Glycine/serine ratio in amniotic fluid is elevated in this disease,[24] but cannot be used as a reliable indicator because there is overlap with the ratios determined in normal controls.[25]

The variability in enzyme activities or in the levels of other proteins and metabolites that is frequently observed in cultured amniotic fluid cells and trophoblasts can be minimized by a careful choice of control cell cultures of similar confluency and morphology. For example, arylsulfatase A activity is normally low during the log phase of cell growth, and increases significantly only after the cultured cell monolayer has reached confluency. Therefore, in prenatal evaluation for metachromatic leukodystrophy careful attention must be paid to cell culture conditions and time of harvest.[26] The choice of control cell cultures, with respect to confluency and morphology, is crucial when amniotic fluid cells are assayed for argininosuccinate synthase (citrullinemia) and argininosuccinate lyase (argininosuccinuria) activities. The proportion of epithelioid (epithelial-like) to fibroblastic (fibroblast-like) cells in the control culture(s) should match closely that of the fetus at risk because the fibroblastic cell type is remarkably more active than the epithelioid one.[27-29]

Amniotic fluid supernatants should be aliquoted to avoid loss of activity with repeated freezing and thawing. Determinations of amniotic fluid concentrations of specific metabolites, as well as enzymes and other proteins, usually serve as supporting findings in prenatal diagnoses. The final diagnosis preferably should rely on demonstration of the underlying biochemical defect in cells or tissues. In propionic acidemia (ketotic hyperglycinemia), for example, prenatal diagnosis has been accomplished reliably by measuring propionyl-CoA carboxylase activity in cultured amniotic fluid cells,[30] by measuring [^{14}C]-propionate fixation in amniotic fluid cells,[31] or by measuring methylcitrate in amniotic fluid.[32] Methylcitrate is probably formed from the intramitochondrial condensation of propionyl-CoA with oxaloacetate.[33] In some acidurias, the basic biochemical defect is unknown and prenatal diagnosis must rely on measurement of amniotic fluid metabolites. This is the case in 3-methylglutaconic aciduria without 3-methylglutaconyl-CoA hydratase[34] and in 3-hydroxy-3-methylglutaric aciduria without 3-hydroxy-3-methylglutaryl-CoA lyase.[35] It is possible that a defect in cholesterol biosynthesis and overload of the leucine catabolic pathway could make the limiting enzyme to be the hydratase in some patients and the lyase in others.

Fetal blood sampling and fetal liver biopsy should be considered only as a last resort because of the high risk for pregnancy loss with these invasive procedures. In glycogenoses 1a, 1b, and 1c, the respective enzyme (glucose-6-phosphatase) and transporter proteins (glucose-6-phosphate translocase and phosphate translocase) involved are expressed only in liver and kidney. If the mutations are identified, DNA techniques may provide a simpler diagnostic tool. In cases in which DNA technology is not available, the only option left for prenatal diagnosis is fetal liver biopsy in which glucose-6-phosphatase activity can be measured in the absence and presence of detergent.[36] On the other hand, prenatal diagnosis of hyperargininemia (arginase deficiency), which has been made in the past only by fetal blood, can in many instances be replaced by molecular technique.[37,38] Even when available, DNA methodology is not informative in all cases and families examined. Biochemical techniques must be considered in such instances. Ornithine carbamoyltransferase deficiency with no informative restriction fragment length polymorphism or deletion can be prenatally diagnosed in hemizygous male fetuses by direct enzyme assay on fetal liver biopsy.[39]

To eliminate adverse effects of storage and shipment, it is advisable to keep tissue specimens frozen and ship them on dry ice. This applies to chorionic villus samples (after a portion has been dedicated for culture) and fetal liver biopsies. Cell pellets, amniotic fluid supernatant, and fetal serum or plasma also should be kept frozen and shipped on dry ice. Cell cultures should be almost confluent and should be shipped at room temperature with flasks filled with medium (to avoid foaming). Chorionic villus samples, whole amniotic fluids, and fetal blood to be processed by the receiving laboratory should be sent as soon as possible at room temperature. Whenever possible, appropriate normal controls from the referring physician's facility should accompany the samples to be analyzed.

ENZYME PREPARATIONS

Prenatal diagnosis of an enzymatic defect may be made by direct assay of fetal tissue or cells when the particular enzyme is the product of the gene in question and is expressed in the fetal specimen to be analyzed. Direct demonstration of abnormality or deficiency of the gene (molecular techniques) or gene product (biochemical techniques) is the preferred diagnostic approach. Enzyme assays can be frequently performed on tissue and cell extracts. In some cases, assays must be performed on the cells in culture. Prenatal detection of citrullinemia and argininosuccinuria and characterization of the mutant enzyme (argininosuccinate synthase and argininosuccinate lyase, respectively) are carried out in trophoblast or amniotic fluid cell cultures by measuring the incorporation of ^{14}C from citrulline into arginine residues of newly synthesized protein.[27–29]

Tissue and cell extracts are prepared by homogenization and sonication, respectively. The duration and intensity of these extracting procedures should be adjusted, depending on the nature of the enzyme to be analyzed. Membranous enzymes, such as the lysosomal membrane glucocerebrosidase (Gaucher disease)[40] and the Golgi membrane N-acetylglucosamine 1-phosphotransferase (1-cell disease and pseudo-Hurler polydystrophy)[41] require effective extraction that is often aided by the use of detergents. Milder extraction procedures are required for cytosolic enzymes such as adenine phosphoribosyltransferase (adenine phosphoribosyltransferase deficiency and 2,8-dihydroxyadenine urolithiasis)[42] and prolidase (hyperimidodipeptiduria).[43]

Extraction of labile enzymes such as sialidase (sialidosis) should be performed with special care with respect to the duration of homogenization or sonication.[20] Utilizing fresh chorionic villus tissue and freshly harvested trophoblasts and amniotic fluid cells helps to preserve the activity of such labile enzymes.

ASSAY CONDITIONS

The pH optimum, the apparent K_M values for the substrate(s) and cofactors, and the linear range with respect to incubation time and protein concentration in the enzyme preparations should be established for each assay system and for each tissue, cell, or fluid type. Ideally, reactions should be performed at the pH optimum, at saturating substrate(s) and cofactors concentrations (at least 5 times the respective K_M values), and with enzyme concentration and incubation time within the respective linear ranges. Practical considerations, however, force us to deviate occasionally from these guidelines. For example, α-glucosidase assay for detection of Pompe disease (glycogenosis II) is carried out at a more acidic pH than the pH optimum to avoid interference by neutral β-glucosidase.[44] Saturating substrate concentrations are impossible or unrealistic in some instances owing to solubility limits or economic reasons.

In some assay systems, incubation times must be extended into the nonlinear range to produce detectable product levels. Incubation temperature may deviate from the usual 37°C, as described for the assay of sulfamidase (heparan N-sulfatase), in which improved discrimination between patients with mucopolysaccharidosis III A (Sanfilippo A syndrome) and carriers can be achieved when the assay is conducted at 55°C.[45]

CONTROLS AND BLANKS

A typical test consists of duplicates of reaction mixtures containing appropriate dilutions of enzyme preparations from the fetus in question and from at least 1 normal control, and appropriate concentrations of substrate(s) and cofactors in a buffer of proper composition, ionic strength, and pH. Following incubation, the reactions are terminated and the product is quantitated directly or after its isolation. Blanks are composed of the same mixtures but the reaction is terminated at the start (0 time blanks), and/or boiled enzyme preparations are substituted for native enzyme preparations (boiled blanks). Blanks account for nonenzymatic reaction and interfering substances and are subtracted from the test values.

Additional sets as described are used for the assay of other enzyme activities, which originate from the same subcellular location as the enzymatic activity in question. These additional enzymes are not expected to be altered in the fetus in question, and as such, they serve as controls for viability of the patient specimen and for proper extractability of the enzyme in question. Indirect methods such as the differential heat inactivation of α-galactosidase (Fabry disease)[46] and hexosaminidase A (Tay-Sachs disease)[47] should be calibrated in the appropriate tissue or cell preparation, and when applicable, the findings should be supported by additional means such as use of additional substrates, ion exchange chromatography, or electrophoretic separation and visualization.[48]

SUBSTRATES AND COFACTORS

There are 2 major categories of substrates and cofactors: natural and artificial. In each group, some are commercially available and others must be prepared or at least tagged (e.g., radioactive label) by the testing laboratory. Satisfactory diagnostic assays can be established in many cases by employing artificial substrates and/or cofactors. Such assays are usually simpler and more sensitive than those utilizing natural substrates and cofactors, but they may fail to detect some variants and they are less likely to distinguish between severe and mild forms of a given disease.

These points can be illustrated by the GM_2 gangliosidoses. This is a group of disorders caused by mutations at 3 distinct loci that code the α-chain and β-chain of hexosaminidases and the GM_2 activator protein.[49] The common denominator is the inability to degrade GM_2 ganglioside, a process that requires the combined action of the α-β hetero-oligomeric hexosaminidase A and the G_{M2} activator protein. In Tay-Sachs disease (G_{M2} gangliosidosis B), the defect is in the gene coding the β-chain, and consequently hexosaminidase A is absent and the homo-oligomeric hexosaminidase B is present but is incapable of catabolizing GM_2 ganglioside. In Sandhoff disease (GM_2 gangliosidosis O), the defect is in the gene coding the β-chain, and consequently both hexosaminidases A and B are affected. In GM_2 activator deficiency (GM_2 gangliosidosis AB), the defect is in the gene coding the activator, and both hexosaminidases A and B are unaffected.

The commonly used substrate is an artificial fluorogenic (4-methylumbelliferyl) derivative of β-N-acetylglucosamine that can be cleaved by both hexosaminidases A and B. Discrimination between the 2 isozymes is achieved by heat inactivation of the thermolabile hexosaminidase A. This method can detect Tay-Sachs and Sandhoff diseases, but not the activator deficiency. This method also fails to detect a variant designated GM_2 gangliosidosis B1. In this disorder both hexosaminidases A and B are present, but the α-chain of hexosaminidase A is catalytically defective. The B1 variant, as well as Tay-Sachs disease (GM_2 gangliosidosis B), can be detected by sulfated artificial substrates (p-nitrophenyl or 4-methylumbelliferyl derivative of β-N-acetylglucosamine-6-sulfate), which are specific for hexosaminidase A, but these artificial substrates fail to detect some α-chain defects.[50,51] The sulfated and unsulfated substrates are cleaved by distinct catalytic sites residing on the some α-chain and some β-chain, respectively.[49]

The natural substrate GM_2 ganglioside is commercially available but must be radiolabeled by the testing laboratory to allow its use for diagnostic purposes. All types of GM_2 gangliosidosis, including the activator deficiency, can be detected by this substrate when used with intact cells in culture (trophoblasts and amniotic fluid cells). However, when used with tissue or cell extracts, the concentration of the endogenous GM_2 activator protein becomes insufficient (because it is no longer localized) and the reaction mixture must be supplemented with purified activator protein preparation or with detergent (artificial activator). This assay system cannot detect the activator deficiency but can detect all some α-chain and some β-chain defects, and when the natural activator protein is utilized, the activity levels highly correlate with the severity of the disease.[52]

SEPARATION AND DETECTION METHODS

Elevated concentrations of amino acids and organic acids in amniotic fluid serve as preliminary indications for several inherited disorders such as amino and organic acidopathies and urea cycle defects. In most cases, however, final diagnosis is made by measuring the actual gene product responsible for the metabolic block. Identification and quantitation of amino acids and organic acids in physiologic fluids and in reaction mixtures are performed on amino acid analyzer and gas chromatograph, respectively. Quantities are determined by the ratio between the peak area revealed in the sample and that of the same compound in a calibration mixture of known concentrations. Internal standards are used to correct for any inaccuracies in the amount of sample injected into the instrument. Organic acids must be extracted and derivatized prior to their separation and quantitation by gas chromatography.

Some natural products of enzymatic reactions can be quantitated directly or following their isolation from the reaction mixtures based on their physicochemical properties. In other systems, substrates are tagged with a colored group, a fluorescent group, or a radioactive group, and thus provide products that can be detected by sensitive colorimetric, fluorometric, or radiometric assays, respectively. For example, detection of galactosemia is based on direct measurement of the fluorescence of the reduced natural electron acceptor, NADPH, using a fluorometer with excitation at 340 nm and emission at 460 nm. NADPH is produced from $NADP^+$ by the reaction of UDP-glucose:galactose-1-phosphate uridyl transferase followed by phosphoglucomutase, glucose-6-phosphate dehydrogenase, and 6-phosphogluconate dehydrogenase.[53]

The absorbance of free p-nitrocatechol at a wavelength of 515 nm (spectrophotometer) is a measure for arylsulfatases A (metachromatic leukodystrophy) and B (mucopolysaccharidosis VI or Maroteaux-Lamy syndrome) activities. Under differential conditions with respect to ionic composition and pH these enzymes release p-nitrocatechol from the synthetic chromogenic substrate p-nitrocatechol sulfate.[54] Similarly, the activities of many glycosidases are determined by the release of 4-methylumbelliferone (a fluorescent compound with excitation wavelength at 365 nm and emission wavelength of 448 nm) from the artificial fluorogenic derivatives of the respective sugar in the proper anomeric configuration (e.g., 4-methylumbelliferyl-α-L-fucoside is used for diagnosis of fucosidosis).[20]

The use of commercially available donor (UDP-[^{14}C]-N-acetylglucosamine) and acceptor (α-methylmannoside) substrates for prenatal diagnosis of I-cell disease and pseudo-Hurler polydystrophy requires the separation of the reaction product (N-acetylglucosamine-phospho-α-methylmannoside) from both the uncleaved donor substrate and the unavoidable breakdown product (free N-acetylglucosamine). This is achieved by stepwise elution from an ion exchange column (QAE, Sephadex). The neutral breakdown product is eluted with 20 mmol of NaCl, the negatively charged reaction product with 30 mmol of NaCl, and the highly negative substrate with 200 mmol NaCl.[55]

NONENZYMATIC DEFECTS

Detection of nonenzymatic proteins such as receptors, transporters, and activators is more complex than direct enzyme assays in tissue or cell extracts and usually requires the use of intact cells in culture. Cell cultures have some advantages, including the ability to incorporate radioactive precursors, the ability to carry out repeated studies, and the relative ease with which comparative studies can be performed on different patient and control cell lines.

The development of methods for quantitative assessment of the low-density lipoprotein (LDL) receptor in cultured cells permitted the prenatal diagnosis of fetuses homozygous for the autosomal-dominant disease familial hypercholesterolemia.[56] Four tests are available for quantization of the receptor activity: (1) measurement of the cell surface binding and intracellular uptake of ^{125}I-labeled LDL; (2) measurement of the rate of proteolytic degradation of ^{125}I-labeled LDL; (3) measurement of LDL-mediated suppression of the synthesis of [^{14}C]cholesterol from [^{14}C]acetate in intact cells or of 3-hydroxy-3-methylglutaryl CoA reductase activity in cell extracts; and (4) measurement of LDL-mediated stimulation of the incorporation of [^{14}C]oleate into cellular cholesteryl[^{14}C]oleate. In addition, the number of LDL receptors can be determined by immunoblotting or immunoprecipitation of ^{35}S-labeled receptors.

It should be noted, however, that the feasibility of making prenatal diagnosis has been established only for the severe, receptor-negative homozygous familial hypercholesterolemia. It has not yet been established that the diagnosis can be reliably made in those familial hypercholesterolemia homozygotes with the less severe form who have some detectable receptor activity (5%–30% of normal). It is unlikely that such homozygotes can be distinguished with sufficient certainty from heterozygotes.

Cystinosis, an autosomal recessive lysosomal storage disease in which cystine accumulation is presumably the result of defective transport across the lysosomal membrane, can be diagnosed prenatally by pulse labeling of cultured cells with [^{35}S]cystine or even by direct measurement of cystine content in chorionic villi.[57] Because of the success with cysteamine therapy, many families prefer diagnosis at birth and immediate initiation of therapy if the child is affected. This is done by measuring the cystine content of the placenta or the cord blood leukocytes.[58]

References

1. Scriver CR, Beaudet AL, Sly WS, et al. *The Metabolic Basis of Inherited Disease.* 7th ed. New York: McGraw-Hill; 1995.
2. McKusick VA. *Mendelian Inheritance in Man.* 11th ed. Baltimore, Md: The Johns Hopkins University Press; 1994.
3. Navon R, Lejbkowicz I, Adam A. Fetal hexosaminidase A in mother's serum: Pitfalls for carrier detection and prospects for prenatal diagnosis of GM$_2$ gangliosidoses. *Am J Hum Genet.* 1987;40:60.
4. Ben-Yoseph Y, Pack BA, Thomas PM, et al. Maternal serum hexosaminidase A in pregnancy: effects of gestational age and fetal genotype. *Am J Med Genet.* 1998;29:891.

5. Wenger DA, Riccardi VM. Possible misdiagnosis of Krabbe's disease. *J Pediatr.* 1976;88:76.

6. Dubois G, Harzer K, Baumann N. Very low arylsulfatase A and cerebroside sulfatase activities in leukocytes of healthy members of metachromatic leukodystrophy family. *Am J Hum Genet.* 1977; 29:191.

7. Kihara H, Ho C-K, Fluharty AL, et al. Prenatal diagnosis of metachromatic leukodystrophy in a family with pseudo arylsulfatase A deficiency by the cerebroside sulfate loading test. *Pediatr Res.* 1980;14:224.

8. Ben-Yoseph Y, Mitchell DA. Discrimination between metachromatic leukodystrophy and pseudo-deficiency of arylsulfatase A by restriction digest of amplified gene fragments. *Am J Med Sci.* 1995;309: 88–91.

9. Triggs-Raine BL, Feigenbaum AS, et al. Screening for carriers of Tay-Sachs disease among Ashkenazi Jews. A comparison of DNA-based and enzyme-based tests. *N Engl J Med.* 1990;323:6.

10. Kaback M, Lim-Steele J, Dabholkar D, et al. Tay-Sachs disease: carrier screening, prenatal diagnosis and the molecular era. *JAMA.* 1993;270:2307.

11. Bloomer JR, Morton KO. A radiochemical assay for heme synthase activity. *Enzyme.* 1982;28:220.

12. Labbe P, Camadro JM, Chambon H. Fluorometric assays for coproporphyrinogen oxidase and protoporphyrinogen oxidase. *Anal Biochem.* 1985;149:248.

13. Lyon MF. Possible mechanisms of X chromosome inactivation. *Nature.* 1971;232:229.

14. Broadbent JC, Edwards WD, Gordon II, et al. Fabry cardiomyopathy in the female confirmed by endomyocardial biopsy. *Mayo Clin Proc.* 1981;56:623.

15. Hauser ER, Finkelstein JE, Valle D, et al. Allopurinol-induced orotidinuria: a test for mutations at the ornithine carbamoyltransferase locus in women. *N Engl J Med.* 1990;322:1641.

16. Wapenaar MC, Bassi MT, Schaefer L, et al. The genes for X-Linked ocular albinism and microphthalmia with linear skin defects: cloning and characterization of the critical regions. *Hum Mol Genet.* 1993;2:947.

17. Schmidt M, Du Sart D. Functional disomies of the X chromosome influence the cell selection and hence the X inactivation pattern in females with balanced X-autosome translocations: a review of 122 cases. *Am J Med Genet.* 1992;42:161.

18. Biggs R, Douglas AS, MacFarlane RG, et al. Christmas disease: a condition previously mistaken for haemophilia. *Br Med J.* 1952;2: 1378.

19. Nagel RL, Bookchin RM. Human hemoglobin variants with abnormal oxygen binding. *Semin Hematol.* 1974;11:385.

20. Ben-Yoseph Y, Evans MI, Bottoms SF, et al. Lysosomal enzyme activities in fresh and frozen chorionic villa and in cultured trophoblasts. *Clin Chim Acta.* 1986;101:307.

21. Poenzini L. First trimester prenatal diagnosis of metabolic diseases: a survey in countries from the European community. *Prenat Diagn.* 1987;7:333.

22. Sanguinetti N, Marsh J, Jackson M, et al. The arylsulphatases of chorionic villi: potential problems in the first-trimester diagnosis of metachromatic leucodystrophy and Maroteaux-Lamy disease. *Clin Genet.* 1986;30:302.

23. Tada K, Kure S. Nonketotic hyperglycinemia: molecular lesion and pathophysiology. *Int Pediatr.* 1993;8:52.

24. Applegarth DA, Levy HL, Shih VE, et al. Prenatal diagnosis of non-ketotic hyperglycinemia. *Prenat Diagn.* 1986;6:257.

25. Mesavage C, Nance CS, Flannery DB, et al. Glycine/serine ratios in amniotic fluid: an unreliable indicator for the prenatal diagnosis of nonketotic hyperglycinemia. *Clin Genet.* 1983;23:3, 54.

26. Percy AK, Farrell DF, Kaback MM. Cerebroside sulphate (sulphatide) sulphohydrolase: an improved assay method. *J Neurochem.* 1972;19:233.

27. Fleisher LD, Rassin DK, Desnick RJ, et al. Argininosuccinic aciduria: prenatal studies in a family at risk. *Am J Hum Genet.* 1979;31: 439.

28. Fleisher LD, Harris CJ, Mitchell DA, et al. Citrullinemia: prenatal diagnosis of an affected fetus. *Am J Hum Genet.* 1983;35:85.

29. Ben-Yoseph Y, Mitchell DA. Detection of kinetically abnormal argininosuccinate synthase in neonatal citrullinemia by conversion of citrulline to arginine in intact fibroblasts. *Clin Chim Acta.* 1989;183: 125.

30. Gompertz D, Goodey PA, Thom H, et al. Prenatal diagnosis and family studies in case of propionicacidaemia. *Clin Genet.* 1975;8:244.

31. Willard HF, Ambani LM, Hart AC, et al. Rapid prenatal and postnatal detection of inborn errors of propionate, methyl-malonate, and cobalamin metabolism: a sensitive assay using cultured cells. *Hum Genet.* 1976;34:277–283.

32. Sweetman L, Weyler W, Shafai T, et al. Prenatal diagnosis of propionic acidemia. *JAMA.* 1979;242:1048.

33. Ando T, Rasmussen K, Wright JM, et al. Isolation and identification of methylcitrate, a major metabolic product of propionate in patients with propionic acidemia. *J Biol Chem.* 1972;247:2200.

34. Leopold D, Bojasch M, Jakobs C. 3-Hydroxy-3methylglutaryl-CoA lyase deficiency in an infant with macrocephaly and mild metabolic acidosis. *Eur J Pediatr.* 1982;138:73.

35. Hammond J, Wilcken B. 3-Hydroxy-3-methylglutaric, 3-methylglutaconic and 3-methylglutaric acids can be non-specific indicators of metabolic disease. *J Inherited Metab Dis.* 1984;7: 117.

36. Golbus MS, Simpson TJ, Koresawa M, et al. The prenatal determination of glucose-6-phosphatase activity by fetal liver biopsy. *Prenat Diagn.* 1988;8:401.

37. Grody WW, Klein D, Dodson AE, et al. Molecular genetic study of human arginase deficiency. *Am J Hum Genet.* 1992;50: 1281.

38. Meloni R, Fougerousse F, Roudaut C, et al. Dinucleotide repeat polymorphism at the human liver arginase gene. *Nucleic Acids Res.* 1992;20:1166.

39. Holzgreve W, Golbus MS. Prenatal diagnosis of ornithine transcarbamylase deficiency using fetal liver biopsy. *Am J Hum Genet.* 1984;36:320.

40. Evans MI, Moore C, Kolodny EH, et al. Lysosomal enzymes in chorionic villi, cultured amniocytes, and cultured skin fibroblasts. *Clin Chim Acta.* 1986;157:109.

41. Ben-Yoseph Y, Mitchell DA, Nadler HL. First trimester prenatal evaluation for I-cell disease by *N*-acetylglucosamine 1-phosphotransferase assay. *Clin Genet.* 1988;33:38.

42. Rylance HJ, Wallace RC, Nuki G. Adenine phosphoribosyl transferase: assay using high performance liquid chromatography. *Clin Chim Acta.* 1985;148:267.

43. Myara I, Charpentier C, Lemonneir A. Optimal conditions for prolidase assay by proline colorimetric determination: application for iminodipeptiduria. *Clin Chim Acta.* 1982;125:193.

44. Grubisic A, Shin YS, Meyer W, et al. First trimester diagnosis of Pompe's disease (glycogenosis type II) with normal outcome: assay of acid α-glucosidase in chorionic villous biopsy using antibodies. *Clin Genet.* 1986;30:298.

45. Matalon R, Deanching M, Marback R, et al. Carrier detection for Sanfilippo A syndrome. *J Inherited Metab Dis.* 1988;11:158.

46. Desnick RJ, Allen KY, Desnick SJ, et al. Fabry's disease: enzymatic diagnosis of hemizygotes and heterozygotes. *J Lab Clin Med.* 1973;81:157.

47. Kaback MM. Thermal fractionation of hexosaminidases: application to heterozygote detection and diagnosis of Tay-Sachs disease. *Methods Enzymol.* 1972;28:862.

48. Grabowski GA, Kruse JR, Goldberg JD, et al. First-trimester prenatal diagnosis of Tay-Sachs disease. *Am J Hum Genet.* 1984;36: 1309.

49. Kytzia H-J, Sandhoff K. Evidence for two different active sites on human β-hexosaminidase A. Interaction of G_{M2} activator protein with β-hexosaminidase A. *J Biol Chem.* 1985;260:7568.

50. Fuchs W, Navon R, Kaback MM, et al. Tay-Sachs disease: one step assay of β-*N*-acetylhexosaminidase in serum with a sulfated chromogenic substrate. *Clin Chim Acta.* 1983;133:253.

51. Ben-Yoseph Y, Reid JE, Shapiro B, et al. Diagnosis and carrier detection of Tay-Sachs disease: direct determination of hexosaminidase A using 4-methylumbelliferyl derivatives of β-N-acetylucosamine-6-sulfate and β-N-acetylgalactosamine-6-sulfate. *Am J Hum Genet.* 1985;37:733.

52. Conzelmann E, Kytzia H-J, Navon R, et al. Ganglioside GM_2 N-acetyl-β-D-galactosaminidase activity in cultured fibroblasts of late-infantile and adult GM_2 gangliosidosis patients and of healthy probands with low hexosaminidase level. *Am J Hum Genet.* 1983;35:900.

53. Copenhaver JH, Bausch LC, Fitzgibbons JF. A fluorometric procedure for estimation of galactose-1-phosphate uridyltransferase activity in red blood cells. *Anal Biochem.* 1969;30:327.

54. Baum H, Dodgson KS, Spencer B. The assay of arylsulfatases A and B in human urine. *Clin Chim Acta.* 1959;4:453.

55. Ben-Yoseph Y, Baylerian MS, Nadler HL. Radiometric assays of N-acetylglucosaminylphosphotransferase and α-N-acerylglucosaminyl phosphodiesterase with substrates labeled in the glucosamine moiety. *Anal Biochem.* 1984;142:297.

56. Goldstein JL, Basu SK, Brown MS. Receptor-mediated endocytosis of low density lipoprotein in cultured cells. *Methods Enzymol.* 1983;98:241.

57. Gahl WA, Dorfmarm A, Evans MI, et al. Chorionic biopsy in the prenatal diagnosis of nephropathic cystinosis. In: Fraccaro M, Simoni G, Brambati G, eds. *First Trimester Fetal Diagnosis.* Berlin, Springer-Verlag, 1985:260–265.

58. Smith ML, Clark KF, Davis SE, et al. Diagnosis of cystinosis with use of placenta. *N Engl J Med.* 1989;321:397.

CHAPTER 43

MOLECULAR DIAGNOSTICS FOR PRENATAL DIAGNOSIS

Laura S. Martin / Mark I. Evans

The demand for prenatal diagnosis has increased rapidly over the last 30 years. This chapter illustrates the theory and methods required for this undertaking.

MOLECULAR GENETICS: PRENATAL DIAGNOSIS

Molecular genetics is the study of human variation—mutation—at the level of the gene: its organization, regulation, and expression. The study of the genetic mechanisms for the expression of inherited information and their mutant protein products has been facilitated by investigating experimental bacterial and animal models. Because similar experimental methods, for example, irradiation or chemical exposure, are not suitable in the human, the study of naturally occurring mutations provides models and insight into the structure–function relationship of the gene and its environment. These research methodologies have yielded precise diagnostic testing capabilities for many genetic diseases. In this section we review the development of important recombinant molecular genetic diagnostic techniques with emphasis on the utility of molecular genetics in prenatal diagnosis.

In 1970, H.O. Smith at the Johns Hopkins University School of Medicine isolated and purified the first restriction endonuclease, Hind II, in *Haemophilus influenza,* for which he, D. Nathans, and W. Arber received the Nobel Prize in Medicine and Physiology in 1978. In 1980, Lawn and Maniatis cloned and sequenced the β-globin gene, thereby opening the door for DNA mutational analysis.[1] Fortuitously, the β-globin gene, located on chromosome 11, is only 1600 base pairs (bp) in length (in contrast to the *CFTR* gene, which is 250,000 bp) of which only 438 bp are of coding sequence. In 1978, the first DNA restriction fragment length polymorphism (RFLP), Hpa 1, was found by W.Y. Kan at the β-globin locus. This discovery led to the use of haplotype analysis in prenatal diagnosis as markers for gene mapping, for differentiation of mutant alleles, for the study of the mechanisms of mutation, and in forensic and paternity testing.

It has been estimated that the human genome, 3.0×10^9 bp per haploid copy, contains 50,000–100,000 genes dispersed on 23 chromosomes. Each individual is thought to have 6–10 abnormal genes.

Genes are composed of a variety of elements critical to the normal function of the gene: its expression of the messenger RNA (mRNA) and the processing of that message (its final protein sequence). The sequence of a gene is defined by regions of coding and noncoding domains, called *exons* and *introns.* The coding regions are constructed by a seemingly random sequence of a 4-letter alphabet of nucleotides (guanine, adenine, thymine, and cytosine), which directs the assembly of the protein through an intermediate molecule known as *messenger RNA.* The intervening sequences (IVS), introns, are removed by a nuclear process called *splicing* prior to translation of the mature mRNA to protein in the rough endoplasmic reticulum, located in the cytoplasm. The nucleotides that precede (splice donor-GT) and terminate (splice acceptor-AG) the IVS are critical for proper splicing, although the function of the intron has not been entirely elucidated. At the beginning of every gene is a region called the *5′ untranslated region* containing the promoter that dictates in which tissue the gene is active and at what level. The transport of the mRNA from the nucleus to the cytoplasm is in part conferred by a series of about 200 adenosine residues at their 3′ end (polyadenylation); thereby, protein assembly is completed.

Mutations in DNA—alterations or changes—can occur in any of the regions of DNA described, resulting in a change in the production of the protein, often a reduction or an abnormally functioning protein. This may include an alteration of 1 nucleotide, known as a *point mutation,* in the coding region, which changes the amino acid at that position to a differing amino acid; a *missense mutation;* or a termination signal, which causes translation to stop at that position, a *nonsense mutation.* A mutation may also be a deletion or insertion of DNA resulting in the loss of one to thousands of nucleotides producing a shift in the reading frame assuming a change of a multiple not of 3, termed a *frameshift mutation,* and frequently introducing a premature termination signal. Alterations in the signaling regions, for example, splice junctions or promoter, may result in splicing abnormalities leading to incorrectly modified mRNA, too little or too much mRNA, thus leading to an unstable mRNA and too little or too much protein.

Molecular genetic technology has permitted analysis of the gene. We now discuss a variety of recombinant DNA methodologies, diseases, and the genes that best illustrate them. Table 43-1 provides a list of common terms and abbreviations along with their definitions.

POLYMERASE CHAIN REACTION

In 1987, while "snaking along a moonlit mountain road into northern California's redwood country,"[2] Kary B. Mullis conceived of an idea that would revolutionize the molecular biology world and for which he would ultimately receive the Nobel Prize.[3,4] This discovery is known today as the *polymerase chain reaction* (PCR). A small aliquot of genomic DNA is taken and a specific region of that DNA is enzymatically amplified. That is to say, 2 primers are devised—a short fragment of known DNA sequence surrounding the area of interest—bound to the complementary sequence on the patient's genomic DNA, and with the addition of a DNA polymerase

TABLE 43-1	GLOSSARY OF TERMS AND ABBREVIATIONS
	Meaning
Allele	One of several alternate forms of a gene at any specific locus
ASO	Allele-specific oligonucleotide
bp	Base pair
CFTR	Cystic fibrosis transmembrane regulator gene
CCM	Chemical cleavage of mismatch
DNA	Deoxyribonucleic acid, the molecule of which all eukaryotic life exists
DGGE	Denaturing gradient gel electrophoresis
Exon	The regions of the gene that are transcribed and present in the mature RNA; usually represent the coding portion of a gene
Haplotype	Specific combinations of alleles found in close association—linked—to a gene whereby one defines a genotype, usually inherited as a single group
Heteroduplex	The pairing of homologous double-stranded DNA or RNA from 2 parental molecules, usually wild type and mutant, each being complementary to each other with the exception of a small region of mismatch
Intron	Intervening sequences of DNA found between exons in genes, spliced out of the immature message RNA, prior to translation of the mature RNA into protein
IVS	Intervening sequences
Kb	Kilo bases
Linkage	Describes the predilection for nonallelic genes or segments of genes to be inherited as a unit as a result of their close proximity on the same chromosome
mRNA	Messenger RNA; the template on which polypeptides, proteins, are synthesized
Multiplex PCR	Method whereby multiple exons are amplified in a single reaction tube via the polymerase chain reaction
Mutation	A change or alteration in the sequence of a gene
Nucleotide	Unit of DNA
Normal transmitting male	A male who carries the fragile X mutation and thus can transmit the gene to his daughter, but he himself has a normal phenotype
Polymorphism	Genetic variation in individuals, often seen as an alteration, obliterating or creating, a restriction endonuclease site, or as difference in the number of tandem repeats, eg, triplet repeats
PCR	Polymerase chain reaction
PSM	PCR-mediated site-directed mutagenesis
Restriction endonuclease	Enzymes isolated from a variety of bacteria that are capable of cutting double-stranded DNA at specific sites
RFLP	Restriction fragment length polymorphism
RT-PCR	Reverse transcriptase-polymerase chain reaction
Splice junction	Nucleotide sequences adjacent to the exon–intron boundaries in a gene
SSCP	Single-stranded conformation polymorphism, differences present in single-stranded DNA detected on a nondenaturing gel

the genomic sequence of interest is replicated by theoretically 1 billion fold, practically 1 million fold (Fig. 43-1). These fragments of DNA can then be visualized by electrophoresing them through an agarose gel and staining the gel with the fluorescent dye ethidium bromide, which intercalates between the stacked bases of DNA. The ways in which PCR has been utilized for mutational analysis and diagnostics as it relates to disease genes are multifold.

Recently, a number of diseases (e.g., fragile X syndrome, Huntington disease, Kennedy's disease, spinal cerebellar ataxia, dentatorubral—pallidoluysian atrophy [DRPLA] and myotonic dystrophy) have been found to be the result of an expansion of an region of DNA known as trinucleotide repeats. Analysis of normal individuals reveals length vari-

ation ranging from a low of 6 to a high of 54 repeats in the fragile X gene. Two types of mutations have been described: premutational state in which only a female may pass an allele capable of expanding in an offspring to a full mutation (Sherman paradox), and the full mutation associated with the fragile X syndrome. The PCR conditions are modified to incorporate a radioisotope, which allows direct visualization of PCR-amplified product after electrophoresis through an acrylamide gel, thus revealing the size of the repeat, CGG, found in both the normal and premutation state. However, when hundreds of repeats are present as in the full mutation, the region is often too large to be amplified by PCR. Thus, this potential problem is resolved using the Southern transfer technique.

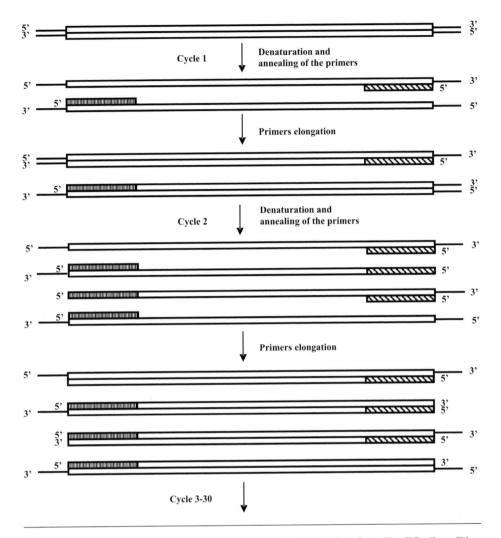

FIGURE 43-1 PCR reaction diagram. (Reproduced, with permission, from Toy EC: *Case Files: Biochemistry.* New York, McGraw-Hill, 2005:54.)

MULTIPLEX PCR

PCR technology allows us to amplify multiple exons simultaneously. This method is known as multiplex PCR. It combines the rapidity and sensitivity of the PCR process and allows the analysis of small or poor-quality samples (i.e., those that might not be sufficient for Southern blot analysis). It requires the development of specific oligonucleotide primer sets unique to each region of the gene of interest, special amplification conditions, and the creation of amplified product of varying length for easy interpretation. This technique has been applied to the Duchenne/Becker muscular dystrophy (*DMD/BMD*) gene; this large—nearly 2400 kb with ~70 exons and 329 deletions—gene may be scanned for deletions in those patients or fetuses at risk for DMD/BMD with detection of over 97% of deletions in DMD and all those with BMD (Fig. 43-2).[5]

This assay has also been performed in the analysis of the 9 exons of the hypoxanthine guanine phosphoribosyltransferase (*HPRT*) gene within 8 fragments for Lesch-Nyan disease[6] and

the identification of 4 point mutations in the cystic fibrosis transmembrane regulator (*CFTR*) gene.[7]

NORTHERN BLOT/REVERSE TRANSCRIPTASE-POLYMERASE CHAIN REACTION

Northern blot is the term given to the procedure whereby RNA is separated according to size by electrophoresis through an agarose gel, transferred to a solid support such as a nylon filter, hybridized to radiolabeled or chemiluminescent probe, and autoradiography is used to locate the position of the band complementary to the RNA:DNA complex. In some instances, the quantity of RNA is insufficient to be detected in this manner; thus, reverse transcriptase-PCR (RT-PCR) methodology permits the scientist to identify and isolate these small quantities of mRNA and thereby analyze genes in a more fastidious manner. Grompe et al.[8] were unable to detect the mRNA in an OTC-deficient patient by northern analysis. Nonetheless, the mRNA was isolated and successfully amplified (after synthesis

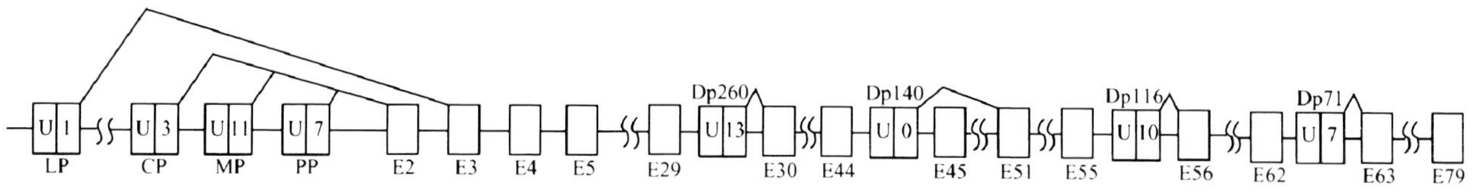

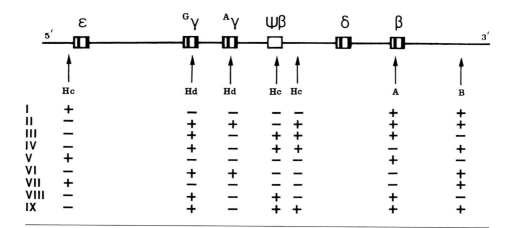

FIGURE 43-2 Structure of the dystrophin gene. Boxes denote exons. LP, CP, MP, and PP indicate first exons of full-length dystrophin transcripts driven by lymphocyte-, cortical (brain)-, muscle-, and Purkinje cell-dystrophin promoters. Dp260, Dp140, Dp116, and Dp71 depict first exons of the short transcripts driven by intronic promoters in full-length dystrophin. A "U" in a box indicates an untranslated sequence; numbers in boxes refer to the numbers of codons in the first exon. (Reproduced, with permission, from Engel AG: *Myology,* 5th ed. New York, McGraw-Hill, 2004:962.)

of a single-stranded cDNA by the utilization of the RNA-directed DNA polymerase, reverse transcriptase) and the mutation responsible for the disease was identified. This technique also isolation of the shorter cDNA fragments corresponding to the coding region of the gene of interest. As in Menkes (kinky hair) disease, a neurodegenerative disorder associated with a disturbance of copper metabolism, exon splicing is the characteristic result of the splice junction mutations seen in this rather large gene.[9] Thus, by utilizing RT-PCR, the exons that are lacking can be discerned by the size of fragment seen on agarose gel or by sequence analysis.

RESTRICTION ENDONUCLEASE ALLELE RECOGNITION

Hemoglobinopathies are the qualitative or quantitative disorders of the globin chains, either alpha or beta. Sickle cell anemia is the most common disease among these disorders. Among the American black population, the frequency of the heterozygous state is 8%; 1 in 500 individuals has the disease. The diagnosis can be readily made on examination of a peripheral blood smear. Hemoglobin electrophoresis confirms

this diagnosis. The β-globin gene is located on chromosome 11; the only mutation responsible is an A to T transition in the second nucleotide of the 6th codon, substituting a valine for glutamic acid. Allelic heterogeneity does not exist for this disease. This alteration of DNA obliterates a sequence that the enzyme Dde1 recognizes, CTNAG, which is present in the normal A, CTGAG, and hemoglobin C, CTAAG, allele but not in the S allele, CTGTG, and thus enables prenatal diagnosis of sickle cell disease or trait by utilizing restriction endonuclease site analysis.

An alternative to relying on naturally occurring phenomena to create or obliterate a restriction endonuclease site is a novel technique called *PCR-mediated site-directed mutagenesis* (PSM), whereby a restriction site is created to facilitate the discrimination of mutations. The general principle is to enzymatically amplify genomic DNA using modified primers containing altered 3' terminal nucleotide to create these sites. After these primers have been efficiently incorporated into the amplified DNA, the PCR products may then be digested with their respective enzyme (Fig. 43-3). This assay has been applied to the analysis of the β-globin gene with respect to the sickle cell mutation, A→T, in the sixth codon of this gene.[10] Another example of similar analysis is the amplification of exon 10 of the *CFTR* gene for ascertainment of those

FIGURE 43-3 Polymorphic restriction enzyme sites in the human β-globin complex and nine of the common haplotypes derived from them. (Reproduced, with permission, from Scriver CR, Beaudet AL, Sly WS, Valle D, Childs B, Volgelstein B: *The Metabolic and Molecular Bases of Inherited Disease,* 8th ed. New York, McGraw-Hill, 2001:4576.)

individuals with the ΔF508 mutation, responsible for approximately 70% of all cystic fibrosis chromosomes, and the use of the restriction endonuclease, Mnl1, resulting in obliteration of the site in the presence of the mutation, resulting in persistence of the 83-bp fragment.[11] This technique allows rapid diagnosis—within hours—and avoids the use of radioisotope and its inherent problem of safety and disposal.

ALLELE-SPECIFIC OLIGONUCLEOTIDE HYBRIDIZATION

ASO hybridization has proven to be a valuable technique which measures the specific binding of short (18-20-mer), radioactively or nonradioactively, labeled oligonucleotide probes that either match the wild-type, normal, DNA sequences exactly or the mutant sequence containing a single base pair substitution under stringent washing conditions. Only the probes that exactly complement the immobilized DNA remain bound, and thus generate a signal seen on autoradiography. This technique was originally described by Conner et al.[12] in 1983 for the detection of sickle cell β^{s-}globin allele without the luxury of PCR amplification of genomic DNA. This technique greatly facilitates the evaluation of genetic disorders in which the gene has to be screened for numerous mutations like thalassemia or cystic fibrosis, or in those where a restriction site is neither created nor obliterated (Fig. 43-4).

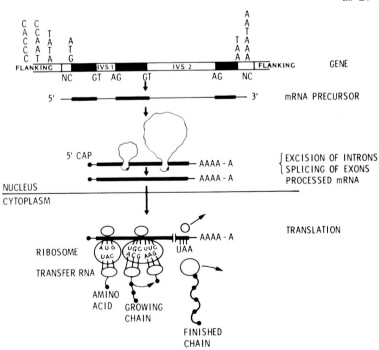

FIGURE 43-4 The expression of a human globin gene. (Reproduced, with permission, from Beutler E, Lichtman MA, Coller BS, Kipps TJ, Seligsohn U: *Williams Hematology,* 6th ed. New York, McGraw-Hill, 2000:550.)

REVERSE DOT BLOT

The reverse dot blot hybridization procedure, which was devised by Saiki et al.[13] in 1989, utilizes membrane-bound oligonucleotides as hybridization targets for amplified genomic DNA. The probe:DNA hybrids may be visualized by nonradioactive chemiluminescent activation or radioactive probes. As one might imagine, it would be more efficient to screen a set of mutations with a sample of amplified genomic DNA rather than screen a patient's DNA sample with a single oligonucleotide as a probe for each of approximately 30 or more allelic mutations. Such a range of potential mutations must be tested to achieve a reasonable level of confidence in a negative test with the unlikelihood of a new mutation.

A prime example for utilization of this methodology would be the diagnosis or screening of the *CFTR* gene.[14] Cystic fibrosis is characterized by elevated sweat electrolytes and thick mucous secretions owing to abnormal chloride permeability in epithelial tissues. In 1989 a consortium headed by L.C. Tsui cloned and sequenced the cystic fibrosis (*CFTR*) gene. The incidence of cystic fibrosis varies dramatically among different populations. In the northern European population, 1 in 2500 individuals is affected with this autosomal recessively inherited disease; however, in Northern Ireland 1 in 1700, in Sweden 1 in 7700, and in the Asian and African ethnic groups 1 in 110,000 individuals are affected.

The *CFTR* gene localized on chromosome 7 encompasses approximately 250,000 base pairs of DNA, and is arranged as 27 exons with 26 introns. Exon 11, which encodes the nuclear binding fold 1, harbors the more common mutations. One region of exon 11 has at least 11 different sequence alterations clustered in 5 codons. In contrast, there are several regions in which no mutation has been identified.

To date 30,000 mutant chromosomes have been examined worldwide and 70% carry the delta F508 mutation; however, more than 325 different mutations have been defined. Only 7 alleles are represented by more than 100 cases and 23 additional mutations by greater than 10 cases. Thus, this is ideally suited to the reverse dot blot method in which multiple alleles need to be examined to determine the parental carrier status and fetal genotype.

SOUTHERN BLOT ANALYSIS

Localization and identification of specific sequences in the genomic DNA is often performed by the transfer technique described by E.M. Southern.[15] In this method, genomic DNA fragments are transferred to a solid support system

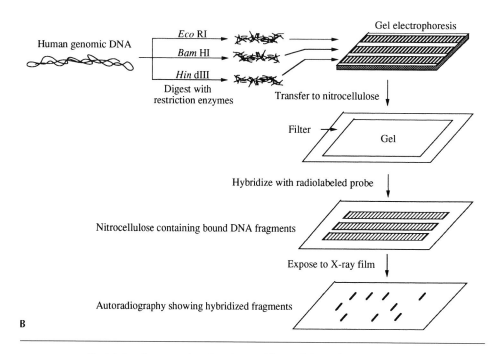

FIGURE 43-5 Restriction fragment length polymorphisms. Schematic of the use of RFLP analysis to detect a point mutation associated with mitochondrial encephalomyopathy, lactic acidosis, and stroke-like episodes (MELAS). An A ↑ G transition in the mitochondrial genome at mtDNA position 3243 creates a *Hae*III polymorphism. PCR of mtDNA with primers (P) generates a 238-bp fragment. Cleavage of normal DNA with *Hae*III (H) yields three fragments that are 169, 37, and 32 bp long. The extra *Hae*III site in MELAS and mtDNA (H) cleaves the 169-bp fragment into two smaller fragments of 97 and 72 bp (arrows on schematic of an electropheretic gel). (Reproduced, with permission, from Engel AG: *Myology,* 5th ed. New York, McGraw-Hill, 2004:936.)

and probe DNA is radioactively labeled. Then by hybridization of the nylon filter with a solution containing then probe DNA, fragment binds to complementary regions in the genomic DNA linked to the nylon support filter. The filter is exposed to an x-ray film and regions in which the binding occurs is discerned by the bands that are visible on the autoradiograph. Figure 43-5 provides a schematic representation of the procedure.

The Southern blot analysis allows for the identification of 2 kinds of mutational differences: (1) single base pair changes that alter—either obliterate or create—a restriction endonuclease site that results in an altered band size and (2) insertions or deletions, resulting in the rearrangement of the gene. Fragile X (Bell) syndrome is the most common inherited form of mental retardation occurring in approximately 1 of 1250 males and 1 of 2500 females. It is inherited in an unusual X-linked fashion;

30% of carrier females are affected and 20% of males (normal transmitting males) who carry a fragile X chromosome are phenotypically normal. Transmission of the fragile X mutation and phenotypic expression thereafter demands that the X chromosome be inherited through a female. This is known as the Sherman paradox. The mutation seen in the fragile X syndrome may be 1 of 2 types, small insertions called *premutations* (~100–600 bp) or large insertions (600–4000 bp) called *full mutations.* It is now apparent from studies analyzing the alteration of the expansion, twinning, and a variety of tissues that this phenomenon is a somatic event occurring after the creation of the zygote. Variation of the length of DNA at the fragile site is found between normal and fragile X individuals and is caused by expansion of a CGG repeat with methylation upstream of the CpG island that appears to correlate with the loss of expression the FMR-1 mRNA. Methylation of the CpG island alters

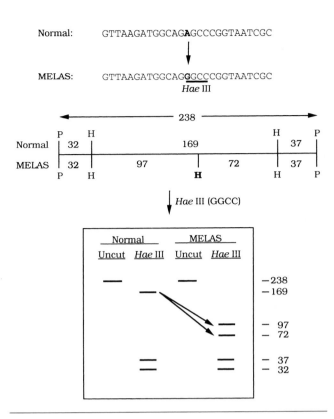

Normal: GTTAAGATGGCAG**A**GCCCGGTAATCGC

MELAS: GTTAAGATGGCAG**GG**CCCGGTAATCGC
Hae III

FIGURE 43-6 Filter hybridization. *A.* Southern blotting of a cloned DNA sequence in a plasmid. (Adapted from Darnell J, Lodish H, Baltimore D: *Molecular Cell Biology.* New York, Scientific American/W.H. Freeman, 1986. Copyright © 1986 by Scientific American Books, Inc. Reprinted with permission of W.H. Freeman and Company.) B. Southern blotting of genomic DNA. Adapted from Watson JD, Hopkins NH, Roberts JW, et al: *Molecular Biology of the Gene.* Menlo Park, CA: Benjamin Cummings, 1987. With permission. Copyright © 1987 by The Benjamin Cummings Publishing Company, Inc.)

(obliterates) the restriction site endonuclease activity of Eag1; thus, the Eag1 and EcoR1 endonuclease restriction digest and Southern transfer is utilized to analyze the methylation pattern and presence or absence of the mutation (Fig. 43-6).[16–18]

LINKAGE

Most variation in DNA is inconsequential with respect to causing disease. The majority of sequences of DNA are not known to be coding regions; only about 5% of a gene is made up of protein-coding sequence. Within IVS, noncoding regions, there is a mutation approximately every 200 base pairs. Often, these changes alter or create a restriction endonuclease site, thereby allowing the change in band size on Southern blot to be determined. These variations in sequence are known as *DNA polymorphisms.* By definition, these alterations should occur in less than 1% of the population. These fragments created by restriction enzymes are termed *restriction fragment length*

polymorphisms (RFLP) and their analysis of association with the disease gene, *linkage analysis.* The closer the polymorphism is to the disease gene, the less likely recombination is to occur between the two and hence increasing the likelihood that they will be inherited together. This is known as *linkage.* If an alteration were in close proximity to the disease causing gene, but not necessarily in that gene, one could track the associated fragment (the band on Southern blot) in a given family pedigree. Today, RFLP analysis is used primarily in the diagnosis for diseases in which the gene has yet to be cloned, the mutations are "private," or DNA sequencing is not practical.

SEQUENCE ANALYSIS

Direct sequencing of the amplified product of a segment of genomic DNA is often the only method for analysis of mutations.[19] This may be because of a previously unrecognized mutation in an affected individual, or in certain diseases for which the no allele is predominant, in contrast to the single mutation responsible for sickle cell anemia, or definable but heterogeneous alleles as in the *CFTR* gene in cystic fibrosis. Manual methods of sequence analysis have been developed and are routinely employed; however, new automated techniques have been exploited to speed the process.

MUTATIONAL SCANNING

In *mutational scanning,* exons and intron borders are scanned to identify alterations, primarily point mutations, in those genes with a high frequency of sporadic mutation (e.g., X-linked or dominant disorders). Single-stranded conformation polymorphism analysis (SSCP), chemical cleavage of mismatch (CCM), and denaturing gradient gel electrophoresis (DGGE) are 3 modalities of this kind. These applications allow detection of point mutations that alter electrophoretic mobility of radioactively labeled single-stranded DNA in nondenaturing polyacrylamide gels or heteroduplex/homoduplex formation in denaturing gradient gels, respectively.[20–25] These methods have been employed in the prenatal diagnosis of such conditions as hemophilias A and B,[26,27] α-1-antitrypsin deficiency,[28,29] β-thalassemia,[30] and cystic fibrosis.[31] Detection rates vary between 30–100% depending on the method, type of nucleotide change present, and gel conditions adopted.

References

1. Lawn RM, Efstratiadis A, O'Connell C, et al. The nucleotide sequence of the human β-globin gene. *Cell.* 1980;21:647–651.

2. Mullis KB. The unusual origin of the polymerase chain reaction. *Sci Am.* 1990;April:56–65.

3. Mullis KB, Faloona FA. Specific synthesis of DNA in vitro via a polymerase-catalyzed chain reaction. *Methods Enzymol.* 1987; 155:335.

4. Saiki RK, Scharf S, Faloona F, et al. Enzymatic amplification of β-globin genomic sequences and restriction site analysis for diagnosis of sickle cell anemia. *Science.* 1985;230:1350–1354.

5. Beggs AH, Koenig M, Boyce FM, et al. Detection of 98% of DMD/BMD gene deletions by polymerase chain reaction. *Hum Genet.* 1990;86:45–48.

6. Gibbs RA, Nguyen PN, Edwards A, et al. Multiplex DNA deletion detection and exon sequencing of the hypoxanthine phosphoribosiftransferase gene in Lesch-Nyhan families. *Genomics.* 1990;7: 235.

7. Fortina P, Conant R, Monokian G, et al. Non-radioactive detection of the most common mutations in the cystic fibrosis transmembrane conductance regulator gene by multiplex allele-specific polymerase chain reaction. *Hum Genet.* 1992;90:375–378.

8. Grompe M, Muzny DM, Caskey CT. Scanning detection of mutations in human ornithine transcarbamoylase by chemical mismatch cleavage. *Proc Natl Acad Sci USA.* 1989;86:5888–5892.

9. Das S, Levinson B, Shitney S, et al. Diverse mutations in patients with Menkes disease often lead to exon skipping. *Am J Hum Genet.* 1994;55:883–889.

10. Hatcher SLS, Trang QT, Robb KM, et al. Prenatal diagnosis by enzymatic amplification and restriction endonuclease digestion for detection of haemoglobins A, S and C. *Mol Cell Probes.* 1992;6:343–348.

11. Friedman KJ, Highsmith WE Jr, Prior TW, et al. Cystic fibrosis deletion mutation detected by PCR-mediated site-directed mutagenesis. *Clin Chem.* 1990;36:695–696.

12. Conner BJ, Reyes AA, Morin C, et al. Detection of sickle cell β^{S}-globin allele by hybridization with synthetic oligonucleotides. *Proc Natl Acad Sci USA.* 1983;80:278–282.

13. Saiki RK, Walsh S, Levenson CH, et al. Genetic analysis of amplified DNA with immobilized sequence-specific oligonucleotide probes. *Proc Natl Acad Sci USA.* 1989;86:6230–6234.

14. Chehab FF, Wall J. Detection of multiple cystic fibrosis mutations by reverse dot blot hybridization: a technology for carrier screening. *Hum Genet.* 1992;89:163–168.

15. Southern EM. Detection of specific sequences among DNA fragments separated by gel electrophoresis. *J Mol Biol.* 1975;98:503–517.

16. Oostra BA, Jacky PB, Brown WT, et al. Guidelines for the diagnosis of fragile X syndrome. *J Med Genet.* 1993;30:410–413.

17. Fu PH, Kuhl DP, Pizzuti A, et al. Variation of the CGG repeat at the fragile X site results in genetic instability: resolution of the Sherman Paradox. *Cell.* 1991;67:1047–1058.

18. Warren ST, Nelson DL. Advances in molecular analysis of fragile X syndrome [special communication]. *JAMA.* 1994;271:536–542.

19. Maxam AM, Gilbert W. A new method for sequencing DNA. *Proc Natl Acad Sci USA.* 1977;74:560.

20. Sekiya T. Detection of mutant sequences by single-strand conformation polymorphism analysis. *Mut Res.* 1993;288:79–83.

21. Cotton RG, Rodrigues NR, Campbell RD. Reactivity of cytosine and thymine in single-base-pair mechanisms with hydroxylamine and osmium tetroxide and its application to the study of mutation. *Proc Natl Acad Sci USA.* 1988;85:4397–4401.

22. Smooker PM, Cotton GH. The use of chemical reagents in the detection of DNA mutations. *Mut Res.* 1993;288:65–77.

23. Rossiter BJF, Caskey CT. Molecular scanning methods of mutation detection [mini-review]. *J Biol Chem.* 1990;265:12753–12756.

24. Fan E, Levin DB, Glickman BW, et al. Limitations in the use of SSCP analysis. *Mut Res.* 1993;288:85–92.

25. Myers RM, Lumelsky N, Lerman LS, et al. Detection of single base substitutions in total genomic DNA. *Nature.* 1985;313:459–468.

26. Schwartz M, Cooper DN, Millar DS, et al. Prenatal exclusion of haemophilia A and carrier testing by direct detection of a disease lesion. *Prenat Diag.* 1992;12:861–866.

27. Caprino D, Acquila M, Mori PG. Carrier detection and prenatal diagnosis of hemophilia B with more advanced techniques. *Ann Hematol.* 1993;67:289–293.

28. Dubel JR, Fenwick R, Hejtmancik JF. Denaturing gradient gel electrophoresis of the alpha 1-antitrypsin gene: application to prenatal diagnosis. *Am J Med Genet.* 1991;41:39–43.

29. Forrest SM, Dry PJ, Cotton RGH. Use of the chemical cleavage of mismatch method for prenatal diagnosis of alpha-1-antitrypsin deficiency. *Prenat Diag.* 1992;12:133–137.

30. Ghanem N, Girodon E, Vidaud M, et al. A comprehensive scanning method for rapid detection of beta-globin gene mutations and polymorphisms. *Hum Mut.* 1992;1:229–239.

31. Desgeorges M, Boulot P, Kjellberg P, et al. Prenatal diagnosis for cystic fibrosis using SSCP analysis [letter]. *Prenat Diagn.* 1993;13:147–148.

CHAPTER 44

MOLECULAR SCREENING

Roderick F. Hume, Jr.

INTRODUCTION

Molecular screening has emerged from the realm of the possible to the actual[1] within the gestational period of this text's second edition.[2] The rapid growth and development of biotechnology has allowed the more accurate molecular laboratory methods to replace previous methods, expanding classic texts and changing titles.[3] Most of these methods were developed in the research laboratory in the effort to more rapidly search for possible mutations associated with a specific disease.[4,5] When proven, these tests become available to the clinical geneticist.[6] In general, genotype based laboratory methods offer several advantages compared to the more cumbersome and imprecise phenotypic tests. One needs only to recall the difficulties of sweat testing for cystic fibrosis when compared to the widespread, and cost-efficient, molecular methods in current use to recognize the remarkable impact of the molecular genetic advance.[7] Genotypic characterization may also facilitate the more accurate prediction of phenotype for some inherited disorders, such as is the case for cystic fibrosis, congenital absence of the vas defferens, Gaucher, and other disorders. The capacity to perform automated, repeated, or sequential testing on a minuscule quantity of biologic specimen enables the application of molecular screening methods to several clinical situations. We will explore this new realm through the discussion of several current examples of the use of molecular screening methods in a variety of clinical situations and for a variety of specific diseases. Pertinent in our discussion will be a consideration of the ethical challenges posed by the assessment of genetic risk through molecular screening.[8] Questions remain, however. Who may benefit from these advances in our ability to detect the actual from the among possible diagnoses: potential insurers, employers, prospective parents, or the individual?[9]

PRESYMPTOMATIC DETECTION

Neonatal screening programs have proven very effective in the preclinical detection of disease. Most appropriate diagnoses for neonatal screening are severe life-threatening disorders which have a proven therapeutic intervention. This is certainly the case for congenital hypothyroidism and phenylketonuria (PKU).[10] Sickle cell anemia and cystic fibrosis may benefit from preclinical diagnosis by aggressive vaccination and antibiotic therapy programs. Novel therapeutic approaches may offer even greater potential benefit. Hydroxyurea (HU) treatment has been shown to increase the expression of fetal hemoglobin which has a favorable influence on prognosis for sickle hemoglobinopathy. Molecular screening has been shown to be more efficient for the detection for many

hemoglobinopathies.[11-14] The molecular characterization of the ethnic and geographic distribution of mutations provides the basis for molecular screening programs. Such programs have been suggested for CF, DMD, and BMD.[15] A known risk population with proven molecular methods for a specific disease is required. Cost-effective programs can then be selected for each specific disease. In this regard, neonatal screening refers to the identification of an affected individual from among a population without any specific known family risks. The goal is the prevention of any avoidable sequelae resultant from the preclinical phase of the disease.

Presymptomic detection in adults for autosomal dominant disease of late onset poses a major medical-ethical problem, especially for cancer genes.[16-21] The lessons learned with Huntington disease (HD) are being tested with the many cancer susceptibility genetic screening programs currently being deployed with great rapidity. Such screening projects may create a greater need than currently exists for genetic counseling. It remains critical for the success of any molecular screening program that the genetic counseling capability be in place prior to the implementation of the program. This advance may mean that more reproductive geneticists are drawn into cancer genetics and family counseling. The prenatal diagnosis setting in which the reproductive geneticist may become involved in the presymptomic detection of parental disease include adult polycystic kidney disease (APDK),[22] bilateral renal agenesis (BRA),[23] or breast cancer (BRCA1/2).[24]

CARRIER DETECTION

Carrier detection for an autosomal recessive life-threatening disorder has generally been based on pedigree analysis or ethnicity. Molecular screening can now be offered based on ethnicity and population risks for many of the classic genetic diseases.[25-27] This includes cystic fibrosis for individuals of Northern European descent, Tay-Sachs, tyrosinemia in French Canadians, familial dysautonomia, and Gaucher among Ashkinazim. Also hemoglobinapathies and thalassemias for those with asian and/or mediterranean ancestry.[28] The natural outgrowth of the recent advances in molecular diagnosis provides a more accurate assessment of carrier status for prospective parents. If a couple is found to both be carriers for a disease then the specific homozygous or compound heterozygous state predicted provides a more accurate basis for prenatal diagnosis, genetic counseling, and prognostic estimation. Molecular characterization makes the genetic counseling more straightforward. For the perinatologist or reproductive geneticist molecular screening for carrier detection most often occurs for the couple who present in a current pregnancy with a family history, or an ethnic risk, for a specific disease. It should be our goal to move this point of mutational analysis, or molecular recognition, away from the prenatal and into the preconceptional period. Preconceptional counseling, with an emphasis on ethnic and pedigree analysis, affords the reproductive geneticist the time to ascertain the specific risks for the couple, pursue the educational requirements and proceed with the most appropriate testing. Molecular screening has its greatest potential benefit in this clinical situation.[29,30]

NONCLASSICAL APPLICATIONS

There are several scenarios in which the element of mystery can be lifted through molecular screening. The most common will be the pregnancy with a remote family history, or a previously uncharacterized mutation in a sibling with a specific disorder such as cystic fibrosis. In such a setting sequential mutational analysis may refine the risks such that prenatal testing is unnecessary, impossible or very specific. It gives a clear yes or no answer to a very specific genetic question. Such risk modification is well within the scope of normal practice for a geneticist. Another example would be seeking the genetic basis of male infertility.[31] Among the more bizarre uses reported for molecular screening has been its application to the identification of decedents following a mass disaster.[32] In general, DNA testing has greatly advanced the precision of forensic science.

A similar stretch of genetic testing, and one that may take on a greater importance in fetal therapy, is the use of molecular screening to identify matching donors for bone-marrow or organ transplantation.[33]

In both of these novel examples the speed and accuracy of DNA tests are amplified by the ability to perform repetitive tests on the same minuscule sample via PCR and reverse dot blot methods. The cost-efficiency of these methods also provide the potential employer or insurer with the capability to apply genetic discrimination in decisions which may adversely impact the individual. The routinely collected blood sample can be tested for presymptomatic diagnosis of "pre-existing" disease, or identification of genotypes which should avoid certain occupational exposures.[34] The balance between potential benefits or harm for the individual remains problematic. The same technology that offers a clear benefit for the molecular recognition of ethnic disease, carrier detection in a couple for Tay-Sachs or cystic fibrosis prior to in vitro fertilization, becomes a potential nightmare of unintended consequences for BRCA, HD, or APKD. The same methodology that is clearly beneficial in the genetic counseling paradigm for a family member undergoing yearly endoscopy for FAP or prophylactic mastectomy for BRCA[35] may be used to exclude another individual from employment or insurability.

SUMMARY

In summary, molecular screening can be utilized to refine the risks for a couple planning pregnancy, define prenatal diag-

nostic accuracy, facilitate the identification of donor-recipient matching for transplantation, provide the molecular recognition of ethnic disease carrier detection in population testing, enhance the accuracy of presymptomatic neonatal screening programs, identify special occupational exposure risk situations, and for individual identification following a mass disaster.

References

1. Jacob F. *The Possible and the Actual.* New York: Pantheon Books; 1982.
2. Evans MI. Reproductive Risks and Prenatal Diagnosis. Norwalk, CT: Appleton & Lange; 1992.
3. Scriver CR, Beaudet AL, Sly WS, et al. The Metabolic and Molecular Bases of Inherited Disease. 7th Ed. New York: McGraw-Hill; 1997.
4. Miller DS, Zoll B, Martinowitz U, et al. The molecular genetics of hemophilia A: screening for point mutations in the factor VIII gene using the restriction enzyme Taq I. *Hum Genet.* 1991;37:607.
5. Feldmann D, Rozet JM, Pelet A, et al. Site specific screening for point mutations in ornithine transcarbamylase deficiency. *J Medical Genet.* 1992;29(7):471–475.
6. Koback M, Lim-Steele J, Dabholkar D, et al. Tay-Sachs disease: carrier screening, prenatal diagnosis and the molecular era. *J Am Med Assoc.* 1993;270:2307.
7. Spence WC, Paulus-Thomas J, Orenstein DM, et al. Neonatal screening for cystic fibrosis: addition of molecular diagnostics to increase specificity. *Biochem Med Metab Biol.* 1993;49:200.
8. Anderson LB, Fullerton JE, Holtzman NA, et al. Assessing Genetic Risk: Implementation for Health and Social Policy. Washington, DC: National Academy Press; 1992.
9. Clayton EW. Ethical, Legal, and Social Implications of Genomic Medicine. *N Engl J Med.* 2003;349:562–569.
10. Giannattasio S, Bisceglia L, Lattanzio P, et al. Molecular screening of the genetic defects with RNA-SSCP analysis: the PKU and cystinuria model. *Molecular and Cellular Probes.* 1995;9(3):201–205.
11. Soria NW, Tulian CL, Plassa F, et al. Beta-thalassemia and hemoglobin types in Argentina: determination of most frequent mutations. *Amer J Hematol.* 1997;54(2):160–163.
12. Rosatelli MC, Tuveri T, Scalas MT, et al. Molecular screening and fetal diagnosis of beta-thalassemia in the Italian population. *Hum Genet.* 1992;89(6):585–589.
13. Thonglairoam V, Winichagoon P, Fucharoen S, et al. Hemoglobin constant spring in Bangkok: molecular screening by selective enzymatic amplification of the alpha 2-globin gene. *Amer J Hematol.* 1991;38(4):277–280.
14. Hsia YE, Ford CA, Shapiro LJ, et al. Molecular screening for haemoglobin constant spring. *Lancet.* 1989;1(8645):988–991.
15. Prior TW, Highsmith WE, Friedman KJ, et al. A model for molecular screening of newborns: simultaneous detection of Duchenne/Becker muscular dystrophies and cystic fibrosis. *Clin Chem.* 1990;36(10):1756–1759.
16. Birrer MJ. Translational research and epithelial carcinogenesis: molecular diagnostic assays now—molecular screening assays soon? *J Nat Cancer Inst.* 1995;87(14):1041–1043.
17. Gazzoli I, De Andreis C, Sirchia SM, et al. Molecular screening of families affected by familial polyposis (FAP). *J Medical Screening.* 1996;3(4):195–199.
18. Hayes VM, Kotze MJ, Grobbelaar JJ, et al. Presymptomatic diagnosis of familial adenomatous polyposis using intragenic polymorphisms and CA repeats flanking the APC gene. *Genetic Counseling.* 1996;7(1):1–7.

19. Elbein SC, Yeager C, Kwong LK, et al. Molecular screening of the lipoprotein lipase gene in hypertriglyceridemic members of familial noninsulin-dependent diabetes mellitus families. *J Clin Endocrinol Metabol.* 1994;79(5):1450–1456.

20. Barret JM, Ernould AP, Ferry G, et al. Integrated system for the screening of the specificity of protein kinase inhibitors. *Biochem Pharmacol.* 1993;46(3):439–448.

21. Easton D. Breast cancer genes—what are the real risks? *Nature Genetics.* 1997;16(3):210–211.

22. Wilson PD. Polycystic Kidney Disease: Mechanism of Disease. *N Engl J Med.* 2004;350:151–64.

23. Fries MH, Holt C, Carpenter I, et al. Guidelines for evaluation of patients at risk for inherited breast and ovarian cancer: recommendations of the Department of Defense Familial Breast/Ovarian Cancer Research Project. *Military Medicine.* 2002;167(2):93–8.

24. Fries MH, Holt C, Carpenter I, et al. Diagnostic criteria for testing for BRAC1 and BRAC2: the experience of the Department of Defense Familial Breast/Ovarian Cancer Research Project. *Military Medicine.* 2002;167(2):99–103.

25. Fellowes AP, Murphy JM, Wesley AW, et al. Molecular screening of cystic fibrosis patients. *New Zealand Medical J.* 1991;104(921):415–416.

26. Choy FY, Linsey J, MacLeod PD. Gaucher disease: molecular screening of the glucocerebrosidase 1601G and 1601A alleles in Victoria British Columbia, Canada. *J Medical Genet.* 1997;34(1):83–85.

27. Shrimpton AE, Brock DJ. Molecular screening of partners of cystic fibrosis heterozygotes. *Genetic Counseling.* 1992;3(1):13–18.

28. American College of Obstetricians and Gynecologists: Committee Opinion Number 238, Genetic Screening for Hemoglobinopathies. Washington, DC: American College of Obstetricians and Gynecologists, 2000.

29. Grody WW, Cutting GR, Klinger KW, et al.: Laboratory standards and guidelines for population-based cystic fibrosis carrier screening. *Genet Med.* 2001;3:149.

30. American College of Obstericians and Gynecologists and the American College of Medical Genetics. Preconception and Prenatal Carrier Screening for Cystic Fibrosis. Washington, DC: The American College of Obstetricians and Gynecologists, 2001.

31. Henegariu O, Hirschmann P, Kilian K, et al. Rapid screening of the Y chromosome in idiopathic sterile men, diagnostic for deletions in AZF, a genetic Y factor expressed during spermatogenesis. *Andrologia.* 1994;26(2):97–106.

32. Corach D, Sala A, Penacino G, et al. Mass disasters: rapid molecular screening of human remains by means of short tandem repeats typing. *Electrophoresis.* 1995;16(9):1617–1623.

33. Rubocki RJ, Wisecarver JL, Hook DD, et al. Histocompatibility screening by molecular techniques: use of polymerase chain reaction products and heteroduplex formation. *J Clin Lab Anal.* 1992;6(5):337–341.

34. Wetmur JG, Kaya AH, Plewinska M, et al. Molecular characterization of the human delta-aminolevulinate dehydratase 2 (ALAD2) allele: implications for molecular screening of individuals for genetic susceptibility to lead poisoning. *Amer J Human Genetics.* 1991;49(4):757–763.

35. Haffty BG, Harrold E, Khan AJ, et al. Outcome of conservatively managed early-onset breast cancer by BRCA 1/2 status. *Lancet.* 2002;359:1471–7.

PRENATAL DIAGNOSIS USING FETAL CELLS FROM MATERNAL BLOOD

Sinhue Hahn / Wolfgang Holzgreve

One of the most promising means for developing a noninvasive method for prenatal diagnosis is the isolation of fetal cells from the blood of pregnant women. In proof-of-concept studies, both fetal aneuploidies and single gene disorders have been detected using such enriched fetal cells. The feasibility of this methodology for the detection of fetal aneuploidies is being investigated in a large scale trial under the auspices of the National Institutes of Child Health and Development (NICHD). Preliminary results from this study have indicated that significantly lower false-positive rates can be attained for the detection of specific fetal aneuploidies than current noninvasive screening methods. However, several improvements, which we address in this chapter, have to be made before this methodology is introduced into a clinical setting.

HISTORICAL AND TECHNICAL OVERVIEW

Although the presence of fetal cells in maternal blood was first reported more than a century ago by Schmorl,[1] who found trophoblasts in the lungs of women who had succumb from eclampsia, a considerable debate has raged over whether the presence of fetal cells in the blood of pregnant women was a common or sporadic event.[2] Several recent reports have, however, demonstrated the reliable and reproducible isolation of fetal cells, in particular fetal erythroblasts, from the blood of pregnant women, thereby refuting reports are otherwise skeptical of their existence.[3]

These successes were only achieved after a considerable period of frustration, partly in the inability to confirm Schmorl's original finding,[4,5] but mainly because the proper tools for enrichment and fetal cell identification were not available yet. Another snag was that researchers had not decided on which fetal cell they should focus their attention. Because such trophoblasts were found to be inadequate candidates and trophoblast deportation does not appear to be a feature common to all pregnancies,[6,7] and furthermore, by their large multinucleate nature, they were determined to be unsuitable for cytogenetic analysis by such technologies as fluorescent in situ hybridization (FISH). A further complication with this cell type was that most efforts to enrich for trophoblast cells, even when using purported specific antibodies, failed.[8]

Fetal lymphocytes were determined to be unsuitable; because of their longevity, the danger existed that cells from a previous pregnancies could be retrieved for analysis.[9,10]

It is for these reasons that most researchers in the field have decided to focus their attention on fetal erythroblasts, also termed *nucleated red blood cells*.[3] These cells have the advantage that they are particularly abundant in the fetal circulation early in gestation and are rare in the normal adult periphery. By their short lifespan of approximately 90 days,

there is no danger of obtaining cells from a previous pregnancy. Furthermore, erythroblasts are readily identified by their well-defined morphology: a small dense nucleus, clear cytoplasm, and the size of an erythrocyte. Additionally, fetal erythroblasts can be tentatively identified by the expression of embryonic and fetal hemoglobins, which are expressed during fetal development. These, and high levels of expression of the transferrin receptor (CD71:TfR), the blood group antigen glycophorin A (GPA) and potential fetal specific antigens, such as the HAE9 antigen have also proven very helpful for the enrichment and isolation of these rare cells.[11]

Arguably, the field benefited most by the introduction of techniques that permitted the enrichment of rare cell populations. The first innovation to facilitate this was the fluorescent activated cell sorter (FACS), and which was first used by Herzenberg et al[12] for the enrichment of fetal lymphocytes from maternal blood using HLA disparities between mother and fetus. This methodology was subsequently used by Bianchi et al for the enrichment of fetal erythroblasts, who used either CD71 or the gamma globin molecule to target erythroblast selection.[13,14]

By using the then novel technique of magnetic cell sorting (MACS)[15] and micromagnetic conjugated antibodies to CD71, our group pioneered the enrichment of fetal erythroblasts form maternal blood by these means.[15]

A further vital development was the ability to genetically identify cells as being fetal. This was provided on the one hand by the advent of FISH,[17] which permitted a specific cytogenetic analysis in interphase cells, and also by the development of polymerase chain reaction (PCR),[18] by which means it was now possible to examine and analyze minute quantities of genetic material, even single cells.

INITIAL SUCCESSES AND THE ADVENT OF THE NICHD NIFTY STUDY

In the early 1990s, 3 publications in rapid succession reported the detection of fetal aneuploidies using fetal erythroblasts enriched from pregnant women.[19–21] Two of these studies had used FACS for the enrichment, and the other from our group used a combination of a triple-density Ficoll gradient and MACS.

These results were so encouraging that the NICHD was prompted to initiate a large-scale study to examine the feasibility of using fetal cells from maternal blood for the detection of fetal aneuploidies.[22] In the National Institute for Child Health and Development Fetal Cell Isolation Study (NIFTY), some 3000 women at risk of bearing an aneuploid fetus will be recruited; that is, maternal age of over 35, abnormal sonogram or serum screening result, or previous instance of a fetal aneuploidy.

The enrichment procedures used by the 4 laboratories include 2 different FACS protocols,[14,23] and 2 forms of magnetic separation, a magnetic colloid system[24] and the traditional miniMacs columns as pioneered in our laboratory.[16] No significant difference in efficacy has been observed between the 2 MACS procedures. Preliminary indications are that fetal aneuploidies can be detected by these means with specificities superior to current noninvasive methods.[25]

An integral part of this study is an evaluation of the psychosocial response of pregnant women to the introduction of a new, noninvasive method for prenatal diagnosis, which is especially aimed at clarifying any feeling of coercion. An intermediate report from this study, which examined the response of a cohort of high-risk pregnant women, has indicated that there is an overwhelmingly favorable response among this cohort for the introduction of such a noninvasive diagnostic test.[26] In our own extensions of this facet, we have interviewed 4 groups of women:

1. Those with a high risk for a fetal aneuploidy and who were about to undergo or have undergone an invasive procedure for prenatal diagnosis.
2. Those with a normal, low-risk pregnancy.
3. Those who required some form of assisted reproduction technology (ICSI, IVF).
4. A control group who were currently not pregnant.

This study indicated that the majority of women favored the introduction of a noninvasive alternative for prenatal diagnosis, even if this test could not cover the entire spectrum of chromosomal abnormalities. This desire was especially high in the group that had sought reproductive assistance and in those women who were currently pregnant with their first child. Very few of the women interviewed felt that they would be coerced to undergo such a test. An interesting aspect of this study was that although women would generally not question results indicating that the fetus was normal, they would invariably opt for an invasive second opinion to confirm that a fetal anomaly was present in those cases where an abnormality was detected using fetal cells.

OPTIMIZATION OF RECOVERY

An observation made by all participants of the NIFTY study and other researchers in the field is that although fetal cells can now be reliably and reproducibly enriched for, several steps of the enrichment procedure need to be optimized, as fetal cells appear to be lost in each step of the enrichment procedure.[11,27,28] If one considers that as few as 20 fetal cells may be present in the maternal blood sample drawn, then it is a foregone conclusion that a loss of these rare cells should be avoided at all costs.

In this manner, even though our laboratory was instrumental in the introduction of differential density gradients for the selective enrichment of erythroblasts prior to the application of the MACS enrichment step,[16,21] our recent work has shown the benefit of using simpler high-density Ficoll or Percoll gradients.[3,11,29] In a large-scale examination of over 300 samples, where fetal cells were scored on the basis of FISH for X and Y chromosomes, we noted that similar efficacies could be attained by using a single 1077 g/L Ficoll density gradient, when compared with the more complex triple-density gradient.[28] The added advantage of this switch in protocol is that it permitted the use of smaller blood samples (16 versus 40 mL), thereby allowing us to recruit more patients.

In addition, we have observed that enrichment could be further enhanced by the use of a single heavy (1119 g/L) Ficoll density gradient, as this allowed for the greatest recovery of erythroblasts,[11] a feature we have also observed with different Percoll density gradients.[29] To obtain the greatest purity, we then showed that it was best to couple an initial gradient separation step to ensure the greatest yield with the most specific antibody obtainable for the subsequent antibody-mediated step.[11] In our investigation comparing different antibodies, which included alleged fetal specific ones such as the anti-fetal liver generated HAE-9 or the i blood group antigen, we observed the best recovery with anti-GPA, which regularly yielded at least a 3- to 5-fold higher yield than our old standard, anti-CD71 (transferrin receptor).[11]

In a similar manner, altering the protocols for enrichment by FACS, by such means as intracytoplasmic fetal hemoglobin staining[30] or new more efficient staining and storing protocols[31,32] has lead to significantly improved yields.

Other promising alternatives that have recently been described include charge flow separation, where near-to-phenomenal recoveries of erythroblasts have been reported,[33] but also step[34] Percoll gradients or minimal enrichment techniques such as explored by Oosterwijk et al.[35] In addition, we recently explored the use of a novel continuous Percoll gradient in a study examining the use of fetal erythroblasts for the prenatal diagnosis of hemoglobinopathies.[36]

A problem with all these approaches is that even after enrichment for fetal cells, the majority of recovered cells are still of maternal origin, which means that only 1 in 100 to 1 in 1000 cells analyzed may actually be fetal. It is for this reason that several groups have voiced the need for fetal-cell–specific markers and for effective automatic recognition systems to locate these cells in the enriched preparations.

IDENTIFICATION OF FETAL CELLS: THE BASIS FOR AUTOMATED SCANNING

A problem that affects all of these enrichment procedures is that all the resulting preparations are heavily contaminated by co-enriching maternal cells. This means that as few as 1 in 1000 of the obtained cells may be fetal. When fetal cells such as erythroblasts are the subject of investigation, the problem is further exasperated by the fact that many of the erythroblasts analyzed are of maternal rather than of fetal origin.[3]

To overcome this problem, a common strategy has been opted for by most groups: identification of fetal cells by immunohistochemical staining using fetal-specific antibodies, such as anti-fetal (HbF) or embryonic—hemoglobin (HbE).[3] In our hands, staining with anti-gamma globin antibodies accurately identified fetal erythroblasts enriched from maternal blood,[3] even though basal levels of gamma globin-positive cells can be detected in the blood of pregnant women. In those pregnancies, where maternal levels of gamma globin may be excessively high, such as for carriers of a hemoglobinopathy, it may be advisable to use anti-zeta or anti-epsilon globin antibodies instead.[36,37]

It should, however, be borne in mind that no antibody is absolutely fetal specific, and that the only way in which a fetal cell can be irrefutably identified as been fetal is on the basis of a genetic marker.

The central idea for being able to identify fetal cells by such means is to use some form of automated recognition device to localize these cells among the myriad of co-enriched maternal cells. This could either be accomplished using laser scanning approaches,[38] fluorescence correlation spectroscopic microscopy,[39] or digital recognition equipped microscopes.[40]

CURRENT EFFICACY IN THE CYTOGENETIC ANALYSIS FETAL CELLS

For simplicity's sake, and because almost half of all pregnant women give birth to boys, many researchers have used to use FISH for the X and Y chromosomes to monitor the efficiency of their fetal cell enrichment and detection procedures. A further advantage of this approach is that because it is easier to recruit a large number of normal pregnancies with male fetuses than those with an aneuploid fetus, it is considerably easier to assess the influence of any potential modifications. For instance, by these means we were able to determine that the switch to a different, less complex primary enrichment step lead to similar or better recoveries than the more complex triple gradient we previously used. Furthermore, by only having to focus on 2 signals per cell, the technicians responsible for the evaluation of the FISH signals are also able to process more samples than if they were required to examine an additional 2 or more signals per cell.

By these means, we were also able to observe subtle differences in efficacy, for instance in the effect of the anticoagulant used during blood sampling, where samples treated with EDTA were consistently superior to those treated with heparin.[41]

This approach also indicated that successful recovery and identification of fetal cells is a multifactorial process and depends on several variables, 1 of which is the ability of the technician to correctly analyze the sample preparation, and not to be mislead by erroneous background hybridization signals.[3] This

also implies that the specificity of the FISH probes is critical, and indeed, we have noticed major fluctuations in the efficacy of fetal cell recognition with FISH reagents of different batches or different manufacturers.

In a recent review of our data, we determined that for the 560 cases we processed in the prior 18 months, the following sensitivities and specificities could be attained: If 1 XY$^+$ cell was used as being indicative of a male fetus then the sensitivity was 57% and the specificity was 77%. By using 2 XY$^+$ cells, an increase in specificity to 87% was noted, which could be increased to almost 95% if 3 XY$^+$ cells were used. Although this level of specificity is comparable to current noninvasive procedures for the determination of fetal aneuploidies, this result indicates of the power of this system; no other noninvasive method is able to determine specific fetal chromosomes with such accuracy. The downside of these investigations was that this high level of specificity was coupled with a decrease in sensitivity to below 20%. This result indicates the need to be able to accurately retrieve and score more than 3 fetal cells to achieve those levels of diagnostic accuracy required for prenatal diagnosis, thereby again raising the need for automatic recognition systems. In a sense, these results parallel our observations made with the analysis of single fetal cells by PCR, where we calculated that to achieve a diagnosis with an accuracy of 98% or greater 4 or more individual fetal cells would have to be analyzed.[42]

DIAGNOSIS OF FETAL ANEUPLOIDIES

Because it is likely that the number of fetal cells recovered will nevertheless be small, regardless of the enrichment procedure, it is of obvious importance to obtain the maximum amount of information from these few cells. For the diagnosis of fetal aneuploidies it is, hence, pertinent to use multicolor FISH procedures, which would be able to identify the most common aneuploidies (X,Y, 13, 18, and 21) simultaneously in a single cell.[43] Consequently such approaches are actively being pursued. This can be accomplished by direct examination of these chromosomes either directly by 5-color FISH in a single cell,[43] or by the sequential hybridization of the chromosomes of interest as pioneered by the laboratory of Ferguson-Smith,[44] which has also been termed *poly-FISH*.[45]

By the use of 3-color FISH for the X, Y, and 18 chromosomes, we have recently been able to correctly determine the fetal genotype for this fetal aneuploidy with a high degree of success.

PCR AND MENDELIAN DISORDERS

Pioneering publications by Sekizawa et al.[46] and from the laboratory of Y.W. Kan[37] demonstrated the feasibility of using

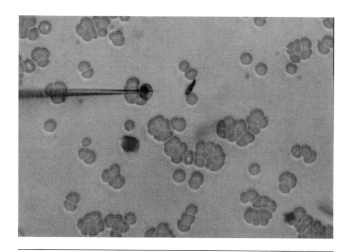

FIGURE 45-1 Micromanipulation of a single erythroblast.

single fetal erythroblasts for the prenatal diagnosis of inherited single gene disorders (Fig. 45-1).

A major problem with such an approach is the need to positively identify fetal erythroblasts. Because we were not of the opinion that an antibody, such as anti-gamma globin or anti-zeta globin is able to provide the degree of discrimination needed, we set out to use another means, namely DNA fingerprinting. This process makes use of pattern generated by microsatellites or short tandem repeats (STRs), which are unique for each individual (Fig. 45-2).

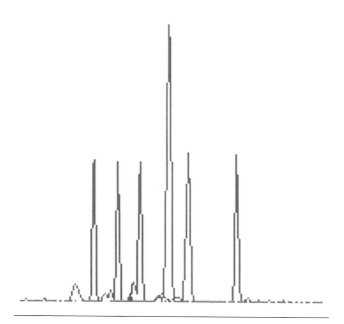

FIGURE 45-2 Single-cell PCR identification of microsatellite loci specific for chromosome 21 using a single lymphocyte. This figure indicates that an uneven ratio is obtained for the 2 loci analyzed (D21S1440: green peaks), thereby implying that this analysis cannot be used for the quantitative analysis of fetal aneuploidies on single cells. The peaks are the molecular weight standard.

A further problem when dealing with limiting amounts of input template for the PCR reaction is *allele drop out* (ADO), whereby only 1 locus of an allele pair is amplified. Obviously this can lead to false diagnoses, when only the mutant or normal allele is amplified from a normally heterozygous state.

We have shown that ADO is best overcome by the sequential analysis of several individual cells, and that by these means a high degree of accuracy can be obtained.[42,47] We also showed that even under conditions of extremely high levels of ADO, an STR analysis can be used to distinguish fetal cells from maternal ones.[42]

This study also indicated that 4–5 fetal cells would have to be individually analyzed to attain those levels of diagnostic accuracy required for prenatal diagnosis.

A further advantage of the use of STRs is that they can be used to give an indication of chromosomal ploidy.[47,48] (Because quantitative fluorescent PCR is not really feasible from single cells, it cannot be reliably used to detect aneuploidies that have arisen from errors in meiosis II, in which 2 copies of the same maternal chromosome are inherited. These, however, only account for up to 28 % of all aneuploidies[49]; therefore, the use of STRs yields valuable additional information concerning ploidy. They should, however, not solely be used for this purpose.

HOW MANY ERYTHROBLASTS ARE OF FETAL ORIGIN?

As pointed out, during pregnancy both fetal and maternal erythroblasts are present in the maternal circulation. To date no reliable data exist to indicate the relative proportion of the 2 populations; most studies used only a single locus as being indicative of fetal origin.

We set out to address this question by using single-cell PCR on isolated fetal cells by turning to a simple model system, namely by examining the fetal rhesus D status in pregnancies where the mother is rhesus D negative.[50] By concentrating on 2 fetal loci, absent from the maternal gene, namely the SRY locus on the Y chromosome and the rhesus D gene, we are able to very rapidly and simply discern between fetal and maternal cells (Fig. 45-3).

In this study, in which we examined 19 cases, we were able to successfully recover erythroblasts in 14 instances. Single morphologically identified erythroblasts were micromanipulated and individually examined by a multiplex PCR reaction that is able to simultaneously detect the presence of the SRY locus on the Y chromosome, the rhesus D gene and the β-globin gene. Because the latter is common to all genomes, it was used as a control to ensure that a cell had been transferred to the reaction vessel and that the PCR amplification had functioned. Because both the Y chromosome and the rhesus D gene are absent from the maternal genome in the cases recruited, their presence indicates a fetal cell. A perhaps surprising outcome

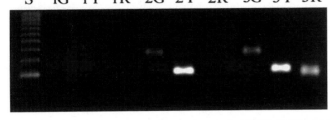

FIGURE 45-3 Simultaneous analysis of fetal sex and rhesus D using a fetal cell enriched from maternal blood. The PCR products are indicated by the following key: **S,** DNA molecular weight marker; **G,** β-globin PCR product, **Y,** SRY PCR product; **R,** rhesus D PCR product. The first cell is, hence, maternal as no amplification occurred for the rhesus D and SRY loci. The second cell is from a rhesus D–negative male fetus, and the third cell is from a male rhesus D–positive fetus (it is positive for all 3 loci).

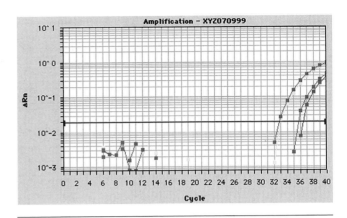

FIGURE 45-4 Real-time PCR quantification of fetal DNA in maternal plasma in a euploid pregnancy and in an aneuploid (47XY + 21) pregnancy. Because fewer PCR amplification cycles are needed to detect the same threshold level of PCR product—33 cycles instead of almost 36—this figure shows that in pregnancies with an aneuploid fetus, more fetal DNA may be present in the maternal plasma.

of this study was that in all 14 cases in which erythroblast could be recovered, we were able to correctly determine the fetal genotype for both loci interrogated. This study, which is currently the largest, for the analysis of any fetal gene by noninvasive means, illustrates both the potential of this system and that there may be instances in which no fetal cells are recovered. This study also showed that approximately half of the erythroblasts examined were of fetal origin.

A similar trend has emerged in a second study we have collaborated with, in which the use of fetal cells for the diagnosis of β-thalassemia was investigated.[36] Here, blood samples were recruited from 6 couples at risk for this disorder. Following enrichment on a novel density gradient, fetal erythroblasts were identified by immunohistochemistry for zeta globin. Strongly staining cells were observed in 4 of the cases examined and by examining these cells by single cell PCR, they were determined to be of fetal origin, as in all these cases the fetal β-globin genotype was correctly determined. A feature that also emerged from this study is that at least 4 fetal cells have to be analyzed to obtain a highly accurate result, thereby supporting the hypothesis we proposed on the basis of earlier work.[42,47]

FETAL DNA IN MATERNAL PLASMA

By extrapolating from the observation that tumor-specific DNA can be detected in plasma of affected patients, Lo et al[51] showed the presence of extracellular fetal DNA, which can be detected by PCR in the plasma and serum of pregnant women. By the use of sensitive real time quantitative PCR technology (Taqman) (Fig. 45-4), they were able to show that in normal pregnancies the quantities of this fetal DNA accounted for almost 5% of the total plasma DNA.[52] Because it is possible to distinguish between free extracellular fetal and maternal DNA except for those loci where disparities exist, the potential applications of this technology are limited. It can, however, be successfully

used to detect the presence of fetal loci absent from the maternal genome, examples again being Y-chromosome–specific loci and the rhesus D gene in rhesus D-negative women.[53] Although the feasibility of this system has been demonstrated for the determination of the fetal rhesus D status, the sensitivity when using samples from the first trimester of gestation was only around 80%,[54,55] thereby indicating that this test may only be suitable for the screening of second trimester samples.

We have extended the scope of this methodology by showing that it is possible to simultaneously analyze several fetal loci by the use of multiplex PCR, in that by employing the same PCR for SRY and rhesus D that we had developed for the analysis of single cells, we were able to determine the fetal genotype for these 2 loci with a high degree of accuracy.[56]

A caveat concerning this test is that no positive control exists to indicate that fetal DNA was indeed present in the plasma sample and that it was correctly amplified. As such, no protective strategies can be developed against obtaining false-positive results. When one bears in mind that considerable fluctuations in fetal DNA levels are detected during pregnancy, this danger can become very real. Similarly, the use of very sensitive nested PCR techniques raises the danger of obtaining false-positive results owing to spurious contaminants.[56]

IN VITRO CULTURE OF ENRICHED FETAL CELLS

Serious limitations when dealing with isolated fetal cells are the small numbers of recovered cells and the inability obtaining information concerning the entire karyotype. The only option to overcome this is by being able to culture the enriched fetal cells, thereby not only increasing their initial number but perhaps also permitting the metaphase chromosome analysis.

Although attempts in such a direction have been made for a considerable time,[57,58] these have largely been unsuccessful as the few fetal cells in the culture inoculum were generally out-competed by the abundance of maternal cells present in the enriched fraction. This may, however be redressed by the availability of new cytokines, which in combination with better culture conditions may favor the selective proliferation of fetal progenitor cells over maternal ones.[59]

In examinations we carried out on early fetal progenitor cells, we observed that these cells displayed a much higher basal proliferative capacity than comparable mature progenitor cells, but that marked differences in the response of these cells to different cytokine cocktails, in particular to flt-3 ligand and thrombopoietin occur.[60] Other similar approaches have revealed that alterations in serum conditions may favor the outgrowth of fetal erythrocytic progenitors.[59]

To ascertain the optimal culture conditions for maternal blood derived fetal progenitor cells we have turned to the Taqman real-time qPCR system. By choosing only pregnancies bearing a male fetus, we quantitated the number of male fetal cells after enrichment and compared this to the number obtained after in vitro culture. This system permits a very rapid and accurate assessment of those culture conditions that truly favor the selective expansion of fetal cells. This system can now be applied to individual colonies to determine which cell types are most frequently generated.

It is hoped that once the ideal conditions have been derived that enhanced numbers of fetal cells will be available for numerous examinations. In the instance of PCR, this greatly facilitates more simple forms of analyses, because the problem of ADO is no longer a concern. Second, the genome of pools of cells is much more amenable to whole genome amplifications methods, thereby generating sufficient DNA for dozens if not hundreds of analyses.

The big hope is of course that this will permit direct metaphase karyotype analysis, either by traditional or modern molecular genetic means, such a comparative genome hybridization or multicolor spectral karyotyping.[61] It is most likely that many researchers will opt for the latter more sensitive approach, which allows for the detection of translocations and other chromosomal abnormalities which would usually be missed. A factor that should be borne in mind, though, is that any form of culture requires a period of time, and that hence, the idea of a quick screening test is somewhat compromised.

FETAL CELLS AND DISEASE

The observation by Bianchi et al[10] that certain fetal cells, with a stem cell–like phenotype could persist for several decades in the maternal circulation raised the question of what the consequence could be of such a long-term microchimerism. This

has been answered to some extent by 2 recent papers highlighting the possible involvement of persisting fetal cells in autoimmune disorders, such as systemic sclerosis.[62,63] Interestingly, evidence for fetal cells has also been observed in polymorphic eruptions of pregnancy, a disorder of pregnancy with autoimmune-like characteristics.[64]

We made a separate novel observation regarding fetal cells and the pregnancy-related disorder, preeclampsia, in that we observed that the levels of erythroblasts are significantly elevated in pregnancies affected by preeclampsia,[65,66] an observation that we have been able to reproduce in 2 separate case control studies. Furthermore, by conducting a case-controlled study in which we only used pregnancies bearing male fetuses, we were able to show that a large proportion of these erythroblasts were fetal.[65] Interestingly, in an independent examination in which they examined the levels of fetal DNA in maternal plasma in normal and preeclamptic pregnancies, Lo and colleagues obtained results closely paralleling ours regarding the number of fetal cells.[67,68] Currently, we are carrying out further studies to confirm these findings, and are also investigating whether our findings can serve as a prognostic marker for those at risk for preeclampsia. In this context, it will be interesting to examine if any association exists between the incidence of preeclampsia and subsequent autoimmune disorders.

CONCLUSION

Although the prime concern regarding fetal cells from maternal blood remains the issue of a noninvasive form of prenatal diagnosis, the recent observations that such cells may play a role in the etiology of diseases such as scleroderma and perhaps preeclampsia has widened the spectrum of interest considerably.

On the diagnostic front, advances both in enrichment techniques but also in multicolor FISH and automated recognition systems are bringing the goal of a reliable noninvasive screening method for fetal aneuploidies closer.

Regarding the involvement of fetal cells in disease etiology, it is highly likely that we are standing on the threshold of a new level of understanding.

ACKNOWLEDGMENTS

This work was supported in part by Swiss National Science Foundation Grant Number:3200-047112.96 and NIH (USA) Contract Number: N01-HD-4-3202.

References

1. Schmorl G. *Pathologisch-anatomische Untersuchungen ueber Pubereklampsie*. Leipzig: Vogel; 1893.

2. Covone AE, Johnson PM, Mutton D, et al. Trophoblast cells in peripheral blood of pregnant women. *Lancet.* 1984;2:841–843.

3. Hahn S, Sant R, Holzgreve W. Fetal cells in maternal blood: current and future perspectives. *Mol Hum Reprod.* 1998;4:515–521.

4. Douglas GW, Thomas L, Carr M, et al. Trophoblasts in the circulating blood during pregnancy. *Am J Obstet Gynecol.* 1959;58:960–973.

5. Covone AE, Kozman R, Johnson PM, et al. Analysis of peripheral maternal blood samples for the presence of placental-derived cells using Y-specific probes and mAb H315. *Prenat Diagn.* 1988;5:591–607.

6. Sargent IL, Johansen M, Chau S, et al. Clinical experience: isolating trophoblasts from maternal blood. *Ann N Y Acad Sci.* 1994;731:154–161.

7. Attwood HD, Park WW. Embolism to the lungs by trophoblast. *J Obstet Gynaecol Br Commonw.* 1960;68:611–617.

8. Bertero MT, Camaschella C, Serra A, et al. Circulating "trophoblast" cells in pregnancy have maternal genetic markers. *Prenat Diagn.* 1988;8:588–590.

9. Schröder J, Tilikainen A, De La Chapelle A. Fetal leucocytes in maternal circulation after delivery. *Transplantation.* 1974;17:346–360.

10. Bianchi DW, Zickwolf GK, Weil GJ, et al. Male fetal progenitor cells persist in maternal blood for as long as 27 years postpartum. *Proc Natl Acad Sci U S A.* 1996;93:705–708.

11. Troeger C, Holzgreve W, Hahn S. A comparison of different density gradients and antibodies for enrichment of fetal erythroblasts by MACS. *Prenat Diagn.* 1999;19:521–526.

12. Herzenberg LA, Bianchi DW, Schröder J, et al. Fetal cells in the blood of pregnant women: detection and enrichment by fluorescence-activated cell sorting. *Proc Natl Acad Sci U S A.* 1979;76:1453–1455.

13. Bianchi DW, Flint AF, Pizzimenti MF, et al. Isolation of fetal DNA from nucleated erythrocytes in maternal blood. *Proc Natl Acad Sci U S A.* 1990;87:3279–3283.

14. Zheng YL, Demaria M, Zhen D, et al. Flow sorting of fetal erythroblasts using intracytoplasmic anti-fetal haemoglobin: preliminary observations on maternal samples. *Prenat Diagn.* 1995;15:897–905.

15. Miltenyi S, Müller W, Weichel W, et al. High gradient magnetic cell separation with MACS. *Cytometry.* 1990;11:231–238.

16. Holzgreve W, Garritsen HS, Ganshirt Ahlert D. Fetal cells in the maternal circulation. *J Reprod Med.* 1992;37:410–418.

17. Klinger KW. FISH: sensitivity and specificity on sorted and unsorted cells. *Ann N Y Acad Sci.* 1994;731:48–56.

18. Saiki RK, Scharf S, Faloona F, et al. Enzymatic amplification of beta-globin genomic sequences and restriction site analysis for diagnosis of sickle cell anemia. *Science.* 1985;230:1350–1354.

19. Elias S, Price J, Dockter M, et al. First trimester prenatal diagnosis of trisomy 21 in fetal cells from maternal blood. *Lancet.* 1992;340:1033.

20. Bianchi DW, Mahr A, Zickwolf GK, et al. Detection of fetal cells with 47,XY,+21 karyotype in maternal peripheral blood. *Hum Genet.* 1992;90:368–370.

21. Gänshirt-Ahlert D, Börejesson-Stoll R, Burschyk M, et al. Detection of fetal trisomies 21 and 18 from maternal blood using triple gradient and magnetic cell sorting. *Am J Reprod Immunol.* 1993;30:194–201.

22. de la Cruz F, Shifrin H, Elias S, et al. Prenatal diagnosis by use of fetal cells isolated from maternal blood. *Am J Obstet Gynecol.* 1995;173:1354–1355.

23. Lewis DE, Schober W, Murrell S, et al. Rare event selection of fetal nucleated erythrocytes in maternal blood by flow cytometry. *Cytometry.* 1996;23:218–227.

24. Steele CD, Wapner RJ, Smith JB, et al. Prenatal diagnosis using fetal cells isolated from maternal peripheral blood: a review. *Clin Obstet Gynecol.* 1996;39:801–813.

25. de la Cruz F, Shifrin H, Elias S, et al. Low false-positive rate of aneuploidy detection using fetal cells isolated from maternal blood. *Fetal Diagn Ther.* 1998;13:380.

26. Zamerowski S, Lumley M, Arreola RA, et al. The psychosocial impact on high-risk pregnant women of a noninvasive prenatal diagnostic test. *Fetal Diagn Ther.* 1999;14:125–126.

27. Bianchi DW, Shuber AP, Demaria MA, et al. Fetal cells in maternal blood: determination of purity and yield by quantitative polymerase chain reaction. *Am J Obstet Gynecol.* 1994;171:922–926.

28. Hahn S, Kiefer V, Brombacher V, et al. Fetal cells in maternal blood. An update from Basel. *Eur J Obstet Gynecol Reprod Biol.* 1999;85:101–104.

29. Smits G, Holzgreve W, Hahn, S. An examination of different Percoll density gradients in combination with MACS for the enrichment of fetal erythroblasts. *Arch Gyn Obstet.* 2000;263:160–163.

30. Bianchi DW, Zickwolf GK, Yih MC, et al. Erythroid-specific antibodies enhance detection of fetal nucleated erythrocytes in maternal blood. *Prenat Diagn.* 1993;13:293–300.

31. Oosterwijk JC, Mesker WE, Ouwerkerk-van Velzen MC, et al. Fetal cell detection in maternal blood: a study in 236 samples using erythroblast morphology, DAB and HbF staining, and FISH analysis. *Cytometry.* 1998;32:178–185.

32. Murrell-Bussell S, Nguyen D, Schober WD, et al. Optimized fixation and storage conditions for fish analysis of single-cell suspensions. *J Histochem Cytochem.* 1998;46:971–974.

33. Wachtel SS, Sammons D, Twitty G, et al. Charge flow separation: quantification of nucleated red blood cells in maternal blood during pregnancy. *Prenat Diagn.* 1998;18:455–463.

34. Takabayashi H, Kuwabara S, Ukita T, et al. Development of noninvasive fetal DNA diagnosis from maternal blood. *Prenat Diagn.* 1995;15:74–77.

35. Oosterwijk JC, Mesker WE, Ouwerkerk-van Velzen MC, et al. Prenatal diagnosis of trisomy 13 on fetal cells obtained from maternal blood after minor enrichment. *Prenat Diagn.* 1998;18:1082–1085.

36. Di Naro E, Ghezzi F, Tannoia N, et al. Prenatal diagnosis of fetal β-thalassemia using fetal cells from maternal blood. *Am J Obstet Gynecol.* 1999;180:S179.

37. Cheung MC, Goldberg JD, Kan YW. Prenatal diagnosis of sickle cell anaemia and thalassaemia by analysis of fetal cells in maternal blood. *Nat Genet.* 1996;14:264–268.

38. Mignon-Godefroy K, Guillet J, Butor C. Solid phase cytometry for detection of rare events. *Cytometry.* 1997;27:336–344.

39. Eigen M, Rigler R. Sorting single molecules: application to diagnostics and evolutionary biotechnology. *Proc Natl Acad Sci U S A.* 1994;91:5740–5747.

40. Oosterwijk JC, Knepfle CF, Mesker WE, et al. Strategies for rare-event detection: an approach for automated fetal cell detection in maternal blood. *Am J Hum Genet.* 1998;63:1783–1792.

41. Brombacher V, Kiefer V, Troeger C, et al. Choice of anticoagulant can influence the analysis of fetal cells enriched from maternal blood. *Prenat Diagn.* 2000;20:257–259.

42. Garvin AM, Holzgreve W, Hahn S. Highly accurate analysis of heterozygous loci by single cell PCR. *Nucleic Acids Res.* 1998;26:3468–3472.

43. Bischoff FZ, Lewis DE, Nguyen DD, et al. Prenatal diagnosis with use of fetal cells isolated from maternal blood: five-color fluorescent in situ hybridization analysis on flow-sorted cells for chromosomes X, Y, 13, 18, and 21. *Am J Obstet Gynecol.* 1998;179:203–209.

44. Zheng YL, Carter NP, Price CM, et al. Prenatal diagnosis from maternal blood: simultaneous immunophenotyping and FISH of fetal nucleated erythrocytes isolated by negative magnetic cell sorting. *J Med Genet.* 1993;30:1051–1056.

45. Zhen DK, Wang JY, Falco VM, et al. Poly-FISH: a technique of repeated hybridizations that improves cytogenetic analysis of fetal cells in maternal blood. *Prenat Diagn.* 1998;18:1181–1185.

46. Sekizawa A, Kimura T, Sasaki M, et al. Prenatal diagnosis of Duchenne muscular dystrophy using a single fetal nucleated erythrocyte in maternal blood. *Neurology.* 1996;46:1350–1353.

47. Hahn S, Garvin A, Di Naro E, et al. Allele drop out can occur in alleles differing by a single nucleotide and is not alleviated by preamplification nor minor template increments. *Genetic Testing.* 1998;2:351–355.

48. Pertl B, Kopp S, Kroisel PM, et al. Quantitative fluorescence polymerase chain reaction for the rapid prenatal detection of common aneuploidies and fetal sex. *Am J Obstet Gynecol.* 1997;177:899–906.

49. Ballesta F, Queralt R, Gomez D, et al. Parental origin and meiotic stage of non-disjunction in 139 cases of trisomy 21. *Ann Genet.* 1999;42:11–15.

50. Troeger C, Zhong XY, Burgemeister R, et al. Approximately half of the erythroblasts in maternal blood are of fetal origin. *Mol Hum Reprod.* 1999;5:1162–1165.

51. Lo YMD, Corbetta N, Chamberlain PF, et al. Presence of fetal DNA in maternal plasma and serum. *Lancet.* 1997;350:485–487.

52. Lo DYM, Tein MSC, Lau TK, et al. Quantitative analysis of fetal DNA in maternal plasma and serum: implications for noninvasive prenatal diagnosis. *Am J Hum Genet.* 1998;62:768–775.

53. Faas BH, Beuling EA, Christiaens GC, et al. Detection of fetal RHD-specific sequences in maternal plasma. *Lancet.* 1998;352:1196.

54. Lo YMD, Bowell PJ, Selinger M, et al. Prenatal determination of fetal RhD status by analysis of peripheral blood of rhesus negative mothers. *Lancet.* 1993;341:1147–1148.

55. Bischoff FZ, Nguyen DD, Marquez-Do D, et al. Noninvasive determination of fetal RhD status using fetal DNA in maternal serum and PCR. *J Soc Gynecol Invest.* 1999;6:64–69.

56. Zhong XY, Holzgreve W, Hahn S. Detection of fetal rhesus D and sex from fetal DNA in maternal plasma by multiplex PCR. *BJOG.* 2000;107:766–769.

57. Lo YMD, Morey AL, Wainscoat JS, et al. Culture of fetal erythroid cells from maternal peripheral blood. *Lancet.* 1994;344:264–265.

58. Valerio D, Aiello R, Altieri V, et al. Culture of fetal erythroid progenitor cells from maternal blood for non-invasive prenatal genetic diagnosis. *Prenat Diagn.* 1996;16:1073–1082.

59. Bohmer RM, Zhen D, Bianchi DW. Differential development of fetal and adult haemoglobin profiles in colony culture: isolation of fetal nucleated red cells by two-colour fluorescence labelling. *Br J Haematol.* 1998;103:351–360.

60. Wyrsch A, dalle Corbonara V, Jansen W, et al. Umbilical cord blood from preterm human fetuses is rich in committed and primitive hematopoietic progenitors with high proliferative and self-renewal capacity. *Blood.* 1999;27:1338–1345.

61. Macville M, Veldman T, Padilla-Nash H, et al. Spectral karyotyping, a 24-colour FISH technique for the identification of chromosomal rearrangements. *Histochem Cell Biol.* 1997;108:299–305.

62. Artlett CM, Smith JB, Jimenez SA. Identification of fetal DNA and cells in skin lesions from women with systemic sclerosis. *N Engl J Med.* 1998;338:1186–1191.

63. Nelson JL, Furst DE, Maloney S, et al. Microchimerism and HLA-compatible relationships of pregnancy in scleroderma. *Lancet.* 1998;351:559–562.

64. Aractingi S, Berkane N, Bertheau P, et al. Fetal DNA in skin of polymorphic eruptions of pregnancy. *Lancet.* 1998;352:1898–1901.

65. Holzgreve W, Ghezzi F, Di Naro E, et al. Disturbed Fetomaternal cell traffic in preeclampsia. *Obstet Gynecol.* 1998;91:669–672.

66. Gänshirt D, Smeets FW, Dohr A, et al. Enrichment of fetal nucleated red blood cells from the maternal circulation for prenatal diagnosis: experiences with triple density gradient and MACS based on more than 600 cases. *Fetal Diagn Ther.* 1998;13:276–286.

67. Lo YM, Leung TN, Tein MS, et al. Quantitative abnormalities of fetal DNA in maternal serum in preeclampsia. *Clin Chem.* 1999;45:184–188.

68. Holzgreve W, Hahn S. Novel molecular biological approaches for the diagnosis of preeclampsia. *Clin Chem.* 1999;45:451–452.

CHAPTER 46

CLINICAL PROTEOMICS

Chris Shimizu / Kevin P. Rosenblatt / Peter K. Bryant-Greenwood

With the sequencing of the human genome came significant advances in the field of obstetrics. The entirely new field of prenatal diagnostics was born, which subsequently gave way to the field of preimplantation diagnostics. With the development of these 2 fields, obstetrics has assumed a natural leadership position in molecular diagnosis, not only in terms of applied technology but also in the social, clinical, economic, and political ramifications of these technologies.

Despite the advances that came with the sequencing of the human genome, diagnostic testing in obstetrics is far from being complete or reliable. The advances that have been made are mostly in the areas of single gene abnormalities or infectious diseases. Although these developments have had an important impact, early diagnoses such as predicting preterm birth, intrauterine growth restriction, preeclampsia, or the initiation of labor remain elusive.

The problem with DNA-based diagnosis results from the small number of only 40,000 genes that make up the human genome. Mutations in single genes rarely correlate with disease status. The diagnosis of complex diseases requires much more than the ability to monitor mutations in multiple genes.

Accurate diagnostic tests for complex diseases will instead be made at the protein level. The 40,000 genes in the human genome encode for 1,000,000 different proteins, whose synthesis is regulated by 10,000 different transcription factors. To detect, monitor, and analyze this proteome requires 3 critical components: (1) clinical serum and tissue samples linked to clinical data, (2) mass spectrometry, and (3) bioinformatics. In this chapter, we overview mass spectroscopy and bioinformatics and then discuss the application of these 2 tools to a broad array of clinical questions.

MASS SPECTROMETRY

The technique of mass spectrometry was developed in the early 1900s, with J.J. Thompson's invention of the first spectrometer.[1] These instruments consist of 3 basic components: the source, mass analyzer, and detector (Fig. 46-1). The source produces ions from a sample to be separated by the analyzer by their mass/charge (m/z) ratios. The detector then quantifies the separated ions and allows the interpretation of these data. Although different types of sources, analyzers, and detectors have been developed, they all work the same way, separating ions by their m/z ratios. The advances made in mass spectrometry equipment over the past 2 decades allow for the analysis of larger, more fragile biomolecules that would fragment under analysis by earlier instruments.

There are 3 modern source types that can be used for the analysis of larger peptides and proteins: electrospray ionization (ESI), matrix-assisted laser desorption/ionization (MALDI), and surface-enhanced laser desorption/ionization (SELDI).

These ionizing techniques are most often paired with either a time-of-flight or quadrupole analyzer. These ionizing sources allow for soft ionization, a process that leaves large molecules such as proteins and peptides intact. Both ESI and MALDI were developed in the late 1980s, and for the first time, mass spectrometry could be used for the analysis of biological samples. SELDI, a variation of MALDI, ionization was developed in the early 1990s. These ionization techniques are sensitive to the picomole-to-femtomole range required for application to biological samples, including carbohydrates, oligonucleotides, small polar molecules, and peptides, proteins, and posttranslationally modified proteins, such as glycoproteins and phosphoproteins.[2]

In the MALDI technique, biological samples are first mixed with energy-absorbing compounds, known as a *chemical matrix,* then are spotted onto a solid surface, sometimes called a *probe.* The matrix contains small chromophores that absorb light at a particular wavelength. Commonly used matrix chemicals include α-cyano-4-hydroxycinnamic acid, 3,5-dimethoxy-4-hydroxycinnamic acid, and 2,5-dihydroxybenzoic acid. After the matrix and samples have been mixed, water is evaporated off of the probe, and sample proteins become embedded in a crystalline lattice made up of matrix molecules. The probe is then subjected to the source laser, which fires at the matrix's set wavelength. The matrix molecules absorb energy and then transfer it to the sample molecules. This transmission of energy causes both the matrix and sample to vaporize. Positive sample ions are then produced when protons are transferred from the matrix to the sample. This process allows for the ionization of the sample particles, and causes little fragmentation because most of the energy is absorbed by the matrix. The ion gas cloud is subsequently accelerated into the mass analyzer electrostatically.

The SELDI technique is similar to MALDI, except that selective surfaces are used in SELDI to separate out unwanted proteins from the very start. The probe is washed to remove unbound proteins and other impurities. Also, the use of a chemical matrix is not required for the SELDI process. Surfaces with diverse affinities for different proteins of interest can be generated to carry out on-probe chromatography, including cation/anion exchange, reverse phase (for hydrophobic interactions), and metal affinity chromatography, among others. This chromatography method is advantageous over other methods such as column chromatography and electrophoresis; it is fast, simple, inexpensive, and versatile. It is sensitive to the femtomole range and reproducible. These traits give SELDI potential for high-throughput diagnostics.

The ESI process does not require probes as MALDI and SELDI do. Instead, ESI creates an ion vapor by sending high voltage through a stream of aqueous sample solution. The sample is then electrostatically driven through drying agents to evaporate off water. The charges are left behind on the sample molecules as solvent evaporates off. This method of ionization is gentler than MALDI and SELDI and produces less

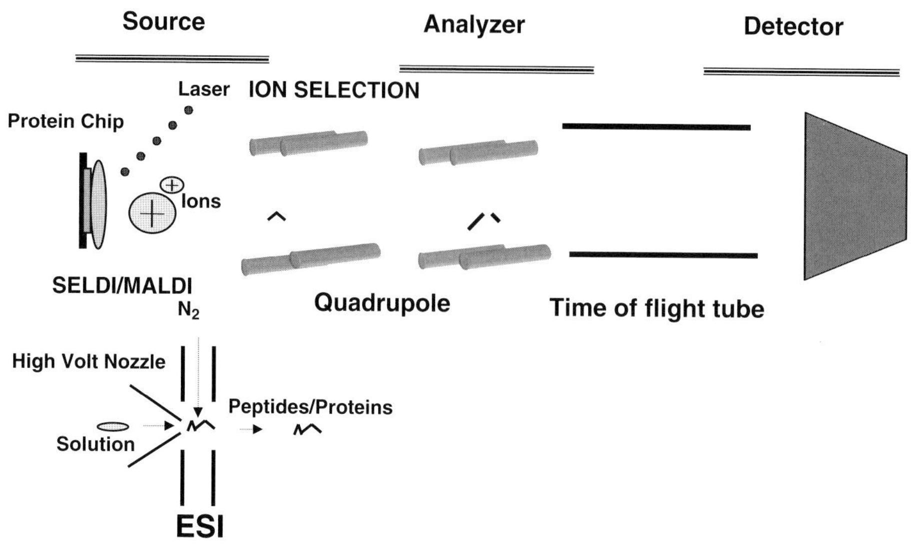

FIGURE 46-1 The basic components of a spectrometer.

protein fragmentation, but produces ions in the m/z range of ESI-coupled analyzers that have a smaller mass range than TOF analyzers.

MALDI and SELDI ionization sources are usually connected to TOF analyzers that have a mass limit between 150,000 and 300,000 Da. The ESI ionization method has a mass limit of 70 kDa, and is usually paired with a quadrupole or other analyzer. TOF analyzers are able to determine the m/z ratio of a sample particle by using the measurement of time for the particle to travel from source to detector. Following ionization, proteins are accelerated into the analyzer with equal kinetic energy (KE). The KE gained by an ion depends on its charge. The relationship between KE, mass (m), and velocity (v) is $KE = \frac{1}{2} mv^2$. This means that smaller particles travel through the analyzer with a greater velocity than larger particles, and reach the detector sooner. By knowing the time required for a sample particle to travel from source to detector, the particle's mass can be calculated. TOF analyzers have a lower resolution than other analyzers because of the KE spread of ions reaching the detectors. This causes broadened peaks for each m/z value, but resolution can be improved in TOF analyzers by the addition of reflectron components within analyzers that reduce the variation in KE for each ion species hitting the detector (Fig. 46-2).

BIOINFORMATICS

Mass spectrometry creates serum fingerprints (Fig. 46-3) that can be analyzed with complex bioinformatics algorithms and used to develop diagnostic tests for disease. The Proteome Quest software application uses a 2-phase process to create a diagnostic test. The first step requires a genetic algorithm, a parallel to the natural selection process. Proteome fingerprints are collected from both diseased and nondiseased patients, and the 15,500 m/z values produced by the SELDI-TOF technique are analyzed to determine which proteins are indicative of disease. In this process, the computer creates hundreds to tens of thousands of "virtual" chromosomes, which are simply small sets of m/z values randomly selected from the x-axis of the data input.

Each candidate subset of m/z values contains from 5–20 of the 15,500 potential x-axis values from the spectra, which can be likened to combinations of genes or alleles on a chromosome. A cluster-analysis method is then used as a fitness test of the genetic algorithm; it plots the pattern formed by the combined y-axis amplitudes of the candidate m/z subsets in N-dimensional space, where N is the number of m/z values in the test set. The pattern formed by the relative amplitude of a particular m/z value subset is then rated for its ability to distinguish between disease and nondisease; only the best discriminator sets are saved. The m/z values within the highest rated sets are recombined to form new subsets (Fig. 46-4). These new subsets are then rerated accordingly until a set of m/z values emerges that fully discriminates diseased from the nondiseased serum samples. Literally trillions of iterations can be run until the best combination of m/z values surfaces. The final output of the bioinformatics tool is a diagnostic pattern defined by the relative combination of m/z amplitudes; this pattern of amplitudes acts as a discriminator for the training set cohorts. This completes the initial step in developing the diagnostic pattern, deriving a set of m/z values and relative amplitudes that distinguish 1 study set (disease) from another (nondisease).

The second step of the bioinformatics process uses the diagnostic pattern to analyze unknown patient serum samples (Fig. 46-5). The set of m/z values determined in the first phase is analyzed for each sample. The unknown patterns

A

LOW RESOLUTION

- •15,000 data points
- •Low Resolution
- •No protein peak ID
- •MALDI-TOF ions do not necessarily reflect relative abundance in sera

B

HIGH RESOLUTION

450,000 data points

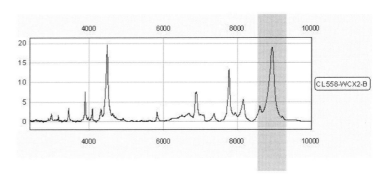

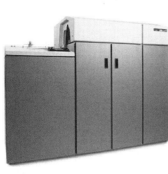

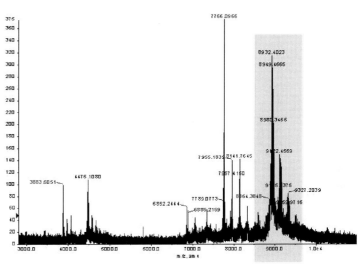

FIGURE 46-2 Comparison of low (**A**) and high (**B**) resolution spectrometers.

are matched against the optimum values of the training set, and are then classified as either cancer, unaffected, or unknown.

In the testing of this platform, all 18 patients with stage I ovarian cancer were correctly identified. Of the 66 patients without cancer, 63 were diagnosed correctly. The sensitivity and specificity of this platform are, respectively, 100% and 95%.[3] Using the high-resolution QSTAR instrument, the serum diagnostic test was improved, and an optimal 100%

was reached for both specificity and sensitivity; every stage I ovarian cancer was correctly identified and no benign cases were misinterpreted as cancer. These results suggest that this bioinformatics platform has the potential to develop both early screening and diagnostic tests. Similarly high sensitivities and specificities have been achieved for the early diagnosis of non-neoplastic diseases as well. The detection of preclinical graft-versus-host disease (GVHD) was successful with 100% sensitivity and specificity; detection of labor in the term and preterm period was 100% sensitive and more than 90% specific.[4,5] This system is only 1 of the bioinformatics programs available in serum proteomics. Recent software includes hierarchical-clustering algorithms, neural networks, and other statistical algorithms used previously in the analysis of DNA microarrays.

APPLICATIONS

SERUM DISEASE DIAGNOSIS

For many patients, disease is diagnosed too late, after the tumor has already metastasized throughout the body. Perhaps more than 60% of patients with breast, colon, lung, or ovarian

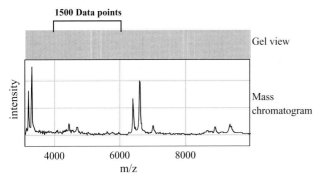

Data analysis window: 0-20,000 Daltons = 15,500 data points

FIGURE 46-3 Typical serum profile from SELDI analysis.

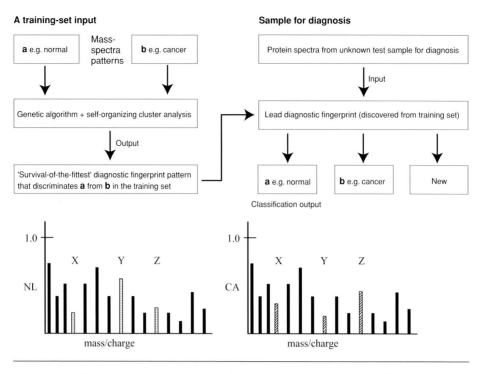

FIGURE 46-4 The process of creating subsets for gene analysis, or a proteomic "fingerprint."

carcinoma have microscopic or obvious metastatic disease at the time of diagnosis; the success of therapy after distant disease is often very limited. Early detection of disease often translates into higher cure rates. Ovarian cancer is an excellent example of the benefits of early disease detection. Greater than 80% of patients present at an advanced clinical stage, when tumor cells have left the ovary and disseminated throughout the pelvic and peritoneal cavities or beyond.[6] The 5-year survival rate for these late-stage patients is about 35%, even for patients receiving the most advanced surgical and pharmacologic treatments. In contrast, early stage ovarian cancer is associated with 5-year survival rates in excess of 90% when conventional treatment is given.[6] It is clear that an early detection method that identifies disease well in advance of the symptoms, when the tumor is confined to the ovary, will have a profound effect on patient survival.

The present schematic for the diagnosis of disease using an initial screening test is born out of necessity. The inherent inaccuracy of our present screening modalities for disease, whether it is the Pap smear, the triple screen for Down syndrome, or a serum cancer marker such as CEA demand a confirmatory gold standard test. These gold standard tests represent the second layer of problems inherent in our present disease diagnosis strategy. The most common gold standard cancer test is really a combination of 2 completely different tests—imaging followed by biopsy. Correct diagnosis in this context requires multiple types of equipment and multiple experts. The inaccuracy inherent in this process is the first problem with our gold standard modalities. The inevitable false-positive and false-negative results lead to unnecessary treatment with its associated morbidity and mortality, or premature death from undiagnosed or misdiagnosed diseases. The second problem with our confirmatory tests is that they are invasive. Invasive tests result in their own morbidity, whether

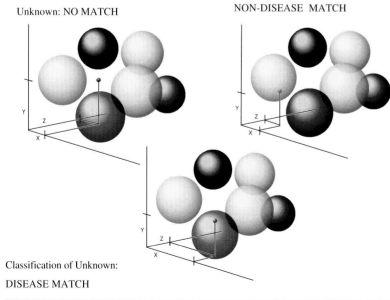

Classification of Unknown: NO MATCH

Classification of Unknown: NON-DISEASE MATCH

Classification of Unknown: DISEASE MATCH

FIGURE 46-5 Analysis of unknown serum samples.

it is a lung biopsy resulting in a pneumothorax or an allergic reaction to radiologic contrast material. The error rate and the invasive nature of our confirmatory tests result in increased cost and patient avoidance of the initial screening test.[7] Patient avoidance, combined with the error rates inherent in our present modalities, represents a glass ceiling for disease survival rates.

The ovarian cancer data described previously are important because they provide us with insight into the kinetics of the serum proteome. First, small molecules that would otherwise be cleared by the body must be shed into the serum, to the point where they achieve a steady-state concentration. Rapid changes in disease may not be detected, or may be more difficult to diagnose because the small molecules fail to achieve the required steady-state concentration in the patient's serum compartment. Thus, potentially important proteins or peptides are missed in the platform currently under development. A second, and related, problem is protein or peptide half-life. A cohort of proteins or peptides, even if they attain steady-state concentrations in the serum, may have such short half-lives that they elude detection. They degrade to the point of spectral noise in the time it takes to get the sample from the patient to the mass spectrophotometer. These reasons perhaps explain why the same platform that is 100% sensitive and 95% specific for stage I ovarian cancer can only tell the difference between a woman in labor and not in labor with 100% sensitivity and 90% specificity. The third weakness of the ovarian platform is that a protein's activity state cannot be detected directly. For example, a protein may have the same m/z value in the serum from a cancer patient versus a normal individual, but may be phosphorylated. This imparts significant changes in biologic activity outside of the spectral range of the SELDI-TOF system, thus escaping detection and analysis.

The diagnostic bioinformatics platform used for early diagnosis can also be applied to a number of other disease management issues. These include diagnosis of minimal residual disease and microscopic disease to specific tissues before radiologic detection, for example, liver, brain, or cancer cell signal pathway profiling (outlined below). Application to non-neoplastic disease processes such as infectious agents, autoimmune disease, prenatal diagnostics, or dementia is underway.

SERUM SURROGATES FOR DISEASE PATHWAY PROFILING

The molecular classification of disease serves a singular purpose; the identification of cell-signaling and growth pathways specific to cancer, independent of cell origin. This represents an important evolution in our research endeavor. The present clinical trial model requires accurate identification of cell of origin (eg, ovarian, breast duct, thyroid, etc.), pathologic stage, and histologic grade. Some trials even require some level of immunohistochemical detection of protein expression, such as ER/PR, Her-2-neu or C-kit expression. The types of trials that are now possible are those that attempt to map out the protein cellular circuitry of the diseased cells in addition to therapy evaluation. These trials would demonstrate that

1. diseases of the same morphologic type use different pathways.
2. diseases of different morphologic types use the same pathways.
3. therapies can be developed to the specific pathways used by a patient's disease, thereby individualizing a patient's treatment regimen.
4. specific therapies improve response and cure rates and reduce toxicities.
5. specific therapies allow the rational treatment of disease recurrence or resistance.

Customizing therapy to the individual and the individual's disease process is the next step in realizing improved outcome for cancer patients. Our aim is to use a combination of proteomic techniques to not only dissect and evaluate the pathways of importance, but to be able to do this from the patient's serum.

Reverse phase protein arrays have been pioneered by the National Cancer Institute for this purpose. Briefly, microdissected pure abnormal cells from frozen biopsy tissue are lysed and arrayed in miniature dilution cures onto nitrocellulose slides (Fig. 46-6). These lysates are nondenatured and do not require antigen retrieval. The dilution curve allows the direct quantitative measurement of protein expression. Because there is no direct labeling or tagging of the protein of interest, the assay has markedly improved sensitivity and reproducibility. From 3000 microdissected cells, 30 or more arrays can be made and probed with a wide range of antibodies. Reverse-phase arrays can now be used to study key "nodes" in the cellular circuitry of a disease cell and monitor a patient in real time for the purpose of therapy customization.

In addition to being relatively laborious, reverse phase arrays require biopsy material to be procured from the patient. Even if the array manufacturing process was automated, reverse phase arrays would be prohibitively expensive—procuring tissue from every cancer recurrence by minimally invasive surgery or interventional radiology would place an enormous fiscal burden on patients and our health care system. However, linking the data derived from reverse phase arrays in clinical trials with serum proteomics offers an exciting and much more cost-effective modality (Fig. 46-7). Serum is drawn from the patient before biopsy. Biopsy material is microdissected, arrayed, and probed with antibodies to selective cell circuitry nodes. The patient's serum is run on the SELDI platform and interrogated with the same bioinformatics tool utilized for early diagnosis. In this case the training sets are not cancer versus noncancer, but more sophisticated.

Cells from both tumors would stain positive by immunohistochemistry for EGFR. However, because of the complexity of the signaling system and pathway–pathway interactions, positive immunohistochemistry does not accurately reflect biologic behavior. Study set 1 shows a subtly altered pathway utilized by a cohort of 50 patient's lung cancers in which an EGFR-mediated activated pathway resulted in both cell cycle activation and angiogenesis, but not in the usual, expected

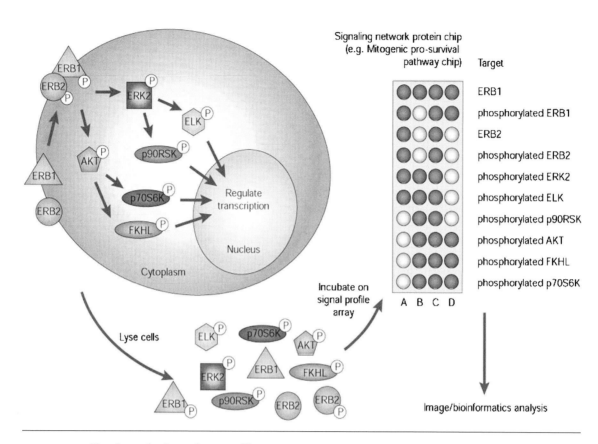

FIGURE 46-6 Signal transduction pathway profiling.

expression of cell motility and metastasis proteins. Study set 2 shows a different cohort of 50 patients who have a block in RAS activation with an expected decrease in angiogenesis proteins but no decrease in either cell-cycle or cell-motility protein expression, suggesting an alternative pathway used by the tumor cells.

Utilizing the same software for early diagnosis as described previously, we can ask the bioinformatics tool to tell us whether a new patient with either a primary process or a cancer recurrence clusters to study set 1, study set 2, or matches to neither based on the patients serum. Non-neoplastic disease would work similarly. In the case of preterm birth, detection of infectious versus noninfectious pathways for premature rupture of membranes could be achieved. Our assumption is that different signaling pathway result in different biologic behavior and is reflected in the patient's serum. To date this is largely unknown, though serum detection of elevated Her-2-neu expression in breast cancer patients offers an exciting hint at the possibilities.[8] In cases where a patient's serum does not match, biopsy can be performed followed by reverse-phase array analysis and a new study cohort can be generated as new "nonfit" patients are biopsied.

Posttreatment biopsies can be analyzed the same way. For instance, assume that study set 2 represents a cohort treated with a small molecule that actively blocks RAS. Ideally, we would like to see angiogenesis, proliferation, and invasion protein pathways turned off. In this case only 1 of the 3 is.

This again suggests RAS-independent proliferation and invasion pathways at work. If a new patient is given the small molecule or biologic that blocks RAS, we can draw serum at midtreatment and assess through our bioinformatics tool whether the patient's tumor is responding or is partially responding to blockade. Apoptosis in the tumor cells could also be monitored through surrogate serum analysis. Partial responders would have a second treatment added, and nonresponders would have this otherwise unnecessary treatment discontinued.

SERUM MANAGEMENT OF THERAPY TOXICITY: REAL-TIME MANAGEMENT OF THE THERAPEUTIC WINDOW

Toxic side effects are an inherent component of all medical interventions, whether they are traditional small-molecule pharmacologic agents, monoclonal antibodies, or clonally expanded lymphocytes. In addition to dose, the toxicity profile of an agent depends on host response. Analysis of this host response includes prediction of toxicity and monitoring for end-organ damage.

Pharmacogenomics represents an initial attempt at toxicity prediction. Individuals with specific mutations in genes responsible for drug metabolism, such as those involved in the p450 system, are at higher risk for either reduced metabolism of the drug, and hence toxicity, or in some cases increased metabolism and a subsequent subtherapeutic response. In being able to predict response, pharmacogenomics is

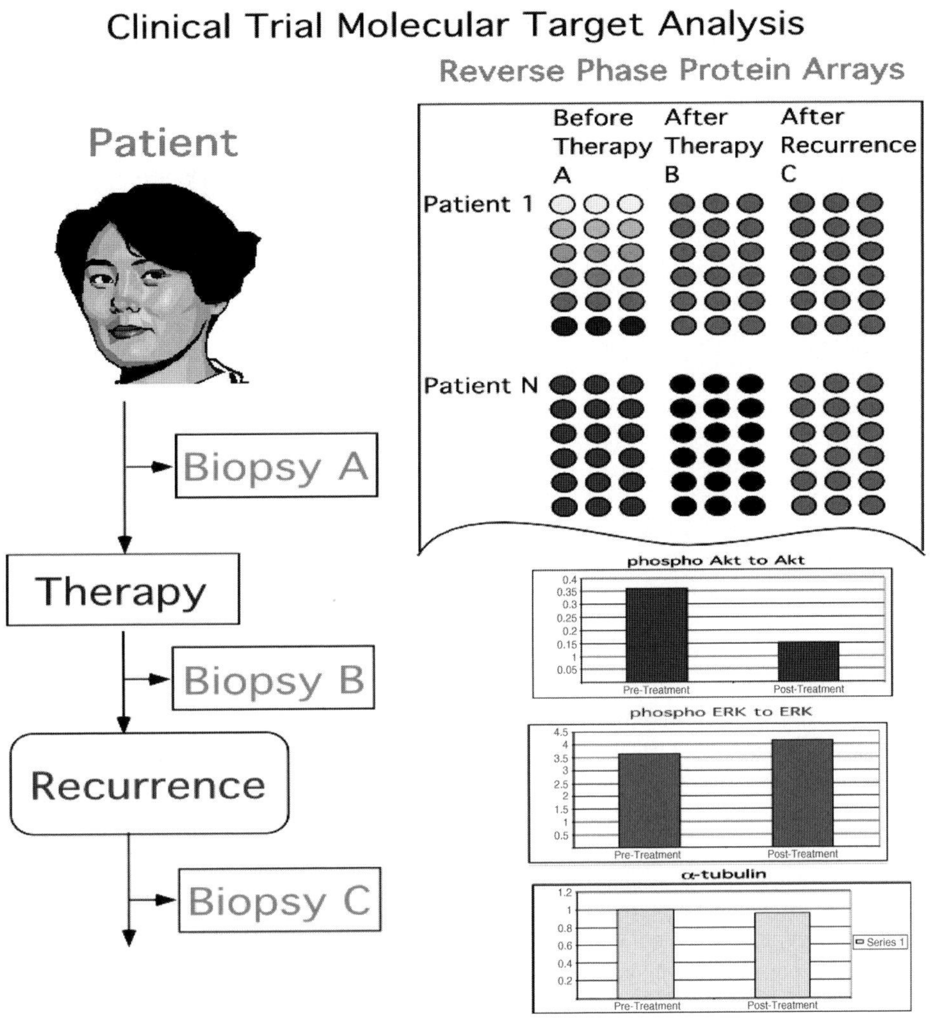

Clinical Trial Molecular Target Analysis

Reverse Phase Protein Arrays

FIGURE 46-7 Real-time monitoring of disease.

fundamentally different from our traditional modalities fused to monitor drug toxicity and its corollary, drug efficacy.

Traditionally, clinical trials define the toxic ranges for a drug. This requires the drug to be administered to a standardized cohort of patients at a number of different doses. Patients are then monitored clinically for drug toxicity and correlated with serum, blood, tissue, or plasma levels of the drug. Clinical monitoring becomes the critical process for toxicity evaluation. Clinical monitoring requires a number of different instruments. These include patient questionnaires, blood tests, urinalysis, imaging studies, physical examinations, and even interventional procedures such as angiogram or colonoscopy. Although clinical monitoring is the gold standard for determining toxicity, it is far from being a perfect modality:

1. *Variation.* Multiple tests are available that attempt to define the same toxic event, each having its own test sensitivity and specificity. For example, serum troponins and cardiac echocardiography can both be utilized to define cardiac toxicity. Troponins are more sensitive, and allow

for monitoring for subclinical toxicity, but are not as specific as direct imaging. Troponins, as a laboratory test, may be more standardized than imaging studies that require a physician's subjective interpretation, but intra- and interlaboratory variation may still be problems. The question is not only which test to use, but also how to use them together for a given clinical trial. Unfortunately, the answer to the latter question differs from 1 clinical trial to the next. Multiple test modalities results in a process variation that prevents data collected from a clinical trial to be either transferred to another trial (e.g., the same type of cardiotoxicity caused by completely different medications) or worse, from being directly applied to real clinical practice.

2. *Expense.* Combining multiple test modalities, whether it is a physical examination, laboratory test, or imaging study, requires physician interpretation. This is a laborious, expensive process.

3. *Time.* The complexity and expense of toxicity/efficacy evaluation means shortened time frames for this evaluation. Many toxic events are subsequently missed.

At a fundamental level, pharmacogenomics attempts to address the problems encountered in clinical monitoring for toxicity and efficacy. Individuals with known mutations that result in toxicity from certain classes of medications are excluded from study at the outset. This reduces one of the greatest sources of variation in the clinical trial setting—that of the patients themselves. Clinical trials become more accurate and less costly as a result: by narrowing the range of toxic side effects of the study population, fewer test modalities are required to detect toxicity or gauge toxic severity.

Monitoring the expression of 35,000 genes in the pretrial state or using high-throughput single nucleotide polymorphisms to predict toxicity is neither cost effective nor accurate. Pharmacogenomics does not replace clinical monitoring; it only reduces the magnitude of its inherent inaccuracies. In serving as a direct, real-time surrogate marker for specific end-organ dysfunction, serum proteomics directly addresses the problem of clinical monitoring.

Serum proteomics will be used as a pretrial predictor of toxicity. The goal of 100% specificity and 100% sensitivity for predicting toxicity is only possible with the 450,000 data points and bioinformatics interrogation algorithms of serum proteomics. The 35,000 genes in the human genome are not reflective of the biologic state of the organism because they correlate poorly with protein expression and activity, are not as responsive to the cellular environment as their protein counterparts, and do not represent enough data points for accurate prediction. Serum proteomic prediction will use the same bioinformatics tool utilized for the yes-no–type diagnostics described. The use of the serum proteome for clinical trial and post trial monitoring, however, requires a completely different, more complicated kind of bioinformatics tool currently under development. This tool attempts to place an individual on the curve or spectrum of toxicity.

The application of serum proteomics to diagnosis and monitoring of toxicity and disease state is a daunting challenge. It requires a host of very disparate disciplines to work together to input meaningful data into the system. This data may be in the form of clinical information, tissue samples, pathologic diagnosis, clinical pharmacology, or mass spectrometry–derived data points. This challenge is no longer just the development of new technologies, but rather the best use and integration of these technologies for the diagnosis and treatment of disease.

References

1. Siuzdak G. *Mass spectrometry for biotechnology*. San Diego: Academic; 1996, pp. XVI, 161.
2. Fenn JB, Mann M, Meng CK, et al. Electrospray ionization for mass spectroscopy of large molecules. *Science*. 1989;246:64–71.
3. Petricoin EF, Ardekani AM, Hitt BA, et al. Use of proteomic patterns in serum to identify ovarian cancer. *Lancet*. 2002;359:572–577.
4. Killian J, Geho D, Quesado M, et al. Use of serum proteomic patterns to help diagnose acute graft vs. host disease [abstract]. US–Canadian Academy of Pathology; 2003.
5. Weil R, Millar L, Shimizu C, et al. Identification of preterm labor from the maternal serum proteome [abstract]. Society for Maternal Fetal Medicine; 2005.
6. Ozols RF, Rubin SC, Thomas GM, et al. Epithelial ovarian cancer. In: Hoskins WJ, Perez CA, Young RC, eds. *Principles and Practice of Gynecologic Oncology*. 3rd ed. Philadelphia: Lippincott Williams & Wilkins; 2000:981–1058.
7. Sung NS, Crowley WF Jr, Genel M, et al. Central challenges facing the national clinical research enterprise. *JAMA*. 2003;289:1278–1287.
8. Carney WP, Neumann R, Lipton A, et al. Potential clinical utility of serum Her-2/neu oncoprotein concentration in patients with breast cancer. *Clin Chem*. 2003;49:1579–1598.

Management of Problems

CHAPTER 47

PSYCHOLOGICAL REACTION TO PRENATAL DIAGNOSIS AND LOSS

Natalie Gellman

Preparing oneself to work with individuals who possess medical problems involves extensive training. Too often there is a focus on the science and technical aspects of medicine, which incorporates a massive amount of material. There is less study regarding the experience of working with patients, and preparing for the emotional aspects of practicing medicine.

Most physicians are accustomed to information being collected and presented in an analytical, statistically based fashion. While there are numerous psychological studies that follow such a model, there is very little literature on the experiential nature or psychological reaction to a defective pregnancy. In order to fully understand and appreciate the prenatal diagnostic experience, it is necessary to listen to the people involved. Through words their thoughts and feelings become clear. The material in this chapter has been gathered *phenomenologically*. It has emerged from the self-reporting of couples who have gone through prenatal testing. Some have chosen to terminate their pregnancy in light of a positive diagnosis, and others have chosen to have their baby.

The technology and science of reproduction are progressing at a remarkable pace. Innovations have afforded many people the opportunity not only to give birth, but also to give birth to babies with fewer medical problems. However, this entire field has precipitated debate in the ethics community. Also, it has created a new focus in the field of psychology because the emotional impact experienced by the patients involved in the diagnosis and treatment of birth defects is being recognized.

Clearly there is an intense response from a pregnant woman when she is told her fetus may be defective.[1] The emotional consequences of contemplating and, perhaps, experiencing an abortion are even greater.[2] It is imperative for professionals to understand a woman's experience; similarly, it is important to understand the emotional responses of the father and the doctors involved with treatment.

For most couples, it is unfathomable not to see a pregnancy to term. From the start, each member of the couple begins to fantasize about her or his role as a parent. Sometimes the decision is made to seek housing that is more conducive to the growing family. Others prepare for career changes and financial needs to accommodate a baby.

Thus, for those who have not miscarried or anticipated problems for other reasons, the news of a possible defect are shocking. However, people who have been through or have reason to suspect they are at risk find a loss or defect no easier to bare. Those who are advised to have prenatal diagnosis are typically unprepared for the experience.

When patients seek prenatal diagnosis, they are entering into processes of evaluating disabilities, and deciding which disabilities make life not worth living as well as which disabilities demand too many resources or strain their competence as parents. Often an individual woman entering the process does not fully appreciate how difficult these decisions will be. Most are not adequately informed to anticipate the range of possible diagnoses or the ambiguity inherent in the diagnostic process.[1]

Women, who are confronted by the prospect of prenatal testing, report that the suggestion of a defect creates feelings of disbelief, confusion, and bewilderment. In essence, they are thrust into an experience of grief as they also seek to reconcile a sense of loss, in particular the belief that they would have a healthy baby. Countless thoughts and feelings converge on them. Initially, they are shocked by the prospect that something could be wrong. The fantasy of family, so quickly in place after conception is confirmed, is suddenly threatened. Even those who conceive with the knowledge of possible genetic problems experience a sense of disappointment. Most women fear initiating a miscarriage during the diagnostic procedure.

For many women, the initial awareness of a possible birth defect marks the beginning of a set of emotional polarities, which many people never understand. Often these women have 2 contradictory feelings simultaneously. They try to convince themselves that 1 of the feelings is legitimate, and are often tormented as they struggle with the opposing feelings. In reality, both feelings are genuine and reflect the intensity of the struggle within the woman. This polarity is very common for women who are at risk with their pregnancies. On the one hand, a woman may tell herself she should accept this baby no matter what, for that is the stereotypical image of a mother. On the other hand, the anticipation of having a defective child precipitates feelings of anger, resentment, and fear. Too often, women are not allowed to express these latter feelings even to themselves. They feel they are betraying their role as mothers who are supposed to feel unconditional love and acceptance of their children. The result can be a pervasive feeling of guilt, which can color every decision including her decision to pursue prenatal testing.

There are some women, so frightened of the prospect of a birth defect, who will employ denial as a means of coping with their fear.[3] A small number of women will deny the reality of their pregnancy until the results of the prenatal tests are known. Some claim that at this time they cease to be aware of fetal movement. Other women will avoid discussing the prospect of a birth defect. One, under this form of denial, believes that if something is not validated, it does not exist. For women who are terrified of the truth this is their coping mechanism.

Women choose not to have prenatal testing for other reasons. Those who are committed to having the baby despite its problems do not always see the value of prenatal testing. Those opposed to abortion question the necessity of learning about a defect. However, some choose to have prenatal testing and hope the results will show a healthy fetus. This enables them to feel reassured during the remainder of the pregnancy. Others will agree to do so to be prepared for interventions at birth.

Women, who are at high risk for complications and choose not to have prenatal testing, report a high level of anxiety through duration of the pregnancy. Their fears and fantasies remain unconfirmed; this is a stressful and lonely position. It is advisable that women who forego prenatal testing receive some type of psychological counseling. However, it is often harder to find support for their decision because they are often going against medical advice.

Anxiety and guilt are highly pervasive in women confronted by suspected birth defects.[4] Initially, there is a tendency to impose self-blame. Desperate to control what feels like an out-of-control situation, women will conjure up explanations for the problem. If there is reason to believe there is a genetic link, they will feel responsible for having conceived this less-than-perfect-baby. Women who had problems conceiving blame their bodies. Those who were uncertain about wanting children blame their psychological resistance. Sometimes there is guilt over past behavior.

These types of "irrational" fantasies are very rational responses to these difficulties. Physicians must accept these fantasies as a manifestation of fear and anxiety and not as a statement of fact. Women should be encouraged to express these thoughts and *not* repress them. Repression usually leads to a heightening of emotions rather than a dissipation of them. Reassurance and support, blended with an interspersion of facts, will help a woman healthily move through these feelings.

The decision whether to proceed with medical tests or procedures can be very stressful. Most women are still suffering from the shock, guilt and fear provoked by the discovery that there may be a birth defect. The response is typically exacerbated by the confirmation of a problem. Thus, the decision of whether to test becomes replaced with the decision of how to proceed if a problem has been identified. There are cultural variations as well as religious differences in how the information is received and processed by couples before they make their choice.[5,6,7]

A woman with suspected or confirmed problems has entered a strange world of technical jargon and emotional difficulty. They usually have no information or understanding of how to proceed. For those professionally involved in this field—doctors, genetic counselors and mental health workers—there is a tendency to be desensitized to a woman's experience. What may be routine for a professional, such as testing older women or performing selective termination, is not routine for the particular woman.

In *The Tentative Pregnancy*, Barbara Katz-Rothman described this stage when she said, "Initially, I felt this alienation-from the pregnancy, from the fetus. I didn't want to put my hands down on my stomach."[8] Rothman makes another poignant observation:

In choosing between the tragedy of a disabled, defective damaged, hurt, "in-valid" child, and the tragedy of aborting a wanted pregnancy, a woman becomes responsible for the tragedy of her choice. Whichever "choice" she makes, it is all the worse for having been chosen. If she chooses to keep the pregnancy and have the baby, she is responsible for its suffering. After all, she chose to have the baby; she could have avoided this tragedy, but chose not to. If she chooses to abort it, if she chooses a fetal loss, then she grieves for the loss

of a baby nonetheless because she has chosen its loss. In adding in the element of choice, her burden grows no lighter. Yes, we can sit here and weigh tragedies and say that the tragedy of a baby's death is less than the tragedy of disability. Or the other way around. And whichever tragedy one chooses as the lesser is the one you get. The chosen tragedy.[5] (p. 180)

First, such feelings must be addressed and expressed. Different women require different lengths of time to go through this stage. How this is facilitated depends on the needs of each person. One may want time to herself. Another might seek support from family and friends and others may crave information and ask for material to read or professional help. Some women want to see the fetus on ultrasound; others do not, and, are devastated at the experience. Many women have expressed an interest in talking to others who have gone through similar experiences. For some, meeting mothers of children with a birth defect helps them reconcile their decision. It is mandatory to listen to the patient and, based on their unique needs, to be prepared with a variety of interventions, rather than predetermine what will be in their best interest.

Many women describe the experience of making a decision as feeling caught, trapped, or involved many, this fetus is a real in a nightmare. It is not easier for those who have been told their fetus eventually will die. The mother is involved in a life-and-death decision that she must live with forever. There is evidence that women are less bonded to a fetus earlier in the pregnancy and, thus, are more likely to select abortion during the first trimester, although recent data suggest similar decisions in the first and second trimester.[2]

Women who have been taught to believe that abortion is murder feel like villains as they decide whether to terminate a pregnancy. It is difficult for them to validate their own needs and wants. Some women will encourage the father to make the decision in order to lessen their own guilt.

The position of choice can be devastating. There is a feeling of bitterness about being put in this position. And yet, there is no alternative.

I just went crazy with it. Hysterical....I could not stand for the baby to move, just could not stand it. My emotional rejection of the child came early—embracing her and rejecting her at the same time. Crying for her. Not knowing if I could deal with birthing her knowing what I knew about her.[5] (p. 166)

For those who choose to abort or have selective termination the grief process intensifies. What was the anticipation of the loss of a healthy baby becomes a real loss. In reviewing the experiences of women who have had miscarriages, there is a significant difference in the minds of the women: these women *choose to* terminate a pregnancy. Though a miscarriage is an intensive painful experience, women who miscarry are not responsible for having made the choice that led to the death of the fetus. The factor of choice is a tremendous, emotional burden for women who choose to abort.

Another feeling is anger, which manifests in a variety of ways. A woman may express anger toward the doctor and the hospital by indicating that the staff or facility are somehow responsible for what has happened. She may also blame God for causing her to conceive a defective baby. Some women blame themselves and may display self-destructive behavior as punishment for having conceived and/or chosen to abort the baby. They may withdraw from family and friends because they feel unworthy of relationships and support. They may gain or lose significant amounts of weight, drink excessively, abuse drugs, and set themselves up to be fired at work.

Marriages and partnerships can undergo tremendous stress at this time. A woman may focus her anger at her mate. Rather than confront the guilt over her choice, she will blame her partner. It was his gene. It was the pressure he imposed to conceive or abort. Undeniably, there are men who do exert these intense pressures and there is validity for the anger, but emotionally she accepts the blame because she is aware that the final decision was hers.

A man's expressed feelings of shock, hurt and disappointment contribute to stress in the relationship. Often their pain is overlooked as doctors as well as family and friends seek to counsel and support the woman. It is also a lonely experience for a man. He feels very helpless and scared. Nothing he can do or say can fix the situation. He feels responsible; he reflects on the pressure he exerted on his partner to conceive or abort; he thinks about time he spent away from home; or he perceives of himself as failing to understand. Perhaps he believes it was his gene that contributed to the defect, or possibly he blames his mate and is confused by his anger toward her.

Often a man will feel he is not entitled to his grief. He tells himself that he is going through less than his partner is and tries to discount his pain. It is important to not abandon a man during this experience. There is a very strong tendency to ignore the man, even though he is the parent of the fetus, because most of the focus is on the woman. Such a focus is facilitated by the fact that women often show their feelings more easily. A woman may cry when she is frightened, angry or sad, whereas a man often withholds his feelings and may be reluctant to let others see his discomfort.

Consider the following example. A couple was told that the ultrasound showed fetal demise. The couple had come to the hospital for CVS because of advanced age. They had reported during the intake that there was light spotting for 2 days, but the woman was not alarmed since she had also had spotting during a prior successful pregnancy. When the doctor informed them of the demise the man sat without moving and stared into space. He then reached over to his wife and attempted to touch her shoulder. She seemed oblivious. They decided to proceed with the CVS to gain information about the death. As the procedure progressed, he sat frozen in the chair and said nothing. When the procedure was finished, he accompanied his wife out of the room and she went to change her clothes. When I walked out into the hallway, the man continued to sit in the chair with a blank look on his face. In other circumstances his pain might have been overlooked because of his silence and not so visible signs of grief.

On another occasion there was a man who had anguished over the termination of a pregnancy for 2 years. When it was determined through amniocentesis that the baby had Down syndrome, he and his wife had readily agreed to terminate. Because he was afraid of precipitating more sadness in his wife who was already in distress, he decided to withhold his feelings. He had never expressed any of his feelings, but had provided his wife with emotional support. In the 6 months prior to seeking counseling, he had been to 3 medical doctors with somatic complaints. Each encouraged him to seek psychological help when their tests revealed no physical illness. At the start of counseling, he was very depressed and unable to explain the source of his sadness. After a few questions that prompted him to talk about the abortion he was able to get to the root of the problem. As he described the experience, relating his knowledge about the results of the amniocentesis and going through the abortion, he was overcome by sobbing. He later said he was shocked by his response.

All of the feelings of the partners can contribute to estrangement in the relationship if they do not openly and honestly express themselves.

It is important not to discount the effects of this experience on the siblings. At an early age, children are capable of understanding that they will be having a brother or sister. They will often announce to perfect strangers that "Mommy has a baby in her tummy." Just as they are invited to share in the excited anticipation of a baby, so should they be included in the process of grieving the loss. Children are very aware of their parents' feelings, and it is wise to validate the perception that something is wrong and that the parent is sad. Because of their self-centered tendencies, a child needs to be reassured that they did not cause the sadness or the death of the baby.

It is a loss for the sibling too. Often they eagerly await an anticipated playmate, and other times they reluctantly await an anticipated competitor. In either case, it is a loss, and it is important to respect their right to know. Children can become very distrusting of their parents if someone else reveals the loss of the baby to them. Their need to grieve should be respected. They will likely ask many questions, some arising from a natural curiosity and others resulting from anxiety. The idea of a baby dying may feel threatening, and they need to be reassured that they will be all right.

Parents should be honest with children, but not flood them with too much information. Usually, it is best to present a basic outline of the events, and then allow the child to indicate the best way to proceed. Questions will reflect what knowledge a child is ready to receive. Emotional responses can vary. It is possible that a child will not feel terribly upset, but possible that a child will be frightened and sad. Either response should be respected, and there should be an opportunity to discuss feelings. It is very appropriate to include a sibling in whatever ritual the parents may choose to denote the termination of the pregnancy.

In some situations, an unborn or aborted child becomes the ghost of the "perfect child" in a family, i.e., the fetus becomes idealized. The parents may imagine what this child would have been in life if he or she had lived, and often the imagined characteristics become hyperbolized. In these cases, the living siblings often find that they are competing with a ghost. Because the unborn child is imagined in such idealistic ways, the siblings can never win. Parents are typically unaware of the fact that they have idealized the unborn baby, and are less aware of its impact on the surviving children. Siblings will describe a feeling of never being quite good enough for their parents, yet are unaware of how the standard was set.

It is best to confront this issue directly, perhaps by discussing the possibility of the "perfect child" phenomenon to the parents. This precipitates a conscious awareness and reduces the likelihood of it occurring.

Women often feel reticent, embarrassed or awkward about sharing their feelings. This contributes to a strong sense of isolation or emotional withdrawal. Some women intentionally do not announce their pregnancies if they are concerned about possible defects. Thus, support is often not offered because people do not know what has happened. Women may also seek to avoid people who are pregnant or who have children: it is too painful to confront what might have been. They are often afraid that people are judging what they have done or what has occurred.

Each stage of this experience involves a grief response. When a person learns that there is suspicion of a problem in the fetus, there is fear for the loss of one's dream about one's child. For those who decide not to proceed with prenatal testing, and are left wondering until the baby is born, the experience of uncertainty is very stressful and lonely. If prenatal diagnosis indicates a problem, grief is again experienced because the diagnosis confirms loss of a dream; and, if the testing is followed by abortion, there is the grief of the baby's death. Each stage is anguishing; time seems slowed. There is a feeling of disconnection from everyone and everything. A person feels alone. There is the hope of "waking up and discovering it is all a bad dream." Many fantasize about committing suicide rather than having to feel the pain.

The symptoms of going through this grief process vary from one person to the next. As one moves through stages of shock, denial, bewilderment, confusion, anger, sadness, guilt and, hopefully, reconciliation or acceptance, one's behavior varies. There are stages of emotional incubation as women withdraw into themselves as they work to reconcile their pain or decision. Withdrawal from people and activities is also symptomatic of depression; also, here may be a loss or increase of appetite. Erratic sleeping patterns may develop: a woman may sleep more than usual, less than usual or report interrupted sleep.

A reduced sex drive often accompanies depression, but some women report heightened sexuality, which tends to enhance their need to be validated as women. Alcohol or drugs may be taken to numb the pain. A woman may overreact to other people and events as her emotions become fragile. As mentioned earlier, self-destructive behaviors may ensue as a means of inflicting punishment on herself for having produced an "imperfect" child or for choosing to abort it.

Doctors may also see an increase in physical complaints. It is common for grieving people to become hypersensitive to their bodies. In some cases this may be because a woman is not taking good care of herself and may be more vulnerable physically. Others may translate their emotional pain to physical pain that has no medical origin. Stomach problems, headaches, acidity, muscular tension and nausea are often symptomatic of depression and anxiety. However, it is important to not make that assumption. If no physical source was discovered after an examination, it would be helpful to advise the patient to seek counseling. In all likelihood, with support and understanding, these symptoms may diminish rather quickly.

Valuable interventions that can be made by the people who work in the area of birth defects include:

1. Listen. Not being listened to is a common complaint verbalized by many patients.
2. Recognize and allow the expression of feelings. This is an intense time, and many women do not feel safe communicating with anyone but their doctors.
3. Avoid judgment. It is a woman's right to decide what she needs to do. Often what is self-destructive for one person is self-constructive for another. Be sensitive to the differences.
4. Avoid giving advice. Give information openly and honestly about the causes, options and potential for the future. This will enable a woman to make her own decision.
5. Do not patronize a woman with comments such as, "I understand what you are going through." You will be trusted more if you acknowledge her suffering and not try to sympathize.
6. Avoid comments meant to lessen the pain such as, "You can try again," "It is nature's way....It is the best thing for the baby." This type of statement does not respect a woman's struggle. Pain is a part of the experience.
7. If she wishes, allow a woman to see an ultrasound. Do not make a decision for her despite how upset she may become. She is entitled to the pain and may need to see the ultrasound in order to take the next step.
8. Let the woman know that she can have access to the pictures, if she so chooses.
9. Do not discourage a woman from wanting to bury the fetus if she chooses. It may be wise to let her know that this is an option and not an expectation.
10. Encourage some ritual or action to acknowledge the death. It is a way of providing some validation and closure.
11. Do not tell a woman she will get over it; most never do.
12. Encourage therapy or a self-help group. It is important to express the feelings precipitated by this experience. Often a trained professional or people who have been through the experience can provide support. Have a referral list available.

This chapter has thus far addressed the emotional impact in the field of genetic reproduction. It is also imperative to recognize the emotional effects on the professionals involved in the field. Many doctors experience conflicting feelings about their work, not unlike the polarities mentioned earlier for the women. Doctors experience fear also. There is the fear of accidentally aborting a healthy fetus or of delivering a defective baby.

Some doctors are opposed to abortion because of religious or moral convictions. It is important to be honest about these beliefs and encourage women to consult with other professionals rather than of biasing their decisions.

There is also the risk of becoming desensitized to the point of debilitating a woman's decision. Clearly, after doing many procedures, a doctor is likely to develop confidence in the test or method. It is possible at these junctures to lose sight of the woman's anxiety and ongoing doubt. However, a woman will not find her experience to be a clear-cut medical problem that is treated in clear-cut ways, and thus the professional staff will be exposed over and over again to a world that involves pain, anger and fear as well as relief and appreciation. If a physician can confront that reality, he or she will truly offer a woman an option to make the right decision for herself. This is the true reward.

References

1. Cole D. It might have been: mourning the unborn. *Psychology Today.* July 1987;64.
2. Drugan A, Greb A, Johnson MP, et al. Determinants of parental decisions to abort for chromosome abnormalities. *Prenat Diagn.* 1990;10:483.
3. Evans ML, Bottoms SF, Carducci TJ, et al. Parental perceptions of genetic risks: it's the spouse's fault. Proceedings of the Society of Perinatal Obstetricians; 1987 Feb 5–7; Orlando, Florida.
4. Evans MI, Bottoms SF, Carducci TJ, et al. Determinants of altered anxiety following abnormal maternal serum alpha-fetoprotein screening. *Am J Obstet Gynecol.* 1988;159:1501.
5. Carnevale A, Lisker R, Villa AR, et al. Counseling following diagnosis of a fetal abnormality: comparison of different clinical specialists in Mexico. *Am J Med Genet.* 1997;69:23–28.
6. Bryar SH. One day you're pregnant and one day you're not: pregnancy interruption for fetal anomalies. *J Obstet Gynecol Neonatal Nurs.* 1997;26:559–566.
7. Bell M, Stoneman Z. Reactions to prenatal testing: reflection of religiosity and attitudes toward abortion and people with disabilities. *Am J Ment Retard.* 2000;105:1–13.
8. Katz-Rothman B. *The Tentative Pregnancy.* New York: Viking Press; 1986.

COUNSELING FOR ABNORMALITIES

Anne Greb / Jane Wegner

INTRODUCTION

Prenatal diagnosis is an important option for many families with an increased risk for having a child with a birth defect or genetic condition. In fact, many of these couples would not consider another pregnancy without the ability to know whether or not their unborn fetus is affected with their family's genetic disorder. Fortunately, the vast majority of families are provided with reassurance that the disorder is not present in their fetus. Consequently, the availability of prenatal diagnosis has actually led to the birth of many healthy babies that would otherwise have not occurred. However, approximately 5% of patients receive abnormal results following prenatal diagnosis and require skillful and timely counseling from the health care team.[1] The purpose of this chapter is to describe a protocol for counseling this group of patients, their partners and families. This chapter is written by a genetic counselor, who has worked for many years with families that have received abnormal prenatal diagnostic results. The chapter also incorporates the perspective of a patient who relates her experiences and has had to deal with the issues associated with the prenatal diagnosis of a chromosome abnormality.

The ability to diagnose chromosome abnormalities prenatally became a reality in the early 1970s, which helped to spark the initial interest in clinical genetics that ultimately resulted in the current genetic revolution. In the 1980s, maternal serum alphafetoprotein screening for neural tube defects became routine, and its usefulness in screening for Down syndrome was recognized. Also during this time, chorionic villus sampling (CVS) moved the application of prenatal diagnosis to the first trimester and work was done to develop in utero therapies for specific birth defects. The Human Genome Project (HGP) began in 1990 and achieved its goal of obtaining a draft sequence of the entire human genome in February 2001. Laboratory methods continued to improve, which made molecular diagnosis more efficient and cost effective. Because of these successes, prenatal diagnosis has become common for a wide range of birth defects and genetic conditions as well as a fundamental part of routine obstetrical care and management.

INDICATION FOR PRENATAL DIAGNOSIS

In general there are 2 groups of patients who may be offered prenatal diagnosis: those at risk of recurrence and those at risk of occurrence. Couples at risk of recurrence include patients who have had recurrent and unexplained pregnancy losses resulting from a genetic cause and those who have a family member with any of the following conditions: multiple congenital anomalies (including chromosome abnormalities), isolated birth defects, single gene disorders, skeletal dysplasias,

visual and/or hearing impairments or mental retardation. Couples at risk of occurrence include those in the following circumstances: couples who are related or consanguineous, of increased maternal or paternal age, women of a specific ethnic background in which there is an increased frequency of harmful autosomal recessive genes, exposed to a potential teratogen during pregnancy, women with an abnormal maternal serum screen, and women who have had an ultrasound evaluation that revealed a specific fetal abnormality or more subtle ultrasound findings that may be associated with an underlying fetal anomaly. It is important, however, to realize that the majority of birth defects occur "out of the blue" to couples with no known risk factors. This latter group of patients usually has no reason to suspect a problem in their fetus and consequently is completely unprepared to deal with the complex issues, emotions and decision making that surrounds the prenatal diagnosis of a fetal anomaly.

Rebecca was our third pregnancy. We had a miscarriage with our first pregnancy and then a healthy baby girl who was two years old at that time. Aside from being exposed to chicken pox and needing to get a vaccination, this pregnancy seemed to be going along normally. I was 30 years old and had no reason to be concerned about any problems with my pregnancy or baby. I wasn't offered the MSAFP test, but this didn't worry me since I did not have that test with my last pregnancy and everything turned out fine. I was looking forward to having an ultrasound done, which my doctor scheduled during my sixth month. The ultrasound examination in my doctor's office at 25 weeks showed that the baby was smaller than expected. At the time, my obstetrician put my due date back by one month even though I was sure of my menstrual dates. I was frustrated that she didn't trust the accuracy of my information. I was just told to come back one month later. I was concerned because I was certain about my dates. My obstetrician did another ultrasound the next month and again the baby's growth wasn't keeping up with the previous ultrasound measurements. I was told I would just have a "petite" baby. Finally she realized something else might be going on and referred me to a maternal fetal medicine specialist.

I saw the specialist and had another ultrasound. He wasn't initially concerned with the baby's growth until he did a follow-up ultrasound a few weeks later and compared both measurements. During that first ultrasound he also noticed something about the baby's heart that wasn't completely normal. He thought it was just a normal variation, but wanted to look at the heart in a couple weeks. At the next follow-up ultrasound it was now obvious that the baby's growth was lagging behind and something wasn't right with the heart. A fetal echocardiogram and amniocentesis was suggested and both were performed the next week.

PRENATAL DIAGNOSTIC TECHNIQUES AND COUNSELING

There are several techniques that can be utilized in the prenatal diagnosis of birth defects and genetics conditions, which are discussed in detail elsewhere in this textbook. These include standard invasive procedures such as amniocentesis, CVS, and cordocentesis, as well as noninvasive procedures such as ultrasonography. Other procedures such as embryoscopy, 3-D ultrasonography, ultrafast MRI, and specific fetal tissue biopsies are available at more comprehensive prenatal diagnostic centers. Pre-implantation genetic diagnosis is becoming more readily available as a diagnostic technique that allows those couples at an increased risk for certain disorders to undergo in vitro fertilization (IVF) with the implantation of unaffected embryos. It is usually recommended that these couples undergo subsequent prenatal diagnosis to confirm the predicted result. For more common chromosome abnormalities efforts are currently underway to isolate and characterize fetal cells in the maternal circulation as a first trimester screening method. Once available, although much more needs to be done before this is clinically useful, it will greatly increase the ability to detect certain chromosome abnormalities antenatally.

Prenatal diagnostic techniques should be differentiated from prenatal screening methods. Screening tests, such as maternal serum screening and routine ultrasound screening, are usually not intended to provide a definitive diagnosis. Instead screenings identify a subset of the population for whom prenatal diagnostic tests should be offered. Unless properly counseled prior to the screening test, a patient will inevitably interpret a positive screening test as meaning that there *is* a problem with their unborn baby and endure unnecessary panic and stress.

The importance of counseling and informed consent prior to any prenatal diagnostic procedure cannot be over emphasized. *Time taken at this point will greatly reduce unnecessary confusion and frustration in the event that an abnormal result occurs.* During this initial genetic-counseling session, the topics that should be discussed include information about the risks and characteristics of the condition being tested should be discussed, the nature of the procedure and risk of complications, method, accuracy and limitations of the specific laboratory tests being performed. The counselor should also mention the possible options available to the couple if an abnormal result is found—*at the time of counseling the couple does not need to know their course of action, only what decision making they could face in the event of an abnormal result.* Finally, the counselor should explain how the results will be relayed to the couple as well as mention any other unrelated conditions that are being tested for (e.g., the measurement of alphafetoprotein levels to test for open neural tube defects even though there is not an increased risk in patients of advanced maternal age).

FACILITATING THE WAITING PERIOD, INFORMING THE PATIENT OF THE RESULTS, AND PROVIDING THE NECESSARY INFORMATION AND SUPPORT

Waiting for test results can be extremely difficult for patients, especially if there is already suspicion of a problem. During this time, it is important to encourage the patient to call for support and to check on the status of their results. Even though results are normally relayed to the patient as soon as they are available, if patients feel it is all right to call periodically, then they have a sense of control and purpose. Also, offering to check with the laboratory—even if just to report that everything is progressing along as anticipated and to confirm when the result is expected—can be very helpful and reassuring. The health care provider can supply tremendous comfort and help to patients, who oftentimes must wait weeks for the results, by simply validating that the waiting period is hard, and reassuring the patients that they will be contacted as soon as the results are available.

Giving bad news is difficult and stressful for any health care provider. However, what the patient hears and understands, and how she integrates and reacts to the news depends on how the information is conveyed. Usually, nothing can be offered in terms of a cure or effective treatment for a diagnosed fetal anomaly. However, health care providers can offer empathy, time and resources to the patient and her family as they try to make sense out of what has happened and cope with the diagnosis. There are certain techniques and strategies for conveying abnormal prenatal diagnostic results that are better than others.[1]

Often the initial information about an abnormal result must be given over the telephone. In this circumstance, the call should be made in the evening when both the patient and her partner are likely to be home. Also, it should be when the health care professional can spend time on the telephone to provide support and answer questions. The important information to relay initially is that *yes* there is a problem and it is important to meet as soon as possible to discuss the details of the diagnosis. *Do not beat around the bush:* be direct, yet caring, with information that is straightforward, accurate, and not technical. The patient is often in shock and not able to remember specific details. Let her determine how much information she is ready for at this point. Make sure there is a support person either present or that she can contact immediately. Have specific information about the time and place for the follow-up appointment the next day. Be sure to inform any other health care providers associated with the case about the diagnosis— often patients call others involved in their care to get additional input and opinions.

If the problem is identified during a routine ultrasound evaluation, then the approach should be similar. Inform her that a problem has been identified and be prepared to answer questions. *Do not have a lengthy discussion* while the patient is lying on the ultrasound table—finish the scan, let her dress, ask whether or not a support person came with her and find a quiet place to sit down for the discussion. Again, the patient can absorb very little information at this point. It is probably most helpful to give the patient some time to realize there is a problem, gather her support system together and schedule a followup visit for the next day, when the ultrasound findings can be described in more detail and indicate any specific invasive testing. Conveying a sense of empathy and willingness to do what ever is needed to help is a critical contribution made on the part of the healthcare team.

When the patient and her family are ready, it is important that they have accurate and complete information about the diagnosis in order to make informed decisions about any subsequent testing that might be indicated, pregnancy and neonatal management, and the option of pregnancy termination. Providing written information that is not too technical will be important. This augments the counseling process by allowing the patient to absorb information. A referral to a medical subspecialist who cares for individuals with the specific diagnosis can be helpful and should *always* be offered if indicated and available. Other resources some families find helpful are disease specific support groups. It is important to be familiar with all referral sources and to know that the information provided is accurate, appropriate and balanced. For example, the patient may be given very different (and often optimistic) information about a certain condition from a pediatric specialist. This is usually because the prenatal natural history of the condition is different than the natural history of those neonates who survive to be seen by the pediatric specialist. It is important that all information be provided in a manner that is *not* judgmental or directive. Lastly, patients may utilize the Internet as a way to gather information and/or seek out other specialists. It is important to be familiar with information available on the Internet and to encourage patients to share the information with the healthcare team so it can be reviewed for accuracy.

If possible, encourage the family to take as much time as necessary to gather and digest all the information they need before making a decision about whether or not to continue the pregnancy. However, these decisions, which require the integration of complex medical information, often must be made within pressing time constraints.

Families often ask if there is any chance that the diagnosis could be wrong. An explanation of the testing procedure, how the diagnosis was made and the accuracy of the test results should be given again. For some couples, actual confirmation by a repeat procedure and/or a second opinion may be important and should be supported if time allows.

In some situations, the prenatal findings, or the implications of the findings, are uncertain. For example, this can happen with particular ultrasound findings and unusual or subtle chromosomal findings. It is important that the healthcare team do a comprehensive literature search and consult with recognized experts in the field. They need to be honest with the patient about the lack of, or limited information available. As a consequence, the patient and her family are left knowing there is a problem (or potential problem), but they do not have specific information. The lack of information is very confusing for the patient who is not sure whether to continue hoping or start grieving. In some circumstances, further tests may be helpful to clarify the findings. Other times, it is not until the fetus can be examined after birth that light is shed on the prenatal findings. Needless to say, the decision-making task becomes even more burdensome in the case of diagnostic uncertainty.

In the face of an abnormal or potentially abnormal result as the consequence of prenatal diagnosis, the patient and her family are likely to be in a psychological state of shock.[2] As they begin to absorb the reality of the diagnosis, their emotional state will continue to reflect other stages of grief and mourning such as: denial, sadness or anger. Families should be encouraged to express these feelings. Support, time and privacy should be provided to them as they begin to work through the grieving process.

Fourteen days passed by before the doctor called with the amniocentesis results. This was the longest two weeks of my life. I met with my obstetrician while waiting for results and expressed my concerns as to why it was taking so long. I was hoping she would be willing to call the laboratory and see if she could obtain any information. However, she was not willing to make the phone call.

The specialist finally called and confirmed my worst nightmare. Our little girl had Wolf-Hirschhorn or 4p-syndrome. Over the telephone, the doctor explained in medical terms—as though he was reading from a medical textbook—about Wolf-Hirschhorn syndrome. When you hear this type of news about your child it is extremely difficult to comprehend what the doctor is telling you. I started asking him several questions and he basically told me to give my sister a call and 'that she can probably explain it to me better.' My sister, who lives in a different state, just happened to be a genetic counselor and was already doing a lot to try and help me through this whole ordeal. The specialist ended the phone call by asking me to give him a call in the morning to come in and talk. After I hung up the phone I called my sister to find out what was really wrong with our child. I desperately needed more information, but felt bad putting my sister in the position that she would be the one to have to do this. She gave me some information, but told me I really needed to meet in person with a genetic counselor who could explain what this condition meant and what my options were. I asked her what she meant by options. She told me that even though I was in my third trimester, pregnancy termination was still an option in a few states. My sister had worked with many families in similar situations before, however, this time she wanted to be in the role of sister and not genetic counselor.

The next morning I called to set up a meeting with the MFM specialist. I was told he was not available and was at another hospital that day. At my sister's urging I called again and insisted he see us that day and we would be willing to meet him at the other hospital.

We went in and talked with him and he went over what our options were. He mentioned we could proceed with the pregnancy as high risk or basically let nature take its course. I then brought up the option of termination. He said yes this was also something we could do. At my request, he called to set up an appointment for us in the genetics clinic at our city's children's hospital. They were willing to see us immediately.

When we met with the geneticist and genetic counselor they right away made us feel as though they really were concerned about our situation and would do what they could to help. They took the time to really explain what the chromosome abnormality would mean for our child's health and development, and what the quality of life would be like for her and the rest of our family. They talked from their own experiences of taking care of children with Wolf-Hirschhorn syndrome and not from just reading information out of a medical textbook. I finally felt like I had enough information to begin to make decisions about my options. We also discussed the option of pregnancy termination and they reassured us that this was a reasonable option given the severity of the condition. They told me they would facilitate the arrangements and would support us if this is what we chose to do. I finally felt like there were people out there who truly cared. We left and went to my parents' house to pick up our daughter and to inform them about what was going on.

Each morning I woke up hoping this was not true and was all a nightmare. But it was not. After going over everything we had learned the past few days about Wolf-Hirschhorn syndrome, we now needed to make the most difficult decision of our lives. We chose to terminate the pregnancy. We informed the genetic counselor of our decision and she made the necessary arrangements. Because we were in our third trimester, we needed to go out of state.

As I look back, I remember how devastated I felt throughout this whole experience; how in less than a week our entire lives had been turned upside down. One day life was wonderful and the next we learned about Wolf-Hirschhorn syndrome—something we had never even heard about before, now suddenly consuming our every waking moment. We were getting on an airplane, going out of state, away from our family and friends to end the hopes and dreams of bringing home a child to love. We were going someplace strange and far away. I had never felt so heartbroken in my life. I remember thinking over and over "This is not the way it was supposed to be."

THE DECISION-MAKING PROCESS

Families need information and support so they can make an informed decision about whether or not to continue a pregnancy in which a fetal abnormality is found. Seldom is there a cure or effective treatment so families grapple with trying to decide which painful outcome is "less worse." Decisions are made not only based on the medical facts surrounding the diagnosis;[3,4] but also on how the diagnosis will impact the rest of the family, particularly the couple's other children, and financial constraints as well as moral, religious and cultural values.[5] The field of medical genetics is deeply committed to patient autonomy and informed decision-making. The fact that families faced with the same diagnosis make different decisions and utilize different coping mechanisms must be respected and valued. Individuals and their families react differently because of the spectrum of belief and value systems that exist within our society.

THE DECISION TO TERMINATE THE PREGNANCY

The health care team should recognize the distinction between choosing to end a pregnancy for social reasons and making a decision to end a pregnancy because of the knowledge of the poor prognosis. To help reduce the stigma of abortion, the health care provider must be nonjudgmental and supportive of the patient's decision. The next step in the counseling process is an exploration and explanation of the available pregnancy termination procedures. The types of procedures available are based on the diagnosis and whether or not there is a need for a postmortem evaluation, gestational age, health of the mother, experience and preference of the physician, preference of the patient, and any hospital rules and regulations.

Another important issue to discuss when describing the pros and cons of different pregnancy termination procedures is the potential psychological ramifications. Many patients may prefer a dilatation and extraction (D&E) procedure to an induction of labor because it is performed in the operating room under general anesthesia and is over relatively quickly. However, patients need to be cautioned that the grieving process will not end as easily. Patients should be encouraged to gather mementos of the pregnancy such as ultrasound pictures in order to remind them that the pregnancy and fetus did exist.

Other couples prefer an induction of labor procedure because it leads to the birth of an intact baby. This not only allows them to see and acknowledge the wanted child, whom they have lost because of its medical problems; but also allows the family to see the anomalies, which helps to validate their decision. Besides seeing the baby, the patient should be encouraged to hold, photograph, and name the baby. Many couples decide to have their baby baptized and/or plan a funeral or memorial service. If necessary, a postmortem evaluation should be performed to try and determine the etiology and subsequent recurrence risks. In arranging for an induction of labor procedure, every effort should be made to provide the patient with a private room on a nonmaternity floor.

Regardless of the method of pregnancy termination there are other things that should be provided to the couple to facilitate the grieving process.[6] A referral to a professional such as a social worker, psychologist and/or clergy member, who deals with grief and loss issues, is very helpful and should routinely be made. Other ways of memorializing the baby, such as planting a tree or donating to a charity, can be valuable to the family.

Before discharge, it will be important to discuss with the patient what physical (e.g., hormonal changes and possible lactation) and emotional changes she should expect. Talk with her about some of the emotional reactions that others who have had a similar experience report. These include: how emotional recovery is much more difficult than anticipated, difficult it will be to see other pregnant women and baby-related items in store aisles, difficult the time surrounding the baby's due date will be, male partners react and grieve differently, family members and friends may have difficulty knowing how to react to the loss and that, unfortunately, some individuals might make insensitive comments. Explain that they can expect to feel many emotions, and that this is a normal and important part of the grieving process. Many patients report that journaling can be extremely therapeutic in both the short term and long term. It not only helps to express feelings, document the events and serve as a reminder about how and why they arrived at their decision.

Tips on how to talk to family, friends and young children about the loss will also be helpful. Encourage the couple to find individuals whom they know will be supportive of the events surrounding their loss. Having a few nonjudgmental and caring people to listen will be invaluable. It is difficult for spouses to rely on each other because they are each on different emotional roller coasters and not in a position to be each other's sole support. It is not easy to know how or what to tell the rest of the world about the loss. Some patients simply state that there were problems with the pregnancy and that they lost the baby. For others, they feel it is important to be forthcoming about the events surrounding the loss, even if it means having to cope with some unpleasant reactions. Encourage the patient to ask close family and friends for help with this task. The couple needs to be very selfish during the initial period of grief and not worry about the needs or concerns of others. If necessary, they should be given several weeks of medical leave from work.

When dealing with other children, it is important to be honest; but keep explanations simple, and at a level appropriate with their ability to understand. Children should be included in the grieving process. Even if the parents pretend that everything is fine, the children will still sense that things are not; and, consequently, may be denied their need to grieve. Children should be encouraged to express their feelings and be reassured that they and the rest of the family will be all right. They need to be told that they were not the cause of the problem and that nothing they thought or did made this happen.

Specific resources for families who have made the decision to terminate a wanted pregnancy because of the presence of a fetal abnormality are available and should be utilized routinely. They include written information in the form of booklets, Internet sites and support groups specific for families in this circumstance. The health care provider should keep an updated file with current available resources and pass the information on to the patient. *A Heartbreaking Choice* is an Internet site (*www.aheartbreakingchoice.com*) that is designed for families who have chosen pregnancy termination in the face of a fetal anomaly. Besides the valuable written information for families, the site also maintains a listserv and has a list of regional support groups. Referral to more general pregnancy loss support groups or Internet sites is usually *not* appropriate for these families.

We arrived at the clinic where the pregnancy termination would take place to find abortion protestors. We had been warned about this, however, actually seeing the protestors was difficult. All I could think was that these people have no idea what we are going through. Once inside the clinic we filled out the necessary paperwork and began the next phase of our nightmare—actually going through with the termination. It turned out that there were seven other couples going through what we were. On one hand it was comforting to know we were not alone; but on the other hand hard to know that others were also suffering as we were. Our experience at the clinic was as positive as can be expected under the circumstances. The personnel there were caring and emotionally supportive. The opportunity to talk with other couples helped immensely. More decisions needed to be made: whether to see and hold our child, whether to have her baptized, and whether to have her cremated there or have her body delivered back home.

Rebecca Lynn was born on February 14th—Valentine's Day. Valentine's Day in our family would never be the same. We were able to see her and hold her that day. Right away I was able to see the physical signs that are apparent with Wolf-Hirschhorn syndrome. We held her for only a few moments. It was difficult because there was no family support available. We felt very alone at the most difficult time of our lives. After the actual termination, we did feel very relieved that the medical procedure was over. I ended up meeting another woman who was also going through the same thing while at the clinic and I have kept in contact with her over the years since the termination. I am grateful for her friendship and support, as the difficult months and years have passed.

As we left the clinic to return back home, we were given photographs of our daughter, handprints, footprints, and a certificate to take home. Once home we began the very long road to emotional recovery. We needed to let family and friends know that our baby had died. How do you tell people you have terminated your pregnancy? How do you tell people that the medical condition of your unborn child is horrifying enough to want to end her life before it even began—especially in a society where this is not an acceptable action? How do you make people understand what it is like, as a parent, to be forced to make that type of decision for a child you very much wanted and already loved? When people have a hard time talking about grief in general, how does someone comfort you in your grief when they have never even seen the person you are grieving for?

My six-week postpartum check-up was very difficult. Just walking into the office was hard. I remember thinking 'the last time I was here I was pregnant.' Also, seeing all the other pregnant women sitting there was very hard. I had all along sensed that my obstetrician was not supportive of our decision to terminate the pregnancy. After the exam was over, she needed to sign some papers from the clinic where I had the termination procedure performed to say she had examined me, which she reluctantly did. She never really seemed to care about how I was doing, although, she did hand me a piece of paper with a phone number on it for a pregnancy loss support group named RESOLVE Through Sharing. I just threw the number away when I got home. I never went back to see her. I was often tempted to write her a letter expressing my disappointment with how she handled our situation, but never did. I just started looking for a new obstetrician.

The next several months were very difficult. People stopped calling to see how I was doing. Life for everyone else was pretty much back to normal. Somehow I seemed to get through each day one at a time. Having my older daughter to care for seemed to be the only reason to get up in the morning.

The next difficult hurdle to tackle was preparing for Rebecca's memorial service. We met with the funeral home to start preparing for the service. The woman at the funeral home was very nice and I felt comfortable telling her that we had terminated the pregnancy. We went over some ideas for songs, poems, etc. I just kept thinking 'In a million years I would have never thought that at the age of 30 I would be preparing a memorial service for my own child.' The memorial service was scheduled for May 18th. It was probably one of the most difficult days of my life.

The hardest part about dealing with the loss of a child whose life you decided to end because of a serious medical problem is that you just feel so alone. Nobody around you has any idea what you are going through. All you want is for people to acknowledge how painful and real your grief is. There are very few support groups or books available specifically related to pregnancy termination. We ended up getting connected with a support group about an hour away that was specifically for people who had terminated a pregnancy because of problems with the baby. Here, we were finally able to talk to people who had to make the same decisions as we did.

I have also remained in contact with the woman I met at the clinic where the termination took place. She had also terminated her second pregnancy, a little girl. I can truly say she is the only person on earth I can talk to who really understands what I have been through. She has been a great source of support over the four years since we met.

THE DECISION TO CONTINUE THE PREGNANCY

The decision to continue with a pregnancy, when a fetal abnormality has been diagnosed, takes into consideration many complex factors. Sometimes the decision is made because of a more favorable prognosis,[4] and other times a prenatal or neonatal intervention can be offered to improve the outcome. Just as the healthcare provider must be nonjudgmental and supportive of the decision to terminate a pregnancy, they must likewise support the decision to continue a pregnancy in which a fetal anomaly has been diagnosed.

After the decision to continue with the pregnancy has been made, the couple will continue to deal with the emotional issues surrounding the loss of a "normal" baby. These include feelings associated with loss and grief such as sadness and anger. The family is faced with working through the grieving process as they also anticipate and prepare for the birth of a baby with special medical needs. The opportunity for the patient and her family to talk with a therapist should be encouraged.

Prenatal diagnosis of fetal abnormalities allows parents the opportunity to be prepared for the birth of their child by having time to learn about the condition as well as issues related to delivery, treatment and postnatal management.[7] If surgical intervention is indicated following delivery, the parents should meet with the pediatric surgeon to better understand the details of the surgery and recovery.[8] In fact, a big advantage of prenatal diagnosis is the ability to be able to plan and prepare for postnatal surgical treatment following delivery in a tertiary carecenter.[9] Prior to delivery, many families find it helpful to meet with the neonatal intensive care unit (NICU) staff in order to become familiar with technical aspects of the nursery and other issues such as infant feeding and visiting hours. Also, families should become acquainted with community and financial resources.

Usually the involvement of a maternal fetal-medicine specialist, who assists in or takes over the prenatal care, is necessary. Serial ultrasound evaluations may be needed to monitor the status of a specific fetal anomaly (e.g., hydrocephalus). Input from a reproductive and/or pediatric geneticist may be important to clarify the diagnosis, etiology and natural history of a particular condition. The neonatology staff needs to be consulted and told of the pending birth of a baby with medical problems. During this period, families often benefit from speaking to other families who have children with the same diagnosis for information and support.

In some situations, a couple may decide to continue with a pregnancy in spite of an extremely poor (e.g., trisomy 13) or even lethal (e.g., anencephaly) prognosis. This decision may have been made because of religious beliefs or perhaps the couple wants the time during pregnancy and after delivery to spend with their wanted, although very sick, child. These pregnancies are usually expectantly managed. In other words, no technical intervention for the sake of the fetus; nature is allowed to take its course. The family and healthcare team need to work closely together to ensure that the experience is as positive as possible, and that the family has input into how the pregnancy, delivery and neonatal care are managed.

As is the case with couples that have chosen to terminate a wanted pregnancy in the face of a fetal abnormality, it is important that families who continue a pregnancy with a poor fetal prognosis have time after delivery to see, hold and take photographs of their baby. If the baby dies, then a discussion about whether or not to have the baby baptized and to have a funeral or memorial service needs to take place. A postmortem evaluation is important in most cases to document the prenatal findings and identify any other anomalies in an attempt to make diagnosis. During delivery, it will be important that the patient has a private room and that the nursing and NICU staff be told about the situation. The same psychosocial issues that are relevant following a couple's decision to terminate a pregnancy also apply to couples that continue a pregnancy associated with a poor fetal outcome, and these issues will need to be addressed. Again, these include a discussion about what physical and emotional changes to expect, how to talk to family and friends and the available support services in the area and on the Internet. If the patient has not yet spoken with a grief counselor, this issue should be brought up again and followup encouraged.

Although the option of prenatal treatment of a fetal anomaly is not common, the list of birth defects that can be considered for in utero treatment is growing, and currently includes diaphragmatic hernia, obstructive uropathy, cardiac arrhythmia, congenital cystic adenomatoid malformation (CCAM), sacrococcygeal teratoma, neural tube defect, certain metabolic disorders such as congenital adrenal hyperplasia and vitamin-B_{12} responsive methylmalonic aciduria, and certain inherited disorders that are amenable to stem cell therapy such as X-linked severe combined immunodeficiency syndrome (SCIDS). Some treatments are moderately invasive, whereas others involve open fetal surgery and present a considerable risk to the mother and fetus. If a birth defect is identified prenatally and fetal treatment is an option, then the patient needs to be referred to one of the few worldwide centers that have the appropriate experience and expertise to counsel the patient and her family about the risks, benefits and limitations of in utero treatment.[10]

FOLLOWUP COUNSELING

The months following the loss of a baby are emotionally difficult, especially after the diagnosis of a fetal abnormality. Supportive phone calls during the weeks following the delivery will be important. Also important within the first few months is a follow-up appointment to review the diagnosis, etiology, recurrence risks and prenatal diagnostic options available during possible subsequent pregnancies.[11] If a postmortem evaluation was performed, then at this time the results need to be reviewed with the couple. Time must be provided in order to answer questions and help the couple understand the genetic and medical aspects surrounding what has happened. This is a very important part of helping the family make some sense out of their difficult situation.

A discussion about how the couple is coping emotionally needs to continue during this time. Inquire about their support systems: how the experience has affected their relationship with each other, how their children have reacted to what has happened and how have other family members and friends responded to the situation. They need to know that the situation is difficult and being emotional is expected and normal. Encourage them to express their feelings and remind them again about local support groups and Internet sites that are applicable to their situation. Talk with them again about journaling as a method of documenting and validating their feelings and situation. Again, bring up the importance of seeing a psychotherapist for ongoing support and counseling. Finally, a letter should be sent to the patient summarizing all the information discussed at the follow-up counseling session.

THE NEXT PREGNANCY

When someone decides to have a child it is because they have a certain desire to bring a child into the world. I was one month from what was supposed to be a normal delivery that would result in a healthy baby to bring home. Suddenly all those hopes and dreams were shattered. After the termination, that feeling of wanting to bring another child into the world did not go away. Now I was faced with grieving for the child I thought I would bring home and also faced with the questions of when or if I will ever have another child to love. Part of me wanted to get pregnant right away because my desire to have a child was so great. But part of me was scared to death to ever be in the situation again where something so terrible could go wrong.

I chose to find a new obstetrician and that meant starting over with a new doctor. I needed to find someone who I could trust, someone who would understand how scared I felt at the thought of another pregnancy. It also meant that I had to tell my story again.

Six months after we terminated the pregnancy with Rebecca, I was pregnant again. I had found a new obstetrician with whom I felt comfortable. That was the easy part, now I had to make it through the next nine months. As I soon discovered, a subsequent pregnancy is an emotional roller coaster. I was still grieving over the loss of Rebecca, yet excited that a new life was upon us. Feelings of guilt, anger and sadness were part of everyday life. I felt guilty that I was excited about having another child. I felt like Rebecca was being even more and more forgotten. I wondered if I would feel resentment towards the new baby because Rebecca did not have a chance at life.

We had an early ultrasound done so we could date the pregnancy accurately. This time the due date would not change and not be an issue. We also scheduled another amniocentesis. This was a major hurdle. We were once again faced with the fact that something could be wrong with this child. A whole flood of emotions came back with having to go to the same hospital, the same high-risk doctor, the same hospital floor, the same office, and the same examining table where we were first told that our unborn child was not healthy.

The amniocentesis results came back with good news this time. After hearing the news one would think all is well. We knew the baby's chromosomes were normal, however, we still worried about the so many other things that could go wrong. I also realized that for me pregnancy was a time of worry and not a time of joyous anticipation. Friends and family all talked with excitement of a new baby arriving; I was scared to death. I got through this pregnancy one day at a time. Not until the very end of the pregnancy was I able to buy a new outfit and blanket for the baby for fear that once again, this baby would not come home with us.

Once we got closer to the actual due date, more emotions and fears began to erupt. Now I was faced with how would I react when I actually see the new baby? Would I be able to control my emotions in the delivery room? My last experience with delivering a child resulted in a dead baby. I really felt very alone at this point of the pregnancy. Those around me were excited because the new baby would be arriving soon and I was becoming an emotional wreck. This is a time I really could have used some emotional support.

Our third child arrived on her due date. She was a beautiful healthy little girl. The next few weeks were difficult—very bittersweet. I knew that I would not be holding my third daughter in my arms, had my second daughter lived. I felt guilty because I was feeling happy once again. Did I have the right to smile when Rebecca was not able to live a healthy life?

My third child is now three years old. As I sit here writing this, my fourth beautiful little eight-week-old daughter is at my side.

CONCLUSION

Modern technology, along with advances in science and medicine, has produced techniques that prenatally diagnose a wide spectrum of congenital anomalies and genetic conditions. The ability to diagnose fetal problems antenatally has resulted in greater successes for the treatment and management of an increasing number of fetal anomalies. This is truly an exciting time, and there is every reason to be optimistic that prenatal diagnosis and targeted intervention will decrease the morbidity and mortality associated with many serious conditions. However, the provision of appropriate counseling and support to families faced with the diagnosis of a fetal anomaly will be essential to the successful use of prenatal diagnosis and the further development of utero therapies.

DEDICATION

This chapter is dedicated to Rebecca Lynn Wegner. We will always remember you.

ACKNOWLEDGMENT

The authors would like to thank Peggy Rush, MS, CGC for reading this chapter and contributing her valuable comments and insightful perspective.

References

1. Fertel P, Reiss RE. Counseling prenatal diagnosis patients: the role of the social worker. *Soc Work Health Care*. 1997;24:47–63.
2. Matthews AL. Known fetal malformations during pregnancy: a human experience of loss. *Birth Defects*. 1990;26:168–175.
3. Drugan A, Greb A, Johnson MP, et al. Determinants of parental decisions to abort for chromosome abnormalities. *Prenat Diagn*. 1990;10:483–490.
4. Pryde PG, Drugan A, Johnson MP, et al. Prenatal diagnosis: choices women make about pursuing testing and acting on abnormal results. *Clin Obstet Gynecol*. 1993;36:496–509.
5. Punales-Morejon D. Genetic counseling and prenatal diagnosis: a multicultural perspective. *JAMWA*. 1997;52:30–32.
6. Furlong RM, Black RB. Pregnancy termination for genetic indications: the impact on families. *Soc Work Health Care*. 1984;10:17–34.
7. Clark SL, DeVors GR. Clinical Commentaries: Prenatal diagnosis for couples who would not consider abortion. *Obstet Gynecol*. 1988;73:1035–1037.
8. Crombleholme TM, D'Alton M, Cendron M, et al. Prenatal diagnosis and the pediatric surgeon: the impact of prenatal consultation on perinatal management. *J Pediatr Surg*. 1996;31:156–163.
9. Kemp J, Davenport M, Pernet A. Antenatally diagnosed surgical anomalies: the psychological effect of parental antenatal counseling. *J Pediatr Surg*. 1998;33:1376–1379.
10. Thomassen-Brepols, LJ. Psychological implications of fetal diagnosis and therapy. *Fetal Ther*. 1987;2:169–174.
11. Kenyon SL, Hackett GA, Campbell S. Termination of pregnancy following diagnosis of fetal malformations: the need for improved follow-up services. *Clin Obstet Gynecol*. 1988;31:91–100.

CHAPTER 49

TERMINATION OF PREGNANCY

Rony Diukman / James D. Goldberg

Many couples, when faced with the prenatal diagnosis of a genetic defect in their fetus, consider the option of pregnancy termination. It is important to provide these couples with accurate information concerning the various approaches to pregnancy termination in order for them to make an informed decision. It addition, it is critically important to have an understanding of studies that can be performed on the abortus to establish an accurate diagnosis and define a potential recurrence risk for the couple. This chapter will provide an overview of existing methods of pregnancy termination in the first and second trimester including selective termination of multiple gestations. The proper evaluation of the aborted fetus and psychological support for the couple will also be discussed.

FIRST TRIMESTER TERMINATION OF PREGNANCY

SURGICAL TECHNIQUES

Suction curettage and to a lesser extent sharp curettage are by far the most frequently used techniques for pregnancy termination in the first trimester.[1]

Suction Curettage and Dilation and Curettage (D&C)

Abdominal and bimanual examination are initially performed to determine the shape, position, and size of the uterus. Any questionable finding at this point, especially a discrepancy between dates and size, should be verified by ultrasound examination. A speculum examination is then performed at which time cervical cultures and a pap smear may be obtained. If laminaria are to be used they are inserted transcervically as sterilely as possible after povidone-iodine cleansing of the vagina and cervix. Laminaria tents, which are made from seaweed root, are tampon-like objects that can be inserted into the cervical canal through the internal os. They swell to 4–5 times their dry diameter without lengthening, resulting in cervical dilation. For first trimester abortion, laminaria can be left for several hours, although some physicians prefer overnight placement. The use of laminaria provides adequate dilatation and facilitates further mechanical dilation if needed. The number of tents used depends on the size of the cervical canal and the gestational age.

Those who advocate the use of laminaria believe that gradual dilatation of the cervix reduces the risk of cervical laceration, uterine perforation and the duration of the transcervical procedure is shorter and less painful.[2–4] The disadvantages are pain at insertion, infection and rupture of membranes. Synthetic hydrophilic dilators made of hydrogel polymer dilators have been recently introduced.[5] They have the advantage of complete sterilization and more rapid action. Prostaglandin preparations applied intracervically or intravaginally prior to first trimester termination have also been successfully used to facilitate the abortion procedure.[6,7]

After laminaria tents have been removed, the vagina is recleansed with a povidone-iodine solution. A paracervical block or general anesthesia may be used for the procedure. If a paracervical block is used, diazepam and meperidine may also be given by slow intravenous injection. The cervix is grasped with a tenaculum and the direction of the canal is ascertained with a uterine sound. If additional dilatation is required, manual dilatation is done by using steel dilators increasing by 0.5 mm between dilators. The dilator should be introduced slowly and carefully because at this stage serious perforation can occur.

At this point, suction curettage with a vacuum cannula is performed. The canula is introduced in the direction of the uterine curve. The principle motion of the suction handle is rotation with occasional in and out movements, while avoiding movement of the suction tip into the cervical canal. The vacuum aspiration is usually followed by a brief sharp curettage to verify that the uterus is empty.

The operator must perform a careful examination of the aspirated tissue by looking for fetal parts and placental villi. If no villi are seen, then the diagnosis of a failed abortion or ectopic pregnancy should be considered. Failed abortion can occasionally occur even when chorionic villi are histologically verified. Thus, making identification of gestational sac or fetal parts important.

COMPLICATIONS

First trimester terminations can result in a number of early or late complications, including uterine perforation, bleeding, laceration of the cervix, anesthesia-related problems, infection, and retention of gestational products. The overall rate of major complication such as severe hemorrhage, prolonged infection, and laparotomy/hysterectomy is estimated to be less than 1% (0.5–0.7%).[8] Failure to interrupt the pregnancy occurs in less than 0.5% of suction curettage procedures, and most commonly when the termination is attempted before 6 menstrual weeks.[8] Late complications such as tissue retention, anemia, infection and bleeding occur in about 2–3% of early abortions.

MEDICAL METHODS

A nonsurgical, outpatient, possibly self-administered method for termination of early pregnancy would be an attractive alternative to vacuum aspiration in early pregnancy.

PROSTAGLANDINS

The use of prostaglandins as abortifacients is based on their unique ability to stimulate uterine contractility even during early pregnancy. Unfortunately, naturally occurring prostaglandins, such as PGE2 and PGF2a, intravenously or intravaginally given in doses necessary to terminate pregnancy have a very high frequency of gastrointestinal and other side effects.[9] Prostaglandin analogues, such as 15-methyl PGE2, 15-methyl PGF2a, 16,16 dimethyl-trans-D2-PGE1 methylester, and others are effective when vaginally or intramuscularly given and are sufficiently stable to allow routine clinical use.[10] Gastrointestinal side effects, following treatment with PGE analogs, while reduced as compared to the natural prostaglandins, are still common. Vomiting and diarrhea occur in approximately 50% of patients.[7] The incidence of strong uterine pain is significantly higher (12%) than after vacuum aspiration. Prostaglandins can be used alone or in combination with antiprogestins such as RU486.[11,12] The frequency of complete abortion with prostaglandin E analogs varies between 92 and 94%.[10,13] The efficacy of vaginally administered PGE analogs has been compared with vacuum aspiration and found to be almost as effective as the surgical procedures.[14–16]

Vaginal suppositories and cervical pessaries are the preferred routes of prostaglandin administration. Therapy is available as PGE2 in 20 mg suppositories for vaginal application. A gel containing prostaglandins for cervical effacement is also available. PGE2 gel can be used in intracervical application prior to first trimester abortion. Using this approach resulted in cervical ripening and dilation (mean Hegar dilation of 11.8) with 80% of patients having a complete abortion.[6]

Prostaglandins currently are the most effective medical method for first trimester abortion. They produce complete evacuation in over 90% of cases. Unfortunately, side effects such as nausea and vomiting (40–50%) bleeding and pain that require analgesia (40%) and fever (5%) are significant complications.[13]

ANTIPROGESTINS

The antiprogestins listed in Table 49-1 are a class of drugs whose administration creates progesterone withdrawal conditions. They convert the uterus into an organ of spontaneous activity and reactivity and lower the threshold of myometrial response to prostaglandins.[10,17]

The various antiprogestins have different modes of action. Epostane is a progesterone synthesis inhibitor and Mifepristone (RU486) is a progesterone receptor blocker. Epostane inhibits the 3 β-hydroxysteroid dehydrogenase activity and blocks the conversion of pregnenolone to progesterone as well as that of dehydroepiandrosterone to androstenedione. RU-486 blocks progesterone receptors of the myometrium,

endometrium, and the decidua. Twenty-four to 36 hours following administration of an antiprogestin, regular uterine contractions appear. The increased sensitivity to prostaglandins starts at the same time. Studies show that RU486 used in early pregnancy causes complete abortion in 87% of patients using a single dose of 600 mg.[18] A higher success rate can be achieved if RU486 is given repeatedly over 2–4 days.

The efficacy of RU486 given in combination with different prostaglandins for termination of early pregnancy has been evaluated in several clinical studies.[10,11] Most commonly, a PGE2 analog was given as a vaginal suppository 48 hours after starting RU486. RU486 was given in a daily dose of 50 to 150 mg for 4 days or a single 400-600 mg dose. The complete abortion rate was 90–100% for pregnancies up to 7 weeks amenorrhea. Another similar combination uses RU486 and oral PGE2 with a frequency of complete abortion of 85%.

The use of the progesterone synthesis inhibitor, Epostane, requires repeated doses for several days.[17] The drug is given in a dose of 200 mg 4 times a day for 7 days. Two large efficacy trials showed an 84% complete abortion rate.[19,20]

There is a significant relationship between the efficacy of the antiprogestins and gestational age. The current medical methods—PG analogs, Epostane, RU486 alone and in combination with PG analogs—can be used most successfully during early pregnancy (7–8 weeks). At later stages their ability to induce complete abortion declines dramatically. They may be used in later pregnancy to shorten the induction-delivery interval with PG induced abortions.[17]

RU486 is well tolerated with few side effects. While the mean blood loss is 50 to 90 mL, heavy bleeding does occur in 5.6% of cases when RU486 is used alone. This risk is significantly reduced when used in combination with prostaglandins. Nausea, vomiting, dizziness, and fatigue can occur following antiprogestin use, but diarrhea, which is a typical PG side effect, very rarely occurs. Strong uterine pain is also a rare side effect with antiprogestin use alone, but occurs slightly more when used in combination with PG.

ANTIMETABOLITES

The use of methotrexate and misoprostol, a synthetic prostaglandin structurally related to prostaglandin, E1 has been shown to be an effective first trimester abortifacient. In a small preliminary study, 96% of women had a successful first trimester abortion following administration of methotrexate (50 mg per sq meter of body surface area) followed 5–7 days later with a 800 microgram intra-vaginal dose of misoprostol.[21] The incidence of side effects was extremely low.

SECOND TRIMESTER TERMINATION TECHNIQUES

The various methods of midtrimester pregnancy termination can be grouped into 3 general approaches; instillation

TABLE 49-1	ANTIPROGESTINS	
	Mode of Action	*Dose*
Mifepristone (RU486)	Progesterone receptor blocker	50–150 mg × 4 day 600 mg single dose
Epostane	Progesterone synthesis inhibitor	4 × 200 mg/day for 7 days

TABLE 49-2 | **PERCENTAGE OF REPORTED LEGAL ABORTIONS, BY WEEKS OF GESTATION AND TYPE OF PROCEDURE, 1995**

Weeks of Gestation	Procedure				
	Curettage (Suction and Sharp)	Intra-amniotic Saline	Intra-amniotic Prostaglandin	Hysterectomy/Hysterotomy	Others
< 8	99.6	0	0	0	0.3
9–10	99.9	0	0	0	0.1
11–12	99.7	0	0.1	0	0.2
13–15	99	0.3	0.2	0	0.5
16–20	90.4	3	2.3	0	4.2
> 21	81.6	1.9	5.0	0	11.4
Total	99	0.2	0.2	0	0.6

Centers for Disease Control Surveillance Summaries Abortion surveillance, United States 1995: *Morbidity and Mortality Weekly Report.* US Department of Health and Human Services, 47(ss-2):31, 1998.

techniques or medical induction, dilatation and evacuation (D&E), and hysterotomy/hysterectomy. The instillation techniques include the intra- and extra-amniotic instillation of prostaglandin, hypertonic saline, and urea. The choice of method depends primarily on whether an intact fetus is needed for evaluation. If not, a D&E can be performed, provided there are experienced operators available to provide the procedure.

DILATION AND EXTRACTION

D&E has become increasingly popular in the last 20 years and, as shown in Table 49-2, is now more commonly used than other methods. Between 1975 and 1985, the percentage of second trimester abortions performed by intrauterine instillation decreased from 57–16%.[1] In earlier years it was thought that vacuum curettage and D&E could be done only up to 12 weeks gestation. Women presented for abortion at 13 weeks or later were treated by hypertonic saline, amnio-infusion or abdominal surgical methods. A series of papers from the Centers for Disease Control and Prevention (CDC) and other investigators documented that instrumental evacuation through the cervix is the procedure of choice for many of these second trimester terminations.[22,23] As mentioned before, a major disadvantage of this procedure is the inability to examine an intact fetus which may be of diagnostic importance for future reproductive counseling.

Proper surgical technique requires experience and sufficient cervical dilatation. Preoperative evaluation should include ultrasound in all cases to confirm gestational age and to assess fetal position. Some operators have recommended that the procedure be performed with real-time ultrasound guidance to reduce complications.

The D&E can be done with local, regional, or general anesthesia. Local anesthesia, usually intracervical or paracervical block, may be the safest approach since the patient can report any unusual symptoms. Use of laminaria or hydrocele dilators is important and may be used in conjunction with prostaglandin cervical gel. Three or more laminaria tents should be inserted at least 4 hours before the procedure; some physicians customarily use sequential packings of laminaria.

After removing laminaria from the cervix, additional mechanical dilation may be necessary to achieve a diameter equal to the number of weeks of gestation plus 2 mm. The procedure is initiated by rupturing the amniotic sac. As fluid is released, the uterus contracts and brings the products of conception down closer to the cervical os. Most operators use special ovum forceps to remove the fetal tissues. For gestations up to 15 weeks, suction curettage, with a large diameter suction cannula, only can be used. Most operators use oxytocin during the operation to decrease bleeding and lessen the risk of uterine perforation. The use of prophylactic antibiotics is variable.

Before 16 weeks gestation, surgical termination is believed to be safer than instillation techniques. There is no observable difference in maternal mortality after 16 weeks with either of the 2 methods, but a lower risk of complication is associated with D&Es than compared with instillation procedures.[1] Although the upper gestational age limit for D&E abortions may be as high as 24 weeks, the majority of these operations take place earlier in the second trimester.[24]

INSTILLATION TECHNIQUES

All instillation techniques have similar requirements— complete history, physical examination, hematocrit and ultrasonography—that should be done before the injection of a specific agent. These processes can detect systemic disease that can increase complications and may require special management.

The intra-amniotic injection regimens include: intra-amniotic prostaglandins, hypertonic saline and hyperosmolar urea. Amnio-infusion methods are most frequently successful when done after 15 weeks gestation. Care should always be taken to avoid intravenous, intraperitoneal, or intramyometrial injection of abortifacient.

HYPERTONIC SALINE

Usually 200 mL of 20% NaCl solution is slowly injected into the intra-amniotic cavity transabdominally after 100–200 mL of amniotic fluid has been removed. Hypertonic saline will reliably cause midtrimester abortion in most cases although the injection to the abortion interval is somewhat long (16–42 hours with a mean of 19). Frequently an oxytocin infusion is added to augment labor. The use of oxytocin or laminaria reduces the duration of the abortion. Fetal demise usually occurs within a few hours of instillation. A repeat injection can be used in those cases that have not responded within 24 hours. The failure rate at 48 hours is 1–3%.[25–27]

HYPEROSMOLAR UREA

This technique includes the removal of 200 mL of amniotic fluid and injection of 80 grams of urea in 135 mL of 5% dextrose in water (i.e., 60% solution). Adjunctive agents such as laminaria tents, oxytocics, and prostaglandins are used because of prolonged injection to expulsion time (36–48 hours). Hyperosmolar urea is extremely fetotoxic resulting in a fetal demise.[25,26] The routine postinjection protocol includes frequent monitoring of vital signs, careful recording of fluid balance, and ascertainment of bleeding, labor, and abortion.[28]

PROSTAGLANDINS

Intra-amniotic prostaglandins have been used with increasing frequency and considerable success. Prostaglandin preparations can reliably produce uterine contractions at any stage of pregnancy. When prostaglandins are used intra-amniotically, one must take great care to avoid inadvertent myometrial or intravascular injection. A small intra-amniotic test dose should be administered. Efficacy rates using PGF2a range from 54–72% at 24 hours after the start of treatment. The use of PG analogs has significantly increased the percentage of complete abortions at 24 and 48 hours (Table 49-3). Until recently, a dose of 40 mg of PGF2a was used in terminations occurring in the United States. This preparation is no longer available, but an equivalent dosage of 2–2.5 mg of 15 methyl PGF2a may be used.

Using a combined method of single dose of intra-amniotic PGF2a and PGE2 intracervical gel markedly improves the abortifacient effects. Using this approach, the initiation to abortion time was 17 hours (range 12–19 hours), with a 48-hour failure rate of 14–18%.[26,29–31]

Prostaglandin administration is associated with a high rate (50%) of gastrointestinal side effects. The side effects using only intra-amniotic PG are somewhat lower. The use of prostaglandins in combination with urea shortens the instillation to abortion time, and produces a fetotoxic effect and decreases gastrointestinal side effects.[28] The use of PG alone may result in the expulsion of a live fetus. PG use is superior to hypertonic saline with regard to the number of complications and length of hospital stay. Intra-amniotic prostaglandin F2a instillation can be safely used for termination of pregnancy, even at advanced gestational ages. The induction-to-abortion interval is inversely correlated with the gestational age at the time of the procedure and is the main factor influencing complications.[32]

Our current protocol at the University of California, San Francisco, utilizes the intra-amniotic injection of 2 mg of 15 methyl PGF2a and laminaria insertion. Approximately 6 hours later an oxytocin infusion is started with 50 U of oxytocin in 1 L of D5 1/2 NS at 100 cc per hour. Ten units of oxytocin is added to the IV bag per hour until delivery. If a second liter of fluid is needed, 250 U of oxytocin are added. The mean injection to abortion interval is approximately 16 hours with this approach.

Recently, intravaginal misoprostol has been shown to be effective in second trimester pregnancy termination. In a study comparing misoprostol with gemprost, patients received 200 μg of misoprostol intravaginally every 6 hours for 4 doses.[33] This was repeated if the patient was undelivered by 24 hours. The median time from drug delivery to abortion was 16.9 hours with 74.9% of women delivering within 24 hours. The incidence of side effects was significantly reduced with misoprostol as compared with gemprost.

EXTRA-AMNIOTIC PROSTAGLANDINS

The extra-amniotic technique of PG administration for induction of abortion was first introduced in the early 1970s. Since then the method has gained increasing popularity as a reliable method of second trimester termination. Through the years different protocols have been used.[34]

Instillation of prostaglandins into the extra-amniotic space produces adequate myometrial stimulation while maintaining low plasma levels of the drug. Extra-amniotic administration of PGE2 or PGF2a can be accomplished with total doses one tenth fewer than those required by the intravenous

TABLE 49-3	INTRA-AMNIOTIC INSTILLATION OF PROSTAGLANDIN ANALOGS: DOSE, EFFICACY, AND INSTILLATION ABORTION TIME (IAT)		
	Dose	*Efficacy*	*Mean IAT(h)*
15 methyl PGE2	100 mg repeated 24 h	90% in 24 h 100% in 46 h	16.5
15 methyl PGF2a	2.5 mg (single)	95% in 48 h	18–20
Sulprostone (PGE2 derivative)	1–4 mg (single)	90–96%	5–17

Amy JJ. Intra-amniotic prostaglandins for mid-trimester abortion. In: Toppozada M, Bydgeman M, Hafez ESE, eds. *Prostaglandins and Fertility Regulation*. Lancaster, Boston, MTP Press Ltd. 1984:107–118.

TABLE 49-4	**EXTRAAMNIOTIC INSTILLATION OF PROSTAGLANDINS: INDUCTION ABORTION TIME (IAT) AND SUCCESS RATE (36H)**	
	IAT (h)	*Success Rate (%)*
PGF2a	22.4	85–96
PGE	19.3	93
15 methyl PGF2a	14.1	80–82

Bydgeman MA. Prostaglandin Procedures in Second Trimester Abortion. Boston, John Wright PSG Inc, 1981:89–106.

TABLE 49-5	**MAJOR COMPLICATION RATES (PERCENTAGE): JOINT PROGRAM FOR STUDY OF ABORTION (JPSA) 1970–1978**	
Suction curettage	< 6 weeks	0.2–0.6
	7–8 weeks	0.2–0.3
	9–10 weeks	0.3–0.4
	11–12 weeks	0.4–0.5
Saline instillation	13–16 weeks	1.6–1.8
	> 17 weeks	1.7–2.8
Prostaglandin instillation	13–16 weeks	2.7–3.0
	> 17 weeks	2.2–2.8
D&E	13–16 weeks	0.6–0.8
	> 17 weeks	0.7–0.9

Tietze C. Fertility Regulation and the Public Health—Selected Papers of Christopher Tietze. Tietze SL, Lincoln R, eds. New York, Berlin, Springer-Verlag. 1987:227–267.

route and, as a result, with markedly reduced systemic side effects.[34–36]

Both PGE2 and PGF2a have been used in a variety of different dosage regimens including intermittent injection of PGF2a gel, a continuous rate infusion pump and a single extra-ovular injection of 15-methyl PGF2a.[37] Most operators use a Foley catheter or a specially designed double balloon catheter that is placed in the extra-ovular space.[35,36]

The success rate after 24 hours is 72–96%, with an induction to abortion time of 12.9–22.4 hours (Table 49-4). A relatively low incidence of side effects has been reported, in particular gastrointestinal.[36] Continuous instillation of extra-ovular PGF2a has been reported for pregnancy termination with a high success rate and no complications in patients who have had previous cesarean sections.[35] Extra-amniotic administration of PG has the following advantages: a low total dose of PG, which results in a lowered incidence of side effects, and the need for less operator skill than the intra-amniotic methods.[38] Pretreatment with a single dose of 200 mg of the antiprogestogen mifepristone, given 24 hours before starting an extra-amniotic prostaglandin E2 infusion, has been shown to shorten significantly the interval between prostaglandin administration and expulsion of the fetus.[39] The amount of prostaglandin E2 needed was also reduced. Most likely, the observed effects were due to an increased sensitivity of the mifepristone primed myometrium to prostaglandins and antiprogestogen-induced ripening of the cervix. It seems pretreatment with mifepristone will become an established practice in second trimester pregnancy terminations as the drug becomes more available.

COMPLICATIONS

The risks associated with late abortions are 3–4 times higher than those associated with abortions performed in early pregnancy.[8,40] Second trimester abortions are responsible for 67% of all complications and for 57% of abortion mortality, even though second trimester abortions account for only 12.4% of all legal abortions in the United States.[41] Fortunately, the case fatality rate has been reduced by a factor of 10, from 4 in 100,000 in 1972 to 0.4 in 100,000 in 1987. Complication rates are lowest for abortion by suction curettage followed in ascending order by classical D&C, saline instillation, hysterotomy, and hysterectomy.[8] Complication rates in the sec-

ond trimester increase with the age of the woman and parity, while for the first trimester there is no association with parity and a slight downward trend with the age of the woman.[8]

The urea-prostaglandin procedure results in a significantly higher rate of serious complications than D&E (1.09 vs. 0.49 per 100 abortions).[4] Saline instillation has a significantly higher risk of serious complication than urea-prostaglandin.[4] Major and minor complications are summarized in Table 49-5.

UTERINE PERFORATION

Uterine perforation is a major, but rare (3 in 1000) complication of D&E.[42] Perforations in the second trimester procedure are usually more severe than those in the first trimester and may be associated with extensive blood loss and injury to other abdominal structures. Perforations are extremely rare with the current instillation techniques. Sudden pain, increased bleeding or extraction of maternal tissue are indications of perforation.

Data suggest that a prior cesarean section is a risk factor for uterine rupture and blood transfusion in women having a midtrimester pregnancy termination. Chapman et al. found a significantly increased risk of uterine rupture (3.8% vs. 0.2%) and an increased need for blood transfusion (11.4% vs. 5.3%) in women who had a prior cesarean section.[43]

INFECTION

The risk of infection and fever following D&E is small (1%). For instillation procedures the infection rate is 3–8% and is increased with the prolongation of the instillation to abortion interval.[42]

RETAINED PRODUCTS OF CONCEPTION

Retained products of conception are less common with D&E than with medically induced abortions. Retained placental products, postabortion fever, bleeding, and pelvic infection are all managed by re-exploring and emptying the uterine cavity. Oxytocin and ergot products may be helpful.

BLEEDING

The loss frequency of more than 500 ml of blood is 5–10% following instillation procedures with an increasing incidence as pregnancy progresses. Coagulopathy is associated with all forms of pregnancy termination with an incidence of 191 in 100,000 for D&E and 658 in 100,000 for saline procedures.[44] Cervical lacerations are rare (1%) secondary to D&E but may result in severe hemorrhage. With intra-amniotic techniques lacerations are more frequent (3%) although laminaria use has lowered the frequency to about 1%.[26]

HYPERTONIC SALINE

Sudden death from hypernatremia and necrosis of the uterine wall have been reported at 1 in 14,000. The sudden onset of tachycardia, hypotension, headache, or salty taste warns the operator of probable intravascular absorption of hypertonic saline, which can lead to cardiovascular collapse, cerebral edema, convulsion and death. Infusion should be stopped immediately and water/dextrose given via IV. Another uncommon but serious complication of this method is disseminated intravascular coagulation (DIC).

Rh ISO-IMMUNIZATION

One of the relatively serious potential outcomes of pregnancy termination is Rh-Iso-immunization. The incidence of Rh-sensitization in early abortions is less than that at term, but it is still significant.[45,46] In first trimester terminations fetal blood may enter the maternal circulation. The estimate of the frequency of this event in the first trimester is 7.2%.[47] Overall, it has been estimated that approximately 4% of susceptible women would become sensitized from early abortion if they were not given immunoprophylaxis. The likelihood of sensitization may increase with instrumentation in the uterine cavity. First trimester patients should receive 50 μg of Rh immune globulin.

The second trimester abortion incidence of Rh-sensitization, in absence of prophylaxis, is approximately the same as in term deliveries. Rh-negative women undergoing midtrimester termination should get 300 mg of Rh immune globulin unless the fetus can be shown to be Rh-negative or if the spouse is Rh-negative. A high frequency of fetal blood entering the maternal circulation during first and second trimester abortion (58% and 96%, respectively) has been demonstrated by measurement of an alpha-fetoprotein rise in maternal blood.[48]

MORTALITY

Since the CDC's surveillance of abortion mortality began in 1972, 93% fewer deaths have occurred. The case fatality rate in 1985 was 0.5 deaths per 100,000 legally induced abortions, which was down from the 0.8 per 100,000 reported in 1982 through 1984, and a 75% drop in number of deaths from 1972 (case fatality rate of 4.1).[1]

SUBSEQUENT PREGNANCIES

Many women undergoing termination of pregnancy are not at the end of their reproductive years. For women desiring further children after their abortion the question of subsequent fertility and pregnancy complications is a crucial one.

Among the problems that can jeopardize future pregnancies and term deliveries, the most critical ones are postabortion infertility, ectopic pregnancies, cervical incompetence leading to spontaneous abortions, premature deliveries, and low birthweight babies.

SECONDARY INFERTILITY

Early reports of postabortion infertility raised the question of the potential harmful effects of abortion on fertility. Currently, most studies show that there is no increased risk of secondary infertility following induced abortion. Some have even shown that the interpregnancy interval is shorter. Prospective and case control studies show that, while secondary infertility may be a rare complication of a complicated termination, the overall risk is not significantly elevated.[8,49]

ECTOPIC PREGNANCY

Several investigators have examined the relationship between prior induced abortion and ectopic pregnancy. Studies completed outside the United States have shown variable results. The relative risk of ectopic pregnancy in women who had prior induced abortion is 1.3–3 in different studies.[50] In studies carried on within the United States the relative risk was 1.0–2.4. Women whose first pregnancy is terminated by vacuum aspiration are at no increased risk of subsequent ectopic pregnancy, while women who had more than 1 induced abortion or have postoperative pelvic inflammatory disease are at higher risk for ectopic pregnancy.[8,51–53]

ABORTIONS

Women whose first pregnancy is terminated by vacuum aspiration are at no increased risk of subsequent midtrimester spontaneous abortion when compared with women who are pregnant for the first time; the relative risk is 0.56–1.2. The type of abortion is related to the risk of subsequent midtrimester spontaneous abortion. Women terminating by D&C in the first trimester have an elevated risk factor (2.7–3.7) for second trimester spontaneous abortion. This may be consistent with possible increased risk for cervical incompetence secondary to the D&C procedure, and is probably related to the extent of cervical dilatation.[8,49]

PRETERM DELIVERY AND LOW BIRTHWEIGHT

Studies conducted in Britain, Hungary, and Israel have shown decreased mean birthweight among women who had had previous induced abortions, while studies in the United States, Yugoslavia, and Taiwan have not confirmed this finding. The World Health Organization task force on pregnancy following induced abortion observed an increased risk of low birthweight and preterm delivery following vaginal termination of pregnancy by D&C.[54] The Royal College of Obstetricians and Gynecologists joint study supports the finding of other investigators that induced abortion has no significant effect on the overall maternal complication rate of childbearing or on the rate of congenital abnormality or neonatal death in offspring in subsequent pregnancy. There was no difference in the rate of stillbirth, low birthweight, and shortened gestation.[8,55]

The impact of multiple abortions and longterm effects on fertility of midtrimester abortions have not been adequately studied. Studies to date suggest that instillation procedures carry little, if any, excess risk. Dilatation and evacuation technique may have elevated risk depending on the method and extent of cervical dilatation.[49]

SELECTIVE SECOND TRIMESTER TERMINATION OF THE ANOMALOUS FETUS IN MULTIPLE GESTATIONS

Three options are available to couples in cases for which a chromosomal, metabolic or morphological abnormality is detected in 1 fetus of a multiple gestation. The first option is to continue the pregnancy for the sake of the healthy fetuses and accept the possibility that an affected sibling will also be born. A second is to perform a selective termination of the affected fetus. The third option is the termination of both fetuses.

Many ethical, moral, and social problems are associated with the choice of a selective termination. The overall experience with this procedure in the second trimester is limited. Selective termination of pregnancy raises many questions concerning attendant risks and problems. Immediate problems include selection of the wrong fetus, technical failure, premature rupture of the membranes, infection and abortion, and damage to or death of the normal fetuses. There is also the risk of DIC from thromboplastin released after the dead fetus, which can affect the normal fetuses and the mother. A later risk is preterm labor and delivery.

COUNSELING

The couple should be counseled about potential risks that could directly or indirectly result from the procedure including loss of the whole pregnancy, chorioamnionitis, premature delivery, permanent damage to the surviving fetus, and termination of the wrong fetus.

IDENTIFICATION OF THE AFFECTED FETUS

Before beginning the procedure it is critical that the abnormal fetus be correctly identified. A careful and detailed sonographic evaluation should be carried out. If a sonographic marker such as nonidentical sex, anatomical abnormality, or significant size difference is present, then the identification is easy. In the absence of such a marker, information from the previous amnio-

centesis is used; therefore, it is extremely important to make accurate descriptions and drawings when performing an amniocentesis in a multiple gestation pregnancy. Unless there is a clear identification, a fetal blood sampling for rapid diagnosis should be done to re-identify the affected fetus.

TECHNIQUES

Over the past 10 years different methods for selective terminations have been used. These techniques include cardiac puncture with exsanguination, hysterotomy, and removal of the affected fetus, air embolization to the cardiac area and through the umbilical vessels, cardiac tamponade with saline and, finally, injection of calcium gluconate, formaldehyde, and potassium chloride (KCl). Usually the procedure is done using a 20- to 23-gauge needle that is guided into the fetal heart with ultrasound.[56-62]

Currently, the most widely used technique is intracardiac injection of KCl. The other methods are less efficient and have many technical problems. Air embolization has a risk of infection, and on the ultrasound the air shadows the fetal heart making confirmation of asystole difficult. Cardiac puncture and exsanguination is unreliable in achieving asystole and may result in bradycardia, which can later recover.

INTRACARDIAC INJECTION OF POTASSIUM CHLORIDE

In this procedure, 5–15 mEq of KCl is injected into the fetal heart. This is the most effective procedure with the lowest complication and failure rate. In most cases, cardiac arrest occurs almost immediately after injection.[56-62]

MONOCHORIONIC GESTATION

An attempt to determine whether the pregnancy is dichorionic or monochorionic is of critical importance. In many monochorionic pregnancies a significant circulatory exchange takes place through placental anastomoses. Termination of an affected fetus in a monochorionic pregnancy using toxic agents or air is likely to end in the spontaneous demise of the normal fetus. This is due to shared circulation with the dead fetus being a low resistance pool for the blood of the living 1; thus causing exsanguination.[56-58] Interruption of the circulation of the affected fetus is necessary. In the past this was performed by hysterotomy and ligation of the umbilical cord and removal of the affected fetus. More recent studies have demonstrated the success of endoscopic cord ligation of the affected fetus.[63,64]

If there is a question of zygosity, DNA polymorphisms can be evaluated to determine zygosity. These can be performed on any fetal nucleated cell such as amniocytes or lymphocytes.

PREMATURE LABOR

Premature labor and delivery is a major complication in second trimester selective terminations. Decreasing the procedure time of intrauterine manipulations and performance of the procedure as early in gestation as possible may lower the premature labor rate.

INTRAVASCULAR CONSUMPTIVE COAGULOPATHY

This complication is known in singleton pregnancies and has been reported in cases of intrauterine fetal death of 1 fetus in twin and triplet pregnancies.[65,66] D&C related lesions in a living twin of monochorionic pregnancies were reported after spontaneous death of a co-twin.[67] There have been no reported cases of this complication related to selective termination of pregnancy and the risk is probably low.

OUTCOME

Data from a large multicenter collaborative reports suggest that selective termination of a dichorionic abnormal twin is effective and safe.[68,69] Outcome statistics showed that 83.8% of deliveries occurred after 33 weeks with only 4.3% occurring at 25–28 weeks of gestation. The overall loss rate was 12.6%. Gestational age at the time of the procedure was found to correlate positively with loss rate and inversely with gestational age at delivery. This emphasizes the need for early diagnosis.

DIAGNOSTIC EVALUATION OF THE ABORTED FETUS

Contrary to general perceptions, loss of an embryo or fetus carries for the parents a feeling of grief and loss as if a living child had died. Prevention of recurrence is uppermost in their minds. Genetic counselors, obstetricians, and perinatologists sometimes are unable to answer parents' questions as to probable cause of death, recurrence risk and potential for prenatal diagnosis in the next pregnancy because of the lack of anatomical, pathological, and other data on the fetus.[70]

The importance of a thorough study of the aborted fetus has been reinforced by the growth in the ability to prenatally diagnose birth defects and genetic disorders as well as the development of antenatal therapies for some of them. The information obtained from autopsy and other studies done on the fetus also serves to confirm the accuracy of ultrasound diagnosis, amniocentesis, CVS, and the efficacy of antenatal therapy.[71] This information is invaluable to the families as well as to the clinicians.

Available tools, such as cytogenetical, enzymological, and molecular methods of diagnosis and imaging techniques, should be used in the investigation of the aborted fetus and products of conception.

ROLE OF THE CLINICIAN

It is important to give the pathologist performing the autopsy all the clinical information available before commencing the postmortem examination. Such clinical information should include data on prenatal age, health, race, family history, prior obstetric history, and history of present pregnancy including last menstrual period (LMP), expected date of confinement (EDC), date of termination, and method of collection. Other important information should include diagnosis considered before the termination and whether proved or not as well as desirable studies (e.g., blood or tissue cultures for chromosomes, mi-croorganisms, serologic, or enzymologic studies). It is advisable to discuss the case with the pathologist. This preliminary discussion can help the pathologist define the most important areas of study and plan the investigation. The refusal of consent for necropsy does not preclude performance of certain diagnostic tests. Physical examination, weight and measurement, whole body photographs, x-rays, ultrasound, blood and tissue (e.g., skin and liver needle biopsy) specimens for cell culture and other studies may still be performed.[72]

ROLE OF THE PATHOLOGIST

The primary role of the pathologist is to supplement the observation of the clinician by carrying out external examination, measurements, dissection, and histological examination as well as any additional studies that are indicated.

SAMPLES

Tests that require fresh tissue or body fluids include muscle biopsies, metabolic and toxicologic studies, chromosome analyses, electron microscopic studies, and microbiologic cultures. All specimens should be taken prior to subjecting the fetus to formalin fixation.

Several types of tissue can be used for chromosome studies. Lymphocytes from blood are preferred and can be cultured if obtained within 12 hours of fetal death. If fetal blood is not available, samples of skin, diaphragm or kidney can be taken by sterile technique, placed in separate containers of sterile physiological saline and transported at room temperature. Sending several tissue-type samples will maximize the chance of obtaining results. If more than 12 hours have elapsed since fetal death, tissue should still be sent, although the likelihood of being able to culture the tissue for karyotype analysis is significantly reduced. Samples should be sent as quickly as possible to the laboratory.

A variety of other tissue samples may be needed depending on what diagnoses are being considered. Samples for metabolic studies include serum and urine which should be refrigerated. Liver and skin should be obtained and immediately frozen, preferable at −70°C. These samples can be analyzed for organic and amnio acids, mucopolysaccharidoses and enzymatic assays. Fresh tissue for DNA extraction and analysis should be frozen. A good source can be the placenta. Tissue for electron microscopic studies should be obtained rapidly and placed in cold fixative (i.e., glutaraldehyde).

Consultation with the laboratory that performs the test can be of great help in deciding what tissues are needed and how they should be stored. Labeling is mandatory for proper processing. It is generally easier to obtain enough samples of all kinds and later discard the unnecessary ones than to try to recover them later.

PHYSICAL EXAMINATION

A careful assessment should be done of prenatal growth, maturation and development. Weight and measurements (i.e., crown rump, total body and head circumference) should be recorded.

Other characteristics that should be described include hair texture, color and pattern; fontanels and sutures; shape of the skull; ear formation, shape and position; eye position, shape, and measurements; nose shape; mouth anomaly, lips, and palate; general shape of neck, chest, abdomen, genitalia and extremities. The participation of a dysmorphologist at this stage can be of great advantage.

The external features should be photographed. This is particularly important for dysostoses, skeletal dysplasias, and in cases of multiple congenital anomaly syndromes.[73]

The examination of the fetus and pregnancy products after termination of the pregnancy, the performance of a necropsy, and obtaining the necessary samples for confirmation of the diagnosis should be an integral part of the management of the aborted fetus.

PSYCHOLOGICAL ASPECTS OF PREGNANCY TERMINATION

With the increasing incidence of prenatal diagnosis, greater numbers of women will be requesting termination of otherwise much wanted pregnancies. The psychological difference between elective and medically indicated abortion is extreme. While women going through elective abortion will primarily feel relieved, when a genetic abnormality or major malformation is the cause for abortion, a grief response by both parents is to be expected.

Women who have a wanted pregnancy and have established some sort of psychic relationship to the fetus are at a higher risk and may require prolonged psychiatric treatment or even hospitalization within the 12 months following termination. The grief reaction following abortion of a malformed, but otherwise desired fetus, can be similar to the death of a living child. Questions such as "What was the baby like?" "Did he have a chance?" "Will it happen again?" are often asked.

Reaction to abortion may vary depending on the age of the patient, her religious background, gestational age, degree of social support and other factors such as premorbid psychiatric status. Second trimester abortions generally produce more difficulty. At later stages of pregnancy women are more likely to have felt fetal movements and to have a greater psychological investment in the pregnancy.

Depending on the specific procedure selected, the procedure itself is emotionally stressful. Women who undergo midtrimester instillation-abortion techniques face a long stressful labor and delivery, side effects of medication and sometimes complications that may potentiate reactions such as anger and depression. Many couples, however, having realized the destructive nature of a D&E will request an instillation procedure. The procedure for the patient is relatively quick, painless and less stressful using the D&E method, but the operator must deal with the stressful situation of removing fetal parts.

Long-term psychological stress in women whose pregnancy is terminated following ultrasonographic detection of fetal anomalies does not differ from the stress response seen in women experiencing a perinatal loss.[74] A possible adverse effect on the psychological response of women having to decide themselves about the continuation of pregnancy was not found. Women undergoing pregnancy termination following ultrasonographic detection of fetal anomalies are more likely to try to become pregnant again in the year following the loss than women having a late spontaneous abortion or perinatal death.

There is a positive correlation between the premorbid psychological status and the amount of postabortion psychiatric difficulty. Postabortal psychoses occur in women who have pre-abortal emotional disturbances. Preoperative evaluation should include a discussion of how the decision to terminate the pregnancy was made, and the patients' feelings about the decision. Abortion patients require counseling and emotional support before, during and after their procedure. Psychiatric evaluation should be requested if the patient exhibits signs and symptoms of psychiatric illness, has a history of postpartum psychosis or exhibits ambivalence over the decision.[75]

Management of grief, following a loss, involves facilitating the normal processes that occur rather than attempting to isolate or protect a family from the consequences of the loss. Perhaps the most important task for the parents is to recognize both the reality of the fetus's existence and of its death. Some investigators recommend encouraging the parents to see the fetus, if the parents need to make the death a reality. While hospital staff are often reluctant to show a macerated or grossly abnormal baby to the family, parents tend to focus on the baby's normal features. Often, the parents' conception of the abnormality are much worse than reality. Studies show that 90% of parents choose to see the fetus.

A grief response of the father has been less well documented but should be considered. He should be seen during the hospitalization of the mother and asked to return during followup visits with his partner.[76]

There are many different recommendations for the number and timing of followup appointments. In addition to increasing the level and understanding of information, followup visits have been shown to increase satisfaction with medical care. Facilitation of the grieving process during the initial 6 weeks after the procedure should decrease the incidence of longterm depression.[77]

After perinatal loss, a waiting period of from 6–12 months is usually advised before attempting another pregnancy. There is an emotional drive to become pregnant again as soon as possible, but this can put the parents and the new child at increased psychological risk. Inappropriate grief, morbid grief reactions and psychiatric problems occur with increased frequency in couples who attempt pregnancy at an early interval. Self-help groups in which parents can receive help and support from couples with similar experiences are highly recommended.

It should be remembered that feelings of sadness, depression and guilt are common and that a period of mourning after abortion is considered normal. In most cases, grieving is resolved without complications, but some will have abnormal grief reactions. It is the goal of the health providers to facilitate this painful process.[78]

References

1. Lawson HW, Atrash HK, Satflas AF, et al. for the Centers for Disease Control. Abortion surveillance, United States 1984–1985. *MMWR Morb Mortal Wkly Rep.* 1989;38:11.

2. Schultz KF, Grimes DA, Cates WJ. Measurements to prevent cervical injury during suction curettage abortion. *Lancet.* 1983;1:1182.

3. Cates W, Schultz KF, Grimes DA. The risk associated with teenage abortion. *N Engl J Med.* 1983;309:621.

4. Centers for Disease Control Surveillance Summaries. Abortion surveillance, United States 1984–1985. *MMWR Morb Mortal Wkly Rep.* 1989;38:10.

5. Darney PD. Preparation of the cervix: hydrophilic and prostaglandin dilators. *Clin Obstet Gynaecol.* 1986;13:43.

6. Shalev E, Tsabari A, Edelstein S, et al. Intracervical administration of prostaglandin E2 gel prior to therapeutic abortion: a prospective randomized double-blind study. *Int J Gynaecol Obstet.* 1988;27:119.

7. Chen JK, Elder MG. Preoperative cervical dilatation by vaginal pessaries containing E1 analogue. *Obstet Gynecol.* 1983;62:339.

8. Tietze SL, Lincoln R, ed. *Fertility Regulation and the Public Health: Selected Papers of Christopher Tietze.* New York: Springer-Verlag; 1987:227–267.

9. Lippert TH. *Side effects of Natural Prostaglandins in Prostaglandins and Fertility Regulation.* Lancaster, England: MTP Press, Ltd; 1984:129–139.

10. Bygdeman MW, Baird DT. Induction of therapeutic abortion in early pregnancy with mifepristone in combination with prostaglandin pessary. *Lancet.* 1987;2:1415.

11. Rodger MW, Baird DT. Induction of therapeutic abortion in early pregnancy with mifepristone in combination with prostaglandin pessary. *Lancet.* 1987;2:1415.

12. Cameron IT, Michie AF, Baird DT. Therapeutic abortion in early pregnancy with antiprogesterone RU486 alone or in combination with prostaglandin analog. *Contraception.* 1986;34:459.

13. Bydgeman M, Christensen NJ, Green K, et al. Termination of early pregnancy; future development. *Acta Obstet Gynecol Scand.* 1983;113 Suppl 1:125.

14. Rosen AS, Von Knorring K, Bygdeman M, et al. Randomized comparison of prostaglandin treatment in hospital or at home with vacuum aspiration for termination of early pregnancy. *Contraception.* 1984;29:423.

15. Cameron IT, Baird DT. Early pregnancy termination: a comparison between vacuum aspiration and medical abortion using prostaglandin (15.15 dimethyl-trans-delta 2-PGE1 methyl ester) or the antiprogesterone RU486. *Br J Obstet Gynaecol.* 1988;95:271.

16. World Health Organization, Task force on post ovulatory methods for fertility regulation. Menstrual regulation by intramuscular injection of 16-phenoxy-tetranor-PGE2 methyl sulfanilamide or vacuum aspiration: a randomized multicenter study. *Br J Obstet Gynaecol.* 1987;94:949.

17. Selinger M, Mackenzie IZ, Gillmer MD, et al. Progesterone inhibition in the mid-trimester termination of pregnancy: physiological and clinical effects. *Br J Obstet Gynecol Reprod.* 1987;94:1218.

18. Maria B, Stampf F, Goepp A, et al. Termination of early pregnancy by a single dose of mifepristone (RU-486), a progesterone antagonist. *Eur J Obstet Gynecol Reprod.* 1988;28:249.

19. Bigerson L, Olund A, Odlind V, et al. Termination of early human pregnancy with epostone. *Contraception.* 1987;35:111.

20. Crooij MJ, de Nooyer CC, Rao BR, et al. Termination of early pregnancy by the b-hydroxysteroid dehydrogenase inhibitor epostane. *N Engl J Med.* 1988;319:813.

21. Hausknecht RU. Methotrexate and misoprostol to terminate early pregnancy. *N Eng J Med* 1995;39:537.

22. Grimes DA, Cates W Jr. Gestational age limit of twelve weeks for abortion by curettage. *Am J Obstet Gynecol.* 1978;132:207.

23. Grimes DA, Hulka JF, McCatchen ME. Midtrimester abortion by D&E versus intraamniotic instillation of prostaglandins F2: a randomized clinical trial. *Am J Obstet Gynecol.* 1980;137:785.

24. Grimes DA, Cates W Jr. *Dilatation and Evacuation in Second Trimester Abortion.* Boston, MA: John Wright PSG, Inc; 1981:119–134.

25. Rayburn WF, LaFerla JJ. Second trimester termination for genetic abnormalities. *J Reprod Med.* 1982;27:584.

26. Castadot RG. Pregnancy termination: techniques, risks and complications and their management. *Fert Steril.* 1986;45:5.

27. Kerenyi TD. Intra-amniotic hypertonic saline instillation in the second trimester. In: Keirse MJ, Gravenhorst JB, Von Lith DAF et al. eds. *Second Trimester Pregnancy Termination.* Boston, MA: Leiden Univ Press; 1982:80.

28. Burkman RT, Atienza MF, King TU, et al. Intraamniotic urea and prostaglandin F2 for midtrimester abortion: a modified regimen. *Am J Obstet Gynecol.* 1976;126:328.

29. Amy, JJ. Intra-amniotic prostaglandins for mid-trimester abortion. In: Toppozada M, Bygdeman M, Hafez ES, eds. *Prostaglandins and Fertility Regulation.* Lancaster, England: MTP Press, Ltd; 1984: 107–118.

30. Anderson LF, Poulson HK, Sorenson SS, et al. Termination of second trimester pregnancy with gamaprest vaginal pessaries and intra-amniotic PGF2 alpha. *A Comparative study. Eur J Obstet Gynecol Reprod.* 1989;31:1.

31. Allen J, Maigaard S, Forman A, et al. Combined intracervical PGE2 and intra-amniotic PGF2 alpha for induction of 2nd trimester abortion. *Acta Obstet Gynecol Scand.* 1987;66:603.

32. Lipitz S, Grisaru D, Libshiz A, et al. Intraamniotic prostaglandin f2a for pregnancy termination in the second trimester and early third trimester of pregnancy. *J Reprod Med.* 1997;42:235.

33. Dickinson JE, Godfrey M, Evans SF. Efficacy of intravaginal misoprostol in second-trimester pregnancy termination: A randomized controlled trial. *J Maternal Fetal Med.* 1998;7:115.

34. Embrey MP, Mackenzie IZ. Extraamniotic prostaglandins for every second trimester abortion. In: Hafez ES, ed. *Voluntary Termination of Pregnancy.* Lancaster, England: MTP Press, Ltd; 1984:57.

35. Atad J, Lissak A, Calderon I, et al. Continuous extraovular prostaglandin F2 alpha instillation for late pregnancy termination in patients with previous cesarean section delivery. *Int J Gynaecol Obstet.* 1986;24:315.

36. Atad J, Lissak A, Sorokin Y, et al. Continuous extraovular prostaglandin F2 alpha instillation for second trimester pregnancy termination. *Isr J Med Sci.* 1985;21:935.

37. World Health Organization Task Force on the Use of Prostaglandin and Abortion. An international multicentric study. *Am J Obstet Gynecol.* 1977;129:597.

38. Bygdeman MA. *Prostaglandin Procedures in Second Trimester Abortion.* Boston, MA: John Wright PSG, Inc; 1981:89–106.

39. Van Look PA, Von Hertzen H. Clinical uses of antiprogestogens. *Hum Reprod Update.* 1995;1:19.

40. Tyler CA Jr. Epidemiology of abortion. *J Reprod Med.* 1981;26:459.

41. Laron E, Mazor M, Leiberman JR. Prostaglandins and termination of second trimester pregnancy. *Hraefuah.* 1998;134:136.

42. Grimes DA, Schulz KF, Cates W Jr, et al. Mid-Trimester abortion by dilation and evacuation. *N Engl J Med.* 1977;296:1141.

43. Chapman SJ, Crispens M, Savage K. Complications of midtrimester pregnancy termination: the effect of prior cesarean delivery. *Am J Obstet Gynecol.* 1996;175:889.

44. Kafrissen ME, Banke MW, Workman P, et al. Coagulopathy and induced abortion methods: rates and relative risks. *Am J Obstet Gynecol.* 1983;147:346.

45. Katz J. Transplacental passage of fetal red blood cells in abortion: increased incidence after curettage and effect of oxytocic drugs. *BMJ.* 1969;4:84.

46. Voift JC, Britt RP. Feto-maternal hemorrhage in therapeutic abortion. *Brit Med J.* 1969;4:395.

47. Queenan JT, Kubaryet SF, Shah S, et al. Role of induced abortion in rhesus isoimmunization. *Lancet.* 1971;1:815.

48. Naik K, Kitau M, Satchell ME, et al. The incidence of fetomaternal hemorrhage following elective termination of first-trimester pregnancy. *Eur J Obstet Gynecol Reprod.* 1988;27:355.

49. Hogue CJ. Impact of abortion on subsequent fecundity. *Clin Obstet Gynaecol.* 1986;13:95.

50. Burkman RT, Mason KJ, Gold EB. Ectopic pregnancy and prior induced abortion. *Contraception.* 1988;37:21.

51. Levin AA, Schoenbaum SC, Stubblefild PG. Ectopic pregnancy and prior induced abortion. *Am J Public Health.* 1982;72:253.

52. Chung CS, Smith RG, Steinhoff PG. Induced abortion and ectopic pregnancy in subsequent pregnancies. *Am J Epidemol.* 1982;115:879.

53. Daling JR, Chow WH, Weiss NS, et al. Ectopic pregnancy in relation to previous induced abortion. *JAMA.* 1985;253:1005.

54. World Health Organization Task Force on Sequelae of Abortion, Gestation, Birth Weight, and Spontaneous Abortion in Pregnancy After Induced Abortion. *Lancet.* 1979;1:142.

55. Frank PI, Kay CR, Scott LM, et al. for the Royal College of General Practitioners/Royal College of Obstetricians and Gynaecologists Joint Study. Pregnancy following induced abortion: maternal morbidity, congenital abnormalities and neonatal death. *Br J Obstet Gynaecol.* 1987;94:836.

56. Chitkara U, Berkowitz RL, Wilkins IA, et al. Selective second-trimester termination of the anomalous fetus in twin pregnancies. *Obstet Gynecol.* 1981;73(5 pt 1):690.

57. Golbus MS, Cuningham N, Goldberg JD, et al. Selective termination of multiple gestations. *Am J Med Genet.* 1988;31:339.

58. Donnenfeld AE, Glazerman LR, Cutillo DM, et al. Fetal exsanguination following intrauterine angiographic assessment and selective termination of hydrocephalic, monozygotic co-twin. *Prenat Diagn.* 1989;9:301.

59. Abery A, Miterian F, Cantz M, et al. Cardiac puncture of fetus with Hurler's disease avoiding abortion of unaffected co-twin. *Lancet.* 1978;2:990.

60. Rodeck C, Mibashan R, Abramowitz J, et al. Selective feticide of the affected twin by fetoscopic air embolization. *Prenat Diagn.* 1982;2:189.

61. Antsaklis A, Politis J, Karangiannopoulos C, et al. Selective survival of only the healthy fetus following prenatal diagnosis of thalassanemia major in binovular twin gestation. *Prenat Diagn.* 1984;4:289.

62. Petres R, Redwine F. Selective Birth in twin pregnancy. *N Engl J Med.* 1981;305:1218.

63. Quintero RA, Romero R, Reich H, et al. In utero percutaneous umbilical cord ligation in the management of complicated monochorionic gestations. *Ultrasound Obstet Gynecol.* 1996;8:16.

64. Deprest JA, Evraad VA, Van Schoubroeck D, et al. Endoscopic cord ligation in selective feticide. *Lancet.* 1996;348:890.

65. Skelly H, Marivate M, Normal R. Consumptive coagulopathy following fetal death in a triplet pregnancy. *Am J Obstet Gynecol.* 1982;142:595.

66. Romero R, Duffy TP, Berkowitz RL, et al. Prolongation of a preterm pregnancy complication by death of a single twin in utero and DIC. *N Engl J Med.* 1984;310:772.

67. Enbom JA. Twin pregnancy with intrauterine death of one twin. *Am J Obstet Gynecol.* 1987;152:426.

68. Evans MI, Goldberg JD, Dommergues M, et al. Efficacy of second trimester selective termination for fetal abnormalities: international collaborative experience among the world's largest centers. *Am J Obstet Gynecol.* 1994;171:90–94.

69. Lipitz S, Shalev E, Meizner I, et al. Late selective termination of fetal abnormalities in twin pregnancies: a multicentre report. *Br J Obstet Gynecol.* 1996;103:1212–1216.

70. Opitz JM, Fitzgerald JM, Reynolds JR, et al. The Montana Fetal Genetic Pathology Program and a review of prenatal death in humans. *Am J Med Genet.* 1987;3 Suppl:93.

71. Murphy JL, Mendoza SA, Griswold WR, et al. Severe bilateral renal disease: correlation of antenatal and autopsy findings. *Prenat Diagn.* 1989;9:119.

72. Wigglesworth JS. Investigation of perinatal death. *Arch Dis Child.* 1987;62:1207.

73. Tyson W, Manchester DI. Pathologic aspects of fetal death: diagnostic evaluation of perinatal death (part II). *Clin Obstet Gynaecol.* 1987;30:331.

74. Salvesen KA, Oyen L, Schmidt N, et al. Comparison of long term psychological responses of women after pregnancy termination due to fetal anomalies and after prenatal loss. *Ultrasound Obstet Gynecol.* 1997;9:80.

75. Lazarus A, Stern R. Psychiatric aspects of pregnancy termination. *Clin Obstet Gynecol.* 1986;13:125.

76. Blumberg BD, Golbus MS, Hanson KH. The psychological sequelae of abortion performed for genetic indication. *Am J Obstet Gynecol.* 1975;122:799.

77. Stierman ED. Emotional aspects of perinatal death. *Clin Obstet Gynecol.* 1987;30:352.

78. Llewelyn SP, Pytches R. An investigation of anxiety following a termination of pregnancy. *J Adv Nurs.* 1988;13:468.

THE FETAL AUTOPSY

Faisal Qureshi / Suzanne M. Jacques

INTRODUCTION

Interest in perinatal and fetal autopsies has grown in recent years, as the number of deaths in the perinatal period has declined and as the size of families has decreased. More stress is placed on smaller families and, in the event of poor pregnancy outcome, the desire of the parents to have an explanation for the loss has grown. The parents want to know not only the reason for their loss, but how it will affect any future pregnancy and if it can possibly be prevented from happening again. In cases where prenatal examination has demonstrated fetal anomalies, it is important to confirm these findings, obtain tissue or other material for special studies, as indicated, or look for additional abnormalities. The perinatal or fetal autopsy (fetopsy) is an important adjunct to the prenatal examination and is considered a standard for determining the cause of perinatal loss and in the confirmation and further delineation of perinatal diagnoses.[1] This chapter is not meant to provide details on how to perform a complete and thorough fetopsy or to describe the pathology of various disorders, since there are excellent textbooks on these subjects.[2,3,4] However, it is meant to provide a sense of the usefulness of the fetopsy, to outline basic guidelines on how to perform the fetopsy, and utilize tissue preserved during autopsy for diagnosis and research. The importance of a pathologist interested in fetal and perinatal pathology is also discussed.

Fetal and perinatal pathology is largely concerned with the pathogenesis of reproductive loss and malformations. Much of fetal and perinatal pathology involves either a fetopsy or examination of specimens obtained at dilatation and evacuation (D&E). The information sought in a fetopsy is different from that in an adult autopsy. This information is not only useful in documenting disease, but also requires consideration of disorders unique to the maternal-fetal-placental unit, assessment of anatomical maturity of the fetus and its individual organs, assessment of the type of malformations and syndromes, assessment of possible recurrences in future pregnancies, and recognition of unsuspected complications of medical care. As Rushton[5] has noted "the perinatal autopsy is unique in that the results may affect not only future reproductive behavior of the parents and their close relatives, but may influence subsequent generations in whom genetically determined disorders are identified. It is sometimes forgotten that it is equally important to exclude as to confirm diagnoses in perinatal deaths, and the recording of negative findings is of paramount importance." Macpherson[6] has also affirmed that it is important to recognize the value of the so-called "negative" findings, since at a minimum they indicate the absence of identifiable recurrence risks. The fetopsy is important to clinicians who must develop a strategy for the management of future pregnancies in the family, but can also benefit other families in similar situations. It can also be used as an important tool in medical education and the data obtained is important for registries and databases. These roles of a fetopsy are best fulfilled when performed by a pathologist interested and knowledgeable in perinatal and developmental pathology.[7] For an adequate fetopsy, good clinical information, external examination, good dissection, adequate sampling of tissues, special studies (including radiology and photography), and placental examination are vital.

It also appears that the rate of the fetal autopsy has not dropped as has the rate of the adult autopsy; this is partly the result of increased utilization of new diagnostic techniques during pregnancy and partly the result of increased desire of the parents to know about future pregnancies. However, even so, the perinatal and fetopsy rates remain low, suggesting the ambivalence of clinicians about the value of the autopsy.[8] This is partly because it is assumed that new methodologies allow a better identification and understanding of the disease process, and partly because of poorly performed or untimely reporting of autopsies.

The ultrasound examination has become a tool to provide an in utero "physical examination."[9] However, despite the advances made in prenatal fetal testing and ultrasound diagnosis, the perinatal autopsy remains the standard for determining the cause of perinatal loss and in the confirmation and further delineation of perinatal diagnoses.[1,10] This is partly because, despite the sophistication of the ultrasound, only major anomalies are diagnosed, with most of the minor abnormalities—facial, extremity, and the like—not being suspected clinically.[11] These minor abnormalities, although not significant enough to cause fetal problems, serve as markers for the major anomalies and may be useful in changing the diagnosis and lead to a proper diagnosis.[11] It should also be noted that prenatal diagnostic techniques do not provide the proper diagnosis in a significant percentage of the cases.[1,9,10,12] The autopsy confirmed the clinical diagnosis in 52 (55.3%) of 94 conclusive perinatal autopsies examined by Saller et al.,[1] while in the remaining 42 (44.7%) the autopsy changed or significantly added to the diagnosis. These investigators also noted that in 48 fetal autopsies, the clinical diagnosis was changed or added to in 26 (54.2%) of the cases. The major diagnoses that were changed were anencephaly due to early amnion rupture sequence, congenital diaphragmatic hernia to cystic adenomatoid malformation, and premature rupture of membranes to bilateral renal agenesis. It also appeared that congenital heart disease and renal anomalies were among the unexpected but significant findings identified at autopsy but not diagnosed prenatally. Sun et al.[13] found minor differences between the ultrasound diagnosis and fetopsy in 14.8% of cases with a central nervous system abnormality and 23% in somatic abnormalities; major differences were noted in 6.5% of cases with central nervous system abnormalities and 27.9% of somatic abnormalities. These investigators concluded that the limitations of ultrasound examination necessitated a thorough perinatal autopsy after fetal demise or abortion to confirm the prenatal diagnosis and allow proper management and counseling. In a study comparing the accuracy of prenatal ultrasonography, Chescheir and Rietnauer[9] found that the ultrasound correctly identified over 80% of all abnormalities of the brain, skull, spine, neck, and skeleton and cases of hydrops, while missing approximately 50% of abnormalities involving the extremities, heart, face, and external genitalia, Meier et al.[12] noted that among 139 perinatal deaths, despite careful clinical review, the autopsy was the only means by which a cause of death could be assigned in 36 (26%) of the cases. Also in the same study, autopsy was the only means by which information essential to follow-up was obtained in 30 (48%) of 62 cases, in which genetic counseling or evaluation was indicated.

IMPORTANCE OF THE PERINATAL PATHOLOGIST

In the past the fetopsy was generally not considered demanding of pathological skills and was performed by junior residents. It has only been recently recognized that the performance of a good fetopsy requires special skills and knowledge of a pathologist with interest and experience in this area of pathology; such specialists are usually available only in specialized centers. That a pathologist interested in perinatal or fetal pathology can better perform and document fetal and perinatal problems has been demonstrated in various studies. Wigglesworth[14] notes that when an autopsy is requested, that "Too often the response is a hurried and meaningless ritual by an uninterested pathologist that leaves the clinician looking embarrassed that he requested permission from the parents for such an unproductive mutilation of their deceased infant." Part of the need for a pathologist trained in perinatal pathology stems from the need to stay abreast of the increasing knowledge in the fields of reproductive medicine and genetics; this requires close contact with other clinical specialists with similar interests and also necessitates an adequate exposure to case material.[5] An inadequate fetopsy may also result in failure to document and classify lesions appropriately, leading to inappropriate counseling of the parents and a totally erroneous prognosis.[5]

PERMISSION FOR THE AUTOPSY

It is extremely important in the current medico-legal climate to make sure that proper permission is obtained before the start of the autopsy, and the pathologist must have a working knowledge of the laws pertaining to the performance of the autopsy. Since laws regarding autopsies differ from state to state, an understanding of the local laws and guidelines pertaining to the autopsy is useful. The state health authorities can usually provide information regarding the appropriate laws; information can also be obtained from the College of American Pathologists regarding these laws. The first thing a pathologist does before performing the autopsy is carefully check the permission papers and adhere to any restrictions. Once the papers have been checked, proper identification of the body is necessary prior to starting the autopsy. In some cases the parents may only grant permission for an autopsy limited to certain organ systems or they may deny the autopsy for religious or personal reasons. In such cases, these limitations should not preclude a proper and thorough external examination; in such instances photography and radiology provide invaluable help.[15]

CLINICAL INFORMATION

An essential of a good and complete perinatal autopsy is a review of the clinical information available. Since this is a retrospective look, it allows the perinatal pathologist to have access to complete information about the fetus. Clinical information can not only be obtained by reviewing the physician's case records, but can also be gleaned from the nurses' notes, since these may provide invaluable information about specific therapies or diagnostic procedures. Some investigators recommend using a clinical data sheet to record useful clinical information.[16] Discussion about the case with the clinician requesting a fetopsy can also be useful, since information that may not be on the clinical records can be obtained this way; this also establishes closer links between the pathologist and the clinician. Information most useful in a fetopsy includes maternal medical and obstetrical history, particularly as it relates to previous pregnancy losses or genetically abnormal fetuses. A history of previous maternal exposure to known teratogens or social drugs such as cocaine, alcohol, smoking, and so on is also helpful.

RADIOLOGICAL EXAMINATION

With the increasing use of high-resolution ultrasonography there is an increasing identification of abnormalities of the fetus. Radiography remains a simple yet informative means of examination of stillborn fetuses.[17] Its several uses include a refinement of the autopsy technique and diagnosis. The bony skeleton and bony abnormalities of the spine and limbs are more often seen radiographically and with more clarity leading to enhanced genetic counseling[17,18]; this also saves the grueling and laborious task of dissecting the bones.[17] Radiographic examination of the fetus along with a good external examination can lead to a correct postmortem diagnosis even in those cases where a fetopsy is not feasible. It serves as a permanent documentation of the autopsy findings and as instructional material and may be of value in those cases where a regular autopsy cannot be performed.[19] It also allows for observation of normal development and consequently a better

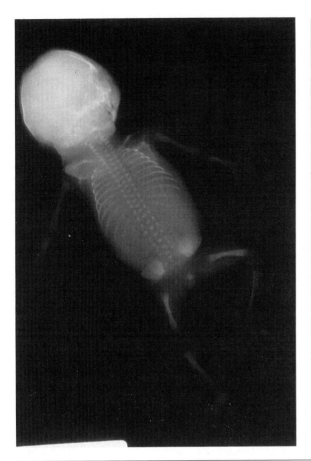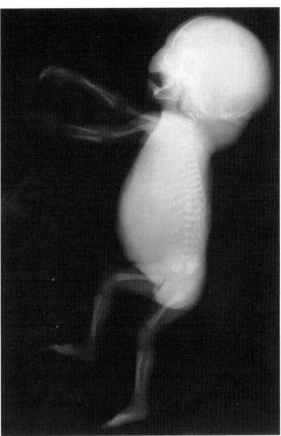

FIGURE 50-1 Routine radiological examination includes an anteroposterior (left) and lateral views (right) of the body.

understanding of disease processes. Radiologic examination is useful in assessing fetal bone age, identifying pathological calcifications of soft tissues and air in the thorax or peritoneum. It can help in determining the gestational age of the fetus and is essential for diagnosing skeletal malformations, especially osteochondrodysplasias.[19]

Griscom and Driscoll[17] have suggested certain guidelines for radiological examination of fetuses. These include: (1) all fetuses greater than 20 weeks EGA with gross abnormalities, (2) fetuses with a positive family or pregnancy history (abnormal ultrasound or chromosomal analysis) suggesting malformation, and (3) fetuses where fetopsy is refused. Routine radiologic examination consists of the anteroposterior and lateral views of the body and is obtained before the autopsy is performed. Slight angulation of the head, arms by the side, and legs extended at the knees are best for anteroposterior view. For the lateral film, the arms are in the front of the chest and the knees are slightly flexed for the best view (Fig. 50–1).

Many investigators have also utilized the injection of radio-opaque material into the blood vessels or body cavities of the fetus to identify abnormalities.[18,20,21] Talamo et al.[20] utilized injection of radio-opaque dye to demonstrate the vascular anomalies in a sirenomelic fetus. Arteriography is carried out by injecting the contrast medium into the umbilical or femoral arteries; the contrast medium can be barium sulphate or a radio-opaque dye. Böhm[21] has shown that postmortem arteriography is particularly useful for the demonstration and documentation of anomalies in the pulmonary and systemic circulations; in fact it may provide more useful information than a fetopsy in such instances.[21] The conditions that can be identified are supernumerary vessels, absent, hypo- or hyperplastic arteries, stenoses, and aortic abnormalities. Injection studies can also be used to display vessel course and blood supply in acardiac fetuses, sacrococcygeal teratoma, and conjoined twins. At our institution we have also used radio-opaque dye in the urinary bladder in cases of fetal obstructive uropathy to demonstrate the site of the obstruction (Fig. 50–2). Other investigators have suggested using magnetic resonance imaging, plain X-ray films, and ultrasound examination in cases where the permission for an autopsy is refused.[15]

PERFORMANCE OF THE FETOPSY

The performance of a good fetopsy demands attention to detail, a knowledge of normal and abnormal development, and variations from the normal. The fetopsy includes both

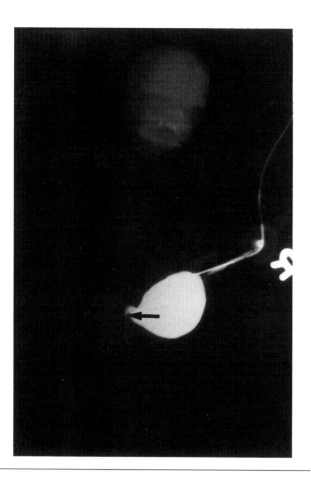

FIGURE 50-2 Injection of radio-opaque dye into the urinary bladder effectively demonstrates the marked narrowing of the urethra (arrow). The obstruction was present at the meatus.

an external examination and an internal examination with histopathological sectioning for microscopic evaluation and clinico-pathologic correlation.

The external examination includes a thorough evaluation of the external features of the fetus and recording of certain weights and measurements. Both major and minor abnormalities are noted and recorded on external examination, since they are of great importance. Major structural abnormalities have social and medical consequences and their incidence appears highest among abortions, intermediate in stillborn infants, and lowest in liveborn infants.[11] These include major cardiac defects or renal defects such as absent kidney. Minor anomalies such as frontal bossing, microtia, bifid earlobe, synophrys, epicanthal folds, microstomia, and macrostomia are relatively frequent structural abnormalities that pose no significant health or social burdens (for a list of minor abnormalities see ref. 11. Approximately 15% of newborn infants have 1 or more minor anomalies; however, they are important because their presence should prompt a search for co-existent major anomalies. Infants free of minor defects have a low incidence (approximately 1%) of major malformations. Infants with 1 minor defect have a 3% risk of major defects, those with 2

minor defects a risk of 10%, and those with 3 or more have a 20% risk of major defects.[11]

WEIGHTS AND MEASUREMENTS

The measurements most useful in a fetopsy or perinatal autopsy include crown-rump (CR) length, crown-heel (CH) length, foot length, and hand length. These measurements provide a useful indicator of the gestational age of the fetus. The foot length is of particular help in fetuses presenting with major head and spinal malformations such as anencephaly, cranio-spinal rachischisis, or amniotic band syndrome; it is also useful when the fetus is macerated and autolyzed. It should be remembered that in cases of osteochondrodysplasias (dwarfism), measurements of all 4 extremities including both distal and proximal portions should be taken, since these give an idea if there is mesomelic or rhizomelic dwarfism. Other measurements that are useful and necessary include the head circumference, chest circumference, and abdominal circumference. The head circumference, along with measurements of the anterior and posterior fontanelles, serves as a useful guide to the degree of hydrocephaly or microcephaly. The abdominal circumference is increased in cases of obstructive uropathy associated with megacystis and in cases of abdominal organomegaly. The chest circumference may be decreased in pulmonary hypoplasia associated with the oligohydramnios sequence, or in cases of short rib and thoracic dystrophy syndromes (Jeune's asphyxiating thoracic dystrophy). The fetus should always be weighed since this provides a guide to the nutritional status of the fetus. The weights and measurements of fetuses at different gestational ages have been published in previous monographs.[2,3,22,23]

GROSS EXTERNAL EXAMINATION

After the weight and other measurements of the fetus have been taken, a thorough external examination is performed to identify abnormalities, both major and minor. It should be stressed here that since genetic terminations are performed in early fetuses, features normally associated with the fully developed syndromes may not be present, namely Down syndrome.[24] A systematic external examination according to established guidelines is important.

The external examination starts with examining the craniofacial region and proceeding caudally in a systematic manner. The shape of the head is examined and may be dolichocephalic (long, keel-shaped skull with prominent forehead and occiput), brachycephalic (high, wide, and short skull due to premature closure of coronal sutures), or asymmetric; the head may be microcephalic, macrocephalic, or hydrocephalic. Abnormalities of closure of the neural tube such as anencephaly or an encephalocele are noted. In the case of an encephalocele, it should be recorded if it is anterior, posterior, or lateral; lateral encephaloceles are associated with the amniotic band syndrome. The status of the sutures, whether closed (synostosis) or overlapping is noted. Abnormalities of the eyes such as microphthalmia, anophthalmia, cyclopia, abnormal spacing (hypertelorism or hypotelorism), and epicanthal folds are recorded, along with abnormalities of the eyebrows, such as synophrys. Features of the nose of genetic interest are patent choanae, abnormal bridge, anteversion, or abnormal length. Examination of the mouth includes size (microstomia), abnormal length of the philtrum, cleft lip, hypoplastic mandible (micrognathia), abnormal teeth or gums, and cleft or high-arched palate.

In the neck the most significant finding is the presence of a cystic hygroma. It is important to determine whether it is septated or not, since septated cystic hygromas are usually larger and commonly progress to nonimmune hydrops.[25] Abnormalities of the shape of the chest including a small chest are noted. A small chest may be seen in pulmonary hypoplasia or short rib polydactyly syndromes. A protuberant abdomen is a sign of an obstructive uropathy, abnormally large cystic kidneys (if symmetric, this indicates infantile polycystic kidney disease), or other organomegaly. The size and site of abdominal wall defects such as gastroschisis or omphalocele are noted. Abnormalities of genital differentiation may be seen in some syndromes and include hypospadias, epispadias, undescended testes, abnormal labia or scrotum, and an abnormally sized penis or clitoris. It should be determined if the anus is patent or not and associated with a smooth perineum; this finding is a sign of the more serious cloacal dysgenesis. Examination of the extremities includes the recording of abnormal length, polydactyly (postaxial or preaxial), syndactyly, reduction deformities, arthrogryposis, abnormal clenching or overlapping digits, and rocker-bottom feet. Abnormal nails may be associated with certain syndromes—hypoplastic nails in trisomy 18 and in the Ellis-van Creveld syndrome (chondro-ectodermal dysplasia). Although dermatoglyphics are of importance in many chromosomal syndromes, it is impossible to record them at an early gestational age. The only findings that we have been able to identify in genetic fetopsies (gestational age of 20–22 weeks) are the simian crease or the Sydney line. Finally the skin is examined for any lesions or subcutaneous edema. Cutaneous lesions such as hemangiomas or pigmented lesions should be noted, along with signs of maceration or constriction bands. An important aspect of external examination is the detection of hydrops fetalis associated with subcutaneous edema and effusions. Once this diagnosis is made, an effort should be made to identify the cause, whether immunologic or nonimmunologic.[26,27]

INTERNAL EXAMINATION

In Situ Examination

Although the precise order and manner of dissection of the organs is secondary to the thoroughness of the autopsy, it is best to follow an individual routine to prevent any important pathology being missed.[16] After the initial skin incisions have been made and the body cavities have been exposed, an in situ examination of the organs is made to assess proper situs of the organs, any organomegaly, and abnormalities. In the abdominal and pelvic regions, the peritoneal surfaces are examined for calcifications, possible meconium spillage, or hemorrhage.

The diaphragm is examined for hernias and the size of the hernias recorded. Any abnormality of the mesenteric attachments is noted, since this is associated with malrotation of the intestines. The size of the liver and extension below the diaphragm is measured. It is also important to note if the liver and gallbladder are in the midline, since these are part of the heterotaxy syndromes (asplenia and polysplenia). Abnormalities of the genitourinary tract such as a dilated bladder and ureters, hydronephrosis, and cystic change of the kidneys is recorded. In both the pleural and peritoneal cavities, the volume and type of fluid is measured. In the thoracic cavity, situs of the heart and lungs, abnormal lobation of lungs, and presence of abdominal contents (in cases of diaphragmatic hernia) is important. This initial in situ examination also allows the pathologist to prepare for any special studies, if needed.

EXAMINATION OF INDIVIDUAL ORGANS

CNS

It appears that central nervous tissue is not well preserved in most cases in which labor is induced by prostaglandins for termination of the pregnancy. The central nervous system tissue is poorly myelinated at gestational ages when induction is performed, making it impossible to assess structural abnormalities of the brain in many of these cases. Moreover, abnormalities such as the Arnold-Chiari malformation, a common association of meningomyelocele, are not fully developed at this stage, adding to the difficulty in diagnosing such conditions. Other developmental migrational defects such as lissencephaly or polymicrogyria are also difficult to diagnose on gross examination, since the brain normally appears lissencephalic at 20–22 weeks gestation.

The usual method of removal of fetal and neonatal brains involves creating lateral flaps of calvarium thereby exposing the brain. The brain is then inspected in situ for intracranial hemorrhages and tears of the tentorium or falx cerebri. When a Dandy-Walker anomaly is suspected, the posterior fossa is exposed after removing the occipital bone. Since the cyst is liable to be lost during removal, it is advisable to photograph the cyst wall before removing the brain. It has been suggested that the brain be removed by floating it under water using a "no-touch" approach and trying to keep the leptomeninges intact. Despite such precautions, removal of the intact fetal brain is difficult in induced cases, necessitating other methods to examine or fix the brain in situ. Kent et al.[28] employed an unusual method for neuropathologic examination of abortuses suspected of having cerebral malformations involving the ventricular system. Their method involves decapitation and freezing of the head at −4°C. The specimen is then serially sectioned using a bandsaw, followed by photography. However, this method of examination causes marked artifactual changes, rendering it unsuitable for histopathologic evaluation. Other methods that we have used include injection of formalin directly into the subdural region, or into the carotid arteries in the neck, at least 1–2 hours before the performance of the fetopsy. However, these methods also show limited success in cases where the brain is markedly autolyzed.

In cases of neural tube defects such as anencephaly or spinal dysraphia (meningomyeloceles), histopathological examination is of limited diagnostic use, since the defect is grossly recognizable. However, Kronz and Hutchins[29] have proposed serial sectioning and histopathologically examining the entire defect, and have suggested on the basis of these studies that these defects are homologous and a consequence of a musculoskeletal disorder or a secondary injury, rather than failure of the neural tube to close.

Heart

The heart is examined after first removing the thymus and pericardium. Before removing the heart from the thoracic cavity, the normalcy of the heart's position and shape, the pattern of all venous return, and the orientation of the great vessels is recorded. This initial examination provides useful clues to underlying congenital heart disease. When the left anterior descending branch of the left coronary artery lies toward the left it indicates a hypoplastic left ventricle. Transposition of the great vessels can be appreciated by observing the reversal of the normal pulmonary trunk and aortic positions. A right sided aortic arch and coarctation are easily appreciated. If a congenital cardiac anomaly is suspected on clinical grounds, the heart is removed along with the lungs, inferior vena cava, and a portion of the liver; this is to allow recognition of anomalous pulmonary venous return.

After removing the heart, standard dissection techniques are employed to optimally examine the heart.[30] In complex congenital heart disease, it is important to identify each chamber as right or left according to established morphologic criteria, to better define the defect. The right atrium is recognized by the wide based appendage (dog ear), crista terminalis, and a fossa ovalis, while the left atrium is recognized by a narrow based appendage (bent finger) and a crenelated border. The right ventricle shows the presence of coarse trabeculations, poorly defined papillary muscle bundles, scattered chordae, separation of the pulmonary and tricuspid valves by the presence of a septal band, and a pulmonary conus. The left ventricle shows a smooth septal and endocardial surface, well-defined papillary muscles, prominent chordae attached to the mitral valve and mitral-aortic valve fibrous continuity.

Lungs

The lungs are weighed and inspected for normal lobation, masses, and petechiae. The weight of the lungs is used as guide to determine pulmonary hypoplasia, if present. To determine if the lungs are hypoplastic, the lung to body-weight ratio is used. Wigglesworth et al.[31] have suggested that in fetuses with a gestational age of 28 weeks or less, a ratio of 0.015 and in fetuses 28 weeks or more a ratio of 0.012 or less should be considered consistent with hypoplasia; however, Page and Stocker find that a lung to body weight ratio of 0.010 identifies pulmonary hypoplasia in most instances.[32] The masses usually identified in the lungs are congenital cystic adenomatoid malformations

or sequestrations. In such cases angiography of the pulmonary and bronchial arterial systems is of great diagnostic help.

Genito-Urinary Tract

The entire genito-urinary tract, from the kidneys to the urethra, is removed in a single block. This is particularly important in males since obstructive uropathies from any cause—posterior urethral valves, urethral atresia, or stenosis—are more common in males. Hoagland and Hutchins[33] documented a case of "kinking" of the urethra and not urethral atresia, as a cause of the prune-belly syndrome, and recommended that serial sectioning of the intact lower urinary tract be performed. This technique allowed histopathologic examination of the entire urinary tract and ensured identification of short segmental lesions within the urethra.

Gastrointestinal Tract

The gastro-intestinal system is examined from the esophagus to the anorecturm. Anomalies of interest in the esophagus include tracheo-esophageal fistulas, webs, and stenoses. Duodenal atresia and an annular pancreas may be seen in Down syndrome. Atresias and stenoses of the small intestine suggest a possible diagnosis of cystic fibrosis. Recognition of other abnormalities such as Meckel diverticulum is important since these may be syndromic. The length of the colon (short colon syndrome) may be an indicator of maternal diabetes mellitus. Meconium peritonitis with calcification and matting of intestines may be seen in cytic fibrosis. In cases of anal atresia (a manifestation of abnormal cloacal development) other features associated with abnormal cloacal development, such as colon ending in the bladder, absent urethral and vaginal openings, should be carefully searched for.

Skeletal System

Although radiological examination is the best tool available for examining the skeletal system, histopathological evaluation of the skeletal system has been of significance in defining various osteochondrodysplasias.[34] For the most appropriate histopathological examination of the skeletal system, the method of Yang et al. is recommended.[34] These investigators recommend sections of the ribs, vertebral bodies, and proximal or distal femur or humerus as a minimum requirement for adequate evaluation. Additional sections from bones with significant radiologic changes may also be used.

Lymphatic System

The weight, location, and presence of the thymus are noted; absence of the thymus is associated with the DiGeorge syndrome. Examination of the spleen involves location and number. It is located on the right in cases of situs inversus and in heterotaxy syndromes (asplenia, polysplenia). Normally 2–3 small splenic masses (spleniculi) in association with a normal-sized spleen may be present occasionally. Multiple small spleniculi without a single large spleen (polysplenia) or absence of the spleen (asplenia) are associated with severe cardiac malformations. Lymph nodes are not generally appreciated in second trimester fetuses; however, enlarged nodes, when present, signify an infectious process.

Microscopic Evaluation

After a thorough gross examination, tissue can be submitted for microscopic evaluation. Appreciation of normal histology at various stages of development is important. Usually one section is taken from each organ and one from each side for the paired organs. Sections from each cardiac ventricle are appropriate, although some investigators recommend serially sectioning the entire heart when it is small. In most early genetic fetopsies, although histopathological findings of interest can be found in any organ, the most important are frequently the central nervous system, kidneys, and the skeletal system. In the central nervous system, migrational defects, such as heterotopias and abnormalities of gyration (polymicrogyria and lissencephaly) and changes associated with hypoxic/ischemic damage can only be identified by microscopy. In the kidney, differentiation of cystic disease into multicystic dysplastic, infantile recessive polycystic, or "adult" type of polycystic kidney disease is important, since the genetic implications are different. On occasion we have noted calcifications in the liver and papillary muscles of the heart. Recently, Faquin et al.[35] have suggested that fetal liver calcifications may be associated with chromosomal abnormalities and not infections. The significance of cardiac calcifications is not known; however, it is possible that these may represent hypoxic events. Although radiological examination remains of prime importance in osteochondrodysplasias, histopathological examination has helped define many of these disorders.[34] It is important to save tissue in paraffin since this can serve as an important resource for molecular biological studies.

EXAMINATION OF DILATATION AND EVACUATION SPECIMENS

Elective termination of pregnancy is being performed with increasing frequency for cases in which major chromosomal abnormalities or complex fetal anomalies are identified on prenatal examination. After a major fetal anomaly or chromosomal abnormality has been identified, and the parents appropriately counseled, the pregnancy can be terminated by prostaglandin induction or by D&E. While prostaglandin induction allows for delivery of an intact fetus, which can be examined in detail and the prenatal diagnoses confirmed, it carries certain disadvantages.[36] It is prolonged, may be associated with labor discomfort,[36] and may be accompanied by vomiting or diarrhea. D&E offers certain advantages over prostaglandin induction which include rapidity, less pain, and in this day of cost containment, a much shorter stay in hospital resulting in saving hospitalization costs. Consequently, it is the most common method of termination of second trimester pregnancies. However, there is disruption and fragmentation of fetal tissue

making gross examination of the fetus difficult. There is also a possibility of microbial contamination of the tissues from the vaginal flora, precluding cell culture growth.[37,38] Klatt[36] has proposed a method for examining the D&E specimen; this involves the separation of fetal from placental tissue and sorting of the fetal tissue into separate regions with proper anatomic relationship. After an initial radiologic examination, the fetal tissue is weighed and examined in detail, region by region, to identify abnormalities, if any. Photographs of any unusual or characteristic features are taken for teaching and documentation. If cytogenetic or biochemical testing is to be performed, the tissue is submitted fresh and appropriate samples taken in a sterile fashion. Using the above method, Klatt[36] identified a major fetal abnormality in 92% of the 37 cases examined. In 46% of cases, pathological examination provided a specific diagnosis not previously made. However, the procedure did not allow for identification of intracranial abnormalities such as Dandy-Walker malformation, Arnold-Chiari malformation, or encephalocele because of the softness of the brain. Identification of herniation and abdominal wall defects was also difficult, since fragmentation hampered proper relationships of body parts. This experience was not shared by Sun et al.,[39] who noted that in D&E specimens pathologic examination was confirmatory in most neural tube defects, but was of very limited value in detecting most other fetal anomalies.

THE IMPORTANCE OF PLACENTAL EXAMINATION

Pregnancy represents a complex biologic interaction of the fetus, placenta, and the mother, and an accurate assessment of events during abnormal pregnancy requires knowledge of all 3. The placenta is a fetal organ and mirrors fetal disease and in recent times there has been an increased interest in studying the placenta as it reflects on the health of the fetus. With increasingly sophisticated tools being used for assessing the health of the fetus, both clinicians and pathologists have shown an increased awareness of the fetoplacental unit. The placenta can also provide valuable information in genetic and infectious diseases of the fetus. Most of the diseases of the mother and other placental problems associated with fetal loss later in gestation are not seen in the early conceptus and will only be alluded to in this chapter. In this chapter we will cover only some of the basic aspects of placental pathology as it refers to genetic, chromosomal and infectious diseases of the placenta; for more understanding of placental pathology, refer to monographs in placental pathology.[40,41,42]

As the placenta is a fetal organ, it is essential to examine it as part of any pathologic evaluation of an abnormal pregnancy outcome, and it has been argued that all placentas should be examined.[43] Much has been learned about placental morphology and pathology and it is incumbent upon the perinatal pathologist to be familiar with the placenta, its variations, and pathological changes caused by various fetal and maternal disorders. In many cases of placental examination, morphologic lesions simply confirm clinical events during pregnancy (antepartum hemorrhage, meconium staining), and recording them serves important quality assurance and medico-legal issues.[44] Placental examination is important in cases of multiple gestations, not only for zygosity determination but also for possible causes of discordant growth—i.e., determination of anastomoses in twin-to-twin transfusion. Detailed placental study is recommended in cases of invasive procedures, such as selective termination in multiple pregnancies, fetal surgery, or ablation of anastomoses in twin-to-twin transfusion. Other placental lesions of interest from a clinico-pathological and legal standpoint include abruption, retroplacental hemorrhage, maternal floor infarct, placental infarcts, meconium staining, maternal disorders including hypertension, diabetes mellitus, autoimmune diseases, and rhesus incompatibility.

In fetal genetic disorders and structural abnormalities, the placenta generally shows morphologic abnormalities that do not appear to be very specific. Microscopically, these placentas generally show large immature villi, which appear to be hypovascular, with decrease in the number of small arteries and arterioles;[45,46] growth as measured by proliferation markers tends to be comparable to normal controls.[47] These findings correlate with abnormal Doppler findings on ultrasound examination, suggesting that abnormal placental morphology and fetoplacental blood flow may contribute to disturbed fetal growth.[45] It has been suggested that most cases of triploidy are associated with a partial hydatidiform mole and associated with diandry (2 sets of paternal chromosomes); however, McFadden and Pantzer[48] have shown that most cases of triploidy show digyny (2 sets of maternal chromosomes) and that only 15% of triploid conceptions show a partial hydatidiform mole. Of interest is the finding of confined placental mosaicism (CPM), where the chromosomal abnormalities are present in the placenta and not in the fetus; these have been shown to have a worse prognosis.[49] Since it is limited to the placenta, CPM is not detectable by gross, histopathologic, or cytogenetic studies of the fetus. The introduction of fluorescent in situ hybridization (FISH) has made the assessment of CPM in the fetus and placenta feasible. The most common karyotypic abnormality in CPM involves chromosome 16, although other chromosomes such as 2,3,7,9,12,13,15, and 18 may also be involved.[49]

Other genetic abnormalities may be associated with abnormal placentas; these include conditions associated with fetal hydrops. Of these the hemoglobinopathies are generally associated with large placentas showing villous edema and intracapillary hematopoesis.[44] Although many of the inherited metabolic disorders are diagnosed in utero using assays of cultured amniotic cells, these changes are not generally appreciated by light microscopy.

However, in many of these conditions vacuolation of trophoblast epithelium and villous stromal and Hofbauer cells in various combinations occurs;[50] biochemical means aided by electron microscopy is essential for a definitive diagnosis.[51]

In most structural abnormalities of the fetus, the placental findings are generally nonspecific and not helpful in arriving at a diagnosis. In most of these conditions, the placenta shows nonspecific findings including villous immaturity and edema, with atrophy of trophoblast and occasional trophoblast inclusions; these findings have been described in anencephaly and we have seen them in other fetal conditions. However, in certain conditions, placental examination provides a clue to the diagnosis. A typical example of this is the early amnion rupture sequence (amniotic band syndrome), which may be associated with anencephaly, limb-body wall malformations, and limb amputations and constrictions. The diagnosis is sometimes confirmed only after placental examination, with the pathological findings including a thickened and attenuated fetal surface, vernix granulomas, chronic inflammation, and fibrosis.[52] Another fetal abnormality that is associated with specific placental pathological changes is the oligohydramnios sequence in which the classical finding of amnion nodosum is present.

Many maternal infections can also involve the placenta, and may have severe consequences for the fetus. These infections may be acquired as an ascending infection from the cervix, through hematogenous spread, or by extension from the endometrium. With newer diagnostic modalities, other possible routes of infection include amniocentesis, chorionic villous sampling, and fetal biopsy. While viral infections are less common than bacterial infections, they are more often teratogenic. The most common viral infection of the placenta is the cytomegalovirus (CMV); other viral infections include herpes simplex virus (HSV), varicella zoster virus (VZV), and rubella. The hallmarks of CMV infection are the characteristic intra-nuclear inclusions and intra-cytoplasmic inclusions, lymphoplasmacytic villitis, and necrosis of villous tissue; however, this histopathologic picture may vary depending on the age of the fetus.[53] In cases where histopathology is nondiagnostic, special techniques such as the polymerase chain reaction (PCR), immunoperoxidase, and in situ hybridization are of help.[54,55] HSV gives rise to an acute and chronic villitis if the infection is acquired from the endometrium or a necrotizing chorioamnionitis associated with plasma cells, if it is an ascending infection.[42] Although varicella infection of the mother in the third trimester is rarely associated with fetal or placental involvement, infection in the first trimester may be associated with the "congenital varicella syndrome" with cutaneous scars, limb hypoplasia, and ophthalmologic problems. The placenta shows chronic villitis with granuloma-like changes.[56] The fetal rubella syndrome is acquired through transplacental infection; however, the associated placental changes including focal trophoblastic necrosis and decidual perivascular infiltration, abnormal villous vasculature, and fibrosis, appear to be nonspecific.[42] Of the bacterial infections, syphilis, and listeria are associated with specific placental pathology. In syphilis there is chronic villitis, villous immaturity, proliferative vascular changes, and acute villitis.[57] Confirmation depends on identifying the organism in the placenta, using special stains such as Steiner and Steiner stain to identify the organisms. Listeria gives rise to intraplacental abscesses.

Single umbilical artery is the most common true congenital abnormality in humans and can be detected by ultrasound examination, and confirmed by microscopic examination.[42]

SPECIAL STUDIES

Since the earliest times the principal use of the autopsy has been as a research tool to understand the changes induced by disease on the whole organism; the increasing usage of complex molecular techniques provides such an opportunity to understand the molecular basis of disease.[58] The autopsy serves as a useful resource to preserve tissue for further studies, since in many cases fresh tissue from biopsies or surgically excised material may not be available from all organs, such as the brain and heart.[58] In this regard tissue obtained from a fetopsy may be of more value, since it can be used to study developmental genes and processes. However, in many cases the fetopsy may be performed several hours to possibly days after the death or delivery of the fetus raising the question of preservation of DNA and RNA in tissue. Larsen et al.[59] studied the preservation of tissues obtained at autopsy and their usefulness in molecular biological techniques. They showed that RNA was sufficiently preserved in tissues obtained less than 2 days postmortem, to give signals on Northern blot analysis, while DNA could be extracted 3–5 days postmortem as demonstrated by Southern blot analysis. DNA stability was documented in the liver 24–36 hours postmortem, up to 5 days postmortem in the spleen, kidney, and thyroid and up to 3 weeks in brain tissue.[60] DNA preservation is good in paraffin-embedded tissue previously stored in buffered formalin, but not if stored in nonbuffered formalin; however, the genetic material obtained at autopsy may be used for qualitative and not quantitative determination, since partial degradation of signal may occur because of autolysis.[59] Humphreys-Beher[61] et al. identified mRNA in tissue obtained postmortem from patients with cystic fibrosis. Significant quantities were obtained from the lung, but not from the pancreas or stomach, suggesting that the pancreas and stomach could be producing RNase. The authors stressed the importance of time as a critical factor in the recovery of RNA and the utility of this methodology to study not only cystic fibrosis but other genetic diseases as well.

With the advent of the PCR, the identification of even small strands of DNA and oligonucleotides is possible. PCR has been used for the identification of infectious organisms, including viruses and bacteria from tissue obtained at autopsy. Utilizing PCR, Dong et al. identified congenital cytomegalovirus infection in 23.5% of first trimester pregnancies.[54] For the best results it is preferable to use fresh or frozen tissue for PCR analysis; however, PCR has been used to identify appropriate DNA in formalin-fixed, paraffin-embedded archival tissue. Turner et al.[62] identified adenovirus DNA in formalin-fixed, paraffin-embedded tissue obtained at postmortem, while Nakamura et al.[63] were able to identify the human CMV gene in placental chorionic villitis in formalin-fixed paraffin-embedded tissue, even in cases where the typical intra-nuclear inclusions were not identified on light microscopy or by immunohistochemistry.

FISH has been used to identify specific chromosomes in interphase and metaphase cells for rapid prenatal diagnosis from uncultured amniocytes, single cells from blastomeres, and fetal cells extracted from maternal blood.[64]

Although routinely performed on cells taken from fresh tissue, it has been used to identify the abnormal chromosomal complement in formalin-fixed, paraffin-embedded tissue.[64] These investigators correctly identified the chromosomal complement in 15 of 19 placental tissues examined, including all cases of trisomy 18 and 13; probes for trisomy 21 were less reliable. Drut et al.[65] also identified trisomy 13 in archival tissue obtained at autopsy. Although most structural chromosomal abnormalities cannot be identified by this technique, FISH may be used to identify specific cytogenetic abnormalities in formalin-fixed, paraffin-embedded tissues, especially in cases where tissue is not submitted fresh for genetic analysis or the cells fail to grow in culture. FISH offers many benefits compared with traditional cytogenetic analysis of cultured tissue: (1) it eliminates the difficulty associated with culture of fetal tissue from macerated fetuses which often fails to grow; (2) it eliminates the tissue culture-induced bias of variable viability of diploid and aneuploid cells and their ability to yield analyzable metaphases; and (3) a large number of cells from multiple tissue samples can be analyzed rapidly, permitting effective detection of chromosomal mosaicism especially in cases of CPM.[49] One of the most powerful tools in molecular biology and wherein lies one of the greatest uses of the autopsy, is the prospective planned necropsy-based research, where tissue is gathered in a systematic and uniform manner for all cases. This has the advantage of uniform sampling with optimum preservation.[58,66]

Microbiologic studies involving both viral and bacterial cultures are recommended on selected cases.[44,67] These have to be done before the autopsy is completed. Infection can be suspected on the basis of maternal history or potential exposure to an infectious agent. The external appearance of the fetus may be help in a few cases; hydrops fetalis may have an infectious cause. If the internal examination reveals hepatosplenomegaly and enlarged lymph nodes in the absence of a hematologic problem, an infection may be the cause. Bacterial infections are more important in cases of abortions, stillbirths, and preterm delivery;[44] however, both viral and bacterial cultures are recommended in select cases. For identification of viruses, tissue culture is variably successful; however, more recently PCR, FISH, and immunohistochemistry have been very useful.

PHOTOGRAPHY

The importance of photography in the performance of a good perinatal autopsy cannot be stressed enough. Although in an ideal situation all fetopsies should be photographed, reality dictates that only those cases in which anomalies are present be photographed. All external anomalies are photographed at our institution and as the fetopsy proceeds additional photographs are taken as the need arises. These photographs not only provide a permanent record of the autopsy for future reference, but also serve as a powerful teaching tool for residents and other health care providers and can also aid in better parental counseling. If properly taken, photographs provide a more accurate record than a lengthy written description and they are particularly useful when further consultation is needed.[67]

AUTOPSY SUMMARY

Finally, the autopsy report should include a final diagnosis, which is a compilation of all the findings noted during performance of the autopsy, whether these are macroscopic or microscopic. This should be accompanied by a clinico-pathologic correlation or autopsy summary, which summarizes the gross and microscopic findings and any special studies that were performed, and correlates them with the clinical findings. The summary allows the pathologist to describe and interpret the findings in an objective manner, and provides others with an understanding of the pathological findings.[68] This summary should be concise and directed and should include references pertinent to the case, since these serve as important teaching tools.

References

1. Saller DN, Lesser KB, Harrel U, et al. The clinical utility of the perinatal autopsy. *JAMA.* 1995;273:663–665.
2. Wigglesworth JS, Singer DB. *Textbook of Fetal and Perinatal Pathology.* Blackwell Scientific Publications: Boston, 1991.
3. Stevenson RE, Hall JG, Goodman RM. *Human Malformations and Related Anomalies.* Oxford Monographs on Medical Genetics # 27. Oxford University Press: New York, 1993.
4. Dimmick JE, Kalousek DK. *Developmental Pathology of the Embryo and Fetus.* Lippincott: Philadelphia, 1992.
5. Rushton DI. Should perinatal post mortems be carried out by specialist pathologists? *Br J Obstet Gynecol.* 1995;102:182–185.
6. Macpherson TA. The role of the anatomical pathologist in perinatology. *Semin Perinatol.* 1985;9:257–262.
7. Macpherson TA, Valdes-Dapena M, Kanbour A. Perinatal mortality and morbidity: the role of the anatomical pathologist. *Semin Perinatol.* 1986;10:179–186.
8. Cartlidge PHT, Dawson AT, Stewart JH, et al. Value and quality of perinatal and infant postmortem examinations: cohort analysis of 400 consecutive deaths. *Br Med J.* 1995;310:155–158.
9. Chescheir NC, Reitnauer PJ. A comparative study of prenatal diagnosis and perinatal autopsy. *J Ultrasound Med.* 1994;13:451–456.
10. Shen-Schwarz S, Neish C, Hill LM. Antenatal ultrasound for fetal anomalies: importance of perinatal autopsy. *Pediatr Pathol.* 1989;9:1–9.
11. Stevenson RE, Hall JG. Terminology. In: Stevenson RE, Hall JG, Goodman RM, eds. *Human Malformations and Related Anomalies.* Oxford University Press: New York. 1993;21–30.
12. Meier PR, Manchester DK, Shikes RH, et al. Perinatal autopsy: its clinical value. *Obstet Gynecol.* 1986;67:349–351.
13. Sun C-C, Grumbach K, Decosta D, et al. Correlation of prenatal ultrasound diagnosis and autopsy findings in fetal anomalies: importance of the perinatal autopsy. *Lab Invest.* 1997;76:177A (abstract).
14. Wigglesworth JS. Quality of the perinatal autopsy. *Br J Obstet Gynecol.* 1991;98:617–623.
15. Raffles A. Ropel C. Non-invasive investigations are also helpful if permission for a necropsy is refused. (Letter) *BMJ.* 1995;310:870.
16. Macpherson TA, Valdes-Dapena M. The Perinatal Autopsy. In: Wigglesworth JS, Singer DB, eds. *Textbook of Fetal and Perinatal Pathology.* Blackwell Scientific Publications: Boston, 1991.
17. Griscom NT, Driscoll SG. Radiography of stillborn fetuses and infants dying at birth. *Am J Roentgen.* 1980;134:485–489.
18. Barson AJ, Langley FA, Russell JGB. Uses of routine postmortem radiography. *Arch Dis Child.* 1974;49:74.
19. Grønvall J, Græm N. Radiography in postmortem examinations of fetuses and neonates. *APMIS.* 1989;97:274–280.
20. Talamo TS, Macpherson TA, Dominguez R. Sirenomelia: angiographic demonstration of vascular anomalies. *Arch Pathol Lab Med.* 1982;106:347–348.
21. Böhm N. Documentation of vascular malformations by postmortal angiography of the fetus and the newborn. *Pathol Res Pract.* 1981;171:423–426.
22. Kalousek DK, Fitch, Paradice BA. *Pathology of the Human Embryo and Previable Fetus: An Atlas.* Springer-Verlag; New York, 1990.
23. Stocker JT, Dehner LP. *Pediatric Pathology.* Lippincott, Philadelphia, 1992.
24. Baldwin VJ, Kalousek DK, Dimmick JE, et al. Diagnostic pathologic investigation of the malformed conceptus. *Persp Pediatr Pathol.* 1982;7:65–108.
25. Bronshtein M, Bar-Hava I, Blumenfeld I, et al. The difference between septated and nonseptated nuchal cystic hygroma in the early third trimester. *Obstet Gynecol.* 1993;81:683–687.
26. Poeschmann RP, Verheijen RHM, Van Dongen PWJ. Differential diagnosis and causes of nonimmunological hydrops fetalis: a review. *Obstet Gynecol Surv.* 1991;46:223–231.
27. Van Meldergem L, Jauniaux E, Fourneau C, et al. Genetic causes of hydrops fetalis. *Pediatrics.* 1992;89:81–86.
28. Kent SG, Isada NB, Larsen JW. A simple method for gross examination of the brain in abortuses and macerated fetuses. *Obstet Gynecol.* 1987;70:946–947.
29. Kronz JD, Hutchins GM. Homologies between cranial and spinal dysraphia: evidence of a primary mesenchymal defect. *Lab Invest.* 1997;76:11A.
30. Donelly WH, Hawkins H. Optimal examination of the normally opened perinatal heart. *Hum Pathol.* 1987;18:55–60.
31. Wigglesworth JS, Desai R, Guerrini P. Fetal lung hypoplasia: biochemical and structural variations and their possible significance. *Arch Dis Child.* 1981;56:606–615.
32. Page DV, Stocker JT. Anomalies associated with pulmonary hypoplasia. *Am Rev Respir Dis.* 1982;125:216–221.
33. Hoagland MH, Hutchins GM. Obstructive lesions of the lower urinary tract in the prune belly syndrome. *Arch Pathol Lab Med.* 1987;111:154–156.
34. Yang SS, Kitchen E, Gilbert EF, et al. Histopathologic examination in osteochondrodysplasia: time for standardization. *Arch Pathol Lab Med.* 1986;110:10–12.
35. Faquin WC, Pflueger S, Roberts DJ. Histologic evaluation of fetal liver calcifications in fetopsy specimens: possible association with chromosomal abnormalities. *Lab Invest.* 1997;76:156A (abstract).
36. Klatt EC. Pathologic examination of fetal specimens from dilatation and evacuation procedures. *Am J Clin Path.* 1995;103:415–418.

37. Shulman LP, Ling FW, Meyers CM, et al. Dilation and evacuation for second-trimester genetic pregnancy termination. *Obstet Gynecol.* 1990;75:1037–1040.

38. Hern WM, Zen C, Ferguson KA, et al. Outpatient abortion for fetal anomaly and fetal death from 15-34 menstrual weeks' gestation: techniques and clinical management. *Obstet Gynecol.* 1993;81:301–306.

39. Sun C-C, Grumbach K, Decosta D, et al. Correlation of prenatal ultrasound diagnosis and pathology findings in dilatation and evacuation specimens. *Lab Invest.* 1997;76:177A (abstract).

40. Fox H. *Pathology of the Placenta. Major problems in Pathology*, Vol. VII. W. B. Saunders: Philadelphia, 1978.

41. Perrin EVDK. *Pathology of the Placenta. Contemporary Issues in Surgical Pathology*, Vol. 5, Churchill Livingstone: New York, 1984.

42. Benirschke K, Kaufmann P. *Pathology of the Human Placenta*, 3rd ed. Springer-Verlag: New York, 1995, 268–318, 319–377, 537–623.

43. Salafia CM. Ventzileos AM. Why all placentas should be examined by a pathologist in 1990. *Am J Obstet Gynecol.* 1990;163:1282–1293.

44. Baldwin VJ. Placenta. In: Dimmick JE, Kalousek DK, eds. *Developmental Pathology of the Embryo and Fetus.* Lippincott: Philadelphia, 1992;271–319.

45. Rochelson B, Kaplan C, Guzman E, et al. A quantitative analysis of placental vasculature in the third-trimester fetus with autosomal trisomy. *Obstet Gynecol.* 1990;75:59–63.

46. Kuhlmann RS, Werner AL, Abramowitz J, et al. Placental histology in fetuses between 18 and 21 weeks' gestation with abnormal karyotype. *Am J Obstet Gynecol.* 1990; 163:1264–1270.

47. Qureshi F, Jacques SM, Johnson MP, et al. Trisomy 21 placentas: a histopathological and immunohistochemical study using proliferating cell nuclear antigen. *Fetal Diagn Ther* 1997;12:210–215.

48. McFadden DE, Pantzar JT. Placental pathology in triploidy. *Hum Pathol.* 1996;27:1018–1020.

49. Kalousek DK, Barrett I. Confined placental mosaicism and stillbirth. *Pediatr Pathol.* 1994;14:151–159.

50. Clarke LA, Dimmick JE, Applegarth DA. Pathology of metabolic diseases. In: Dimmick JE, Kalousek DK, eds. *Developmental Pathology of the Embryo and Fetus.* Lippincott: Philadelphia. 1992;199–234.

51. Hug G, Chuck G, Chen Y-T, et al. Chorionic villus ultrastucture in type II glycogen storage disease (Pompe's disease) (Letter). *N Engl J Med.* 1991;324:342–343.

52. Yang SS. ADAM sequence and innocent amniotic band: manifestations of early amnion rupture. *Am J Med Genet.* 1990;37:562–568.

53. Garcia AGP, Fonseca EF, Marques RLS, et al. Placental morphology in cytomegalovirus infection. *Placenta.* 1989;10:1–18.

54. Dong ZW, Yan C, Yi W, et al. Detection of congenital cytomegalovirus infection by using chorionic villi of the early pregnancy and polymerase chain reaction. *Int J Gynecol Obstet.* 1994;44:229–231.

55. Sachdev R, Nuovo GJ, Kaplan C, et al. In situ hybridization analysis for cytomegalovirus in chronic villitis. *Pediatr Pathol.* 1990; 10:909–917.

56. Qureshi F and Jacques SM. Maternal varicella during pregnancy: correlation of maternal history and fetal outcome with placental histopathology. *Hum Pathol.* 1996;27:191–196.

57. Qureshi F, Jacques SM, Reyes MP. Placental histopathology in syphilis. *Hum Pathol.* 1993;24:778–784.

58. Kleiner DE, Emmert-Buck MR, Liotta LA. Necropsy as a research method in the age of molecular pathology. *Lancet.* 1995;346:945–948.

59. Larsen S, Rygaard K, Asnæs S, et al. Northern and southern blot analysis of human RNA and DNA in autopsy material. *APMIS.* 1992;100:498–502.

60. Bär W, Kratzer A, Mächler M, et al. Postmortem stability of DNA. *Forensic Science Intern.* 1988;39:59–70.

61. Humphreys-Beher MG, King FK, Bunnel B, et al. Isolation of biologically active RNA from human autopsy for the study of cystic fibrosis. Biotech *App Biochem.* 1986;8:392–403.

62. Turner PC, Bailey AS, Cooper RJ. The polymerase chain reaction for detecting adenovirus DNA in formalin-fixed, paraffin-embedded tissue obtained post mortem. *J Infect.* 1993;27:43–46.

63. Nakamura Y, Sakuma S, Ohta Y, et al. Detection of the human cytomegalovirus gene in placental chronic villits by polymerase chain reaction. *Hum Pathol.* 1994;25:815–818.

64. Cowles TA, Elder FFB, Taylor S. Identification of abnormal chromosomal complement in formalin-fixed, paraffin-embedded placental tissue. *Prenatal Diagnosis.* 1995;15:21–26.

65. Drut RM, Harris CP, Drut R, et al. Use of fluorescent in situ hybridization to detect trisomy 13 in archival tissues for cytogenetic diagnosis. *Pediatr Pathol.* 1992;12:799–805.

66. Offerhaus GJA. Molecular and epidemiologic necropsy: two of a pair? *Lancet.* 1996;347:346.

67. Keeling JW. The Perinatal Necropsy. In: ed Keeling JW, Fetal and Neonatal Pathology, 2nd ed. Springer-Verlag, New York: 1993;1–46.

68. Hutchins GM and the Autopsy Committee of the College of American Pathologists. Practice guidelines for autopsy pathology. *Arch Pathol Lab Med.* 1995;119:123–130.

CHAPTER 51

REDUCTION IN MULTIPLE PREGNANCIES

Mark I. Evans / Doina Ciorica / David W. Britt / John C. Fletcher

INTRODUCTION

Since Louise Brown's birth in 1978, more than 1 million IVF babies have been born. Several million more have been born from less aggressive fertility treatments. These positive family outcomes have not come without a price. However, the recent epidemic of multifetal pregnancies, in particular the twin pregnancy rate, which was described for decades as 1 in 90, now has doubled to more than 1 in 45. Even in the past decade, twin pregnancies have continued to rise by 20% and triplets or larger multiples by nearly 200% (Table 51-1).[1] The ratio of observed to naturally expected multifetal pregnancies shows that twins are more than double the expected rate, and quintuplets occur more than 1,000-fold compared to expected numbers without infertility therapies (Table 51-2). More than 70% of all twins and 99% of higher-order multiples derive from infertility treatments. There are some suggestions that the incidence of triplets and higher is slowly diminishing, but the incidence is still very high and may, in fact, only reflect increasing use of production.

The inherent risks of multifetal pregnancies are not always understood.[2–11] The major criteria for the extent of appreciated pregnancy losses relates to the gestational age at that one begins counting. Some reports by perinatologists are overly optimistic because these physicians do not start counting until they begin to see patients at nearly 20 weeks, and at that time most losses have already occurred.[13] We previously estimated losses before viability from attempting to carry twins at 10%, triplets 18%, quadruplets slightly higher than 25% and quintuplets at 50%.[3,12] Serious morbidity rates also correlate with starting numbers. Recent data suggest that the risks to twins is higher in those conceived with fertility treatments than naturally.[15–18]

In the 1980s, pregnancies were initiated with ovulation induction agents such as Pergonal in about 75% of multifetal pregnancy patients seeking reduction.[19] However, even with the first month of the lowest dose of Clomid, quintuplets can occur. Over the years, cases induced by assisted reproductive technologies (ARTs), such as IVF, have become increasingly common. Currently, about 70% of multifetal cases are generated by ARTs (Table 51-3).[19–22]

Despite the increase utilization of ARTs,[19–22] the proportion of cases significantly hyperstimulated and resulting in quintuplets or more has dramatically decreased to less than 10% of all cases relevant to us. Regardless, the 2000 report of the Society of Assisted Reproductive Technologies (SART) suggests that of all pregnancies achieved in the United States by ARTs 58.5% are singletons, 28% twins, 7.5% triplets or higher, and 5.9% unknown.[23,24] In our experience with referred cases of ovulation stimulation, particularly those using FSH analogues, the proportion of cases that are quintuplets or more has fallen, but not dramatically.[25] Such data continue to emphasize the significant role of vigilance in monitoring infertility therapies. The vast majority of multifetal cases occur to physicians, with the best equipment and intentions, who have an unfortunate and reasonably unpredictable or unpreventable mal-occurrence. Despite this, some cases might have been prevented by increased vigilance.[12,25,26]

Media hype associated with multifetal pregnancies extends back to the 1930s with the birth of the Dionne quintuplets in Ontario, Canada.[27] In the 1980s, quintuplets would raise national attention, but the bar is set higher and higher for press interest. In the early 1990s, sextuplets, such as the Dilly family in Indiana, drew intense media attention. This family received help from diaper, formula and crib companies as well as the tremendous support of neighbors in their small town. The ultimate media circus was the Iowan MacCaughy septuplets, where virtually the entire town was marshaled to help the family deal with the rigors of so many children. The state of Iowa bought them a house, and a local automotive dealer gave the family a van. At the time, some commentators remarked that there were already thousands of children in Iowa without adequate housing and questioned why they were less deserving. Miraculously, the MacCaughy pregnancy lasted until about 31 weeks, and the national media reported all was doing well. However, closer inspection revealed that the presenting fetus was a transverse lie, who rather than acting as the usual wedge to cause dilatation actually blocked the cervix from opening. What the media presently glosses over is that 2 of the children, now 8 years old, have been diagnosed with cerebral palsy and a third is said to have epilepsy. Three had required feeding tubes for several of their first years. The Houston octuplets, born in 1998, received much less attention. Whether media disinterest was due to the saturation of stories about multifetal pregnancies or (more likely) to the African origin of the couple is open for speculation. One of the fetuses died shortly after birth and the other 7 are said to be doing reasonably well.

PROCEDURES

Multifetal pregnancy reduction (MFPR) is a clinical procedure that began in the 1980s when a small number of centers in both the United States and Europe attempted to ameliorate the usual and tremendously adverse sequelae of multifetal pregnancies by selectively terminating or reducing the number of fetuses to a more manageable number. The first European reports by Dumez[28] and the American reports by Evans et al.,[25] Berkowitz et al.,[30] and later Wapner et al.[31] described a surgical approach in order for physicians to improve the outcome in such cases.

Even these early reports recognized the ethical conundrum faced by couples and physicians under such difficult circumstances.[29] In the mid-1980s, despite mediocre

TABLE 51-1	MULTIPLE BIRTHS IN THE UNITED STATES			
Year	*Twins*	*Triplets*	*Quadruplets*	*Quintuplets and Higher Multiples*
2003	128,665	7,110	468	85
2002	125,134	6,898	434	69
2001	121,246	6,885	501	85
2000	118,916	6,742	506	77
1999	114,307	6,742	512	67
1998	110,670	6,919	627	79
1997	104,137	6,148	510	79
1996	100,750	5,298	560	81
1995	96,736	4,551	365	57
1994	97,064	4,233	315	46
1993	96,445	3,834	277	57
1992	95,372	3,547	310	26
1991	94,779	3,121	203	22
1990	93,865	2,830	185	13
1989	90,118	2,529	229	40
% Increase from 1989–2003	34.5% / 32.7%	172.2% / 181.1%	118.8% / 104.4%	212.5% / 112.5%

ultrasound visualization, needles were inserted transabdominally and maneuvered into the thorax for KCL injections, air embolization, or mechanical disruption of the fetus. Transcervical aspirations initially were tried, but without much success. Some centers also used transvaginal mechanical disruption, but data suggested a significantly higher loss rate than the transabdominal route.[32,33]

Today, virtually all experienced operators perform the procedure inserting needles transabdominally under ultrasound guidance. We find it best to line up the needle with the thorax first in the longitudinal plane. Under transverse visualization, the needle is carefully thrust into the thorax and a syringe attached to the needle. KCl is then injected slowly so as not to dislodge the needle tip. A pleural effusion should be seen as well as cardiac asystole (Fig. 51-1).

OUTCOMES

Several centers with the world's most experience began collaborating to leverage the power of their data. In 1993 the

TABLE 51-2	RATIO OF OBSERVED TO EXPECTED MULTIPLES		
Births	*Observed*	*Expected*	*Ratio*
Twins	128,665	45,444	2.83:1
Triplets	7,110	505	14.7:1
Quadruplets	468	6	78.0:1
Quintuplets & higher multiples	85	6	1416:1

Total births in 2003: 4,089,950.

first collaborative report showed a 16% pregnancy loss rate through 24 completed weeks.[19] This was a major improvement compared to expectations of higher order multiple pregnancies, particularly quadruplets and higher-order multiples. Further collaborative efforts were published 1994, 1996, and 2001, and show continued dramatic improvements in the overall outcomes of such pregnancies (Table 51-4).[25,33,34] The 2001 collaborative data demonstrated that the outcome of triplets reduced to twins and quadruplets reduced to twins now perform essentially as if they started as twins (Fig. 51-2).[25] Even with tremendous advances in neonatal care for premature babies, the 95% take-home-baby rate for triplets and the 92% for quadruplets clearly represent dramatic improvements over natural statistics. Not only has the pregnancy-loss rate been substantially reduced, but so has the rate of dangerous prematurity. Both the loss and prematurity rates continue to be correlated with the starting number. Data from the past few years show that the improvements are, not surprisingly, greatest in cases with higher starting numbers (Fig. 51-3).

Finishing number data also showed the lowest pregnancy-loss rates for those cases reduced to twins and increasing losses for singletons that follow from triplets. Not surprisingly, the rate of early premature delivery has been highest with triplets

TABLE 51-3	CHANGES IN ETIOLOGY OF MULTIFETAL PREGNANCIES	
	Ovulation Induction	*Assisted Reproductive Technologies*
1980s	75%	25%
1990s	50%	50%
2000s	70%	30%

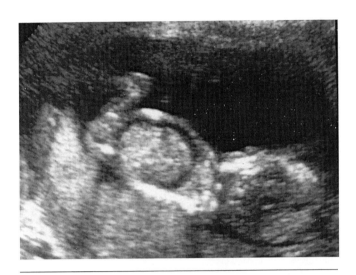

FIGURE 51-1 Pleural effusion following KCl injection.

followed by twins and lowest with singletons. Mean gestational age at delivery was also lower for higher order cases.

Birthweights following MFPR decreased with starting and finishing numbers reflecting increasing prematurity.[35] However, analysis of birthweight percentiles, particularly for singletons, reflects falling percentiles with starting number, from 51.75 percent for 2→1, to 31.26 percent for 4→1.[25] Furthermore, in remaining twins, the rate of birthweight percentile discordancy among the twins increased from 0.57% for starting triplets to 4.86% for starting 5+. For remaining triplets, the percentile differences were even greater. Analysis of the data show that the improvements in multifetal pregnancy reduction outcomes are a function of extensive operator experience combined with improved ultrasound.

Historically, most observers, except for those completely opposed to intervention on religious grounds, have accepted MFPR with quadruplets or more and saw no need to use it for twins.[36] The debate has been over triplets. While data in the literature conflicts, our experiences suggest that triplets reduced to twins do much better in terms of loss and prematurity than do unreduced triplets.[37–42] We believe that if a patient's primary goal is to maximize the chances of healthy children, then the reduction of triplets to twins achieves the best live born results.

Political and ethical questions about triplets have been addressed by several recent papers, which have argued whether or not triplets have better outcomes when reduced. Yaron et al.[37] compared triplets to twins (3→2) data with unreduced triplets within 2 large cohorts of twins. The data show substantial improvement of reduced twins as compared to triplets. Data from the most recent collaborative series suggest that pregnancy outcomes for cases starting at triplets, or even quadruplets, and reduced to twins do fundamentally as well as pregnancies starting as twins. Therefore, the data support some cautious aggressiveness in infertility treatments to achieve pregnancy in difficult clinical situations. However, when higher numbers occur good outcomes clearly diminish. A 2001 paper suggested that reduced triplets did worse than continuing ones.[38] Analysis of that series showed a loss rate following MFPR twice that seen in our collaborative series[25,42] and poorer outcomes in every other category for remaining triplets. Several other recent papers have likewise shown higher risks for unreduced triplets than for reduced cases.[39–44] It is clear that one must use extreme caution in choosing comparison groups (Table 51-5). An ever-increasing situation involves the inclusion of a monozygotic pair of twins in a higher-order multiple (Fig. 51-4).[43] Our experience suggests that provided the "singleton" seems healthy, the best outcomes are achieved by reduction of the monozygotic twins. Obviously, if the singleton is not healthy, then keeping the twins is the next choice.

Pregnancy loss is not the only poor outcome. Very early preterm delivery correlates with the starting number. It is not well appreciated that about 20% of babies born at less than 750 g develop cerebral palsy.[46,47] In Western Australia, Petterson et al. showed that the rate of cerebral palsy was 4.6 times higher for twins than singletons per live births, but 8.3 times higher when calculated per pregnancy.[48] Pharoah and Cooke calculated cerebral palsy rates per 1000 first year survivors at 2.3 for singletons, 12.6 for twins, and 44.8 for triplets.[49] The data on diminishing birthweight percentile in singletons from high starting numbers and discordancy in twins are of concern, and are consistent with a belief that there is perhaps a fundamental "imprinting" of the uterus early in pregnancy that is not completely undone by MFPR.[25]

In the 2001 collaborative report, the subset of patients who reduced from 2 to 1, (not for fetal anomalies) included 154 patients. The data suggested a loss rate comparable to 3 to 2,

TABLE 51-4	**MULTIFETAL PREGNANCY REDUCTION—LOSSES BY YEARS**						
		Losses (Weeks)		*Deliveries (Weeks)*			
	Total	*% <24*	*% >24*	*% 25–28*	*% 29–32*	*% 33–36*	*% 37+*
1986–1990	508	13.2	4.5	10.0	21.1	15.7	35.4
1991–1994	724	9.4	0.3	2.8	5.4	21.1	61.0
1995–1998	1356	6.4	0.2	4.3	10.2	31.5	47.4

Data from reference 11.

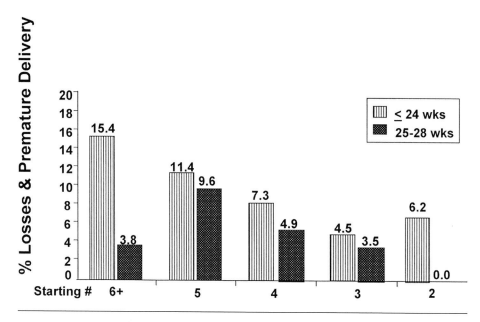

FIGURE 51-2 Multifetal Pregnancy Reduction: Losses and very prematures by starting number. Adapted from reference 11.

but, in about one third of the 2 to 1 cases, there was a medical indication for the procedure—for example, maternal cardiac disease, prior twin pregnancy with severe prematurity or uterine abnormality.[25] In recent years, however, the demographics have changed and the vast majority of such cases are from women in their 40s and 50s, some of whom are using donor eggs and, more for social than medical reasons, only want a singleton pregnancy.[50,51] Recent data suggest that twins reduced to a singleton do better than remaining as twins.[52] Consistent with the above, more women are desiring to reduce to a singleton. In a recent series of triplets, we found the average age of

outpatients reducing to twins to be 37 years and to a singleton 41 years.[53] While the reduction in pregnancy-loss risk for 3 to 1 is not as much as 3 to 2 (15% to 7% and 15% to 5%, respectfully), the gestational age at delivery for the resulting singleton is higher, and the incidence of births <1500 grams is 10 higher for twins than singletons.[36] Consequently, the data have made the counseling of such patients far more complex than before (Fig. 51-5). Not surprisingly, there are often differences between members of the couple as to the desirability of twins or singleton.[53] There are also profound public health implications to these decisions, as recent United States data

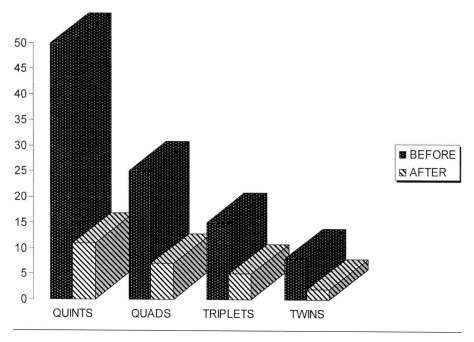

FIGURE 51-3 Risk reduction as a function of starting number.

| TABLE 51-5 | REDUCED VERSUS "UNREDUCED" TRIPLETS COMPARISON |

Years	MFPR Cases Losses <24 Wks	Deliveries (Weeks)			
		24–28 Wk	29–32	33–36	37+
1980s	6.7%	6.1%	9.1%	36.9%	47.9%
90–94	5.7%	5.2%	9.9%	39.2%	45.2%
95–98	4.5%	3.2%	6.9%	28.3%	55.1%
98–02	5.1%	4.6%	10.8%	41.8%	37.6%
Mean GA 35.5	**PMR**	**10.0/1000**			
98–02(3→1)	8.0%	4.0%	12.0%	4.0%	72.0%
	Mean GA 39.5 NON-REDUCED TRIPLETS	PMR	0/1000		
98 (Leondires)	9.9%	Mean GA 33.3	PMR 55/1000		
99 (Angel)	8.0%	Mean GA 32.3	PMR 29/1000		
99 (Lipitz)	25.0%	Mean GA 33.5	PMR 109/1000		
02 (Francois)	8.3%	Mean GA 31.0	PMR 57.6/1000		

Data from reference 37.

show that of $10.2 billion spent per year on initial newborn care, 57% of the money is spent on the 9% of babies born at <37 weeks.[54,55]

In 2003, more than $10 billion was spent on the 12.3% born preterm.[56] Data are now also emerging that there is considerably higher neurologic and developmental disability in six year olds who survived birth at 26 weeks or less. The rates of severe, moderate, and mild disability were 22%, 24%, and 34% respectively. Significant cerebral palsy was present in 12%.[57] Hack et al. also have now shown that in babies born at less than 1000 g, the rate of cerebral palsy was 14% as opposed to controls, and asthma, poor vision, IQ <85 and poor motor skills were substantially higher.[58]

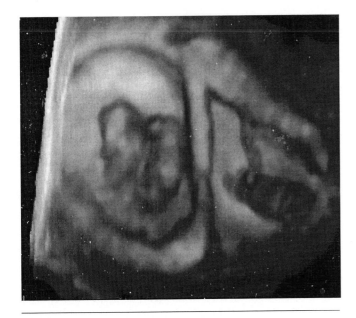

FIGURE 51-4 Monozygotic twin pair as part of multiple.

As a result of all of the above and the changing demographics of who is having infertility and desiring reductions, we believe that reduction of twins to a singleton is likely to become more common over the next several years.

PATIENT ISSUES

The demographics of patients seeking multifetal pregnancy reduction have evolved over the past decade.[25,49] With the availability of donor eggs, the number of "older women" seeking MFPR has increased dramatically. More than 10% of all patients seeking MFPR are over 40 years of age in several programs and most are using donor eggs. A consequence of the shift to older patients, many of whom already had previous relationships and children, is an increased desire by these patients to have only 1 further child and will increase as a percentage of cases. The number of experienced centers willing to do 2 to 1 reductions is still very limited, but we believe it can be justified in the appropriate circumstances.[36]

For patients who are older and using their own eggs, the issue of genetic diagnosis comes into play. By 2001, more than 50% of patients in the United States having ART cycles were over the age of 35 (Table 51-6).[1,23,24,51] In the 1980s and early 1990s, the most common approach was to offer amniocentesis on the remaining twins at 16–17 weeks. A 1995 paper suggested an 11% loss rate in these cases, which caused considerable concern.[59] However, in 1998, a much larger collaborative series settled the issue by showing that loss rates were no higher than comparable controls of MFPR patients who did not have amniocentesis.[60] The collaborative data showed a loss rate of 5%, which was certainly no higher than the group of patients post-MFPR who did not have genetic studies.

Since the centers with the most MFPR experience also happen to be the ones that had the same accomplishments

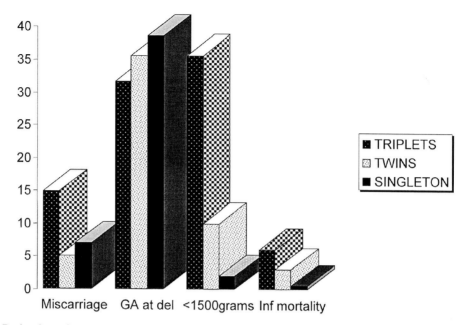

Reduction of triplets to twins has lower loss rates but higher incidence of prematurity, low birth weight and infant mortality than reducing to a singleton.

FIGURE 51-5 Risks starting with triplets.

with chorionic villus sampling (CVS), combinations of the procedures were very logical. There are 2 main schools of thought as to the best approach for first trimester genetic diagnosis: should it be before or after the performance of MFPR? Published data in the early 1990s in which CVS was done first and followed by reduction suggested a 1–2% error rate as to which fetus was which, particularly if the entire karyotype is obtained before going on to reduction.[61] Therefore, for the first 10–15 years, the approach we used was to generally do the reduction first at approximately 10.5 weeks in those patients who reduced down to twins or triplets and then followed with CVS approximately 1 week later.[49] However, in patients going to a singleton pregnancy, i.e. essentially putting "all of their eggs in 1 basket," we believed the best approach was to know what was in the basket before reducing the number of embryos.[25,49] In these cases we usually performed a CVS on all the fetuses, or 1 more than the intended stopping number, and performed a fluorescent in situ hybridization (FISH) analysis with probes

for chromosomes 13, 18, 21, X, and Y. Whereas about 30% of anomalies seen on karyotype would not be detectable by FISH,[62] there is always residual risk.[63] The absolute risk given both a normal FISH and a normal ultrasound including nuchal translucency[64] is only about 1 in 450. We believe this risk is lower than the increased risk from the 2-week wait necessary to receive the full karyotype. We have now extended this approach to all patients who are appropriate candidates for prenatal diagnosis regardless of fetal number. Over the past few years, more than 80% of our patients have combined CVS and MFPR procedures (Fig. 51-6). With data now suggesting increased risks of chromosomal and other anomalies in patients conceiving by IVF, especially with ICSI, the utilization of prenatal diagnosis will likely increase.[65–79]

The other approach used by another group was to perform the CVS and complete karotype first, and then have the patient come back for reduction. Although "mistakes" were common 10 years ago, the chance of error has been considerably reduced and the group believed the benefits of the full karyotype justified the wait. The issue as to the better of these 2 approaches is currently unsettled.

SOCIETAL ISSUES

MFPR will always be controversial. Opinions on MFPR, in our experience have never followed the classic "pro-choice/pro-life" dichotomy.[2,19,25,49,51] We believe that the real debate over the next 5–10 years will not be whether or not MFPR

TABLE 51-6	MATERNAL AGE AND ART (SART DATA—2001)	
	All cases	81,915
	Fresh non-donor	60,780
	<35	28,778
	35–37	14,416
	38–40	11,301
	41–42	4,365
	42+	2,190

Wright VC, Schieve LA, Reynolds MA, Jeng G: Assisted reproductive technology surveillance *Pub Med, MMWR Surveill Summ.* 2003;52:1–16.

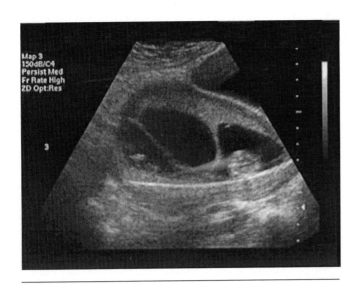

FIGURE 51-6 CVS prior to fetal reduction in triplet pregnancy. Catheter is inserted to reach posterior fundal placenta. Low anterior placenta would likewise be reached transcervically, and anterior fundal placental would be done transabdominally.

should be performed with triplets or more. A serious debate will emerge over whether or not it will be appropriate to offer MFPR routinely for twins, even natural ones for whom the outcome has commonly been considered "good enough."[52] Our data suggest that reduction, of twins to a singleton actually improves the outcome of the remaining fetus.[52] No consensus on appropriateness of routine 2→1 reductions however, is ever likely to emerge. We do, however, expect the proportion of patients reducing to a singleton to steadily increase over the next several years.

Over the years, much has been written on the subject. Opinions will always vary substantially from outraged condemnation to complete acceptance. No short paragraph could do justice to the subject other than to state that most proponents do not believe this is a frivolous procedure, but see it terms of the principle of proportionality, i.e., therapy to achieve the most good for the least harm.[71–73]

How patients "hear" and internalize data and make decisions with respect to reduction have been fascinating to us over the years. Much of the literature on medical decision-making has emphasized a rational choice model in which emotions, feelings and values are treated as complications that must be considered as a second stage of an analysis that puts hard data regarding relative risks center stage.[74,75] Even the literature that talks about genuine alternative models of decision making (systematic versus heuristic, for example), a central assumption is that these are individual differences in style that can be identified through what people say.[76,77]

We have approached this problem from a different direction, arguing that where controversial, high-anxiety decisions are concerned, patients treat these decisions as an ongoing part of the social reality that they are creating to live in and raise a family.[78] This reality construction process is proactive, with couples aware of the potential consequences of sharing with others what they are going through. In a recent study of sharing strategies, strategies for sharing ranged from a defended-relationship approach in which only the partner and patient knew about the problems the patient was facing and the decision to reduce (16/50, or 32%), through a limited-risk strategy of sharing only with "qualified" family and friends (20/50, or 40%), to both sets of parents knowing (9/50, or 18%), and finally to an extended, open network of family, friends and colleagues knowing (5/50, or 10%). No sharing strategy was completely free of risk. Even a defended-relationship strategy between partners broke down if the partners disagreed over the ethics of reduction or the continuation of efforts to become pregnant (2/16, or 12.5% of cases). Partner conflict was also the only factor that undermined the limited-risk strategy (2/20, or 10% of cases). These two strategies were more successful in minimizing hostility than either that in which both sets of parents know or there is a more extended sharing network. These latter two result in hostile or lack-of-support responses in 5/14 (36%) cases.[79]

The realities people construct, composed of supportive people and institutions together with complexes of supportive values, norms and attitudes, are the source of frames that the patients use to view the data.[56–59] The decisions they make and how they justify those decisions may help resolve incompatible elements in the realities in which they find themselves enmeshed. It may often happen, for example, that parents who have gone through reduction to two or one live in families and/or work in communities where having engaged in reduction would be considered as something shameful. The less control they have over the selection of family, friends and workplaces, given the prospect of such stigma, the more likely they are to simply present their pregnancies to these publics as if their pregnancies had always involved twins or singleton. Where they have more control over the situation—as typically happens with friends versus family—they may be more likely to selectively share their experiences.

The one thing all such patients have in common is a very strong desire to have a family (Table 51-6). But there does not appear to be a single set of supportive institutions, people and norms that is conducive to going through the pain, stress and resource expenditure of IVF I are three viable alternative resolutions. The first of these, a rational Medical Model, looks superficially like what one would expect from the rational analysis model. But the commitment to factual analysis comes from their having selected themselves into the hard sciences, medicine, dentistry, engineering or the law—disciplines in which the "facts" are crucial. Such women will want to see the numbers regarding the relative risk associated with different reduction choices and will want to engage in a rigorous discussion of the data and their implications. And they will be likely to choose a final number for reduction that maximizes the chances of a "take-home" baby.

The lens of scientific objectivity is not the only frame through which women who have gone through IVF in order to have a child will examine these data. For those who have immersed themselves in a social reality that has a strong emphasis on norms against abortion and/or reduction—such that they themselves have such normative beliefs and are heavily involved in churches who reinforce similar beliefs—a detached examination of the "facts" is simply not possible. These "facts" hold no special moral authority. Their beliefs and those of the individuals and social institutions in which they have selected themselves have a moral authority as well. The balance that such women will likely seek is one that reduces their relative risk to acceptable limits. So, unless the consequences are dire, they will not reduce or choose to reduce only to three. We labeled such a resolution a Fundamentalist Model.

Finally, there are those for whom the demands of career and/or existing children constitute powerful elements in their constructed realities. For such women—and this includes many of the older patients we encountered—the essential balance that they seek is a more secular one, a Lifestyle Model, one that emphasizes creating a family situation in which having a family can be balanced with having a career. Such women will more than likely choose reduction to two or even one embryo, depending on the number of other children they have and the level of resources that the family has.

Where women have selected themselves into and/or been trained to accept the legitimacy of rigorously-determined statistics regarding relative risk (a Medical Frame), reduction choices *can* be straightforward—or at least they can appear to be relatively straightforward. This is usually not the case, however, for women who must forge a resolution amongst potentially incompatible elements, as for women who are struggling to reconcile the potentially oppositional elements of religious beliefs and involvement with risks associated with higher-level pregnancies (Fundamentalist Frame) or those who are struggling to reconcile the potentially-conflicting identities of home and career (Lifestyle Frame). We have been able to examine some of these issues in a few studies to date. In one we were able to trace the extreme fluctuations in anxiety and stress as women progress through IVF and then must confront the painful choice of reduction.[48] In a second, we were able to show that the meaning of detecting a fetal anomaly changes depending on the needs of the patient and her spouse for some confirmation regarding their choice.[72]

SUMMARY

Over the last two decades MFPR has become a well-established and integral part of infertility therapy and the attempts to deal with sequelae of aggressive infertility management. In the mid-1980's and 90's, the risks and benefits of the procedure could only be guessed.[29-33] We now have very clear and precise data on the risks and benefits as well as an understanding that the risks increase substantially with the starting and finishing number of fetuses in multifetal pregnancies. The collaborative loss rate numbers, i.e., 4.5% for triplets, 8% for quadruplets, 11% for quintuplets, and 15% for sextuplets or more, seem reasonable ones to present to patients for the procedure performed by an experienced operator. Our own experience and anecdotal reports from other groups suggest that less experienced operators have worse outcomes.

Pregnancy loss is not the only poor outcome. The other main issue with which to be concerned is very early preterm delivery and the profound consequences to such infants. Here again there is an increasing rate of poor outcomes correlated with the starting number. The finishing numbers are also critical, with twins having the best viable pregnancy outcomes for cases starting with three or more. Triplets and singletons do not do as well. However, an emerging appreciation that singletons have prematurity rates less than twins is making the counseling far more complex. We continue to hope, however, that MFPR will become obsolete as better control of ovulation agents and assisted reproductive technologies make multifetal pregnancies uncommon.

References

1. Martin JA, Hamilton BE, Sutton PD, et al. *Births: Final Data for 2003.* Hyattville, MD: National Center for Health Statistics; 2003. *National Vital Statistics Reports* 54(2).
2. Evans MI, Rodeck CH, Stewart KS, et al. Multiple gestation: genetic issues, selective termination, and fetal reduction. In: Gleisher N, Buttino L Jr, Elkayam U, et al., eds. *Principles and Practices of Medical Therapy in Pregnancy.* 3rd ed. Norwalk, CT: Appleton and Lange Publishing Co; 1998:235–242.
3. Evans MI, Ayoub MA, Shalhoub AG, et al. Spontaneous abortions in couples declining multifetal pregnancy reduction. *Fetal Diagn Ther.* 2002;17:343–346.
4. Blickstein I, Keith LG: Multiple Pregnancy: Epidemiology, Gestation, and Perinatal Outcome 2005. Taylor and Francis, London.
5. Alexander GR, Salihu HM: Perinatal outcomes of singleton and multiple births in the United States, 1995–98. In: Blickstein I, Keith LG: Multiple Pregnancy: Epidemiology, Gestation, and Perinatal Outcome 2005. Taylor and Francis, London, pp 3–10.
6. Hajnal BL, Braun-Fahrlander C, von Siebenthal K, et al: Improved outcome for very low birth weight multiple births. *Pediatr Neurol* 2005;32:87–93.
7. Magee BD. Role of multiple births in very low birth weight and infant mortality. *J. Reprod Med* 2004;49:812–6.
8. Li SJ, Ford N, Meister K, et al. Increased risk of birth defects among children from multiple births. *Birth Defects Res A Clin Mol Teratol* 2003;67:879–85.
9. Blondel B, Kogan MD, Alexander GR, et al: The impact of the increasing number of multiple births on the rates of pretenn birth and low birthweight: an international study. *Am J. Public Health* 2002;92:1323–30.
10. Tang Y, Ma CS, Cui W, et al: The risk of birth defects in multiple births: a population based study. *Matern Child Health J.* 2005;21:1–7.
11. Alexander GR, Slay Wingate M, Salihu H, et al: Fetal and Neonatal mortality risks of multiple births. *Obstet Gynecol Clin North Am* 2005;32:1–16.
12. Evans MI, Ciorica D, Britt DW: Do Reduced Multifetal Pregnancy Reduction. In: Blickstein 1, Keith L: *Multiple Pregnancies: Epidemiology. Gestation and Perinatal Outcome (2nd ed) Taylor and Francis.* Abingdon 2005 pp 535–543.
13. Keith LG & Blickstein I, eds. *Triplet Pregnancies.* London, England: Parthenon Press; 2002.

14. Luke B, Brown MB, Nugent C, et al. Risks factors for adverse outcomes in spontaneous versus assisted conception twin pregnancies. *Fertil Steril.* 2004;81:315–319.

15. Anwar HN, Ihab MU, Johnny BR, et al. Pregnancy outcomes in spontaneous twins versus twins who were conceived through in vitro fertilization. *Am J Obstet Gynecol.* 2003;189:513–518.

16. Garite TJ, Clark RH, Elliott JP, et al. Twins and triplets: the effect of plurality and growth on neonatal outcome compared with singleton infants. *Am J. Obstet Gynecol* 2004;191:700–7.

17. McDonald S, Murphy K, Beyene J, et al. Perinatal Outcomes of in vitro fertilization twins: a systematic review and meta-analyses. *Am J. Obstet Gynecol* 2005;193:141–52.

18. Shinwell ES. Neonatal morbidity of very low birthweight infants from multiple pregnancies. *Obstet Gynecol Clin North Am* 2005;32:29–38.

19. Evans MI, Dommergues M, Wapner RJ, et al. Efficacy of transabdominal multifetal pregnancy reduction: collaborative experience among the world's largest centers. *Obstet Gynecol.* 1993;82:61–67.

20. Russell RB, Petrine JR, Damus K, et al. The Changing epidemiology of multiple births in the United States. *Obstet Gynecol* 2003;101:129–35.

21. Kissin DM, Schieve LA, Reynolds MA. Multiple-birth risk associated with IVF and extended embryo culture: USA 2001. *Human Reprod* 2005;20:2215–23.

22. Reynolds MA, Schieve LA, Martin JA, et al. Trends in multiple births conceived using assisted reproductive technology: United States, 1997–2000. *Pediatrics* 2003;111:1159–62.

23. Toner JP. Progress we can be proud of: U.S. trends in assisted reproduction over the first 20 years. *Fertil Steril.* 2002;78:943–950.

24. Wright VC, Schieve LA, Reynolds MA, et al. Assisted reproductive technology surveillance—United States, 2001. *MMWR CDC Surveill Summ.* 2004;53:1–20.

25. Evans MI, Berkowitz R, Wapner R, et al. Multifetal pregnancy reduction (MFPR): improved outcomes with increased experience. *Am J Obstet Gynecol.* 2001;184:97–103.

26. Adashi EY, Barri PN, Berkowitz R, et al. Infertility therapy-assisted multiple pregnancies (births): an on-going epidemic. *Reprod Biomed Online.* 2003;7:515–542.

27. Evans MI, Littman L, St Louis L, et al. Evolving patterns of iatrogenic multifetal pregnancy generation: implications for aggressiveness of infertility treatments. *Am J Obstet Gynecol.* 1995;172:1750–1753.

28. Dumez Y, Oury JF. Method for first trimester selective abortion in multiple pregnancy. *Contrib Gynecol Obstet.* 1986;15:50.

29. Evans MI, Fletcher JC, Zador IE, et al. Selective first trimester termination in octuplet and quadruplet pregnancies: clinical and ethical issues. *Obstet Gynecol.* 1988;71:289–296.

30. Berkowitz RL, Lynch L, Chitkara U, et al. Selective reduction of multiple pregnancies in the first trimester. *N Engl J Med.* 1988; 318:1043.

31. Wapner RJ, Davis GH, Johnson A. Selective reduction of multifetal pregnancies. *Lancet.* 1990;335:90–93.

32. Timor-Tritsch IE, Peisner DB, Monteagudo A, et al. Multifetal pregnancy reduction by transvaginal puncture: evaluation of the technique used in 134 cases. *Am J Obstet Gynecol.* 1993;168:799–804.

33. Evans MI, Dommergues M, Timor-Tritsch I, et al. Transabdominal versus transcervical and transvaginal multifetal pregnancy reduction: international collaborative experience of more than one thousand cases. *Am J Obstet Gynecol.* 1994;170:902–909.

34. Evans MI, Dommergues M, Wapner RJ, et al. International collaborative experience of 1789 patients having multifetal pregnancy reduction: a plateauing of risks and outcomes. *J Soc Gynecol Invest.* 1996;3:23–26.

35. Torok O, Lapinski R, Salafia CM, et al. Multifetal pregnancy reduction is not associated with an increased risk of intrauterine growth restriction, except for very high order multiples. *Am J Obstet Gynecol.* 1998;179:221–225.

36. Evans MI, Drugan A, Fletcher JC, et al. Attitudes on the ethics of abortion, sex selection & selective termination among health care professionals, ethicists & clergy likely to encounter such situations. *Am J Obstet Gynecol.* 1991;164:1092–1099.

37. Yaron Y, Bryant-Greenwood PK, Dave N, et al. Multifetal pregnancy reduction (MFPR) of triplets to twins: comparison with non-reduced triplets and twins. *Am J Obstet Gynecol.* 1999;180:1268–1271.

38. Leondires MP, Ernst SD, Miller BT, et al. Triplets: outcomes of expectant management versus multifetal reduction for 127 pregnancies. *Am J Obstet Gynecol.* 1999;72:257–260.

39. Lipitz S, Shulman A, Achiron R, et al. A comparative study of multifetal pregnancy reduction from triplets to twins in the first versus early second trimesters after detailed fetal screening. *Ultrasound Obstet Gynecol.* 2001;18:35–38.

40. Angel JL, Kalter CS, Morales WJ, et al. Aggressive perinatal care for high-order multiple gestations: does good perinatal outcome justify aggressive assisted reproductive techniques? *Am J Obstet Gynecol.* 1999;181:253–259.

41. Sepulveda W, Munoz H, Alcalde JL. Conjoined twins in a triplet pregnancy: early prenatal diagnosis with three-dimensional ultrasound and review of the literature. *Ultrasound Obstet Gynecol.* 2003;22:199–204.

42. Francois K, Sears C, Wilson R, et al. Twelve year experience of triplet pregnancies at a single institution. *Amer J Obstet Gynecol.* 2001;185 Suppl:S112.

43. Antsaklis A, Souka AP, Daskalakis G, et al. Embryo reduction versus expectant management in triplet pregnancies. *J Matern Fetal Neonatal Med* 2004;16:219–22.

44. Evans MI, Shalhoub A, Nicolaides KH. Triplets: outcomes of expectant management versus multifetal reduction for 127 pregnancies. *Am J Obstet Gynecol* 2001;184:1041–3.

45. Yakin K, Kahraman S, Comert S. Three blastocyst stage embryo transfer resulting in a quintuplet pregnancy. *Hum Reprod.* 2001;16:782–784.

46. Task Force of American College of Obstetricians and Gynecologists. Neonatal encephalopathy and cerebral palsy: defining the pathogenesis and pathophysiology. ACOG Washington DC, 2003.

47. Pharoah PO. Risk of cerebral palsy in multiple pregnancies. *Obstet Gynecol Clin North Am* 2005;32:55–67.

48. Petterson B, Nelson K, Watson L, et al. Twins, triplets and cerebral palsy in births in Western Australia in the 1980s. *BMJ.* 1993;307:1239–1243.

49. Pharoah PO, Cooke T. Cerebral Palsy and Multiple Births. *Arch Dis Child Fetal Neonatal Ed.* 1996;75 Suppl: F174–177.

50. Evans MI, Hume RF, Polak S, et al. The geriatric gravida: multifetal pregnancy reduction (MFPR) donor eggs and aggressive infertility treatments. *Am J Obstet Gynecol.* 1997;177:875–878.

51. Templeton A. The multiple gestation epidemic: the role of the assisted reproductive technologies. *Am J Obstet Gynecol.* 2004;190:894–898.

52. Evans MI, Kaufman MI, Urban AJ, et al. Fetal reduction from twins to a singleton: a reasonable consideration. *Obstet Gynecol.* 2004;104:102–109.

53. Evans MI, Krivchenia EL, Kaufman M, et al. The optimal management of first trimester triplets: reduce. Proceedings of the Central Association of Obstetricians and Gynecologists; 2002 October 27–30; Las Vegas, Nevada.

54. St. John EB, Nelson KG, Oliver SP, et al. Cost of neonatal care according to gestational age at birth and survival status. *Am J Obstet Gynecol.* 2000;182:170–175.

55. Henderson J, Hockley C, Petrou S, et al. Economic implications of multiple births: inpatient hospital costs in the first 5 years of life. *Arch Dis Child Fetal Neonatal Ed* 2004;89:F542–5.

56. Cuevas KD, Silver DR, Brooten D, et al. The cost of prematurity: Hospital charges at birth and frequency of re-hospitalizations and acute care vistis over the first year of life: a comparison by gestational age and birth weight. *Am J Nurs* 2005;105:56–64.

57. Marlow N, Wolke D, Bracewell MA, et al. Neurologic and developmental disability at six years of age after extremely preterm birth. *N Engl J Med* 2005;352:9–19.

58. Hack M, Taylor HG, Drotar D, et al. Chronic conditions, functional limitations, and special health care needs of school-aged children born with extremely low birth weights in the 1990's. *JAMA* 2005;94:318–325.

59. Tabsh KM, Theroux NL. Genetic amniocentesis following multifetal pregnancy reduction twins: assessing the risk. *Prenat Diagn.* 1995;15:221–223.

60. McLean LK, Evans MI, Carpenter RJ, et al. Genetic amniocentesis (AMN) following multifetal pregnancy reduction (MFPR) does not increase the risk of pregnancy loss. *Prenat Diagn.* 1998;18:186–188.

61. Brambati B, Tului L, Baldi M, et al. Genetic analysis prior to selective termination in multiple pregnancy: technical aspects and clinical outcome. *Hum Reprod.* 1995;10:818–825.

62. Evans MI, Henry GP, Miller WA, et al. International, collaborative assessment of 146,000 prenatal karyotypes: expected limitations if only chromosome-specific probes and fluorescent in situ hybridization were used. *Hum Reprod.* 1999;14:1213–1216.

63. Homer J, Bhatt S, Huang B, et al. Residual risk for cytogenetic abnormalities after prenatal diagnosis by interphase fluorescence in situ hybridization (FISH). *Prenat Diagn.* 2003;23:556–571.

64. Greene RA, Wapner J, Evans MI. Amniocentesis and chorionic villus sampling in triplet pregnancy. In: Keith LG, Blickstein I, Oleszcuk JJ, eds. *Triplet Pregnancy.* London, England: Parthenon Publishing Group; 73–84.

65. Zadori J, Kozinszky Z, Orvos H, et al. The incidence of major birth defects following in vitro fertilization. *J Assist Reprod Genet.* 2003;20:131–132.

66. Pinborg A, Loft A, Schmidt L, et al. Morbidity in a Danish national cohort of 472 IVF/ICSI twins, 1132 non-IVF/ICSI twins and 634 IVF/ICSI singletons: health-related and social implications for the children and their families. *Hum Reprod.* 2003;18:1234–1243.

67. Place I, Englert Y. A prospective longitudinal study of the physical, psychomotor, and intellectual development of singleton children up to 5 years who were conceived by intracytoplasmic sperm injection compared with children conceived spontaneously and by in vitro fertilization. *Fertil Steril.* 2003;80:1388–1397.

68. Retzloff MG, Hornstein MD. Is intracytoplasmic sperm injection safe? *Fertil Steril.* 2003;80:851–859.

69. Kurinczuk JJ. Safety issues in assisted reproduction technology: from theory to reality—just what are the data telling us about ICSI offspring health and future fertility and should we be concerned? *Hum Reprod.* 2003;18:925–931.

70. Tournaye H. ICSI: a technique too far? *Int J Androl.* 2003;26:63–69.

71. Britt DW, Risinger ST, Mans M, et al. Devastation and relief: conflicting meanings in discovering fetal anomalies. *Ultrasound in Obstetrics and Gynecology.* 2002;20:1–5.

72. Britt DW, Risinger ST, Mans M, et al. Anxiety among women who have undergone fertility therapy and who are considering MFPR: Trends and Scenarios. *Journal of Maternal-Fetal and Neonatal Medicine* (In press).

73. Britt DW, Evans WJ, Mehta SS, et al. Framing the decision: Determinants of how women considering MFPR as a pregnancy-management strategy frame their moral dilemma. *Fetal Diagnosis and Therapy* 2004;19:232–240.

74. Redelmeier DA, Rozin P, Kahneman D. Understanding patients' decisions: cognitive and emotional perspectives. *Journal of the American Medical Association,* 1993;270:72–76.

75. Chapman GB and Elstein AS. Cognitive processes and biases in medical decision making. In: Chapman GB, and Sonnenberg, FA (Eds.). Decision Making in Health Care: Theory, Psychology and Applications. Cambridge University Press; New York; 2000;183–210.

76. Steginga SK and Occhipinti S. The application of the heuristic-systematic processing model to treatment decision making about prostate cancer. *Medical Decision Making,* 2004;24.

77. Hamm RM. Theory about heuristic strategies based on verbal protocol analysis: The emperor needs a shave. *Medical Decision Making,* 2004;24:681–686.

78. Britt DW and Campbell EQ. Assessing the Linkage of Norms, Environments and Deviance. *Social Forces* (December), 1977;532–549.

79. Britt DW, Evans MI (2005). Sharing and risk of negative reactions: preliminary examination of four alternative strategies used by patients facing a fetal reduction. *American Society of Reproductive Medicine, Montreal Canada,* October 2005.

CHAPTER 52

SELECTIVE TERMINATION

Mark I. Evans / Charles H. Rodeck / Mark Paul Johnson / Richard L. Berkowitz

INTRODUCTION

Prenatal diagnostic techniques were first developed in the early 1970s. Amniocentesis was the first invasive test and followed by the development of fetoscopy, sophisticated ultrasound, and ultimately, in the 1980s, by chorionic villus sampling (CVS) and fetal blood sampling.[1] These techniques along with concomitant laboratory tests have allowed couples the option of considering termination of pregnancy when fetal abnormalities are detected.

In the United States during the late 1960s, the very restrictive abortion laws, which were on the books throughout most of the 20th century, began to be repealed. However, in 1973, the United States Supreme Court removed the then existing state regulations against the termination of pregnancy. Two Supreme Court decisions, *Roe v. Wade*[2] and *Doe v. Bolton*,[3] declared a right of privacy that allowed women in the first trimester the ability to decide upon the continuation or termination of pregnancy. The state's only interest, in the second trimester (i.e., prior to fetal viability), was to insure that such procedures were done under safe and acceptable conditions. During the third trimester, corresponding to fetal viability, abortions could only be performed for the health and welfare of the mother. Laws in many other countries underwent similar changes in the 1970s, although in a few countries such as the Federal Republic of Germany, laws tended to become more restrictive in the 1980s and early 1990s. Even after 30 years, legal attacks against the availability of abortion services occur regularly. These have been fought recently both in the national level (e.g., *Carhart v. Stenberg* and *National Abortion Federation et al. v. Ashcroft*[4]) and at state levels (e.g., *Evans v. Granholm*[6] [Michigan]) in which ever increasing restrictions been turned back by the courts.[1,2] It is unlikely that this trend will continue in the United States as more conservative juries get appointed to high courts.

In cases of multifetal pregnancy, the development of prenatal diagnostic techniques has created a new dilemma. Confronted with the diagnosis of an abnormality in 1 twin and presumed normality in the other twin, couples had the unenviable choice of either continuing with both or terminating both fetuses. Faced with such quandaries, couples were forced to choose between 2 very difficult options—either to keep to preserve the normal one, but therefore have a baby with an abnormality, or to terminate both to prevent having a baby with a problem but thereby losing a normal one.

RISKS OF ABNORMALITIES

It has long been recognized that the incidence of certain structural abnormalities such as neural tube, cardiac, and chromosomal defects are more common in twin gestations than in singletons (Table 52-1).[7,8] Monozygotic twins are especially prone to defects of laterality such as situs inversus. Monoamniotic twins have an even higher incidence of abnormalities than do monochorionic/diamniotic fetuses.

The incidence of chromosome abnormalities in monozygotic twins should essentially parallel age-related risks for singleton gestations. Furthermore, 100% concordance should occur between twins with only 1 egg fertilized by 1 sperm and the divergence to twins occurring postfertilization. For dizygotic twins, however, 2 eggs are fertilized by 2 sperm. Thus, the risk of either twin being aneuploid is essentially an independent probability. For example, the risk of having a baby with a chromosome abnormality at maternal age 35 at delivery is approximately 1 in 190.[9] If there are 2 fetuses, the risk is essentially doubled: 2 in 190 or 1 in 95. A 1 in 95 risk corresponds to the risk of a singleton for a 38-year old woman. Similarly, the risk for a 30-year old woman with a singleton is 1 in 380. With twins the risk is approximately 2 in 380 or 1 in 190, which is the risk of a 35-year old woman (Table 52-2).

TERMINOLOGY

Selective termination has been the term used for 2 slightly different procedures. Selection termination usually referred to a second trimester procedure performed on gestations with 1 abnormal twin. Accordingly, selective termination, selective reduction and multifetal pregnancy reduction are terms that describe a first trimester technique to reduce the number of embryos in a multifetal pregnancy usually of triplets or larger multiples.[10–13] These are usually seen in infertility patients as a result of the use of ovulation induction agents, such as *in vitro* fertilization and other assisted reproductive technologies.[10–13] A consensus has emerged to define the term *multifetal pregnancy reduction* for first trimester procedures that reduce the number of fetuses when shear number places the pregnancy at risk. Alternatively, the term *selective termination* is used for procedures performed when a fetal abnormality has been diagnosed.[13]

TECHNIQUES FOR SELECTIVE TERMINATION

There are several techniques by which selective termination has been accomplished. Since the early 1990s, there has been general agreement that hysterotomy was a last-resort procedure, although multiple technologies were used in series of variable sizes and quantities (Table 52-3). Clearly, with all techniques, the major issue is to make sure one is terminating the correct fetus. In a multifetal pregnancy reduction in which

TABLE 52-1

TABLE 52-1 | INCIDENCE (%) OF MALFORMATIONS IN MONOZYGOTIC, DIZYGOTIC, AND SINGLETONS

| | Twins | | | | Singletons | |
| | MZ | | DZ | | | |
Race	Major	Minor	Major	Minor	Major	Minor
White	10.49	9.09	6.06	3.41		
Black	11.54	12.50	8.56	7.65		
Total	10.72	10.99	7.78	5.51	7.10	7.26

the shear number of fetuses *per se* is the indication for the procedure, it probably does not matter which fetuses are terminated. In selective termination, the procedure is specifically performed because of a fetal abnormality in 1 twin. Documentation of which fetus is abnormal can be very easy in cases with obvious structural defects or a chromosome abnormality in discordant sex twins, but can certainly become difficult when the defect is a subtle anatomic abnormality, Mendelian disorder or chromosomal aneuploidy in like-sex twins. Such issues point to the importance of placentation documentation and fetal position when prenatal diagnostic procedures are undertaken (Fig. 52-1). If there is doubt about which fetus is which, then the diagnostic procedure should be repeated.

Consistent with the data of Golbus et al., one must use extreme caution if considering a selective termination on monozygotic/monoamniotic twins or there clearly appears to be a single shared placenta without differentiation between the 2 fetuses. Data from a number of centers suggest that the risk of the normal twin's death are considerably increased under these circumstances when using the techniques described below.[14] Anderson et al. reported 4 cases of neurologic damage in the surviving monochorionic twin of those naturally dying and selectively terminated fetuses.[15,16] It is for this reason that newer methods of umbilical cord ligation and bipolar cautery were developed.[17] These will be described in a separate section.

KCL

All percutaneous techniques have in common the necessity for the accurate placement of a needle into the fetal cardiac chambers (Fig. 52-2). Unlike multifetal pregnancy reduction in the first trimester when placement of the needle within the chest cavity is sufficient for success, in cases of second trimester techniques low-resistance blood return in the operating needle is critical to guarantee vascular access and subsequent success of the procedure. We generally use a 20-gauge needle which is positioned carefully above the fetal thorax. The optimal target is the left ventricle as flow will then go into the coronary articles and require less volume of KCl to achieve cardiac standstill. Position on ultrasound is confirmed in both longitude and transverse planes. Once positioning is believed to be satisfactory, the needle is inserted into the cardiac chamber with a sharp thrust, the stylet removed and blood flow drawn into the syringe. Rotation of the bevel of the needle helps to increase blood return. Once satisfactory blood flow has been confirmed, a fetal blood sample can be obtained and used for confirmation of abnormality. Following blood sampling, another syringe containing 5 or 10 cc of potassium chloride is attached and 2 ml of KCl are injected steadily into the fetal heart. With proper placement, an immediate decrease in fetal heart rate should be noted with complete cessation occurring in approximately 1 minute. The absolute amount of KCl varies from as little as 1 cc to as much as 10 cc, depending upon gestational age and proper needle positioning. The needle should not be removed until the operator is absolutely convinced that cardiac activity has ceased. Anecdotal reports have suggested reinitiation of fetal cardiac activity within a few minutes if the dose of KCl has been insufficient.

Some centers perform the procedure via intrafunic injection of KCl. This technique commonly requires a greater amount of KCl than intracardia and has been associated with anecofotyly failures. A repeat scan 30–60 minutes after cord injection would seem prudent. Rodeck also described air injection via the umbilical cord. He used this procedure for a number of years with good technical success in over 20 cases with only 2 losses (unpublished data).

AIR EMBOLIZATION

Another technique formerly used was air embolization.[18] The position and placement of the needle is the same as for KCl,

TABLE 52-2 | INCIDENCE OF CHROMOSOMAL ABNORMALITIES IN AT LEAST ONE FETUS IN A MULTIFETAL GESTATION

Maternal Age	Singleton	Twin	Triplet
20	1/526	1/263 ≈age 34	1/175 ≈age 36
25	1/476	1/238 ≈age 34	1/150 ≈age 36
30	1/385	1/192 ≈age 35	1/128 ≈age 37
35	1/192	1/96 ≈age 38	1/64 ≈age 40
40	1/66	1/33 ≈age 43	1/22 ≈age 45

TABLE 52-3 | TECHNIQUES OF SELECTIVE TERMINATION IN DICHORIONIC GESTATIONS

Potassium chloride
Air embolization
Exsanguination
Cardiac tamponade
Hysterotomy

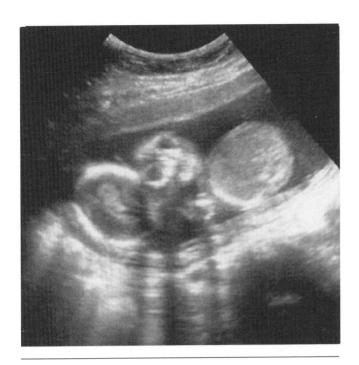

FIGURE 52-1 Anencephalic and normal dichorionic twins.

however, once the needle is in place, 5–10 cc of air was injected directly into the fetal heart. A significant disadvantage of this technique, however, is that the air obscures ultrasonic visualization making confirmation of cardiac asystole sometimes very difficult.[1] Some authors have advocated injecting the air via a Millipore filter to "guarantee" its sterility.[14] It is

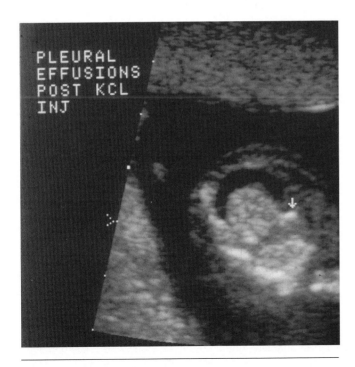

FIGURE 52-2 Needle injected into cardiac chamber.

unclear whether such a precaution is necessary. We have concerns that the extra pressure and manipulations necessary to inject sterile air may increase the risk of needle displacement and an unsuccessful procedure.

EXSANGUINATION

A technique used in the early 1980s was exsanguination: continuing to draw fetal blood until circulatory collapse occurred with subsequent fetal death. However, this technique had a relatively high risk of failure as third-spaced fluid and placental reserves often were sufficient to permit fetal survival, and therefore, the technique has generally been abandoned.[7] We are aware of several instances particularly in the early 1980s, in which this technique failed, and the patient subsequently chose to terminate both fetuses. In fact, some patients were often offered selective termination if they agreed to terminate the entire pregnancy should the procedure fail because of the concern of fetal trauma inflicted by the procedure.

CARDIAC TAMPONADE

Cardiac tamponade, particularly in monochorionic twins, has been successful in a number of cases. After cardiac puncture has been performed to obtain a fetal blood sample, 60 cc of sterile saline can be injected into the pericardial space. An additional 100 cc has often been placed into the pleural cavity to provide further tamponade of heart until asystole has been achieved. Golbus reported 1 case in which 3 attempts at tamponade were necessary, but only temporary bradycardia was achieved. Air embolization was then performed to achieve cardiac asystole.[14]

HYSTEROTOMY

Hysterotomy of 1 abnormal twin has been utilized in some cases, but has the obvious disadvantage of being a major surgical procedure requiring general anesthesia, a classical uterine incision, opening and closure of the uterus and membranes and a high risk of premature labor. Furthermore, because of the "classical" incision, the patient would require cesarean sections in all future pregnancies. As a procedure of last choice, it certainly could be considered an option, particularly if there is a shared placental circulation which would significantly raise the risks of embolization, coagulopathy and damage to the remaining normal twin.

Technically, the procedure is somewhat difficult and requires a high dose of tocolysis to prevent labor. After the maternal abdomen is opened, intraoperative ultrasound should be used to precisely define the optimal point of uterine incision. Experience from the University of California San Francisco Fetal Treatment group suggests the use of a bovie hot knife for entry to minimize bleeding.[19] The fetus can then be removed, the cord clamped and left inside. The membranes and uterus are closed in a "Smead-Jones" combined layered suture with synthetic "super glue" adhesive/sealant instilled to reduce amniotic fluid leakage.

HISTORICAL DATA

In 1978, Aberg et al. was the first to report successful selective birth from a twin pregnancy discordant for Hurler Syndrome.[20] With the poor ultrasound diagnostic technology available at that time, there was considerable concern of possible mistaken identification of the affected fetus, damage or death to the normal fetus, and a risk of disseminated intravascular coagulopathy (DIC) affecting the remaining fetus and/or the mother and inducing preterm labor. Following the original report, a number of other cases have been published which usually drew little attention, yet some have created a considerable stir in the media. In 1981, Kerenyi and Chicaro reported selective birth in a twin pregnancy discordant for Down syndrome.[20] As a justification the authors stated that they were "blackmailed" by the mother, who would terminate both fetuses if they did not attempt to terminate the fetus with Down Syndrome. In 1981, Petres and Redwine reported 2 failed attempts at selective termination by exsanguination of a fetus with Down syndrome.[21] Concerns were appropriately raised that the fetus was now even more compromised by the trauma of the failed attempts than by its genetic disorder. A third attempt was then made with intracardiac air embolization. The affected fetus was successfully terminated, but subsequently chorioamnionitis developed. Preterm labor ensued and neonatal delivery of the normal child at 28 weeks resulted in subsequent death from prematurity. In 2 reports in the early 1980s, Rodeck et al. published 6 cases of second trimester selective termination.[18,22] Under fetoscopic guidance, intrafunic, sterile air embolization was performed. Five of the 6 cases resulted in a normal liveborn twin. In the 6th case, delivery at 29 weeks occurred and the fetus died at 1 month of age from necrotizing enterocolitis. In 1988, Golbus et al. reported selective termination procedures on 22 patients of whom 19 were for a fetal abnormality found in a twin pregnancy.[14] In 17 dichorionic pregnancies there was successful delivery of surviving singletons. However, for twins in 5 monochorionic pregnancies, there was successful delivery of only 1 and pregnancy loss occurred in the other 4. Six of 18 delivered pregnancies in their study were complicated by premature labor and delivery. The general assessment as of the 1980s was that selective termination was a difficult procedure with a high complication rate. The difficulty is now understood to be secondary to poor understanding of monozygotic twin risks, diagnosis and poor ultrasound with a concomitant inability to correctly perform the procedure.

OVERALL RESULTS

Data on second trimester selective terminations have not been as extensively catalogued as those of first trimester multifetal pregnancy reduction. However, reports from a few centers and 2 collaborative series that we have put together suggest that the procedure can be successfully accomplished in the vast majority, if not all cases.[23-28] Concerns that must be considered include: (1) the risk of losing the remaining fetus prior to viability, (2) long-term neonatal morbidity and mortality of the normal twin secondary to prematurity, and/or (3) damage from disseminated intravascular coagulopathies and/or embolizations from the decomposing, dead twin.

Experience has shown that the risks of the procedure are considerably higher in monochorionic/diamniotic twins because of vascular anastomoses.[15] We have also, although rarely, seen vascular connections when there appears to be 2 distinct placentas. We know of 1 case in which a 14-week fetus with an encephalocele was terminated without difficulty, but on a followup ultrasound scan the following day the normal fetus was found to be hydropic and dead. One must, therefore, proceed with extreme caution before declaring that there are no vascular communications between twin fetuses. In a couple of unpublished reports there has been evidence of coagulopathies found in the normal twin of a monochorionic pregnancy which were felt to be secondary to the demise and decomposition of the abnormal twin. Currently, the general opinion is that the damage is more likely to be secondary to hemodynamic imbalance. Regardless of the specific pathophysiology, bipolar cauterization would be the best option in these circumstances.

Two collaborative series have been published by Evans et al. in 1994 and 1999.[23,24] In the later report 402 completed cases of selective termination from 8 centers (Detroit, San Francisco, Philadelphia, Los Angeles, New York, Tel Aviv, Basel, Milan) in 4 countries were combined. Data were collected on procedure indications, methods employed, week the procedure was performed, pregnancy losses, gestational age at delivery, and neonatal outcome. Indications were divided into chromosomal aberrations, structural anomalies, and Mendelian disorders. Techniques included intracardiac and intrafunic potassium chloride.

Of the 402 completed cases there were 345 twins, 39 triplets, and 18 quadruplets or larger multiples. The maternal age distribution of these patients was slightly younger than typically seen in most prenatal diagnosis units reflecting the high proportion of structural abnormalities that are not age related. Of the abnormalities, 56.1% were chromosomal, 40.3% structural, and 3.1% Mendelian disorders. This has changed somewhat over time as more structural cases have now been detected by ultrasound.

Selective termination was technically successful in 100% of the reported cases. Thirty of the 402 cases (7.5%) miscarried before 24 completed weeks. Breakdown of the data by gestational age at procedure shows that from 9–12 weeks there were 5.4% losses. From 13 to 18, 19 to 24, and 25+ weeks, loss rates were 8.7, 6.8%, and 9.1%, respectively. Unlike fetal reduction for multifetal pregnancies, these data did not show the marked improvement in losses or prematurity in time periods over the 15 years. This is, however, partly explained by the number of cases involving triplets or more, which have dramatically increased in the past few years, and partly because these cases have significantly higher loss rates and risks of early prematurity (Tables 52-1, 52-2). When only twins were counted the loss rate was reduced to 7.0%. The inverse correlation between loss or prematurity and gestational age at procedure presented in our

TABLE 52-4	TECHNIQUES USED FOR SELECTIVE TERMINATION IN MONOCHORIONIC GESTATIONS
Absolute alcohol injection	
Alcohol-soaked suture fragments	
Metal coils	
Occlusive substances	
Suture ligation	
Monopolar cauterization	
Laser cauterization	
Bipolar cauterization	
Radiofrequency ablation	

earlier paper does not hold with this larger data set. There were no instances of clinically evident or laboratory appreciated coagulopathies in mothers. Also, no ischemic damage or coagulopathies were observed among the surviving neonates. Eddleman et al. showed a 4% loss rate for twins reduced to a singleton at an average of 19 weeks. However, the loss rate was 5 times higher with triplets consistent with the collaboration data.[24,25]

Premature delivery is a consistent problem which, anecdotally, appears to occur more frequently than with first trimester multifetal pregnancy reductions. One can speculate that the cause of such prematurity is related to the amount of residual fetal tissue that is left in utero. Intuitively, a single 18-week fetus weighs more than several 10-week fetuses added together. As trends in medical practice establish first trimester prenatal diagnosis as the accepted norm, centers that are likely to be involved in selective termination or multifetal pregnancy reduction procedures will no doubt diagnose the presence of fetal anomalies at early gestational ages and such procedures will begin to be undertaken earlier in pregnancies. Such a shift is likely to produce better outcomes with decreased incidence of premature delivery and consequent neonatal morbidity and mortality. As long as there are patients who do not receive first trimester prenatal care or whose ultrasound diagnoses are not made until the late second trimester, the necessity for second trimester procedure will persist and the difficulties associated with such will remain.

SELECTIVE TERMINATION IN MONOCHORIONIC TWIN GESTATIONS

Selective termination may be considered as a management option in monochorionic twin gestations where 1 twin is affected by a significant abnormality such as aneuploidy—a severe malformation that is not compatible with normal ex utero life—particularly if the anomaly is associated with pregnancy complications that can place the normal co-twin at risk or complications caused by the existence of unbalanced vascular anastomoses within the placenta.

Examples include discordant trisomy 18 or anencephaly where the anomalous twin has an increased risk of intrauterine demise and/or, in the case of anencephaly, can develop polyhydramnios resulting in very preterm delivery of the nor-

mal co-twin. Anomalous fetuses, when at an increased risk for intrauterine demise, represent an ongoing danger to their normal co-twins. Monochorionic placentas invariably have vascular communications that hemodynamically link the circulations of both twins.[16] If 1 twin dies, then the co-twin faces a 25–30% risk of demise[19] and, if it survives, a 25–50% risk of severe neurologic morbidity.[25] Postnatal morbidity and neurologic handicap may result from hypoperfusion or thromboembolic complications in various organs, particularly the brain. It has been proposed that acute exsanguination of the surviving twin into the circulation of the dead twin through placental vascular anastomoses is the cause of acute hypotension and irreversible hypoxic brain damage.[29] Thromboplastic proteins transfused from the dead twin to the survivor via placental vascular anastomoses could also result in thrombotic damage to the liver, spleen, kidneys, and brain of the survivor.[30]

The subject of how the death of MZ twins damages the other remains controversial. Undoubtedly vascular collapse, disseminated intravascular coagulation as a result of release of thermoplastic material, or infarction secondary from embolism from the dead co-twin.[30-35]

Hemodynamic complications due to anomalous or unbalanced vascular communications within the chorioangiopagus can threaten survivals as well. One example of this is twin reversed arterial perfusion sequence (TRAP)[30] which places the normal "pump twin" at risk for high output cardiac failure and in utero death, or can lead to early polyhydramnios and premature delivery with its associated morbidity and mortality.[36] Another condition is twin-to-twin transfusion syndrome in which the recipient is hypertensive and hypervolemic, and can develop a progressive hypertrophic cardiomyopathy leading to hydrops and demise.[37]

Conventional feticide techniques with intracardiac injection of potassium chloride are not an option in monochorionic twin gestations because the substance could transfer to the nonaffected twin through the vascular communications within the monochorionic angiopagus. Because of these anastomoses, alternative techniques have been designed that aim at interrupting umbilical cord flow in the anomalous twin completely and permanently.[38] If the occlusion is not complete or becomes patent over time, then persistent fetal-to-fetal transfusion or acute interfetal hemorrhage may occur, both of which are recognized causes of intrauterine fetal death in monochorionic twins.[29] Vascular embolization,[39-45] intrahepatic alcohol injection,[46,47] laser[48,49] and monopolar thermocoagulation,[46,47] radio-frequency ablation,[52] and fetoscopic umbilical cord ligation[53,54] have been used to attempt permanent occlusion, but none have been consistently successful.

More recently, Deprest et al.[53] introduced the use of a 2.7 mm or 3.0 mm bipolar forceps device to thermocoagulate the umbilical cord for selective feticide. Complete occlusion of blood flow to the anomalous fetus was seen in 10 out of 10 cases. However, 2 of these cases experienced premature rupture of membranes within 2 days of the procedure. The remaining 8 pregnancies resulted in the live birth of a healthy baby, with a mean interval between procedure and delivery of 15.1 weeks. Only 1 of these 8 fetuses failed to achieve at least

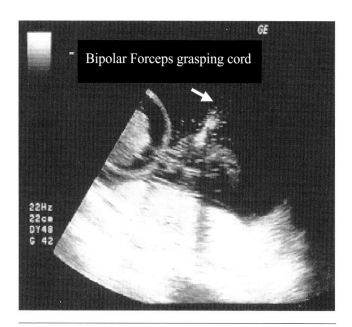

FIGURE 52-3 Selective termination performed by coagulation of umbilical cord using bipolar forceps to sclerose lumen. Care must be used to avoid rupture of the vessel.

36 weeks gestation, and was delivered at 26 weeks because of an unrelated obstetrical complication.

We have adopted this approach with comparable success. In a recent review conducted at Children's Hospital of Philadelphia, of selective feticide procedures using the same 3 mm bipolar cautery devise (Fig. 52-3)—half of the procedures were for TRAP sequence and half for a nonviable anomaly— we were also successful in achieving complete occlusion of umbilical cord blood flow in the selected fetus in all cases. However, our mean gestational age at delivery was 31.2 weeks and mean interval from procedure to delivery was 10.2 weeks. The reason for this difference is unclear, as both centers are experienced in fetoscopic procedures and both contained 2 pregnancies that delivered shortly after the procedure due to premature rupture of membranes (1 at 12 days and 1 at 14 days after the procedure in our series). One possible difference is the gestational age at the time of the procedure: in Deprest et al.[53] a mean age of 20.2 weeks and 21.3 weeks in our series. This suggests that, when the procedure is performed, the gestational age may play a role in outcomes.

We have also used this approach in monochorionic and monoamniotic twin gestations where 1 twin had a significant anomaly that was associated with an increased risk for intrauterine demise. In such cases, however, the umbilical cord is cauterized at 2 closely adjacent locations at both the sites of abdominal cord insertion and placental cord insertion, and the cord transected between cauterization sites at both locations. By severing the cord at both locations, the subsequent risk of cord accidents in the surviving twin due to co-twin cord entanglement and tethering should be markedly reduced. However, this procedure requires the use of 2 fetoscopic ports: 1 for a guiding endoscope and 1 for the operative instruments, but outcomes have been comparable to single port procedures.

We, therefore, believe that selective feticide using bipolar cauterization offers a safe and reliable approach to the selective isolation of the fetal circulations in monochorionic pregnancies, and offers a minimally invasive alternative to suture cord ligation or cord embolization procedures, particularly at later gestations.

ANALYSIS OF DATA

In experienced hands, selective termination for a dizygotic abnormal twin appears to be safe and effective when it is performed by intracardiac or intrafunic injection of potassium chloride. In this collaborative series, the incidence of premature deliveries was relatively low, with 78% of all viable deliveries occurring after 33 weeks and only 6.0% at 25–28 weeks. The gestational age at the time of the procedure did not correlate with the loss rate or with the gestational age at delivery. There does not appear to be the necessity for coagulopathy testing as was done until our first collaborative report.[23] We are unaware of any clinical data consistent with damage from the procedure.

In bichorial pregnancies, the benefits expected from selective termination should be weighed against the potential risk of the procedure concerning the unaffected twin. Pregnancy loss and premature delivery are the major potential obstetrical and perinatal risks associated with selective termination that were identified by our first survey. However, pregnancy losses of up to 30% have been reported in the natural history of twins.[51] Prematurity rates of 40–44% have been reported in twin pregnancies.[42] These figures are comparable with the 37% prematurity rate observed in the first series. Here, following selective termination, 13.7% of potentially viable fetuses were delivered in the 25–32 weeks period, which is slightly higher than the 10.5% rate of severe prematurity observed in the natural history of twins in Britain.[54] This may be due in part to the inclusion of 39 triplets and 18 quadruplets or more in the series of selective termination. When these cases are analyzed separately, the loss rate for 2 to 1 is shown to be lower.[24–26]

ETHICS

To many people, any deliberate termination of a fetus is inherently controversial. There are many parallels when comparing selective termination to multifetal pregnancy reduction in terms of the ethics of the procedure.[55,56] In addition, there are specific ethical differences between selective termination and multifetal pregnancy reduction and that of abortion per se. A woman has an abortion because she has decided that she does not wish to have the child. A woman undergoes selective termination or multifetal pregnancy reduction precisely because she does wish to have a healthy child, and is in circumstances that make this very difficult because either the shear number in cases of multifetal pregnancy or a fetal abnormality has been detected in 1 or more of the fetuses. In the past, the options were to keep both fetuses and commit oneself to care of a potentially severely handicapped infant, or to abort both fetuses and terminate an otherwise healthy, wanted fetus. The development of selective termination has allowed couples to attempt to have a presumably healthy infant while being spared the emotional and financial trauma incurred with a severely handicapped infant. The Ethics Committee of the American College of Obstetricians and Gynecologists has endorsed the ethical probity of offering selective termination under such circumstances.[57] In a society that legally permits abortion, there is no ethical justification for attempting to impose legal sanctions against selective termination as have been proposed but not enacted in a number of jurisdictions in the United States. Shalev et al. have suggested postponing selective termination into the third trimester to reduce the risk of premature delivery.[58]

There certainly is the potential for ethical abuse of the procedure because of its potential use in prenatal diagnosis of a twin pregnancy specifically for the purpose of sex selection. While such cases have been anecdotally suggested, the absolute incidence is probably extremely low.[56,59–61] It is our opinion that sex selection is not routinely appropriate. However, we believe that in a pluralistic society in which abortion can be considered an acceptable option under certain circumstances, selective termination for a significant fetal abnormality is certainly justifiable.

When the risks of performing the procedures are comparable, less important issues such as gender can be a minor consideration.[62] In 1987 Elias and Annas argued that selective termination should only be considered in cases in which there are profound abnormalities, such as Tay-Sachs disease, because of the risk to the normal twin.[63] They specifically felt that Down Syndrome was not a sufficient abnormality to be considered as an indication to offer the procedure. We disagreed then and continue to believe that any aneuploid state is a sufficient indication for the consideration of this procedure, particularly as the data has continued to suggest improving outcomes for the procedures. Others have argued that there is a wide divergence of clinical expression for each aneuploidy, especially cases of trisomy 21 which range from severe psychomotor manifestations to milder degrees that allow sheltered independence in a rare number of individuals. However, there are no present available means that allow prognostic differentiation prenatally; thus, selective reassurance for the expectant parents. We believe that all couples should be allowed to make this difficult choice for themselves based on known clinical facts, and that differing personal perceptions of risk and burden cannot be ethically legislated or imposed. Given that a fundamental tenet of genetic counseling is nondirectional counseling, the imposition of one's view of acceptable versus unacceptable abnormalities is not usually justifiable or ethical.

As with all procedures, as experience increases and the safety of the procedure becomes more appreciated, the appropriate indications for this procedure will likely become clearly delineated. We do not believe that selective termination should ever be considered a frivolous procedure done merely for convenience.[64] However, data suggest a more favorable outcome for twins reduced to a singleton as opposed to continuing twins[62] which makes the 2 to 1 situation even more controversial.

References

1. Evans MI, Quigg MH, Koppitch III FC, et al. First trimester prenatal diagnosis. In: Evans MI, Fletcher JC, Dixler AO, Schulman JD, eds. *Fetal Diagnosis and Therapy: Science, Ethics, and the Law*. Philadelphia: Lippincott Harper Publishing Co; 1989:17–35.
2. U.S. Supreme Court. *Roe v. Wade*. 410 U.S. 113; 1973.
3. U.S. Supreme Court. *Doe v. Bolton*. 410 U.S. 179; 1973.
4. U.S. Supreme Court. *Steinberg v. Carhart*. 530 U.S. 914; 2003.
5. *Evans v. Granholm*. 00-cV-7-586. ED Michigan—permanent injunction 4/26/01.
6. *National Abortion Federation et al. vs Ashcroft*. 03-8695 RCC S.D. NY.
7. Bronsteen RA, Evans MI. Multiple gestation. In: Evans MI, Fletcher JC, Dixler AO, Schulman JD eds. *Fetal Diagnosis and Therapy: Science, Ethics, and the Law*. Philadelphia: Lippincott Harper Publishing Co; 1989:242–66.
8. Luke B: Monozygotic twinning as a congenital defect and congenital defects in monozygotic twins. *Fetal Diagn Ther*. 1990;5:61–69.
9. Verp MS: Antenatal diagnosis of chromosomal abnormalities. In: Sciarra JJ, ed. *Gynecology and Obstetrics*. Vol 5. Philadelphia, PA: JB Lippincott; 1988:1–8.
10. Evans MI, Fletcher JC, Zador IE, et al. Selective first trimester termination in octuplet and quadruplet pregnancies: clinical and ethical issues. *Obstet Gynecol*. 1988;71:289–296.
11. Berkowitz RL, Lynch L, Chitkara U, et al. Selective reduction of multifetal pregnancies in the first trimester. *N Engl J Med*. 1988;318:1043.
12. Evans MI, May M, Drugan A, et al. Selective termination: clinical experience and residual risks. *Am J Obstet Gynecol*. 1990;162:1568–1575.
13. Berkowitz RL, Lynch L. Clinical commentary. *Division of Maternal Fetal Medicine*. 1990;75:873.
14. Golbus MS, Cunningham N, Goldberg JD, et al. Selective termination of multiple gestations. *Am J Med Genet*. 1988;31:339–348.
15. Anderson RL, Golbus MS, Curry CJ, et al. Central nervous system damage and other anomalies in surviving fetus following second trimester antenatal death of co-twin. *Prenat Diagn*. 1990;10:513–518.
16. Bajoria R, Wigglesworth J, Fisk NM. Angioarchitecture of monochorionic placentas in relation to the twin-twin transfusion syndrome. *Am J Obstet Gynecol*. 1995;172:856–863.
17. Quintero RA, Romero R, Reich H, et al. In utero percutaneous umbilical cord ligation in the management of complicated monochorionic multiple gestations. *Ultrasound Obstet Gynecol*. 1996;8:16–22.
18. Rodeck C, Mibashan R, Abramowitz J, et al. Selective feticide of the affected twin by fetoscopic air embolization. *Prenat Diagn*. 1982;2:189–194.
19. Rydhstrom H, Ingemarsson I. Prognosis and long-term follow-up of a twin after antenatal death of the co-twin. *J Reprod Med*. 1993;38:142–146.
20. Kerenyi T, Chitkara U. Selective birth in twin pregnancy with discordancy for Down syndrome. *N Engl J Med*. 1981;304:1525–1527.
21. Petres R, Redwine F. Selective birth in twin pregnancy. *N Engl J Med*. 1981;305:1218–1219.
22. Rodeck C. Fetoscopy in the management of twin pregnancies discordant for a severe abnormality. *Acta Genet Med Gemellol (Roma)*. 1984;33:57–60.
23. Evans MI, Goldberg JD, Dommergues M, et al. Efficacy of second trimester selective term fetal abnormalities: international collaborative experience among the world's largest centers. *Am J Obstet Gynecol*. 1994;171:90–94.

24. Evans MI, Goldberg J, Horenstein J, et al. Selective termination (ST) for structural (STR), chromosal (CHR) and Mendelian (MEN) anomalies: international experience. *Am J Obstet Gynecol.* 1999;181:893–897.

25. Eddleman KA, Stone JL, Lynch L, et al. Selective termination of anomalous fetuses in multifetal pregnancies: two hundred cases at a single center. *Am J Obstet Gynecol.* 2002;187:1168–1172.

26. Yaron Y, Johnson KD, Bryant-Greenwood PK, et al. Selective termination and elective reduction in twin pregnancies. 10 years' experience at a single centre. *Human Reprod* 1998;13:230104

27. Stewart KS, Johnson MP, Quintero RA, et al. Congenital abnormalities in twins: selective termination. Curr Opin Obstet Gynecol: 1997;9:136–9.

28. Challis D, Gratacos E, Deprest JA. Cord occlusion techniques for selective termination in monochorionic twins. J Perinat Med 1999;27: 327–38.

29. van Heteren CF, Nijhuis JG, Semmekrot BA, et al. Risk for surviving twin after fetal death of co-twin in twin-twin transfusion syndrome. *Obstet Gynecol.* 1998;92:215–219.

30. Fusi L, McParland P, Fisk N, et al. Acute twin-twin transfusion: a possible mechanism for brain-damaged survivors after intrauterine death of a monochorionic twin. *Obstet Gynecol.* 1991;78: 517–520.

31. Bilardo CM, Arabin B. Monoamniotic twins in Blickstein I, Keith LG (eds). Multiple Pregnancy: Epidemiology, Gestation, and Perinatal Outcome. 2005. Taylor and Francis. London pp. 574–582.

32. Wada H, Numogami K, Wada T, et al: Diffuse brain damage caused by acute twin twin transfusion during late pregnancy. Acta Paediatr Jpn 1998;40:370–3.

33. Langer B, Boudier E, Gasser B, et al. Antenatal diagnosis of brain damage in the survivor after the second trimester death of a monchorionic monoamniotic co-twin: case report and literature review. Fetal Diagn Ther 1997;12:286–9.

34. van Gemert MJC, Nikkels PG. Placental vasculature in the pathogenesis of fetal mortality and morbidity in multiple pregnancies. In Blickstein I, Keith LG (eds). Multiple Pregnancy: Epidemiology, Gestation, and Perinatal Outcome. 2005. Taylor and Francis. London pp. 586–588.

35. Blickstein I. Management of single fetal death. In Blickstein I, Keith LG (eds) Multiple Pregnancy: Epidemiology, Gestation, and Perinatal Outcome. 2005. Taylor and Francis. London pp 589–593.

36. Van Allen MI, Smith DW, Shepard TH. Twin reversed arterial perfusion (TRAP) sequence: study of 14 twin pregnancies with acardius. *Semin Perinatol.* 1983;7:285–293.

37. Healey MG. Acardia: predictive risk factors for the co-twin's survival. *Teratology.* 1994;50:2051–2053.

38. Naeye RL. Organ abnormalities in a human parabiotic syndrome. *Am J Path.* 1965;46:8–29.

39. Deprest J, Evrard V, Van Schoubroeck D, et al. Fetoscopic cord ligation. *Lancet.* 1996;348:890–891.

40. Porreco R, Barton SM, Haverkamp AD. Occlusion of umbilical artery in acardiac, acephalic twin. *Lancet.* 1991;337:326–327.

41. Grab D, Scheider V, Keckstein J, et al. Twin, acardiac, outcome. *Fetus.* 1992;2:11–13.

42. Holzgreve W, Tercanli S, Krings W, et al. A simpler technique for umbilical cord blockade of an acardiac twin. *N Engl J Med.* 1995;331:57–58.

43. Dommergues M, Mandelbrot L, Delzoide A, et al. Twin-to-twin transfusion syndrome: selective feticide by embolization of the hydropic fetus. *Fetal Diagn Ther.* 1995;10:26–31.

44. Roberts RM, Shah DM, Jeanty P, et al. Twin, acardiac, ultrasound guided embolization. *Fetus.* 1991;1:5–10.

45. Mahone PR, Sherer DM, Abramowicz JS, et al. Twin-twin transfusion syndrome: rapid development of severe hydrops of the donor

following selective feticide of the hydropic recipient. *Am J Obstet Gynecol.* 1993;169:166–168.

46. Denbow ML, Battin MR, Kyle PM, et al. Selective termination by intrahepatic vein alcohol injection of amonochorionic twin pregnancy discordant for fetal abnormality. *Br J Obstet Gynaecol.* 1997;104:626–627.

47. Denbow ML, Overton TG, Duncan KR, et al. High failure rate of umbilical vessel occlusion by ultrasound-guided injection of absolute alcohol or embucrilate gel. *Prenat Diagn.* 1999;19:527–532.

48. Ville Y, Hyett J, Vandenbussche FP, et al. Endoscopic laser coagulation of umbilical cord vessels in twin reversed arterial perfusion sequence. *Ultrasound Obset Gynecol.* 1994;4:396–398.

49. Hecher K, Reinhold U, Gbur K, et al. Interruption of umbilical blood flow in an acardiac twin by endoscopic laser coagulation. *Geburtshilfe Frauenheilkd.* 1996;56:97–100.

50. Rodeck C, Deans A, Jauniaux E. Thermocoagulation for the early treatment of pregnancy with an acardiac twin. *N Engl J Med.* 1998; 339:1293–1294.

51. Lewi L, Van Schoubroeck D, Gratacos E, et al. Monochorionic diamniotic twins: complications and management options. *Curr Opin Obstet Gynecol.* 2003;15:177–194.

52. Tsao K, Feldstein VA, Albanese CT, et al. Selective reduction of acardiac twin by radiofrequency ablation. *Am J Obstet Gynecol.* 2002;187:635–640.

53. Deprest JA, Audibert F, Van Schoubroeck D, et al. Bipolar coagulation of the umbilical cord incomplicated monochorionic twin pregnancy. *Am J Obstet Gynecol.* 2000;182:340–345.

54. Melnick M. Brain damage in survivor after in-utero death of monozygous co-twin. *Lancet.* 1977;2:1287.

55. Evans MI, Fletcher JC, Rodeck C. Ethical problems in multiple gestations: selective termination. In: Evans MI, Fletcher JC, Dixler AO, Schulman JD, eds. *Fetal Diagnosis and Therapy: Science, Ethics, and the Law.* Philadelphia: Lippincott Harper Publishing Co; 1989:266–276.

56. Chervenak FA, McCullough LB, Skupski D, et al. Ethical issues in the management of pregnancies complicated by fetal anomalies. *Obstet Gynecol Surv.* 2003;58:473–483.

57. ACOG Ethics Statement: multifetal pregnancy reduction and selective fetal termination. Proceedings of the Committee on Ethics, American College of Obstetricians and Gynecologists; November 1990.

58. Shalev J, Meizner I, Rabinerson D, et al. Improving pregnancy outcome in twin gestations with one malformed fetus by postponing selective feticide in the third trimester. *Fertil Steril.* 1999;72:257–260.

59. Evans MI, Drugan, Bottoms SF, et al. Attitudes on the ethics of abortion, sex selection, and selective pregnancy termination among health care professionals, ethicists, and clergy likely to encounter such situations. Am J. Obstet Gynecol 1991;164:1092–9.

60. Dorfman SA, Robbins RM, Jewell WH, et al. Second trimester selective termination of a twin with ruptured membranes; elimination of fluid leakage and preservation of pregnancy. Fetal Diagn Ther 1995; 10:186–8.

61. Evans MI, Johnson MP, Quintero RA, et al. Ethical issues surrounding multifetal pregnancy reduction and selective termination. Clin Perinatol 1996;23:437–51.

62. Evans MI, Kaufman M, Urban AJ, et al. Fetal reduction from twins to a singleton: a reasonable consideration. *Obstetrics and Gynecology.* 2004;104:102–109.

63. Elias S, Annas GJ. *Reproductive Genetics and the Law.* Chicago Year Book; 1987:123–129.

64. Evans MI, Berkowitz R, Wapner R, et al. Multifetal pregnancy reduction (MFPR): improved outcomes with increased experience. *Am J Obstet Gynecol.* 2001;184:97–1031.

CHAPTER 53

THE OBSTETRICAL MANAGEMENT OF FETAL ANOMALIES

Peter G. Pryde

INTRODUCTION

Anomalous development of the human embryo and fetus is a common and increasingly relevant clinical problem. It is estimated that as many as 30–50% of human conceptions are lost in early gestation, most of which are thought to be intrinsically abnormal.[1,2] Despite the impact of early spontaneous loss in eliminating the majority of aberrantly developing pregnancies, there remain a significant number who survive. By term an estimated 3% of infants are born with major structural anomalies and 1% have multiple malformations.[3] This clinically significant group of developmentally abnormal neonates contributes increasingly, and disproportionately, to the sum of perinatal mortalities. While recent efforts to reduce perinatal mortality have been effective in reducing deaths related to utero-placental causes, and therefore total perinatal deaths, such a reduction has not been observed with deaths due to fetal anomalies. Therefore fetal anomalies, accounting for only 12% of perinatal deaths in the 1960s,[4] now account for nearly one third of perinatal losses.[5]

Through the application of several rapidly evolving technologies (including high resolution ultrasound, biochemical analyte screening, cytogenetics, and molecular biology), and the development of advanced invasive fetal diagnostic techniques, the obstetricians ability to screen for, accurately diagnose and manage fetal developmental disorders has become quite powerful. Concomitant with the expanding prenatal diagnostic possibilities has been the growing expectation, by prospective parents, that their child will be normal.[6] This has translated into a high uptake of prenatal screening and diagnostic techniques by pregnant women and a high rate of utilization of such technologies by their care providers.[7,8] Thus fetal anomalies are increasingly recognized antenatally allowing evaluation, prognostication, and in some instances intervention to effect outcome.

Although many fetal anomalies carry a dismal prognosis, regardless of efforts at detection and treatment, there are others in which real impact on outcomes can be made. It is the pregnancy management principles for this group of potentially surviving, but anomalous, fetuses on which this chapter shall focus.

DIAGNOSIS OF ANOMALIES: IMMEDIATE MANAGEMENT

When diagnoses of fetal anomalies are made, or suspected, the parents must be informed of the findings in a sensitive but clear and truthful fashion. Education will be the initial priority. Because most parents are quite unprepared for such a discussion it will typically require considerable time. In some instances, particularly when awaiting invasive diagnostic information, serial encounters will be necessary. Several key elements must be conveyed to the parents. First is a frank discussion of the ultrasound findings and the fetal differential diagnosis. As will later be detailed, this must include realistic appraisals of diagnostic certainty and uncertainty. Next, the attendant range of prognostic possibilities is elaborated. And finally, pregnancy management options (including *aggressive* versus *nonaggressive* approaches, or in some cases *abortion*), are sensitively presented (Table 53-1).

As such discussions unfold, parental anxieties naturally arise accompanied by variable levels of grief, guilt, and disbelief. Clinicians commonly observe that the capacity of parents to fully assimilate the information being presented them is often blunted by these emotions. The nonrational component of the parental response must be kept in mind when, despite the shocking news, they may be called upon to consider a variety of medically complicated management options and make decisions.

Before long-term prognosis and pregnancy management can be properly discussed it is essential to establish as precise a fetal diagnosis as is possible (Fig. 53-1). The observation and description of an aberrant ultrasound finding, in most instances, does not constitute a specific diagnosis. It is essential to compile all identifiable abnormalities, acknowledging that high resolution ultrasound continues to have diagnostic limitations,[9] and that varying levels of diagnostic uncertainty are not infrequent. With this information an effort is made to narrow as much as possible the differential etiologic diagnosis. The quality of the counselling very much depends on this effort. In most cases the prognosis for a fetus with the finding of an anatomic defect hinges altogether on the specific etiologic diagnosis. For example observing mild isolated fetal ventriculomegaly during ultrasound tells much less about the fetal prognosis than does this finding when accompanied by the demonstration of associated defects such as a Chiari malformation secondary to a large spina bifida. This is important because difficult parental pregnancy management decisions will depend largely on the fetal prognosis as it is related to them by their physician.[10]

Recall that among fetal diagnoses of structural malformation, the overall rate of aneuploidy can range from 10% (with an isolated defect) to 35% (when 2 or more anomalies are seen).[11] Additionally, one third of newborns having a major congenital anomaly are found to have multiple anomalies.[3] And finally, the organ most commonly affected by structural anomalies, whether in the setting of an isolated defect or in association with multiple congenital anomalies, is the heart. Thus, optimal prenatal diagnostic precision requires minimally (a) a vigilant search for additional extracardiac anomalies,[12] (b) a comprehensive fetal echocardiographic study,[13] and (c) in most instances a fetal karyotype.[11,14] Most prenatal

TABLE 53-1	FETAL MANAGEMENT STRATEGIES	
Strategy	*Methods*	*Clinical Situations*
Abortion	DE versus labor induction techniques	Typically poor prognosis fetal conditions. Available regardless of type of abnormality if gestational age within legal limits.
Nonaggressive	Withhold antepartum testing, intrapartum testing, and any invasive procedures (ie, Cesarean section) which otherwise are performed for fetal benefit alone	Reserved for definitively diagnosed fetal conditions with extremely poor prognosis and little hope for beneficial intervention. Examples include alobar holopros encephaly, anencephaly, large encephalocele, bilateral renal agenesis, lethal congenital heart defects, triploidy, trisomies 13 and 18, etc.
Aggressive	Full provision of appropriate antepartum and intrapartum fetal assessment techniques. Provision of cesarean section for fetal or other obstetrical indications. Fetal therapies where indicated, including invasive fetal procedures for indicated conditions.	Disorders with hopeful outlook by natural history, or in which fetal or neonatal interventions can improve outcomes. Examples are several repairable heart defects, isolated ventral wall defects, many instances of spina bifida, isolated cleft lip and/or palate, selected cases of diaphragmatic hernia or bladder outlet obstruction, and many more.

diagnostic laboratory tests can be performed on fluid obtained by amniocentesis (such as a karyotype, tests for fetal infection,[15] or tests for rare mendellian disorders having structural features shared in the differential diagnosis of the fetal findings). Occasionally, other invasive fetal diagnostic procedures will also be needed such as fetal blood sampling in cases of nonimmune hydrops,[16] and fetal urine sampling in cases of bladder outlet obstruction.[17]

The results of these tests may prove invaluable in refining discussions of prognosis. For example, when there is ultrasound identification of ventricular septal defect (VSD), it is often the underlying cause, or etiology, of that defect (more than

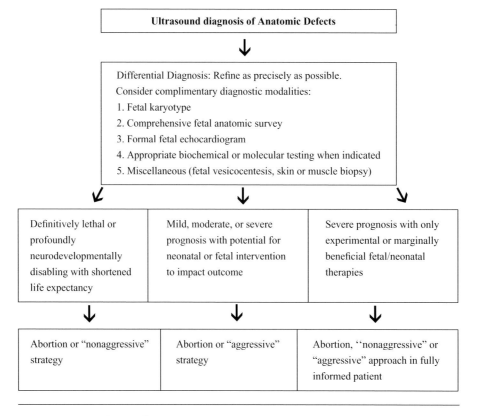

FIGURE 53-1 Fetal anomalies evaluation and management algorithm.

the defect itself) which determines the long-term outlook. The prognosis for truly isolated VSD is, in many cases, excellent. However, if searching the remainder of the fetal anatomy reveals additional structural anomalies then syndromic (Mendellian, sporatic, or chromosomal) causes of VSD must be considered. Not only do the additional anomalies carry their own unique risks, but the presence of multiple defects point to a global, as opposed to single organ specific, abnormality of fetal development. Obviously the aggressiveness of the pregnancy management may be radically different when a poor or lethal prognosis (for example if trisomy 18 is revealed in the work-up of VSD) can be clearly determined, compared to where there is a potentially excellent prognosis (as when the VSD appears to be truly an isolated finding).

THE "PERINATAL TEAM"

Because of the complexity of the maternal and fetal medical issues raised, women having prenatal diagnoses of fetal anomalies are usually referred to, and managed, under the guidance of a perinatal team.[18,19,20] Such a team has multispecialty representation, which typically includes specialists in maternal-fetal medicine, genetics, neonatology, all branches of pediatric surgery, and pediatric cardiology. Other professionals typically involved include genetic counselors, social workers, and at times medical ethics representatives. The team approach, by combining the unique expertise, experience, and viewpoint of many individuals representing a variety of disciplines, often improves diagnostic precision as well as the quality and balance of parental education and counseling. Ultimately, the optimal care of an anomalous fetus may require the input of the entire team.

It is essential that physicians overseeing these pregnancies maintain a reasoned, continuously updated, and as much as possible evidence based approach. However, the reality is that most existing literature in this area is retrospective, uncontrolled and with small numbers of cases. Thus management plans are based not only on a critical appraisal of the available data, but also include consideration of the collaborative experience of the perinatal team.

INFORMED CONSENT

It is essential to maintain utmost sensitivity to the importance of informed consent in managing these patients. Informed consent is perhaps more problematic in fetal medicine than in other medical disciplines due to (a) the frequent pressure of time constraints for decision making, (b) the often considerable levels of diagnostic uncertainty as discussed above, (c) the comparative lack of solid management guidance data sometimes creating legitimate controversy about prognosis as well as management for particular defects, and (d) the available management options may bring maternal and fetal welfare into conflict. Thus, a painstaking effort to elaborate the potential risks (both maternal and fetal), benefits (fetal), as well as alternative options (each with its own risk/benefits), must be made. When the patient has demonstrated sufficient grasp of these issues, she is called upon to choose a course of action. It is the physician's

obligation, then, to devise and follow a mutually acceptable management plan which includes the patients desires (within medical reason) as well as her fully informed and written consent.

ONGOING AND DEFINITIVE MANAGEMENT

ABORTION FOR FETAL ANOMALIES

Before viability, a woman's right to abortion is established through the Supreme Court decision of *Roe v. Wade*.[21] Thus, when abnormalities of most, if not all, types are diagnosed prior to fetal viability the option of pregnancy termination should be presented. When diagnoses are established beyond the limits of viability legal access to abortion becomes more limited. Several centers will provide terminations beyond viability in cases of definitively diagnosed lethal anomalies (i.e., anencephaly, triploidy). Only a few centers, however, allow broader fetal indications for termination beyond viability. Thus for some women who might otherwise prefer abortion, it may not be a realistic option.

AGGRESSIVE MANAGEMENT APPROACH

When the diagnostic evaluation indicates that there is hope for fetal salvage, the pregnant woman and her partner may choose to pursue an *"aggressive"* approach to pregnancy management. Under such circumstances both the maternal patient, and the fetal patient, must be simultaneously considered with the intention of minimizing maternal risk while maximizing fetal outcome. Management will be individualized according to the nature of the fetal disorder (and its anticipated prognosis) as well as a careful consideration of any unique maternal medical and philosophical concerns. Issues to be addressed include (a) where, when and by what route of fetal delivery, (b) what type and intensity of fetal surveillance is indicated, and finally (c) are in utero therapies a consideration.

When aggressive management is chosen, anomalous fetuses should be delivered in a tertiary center equipped with an intensive care nursery and an experienced "perinatal team."[18,19,20] Only in this environment will there be ready access to comprehensive diagnostic, as well as therapeutic interventions. The need for such interventions can arise acutely in the perinatal period, and should be anticipated. Obviously it is best to avoid delivery at a hospital unequipped for complex neonatal problems which are likely to be aggravated by the delay and technical logistics of neonatal transport to a tertiary center.[22]

In most cases full-term delivery is optimal for fetuses affected with malformations.[18] The rationale for this generalization is that larger babies are usually better surgical candidates. Additionally, respiratory problems of prematurity will complicate the already problematic management of the malformed infant and should be avoided whenever possible. Certainly there are exceptions to this rule: For example, occasionally fetuses with obstructive hydrocephally will be noted to have rapidly expanding ventriculomegaly. In these cases delivery, as soon as pulmonary maturity can be established, may reduce progressive cerebral injury by earlier corrective surgery.[23] Other examples would include instances where antepartum testing indicates deteriorating fetal status in anomalous fetuses for whom there remains hope for salvage.[18]

Route of delivery is occasionally a source of controversy in the management of malformed infants. For most anomalies elective cesarean section will provide no demonstrable fetal advantage compared with the vaginal route of delivery, while substantively increasing maternal risks.[18] For these anomalies, therefore, cesarean delivery should only be performed for standard obstetrical indications. Some anomalies, however, will clearly require cesarean section simply due to the near certainty of dystocia (e.g., conjoined twins, sacrococcygeal teratoma, and cases of hydrocephaly with marked macrocephaly when aggressive management is planned thus contraindicating cephalocentesis). There also remain a few relatively common anomalies for which the optimal route of delivery is not yet established, and for which there remains legitimate controversy. Examples are selected cases of meningomyelocele, gastroschisis, and omphalocele.

A final aggressive management option that may be considered in a few relatively uncommon fetal conditions is fetal surgery by either open or percutaneous techniques. These invasive fetal therapies are currently offered only at a handful of "fetal surgery" centers. Current indications include carefully selected cases of obstructive uropathy,[24] isolated congenital diaphragmatic hernia,[25] fetal sacrococcygeal teratoma,[26] congenital cystic adenomatoid malformation of the lung,[27] and isolated fetal hydrothorax.[28] Results have been variable, but techniques are evolving. Prospective studies proving fetal benefit, as well as establishing the level of maternal procedure related risk, are not yet available. Each of these treatments must therefore still be regarded as experimental and, for now, should probably be performed only at the most experienced centers under human investigational protocols.

NONAGGRESSIVE MANAGEMENT APPROACH

Occasionally severe defects are discovered for which the outlook is poor, and interventions are unlikely to be beneficial or entail inordinate maternal risk. For many women abortion, even under such circumstances, is not an option. Alternatively, these defects may be, and often are, diagnosed beyond the local legal limits for abortion. In such instances the pregnant patient and her partner may choose a *nonaggressive* pregnancy management approach. Nonaggressive management, in this context, implies avoidance of obstetrical tests or interventions typically employed strictly for fetal benefit, and in some instances with the potential cost of increasing maternal risk. Such interventions that may be avoided would include (a) antepartum fetal surveillance methods, (b) fetal heart rate monitoring in labor, (c) mandatory delivery in a tertiary care center, and (d) cesarean section for fetal indications. In order to consider the nonaggressive approach there should be a high level of diagnostic certainty predicting either a lethal, or a profoundly neurodevelopmentally and cognitively disabling, fetal condition. Examples of such diagnoses include triploidy, tisomy 18, trisomy 13, anencephaly, alobar holoprosencephaly, hydranencephaly, congenital heart disease with progressive hydrops, and bilateral renal agenesis.

COMMON CLINICAL SITUATIONS

A complete list of fetal anomalies and review of proposed obstetrical management exceeds the scope of this chapter and has been the content of several important textbooks. The following are representative examples of the more common anomalies with which a busy "perinatal team" will be confronted.

CENTRAL NERVOUS SYSTEM ANOMALIES

Structural disorders of the central nervous system (CNS) are comparatively common, and with current ultrasound technology are frequently identified antenataly.[29] As with malformations in other systems, they can occur in isolation or as component of a syndrome involving multiple anomalies including aneuploidy. Additionally, with several of the CNS anomalies, there is a tendency for progression of severity with advancing gestation. Thus, it is imperative that as precise a diagnosis as possible be established including a careful search for associated CNS and non-CNS anomalies as well as chromosome analysis. However, even when an isolated defect is assured, prognostic counseling can be difficult due to problems in predicting the severity of cognitive and neurodevelopmental disabilities for which any given case may be destined. With any previable diagnosis of CNS anomaly abortion must be offered.

NEURAL TUBE DEFECTS

Neural tube defects (NTDS) are the most common CNS anomalies encountered affecting 1–3/1000 live births.[30] Anencephaly and caudal spinal dysraphism are the most frequent among NTD's and occur in nearly equal proportions. Considerably more rare examples include iniencephaly, encephalocele, and craniospinal rachischisis. The prognosis for these disorders is quite variable. While some are predictably lethal (anencephaly and craniospinal rachischisis), or have uniformly poor outcomes (iniencephaly and most instances of encephalocele), the outlook is less predictable in cases of caudal meningocele and myelomeningocele.[31]

In cases with clearly poor prognosis (anencephaly, iniencephally, and craniospinal rachischisis) there is general agreement that a "nonaggresive" approach should be encouraged. Prenatal diagnosis of encephalocele is more problematic: While most instances of encephalocele are in fact cranial meningomyelocele with extremely poor prognoses, there are some instances where the defect is small and contains no neural tissue. In such cases the anomaly is effectively a cranial-meningocele with potentially a much more favorable prognosis.[32] In cases where there is associated microcephaly and neural tissue clearly occupies the encephalocele, the prognosis is predictably poor and "nonaggressive" management is appropriate. However, when such findings are not obvious, the distinction of the two entities may not be possible antenatally. This would lead one toward the "aggressive" approach, which may include cesarean delivery (see meningomyelocele discussion in the following section).

In recent years, attributable mostly to early pediatric neurosurgical and adjuvant medical care, there has been enormous improvement in the outlook for children born with myelomeningocele. Current surveys[33,34,35] report that while most affected individuals have some element of neurologic disability, the majority survive. Among survivors, cognitive abilities (as indicated by intelligence quotient) are within the normal range in 70–80%. Although severity of neurologic disability varies with size and location of the lesion, about 50% of affected individuals are capable of ambulation as adults.

The possibility that obstetrical management may further improve outcomes with meningomyelocele has been debated, and has generated a considerable literature. Following Chervanaks report[36] of 4 fetuses managed by elective cesarean section to allow "atraumatic" delivery, there have been several relatively small series published. Important findings include Hadi's report on 9 fetuses, all having small (≤4 cm in diameter) lesions, that were delivered vaginally from a cephalic presentation.[37] Among these there were no ruptures of the meningocele sacs, no cases of meningitis, and outcomes were not different from abdominally delivered historic controls. Two subsequent retrospective series of 72 and 35 affected infants, respectively, failed to show significant differences in mortality or neurologic outcomes in infancy.[38] However, the former study did show increased numbers of infants developing meningitis among the vaginally delivered group (3 of the total of 4 meningitis complications in the entire series). The later study found a higher incidence of rupture of the meningomyelocele sac (a complication associated with neonatal meningitis which itself is associated with worse overall outcomes) among infants having lesions >6 cm regardless of mode of delivery. Finally, Luthy and associates reported their retrospective experience with 200 meningomyelocele affected infants delivered at the University of Washington.[39] These authors stratified infants by cesarean without labor, cesarean after labor, and vaginal delivery. Although there were no differences in neonatal complications, there were statistically significant, and clinically important, differences in neurologic outcome at 24 months between those exposed and those not exposed to labor. The labored group was 2.2 times more likely to have "severe" paralysis. Similarly, the mean neurologic level of paralysis was higher in the labor exposed compared with the unexposed group.

Each of these studies can be criticized due to their retrospective nature, and the ongoing controversy calls for a prospective study. However, as Hobbins has editorialized, a definitive controlled randomized trial is unlikely to occur.[40] In the absence of such a trial, the available data would support liberal use of cesarean section prior to the onset of labor. Such an approach would allow controlled delivery, into an aseptic environment, in a setting allowing prompt neurosurgical evaluation and repair. A possible exception to this sort of policy may be cephalic presenting fetuses affected with small (<4 cm) lumbosacral lesions in which rupture of the sac appears to be unlikely[37] and outcomes do not appear to be influenced by delivery mode.

VENTRICULOMEGALLY

The term ventriculomegally describes the finding of enlarged cerebral ventricles. It is markedly heterogeneous in etiology including idiopathic, secondary to Chiari malformation associated with spinal dysraphism, infectious, association with aneuploidy, and association with a variety of other developmental disorders. Ventriculomegally thereby has a highly variable prognosis depending very much on the specific etiologic diagnosis.[31] In a series of 267 consecutively diagnosed cases of ventriculomegally, Nicolaides and associates[41] reported that 64% were secondary to open spina bifida, 22% were "isolated" ventriculomegally, and 14% had multiple congenital anomalies. Among cases with multiple defects there were 36% having associated aneuploidy, and 100% mortalities. Among "isolated" ventriculomegally cases there were only 6% with chromosome abnormalities. Additionally the prognosis with mild, static, isolated ventriculomegally in the absence of chromosomal abnormalities was excellent both for survival and for neurodevelopmental outcome.

Thus the presence or absence of associated anomalies and the karyotype, will facilitate discussions about management approach. Abortion should be offered in all instances where ventriculomegally is diagnosed before viability. In poor prognosis cases (those with multiple associated anomalies excepting isolated spina bifida, and/or a serious chromosome abnormality), for which abortion is declined, or the diagnosis is made too late to exercise that option, a "nonaggressive" approach is justified. In these instances decompression cephalocentesis during labor has been considered by some authors, in the attempt to avoid the maternal morbidity of cesarean section, when dystocia occurs due to macrocephaly.[23]

In the early 1980s, efforts at in utero ventriculo-amniotic shunt placement for the treatment of supposedly "isolated" expanding ventriculomegally met with marginal success.[42] Due to an unacceptably high procedure related fetal mortality (12% of reported cases), problems ruling out associated anomalies, and lack of a proper comparison group to demonstrate benefit, the procedure has been abandoned.

In continuing ventriculomegally affected pregnancies which are either isolated, or those cases whose only associated anomaly is spina bifida, an "aggressive" approach is recommended. In these cases serial ultrasound is necessary to observe for progression of the disorder: Occasionally rapidly expanding hydrocephaly may be observed and early delivery recommended.[43] Under these circumstances corticosteroids may be appropriate if delivery is anticipated prior to 34–36 weeks. In all cases fetal lung maturity should be verified prior to delivery. Route of delivery will depend on the presence or absence of attendant macrocephaly. Fetuses having a BPD <100 mm can be allowed a trial of labor for vaginal delivery, with cesarean reserved for obstetric indications.[18] Larger heads will likely lead to dystocia and cesarean section followed by postnatal shunting may optimize outcomes.

MISCELLANEOUS CNS ANOMALIES

There are a variety of less common but important CNS anomalies that come to the attention of the perinatal team and deserve comment.

Miscellaneous disorders of brain development will be discussed together including Dandy-Walker malformation (and its variants also known as "partial agenesis of the cerebellar vermis"), agenesis of the corpus collosum, and the progressively severe varients of holoprosencephaly (lobar, semilobar, and alobar). It is important to recognize that each of these disorders has a high rate of associated CNS and non-CNS anomalies as well as significantly elevated risk for aneuploidy.[29] Additionally, they can have widely variable prognoses depending on the severity of the primary finding, as well as the presence or absence of other abnormalities. As with the other CNS lesions discussed, associated anomalies or chromosomal abnormalities portend poor prognoses. In the absence of associations, however, one needs to be extremely careful in prognosticating, especially in the mild forms of these diagnoses (i.e., isolated partial agenesis of the corpus colossum, partial agenesis of the cerebellar vermis, or lobar holoprosencephaly). These milder forms can, but do not always, have quite normal neurodevelopmental outcomes. Thus, management principles can be generalized to performance of a comprehensive anatomic survey (including fetal echocardiogram) searching for additional anomalies, followed by karyotype evaluation. In clearly poor prognosis cases (multiple anomalies, chromosome abnormality, or alobar holoprosencephaly) nonaggressive management or abortion should be offered. In the remainder of cases, for which prognosis must be considered uncertain, abortion is offered when previable and otherwise "aggressive" obstetrical management is encouraged.

The final group of CNS disorders to be considered together are the fetal brain abnormalities thought to be of a disruptive vascular origin, or of a developmental origin but anatomically resembling a vascular disruption.[44] The former includes hydranencephaly, and type I porencephaly (also known as "false porencephaly"). The later is type II porencephaly (also called "schizencephaly"). From the viewpoint of obstetrical management, the important issue is accurate diagnosis. When type II porencephaly (usually bilateral involving extensive cerebral cortex) is identified, or hydranencephaly is confidently diagnosed, the prognosis is extremely bleak for long-term survival, and neurocognitive development is generally poor in survivors. Abortion is offered and, in continuing pregnancies, a "nonaggressive" approach is encouraged. On one hand for type I porencephaly (usually unilateral and of variable severity) the outlook is less predictable.[44] Mild cystic lesions can be associated with comparatively good outcomes and an "aggressive" approach may be considered. On the other hand "severe" cases tend to follow a course similar to type II porencephally and should be managed accordingly.

CARDIAC ABNORMALITIES

There are multiple well described abnormal patterns of cardiac development. The majority of these can now be diagnosed in the late second trimester fetus, with an impressive degree of confidence, using high-resolution ultrasound and color doppler imaging. The heart is the most common organ to be congenitally anomalous such that nearly 1% of newborns are found to have a cardiac defect.[45] From the viewpoint of obstetrical management, the fetal cardiac disorders can be grouped into (a) those which involve anatomic defects, and (b) those which involve rhythm disturbances.

STRUCTURAL CARDIAC ANOMALIES

As with other fetal anomalies, the observation of a congenital heart defect (CHD) should alert the clinician to the possibility of associated noncardiac anomalies and/or aneuploidy. In published series of antenatally diagnosed CHD multiple anomalies are reported in 25–50% of cases.[46] Similarly, aneuploidy occurs in up to 32% of cases with the prevalence skewed toward those with multiple defects.[47,48] When identified prenatally, the overall survival rate for CHD is reported less than 25%.[49,50] This contrasts with subtler lesions that escape antenatal detection and survive in 80% of cases.[50]

From a prognostic point of view several generalizations can be made. As with many fetal anomalies, the earlier in gestation the diagnosis becomes apparent, the more severe the anomaly and the attendant prognosis. Similarly, those defects that escape prenatal detection, in experienced units, tend to be milder with better outcomes. When associated noncardiac anomalies are noted the prognosis worsens considerably, as is also true with the presence of aneuploidy. Some lesions, even in isolation, are severe and carry predictably poor prognoses (e.g., hypoplastic left heart, and any structural disorders accompanied by evolution of hydrops). Thus, prognostication requires (a) comprehensive fetal anatomic evaluation, (b) fetal karyotype, and (c) serial echocardiagraphic functional evaluation.

When CHD is diagnosed before viability, abortion is offered. For continuing pregnancies, management is dictated by certainty of prognosis. In clearly poor prognosis cases (examples include those with multiple anomalies, severe aneuploidy such as trisomies 13 and 18, or severe primary lesion), the "nonaggressive" approach is recommended. Additionally, lesions which have progressed leading to fetal hydrops have an extremely dismal outlook[51] and should be managed "nonaggressively" as well. On the other hand, when prognosis is regarded as uncertain, or good, the "aggressive" management approach is encouraged. With CHD it is important to keep abreast of pediatric surgical advancements, and to arrange predelivery pediatric cardiology consultation in cases where pediatric outlook is poor but where controversial procedures are available (such as the Norwood procedure[52] for hypoplastic left heart). In such cases the aggressiveness of the obstetrical management will depend on the patient's intentions for management after delivery. For all cases in which aggressive management is chosen, frequent ultrasound fetal evaluation is indicated to watch for signs of fetal decompensation.

FETAL ARRHYTHMIA

The prevalence of fetal arrhythmia is thought to be as common as 1–2% in near term fetuses.[53] Centers seeing large numbers of referrals for the indication of fetal arrhythmia, report that by far the most common arrhythmia is variably frequent extrasystole which in most cases is benign.[53,54] Less common, but of more clinical importance, are the sustained fetal tachyarrhythmias which include in order of frequency: supraventricular tachycardia, atrial flutter, and very rarely atrial fibrillation, or ventricular tachycardia. Also uncommon, but clinically important, is complete congenital heart block manifest as sustained fetal bradycardia. The approach to these disorders requires (a) an investigation to exclude underlying structural heart disease, (b) knowledge about the untreated natural history of the different arrhythmias, as well as which arrhythmias may benefit by therapy, and (c) an understanding of the maternal risks of implementing those treatments.

Whenever a fetal arrhythmia is noted, whether by auscultation in the office, at fetal tocodynamometry, or during ultrasound fetal assessment, it is important that it be thoroughly evaluated. This evaluation includes a comprehensive fetal structural evaluation. Emphasis is given to fetal echocardiography including M-mode doppler imaging to define the nature of the arrhythmia by observing the systolic relationship between the atria and the ventricles. Fetal arrhythmias are associated with structural heart disease in 5% of cases[55] which, when present, is highly associated with aneuploidy.[47,48] Thus when cardiac, or noncardiac, anomalies are seen karyotype is recommended.

EXTRASYSTOLE

Fetal extrasystoles are common.[53] They are rarely associated with CHD, and in the absence of structural abnormalities are typically benign. However, Copel and associates have reported a 0.5% risk of evolution of sustained tachyarrhythmia in such patients.[54] Therefore these pregnancies deserve aggressive obstetrical management and it is recommended that the fetal heart be monitored or auscultated twice weekly until complete resolution of the arrhythmia, or until delivery.

SUSTAINED TACHYARRHYTHMIA

With sustained fetal tachyarrhythmia it is important to sort out the specific arrhythmia both from the standpoint of prognosis and management. Supraventricular tachycardia (SVT), by

far the most frequent tachyarrhythmia, has a 1:1 atrial to ventricular systolic rate (generally 220–260 beats per minute). It is rarely associated with underlying structural heart disease.[54] The major concern for fetuses having sustained unremitting tachycardia in this range is cardiac decompensation and evolution of fetal hydrops (estimated to occur in 40% of untreated fetuses, and an additional 15% of untreated neonates).[56] Often the arrhythmia is intermittent and well tolerated without therapy. However, when unremitting, SVT can be corrected in most instances using antidysrrhythmic therapy. Digoxin is usually employed as the first-line agent, followed by a variety of alternate second-line medications if it fails. Thus, after a full discussion of the potential fetal benefits contrasted with the possible maternal risks of therapy, an aggressive management approach is encouraged. Because conversion to a normal rhythm is not immediate, nor is it guaranteed, very close ultrasound fetal assessment of fetal well being is mandatory. If pulmonary maturity is anticipated and the fetus does not easily convert, delivery is indicated. If the arrhythmia is present during labor it will, in most instances, be impossible to evaluate fetal tolerance of labor. If there is rapidly progressing labor serial scalp pH may allow adequate fetal assessment and vaginal delivery. More typically, a cesarean section will be necessary because of inability to assess fetal wellbeing.

Fetal atrial-flutter and fibrillation are thought to be considerably more rare causes of fetal tachyarrhythmia than SVT.[54] Nonetheless it is important to distinguish them from SVT due to the worse prognostic implications. Both of these arrhythmias have an increased risk of structural heart disease (estimated at 20%).[56] Also these arrhythmias tend to be more recalcitrant to antidysrrhythmic therapy and carry a higher fetal mortality rate than SVT.[54] The distinguishing feature with flutter is atrial rates of 400–460 having variable degrees of AV block such that the ventricular rate is lower. Atrial fibrillation is still more rare and may be difficult to distinguish from flutter but presumably carries a similar prognosis. Management, after excluding underlying structural disease is "aggressive" with a similar approach as in SVT. However, greater fetal risk is acknowledged and accordingly more rapid addition of alternate antidysrrhythmic agents, if digoxin fails, may be advised.

SUSTAINED BRADYARRHYTHMIA

The differential diagnosis for sustained fetal bradycardia includes fetal distress, physiologic sinus bradycardia, blocked atrial bigeminy, second degree heart block, and complete congenital heart block (CCHB).[53] Fetal echocardiography can distinguish these. Obviously fetal distress needs rapidly to be diagnosed followed by in-utero resuscitative efforts and possible delivery if viable. Sinus bradycardia, blocked atrial bigeminy, and second degree heart block, typically are benign if there is no hydrops or structural heart disease.[54] If the biophysical activity is normal, and there is normal heart rate variability expectant management is encouraged. This should include frequent ultrasound evaluation of the fetus including biophysical profile and aggressive management if signs of fetal deterioration. In the case of second degree heart block, this can occasionally progress to complete congenital heart block, which has been reported in mothers with autoimmune antibodies.[57,58] For such fetuses, corticosteroid therapy in effort to reverse or stop progression of evolving immune related damage to the fetal conduction system has been suggested.[57,58]

Fetuses with true CCHB can be sorted into 2 clinically and prognostically discreet groups. The first are those with CCHB and normal cardiac anatomy. These cases appear to have complete heart block as the endpoint of immune-complex–related damage to the fetal cardiac conduction system (secondary to clinical, or preclinical, maternal autoimmune disease).[57,58] The second group has CCHB in face of underlying structural heart disease. This group accounts for 25–63% of fetuses with sustained bradycardia, and it is the structural defect itself which disrupts the conduction system.[59,60] In such cases karyotype abnormality is common, atrial isomerism is frequent, hydrops is typical, and survival rare.[59,60] Management for these cases should be "nonaggressive." In contrast, where there is no evidence of structural disease, and the heart rate is preserved above 50 beats per minute, the outlook is favorable justifying "aggressive" management.

The work-up of newly identified CCHB includes complete maternal autoantibody evaluation including anti-Ro (SSA) and anti-La (SSB) IgG antibodies. At the same time a comprehensive fetal echocardiogram is mandatory to search for structural cardiac defects or evidence of cardiac compromise. When autoantibodies are detected, and structural disease is absent, some authors have advocated weekly dexamethasone in effort to reduce the rare evolution of hydrops in these fetuses.[57] Others have utilized betamimetics to increase fetal ventricular rate also hoping to stave off hydrops.[60] None of these approaches have been tested prospectively against expectant management. Regardless, whether expectant management, dexamethasone, or beta-mimetic regimens are chosen, vigilant fetal surveillance, including weekly biophysical profile and ultrasound cardiac assessment, is indicated for antepartum surveillance. Delivery is recommended if early signs of heart failure evolve in the viable fetus after documenting lung maturity. Regarding route of delivery; some authors have advocated continuous fetal electrocardiography (to monitor fetal atrial rate variability as an indicator of fetal well being) for labor management.[58] The reality is that for most institutions this is not a practical, or even available, solution and cesarean section will be necessary due to inability to assess fetal tolerance of labor.[56]

DIAPHRAGMATIC HERNIA

Diaphragmatic hernia occurs in about 2 in 10,000 live births.[61] The prognosis has been regarded as generally poor when ascertained prenatally, especially when the diagnosis is established before 25 weeks.[62] However, advances in perinatal management (including regionalization and technological advancements in perinatal and neonatal care) seem to have considerably improved the outlook. An 80% mortality rate for prenatally diagnosed cases reported in 1985[63] was reduced to 58% in the extensive experience of one group as published in 1995.[64] Among individuals with "isolated" congenital diaphragmatic hernia (hernia without associated defects), there is a wide range of outcomes ranging from mildly affected to severely disabling and lethal. The principle cause of death in severely affected neonates is related to pulmonary hypoplasia, with attendant pulmonary hypertension, caused by the inadequate growth and expansion of the fetal lungs due to compression by the herniating abdominal viscera. The variable timing and quantity of herniating abdominal viscera create the spectrum of outcomes: Fetuses having large and early developing lesions carry the worst prognosis. Particularly damaging in this regard are right sided hernias with fetal liver extensively occupying the right hemithorax. As with most major congenital anomalies, there is substantial risk of a variety of associated structural (30–50%)[65,66] and/or chromosomal (5–16%)[67,68] abnormalities as well. The presence of associated abnormalities is clearly correlated with worse prognoses than in "isolated" cases.

Thus, it is again important to provide as precise, and complete, a diagnosis as possible which includes a comprehensive search for cardiac and other anatomic defects. A fetal chromosome analysis also should be recommended. A unique caveat regarding procedure of choice for evaluating fetal chromosomes in DH cases is the observation by Donnenfield and associates[69] that mosaic supernumary isochromosome 12p (phenotypically Pallister Killian syndrome) often occurs as tissue line specific mosaisism. In some instances the cytogenetic defect is detectable only in fibroblasts, but not manifest in blood lymphocytes. Pallister Killian affected fetuses, which in 15% of cases have diaphragmatic hernia as part of their anomaly spectrum, might therefore not be detected by fetal blood sampling, while it would be evident on karyotype of cultured amniocytes or villi.

Having exhaustively established a precise diagnosis, that information is used to individualize counselling and management. Prior to viability all cases need to be offered the option of abortion. In continuing pregnancies, where there are associated anomalies and/or severe chromosome anomalies, a nonaggressive management approach typically is encouraged. Perhaps more problematic, from the viewpoint of counselling and management, are those cases with isolated defects. Of concern are the limitations of ultrasound imaging data for prognostication. Even for "isolated" cases neonatal mortality remains high. Despite some reported success in efforts to describe ultrasound predictors of poor prognosis (early gestational age at diagnosis,[62] evolution of polyhydramnios,[70] left heart underdevelopment,[62,72] presence of an intrathoracic stomach,[73] low ratio of right lung area to head circumference,[71] and presence of liver herniation[71]), there remains too much uncertainty to confidently predict lethal outcomes in any given case. Thus, after excluding ultrasound detectable associated anomalies and aneuploidy, an "aggressive" approach is typically utilized acknowledging the uncertain outcome with as much as a 50% chance for a poor or lethal outcome.

The "aggressive" armamentarium for prenatally diagnosed diaphragmatic hernia includes, for selected cases, the controversial approach of open fetal surgery. Endoscopic approaches, also, may be forthcoming. For most patients, currently, these options will not be available or may not be considered. More often, where invasive fetal therapy is declined, "aggressive" management will mean regular ultrasound surveillance, including serial assessment of cardiac function, fetal growth, amniotic fluid volume, and biophysical assessment. In cases where polyhydramnios evolves tocolysis may need to be considered, and in extreme cases amniodecompression might be necessary to maintain maternal comfort as well as in attempt to stave off attendant preterm labor from uterine overdistension. Delivery must be at a tertiary center equipped and staffed for immediate initiation of extracorporeal membrane oxygenation (ECMO) if necessary.[64,74] As with most lesions it is best to deliver as mature a fetus as is possible, and accordingly preterm delivery is discouraged if avoidable. Routine cesarean section will provide no known benefits and therefore is utilized only for standard obstetrical indications. Because of the significant potential for ECMO initiation after delivery it may be best to avoid operative vaginal delivery. In our experience an infant with large diaphragmatic hernia was delivered by uncomplicated vacuum extraction; however, due to ventilation difficulties the child was quickly placed on ECMO. This was followed by the development of a large cephalohematoma (attributed to the attendant need for anticoagulation of ECMO patients), requiring blood transfusion and surgical evacuation.

VENTRAL WALL DEFECTS

The principle ventral wall defects to be considered include omphalocele and gastroschisis occurring in 2/10,000 and 1/10,000 respectively.[75,76] While maternal serum alpha fetoprotein screening facilitates early diagnosis of these disorders (screen positive in more than 75% of cases), each is relatively easy to diagnose by routine ultrasound screening alone. With rare exception they can be clearly distinguished from one another ultrasonographically. This is important because the two entities are etiologically, and pathologically, distinct.[76] Accordingly, they must be approached very differently in the initial diagnostic evaluation and counselling. Omphalocele is a morphogenetic anomaly and as such is highly associated with additional structural anomalies[76,78,79] (40–70%), and/or aneuploidy[76,79,80] (10–40%). In contrast, gastroschisis is thought to be a vascular disruptive process, rather than morphogenetic, and therefore rarely has associated anomalies with the exception of secondary bowel abnormalities.[81]

Thus generalizations about the prognosis for the 2 disorders are dissimilar. The outlook for omphalocele, as a whole, is poor due to the high frequency of severe associated anomalies or aneupoloidy (excluding elective abortion the mortality exceeds 50%).[82] However, in "isolated" omphalocele (absence of associated defects) the outlook is generally excellent with

mortality rates less than 10%.[79] A rare exception to the favorable outlook in "isolated" cases, is "giant omphalocele" in which the huge size of the defect, the large quantity of extruded viscera, and the attendant small size of the remaining abdominal cavity create technical difficulties in repair that in some instances can not be overcome. Gastroschisis, on the other hand, as a typically isolated abnormality, tends to have a good overall prognosis. Most authors report approximately 90% intact survival.[78,79,83] Mortalities in this group relate to surgical complications (including sepsis, and bowel complications) or problems related to prematurity or low birth weight.

The initial management of omphalocele includes a comprehensive fetal anatomic evaluation, including fetal echocardiogram, searching for associated anomalies. A chromosomal analysis is encouraged in all cases. Non-aneuploidy syndomes also must be considered emphasizing the Beckwith-Weidemann syndrome. This is recognized antenatally in some instances by the association of omphalocele with macrosomia, diffuse visceromegally, and macroglossia. After all relevant diagnostic information is gathered, definitive counselling and management decisions are made. Before viability abortion is offered. In continuing pregnancies, the presence of severe associated anomalies or a severe karyotype abnormality will usually be managed "nonaggressively." Cases of "isolated" omphalocele, or Beckwith-Weidemann, with their comparatively good prognoses will be managed "aggressively." In cases of gastroschisis, despite the low likelihood of associated anomalies or aneuploidy, most experts still recommend complete anatomic evaluation and offering chromosomal analysis.[84,85] In virtually all cases of continuing gastroschisis-affected pregnancies, because of the generally good prognosis, management will be "aggressive."

For either of these ventral wall defects aggressive management is similar, but individualized. Both entities are at increased risk for premature delivery as well as intrauterine growth restriction.[77,78] Thus intensification of fetal surveillance in the third trimester is recommended. Additionally, for gastroschisis, serial ultrasound monitoring of the fetal bowel has been advocated watching for signs of evolving bowel injury. As yet no consensus has been achieved but it has been speculated that rapid progressive bowel dilatation is a worrisome feature and may warrant early delivery after demonstrating fetal lung maturity.[85,86,87] Whether this intervention impacts outcomes remains to be proven. In rare cases where fetal bowel perforation is suspected delivery has been recommended.[88]

All cases of ventral wall defect should be managed and delivered in a tertiary center. Mode of delivery remains controversial for both gastroschisis and omphalocele.[18,78,84] In omphalocele cases, most agree that vaginal delivery is appropriate for, and does not present substantive fetal risk, when the sac size and contents are small. When the sac size is large (>5 cm), or when substantial extracorporeal liver is evident within the sac, cesarean section should be considered for obvious reasons.[18] In the case of suspected Beckwith-Weidemann syndrome, the potential for dystocia must be considered when planning delivery route and where significant macrosomia is anticipated liberal use of cesarean delivery is advised. Also the frequent dangerous complication of profound neonatal hypoglycemia must be prepared for and when it occurs must be managed immediately postpartum.

Regarding gastroschisis, there remain advocates firmly maintaining that most cases should be delivered abdominally,[84] while others assert that improved neonatal outcomes data have not been convincingly presented to justify the maternal risk of cesarean delivery.[89] The rationale for elective cesarean section is to avoid bowel trauma at delivery, but also to allow for immediate evaluation and repair of the defect by having the pediatric surgeon standing by. Such rapid repair, it has been hypothesized, improves the neonatal course compared to cases in which there has been delay.[84] Critics of this rationale have noted that this hypothetical benefit remains unproven, and that reasonably early repair should be possible in tertiary centers even if the delivery is unscheduled.

Two other rare but serious ventral wall defects deserve mention. Pentology of Cantrell is the association of omphalocele with peritoneopericardial diaphragmatic hernia resulting in ectopic heart displacement through the anterior chest wall. Cloacal extrophy occurs as a combination of omphalocele and extrophy of the bladder, typically with inperforate anus and variable severity spina bifida. Each of these morphogenetic disorders is highly associated with additional anomalies including aneuploidy.[90,91] Although comparatively mild cases have been described in which there has been survival[90,92] after corrective surgery, it is thought that prenatally diagnosed cases tend to be at the severe end of the spectrum with generally poor prognosis. Previably, the option of abortion is offered to parents. In continuing pregnancies after comprehensive cataloging of associated anomalies and determination of karyotype the aggressiveness of management is individualized according to the anticipated severity of the individual case. When aggressive management is felt to be a reasonable option, close ultrasound follow-up of interval growth, evolution of anomalies, and fetal biophysical assessment should be instituted. Liberal use of cesarean section is encouraged to minimize trauma to the multiple extracorporeal organs. Management must be in a tertiary care center, and predelivery consultation with the pediatric surgeons is prudent.

GENITOURINARY DEFECTS

In aggregate congenital abnormalities of the urinary tract are quite common such that nearly half of all prenatally diagnosed anomalies involve the urinary tract.[93] The urinary tract disorders of prenatal diagnostic relevance can be categorized as renal morphogenetic anomalies (renal agenesis or hypoplasia, ectopic kidney, horseshoe kidney), renal cystic disorders (multicystic dysplastic, adult polycystic, infantile polycystic, and obstructive cystic kidney diseases), extrarenal urinary tract obstructive disorders (urethral, vesicoureteral junction, and ureteropelvic junction obstruction), renal tumors (mesoblastic

nephroma, and Wilms tumor), and genital anomalies (ambiguous genitalia, hydrocolpos, and ovarian cyst).

Because of the fluid production by the kidneys, and conduit function of the collecting system, the fetal urinary tract provides optimal tissue/fluid interfaces for ultrasound evaluation. Using a systematic approach (evaluating each kidney, followed by the collecting system, urinary bladder, and genitalia) one can define anatomic defects, and localize obstructions. Additionally, assessment of the volume of amniotic fluid allows inference about overall urinary systemic function. Thus, when urinary tract anomalies are identified the following generalizations can be made for purposes of prognostication. First, genitourinary defects that are unilateral tend to be associated with good prognoses if associated anomalies are excluded and amniotic fluid volume is preserved.[93,94,95] In contrast, bilateral renal abnormalities, or obstructing conditions involving both kidneys, when accompanied by early onset oligohydramnios, carry a very poor prognosis.[93,94,95,96] Finally, the urinary tract is no exception to the rule that one anomaly elevates the risk for associated defects including nongenitourinary anatomic defect and/or aneuploidy,[93,94,95] the presence of which may considerably alter the prognostic implications.

The initial approach to prenatal diagnosis and management of fetal urinary tract abnormalities begins noninvasively with a comprehensive search for associated structural abnormalities. It is also crucial to define the nature and function of the urinary tract problem. The kidneys are carefully examined for (a) size, shape and location, (b) presence of cysts or abnormalities of echotexture (multicystic? polycystic? microcystic?), (c) urinary collecting system dilatation (hydronephrosis? megaureter? megacystis?), (d) presence or absence of a filling bladder (obstruction proximal or distal to bladder? renal function?), (e) symmetry or asymmetry (unilateral or bilaterality of lesion), and (f) quantification of amniotic fluid volume (indirect assessment of production of urine and egress into the amniotic space).

In most cases optimal diagnostic effort will require invasive techniques. Assessment of the fetal karyotype is usually indicated and can be obtained from amniotic fluid, fetal urine, fetal blood, or villi. Occasionally, imaging will be obscured by the lack of an acoustic window due to anhydramnios of renal dysfunctional origin.[97,98] In these instances percutaneous amnioinfusion and/or fetal peritoneal fluid instillation have been used to improve visualization so that confident anatomic diagnoses can be resolved.[98] In cases of bladder outlet obstruction, with established or evolving oligohydramnios, several authorities have recommended yesicocentesis for urine biochemical evaluation in order to prognosticate regarding salvageability of renal function.[99,100,101] This method has on occasion been reported to be "curative" of the obstruction,[99] but more commonly has been used for selection of fetal surgical candidates.[99,100,101]

Following comprehensive imaging, chromosomal analysis, and serial vesicocentesis where indicated, a specific diagnosis can usually be rendered and the range of prognoses estimated.

In continuing pregnancies the aggressiveness of management will be determined by prognosis. With genitourinary disorders, the prognosis will hinge on the specific etiologic diagnosis, as well as the genitourinary functional assessment described in a previous section.

Some urinary tract congenital disorders are clearly hopeless such as bilateral renal agenesis,[96] early onset infantile polycystic kidney disease,[93,102] or bilateral multicystic dysplastic kidneys with oligohydranios.[93,103] Under these circumstances a nonaggressive approach is encouraged. In some centers, when these anomalies are confidently diagnosed, postviability terminations of pregnancy are offered. Alternatively, "nonaggressive" management is encouraged. In continuing pregnancies with untreated obstructive uropathy having profound megacystis and long-standing anhydramnios, the outlook also is poor. Neonatal death is almost certain due to the pulmonary hypoplasia component of the oligohydramnios sequence.[93,100] For these cases, abortion is offered, or a "nonaggressive" management approach is encouraged. When the "nonaggressive" approach is used in poor prognosis cases with profound megacystis, it should be recognized that fetal abdominal dystocia is likely at vaginal delivery. This should be anticipated and can be averted by performing a percutaneous fetal urinary tract decompression procedure during labor.

When an early diagnosis of bladder outlet obstruction is made in the male fetus a diagnosis of posterior urethral valve is highly likely. This particular lesion is thought to be treatable in selected cases with invasive fetal surgical techniques. Such an "aggressive" management approach is risky both for the maternal and the fetal patient and remains investigational given the comparatively small and quite variable long-term outcome experience.[99,100,101] Accordingly, the counselling and management of candidates for this approach is best done at the most experienced centers having fetal surgery units.

Many times isolated urinary tract abnormalities are seen which have generally good prognoses by virtue of unilaterality, or are bilateral but demonstrate preserved renal and urinary function as indicated by normal amniotic fluid volume. In such cases aggressive management is encouraged and should include close serial ultrasound follow-up to assure continued amniotic fluid production (if bilateral involvement), and if unilateral to assure that bilateral obstructing phenomena do not evolve over time (as can occasionally occur particularly with ostensibly isolated unilateral multicystic dysplastic kidney disease).[93,99] Usually there will be continued adequate amniotic fluid volume and vaginal delivery at term will be appropriate with neonatal management of the urologic disorder. Rarely, however, in late pregnancy there will be evidence of unilateral disease becoming bilateral (due to late onset of obstruction in the normal side of the urinary tract), or with bilateral functional obstruction suddenly worsening (as indicated by progressive decrease in amniotic fluid volume). Under these circumstances early delivery may be indicated.[93,95] Corticosteroids to accelerate fetal pulmonary maturity prior to elective preterm delivery is encouraged in these rare instances.[95]

Cesarean section is reserved for the usual obstetric indications. Regardless of the urinary abnormality noted, even if it is only mild hydronephrosis, neonatal post-hydration urologic evaluation is indicated to confirm diagnosis and allow proper surgical and/or medical follow-up.[104,105] This will avoid many instances of progressive infant urologic diseases, or recurrent occult urinary tract infections, that might have otherwise escaped recognition before irreversible damage if not for their discovery antenatally.[105]

SKELETAL DYSPLASIAS

The birth prevalence of the widely heterogeneous osteochondrodysplasias is 2–4 per 10,000.[106] With the more severe phenotypes abnormal biometry is usually evident early in pregnancy allowing diagnosis in the second trimester.[107] Unfortunately, however, although the prenatal recognition of skeletal dysplasia is increasingly common, establishing confident specific diagnoses remains comparatively infrequent, and is dependent very much on the skill and experience of the sonologist. One particularly experienced group reported accurate prenatal diagnoses in over 50% of skeletal dysplasia with accurate prognoses in about 85% of the cases affected with lethal phenotypes.[108] However, a recent survey, by the International Skeletal Dysplasia Registry, of a broader prenatal diagnosis experience showed accurate specific diagnoses in a minority of cases and an alarming number of normal fetuses misclassified as "dwarfs."[109] Because prognosis relies very much on specific diagnosis, this makes counselling and obstetrical management decisions difficult in many instances.

The initial management approach for skeletal dysplasias focuses on narrowing the differential diagnosis and if possible establishing a precise diagnosis. Obviously, this includes a complete genetic history including ascertainment of consanguinity (because several skeletal dysplasias are autosomal recessively inherited)[110] and history of teratogenic exposures (fetal warfarin syndrome, for example, can present as a phenocopy of nonrhizomelic chondrodysplasia punctata).[111] If the ultrasound findings are borderline for skeletal dysplasia a chromosome analysis should be considered as aneuploidy has been mistaken for osteochondrodysplasia in numerous instances.[109] Frequently, in clinical situations, the ultrasound findings are not specific enough to allow a precise diagnosis, but still provide useful prognostic information. Several details that may provide both diagnostic and prognostic clues deserve systematic ultrasound assessment. These include the following: (a) severity of the long-bone shortening, (b) presence of bone fractures or abnormalities of bone shape, (c) evidence of thoracic dysplasia, (d) suspicion of bone demineralization, (e) appearance of dysmorphic calvaria, (f) abnormalities of hand posture or polydactyly, (g) distribution of long-bone shortening, (h) characteristic spine abnormalities, and (i) assessment of amniotic fluid volume.

When such an evaluation does not elucidate a specific diagnosis, an attempt is still made to prognosticate. Often one can predict lethal versus "probably not lethal" even when the specific skeletal dysplasia can not confidently be established.[112,113] Features thought to be highly correlated with lethality among the skeletal dysplasias include: (a) severe diffuse (micromelic) long bone shortening, (b) presence of hydropic change, (c) evidence of thoracic dysplasia, and (d) marked polyhydramnios. Late onset or comparatively mild limb shortening, in the absence of thoracic dysplasia, bodes well for survival.

With confident diagnoses established in the second trimester, the outlook tends to be poor. Abortion always should be presented as an option. In continuing pregnancies in which clearly lethal disorders such as thanatophoric dysplasia, or osteogenesis imperfecta type II, are diagnosed, a nonaggressive management approach should be encouraged. In prognostically uncertain cases, or confidently good prognosis cases (such as heterozygous achondroplasia), an aggressive management approach is indicated. Usually vaginal delivery can be accomplished in cephalic presenting cases, however some disorders can be complicated by large calvaria (achondroplasia for example)[113] or abnormal shape (Kleblatschatel in thanatophoric dysplasia)[114] such that cesarean is indicated for dystocia. An additional consideration when selecting delivery mode is that of c-spine instability typically observed in infants with achondroplasia. For this reason some authors have suggested pre-labor elective cesarean delivery in confidently diagnosed cases.[115]

NONIMMUNE HYDROPS FETALIS

Nonimmune fetal hydrops is defined as excess total body water resulting in accumulation of fluid in soft tissues and 2 or more serous cavities.[116] It occurs in approximately 2–4 per 10,000 pregnancies.[117] Although episodes of spontaneous resolution are reported,[118] the natural history tends to be characterized by progression with a natural history mortality risk ranging from 40–90%.[119,120] The causes of nonimmune hydrops are myriad including cardiac (structural anomalies and arrhythmias), anemias (thalassemias, transient red cell aplasia, and hemorrhagic), infections (CMV, toxoplasma, syphilis, parvovirus B-19), syndromal (chromosomal, mendellian, sporatic), twins (twin to twin transfusion phenomena, twin reverse arterial perfusion syndrome), and a variety of other miscellaneous disorders.[121] It is important to recognize that hydrops fetalis not only carries risk to the fetus, but substantially increases maternal risk for preclampsia, postpartum hemorrhage, preterm labor, birth trauma, severe anemia, gestational diabetes, and retained placenta.[122]

With recent advances in prenatal diagnostic technologies the ability to establish an etiologic diagnosis in the hydropic fetus continues to improve. Contemporary work-up stratagies incorporate (a) comprehensive ultrasound anatomic evaluation, (b) fetal echocardiogram, (c) fetal karyotype, (d) fetal blood analysis (hemogram and chemistries), (e) maternal blood analysis (Kleihauer Betke and infection serology), as well as (f) amniotic fluid molecular work-up for infectious etiologies. Using this multi-faceted approach recent series have

reported the establishment of an etiologic diagnosis in 50–80% of cases.[123,124]

Although the natural history outlook is generally poor, establishing the etiology will identify many of the cases certain to do poorly, as well as narrrowing the instances which might be considered suitable for *aggressive* obstetrical management. Features which predict a poor prognosis include associated structural anomalies, aneuploidy, severe anasarca, early onset with severe pleural effusions, and marked cardiac enlargement (biventricular outer dimensions >95%).[124,125] Exceptions to this would be instances having treatable diagnoses such as fetal arrhythmia or anemia explaining the "severe" findings. Features associated with the greatest likelihood of response to fetal therapy were fetal tachyarrhythmia,[120,124,126] fetal anemia secondary to fetomaternal hemorrhage[120,124,127] or parvovirus infection,[128] and milder cases having late onset and no identifiable cardiac, anatomic, or syndromal cause.[124]

Obstetrical management, as with other disorders of heterogeneous etiology, will depend on the level of confidence in the diagnosis and attendant prognosis. In previable cases of nonimmune hydrops the outlook is generally poor and abortion is offered. Continuing pregnancies having severe prognostic features mentioned above, will be offered nonaggressive management, unless treatable diagnoses can be identified. In nonaggressively managed fetuses, percutaneous fetal pericentesis may be needed to allow vaginal delivery when ascites is marked. Even when nonaggressive fetal management is elected, very close maternal surveillance is necessary. In cases where associated preeclampsia (sometimes atypical as in "mirror syndrome")[129] or severe anemia evolve, preterm delivery is indicated.

When there remains uncertainty about etiology, or there appears to be a treatable cause, the aggressive management approach is encouraged.[124,126] This approach will include fetal therapy in selected cases including fetal transfusion for severe anemias, antidysrrhythmic therapy for tachyarrhythmias, and indwelling thoraco-amniotic shunt placement in appropriate instances with large pleural effusions. Whether invasive fetal therapy is indicated, aggressive management will also include frequent ultrasound fetal assessment for progression or improvement in the hydropic condition as well as for assessment of biophysical parameters. During this intensive fetal surveillance, as with the nonaggressive approach, the mother also must be closely observed for signs or symptoms of evolving preeclampsia or marked anemia.[122,128] Occasionally premature delivery will be effected for worsening hydrops of undetermined etiology although the outlook in general will be acknowledged as uncertain. In such cases, predelivery corticosteroids for fetal lung benefit should be considered. Recommendations for mode of delivery of hydropic fetuses remain vague in the literature, but several authors suggest liberal use of cesarean delivery.[119,120] Arguments for cesarean include the anticipated limited reserve of the edematous placenta, and to reduce birth trauma which may be sustained by the often severely edematous fetus.

CHROMOSOME ANOMALIES

Chromosomal abnormalities, including both abnormalities of count and abnormalities of structure, occur in 50–80 per 10,000 live-born infants.[130] As a group they are considerably more common than most of the individual disorders so far discussed. There is considerable heterogeneity among the chromosomal abnormalities that are compatible with live-birth and prognoses accordingly are quite variable.

Chromosomal abnormalities often come to prenatal ascertainment by their associations with congenital anomalies detected at ultrasound. In such cases, the prognosis of the underlying chromosomal defect (in effect *the cause* of the observed anatomic defects) often takes on more importance than the defect itself in guiding the optimism or pessimism about counselling. Some chromosomal disorders are lethal in all cases (triploidy[131] for example). Others cause fetal or early neonatal death in most cases but can be compatible with fairly long, albeit profoundly disabled, lives (trisomies 13 and 18 for example.[132,133]) Trisomy 21 affected individuals, on the other hand, can frequently live well into adulthood with comparatively modest severity of disability in many instances.[134] Similarly the sex-chromosomal aneuploidies can have quite mild phenotypic effects.[135]

Thus, while abortion is offered for any of these disorders when identified previably, there is also a place in many cases for the "aggressive" management approach in continuing pregnancies. For lethal and profoundly disabling aneuploidy conditions a nonaggressive approach is encouraged. But, for milder phenotypes (trisomy 21 and sex chromosomal aneuploidy for example), in the absence of life-threatening anomalies, the aggressive approach is suggested. An aggressive approach in these cases would include individualized antepartum, and intrapartum, fetal surveillance. Mode of delivery can generally be by vaginal route, but with standard employment of cesarean section for either maternal or fetal indications. After delivery, current medical practice encourages corrective surgery, within reason, for these milder disorders.

POSTPARTUM MANAGEMENT AFTER DELIVERY OF AN INFANT WITH CONGENITAL ANOMALIES

After an anomalous infant is delivered, and maternal medical issues are stabilized, it is critical to complete genetic counselling about the implications of the neonatal diagnosis. Because of the variable degrees of uncertainty that often accompany a prenatal diagnosis of anomalies, the neonatal period (or post-abortion autopsy) often will allow the definitive evaluations that facilitate unequivocal diagnoses. Of utmost importance to the perinatal or genetics consultant at this point will be education of the family regarding impact of the now refined diagnosis may have on future reproductive planning, decisions, and possible outcomes.

In many cases the diagnosis will prove to be "likely sporadic" and of low recurrence potential. Not infrequently, however, the disorder will have real and quantifiable recurrence risk. For nondysjunctional trisomies a 1% recurrence risk will be quoted, while a variable, but considerably higher, risk will be counselled in cases affected by inherited chromosomal rearrangements. For inherited Mendelian disorders, such as cystic fibrosis (autosomal recessive) or inherited Marfan disease (autosomal dominant), the recurrence risk will be 25% and 50% respectively. In instances of teratogen mediated anomalies the recurrence risk will be variable depending on the agent and potential avoidability of the exposure in future pregnancies.

Included in this discussion will be strategies, where applicable, to reduce or modify recurrence risk. For example in patients with a newborn having diabetic embryopathy, the importance of preconceptional and early pregnancy optimization of glycemic control is emphasized.[136] Women using pharmacotherapeutic teratogens may be candidates for medication adjustment preconceptionally. The mother of a child with NTD needs to be advised about the recurrence risk reduction afforded by preconceptional and first trimester folate supplementation.[137] Parents of infants with Mendelian diseases, or inherited unbalanced chromosomal rearrangements, should be aware of the availability of prenatal diagnosis with selective abortion, or in some cases noncarrier-doner ova or insemination. For these parents pre-implantation diagnosis may soon become a practical reality as well.

References

1. Wilcox AJ, Weinnberg CR, O'Connor JF, et al. Incidence of early pregnancy loss. *N Engl J Med.* 1988;319:189.
2. Miller JF, Williamson E, Glue J, et al. Fetal loss after implantation. A prospective study. *Lancet.* 1980;2:554.
3. Cohen Jr MM. *The Child with Multiple Birth Defects.* New York: Raven Press, 1982.
4. Naeye RL. Causes of perinatal mortality in the United States. Collaborative Perinatal Project. *JAMA.* 1987;238:228.
5. Manning FA. Aspects of fetal life. In: Manning FA. *Fetal Medicine: Principles and Practice*, 1st ed. East Norwalk: Appleton and Lange; 1995.
6. Pryde PG, Drugan A, Johnson MP, et al. Prenatal diagnosis: Choices women make about pursuing testing and acting on abnormal results. *Clin Obstet Gynecol.* 1993;36:496.
7. Hook EB, Schreinemachers DM. Trends in utilization of prenatal cytogenetic diagnosis by New York residents in 1979 and 1980. *Am J Public Health.* 1983;73:198.
8. Evans MI, Drugan A, Koppitch FC, et al. Genetic diagnosis in the first trimester: the norm for the 1990s. *Am J Obstet Gynecol.* 1989;160:1332.
9. Clayton-Smith J, Farndon PA, McKeown C, et al. Examination of fetuses after induced abortion for fetal abnormality. *Br Med J.* 1990;300:295.
10. Pryde PG, Isada NB, Hallak M, et al. Determinants of parental decisions to abort or continue after non-aneuploid ultrasound detected fetal abnormalities. *Obstet Gynecol.* 1990;80:52.
11. Rizzo N, Pittalis MC, Pilu G, et al. Prenatal karyotype in malformed fetuses. *Prenat Diagn.* 1990;10:17.
12. Sabbagha RE, Scheikh Z, Tamura RK, et al. Predictive value, sensitivity, and specificity of ultrasonic targeted imaging for fetal anomalies in gravid women at high risk for birth defects. *Am J Obstet Gynecol.* 1985;152:822.

13. Wladimiroff JW, Stewart PA, Sachs ES, et al. Prenatal diagnosis and management of congenital heart defect: Significance of associated fetal anomalies and prenatal chromosome studies. *Am J Med Genet.* 1985;21:285.

14. Copel JA, Cullen M, Green JJ, et al. The frequency of aneuploidy in prenatally diagnosed congenital heart disease: An indication for fetal karyotyping. *Am J Obstet Gynecol.* 1988;158:409.

15. Isada NB, Paar DP, Grossman JH 3d. TORCH infections. Diagnosis in the molecular age. *J Reprod Med.* 1992;37:499.

16. Nicolaides KH, Rodek CH, Lange I, et al. Fetoscopy in the evaluation of unexplained fetal hydrops. *Br J Obstet Gynecol.* 1985;92:671.

17. Johnson MP, Bukowski TP, Reitleman C, et al. In utero surgical treatment of fetal obstructive uropathy: A new comprehensive approach to identify appropriate candidates for vesicoamniotic shunt therapy. *Am J Obstet Gynecol.* 1994;170:1770.

18. McCurdy Jr CM, Seeds JW. The route of delivery of infants with congenital anomalies. *Clin Perinatology.* 1993;20:81.

19. Harrison M, Golbus M, Filly R. *The Unborn Patient.* New York: Grune and Stratton, 1984.

20. Romero R, Oyarzun E, Sirtori M, et al. Detection and management of anatomic congenital anomalies. *Obstet Gynecol Clin* North Am. 1988;15:215.

21. *Roe v. Wade,* 410 US 113, 1973.

22. Usher R. Changing mortality rates with perinatal intensive care and regionalization. *Semin Perinatol.* 1997;1:309.

23. Chervenak FA, Berkowitz RL, Tortora M, et al. The management of fetal hydrocephalus. *Am J Obstet Gynecol.* 1985;151:933.

24. Harrison MR, Golbus MS, Filly RA, et al. Fetal surgery for congenital hydronephrosis. *N Engl J Med.* 1982;306:591.

25. Harrison MR, Adzik NS, Longaker MT, et al. Successful repair in-utero of a fetal diaphragmatic hernia. *N Engl J Med.* 1990;322:1582.

26. Langer JC, Harrison MR, Schmidt KG, et al. Fetal hydrops and demise from sacrococcygeal teratoma: Rationale for fetal surgery. *Am J Obstet Gynecol.* 1989;160:1145.

27. Adzik NS, Harrison MR, Flake AW, et al. Open fetal surgery for congenital cystic adenomatoid malformation. *J Pediatr Surg.* 1993;28:806.

28. Rodek CH, Fisk NM, Fraser DI, et al. Long-term *in-utero* drainage of fetal hydrothorax. *N Engl J Med.* 1988;319:1135.

29. Hidalgo H, Bowie J, Rosenberg ER, et al. In-utero sonographic diagnosis of fetal cerebral anomalies. *AJR.* 1982;149:143.

30. Greenberg F, James LM, Oakley GP. Estimates of birth prevalence rates of spina bifida in the United States from computer generated maps. *Am J Obstet Gynecol.* 1983;145:570.

31. Edwards MSD, Filly RA. Diagnosis and management of fetal disorders of the central nervous system. In Hoffman HJ, Epstein F, eds. *Disorders of the Developing Nervous System: Diagnosis and Treatment.* Boston: Blackwell Scientific Publications; 1986.

32. Mealy J, Ozenitis AJ, Hockley AA. The prognosis of encephaloceles. *J Neurosurg.* 1970;32:209.

33. Gross RH, Cox A, Tatryrek R, et al., Early management and decision making for the treatment of myelomeningocele. *Pediatrics.* 1983;72:450.

34. McLaughlin JF, Shurtleff DB, Lamers JY, et al. Influence of prognosis on decisions regarding the care of newborns with myelodysplasia. *N Engl J Med.* 1985;312:1589.

35. Hunt GM. Open spina bifida: Outcome for a complete cohort treated unselectively and followed into adulthood. *Devel Med Child Neurol.* 1990;32:108.

36. Chervenak FA, Duncan C, Ment LR, et al. Perinatal management of meningomyelocele. *Obstet Gynecol.* 1984;63:376.

37. Hadi HA, Lot RA, Long EM, et al. Outcome of fetal meningomyelocele after vaginal delivery. *J Reprod Med.* 1987;32:597.

38. Benson JT, Dillard RG, Burton BK. Open spina bifida: Does cesarean section delivery improve prognosis? *Obstet Gynecol.* 1988;71:532.

39. Luthy DA, Wardinsky T, Shurtleff DB, et al. Cesarean section before the onset of labor and subsequent motor function in infants with meningomyelocele diagnosed antenatally. *N Engl J Med.* 1991;324:662.

40. Hobbins JC. Diagnosis and management of neural-tube defects today. *N Engl J Med.* 1991;324:690.

41. Nicolaides KH, Berry S, Snijders RJM, et al. Fetal lateral cerebral ventriculomegaly: Associated malformations and chromosomal defects. *Fetal Diagn Ther.* 1990;5:5.

42. Wilberger JE, Baghai P. Fetal neurosurgery. *Neurosurg.* 1983;13:596.

43. Vintzileos AM, Campbell WA, Weinbaum PJ, et al. Perinatal outcome and management of fetal ventriculomegaly. *Obstet Gynecol.* 1987;69:5.

44. Eller KM, Kuller JA. Fetal porencephaly: A review of etiology, diagnosis, and prognosis. *Obstet Gynecol Surv.* 1995;50:684.

45. Hoffman JIE. Congenital heart disease: Incidence and inheritance. *Pediatr Clin North Am.* 1990;37:25.

46. Copel JA, Pilu G, Kleinman CS. Congenital heart disease and extracardiac anomalies: Associations and indications for fetal echocardiography. *Am J Obstet Gynecol.* 1986;154:1121.

47. Lin AE, Garver KL. Genetic counselling for congenital heart defects. *J Pediatr.* 1988;113:1105.

48. Copel JA, Cullen M, Green JJ, et al. The frequency of aneuploidy in prenatally diagnosed congenital heart disease: An indication for fetal karyotyping. *Am J Obstet Gynecol.* 1988;158:409.

49. Ferrazi E, Fesslova V, Belloti M, et al. Prenatal diagnosis and management of congenital heart disease. *J Reprod Med.* 1989;34:207.

50. Crawford DC, Chita SK, Allan LD. Prenatal detection of congenital heart disease: Factors affecting obstetric management and survival. *Am J Obstet Gynecol.* 1988;159:352.

51. Silverman NH, Kleinman CS, Rudolph AM, et al. Fetal atrioventricular valve insufficiency associated with nonimmune hydrops: A two dimensional echocardiographic and pulsed doppler study. *Circulation* 1985;72:825.

52. Jonas RA, Hansen DD, Cook N, et al. Anatomic subtype and survival after reconstructive operation for hypoplastic left heart syndrome. *J Thorac Cardiovasc Surg.* 1994;107:1121.

53. Reed KL. Fetal arrhythmias: Etiology, diagnosis, pathophysiology, and treatment. *Seminars in Perinatology.* 1989;13:294.

54. Kleinman CS, Copel JA. Fetal cardiac arrhythmias: Diagnosis and therapy. In Creasy RK, Resnik R (eds). *Maternal Fetal Medicine Principles and Practice.* Philadelphia: WB Saunders, 1994.

55. Southall DP, Richards J, Hardwick R, et al. Prospective study of fetal heart rate and rhythm patterns. *Arch Dis Child.* 1980;55:506.

56. Bergsman MGM, Jonker GJ, Kock HC. Fetal supraventricular tachycardia. Review of the literature. *Obstet Gynecol Survey.* 1985;40:61.

57. Bierman FZ, Baxi L, Jaffe I, et al. Fetal hydrops and complete congenital heart block: Response to maternal steroid therapy. *J Pediatr.* 1988;112:646.

58. Schmidt KG, Ulmer HE, Silverman NH, et al. Perinatal outcome of fetal complete atrio-ventricular block: A multicenter experience. *J Am Coll Cardiol.* 1991;17:1360.

59. Wladimiroff JW, Stewart PA, Tonge HM. Fetal bradyarrhythmia: Diagnosis and outcome. *Prenat Diagn.* 1988;8:53.

60. Allan LD, Crawford DC, Anderson RH, et al. Evaluation and treatment of fetal arrhythmias. *Clinical Cardiol* 1984;7:470.

61. Harrison MR, Bjordal RI, Langmark F, et al. Congenital diaphragmatic hernia: The hidden mortality. *J Pediatr Surg.* 1978;13:227.

62. Sharland GK, Lockhart SM, Heward AJ, et al. Prognosis in fetal diaphragmatic hernia. *Am J Obstet Gynecol.* 1992;166:9.

63. Adzick NS, Harrison MR, Glick PL, et al. Diaphragmatic hernia in the fetus: Prenatal diagnosis and outcome in 94 cases. *J Pediatr Surg.* 1985;20:357.

64. Harrison MR, Adzick NS, Estes JM, et al. A prospective study of the outcome for fetuses with diaphragmatic hernia. *JAMA.* 1994;271:382.

65. Wenstrom KD, Weiner CP, Hanson JW. A five-year statewide experience with congenital diaphragmatic hernia. *Am J Obstet Gynecol.* 1991;165:838.

66. Adzick NS, Vacanti JP, Lillehei CW, et al. Fetal diaphragmatic hernia: Ultrasound diagnosis and clinical outcome in 38 cases. *J Pediatr Surg.* 1989;24:654.

67. Benacerraf BR, Adzick NS. Fetal diaphragmatic hernia: Ultrasound diagnosis and clinical outcome in 19 cases. *Am J Obstet Gynecol.* 1987;156:573.

68. Nakavama DK, Harrison MR, Chinn DH, et al. Prenatal diagnosis and natural history of the fetus with a congenital diaphragmatic hernia: Initial clinical experience. *J Pediatr Surg.* 1985;20:118.

69. Donnenfeld AE, Campbell TJ, Byers J, et al. Tissue-specific mosaicism among fetuses with prenatally diagnosed diaphragmatic hernia. *Am J Obstet Gynecol.* 1993;169:1017.

70. Harrison MR, Adzick NS, Nakayama DK, et al. Fetal diaphragmatic hernia: Fatal but fixable. *Semin Perinatol.* 1985;9:103.

71. Metkus AP, Filly RA, Stringer MD, et al. Sonographic Predictors of Survival in fetal diaphragmatic hernia. *J Pediatr Surg.* 1996;41:148.

72. Crawford DC, Wright VM, Drake DP, et al. Fetal diaphragmatic hernia: The value of fetal echocardiography in the prediction of postnatal outcome. *Br J Obstet Gynecol.* 1989;96:705.

73. Hatch EI, Kendall J, Blumhagen J. Stomach position as an in-utero predictor of neonatal outcome in left-sided diaphragmatic hernia. *J Pediatr Surg.* 1992;27:778.

74. Atkinson JB, Ford EG, Humphries B, et al. The impact of extracorporeal membrane support in the treatment of congenital diaphragmatic hernia. *J Pediatr Surg.* 1991;26:791.

75. Baird PA, MacDonald EC. An epidemiologic study of congenital malformations of the anterior abdominal wall in more than a million consecutive live births. *Am J Hum Genet.* 1981;33:470.

76. deVries PA. The pathogenesis of gastroschisis and omphalocele. *J Pediatr Surg.* 1980;15:245.

77. Mabogounje OOA, Mahour GH. Omphalocele and gastroschisis: Trends and survival across two decades. *Am J Surg.* 1984;148:679.

78. Kirk EP, Wah RM. Obstetric management of the fetus with omphalocele and gastroschisis: A review and report of 112 cases. *Am J Obstet Gynecol.* 1983;146:512.

79. Mayer T, Black R, Matlak ME, et al. Gastroschisis and omphalocele. *Ann Surg.* 1980;192:783.

80. Benacerraf BR, Saltzman DH, Estroff JA, et al. Abnormal karyotype of fetuses with omphalocele: Prediction based on omphalocele contents. *Obstet Gynecol* 1990;75:317.

81. Hoyme HE, Higgenbottom MC, Jones KL. The vascular pathogenesis of gastroschisis: Intrauterine disruption of the omphalomesenteric artery. *Semin Perinatol.* 1983;7:294.

82. Hasan S, Hermansen MC. The prenatal diagnosis of ventral abdominal wall defects. *Am J Obstet Gynecol.* 1986;155:842.

83. Caniano DA, Brokaw B, Ginn-Pease ME. An individualized approach to the management of gastroschisis. *J Pediatr Surg.* 1990;25:297.

84. Pryde PG, Bardicef M, Teadwell MC, et al. Gastroschisis: Can antenatal ultrasound predict infant outcomes? *Obstet Gynecol.* 1994;84:505.

85. Sanders RC, Blackmon LR, Hogge WA, et al. Gastroschisis. In: Sanders RC (ed), *Structural Fetal Abnormalities the Total Picture.* St. Louis: Mosby, 1996.

86. Bond SJ, Harrison MR, Filly RA, et al. Severity of intestinal damage in gastroschisis: Correlation with perinatal sonographic findings. *J Pediatr Surg.* 1988;23:520.

87. Langer JC, Khanna J, Caco C, et al. Prenatal diagnosis of gastroschisis: Development of objective sonographic criteria for predicting outcome. *Obstet Gynecol.* 1993;81:53.

88. Concalves LF, Jeanty P. Ultrasound evaluation of fetal abdominal wall defects. In: Callen PW ed, *Ultrasound in Obstetrics.* Philadelphia: WB Saunders; 1994.

89. Lenke RR, Hatch EI. Fetal gastroschisis: A preliminary report advocating the use of cesarean section. *Obstet Gynecol.* 1986;67:395.

90. Toyama WM. Combined congenital defects of the anterior abdominal wall, sternum, diaphragm, pericardium and heart: A case report and review of the syndrome. *Pediatrics.* 1972;50:778.

91. Gosden C, Brock DJH. Prenatal diagnosis of extrophy of the cloaca. *Am J Med Genet.* 1981;8:95.

92. Howell C, Caldimone A, Snyder H, et al. Optimal management of cloacal extrophy. *J Pediatr Surg.* 1983;18:365.

93. Helin E, Perrson PH. Prenatal diagnosis of urinary tract abnormalities by ultrasound. *Pediatrics.* 1986;78:879.

94. Sherer DM, Thompson HO, Armstrong B, et al. Prenatal sonographic diagnosis of unilateral fetal renal agenesis. *J Clin Ultrasound.* 1990;18:648.

95. Golbus MS, Filley RA, Callen PW, et al. Fetal urinary tract obstruction: Management and selection fot treatment. *Semin in Perinatol* 1984;9:91.

96. Dubins PA, Kurtz AB, Wapner RJ, et al. Renal agenesis: Spectrum of in utero findings. *J Clin Ultrasound.* 1981;9:189.

97. Barss VA, Benaceraff BR, Frigoletto FD Jr. Second trimester oligohydramnios, a predictor of poor fetal outcome. *Obstet Gynecol.* 1984;64:608.

98. Fisk NM, Ronderos-Dumit D, Soliani A, et al. Diagnostic and therapeutic amnioinfusion in oligohydramnios. *Obstet Gynecol.* 1991;78:270.

99. Wisser J, Kurmanavicius J, Lauper U, et al. Successful treatment of fetal megavesica in the first half of pregnancy. *Am J Obstet Gynecol.* 1997;177:685.

100. Johnson MP, Bukowski TP, Reitelman C, et al. In utero treatment of obstructive uropathy: A new comprehensive approach to identify candidates for vesicoamniotic shunt therapy. *Am J Obstet Gynecol.* 1994;170:1770.

101. Nicolaides KH, Cheng HH, Snijders RJM, et al. Fetal urine biochemistry in the assessment of obstructive uropathy. *Am J Obstet Gynecol.* 1992;166:932.

102. Reuss A, Wladimiroff JW, Niermeyer MF. Sonographic, clinical, and genetic aspects of prenatal diagnosis of cystic kidney disease. *Ultrasound Med Biol.* 1991;17:687.

103. D'Alton M, Romero R, Grannum P, et al. Antenatal diagnosis of renal anomalies with ultrasound. IV. Bilateral multicystic dysplastic kidney disease. *Am J Obstet Gynecol.* 1986;154:532.

104. Corteville JE, Gray DL, Crane JP. Congenital hydronephrosis: Correlation of fetal ultrasonographic findings with infant outcome. *Am J Obstet Gynecol.* 1991;165:348.

105. Caione P, Zaccara A, Capozza N. How prenatal ultrasound can affect the treatment of ureterocele in neonates and children. *Eur Urol.* 1989;16:195.

106. Orioli IM, Castilla EE, Barbosa-Neto JC. The birth prevalence rates for the skeletal dysplasias. *J Med Genet.* 1986;23:328.

107. Concalves L, Jeanty P. Fetal biometry of skeletal dysplasias: A multicenter study. *J Ultrasound Med.* 1994;13:977.

108. Pretorious DH, Rumack CM, Manco-Johnson ML, et al. Specific skeletal dysplasias in utero: Sonographic diagnosis. *Radiology.* 1986;159:237.

109. Sharony R, Browne C, Lachman RS, et al. Prenatal diagnosis of the skeletal dysplasias. *Am J Obstet Gynecol.* 1993;169:668.

110. McKusick VA. *Mendelian Inheritance in Man,* 10th ed, Baltimore: Johns Hopkins University Press, 1996.

111. Hall JG, Pauli RM, Wilson KM. Maternal and fetal sequelae of anticoagulation during pregnancy. *Am J Med.* 1980;68:122.

112. Escobar LF, Bixler D, Weaver DD, et al. Bone dysplasias: The prenatal diagnosis challenge. *Am J Med Genet.* 1990;36:488.

113. Kurtz AB, Filly RA, Wapner RJ, et al. In utero analysis of heterozygous achondroplasia: Variable time of onset as detected by femur length measurements. *J Ultrasound Med.* 1986;5:137.

114. Chervenak FA, Blakemore KJ, Isaacson G, et al. Antenatal sonographic findings of thanatophoric dysplasia with cloverleaf skull. *Am J Obstet Gynecol.* 1983;146:984.

115. Sanders RC, Blackmon LR, Hogge WA, et al. Achondroplasia. In: Sanders RC, ed. *Structural Fetal Abnormalities the Total Picture.* St. Louis: Mosby, 1996.

116. Platt LD, Devore GR. In utero diagnosis of hydrops fetalis: Ultrasound methods. *Clin Perinatol.* 1982;9:627.

117. Machin GA. Hydrops revisited; literature review of 1,414 cases published in the 1980's. *Am J Med Genet.* 1989;34:366.

118. Pryde PG, Nugent CE, Pridjian G, et al. Spontaneous resolution of nonimmune hydrops fetalis secondary to human parvovirus B19 infection. *Obstet Gynecol.* 1992;79:859.

119. Hutchinson AA, Drew JH, Yu VYH, et al. Nonimmunologic hydrops fetalis: A review of 61 cases. *Obstet Gynecol.* 1982;59:347.

120. Im SS, Rizos N, Joutsi P, et al. Nonimmunologic hydrops fetalis. *Am J Obstet Gynecol.* 1984;148:566.

121. Holzgreve W, Holzgreve B, Curry CJ. Nonimmune hydrops fetalis: Diagnosis and management. *Semin Perinatol.* 1985;9:52.

122. Graves GR, Baskett MB. Nonimmune hydrops fetalis: Antenatal diagnosis and management. *Am J Obstet Gynecol.* 1984;148:563.

123. Castillo RA, Devoe LD, Hadi HA, et al. Nonimmune hydrops fetalis: Clinical experience and factors related to a poor outcome. *Am J Obstet Gynecol.* 1986;155:812.

124. Anandakumar C, Biswas A, Wong YC, et al. Management of nonimmune hydrops: 8 years experience. *Ultrasound Obstet Gynecol.* 1996;8:196.

125. Carlson DE, Platt LD, Meadris AL, et al. Prognostic indicators of the resolution of nonimmune hydrops fetalis and the survival of the fetus. *Am J Obstet Gynecol.* 1990;163:1785.

126. Ayida GA, Soothill PW, Rodek CH. Survival in non-immune hydrops fetalis without malformations or chromosomal abnormalities after invasive treatment. *Fetal Diagn Ther.* 1995;10:101.

127. Cardwell MS. Successful treatment of hydrops fetalis caused by fetomaternal hemorrhage. *Am J Obstet Gynecol.* 1988;158:131.

128. Peters MT, Nicolaides KH. Cordocentesis for the diagnosis and treatment of human parvovirus infection. *Obstet Gynecol.* 1990;75:501.

129. vanSelm M, Kanhai HH, Gravenhorst JB. Maternal hydrops syndrome: A review. *Obstet Gynecol Survey.* 1991;46:785.

130. Hsu LYF. Prenatal diagnosis of chromosome anomalies. In: Milunsky A (ed). *Genetic Disorders and the Fetus*, 2nd ed. New York: Plenum Press, 1986:115–183.

131. Werticki W, Graham JM, Sergivich GP. The clinical syndrome of triploidy. *Obstet Gynecol.* 1976;47:69.

132. Batey BJ, Blackburn BL, Carey JC. Natural history of trisomy 18 and trisomy 13: Growth, physical assessment, medical histories, survival, and recurrence risk. *Am J Med Genet.* 1994;49:175.

133. Root S, Carey JC. Survival in trisomy 18. *Am J Med Genet.* 1994;49:170.

134. Baird PA, Sadovnick AD. Life expectancy in Down syndrome. *J Pediatr.* 1987;110:849.

135. Ratcliffe SG, Butler GE, Jones M. Edinburgh study of growth and development of children with sex chromosome abnormalities. IV. *Birth Defects: Original Article Series.* 1990;26:1.

136. Kitzmiller JL, Gavin LA, Gin GD, et al. Preconception management of diabetes continued through early pregnancy prevents the excess frequency of major congenital abnormalities in infants of diabetic mothers. *JAMA.* 1991;265:731.

137. Centers for Disease Control and Prevention: Recommendations for the use of folic acid to reduce the number of cases of spina bifida and other neural tube defects. *MMWR.* 1992;417:1.

CHAPTER 54

ASSESSMENT AND MANAGEMENT OF NEONATES WITH CONGENITAL ANOMALIES

Seetha Shankaran/Mary P. Bedard

The discovery of a fetal anomaly has a profound impact on the family. They are faced with the loss of their normal infant weeks or months before birth and they must deal with the fear and anger that this brings. The frequency with which this situation arises is increasing dramatically as our ability to evaluate the fetus has improved significantly.

MULTIDISCIPLINARY CONSULTATION

The obstetrician generally has the responsibility of informing the family of the fetal abnormality. It is also his or her responsibility to provide the family with the appropriate information to allow the family to make the best choice for them. This should include the opportunity for the family to meet with a pediatric subspecialist knowledgeable in the care of newborns with that particular anomaly. Ideally, the referral is to a subspecialist practicing in the hospital where the infant will be cared for after birth. In addition to meeting with obstetric and pediatric subspecialists, the family should be given the opportunity to meet with the neonatologist or pediatrician who will be providing pediatric care for the infant at and after delivery.

Communication between the obstetric and pediatric consultants and the family is critically important.[1] The obstetrician should provide written documentation of the prenatal findings to the consultants prior to meeting with the family. The consultants should also provide written feedback to the obstetrician documenting their contact with the family. This information should be readily available at the time the mother delivers to minimize confusion or misinformation to the family.

INTERPRETATION OF DIAGNOSTIC STUDIES

Although prenatal diagnosis is often quite accurate, we must not forget that access to the fetus is limited. Some techniques, such as fetal karyotyping and DNA analysis, are very precise and reliable. Others, such as maternal serum α-fetoprotein or ultrasonography, are less precise. The accuracy of fetal ultrasonography is increased when done in a high-risk center when compared to office scans.[1] However, even under the best of circumstances, misdiagnoses do occur.

In addition, we know that the natural history of some fetal abnormalities may be variable. A good example is fetal cystadenomatoid malformation.[2] Many of these lesions spontaneously regress with the delivery of a healthy infant who may or may not require surgery. Other fetuses develop hydrops with a high likelihood of fetal or neonatal demise. In discussing recommendations for fetal and neonatal manage-

ment, we must keep in mind the limitations of our diagnostic studies.

DELIVERY

Delivery of an infant with a known congenital abnormality should occur in a center that can properly evaluate and care for the infant at and after birth. Ideally the center can care for both mother and baby to avoid the need to transfer the infant to another facility. In many areas, this is not possible and the infant does need to be transferred. This increases the stress on the family with the mother being separated from her infant and the father and other family members torn between staying with the mother and going to the hospital where the baby is. Caregivers at both facilities need to be sensitive to this situation and allow the families easy access to information about the infant and the mother. If at all possible, the mother should be allowed to see her infant prior to transfer. Pictures of the baby should be taken both at the delivery and referral facilities for the mother to have.

Timing of the delivery may be an issue. In general, most infants with congenital abnormalities are not well served by premature delivery. There are circumstances, however, when preterm delivery cannot be avoided. Infants with hydrops, for example, are often at increased risk of fetal demise unless delivered early. This places even more importance on the selection of an appropriate delivery facility. The use of antenatal steroids can be very helpful in reducing the risk of severe hyaline membrane disease for these infants.

Route of delivery also deserves some consideration. With few exceptions, cesarean section delivery should be reserved for the traditional maternal and fetal indications and not done because of the fetal abnormality. There is a report, however, that there is less neurologic deficit in infants with myelomeningocele who are delivered by cesarean section.[3] There are also a number of reports indicating decreased morbidity and shorter hospital stays for infants with gastroschisis who undergo immediate postdelivery repair.[4] In most circumstances, immediate repair is not feasible unless delivery occurs by elective cesarean section.

RESUSCITATION

Infants with congenital abnormalities are at increased risk to require resuscitation in the delivery room. Personnel who are in attendance at delivery should be aware of the antenatal diagnosis. If there is any question of no or limited resuscitation of the infant, discussions between the neonatologist/pediatrician and the family must occur prior to the actual delivery.[5] The parents and the neonatal caregivers should clearly understand what will and will not be done in the course of the resuscitation.

Certain congenital abnormalities should be assumed to require resuscitation in the delivery room. Infants with pulmonary or airway abnormalities, such as diaphragmatic hernia, cystadenomatoid malformation, lung hypoplasia, or cystic hygroma, often present with immediate respiratory distress. Airway management with prompt intubation should be carried out. An orogastric tube should be inserted to keep the intestines decompressed and avoid further pulmonary compromise. The administration of volume expanders and epinephrine may be required. Sodium bicarbonate should be used with great caution unless blood gas analysis is available since many of these infants have severe respiratory acidosis. Infants who fail to respond to resuscitation should be assessed for the presence of a pneumothorax, which needs to be aspirated promptly. The use of oscillatory ventilation may decrease the risk of air leaks in these infants. Once the infant is stabilized, he or she should be evaluated by the appropriate subspecialist. If necessary, transfer to the treating center should be accomplished as soon as possible.

Infants with hydrops of any etiology almost always require delivery room resuscitation. Airway management is the first priority. Once the infant is intubated, drainage of pleural or ascitic fluid may greatly enhance ventilation efforts. There is a report of aspiration of pleural or ascitic fluid from the fetus just before delivery with decreased need for resuscitation.[6] If there is reason to believe that the hydrops is caused by anemia, O-negative packed red blood cells should be available in the delivery room. Placement of an umbilical venous catheter provides ready vascular access. A hematocrit should be obtained at the time of insertion. Despite the fetal edema, many infants have intravascular volume depletion and require volume expansion. After confirmation of venous catheter placement, central venous pressure measurements can guide fluid therapy.

Neural tube and abdominal wall defects generally do not present with life-threatening problems. The defects should be covered with a dressing. Infants with an abdominal wall defect can be placed in a sterile plastic bag to protect the defect from drying out or rupturing. Special attention needs to be paid to thermal management because both the defects and the saline dressings can lead to hypothermia.

PHYSICAL ASSESSMENT

Following delivery and stabilization, the infant should be carefully examined. The presence of 1 congenital anomaly increases the risk of a second. Weight, height, and head circumference should be measured and plotted on growth curves for gestational age. Infants with chromosomal abnormalities, fetal alcohol syndrome, or congenital infections are often small for gestational age. Infants of diabetic mothers or infants with Beckwith-Wiedemann syndrome are *generally* large for gestational age.

The size, shape, and symmetry of the skull should be assessed as well as the fontanels and cranial sutures. Infants with craniosynostosis syndromes often have an unusual skull shape and ridging along suture lines. Large fontanels or split sutures are often signs of underlying hydrocephalus. Microcephaly is found in a large number of syndromes and is frequently associated with mental retardation.

The facies should be examined in a systematic fashion. An initial general impression should assess symmetry of the face. The forehead should be evaluated for prominence, the presence of a metopic suture, or unusual sloping. The eyes should be evaluated for size, spacing, and palpebral fissures. The globes should be examined for the presence of a light reflex, iris colobomas, and unusual pigmentation. In some conditions, such as congenital infection and CHARGE association, the retina should be examined for the presence of chorioretinitis or retinal colobomas. The presence of epicanthal folds and abnormal slanting of the eyes should also be noted. The appearance of the nasal bridge, nose, and philtrum should be noted. The size of the mandible should be assessed. Newborn infants normally have a somewhat small mandible. Micrognathia is seen in a number of syndromes and may be associated with glossoptosis and airway difficulties as is seen in the Pierre Robin malformation sequence. The mouth should be examined for unusual thinness of the lips and clefts. The presence of a high arched palate or clefts of the hard or soft palate should be looked for. The size of the tongue should be assessed. Infants with Down syndrome frequently have a protruding tongue. Infants with Beckwith-Wiedemann syndrome may have macroglossia and may require surgical reduction.

The size, shape, and symmetry of the ears are important. The presence of auricular skin tags or ear pits should be noted. In addition, the position of the ears must be noted. The top of the pinna should be at or above a line that extends from the inner canthus of the eye through the outer canthus. If the top of the pinna is below this line, the ears are low set. In addition, the ears may be posteriorly rotated.

Careful examination of the cardiovascular system should be performed. The location of heart sounds as well as any murmurs should be noted. The quality of the brachial and femoral pulses should be recorded as well as 4 extremity blood pressures. Breath sounds should be assessed for quality and symmetry.

The abdomen should be examined for the presence of hepatosplenomegaly or masses. The most common mass palpated in a newborn is an enlarged kidney. It must be noted, however, that even a very large, hydronephrotic kidney may not present as a palpable mass.

The genitalia deserve careful examination. In female infants the size of the labia majora and minora as well as the clitoris should be noted. Virilization such as that seen in congenital adrenal hyperplasia is usually manifested as enlargement of the clitoris with varying degrees of labial fusion. The presence of separate urethral and vaginal openings should be looked for. In male infants, the size of the stretched penis should be measured before a diagnosis of micropenis is made. The measurement should be compared to published norms for newborn infants of differing gestational age. Hypospadias is a common congenital malformation. Although it may be seen in a variety of syndromes, it most commonly is an isolated abnormality. Cryptorchidism in a full-term infant is also a common finding in many syndromes. Placement and patency of the anus should be noted.

Abnormalities of the skeletal system are common in many syndromes. General note should be made of the proportions and symmetry of the extremities to the trunk. Congenital amputations such as those found with amniotic band syndrome are usually quite obvious. Absent or hypoplastic long bones are most common in the upper extremities and are often accompanied by thrombocytopenia. Polydactyly can be an isolated autosomal-dominant condition, but is also seen in a number of syndromes including Trisomy 13. Syndactyly, especially between the second and third toes is very common as an isolated condition, but can be seen in a number of syndromes. Vertebral and rib anomalies may be present, but may only be apparent on radiographs. The hands should be examined for the presence of simian creases, clinodactyly, and finger position.

Joint mobility should be assessed. Limitation of motion of the joints may be an indication of an underlying neuromuscular problem and is frequently seen in infants with oligohydramnios sequence. Talipes equinovarus is common as an isolated problem and is frequently seen in infants with neural tube defects as well as oligohydramnios sequence.

Abnormalities of the skin should be looked for. The presence of café au lait spots, port wine stains, or other pigmentation abnormalities may be indications of a group of syndromes known as *hamartoses*.

POSTNATAL DIAGNOSTIC STUDIES

The infant with a prenatal diagnosis of a congenital abnormality must have the diagnosis confirmed with postnatal studies if the abnormality is not readily apparent.[7] Many infants in whom 1 abnormality was noted antenatally have additional findings on examination that warrant further diagnostic studies.

Evaluation of structural abnormalities is often best accomplished by x-ray studies and ultrasound examinations. Plain films of the chest allow evaluation of the lungs, heart, ribs, and cervical and thoracic vertebrae. Abdominal films should be evaluated for intestinal gas pattern, masses, intra-abdominal calcifications, as well as the vertebrae. Skull and long bone films are very important in the evaluation of skeletal dysplasias and may also provide clues to the presence of congenital infections.

Cranial ultrasound should be performed in all infants with abnormal head size, neural tube defects, and midline facial de-

T A B L E 54-1	CONDITIONS ASSOCIATED WITH CONGENITAL HEART DISEASE
Omphalocele	
Esophageal atresia with TE fistula	
Congenital diaphragmatic hernia	
Chromosomal abnormalities	
Infant of the diabetic mother	
Fetal alcohol syndrome	
Noonan syndrome	
CHARGE association	
VACTERL association	
Ivemark syndrome	
DiGeorge syndrome	

Abbreviations: CHARGE, *c*olobomas, *h*eart disease, *a*tresia, choanae, *r*etarded *g*rowth and development, *g*enital anomalies, *e*ar anomalies; TE, tracheo-esophageal; VACTERL, *v*ertebral, *a*nal, *c*ardiac, *t*racheal, *e*sophageal, *r*enal, *l*imb.

fects. Cranial magnetic resonance imaging (MRI) is a better choice to evaluate the brain stem and spinal cord and parenchymal abnormalities.

Abdominal ultrasound is indicated in any infant with an abdominal mass, urogenital anomalies, or suspected renal anomalies. Infants with hydronephrosis require a voiding cystourethrogram (VCUG) to look for the presence of vesicoureteral reflux or posterior urethral valves. Mag 3 renal scans are helpful to look at differential renal function or obstruction, although the low renal blood flow limits their use in the immediate neonatal period.

Congenital heart disease is associated with many congenital abnormalities and may not be readily apparent on initial physical examination. Table 54-1 lists conditions with an increased incidence of associated cardiac defects. An echocardiogram is indicated for infants with these conditions as well as any infant with congenital anomalies who has a cardiac murmur or any other evidence suggestive of a cardiac lesion. Pulse oximetry is helpful in detecting cyanotic lesions.

Infants with multiple congenital malformations should have a karyotype done if one was not done antenatally. In addition to chromosome number, banding should be done to evaluate for the presence of more subtle unbalanced chromosomal abnormalities. The presence of microdeletions such as those found with DiGeorge syndrome (chromosome 22) or Prader-Willi syndrome (chromosome 15) can be detected with the use of a fluorescence in situ hybridization assay.

Specific laboratory tests are available for a number of other conditions associated with congenital malformations, such as 7 dehydroxycholesterol for Smith-Lemli-Opitz syndrome.

The ability to make a specific diagnosis is very important. This knowledge focuses additional testing for abnormalities that may not otherwise be looked for. A specific diagnosis provides families with more reliable information regarding life expectancy and physical and neurodevelopmental outcomes. It also allows counseling of families with regard to recurrence risks for future pregnancies. A specific diagnosis can often be made once the results of the physical examination, radiologic and imaging studies, and laboratory testing has been completed. Some conditions, such as Down syndrome, are usually quite typical and relatively easy to diagnose. Other conditions, such as DiGeorge or Smith-Lemli-Opitz syndromes, are less obvious but have specific confirmatory tests available. Many conditions, however, do not have specific testing available and the diagnosis is more difficult to ascertain. Often repeat examinations over time help to clarify the correct diagnosis.

The field of genetic testing is expanding rapidly and it is often difficult for neonatologists and pediatricians to keep abreast of the latest developments in this area. All infants with multiple malformations should be evaluated by a medical geneticist. They can provide valuable assistance in making specific diagnoses. *Smith's Recognizable Patterns of Human Malformation* is a valuable resource to assist in diagnosis of infants with multiple anomalies and should be available in every neonatal intensive care unit.[8] Computer programs, such as POSSUM[9] and BDIS,[10] are also available to assist in the diagnosis of malformation syndromes. These programs are particularly helpful for identification of rare or newly described syndromes.

HYDROPS FETALIS

Hydrops fetalis is one of the more common conditions that is diagnosed antenatally. The cause may be readily ascertainable, as in Rh isoimmunization, or fairly obscure. Table 54-2 lists many of the conditions that have been associated with hydrops. With the development of Rh_o (D) immune globulin (RhoGAM), the majority of cases of hydrops fetalis are now caused by nonimmune factors. In a review of nonimmune hydrops fetalis by Sasidharan et al., 38% of cases were caused by chromosomal or other congenital anomalies.[11] Cardiac lesions accounted for 26%, hematologic causes for 14%, and infectious causes for 3%. In 19% of the cases, no cause could be found and these cases were labeled idiopathic.

The underlying pathophysiology for the development of hydrops is not always clear. Most cases involve either congestive heart failure, hypoproteinemia, tissue hypoxia, or vascular or lymphatic obstruction. These infants are often premature and usually critically ill at birth and require aggressive resuscitation as described.

Once the infant has been stabilized, a diagnostic evaluation needs to be done if the cause of the hydrops is not already known. Table 54-3 lists the studies that should be performed to determine the cause of the hydrops. Not all of the tests may be indicated for an individual patient. The mortality of infants with hydrops fetalis is high. In the previously cited review article, 47% of fetuses were either stillborn or the pregnancy was terminated. Of the infants who were live born, 37% died.

TABLE 54-2	CONDITIONS ASSOCIATED WITH HYDROPS FETALIS

Cardiopulmonary
  Fetal cardiac arrhythmias
  Congenital heart disease
  Premature closure of the foramen ovale
  Cystic adenomatoid malformation
  Pulmonary lymphangiectasia
  Pulmonary hypoplasia
  Arteriovenous malformations
Hematologic
  Blood group incompatibility
  Chronic fetomaternal hemorrhage
  Chronic twin-to-twin transfusion
  Enclosed fetal hemorrhage
  G6PD deficiency
  Homozygous α-thalassemia
  Gaucher disease
Infections
  TORCH infections
  Parvovirus
  Hepatitis
  Coxsackie virus
  Leptospirosis
  Chagas disease
Chromosomal and congenital anomalies
  Trisomies
  Triploidy syndrome
  Turner syndrome
  Achondroplasia
  Noonan syndrome
  Myotonic dystrophy
  Tuberous sclerosis
  Many others
Renal
  Congenital nephrotic syndrome
  Renal dysplasia
  Renal vein thrombosis
Neoplasms
  Neuroblastoma
  Sacrococcygeal teratoma
  Hemangioendothelioma
Placental
  Chorioangioma
  Umbilical vein thrombosis
  Chorionic vein thrombosis
Miscellaneous
  Maternal diabetes mellitus
  Pregnancy-induced hypertension
  Dysmaturity
  Meconium peritonitis
  Idiopathic

Abbreviation: G6PD, glucose-6-phosphate dehydrogenase; TORCH, *t*oxoplasmosis, *o*ther, *r*ubella, *c*ytomegalovirus, *h*erpes simplex.

TABLE 54-3	DIAGNOSTIC WORKUP FOR HYDROPS FETALIS

Placental pathology

CBC, differential, platelet count, and blood smear

Blood type, Coombs test, antibody screen

Hemoglobin electrophoresis

G6PD assay

Maternal Kleihauer-Betke test

TORCH or other viral IgM titers, total IgM level

CMV culture

Karyotype

Total protein and serum albumin levels

Renal and liver function studies

Diagnostic studies on pleural and ascitic fluid

Chest and abdominal x-rays

Skeletal survey

Echocardiogram

Abdominal ultrasound

Cranial ultrasound

Abbreviations: CBC, complete blood count; CMV, cytomegalovirus; G6PD, glucose-6-phosphate dehydrogenase; IgM, immunoglobulin M; TORCH.

CONGENITAL DIAPHRAGMATIC HERNIA

Congenital diaphragmatic hernia (CDH) is estimated to occur in approximately 1 in every 3500 live births.[12] Despite the availability of newer modes of ventilation, extracorporeal membrane oxygenation (ECMO), and inhalational nitric oxide, mortality from this defect remains high. A recent review of 500 articles published between 1990 and 1995 revealed an average mortality of 40%. Several studies suggest that the mortality of infants with a prenatally diagnosed hernia is even higher (mean 65%, range 36–86%).[12] A number of studies have attempted to identify factors, both prenatal and neonatal, that predict survival, without success.

Currently, there does not appear to be any particular strategy for management of the infant with a CDH that is clearly superior.[13] Appropriate management begins with resuscitation in the delivery room as outlined. Administration of exogenous surfactant before the first breath may be useful for those patients diagnosed antenatally. Both conventional and high-frequency ventilation are used. High mean airway pressures should be avoided if at all possible. The goal of ventilatory support should be to maintain a preductal saturation of 85–90%. Attempts at hyperventilation to produce a respiratory alkalosis should be avoided. Infants with evidence of severe pulmonary hypertension may be given a trial of inhaled nitric oxide, although the reported results are inconsistent. Many centers use ECMO for infants who fail to respond to more conventional treatments.

Surgical repair is usually deferred until the infant is stable with resolved or decreased lability of the pulmonary vascula-

ture. Infants who have been placed on ECMO may be repaired after successful decannulation, although some centers elect to defer decannulation until after repair because of concerns of recurrent pulmonary hypertension.

CONGENITAL CYSTIC ADENOMATOID MALFORMATION

Congenital cystic adenomatoid malformation (CCAM) is an uncommon multicystic lung lesion with proliferation of bronchial structures.[14] It is unilobar in the vast majority of cases. Lesions are classified as types I–III depending on the size of the cysts and homogeneity of the mass. Type III lesions are more likely to be associated with fetal hydrops and adverse outcomes. CCAM is usually an isolated defect without other malformations.

Infants with CCAM have a wide clinical presentation ranging from asymptomatic to critically ill with severe respiratory distress. After initial stabilization, a chest x-ray should be obtained. Those infants who require mechanical ventilation are at increased risk for pneumothorax. Very large lesions produce a mediastinal shift and may cause hypoplasia of the uninvolved portions of the lung. Treatment is surgical resection of the mass, which generally entails removing the entire affected lobe.

Infants with antenatally detected lesions who are asymptomatic should also be evaluated. The chest x-ray frequently has subtle abnormalities. Chest computed tomography or MRI may be helpful in detecting small lesions. Some authors recommend resection of even asymptomatic lesions because of the risk of development of later lung tumors. Surgery can be done electively when the child is bigger.

ABDOMINAL WALL DEFECTS

An *omphalocele* is a defect in the ventral abdominal wall with herniation of the intra-abdominal contents. The abdominal contents are covered by a membrane with the umbilical cord inserting into the sac.[15] Most cases are sporadic, although recurrence in families has been reported. Omphaloceles may be associated with a number of syndromes or other malformations including trisomies 13 and 18, Beckwith-Wiedemann syndrome, and pentalogy of Cantrell. Thirty percent may have associated congenital heart disease.

Omphaloceles almost always contain loops of bowel. Larger defects may also contain stomach and liver. The covering membrane may rupture before, during, or after delivery. Prior to surgical repair, the infant should be evaluated for the presence of associated anomalies.

Gastroschisis is a full-thickness defect of the right anterior abdominal wall that is felt to be related to vascular compromise of either the umbilical vein or omphalomesenteric artery. This defect allows herniation of the bowel loops; only rarely are the liver and stomach involved. There is no membrane covering and the bowel loops are usually covered by an inflammatory exudate as a result of exposure to the amniotic fluid.

In contrast to omphaloceles, infants with gastroschisis do not have an increased incidence of abnormalities outside of the gastrointestinal tract. Chromosomal defects have only rarely been reported. Infants with gastroschisis do have a 10–20% incidence of intestinal atresia. Infants with gastroschisis are more likely to be born prematurely.

During delivery room stabilization of an infant with an abdominal wall defect, a nasogastric tube should be inserted and placed to suction to prevent bowel distention. Primary surgical closure is preferable; it is associated with earlier feeding tolerance and shorter lengths of stay. With larger defects, however, primary closure is frequently not possible because of increased intra-abdominal pressure with resultant intestinal and renal ischemia and respiratory compromise. These patients need to be managed with placement of a silo and staged reduction.

Recent reports indicate improved outcomes in infants with gastroschisis who undergo surgical repair immediately after delivery.[4] Infants who underwent immediate repair were more likely to have a primary fascial closure, required fewer days of ventilatory support, were fed earlier, and had shorter lengths of stay.

The outcome of infants with omphalocele is largely dependent on the presence of associated congenital and chromosomal abnormalities as well as the size of the defect. Survival in infants with gastroschisis is higher than those with omphalocele.

RENAL ANOMALIES

Renal abnormalities, especially hydronephrosis, are among the more commonly diagnosed antenatal abnormalities. Of concern is the discrepancy between prenatal and postnatal diagnoses.[16] In 1 study, 62% of infants identified with renal and/or bladder abnormalities on antenatal ultrasound had normal postnatal studies.[17] Other studies report agreement between the prenatal and postnatal diagnoses between 65–74%.

The fetus with severe renal abnormalities and oligohydramnios is at high risk of developing the oligohydramnios sequence. This results from uterine deformation of the fetus owing to decreased amniotic fluid volume, which is the result of absent urine formation in the fetus. These infants have the characteristic "Potter facies" with flattening of the face, creases under the eyes, low-set and posteriorly rotated ears, and multiple joint contractures. They also have pulmonary hypoplasia. The renal abnormality is always bilateral and may

be agenesis, polycystic kidney disease, or severe cystic dysplasia from obstruction. Pulmonary hypoplasia is the major problem and most infants die soon after birth from respiratory failure.

A very high percentage of infants with antenatally diagnosed urinary tract abnormalities have a perfectly normal physical examination. Therefore, all these infants should have a postnatal ultrasound. If the study is done before the third day of life and is normal, a repeat sonogram should be obtained 3–4 weeks later because the low urine output present during the first 2 days of life may mask the abnormality. Some urologists recommend a repeat ultrasound in 6–8 weeks even if the initial ultrasound was done after the third day of life.

Infants with abnormal postnatal renal ultrasounds require further investigation.[16] A VCUG is indicated to evaluate for the presence of posterior urethral valves in male infants with bilateral hydronephrosis and also to look for the presence of vesicoureteral reflux. A renal isotope scan allows assessment of renal function and may help to determine when or if surgical intervention is required. A furosemide washout scan helps to determine the degree of obstruction.

Following confirmation of the urinary tract abnormality, a treatment plan can be formulated. Infants with bilateral obstructive uropathy usually require surgical intervention early to preserve as much renal function as possible. This may involve definitive correction, such as the ablation of posterior urethral valves, or temporary drainage procedures (nephrostomy or vesicostomy) with definitive surgery being performed at a later time. Infants with unilateral disease can often have their surgical treatment performed in later infancy. Infants with vesicoureteral reflux should be placed on antibiotic prophylaxis to minimize the risk of urinary tract infections and subsequent renal scarring.

A significant number of infants with antenatally diagnosed renal abnormalities require surgical intervention at some point during the first year of life. Although many authors believe that antenatal detection is beneficial in improving long-term outcomes, there are no controlled studies that confirm this belief, especially in infants with unilateral disease.[16]

Infants with a nonfunctioning multicystic kidney usually require no intervention in the neonatal period. Many cases undergo spontaneous regression. Others require surgical removal at a later time because of feeding intolerance, systemic hypertension, or fear of malignant degeneration.

Polycystic kidney disease is an inherited disorder and is always bilateral. Infantile polycystic kidney disease is an autosomal recessive trait. The diagnosis is often made antenatally and these fetuses may have oligohydramnios sequence. Infants who are symptomatic at birth have a high mortality related to pulmonary hypoplasia or severe renal insufficiency. Many of these infants require chronic dialysis from a very early age. Adult polycystic kidney disease is an autosomal dominant trait with wide variation in expression. It may be diagnosed antenatally and also present with the oligohydramnios sequence. Infants with this disorder may be difficult to distinguish from the infantile type on the basis of renal ultrasound. Cystic changes of the liver, pancreas, and spleen are often present and help to distinguish between the 2 types. Mortality is high among infants who are symptomatic at birth.

MYELOMENINGOCELE

Myelomeningocele is another commonly diagnosed antenatal anomaly. Elevated maternal serum α-fetoprotein often leads the ultrasound detection of the defect. Hydrocephalus may or may not be present at the time of diagnosis. Although this is most often an isolated anomaly, these infants have many other associated problems. Antenatal diagnosis greatly facilitates providing families with information regarding the problems that will need to be dealt with, both in the neonatal period and beyond. Many families who have an infant with this lesion that was undiagnosed antenatally are overwhelmed with information and faced with making decisions while under a great deal of emotional distress.

Many centers have a team of professionals who are involved in both the immediate and long-term care. Included in this team are neurosurgery, neurology or physical medicine, nursing, urology, orthopedics, and social work. The team should be consulted immediately after admission and can begin to build a relationship with the family.

After initial stabilization, the defect should be covered with sterile, saline-soaked gauze. The infant should be kept prone or on his or her side to avoid pressure on the defect. If the defect is leaking, prophylactic antibiotic coverage is usually begun. All infants should have a cranial and abdominal ultrasound. In addition to hydrocephalus, the majority of infants with a myelomeningocele have an associated Arnold-Chiari malformation. A VCUG is also necessary but may be deferred until after surgical correction. If ventricular size is normal or only minimally enlarged on the preoperative cranial ultrasound, a follow-up study is indicated postoperatively to monitor for the subsequent development of hydrocephalus which may occur days or weeks after surgical closure. Serial head circumference measurements should also be recorded.

Surgery is usually performed within the first 24–48 hours. If hydrocephalus is present at birth a ventriculoperitoneal shunt may be inserted at the time of the initial surgery or within several days.

Postoperatively, the infant's voiding pattern should be documented. Many urologists recommend intermittent postvoid bladder catheterization to check for residual urine. This can also be assessed on VCUG. Infants with significant urine residuals need intermittent catheterization as part of their home management. If vesicoureteral reflux is seen on the VCUG, prophylactic antibiotic treatment is recommended.

Many infants with myelomeningocele have orthopedic problems including talipes equinovarus and hip dysplasia. Treatment of these problems may begin while the infant is in the neonatal intensive care unit or may be deferred until after discharge.

The prognosis for these children is variable, but has improved significantly. The majority have normal or only mildly impaired intellectual function and most can lead very productive lives. Regular follow-up in a multidisciplinary clinic is essential to prevent or deal with complications promptly.

ETHICAL CONSIDERATIONS

The birth of an infant with congenital malformations invariably leads to ethical questions of whether or not and/or how aggressively to treat. Many times, the families have dealt or are still dealing with these issues following the prenatal diagnosis. The decision to continue with the pregnancy of a fetus with congenital anomalies does not necessarily imply that the family wishes to continue treatment in the newborn period. Often, uncertainties as to the exact diagnosis or severity of the problem can be better answered after birth than before.

Before recommendations are made to the family, a thorough evaluation of the infant's problems must be made with appropriate consultation of subspecialists. If the infant has been transferred to a facility other than the birth hospital, discussions to withhold care should be deferred until the mother is able to come to the referral facility. It is extremely difficult to communicate information of this magnitude through family members or by telephone.

Parents remain the best choice for determining what is in the best interest of their child. It is the responsibility of the medical personnel caring for the infant to educate the family regarding the severity of the infant's problems and the prognosis. It is appropriate for the physician to make recommendations regarding the extent of care, but the decision generally rests with the family. If there is conflict between caregivers and the family, Bioethical Review Committees exist in most hospitals that can help to resolve the conflict. The role of these committees is generally to open lines of communication, however, not to make the decisions. If families are refusing treatment that the medical providers feel is clearly in the child's best interest, the legal system can be petitioned to override the parent's decision. The more difficult situation arises when the family insists on continuing care that is clearly not beneficial.[18] There is no ready solution to this dilemma. There are precedents for not instituting treatment that is of no benefit, but withdrawal of ongoing care, such as ventilatory support, remains problematic.

CONCLUSION

The diagnosis of a fetus with a congenital abnormality presents a challenge to all involved. Although it is stressful for families, prenatal diagnosis affords the opportunity to educate the family and make arrangements for appropriate delivery and neonatal management. Optimal management requires communication and cooperation between the obstetrician, perinatologist, geneticist, pediatric subspecialist, and neonatologist.

References

1. Nichols VG, Bianchi DW. Prenatal pediatrics: traditional specialty definitions no longer apply. *Pediatrics.* 97:729, 1996.
2. Adzick NS, Harrison MR, Glick PL, et al. Fetal cystic adenomatoid malformation: Prenatal diagnosis and natural history. *J Pediatr Surg.* 20:483, 1985.
3. Luthy DA, Wardinsky T, Shurtleff DB, et al. Cesarean section before the onset of labor and subsequent motor function in infants with meningomyelocele diagnosed antenatally. *N Engl J Med.* 324:662, 1991.
4. Coughlin JP, Drucker DEM, Jewell MR, et al. Delivery room repair of gastroschisis. *Surgery.* 114:822, 1993.
5. Goldsmith JP, Ginsberg HG, McGettigan MC. Ethical decisions in the delivery room. *Clin Perinatol.* 23:529, 1996.
6. Cardwell MS. Aspiration of fetal pleural effusions or ascites may improve neonatal resuscitation. *South Med J.* 89:177, 1996.
7. Graham JM, Otto C. Clinical approach to prenatal detection of human structural defects. *Clin Perinatol.* 17:513, 1990.
8. Jones KL. *Smith's Recognizable Patterns of Human Malformations.* 6th ed. Philadelphia: WB Saunders; 2005.
9. Bankier A, Danks D. *POSSUM (Pictures of Standard Syndromes and Undiagnosed Malformations).* Victoria, Australia: The Murdoch Institute for Research into Birth Defects; 1987.
10. Buyse ML, ed. *The Computerized Birth Defects Information System.* Dover, Mass: Center for Birth Defects Information Services; 1990.
11. Sasidharan P, Al-Mohsen I, Abdul-Karim A, et al. Nonimmune hydrops fetalis: case reports and brief review. *J Perinatol.* 12:338, 1992.
12. Langham MR Jr., Kays DW, Ledbetter DJ, et al. Congenital diaphragmatic hernia. Epidemiology and outcome. *Clin Perinatol.* 23:671, 1996.
13. Bohn DJ, Pearl R, Irish MS, et al. Postnatal management of congenital diaphragmatic hernia. *Clin Perinatol.* 23:843, 1996.
14. Crombleholme TM. Prenatal diagnosis and management of surgical pulmonary problems. *Neonatal Resp Dis.* 6:1, 1996.
15. Paidas MJ, Crombleholme TM, Robertson FM. Prenatal diagnosis and management of the fetus with an abdominal wall defect. *Semin Perinatol.* 18:196, 1994.
16. Fine RN. Diagnosis and treatment of fetal urinary tract abnormalities. *J Pediatr.* 121:333, 1992.
17. Johnson CE, Elder JS, Judge NE, et al. The accuracy of antenatal ultrasonography in identifying renal abnormalities. *Am J Dis Child.* 146:1181, 1992.
18. Paris JJ, Schreiber MD. Physician's refusal to provide life-prolonging medical interventions. *Clin Perinatol* 23:563, 1996.

Fetal Therapy

FETAL SHUNT PROCEDURES

Mark Paul Johnson

INTRODUCTION

Most congenital malformations do not lend themselves to definitive in utero surgical correction, but the destructive impact of several conditions may be significantly reduced by simple interventions resulting in dramatically improved outcomes in fetuses whose prognosis was otherwise quite dismal. One such intervention involves the use of diverting shunts with the sole purpose of chronically draining fluid-filled spaces. Such diverting shunts, which can be placed percutaneously with a minimum of uterine invasion, have been shown to be safe and reliable, and have resulted in the births of numerous infants who otherwise had little chance of survival. While the actual placement of the shunt is undoubtedly the most challenging aspect of these cases, considerable experience has shown that one must understand the underlying pathologic processes at work, and that careful diagnostic evaluation and patient selection are the most important aspects of this type of in utero therapy. In this chapter we discuss the mechanisms of damage, the prenatal evaluation, criteria for selecting those fetuses who may benefit from intervention, the invasive technique, potential complications, and recommended follow-up after shunt placement for pregnancies complicated by obstructive uropathy, congenital cystic adenomatoid malformation, and idiopathic pleural effusion.

LOWER URINARY TRACT OBSTRUCTION

Fetal obstructive uropathies are a diverse and heterogeneous group of developmental abnormalities that generally involve obstruction of the proximal urethra in the male fetus. The more common etiologies involve urethral atresia, posterior urethral valves, or prune-belly syndrome. Cloacal anomalies may be part of the underlying disorder, reflect the presence of a more complex underlying genetic syndrome, and must be ruled out during prenatal evaluation because such cases have not been found to benefit from shunt therapy. Other etiologies can include anterior urethral valves, chromosomal abnormalities, complex genetic causes such as megacystis/microcolon syndrome, or partial obstructions or strictures that restrict flow through the urethra as may rarely occur in abnormalities of the urethral meatus such as hypo- or epispadius.

Complete urethral obstruction or significant restriction of urethral flow results in accumulation of urine within the fetal bladder, leading to megacystis. Prolonged obstruction results in smooth-muscle hypertrophy and hyperplasia within the bladder wall, and eventual impairment of contractile capacity as well as compliance and elasticity. Bladder distension results in elevated intravesicular pressures, which may overcome the delicate physiologic valve mechanism at the ureterovesical junctions. Bladder wall distortion-associated hypertrophy and hyperplasia may contribute to the loss of these physiologic valves. Reflux eventually results, contributing to the development of hydroureters and hydronephrosis.

Ureteral distension due to reflux also elicits smooth-muscle hypertrophy and hyperplasia, particularly in the distal ureter where smooth muscle is more prevalent. This appears to result in further distortion of the delicate ureterovesical angles as well as diminished elasticity of the ureters.

Experience indicates that there is a subset of male fetuses in which ureteral hypoplasia with patency can be demonstrated on fetal autopsy, although these fetuses appear sonographically identical to those in which complete obstruction is confirmed postnatally. Histologically, these fetuses appear to have a basic underlying defect in the development and response of smooth muscle throughout the upper and lower urinary tract, resulting in dilation of the bladder and subsequent reflux hydronephrosis. In cases of true anatomical obstruction, there is a marked hypertrophic and hyperplastic response of the smooth muscle component in the walls of the bladder and distal ureters to obstruction, which is progressive and reflective of the duration of the obstructive process. In the fetuses without complete anatomical obstructions, we have found no change in the smooth muscle component when compared to age-matched nonobstructed controls,[1] and the long-term prognosis in such cases following shunt intervention appears to be better than outcomes in cases of anatomical obstruction. As such, it would be prognostically helpful to be able to reliably identify these 2 groups prenatally.[2] We have recently introduced the use of fine-needle fetoscopy to perform in utero fetal cystoscopy during the prenatal evaluation to directly examine the bladder mucosa, ureteral orifices, and proximal urethra.[3] In cases of true urethral obstruction, the proximal urethra has been markedly dilated with trabeculations noted in the trigone of the bladder. In cases subsequently confirmed to be urethra-patent prune-belly syndromes, the proximal urethra and bladder neck was much less distended and the trigone was without trabeculations, although sonographically, both groups demonstrated the characteristic "keyhole" sign associated with proximal urethral distention. The capability of differentiating these 2 major groups of fetuses prenatally may allow future changes and refinements in our interventive approaches so as to optimize long-term outcomes.

Hydronephrosis develops from continued urine production in the face of obstructed drainage as well as reflux from the distended bladder. The renal pelvises and calyces systems become progressively distended and compress the renal parenchyma against the distended renal capsule. Histologic studies indicate a progressive dilation of the distal to proximal renal tubules associated with the development of peritubular and interstitial fibrosis. Sonographically, the degree of compression and associated fibrosis is reflected by the echogenic appearance of the parenchyma. Eventually, these processes lead to type IV cystic degeneration of the kidneys and renal insufficiency at birth.

After 14 weeks' gestation, maintenance of amniotic fluid volume is principally from fetal urine production. In cases of obstruction, fetal urine cannot replenish amniotic fluid volume lost by membrane reabsorption and fetal swallowing, and amniotic fluid volume progressively falls. Subsequent severe oligo- or anhydramnios and massive megacystis leads to physical deformations and physiologic changes characteristic of the prune-belly sequence, which include a markedly protuberant abdomen with apparent decrease in skeletal muscle present within the rectus sheath, joint contractures, compressive facial abnormalities, and pulmonary hypoplasia from intrathoracic pressure alterations and inability to take in amniotic fluid during fetal breathing, which may play an important role in lung development and maturation. The presence of severe oligo-hydramnios during the transition from canalicular to alveolar phase of development, which occurs between 18 and 24 weeks' gestation, results in severely underdeveloped lungs and respiratory insufficiency at birth.[4]

PRENATAL EVALUATION

The antenatal evaluation consists of 3 basic steps; high-resolution sonographic survey to rule out additional congenital anomalies, fetal karyotyping, and renal function analysis. Detailed fetal sonographic survey is necessary to rule out the presence of other anomalies, such as neural tube or cardiac defects, which would dramatically affect the long-term prognosis for that fetus. Certainly, in utero intervention would not be warranted when the fetus is afflicted with another life-threatening anomaly. One must also look carefully for other, more subtle phenotypic signs, such as limb shortening or facial abnormalities that may indicate the presence of an underlying genetic syndrome, which might adversely affect the clinical prognosis. The urinary tract is then carefully evaluated from the kidneys to the distal urethra. Long axis measurement of the kidney is useful in evaluating the underlying hydronephrosis and, in general, kidneys that measure large for gestational age and less hyperechogenic are associated with a better prognosis. Kidneys that are hyperechogenic and measure appropriate or small for gestational age are generally found to have poor underlying function due to advanced renal fibrosis. The finding of small kidneys in such cases may reflect the underlying contraction phase of scarring and fibrosis in these severely damaged tissues.

The renal parenchyma is then examined for the degree of echogenicity, compression, and the absence of discreet cortical cysts (Figs. 55-1, 55-2). Care must be taken when possible microcystic changes are noted to ensure that what the sonographer is seeing is not dilated minor calyces. The presence of cortical cysts is associated with irreversible, advanced renal damage, which renders the fetus not amenable to interventive therapy. Occasionally, a large, unilocular cystic structure can be found adjacent to the renal capsule. In many cases, this represents a subcapsular urinoma and must be differentiated from a large pyelectasis or cortical macrocyst. Such urinomas may

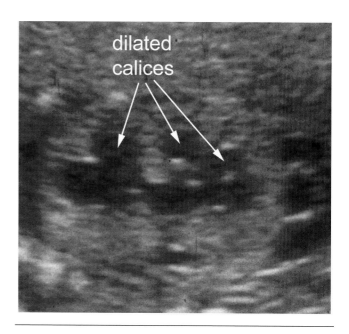

FIGURE 55-1 Ultrasound of obstructed hydronephrotic kidney with mild pyelocaliectasis. Arrows show dilated minor calyces.

result from increased intrarenal pressures from obstructive hydronephrosis and may transiently decrease intrarenal pressure and associated damage, serving a temporary protective function for the kidney.

Next, the ureters are carefully examined for abnormalities. The presence of massive pyelectasis in the absence of hydroureters (Fig. 55-3) may indicate the presence of an obstructive component at the level of the ureteropelvic junction

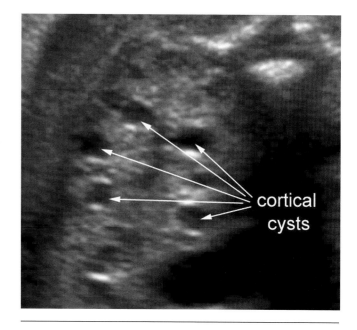

FIGURE 55-2 Ultrasound of obstructed hydronephrotic kidney with renal dysplasia. Arrows show discrete cortical cysts consistent with severe fibrocystic renal dysplasia.

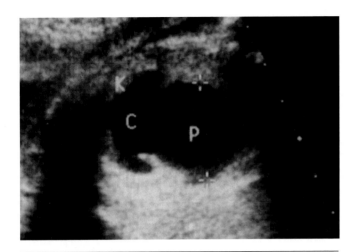

FIGURE 55-3 Ultrasound showing UPJ obstruction with markedly dilated renal pelvis (P) and calyces (C) and compressed renal parenchyma (K).

(UPJ). Successful vesicoamniotic shunting in the presence of a complete or high-grade UPJ obstruction would not allow renal drainage, and bladder shunting would therefore fail to prevent further damage to that kidney.

The bladder is carefully evaluated prior to and following complete drainage by fine-needle vesicocentesis. Prior to drainage, overall size is assessed as well as degree of apparent proximal urethral dilation (i.e., keyhole sign) as an indication of level and etiology of apparent obstruction (Fig. 55-4). In addition, the presence of abnormal bladder shape or urachal abnormalities may indicate the presence of an underlying developmental abnormality of cloacal differentiation, which represent more complex anomalies that have not benefited from simple diverting procedures, such as vesicoamniotic shunting. The penile urethra is also evaluated for dilation or abnormalities indicating a distal etiology, such as stenosis of the urethral meatus or anterior urethral vales. Following vesicocentesis, the extent and uniformity of bladder wall thickening can be assessed.

The second major component of the prenatal evaluation is the fetal karyotype. Female fetuses are rarely found to have simple urethral obstructions and usually have complex developmental abnormalities of the cloaca. Past attempts at in utero shunt therapy have proven unsuccessful in improving the prognosis for these fetuses, and therefore are not indicated. We have also encountered fetuses with trisomy 21, trisomy 18, and Klinefelter syndrome with apparent isolated megacystis, hydronephrosis, and decreased amniotic fluid volume in the absence of other major sonographic markers. As most cases of early onset obstructive uropathy have severe oligohydramnios by the time they are identified, amniocentesis is not an option. We routinely perform chorionic villus sampling via the transabdominal approach, which provides us with a preliminary result in 2–3 days and a final karyotype in 7–10 days. Other options include cordocentesis, which can prove difficult given the typical situation of severe oligohydram-

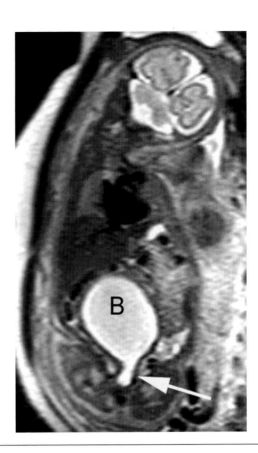

FIGURE 55-4 Ultrafast fetal MRI showing a urethral obstruction with anhydramnios and distended bladder. Arrow points to the "keyhole" sign of proximal urethral obstruction.

nios, as well as vesicocentesis with culturing of the cells from the fetal urine. Although successful in most cases, fetal urine specimens are more difficult to grow and results are therefore delayed.

The last step in the work-up is the evaluation of underlying renal function. We do this utilizing sequential vesicocentesis in which the fetal bladder is completely drained at 48–72 hour intervals on a minimum of 3 occasions.[5] The urine is then analyzed for electrolyte and protein values as a reflection of the level and severity of damage in the fetal kidneys (Table 55-1). Fetuses who demonstrate progressive hypotonicity on sequential urine samples and have final values that fall below recommended thresholds (Fig. 55-5) have been shown to benefit from in utero intervention.[6] Occasionally, especially later

TABLE 55-1	FETAL URINE PARAMETERS
Sodium	≤100 mmol/L
Osmolality	≤200 mOsm/L
Chloride	≤90 mmol/L
Calcium	≤8 mg/dl
Total protein	≤40 mg/dl
B-2 microglobulin	≤6 mg/L

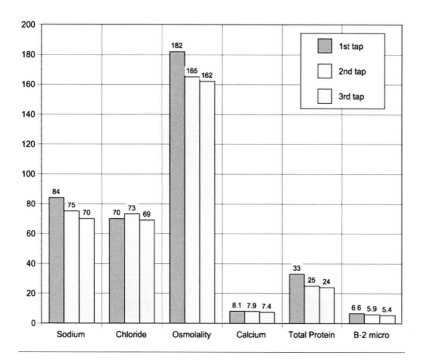

FIGURE 55-5 Fetal urine results showing sequential improvement in values below cutoff thresholds, suggesting potential for renal salvage following successful vesicoamniotic shunting.

in midgestation, it is necessary to perform 4 or 5 bladder drainages in order to establish a clear pattern of improving hypotonicity or increasing hypertonicity prior to final counseling of the patient as to underlying renal status and prognosis. We have been able to demonstrate histologically that there is strong correlation between progressive hypo- or hypertonicity and final urine values in predicting the presence or absence of significant, advanced renal damage.[7] We have found that once electrolyte levels approach threshold values (i.e., sodium >85 mg/dl, osmolality >180 mOsm/L), urinary proteins (total protein, albumin, microglobulins) may provide a better reflection of the degree of underlying damage, and may reflect impairment that has extended past the level of the proximal tubule to involve the glomerulus.[8] With such information, one can reliably counsel the patient about the futility or potential benefits of vesicoamniotic shunt placement.

PATIENT SELECTION

Fetuses with isolated megacystis, bilateral hydronephrosis, decreased amniotic fluid volume, absent associated congenital anomalies, a 46, XY (male) karyotype, and serially improving hypotonicity with values below recommended thresholds would be considered potential candidates for vesicoamniotic shunt placement. Fetuses who meet all other criteria but have urine values demonstrating minimal improvement and cluster about the threshold cutoffs, can be counseled that placement of a vesicoamniotic shunt may help ensure a live birth with a decreased chance of pulmonary insufficiency, but that the infant would be expected to have renal insufficiency, may

require early dialysis, and would likely require early renal transplant if it survives the neonatal period. As with any invasive procedure, the patient must have a clear understanding of the potential risks of the procedure itself to both the mother and the fetus, the level of experience of the operator, as well as the possible complications that may occur later in the pregnancy.

TECHNIQUE

Vesicoamniotic shunting represents a temporary therapeutic intervention allowing simple diversion of fetal urine from the obstructed bladder into the amniotic space. It is essential that patients understand that such therapy is not curative but is, in essence, preventative in nature and the infant will require further evaluation and treatment for the obstruction following birth. Pregnancies complicated by severe oligohydramnios present a sonographic challenge in which visualization is significantly impaired. As such, we routinely utilize amnioinfusion at the time of initiation or our evaluation protocol to restore amniotic fluid volume to assist in sonographic visualization. Because amnioinfusion may carry an increased risk for chorioamnionitis, we routinely give the patient a loading dose and begin a 10-day course of oral antibiotics for prophylaxis.

Vesicocentesis is performed under continuous ultrasound guidance to ensure appropriate needle position throughout. Using a 22-gauge needle, the fetal abdomen is approached just above the pubic rami and lateral to midline. Before entering the bladder, color-flow Doppler is used to ensure that the potential needle track does not pass through the umbilical vessels that course laterally about the bladder. The needle is then passed into the lower bladder and the urine completely emptied while constantly maintaining needle-tip placement within the cavity of the shrinking bladder (Fig. 55-6). Needle placement too high in the megacystis will not allow complete drainage as the bladder drains downward into the fetal pelvis. Paralyzing the fetus with IM pancuronium is generally not necessary during vesicocentesis or vesicoamniotic shunt placement procedures.

Careful sonographic evaluation prior to attempted shunt placement is essential to identify the location and position of the fetus and placenta. It is preferable if the fetus can be approached without having to pass the shunt trocar through the placenta. If a transplacental approach is unavoidable, one must traverse the placenta in a single smooth motion, keeping lateral motion of the trocar to a minimum, utilizing color-flow Doppler prior to passage through the chorionic plate to identify surface vessels that must be avoided. If possible, the fetus should be in the back down, vertex position, allowing a straight approach as high in the fundus as possible. This will significantly reduce the risk of post-procedure fluid leakage. Patient, gentle external manipulation can many times improve and optimize fetal position.

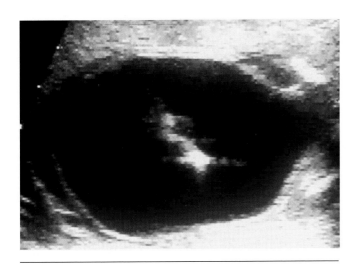

FIGURE 55-6 Ultrasound showing needle within the fetal bladder during vesicocentesis. Note the absence of amniotic fluid around the fetal abdomen due to anhydramnios.

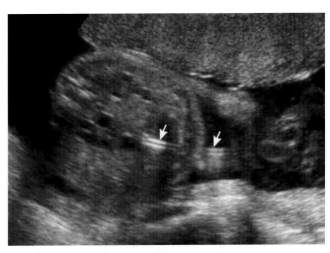

FIGURE 55-7 Ultrasound of fetal pelvis following vesicoamniotic shunt placement. The fetal bladder is no longer distended, and arrows show the coiled ends of the shunt within the bladder and within the amniotic space.

Once the appropriate approach is chosen, the maternal skin is anesthetized with 1% lidocaine and a small 3–5 mm stab wound made to allow easy passage of the shunt trocar. The shunt trocar is then carefully introduced into the amniotic space near the lower fetal abdomen. An adequate pocket of amniotic fluid needs to be present in which to drop the distal end of the vesicoamniotic shunt on exiting the fetal abdomen. If no such space is present, amnioinfusion to create such a fluid pocket can be done through the trocar. The tip of the trocar is positioned in the same manner as the vesicocentesis needle and color-flow Doppler used to confirm the absence of umbilical vessels at that position. The trocar is then quickly inserted into the bladder and positioned into a central location. At this point, the operative assistant should have carefully and gently straightened the vesicoamniotic catheter. The catheter is then threaded into the trocar sheath prior to removal of the internal stylet wire. If the wire is removed prior to threading the catheter, difficulty with kinking and directing the catheter down the shaft of the trocar sheath may be encountered. Once in place, a short push rod is introduced and used to push the proximal segment of the catheter into the fetal bladder. This is then removed and a long push rod gently introduced until it comes in contact with the distal end of the shunt within the trocar sheath. The push rod is then held at this position while the shaft of the trocar sheath is slowly pulled back approximately 1 cm. At this point, the trocar sheath should lie just outside of the fetal abdomen, with the straight segment of the shunt catheter traversing the region between the bladder and amniotic space. Failure to properly perform this maneuver may result in partial displacement of the proximal end of the catheter and increased risk for shunt displacement.

The trocar sheath is now gently directed slightly away from the insertion site and the long push rod advanced to displace the distal end of the catheter into the amniotic space. Positioning of the proximal and distal segments of the catheter as well as subsequent bladder drainage is confirmed sonographically

(Fig. 55-7). The patient is then placed on external fetal/uterine monitoring for approximately 2 hours. Any indication of uterine irritability is aggressively treated with intravenous fluids and tocolytic medications. In addition, the patient is started on a 2-week course of oral antibiotics.

COMPLICATIONS

Counseling of the patient prior to embarking on a course of prenatal evaluation includes discussions of potential complications of any invasive needle procedure such as subsequent chorioamnionitis, premature rupture of fetal membranes, direct trauma to the fetus, and intraplacental bleeding and possible associated onset of preterm labor if transplacental approaches become necessary.

Transient vesicoperitoneal fistulas occasionally occur following vesicocentesis, resulting in urinary ascites (Fig. 55-8). Such fistulas spontaneously close in 10–14 days followed by redevelopment of megacystis. If the urinary ascites results in massive distension of the abdomen, drainage can be accomplished by placement of a peritoneal amniotic shunt. These can be easily placed into either of the lower abdominal quadrants, although care must be taken to avoid traumatic damage to the viscera from the shunt trocar. Once placed, the urinary ascites can be easily diverted to the amniotic cavity until fistula closure is complete.

Shunt displacement is also a fairly common complication, occurring in approximately 40% of cases in our series. Despite the fact that the catheter is designed such that the distal end curls lie flat against the fetal abdomen, it may become dislodged, necessitating replacement with recurrence of the megacystis. If the catheter is placed too high within the megacystis, it may be placed under tension as the bladder shrinks with drainage, and eventually be displaced and pulled within the fetal abdomen, resulting in loss of function.

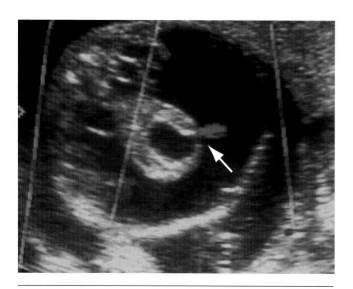

FIGURE 55-8 Ultrasound of a thickened fetal bladder and urinary ascites after displacement of a vesicoamniotic shunt into the amniotic space. Arrow points to the transient fistula in the bladder wall with urine streaming into the abdomen using color-flow Doppler.

Also, we have seen several cases of successful shunt placement at 19 and 20 weeks gestation, in which catheter placement and function was optimal with decreasing hydronephrosis and maintenance of good amniotic fluid volumes. Unfortunately, in these cases, at 26–27 weeks gestation the amniotic fluid volume began to slowly decrease, the renal parenchyma became increasingly echodense, and renal growth as measured from superior to inferior pole stopped and regressed over time. The majority of these cases result in neonatal demise. On autopsy, they demonstrated severe micro cystic dysplasia and fibrosis, however, the catheter was noted to be patent and appropriately positioned within the fetal bladder. The reasons for these occurrences remain unclear.

FOLLOW-UP

Following a vesicoamniotic shunt procedure, we perform a follow-up sonographic evaluation 24–48 hours later to confirm catheter placement and function. Weekly evaluations are recommended for at least the next 4–6 weeks to confirm catheter placement and function, amniotic fluid volume, and progressive resolution of the bilateral hydronephrosis. At that point, evaluations may be spaced to every 10–14 days, depending on maintenance of amniotic fluid volume.

Consultation with the pediatric urologist and neonatologist who will care for the child after birth is recommended so that postnatal management and treatment options can be discussed, a plan formulated, and a relationship established between the family and the postnatal team. This greatly facilitates communication and understanding of postnatal management, significantly reduces family anxiety, and fosters a trusting relationship between the family and medical team.

Route of delivery should be dictated by routine obstetrical indications and not influenced by the presence of

an indwelling catheter. Pregnancies that have undergone shunting in our clinical series[6] have experienced spontaneous rupture of membranes and vaginal delivery at 33–35 weeks gestation; the patient should be counseled about this possibility.

Following delivery, a bag can be placed on the abdomen to catch the urine, which can then be used for renal function studies. Also, the indwelling catheter can be used for retrograde dye studies of the urinary tract prior to simply pulling the catheter once it is no longer necessary for urinary diversion.

CONGENITAL CYSTIC ADENOMATOID MALFORMATION (CCAM)

Congenital cystic adenomatoid malformations are benign, space-occupying tumors of bronchial origin. They are generally classified into microcystic, macrocystic, and mixed types, depending on the size of the cysts they contain (Figs. 55-9 to 55-11). CCAMs can occasionally contain a single or several macrocysts, which fill it with fluid, progressively enlarging until they form very large space-occupying lesions within the fetal chest. Such large lesions, particularly within the lower-left lobe, can cause mediastinal shift and compromise the hemodynamic state of the fetus, resulting in the development of nonimmune hydrops. Once the fetus has developed hydropic changes, the prognosis becomes quite poor and the risk for intrauterine demise high. Early development and enlargement of lesions can result in significant compression of fetal lung tissues, which, if present during the critical transition from canalicular to alveolar stage between 18–24 weeks gestation, may result in lethal pulmonary hypoplasia. In addition, large macrocysts can lead to compression of the fetal esophagus, resulting in decreased fetal swallowing and the development of polyhydramnios and risk of preterm delivery of a compromised infant.

The goal of shunt therapy in such cases focuses on chronic drainage of large macrocysts. Early therapy would be directed at preventing pulmonary hypoplasia, while later interventions would be done for hemodynamic disturbances resulting in evolving hydrops or progressive polyhydramnios due to esophageal compression.

PRENATAL EVALUATION

The differential diagnosis for echogenic, cystic intrathoracic masses includes cystic adenomatous malformation, teratoma, bronchogenic cyst, diaphragmatic hernia, and extralobar pulmonary sequestration (Table 55-2). Prenatal evaluation of such cases includes a complete high-resolution sonographic fetal survey to rule out additional fetal anomalies that may indicate the presence of a more complex genetic syndrome. Detailed fetal echocardiography is necessary because cardiac anomalies may be associated with such lesions; it is also an important component of the evaluation in the presence of fetal hydrops,

Detailed Doppler flow studies of the lesions may help differentiate CCAMs from other masses, such as lung sequestrations which are usually associated with an anomalous artery originating off the fetal aorta while CCAM masses derive their blood supply from pulmonary origin (Fig. 55-12).

Patient Selection Criteria

In utero surgical interventions should be reserved only for those fetuses who have developed secondary complications that worsen the pregnancy prognosis, such as early onset pulmonary compression, evolving hydrops, or progressive polyhydramnios, and in whom simple chronic drainage of a dominant macrocyst would potentially correct the underlying physical disturbances that lead to secondary complications. It must be stressed that such intervention is only temporizing and not corrective in nature, and that the fetus continues to be at risk for subsequent complications and poor outcome due to the primary underlying lesion. The fetus must have the diagnosis of macrocystic CCAM confirmed by high-resolution ultrasound; fetuses afflicted with other potential lesions will not benefit and could be harmed by attempted intervention using transthoracic shunts. In the presence of hydrops, the fetus should be evaluated for other causes of hydrops so as not to overlook an associated anomaly.

TECHNIQUE

Once a fetus is identified who meets the above criteria and intervention holds the potential for benefit, the first step in therapy involves the initial drainage of the macrocyst. The initial step is very important because the cyst may not reaccumulate fluid and this minimally invasive drainage may be the only intervention needed; or the cyst may rapidly reaccumulate fluid demonstrating the need for chronic drainage. The initial cyst drainage is done under continuous high-resolution ultrasound guidance in which a 22-gauge spinal needle is carefully introduced into the amniotic cavity at the appropriate angle to allow a single linear entrance into the fetal thorax between the mid-axillary and mid-clavicular lines. The point of entrance through the fetal chest into the macrocyst should be chosen with careful consideration to how the cyst will predictively shrink during the drainage process such that the cyst can be completely drained of essentially all its fluid while retaining the original position of the needle insertion and eliminating the need for needle repositioning and multiple transthoracic passage. Aspirated fluid may be analyzed for cell count and viral assay to help differentiate a lymphatic (chylous hydrothorax) from an infectious etiology. A >95% mononuclear cell type is highly suggestive of a lymphatic etiology.

Following fine-needle aspiration, we generally re-evaluate the fetus 3–5 days later to determine whether fluid has re-accumulated within the macrocyst or whether there has been a change in secondary complications following the decompression of the macrocyst. If the fluid has not re-accumulated and

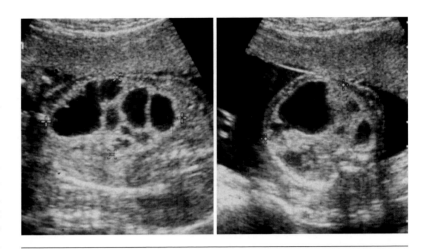

FIGURE 55-9 Sonographic image of a macrocystic congenital cystic adenomatoid malformation of the middle and lower lobes of the right lung. The fetus developed hydrops and had shunts placed into the upper and lower cyst complexes. Child is now 6 years old and developing normally.

secondary complications are resolving, then no further intervention is necessary and weekly sonographic surveillance is suggested to follow the growth of the underlying CCAM and to monitor for additional complications. If the fluid does not return but fetal hydrops or polyhydramnios does not resolve,

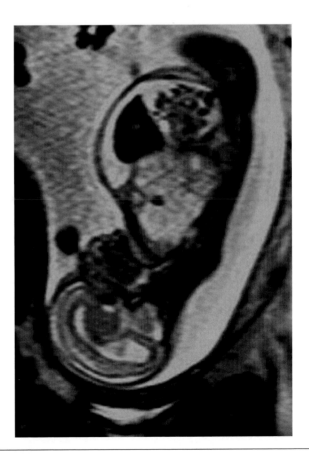

FIGURE 55-10 Ultrafast fetal MRI showing a large, right-sided type II congenital cystic adenomatoid malformation and secondary fetal hydrops. Fetus underwent in utero mass resection and survived.

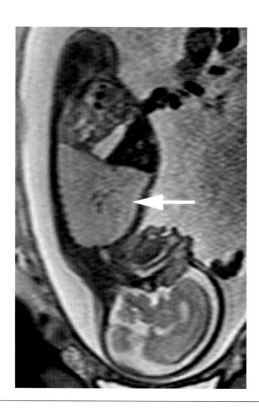

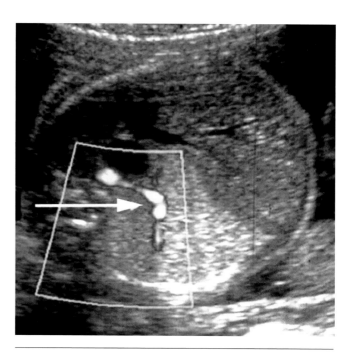

FIGURE 55-12 Sonographic image of a bronchopulmonary seques-tration with color Doppler demonstration of blood supply to the wedge-shaped echogenic mass from the descending aorta.

FIGURE 55-11 Ultrafast fetal MRI showing a large, left-sided type III congenital cystic adenomatoid malformation that is displacing the posterior aspect of the fetal diaphragm into the abdomen and displac-ing the left kidney from the renal fossa. This fetus never developed hydrops, the mass decreased in volume in the third trimester, and the infant delivered using an EXIT-to-mass-resection strategy and survived.

then the prognosis is guarded and alternative etiologies for these problems should be pursued. If the fluid re-accumulates over the course of several days and secondary findings persist, then the fetus should be considered a candidate for chronic shunt drainage.

Prior to attempting shunt placement, the patient should be carefully and thoroughly counseled about the purpose and po-tential benefits of such therapy, as well as the potential risks and complications of the procedure to both the mother and fetus. These include technical failure in placement or function of the shunt, possible infection, preterm labor, traumatic injury, and possible fetal death. In addition, the patient should be aware that the shunt may become displaced into the fetal chest or

TABLE 55-2	DIFFERENTIAL DIAGNOSIS IN CONGENITAL CYSTIC ADENOMATOUS MALFORMATION

Teratoma
Bronchial cyst
Diaphragmatic hernia
Extralobar pulmonary sequestration
Congenital cystic adenomatous malformation

out into the amniotic cavity, which may necessitate the place-ment of an additional shunt if the macrocyst and associated secondary complications recur.

Careful consideration needs to be given to the predicted pattern of cyst involution during drainage based on the previous fine-needle cyst aspiration procedure such that the shunt can be placed at the macrocyst's predicted position on achieving minimum size following successful shunt placement. If this is not done, the macrocyst can potentially move away from the catheter where it enters the fetal chest as the cyst drains, resulting in less of the proximal pigtail within the cyst and a much higher risk of shunt displacement out of the cyst cavity. In addition, when draining a macrocyst within the left thorax, one must position the catheter to enter the fetal chest at the superior and lateral left aspect of the macrocyst to encourage the expected upward and lateral involution of the cyst, thus allowing resolution of mediastinal structures to their normal position within the left chest (Figs. 55-13, 55-14). Placement of the catheter in the mid-clavicular line low within the fetal chest could potentially interfere with restoration of normal cardiac and mediastinal positions and put the catheter at increased risk for displacement.

COMPLICATIONS

If the catheter is not optimally placed initially, it is possible that it will be displaced and drawn into the chest cavity as the macrocyst involutes with drainage. This could result in a poten-tial pleural effusion with its associated complications and may necessitate the placement of a thoracoamniotic shunt. Also, the fetus may actively or passively participate in the displacement

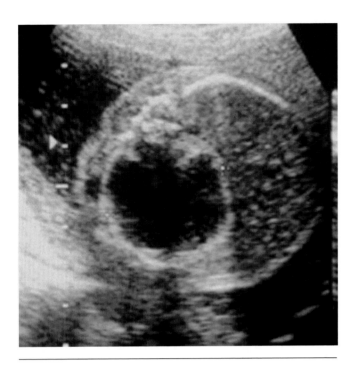

FIGURE 55-13 Macrocystic congenital cystic adenomatoid malformation of the right lung with features of early hydrops.

of the catheter out of the chest such that it is free within the amniotic space necessitating the placement of an additional shunt if the macrocyst and associated secondary complications recur. In our experience, such displaced catheters do not pose a risk to the fetus. Other potential complications include

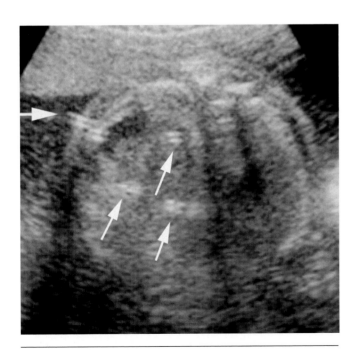

FIGURE 55-14 Macrocystic lesion shown in Fig. 13 following placement of a pleuroamniotic shunt. Following shunt placement, the mass volume decreased by 52% and the hydropic changes resolved.

vascular trauma if one is not careful when choosing a site to place the catheter, and it recommended that color-flow Doppler be used prior to insertion of the catheter into the chest to identify any large vessels along the chosen route of shunt placement. Although not directly contraindicated, all efforts should be made to avoid trocar passage through the placenta; this may result in hematoma formation or vascular damage to the placenta, resulting in fetal death. If no other access to the fetus is available, then the placenta should be traversed in a single pass as far away from cord insertion as possible, using color-flow Doppler to identify and avoid large vessels coursing through the placenta at the chorionic plate. In addition, all insertions should be done as high in the fundal region of the uterus as possible; this will reduce the risk of amniotic fluid leakage and associated risks of oligohydramnios and chorioamnionitis.

FOLLOW-UP

After shunt placement, we routinely have the patient return for follow-up evaluation in 2–3 days to document catheter placement and function. Following this postoperative exam, we recommend weekly sonographic evaluations to document continued shunt function, resolution of associated problems (polyhydramnios/hydrops), and to continue close monitoring of the underlying CCAM lesion and potential additional complications that might arise due to these lesions. Mode of delivery for an infant with an indwelling catheter should be determined by obstetrical indications only, and most would be expected to deliver vaginally. It is highly recommended that the neonatal team be notified well in advance of the delivery as many infants with CCAM have special pulmonary needs in the immediate postnatal period.

IDIOPATHIC PLEURAL EFFUSION

Pleural effusion(s) can present as isolated sonographic findings or as part of a more generalized picture of non-immune fetal hydrops. The etiologies of pleural effusions (Table 55-3) are those of nonimmune hydrops and include association with underlying fetal aneuploidy, in utero infections, cardiovascular malformations, lymphatic anomalies, and hematological perturbations resulting in fetal anemia. Isolated pleural effusions that do not progress to fatal fetal hydrops pose a threat to the developing fetus by intrathoracic compression of the developing lungs, interference with fetal swallowing resulting in

TABLE 55-3	POTENTIAL ETIOLOGIES OF ISOLATED PLEURAL EFFUSIONS
Infectious	
Hematologic	
Chromosomal	
Cardiac anomalies	
Metabolic disorders	
Lymphatic anomalies	

polyhydramnios, and potential disturbances in blood flow secondary to increased intrathoracic pressure or mediastinal shift of the heart and great vessels.

Prenatal Evaluation

Prenatal evaluation focuses on identifying cases of isolated, idiopathic pleural effusion(s) by searching for other etiologies mentioned previously. Detailed, high-resolution study of the fetus is essential to rule out other associated anomalies that may contribute to the effusions or identify the fetus as at risk for a more complex underlying genetic syndrome. A fetal echocardiogram will allow detailed evaluation of the heart and associated major vessels to identify those effusions that may be secondary to cardiovascular malformations. Cordocentesis can be a helpful component of the work-up if the effusions progress to a more generalized picture of hydrops. Fetal blood allows for rapid evaluation of a fetal karyotype, hematological abnormalities by hematocrit and reticulocyte count, and fetal infection by IgG/IgM titers for specific pathogens as well as liver enzymes, albumin, and total protein values.

The interventive goal for a unilateral or bilateral placement of thoracoamniotic shunts would be continuous chronic drainage of idiopathic pleural effusion(s), allowing re-expansion and normal development of compressed pulmonary tissues in fetuses during the critical transition phase from canalicular to alveolar lung development occurring between 18–24 weeks' gestation, the reduction in intrathoracic pressures that may inhibit fetal swallowing leading to polyhydramnios and increased risk for preterm delivery, or the resolution of mediastinal shift and improved hemodynamic status, which may otherwise result in lethal fetal hydrops. Selection criteria for identifying fetuses that may benefit from such intervention are listed in Table 55-4.

An important component of the evaluation involves the performance of a fine-needle thoracocentesis (Fig. 55-15). Under continuous ultrasound guidance, a 22-gauge needle is passed into the lower, lateral aspect of the hemithorax between the midclavicular and midaxillary lines. This entrance point is important in that this is the most dependent portion of the thorax into which the effusion will collect as you aspirate, allowing the maximum amount of fluid to be removed while avoiding intrathoracic structures that may begin to return to their normal anatomic positions during the aspiration. Such drainage also allows for assessment of lung re-expansion following drainage, and evaluation of underlying lung abnormal-

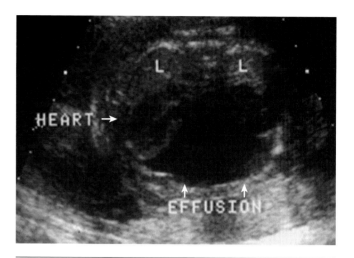

FIGURE 55-15 Sonographic image of congenital hydrothorax. Note the posterior compression of the lungs (L) by the large effusion, body wall edema, and displacement and compression of the heart within the right chest.

ities such as extralobar pulmonary sequestration which can be associated with pleural effusions. Sonographic re-evaluation is then done at 48–72 hours later to evaluate for recurrence of the effusion. In some cases, the effusion(s) will not recur and the single thoracentesis is curative. In others, the effusion(s) will not recur for several weeks. In these cases, therapeutic thoracocentesis may be performed every few weeks as clinically indicated by the volume of effusion present and the development of secondary complications such as polyhydramnios or those suggestive of fetal hydrops. When multiple interventions are necessary during the course of the pregnancy, antibiotic prophylaxis is recommended utilizing an agent known to achieve therapeutic levels in the amniotic fluid. Cases in which the effusion(s) rapidly reaccumulate following thoracocentesis represent those in which the fetus will most likely benefit from chronic drainage through thoracoamniotic shunt placement (Fig. 55-16).

Technique

The approach to placement of thoracoamniotic shunts is similar to that for macrocystic CCAM, except that the shunt only traverses the chest wall. The same technical considerations pertain to shunt placement as discussed with diagnostic effusion drainage. Shunts placed into the left thorax should be positioned into the mid-chest along the axillary line to facilitate drainage and allow the heart to return to its normal anatomical position. Shunts placed into the right thorax should be positioned in the lower one third of the chest between the midclavicular and axillary lines to allow maximal expansion of the right lung with drainage.

COMPLICATIONS

Occasionally the catheter will become displaced into the amniotic cavity and need to be replaced if the effusion(s) recur.

TABLE 55-4	SELECTION CRITERIA FOR PLEURAL EFFUSIONS

Normal karyotype
Negative viral cultures
Normal echocardiogram
Normal laboratory evaluation
Effusion(s) recur following drainage
Normal phenotype on ultrasound exam

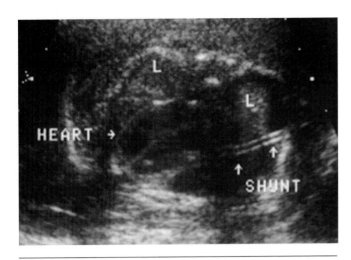

FIGURE 55-16 Sonographic image of the same fetus in Fig. 15 approximately 30 seconds following placement of a thoracoamniotic shunt. Note how the heart is no longer compressed and has shifted to midline, and the lungs (L) are beginning to expand.

Less commonly, if the catheter was improperly placed initially, it may migrate into the thoracic cavity becoming an indwelling foreign body with recurrence of the effusion(s) necessitating a second shunt placement. Care must be taken to stay lateral during catheter insertion as medial insertions may result in placement within the mediastinum, thus isolating the shunt from the pleural space requiring drainage. Also, placement too high or posteriorly in the chest cavity may result in incomplete drainage as the catheter tip may become occluded by the fetal lung as it expands to fill the space made by the draining effusion. Certainly one must stay well away from the paraspinal regions because of the possibility of vascular and nerve-root damage. Lastly, it is possible that the catheter may become occluded by proteinacious material within the effusion or by thrombus if bleeding occurred during shunt placement, resulting in loss of function, although sonographically the catheter appears to be optimally placed.

FOLLOW-UP

Follow-up sonographic evaluation is initially done at 48–72 hours later to confirm successful catheter placement and function as evidenced by the resolving effusion, re-expansion of the fetal lungs, and restoration of normal mediastinal relationships. After, the patient is generally rescanned at weekly intervals to confirm catheter placement and function.

Route of delivery of the infant is dictated by obstetrical factors. If the catheter is not pulled out during the delivery process, it should immediately be clamped to prevent pneumothorax.

Once removed, a chest tube often needs to be placed for transient postnatal chylothorax.

SUMMARY

The era of fetal medicine has become a reality as we have developed methodologies to medically and surgically treat fetuses in utero. Advances in diagnostic technology have improved our capacity to evaluate selectively fetuses with genetic disorders. In many such cases, fetuses that had previously faced a dismal prognosis can now be considered potential candidates for therapeutic intervention. The key to success in such interventions is an appreciation of the diversity of underlying etiologies and pathologic processes, as well as a thorough understanding of the appropriate detailed prenatal evaluation necessary for patient selection. Only then can one reliably predict which fetuses will truly benefit from invasive intervention, and prevent unnecessary procedures in cases where such intervention will not alter the eventual outcome and only serve to place the mother at unnecessary risk for complications.

References

1. Freedman AL, Qureshi F, Shapiro E, et al. Smooth muscle development in obstructed fetal bladder. *Urology*. (submitted).
2. Freedman AL, Bukowski TP, Smith CA, et al. Fetal therapy for obstructive uropathy: diagnosis specific outcomes. *Urology*. (submitted).
3. Quintero RA, Johnson MP, Romero R, et al. In utero percutaneous cystoscopy in the management of fetal lower obstructive uropathy. *Lancet*. 1995;346:537–540.
4. Inselman LS, Mellins RB. Growth and development of the lung. *J Pediatr*. 1981;98:1–15.
5. Johnson MP, Corsi P, Bradfield W, et al. Sequential fetal urine analysis provides greater precision in the evaluation of fetal obstructive uropathy. *Am J Obstet Gynecol*. 1995;173:59–65.
6. Johnson MP, Bukowski TP, Reitleman C, et al. In utero surgical treatment of fetal obstructive uropathy: a new comprehensive approach to identify appropriate candidates for vesicoamniotic shunt therapy. *Am J Obstet Gynecol*. 1994;170:1770–1779.
7. Qureshi F, Jacques SM, Seifman B, et al. In utero fetal urine analysis and renal histology do correlate with outcome in fetal obstructive uropathies. *Fetal Diagn Ther*. (submitted).
8. Johnson MP, Hume P, Quintero R, et al. In utero analysis of fetal proteinuria in obstructive uropathy. Proceedings of the 14th International Fetal Medicine & Surgery Society; 1995 May 3–6; Newport, RI; 1995.

THE EVOLUTION OF FETAL SURGERY FOR TREATMENT OF CONGENITAL DIAPHRAGMATIC HERNIA

George B. Mychaliska / Michael R. Harrison

INTRODUCTION

Managing a fetus with prenatally diagnosed congenital diaphragmatic hernia (CDH) requires an understanding of natural history, pathophysiology, and prognostic factors. Although progress has been made in postnatal management, 58% of fetuses diagnosed with CDH prior to 24 weeks die despite optimal postnatal management including extracorporeal membrane oxygenation (ECMO).[1] Traditionally, a family carrying a fetus with a CDH had 2 options: pregnancy termination or delivery in a tertiary neonatal center. Fetal surgery now offers the possibility of intervention before birth. Fetal surgery is justified if (1) the prenatal diagnosis is certain, (2) the pathophysiology is understood, (3) the prognosis is poor, and (4) maternal safety is assured.

The in utero treatment of CDH has fueled an intensive experimental and clinical research effort. Despite 2 decades of experimental work on animals and a decade of human experience establishing the efficacy of in utero intervention, many hurdles remain. While complete in utero repair of CDH appears to work for fetuses without liver herniation into the chest, this approach has not worked for fetuses with liver herniation because immediate reduction of the viscera and liver cause kinking of the umbilical vein. This devastating problem was the impetus for the PLUG (*P*lug the *L*ung *U*ntil it *G*rows) strategy that creates tracheal occlusion to allow the lungs to expand slowly without disruption of umbilical blood flow. Despite advances in surgical technique and monitoring, pre-term labor remains the nemesis of open fetal surgery. Intractable preterm labor was a major stimulus to develop minimally invasive techniques (Fetendo) to treat CDH in utero.

This chapter chronicles the evolution of in utero treatment of CDH. The rationale for in utero intervention will be presented in the context of the pathophysiology of CDH with reference to animal models. Prior to human application, prenatal diagnosis, prognosis, and maternal-fetal safety had to be assured. We will then present the evolution of open fetal surgery, PLUG strategies, and endoscopic fetal surgery for in utero treatment of CDH.

EXPERIMENTAL RATIONALE FOR IN UTERO INTERVENTION

Initial studies in the fetal lamb were undertaken to unravel the pathophysiology and the reversibility of pulmonary hypoplasia in CDH. Fetal lambs had a silicone-rubber balloon progressively inflated in their left hemithorax during the last trimester to simulate compression by herniated viscera.[2] Lambs with inflated intrathoracic balloons deteriorated rapidly at delivery despite maximal resuscitation and died of severe respiratory failure. At autopsy, the lungs were severely hypoplastic. To determine if pulmonary hypoplasia was reversible, the balloon was deflated at 120 days gestation (simulated correction).[3] All lambs with simulated correction of CDH were easily resuscitated and had normal pulmonary function. Simulated correction produced increased lung weight, air capacity, compliance, and area of the pulmonary vascular bed (Fig. 56-1). Because the fetal lung maintains remarkable plasticity even late in gestation, in utero repair may allow the hypoplastic lung in fetuses with CDH to grow and develop.

While the sheep model demonstrated that in utero correction of CDH allowed the lung to grow and develop enough to ensure survival at birth, it differed from human CDH in several respects. The human diaphragmatic defect is present much earlier in gestation (the first trimester), although the viscera may not herniate until later. Also, although the high mortality of infants with CDH has been attributed to respiratory insufficiency from pulmonary parenchymal hypoplasia, other major physiologic abnormalities are pulmonary hypertension and persistent fetal circulation. These abnormalities lead to muscularized pulmonary arterioles which present a high resistance to the flow of fetal blood.

To address these physiologic differences, CDH was created in fetal lambs early in gestation (60 days; term = 145 days) and morphometric analysis of the pulmonary vascular bed was subsequently performed.[4] The CDH was repaired in experimental lambs at 100 days gestation and an unrepaired group served as controls. The CDH group demonstrated decreased cross-sectional area of the pulmonary vascular bed, decreased number of vessels per unit area of the lung, and increased muscularization of the arterial tree. In utero repair of CDH at 100 days ameliorated this abnormal pulmonary arteriolar muscle hyperplasia, allowed impressive restoration of lung volume, and restored the pulmonary arterial tree almost to normal.[4]

TECHNIQUE OF IN UTERO SURGICAL CORRECTION

After the experimental rationale for in utero treatment of CDH was established, surgical techniques for in utero repair were developed in a fetal lamb model. The diaphragmatic defect was created in the fetal lamb by making a hole in the left diaphragm at 100 days gestation allowing herniation of abdominal viscera and reliably producing pulmonary hypoplasia. At a second operation on day 120, the diaphragmatic hernia was repaired.[5] Initial attempts at repair were unsuccessful because reduction of viscera increased intraabdominal pressure causing decreased umbilical blood flow and subsequent fetal demise. A silastic abdominal silo overcame this problem. In addition, intrathoracic volume displacement also affected umbilical flow, by shifting the mediastinum and impeding venous return. To stabilize the mediastinum and to minimize pressure-volume changes in the chest, the air in the partially empty left side of the chest was replaced with warm Ringer's lactate solution

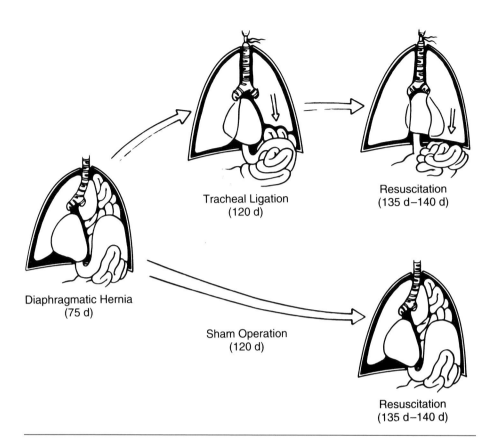

FIGURE 56-1 Fetal lambs with simulated CDH died despite maximal resuscitation and had severely hypoplastic lungs. Lambs "corrected" by balloon deflation in the middle of the last trimester had sufficient lung growth and development to permit survival at birth. Lung weight and air capacity were greater than for lambs with CDH but less than controls. (From Harrison MR, Bressack MA, Churg AM, et al. Correction of congenital diaphragmatic hernia in utero II. Simulated correction permits fetal lung growth with survival at birth. *Surgery.* 1980;88:264; with permission.)

before the diaphragm was closed. When these techniques were used for repair of the diaphragmatic hernia, 6 of 10 lambs were viable after term delivery. At autopsy, the lungs were well expanded, histologically mature, and much larger than those of the controls. These studies showed that correction of diaphragmatic hernia is technically feasible when an appropriate procedure is used. This observation has been confirmed by several investigators in a fetal lamb model.[6]

PRENATAL DIAGNOSIS AND PROGNOSIS

Prior to considering in utero intervention in human fetuses, the accuracy of prenatal diagnosis had to be assured. As a result of advances in prenatal sonography, CDH is frequently diagnosed before birth.[7-9] Fortunately, in our experience, false-positive diagnoses of CDH by ultrasound are rare. However, it is possible that CDH could be misdiagnosed in cases of cystic lung disease (ie, congenital lobar emphysema, cystic adenomatoid malformation) or with mediastinal cystic processes (i.e., neurenteric cysts, bronchogenic cysts, thymic cysts). Although a fluid-filled structure may be present within the chest and may even cause a mediastinal shift, the upper abdominal anatomy should be normal in these fetuses. It is particularly important to exclude large cystic adenomatoid malformations, which may

decrease in size and disappear with time. In cases for which doubt exists, computed tomography or radiography following instillation of contrast material into the amniotic cavity should clarify the anatomy.

Given accurate prenatal diagnosis of CDH, families are faced with difficult choices: termination of pregnancy, standard postnatal therapy, or in utero intervention. Despite our ability to make a prenatal diagnosis and provide intensive care postnatally, the neonatal mortality rate associated with CDH remains high. Retrospective estimates of mortality for CDH vary widely and are flawed by a "hidden mortality" of unknown magnitude because the most severely affected babies never make it to the tertiary center. In a prospective study of 83 fetuses with isolated CDH diagnosed before 25 weeks gestation, 58% died despite optimal postnatal care at an (ECMO) center (Fig. 56-2).[1]

Since the optimal fetal surgery candidate is one who is less likely to survive with standard postnatal care, accurate prognostic indicators would be ideal. Because there is a broad spectrum of severity, some assessment of the degree of pulmonary hypoplasia would be helpful in selecting management. Unfortunately, there is no way to evaluate the functional capacity of the fetal lung because, unlike the fetal kidney which functions before birth, the crucial gas-exchange function of the lung does not become necessary until birth. The degree of pulmonary hypoplasia appears to be affected by the timing and volume of visceral herniation into the chest.[10] Babies who herniate late in gestation or after birth have essentially normal lungs and are guaranteed to live. Babies who herniate very early in gestation have severe pulmonary hypoplasia and are likely to die. Polyhydramnios,[8] detection of CDH before 25 weeks,[9] presence of an intrathoracic stomach,[11–13] small lung-thorax transverse area ratio,[14] and underdevelopment of the left heart region[15,16] have all been associated with poor prognosis, but none of these parameters has been universally accepted or applied.

A new and promising sonographic parameter measures the right lung size compared to head circumference (to correct for gestational age) in order to estimate the degree of pulmonary hypoplasia. The right lung was assessed because the left lung frequently cannot be distinguished sonographically from bowel or liver in fetuses with CDH. The ratio of the right lung area (2-dimensional area at the level of the atria) to head circumference LHR (*L*ung to *H*ead *R*atio) appeared to predict outcome in some cases.[17] In a series of 55 cases, very small right lung size (LHR <0.6) uniformly predicted mortality (5 cases) while large right lung size (LHR >1.35) appeared to ensure survival (14 cases) independent of liver position or gestational age at time of diagnosis. Unfortunately, the majority of cases fell between 0.6 and 1.35. Our results suggest that cases diagnosed before 25 weeks with a small LHR and liver herniation into the chest have the poorest prognosis. This is now confirmed by a large multi-institutional study that defines candidate for treatment before birth: liver herniation and LHR less than 1.0.[18]

In addition to the importance of accurate diagnosis and prognosis of CDH, the presence of multiple associated morphologic and chromosomal abnormalities will influence therapeutic decisions. Studies of prenatally diagnosed CDH suggest that associated anomalies in severe cases of CDH occur in approximately 37% of cases.[9] Current prenatal diagnostic techniques can detect almost all of these defects. Consequently, a thorough sonographic examination of the fetus with CDH is essential to detect the presence of other structural anomalies. Amniocentesis for karyotype analysis is indicated to rule out chromosomal anomalies.

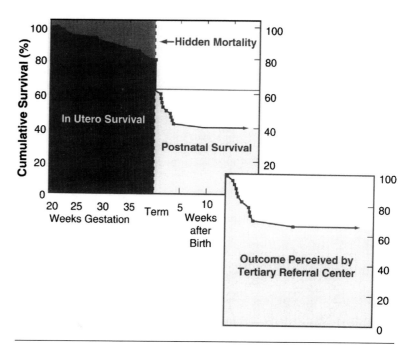

FIGURE 56-2 A cumulative survival plot for 52 fetuses with isolated CDH diagnosed before 25 weeks gestation. Ten fetuses died in utero or from prematurity, and 9 died immediately after birth; most of these would not be recognized as having CDH unless an autopsy was performed. These deaths represent a significant "hidden mortality" that is not perceived when only babies seen at tertiary neonatal referral centers are considered (exploded inset). (From Harrison MR, Adzick NS, Estes JM, et al. A prospective study of the outcome for fetuses with diaphragmatic hernia. *JAMA.* 1994;271(5):383; with permission.)

weighed against the risk of a potentially debilitating or fatal defect. With appropriate selection, benefit to the fetus should dramatically outweigh the risk. Since fetal CDH does not threaten the mother, she must weigh the risk of major surgery against the potential benefits of salvaging her unborn child or alleviating her own burden raising a child with a severe malformation. We believe that for fetal surgery, the rights and safety of the mother must always be placed above those of the fetus. Therefore, any fetal procedure that presented significant risk to the life, function, or future fertility of the mother would be unacceptable. We first demonstrated that hysterotomy and fetal surgery did not adversely affect the mother or her ability to carry subsequent normal pregnancies in the nonhuman primate[20–22] and in our first 17 patients.[23,24] We have had no maternal deaths and few serious maternal complications, but our patients have experienced considerable morbidity, related primarily to preterm labor and its treatment. The choice to proceed with fetal surgery remains highly personal and each mother must weigh these risks and benefits for herself and her family.

MATERNAL AND FETAL CONSIDERATIONS

Ethical Concerns

Fetal therapy raises a number of complex ethical, personal, and societal issues.[19] For the fetus, the risk of surgery must be

Fetal Surgical Procedures

Clinical fetal surgical principles have been derived from more than 1,600 operations in fetal lambs and 400 operations in fetal

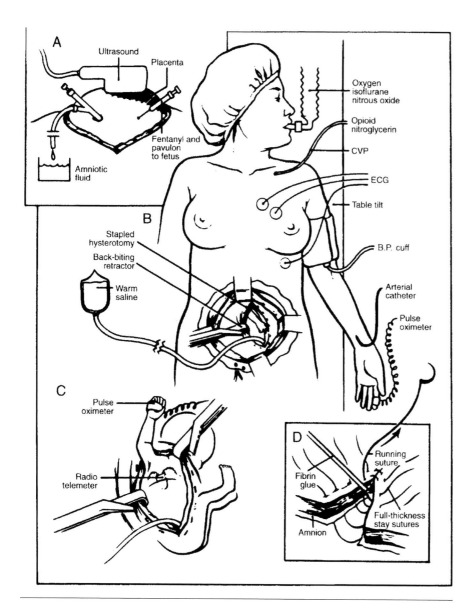

FIGURE 56-3 Fetal surgery techniques. (**A**) The uterus is exposed through a low, transverse abdominal incision. Ultrasound localizes the placenta; (**B**) Maternal positioning includes a leftward tilt to avoid compression of the inferior vena cava by the gravid uterus. The hysterotomy is made away from the placenta using staples that provide hemostasis and seal the membranes. Warm saline is continuously infused around the fetus and the pertinent fetal anatomy exposed. Maternal anesthesia, tocolysis, and monitoring are shown; (**C**) After fetal repair the uterine incision is closed with absorbable sutures and fibrin glue. Amniotic fluid is restored with warm Ringer's lactate; (**D**) (Adapted from Longaker MT, Golbus MS, Filly RA, et al. Maternal outcome after open fetal surgery: A review of the first 17 human cases. *JAMA.* 1991;265:737–741; with permission.)

rhesus monkeys over the past 15 years.[25] For a fetal surgical operation, the mother is supine, with her right side slightly elevated to prevent aortocaval compression by the gravid uterus. The uterus is exposed through a low transverse incision. Sterile ultrasound is used to determine fetal and placental position. Hysterotomy is made at least 6 cm from the placental edge. A specially devised Lactomer uterine stapling device (U.S. Surgical Corp., Norwalk, CT) that fixes the membranes to the myometrium is used for the hysterotomy.[26] Warm saline is

infused constantly into the open uterus. Only the part of the fetus to be operated upon is exposed. Fetal monitoring is achieved with a miniaturized pulse oximeter wrapped around the fetal hand. Periodic sonography monitors heart rate and contractility. During the operation, a radiotelemeter is implanted under the chest wall which transmits continuous electrocardiogram and intrauterine pressure (Fig. 56-3).[27]

After the procedure, the uterine cavity is filled with warm saline and antibiotics. The staples in the hysterotomy edge are excised to permit muscle-to-muscle approximation during closure. The uterus is closed in 2 layers, with an inner running layer for the membranes and myometrium, and an interrupted layer of full-thickness absorbable monofilament sutures. Fibrin glue is placed between the layers to help seal the membranes.

Maternal Perioperative Care

Intraoperatively, mothers are monitored with a central venous pressure catheter and a radial arterial line. For tocolysis, the mother receives preoperative indomethacin and inhalational halogenated anesthesia. Additionally, she may receive intravenous magnesium sulfate, terbutaline, and/or nitroglycerin during the operation. Postoperative tocolysis consists principally of indomethacin, magnesium sulfate, and terbutaline. By 48 hours, she usually requires only subcutaneous terbutaline via a portable pump that continues after hospital discharge. Obstetric ultrasound and fetal echocardiography substitute for the fetal physical exam, and are performed daily in the early postoperative period. On average, the mother is discharged 8 days post-surgery.

In our experience, fetuses who have undergone in utero surgery almost always deliver preterm. The fetus is delivered by cesarean section at a tertiary center when either the membranes rupture or labor cannot be controlled. Because the hysterotomy is performed in the upper segment of the uterine corpus, and thus is comparable to a classic cesarean section, all future deliveries must be accomplished by cesarean section.

The most glaring deficiency in management is our inability to manage the preterm labor induced by hysterotomy and fetal surgery. To date, we have relied on the regimen used (often ineffectively) for spontaneous preterm labor, including external monitoring with a tocodynemometer, bed rest, intravenous magnesium sulfate, IV or subcutaneous betamimetics, and oral prostaglandin synthetase inhibitors. Our experience suggests that the entire regimen is inadequate for fetal surgery. While experimental work with other agents such as IV nitroglycerin looks promising,[28] intractable preterm labor remains the bane of fetal surgery.

COMPLETE IN UTERO CDH REPAIR

For fetuses with no liver herniated into the chest, prenatal repair using a "2-step" technique to reduce the viscera, close the diaphragm, and enlarge the abdomen permits compensatory fetal lung growth and survival after birth.[23,29,30] The traditional subcostal incision used to repair CDH postnatally provided inadequate exposure in the fetus. The solution was a "2-step" approach using both a thoracotomy and a subcostal incision, allowing reduction of viscera using a "push-pull" technique, reconstruction of the diaphragm with a Gore-Tex patch, and enlargement of the abdominal cavity with a Gore-Tex silo (Fig. 56-4).

We recently studied the safety and efficacy of in utero repair of "liver down" CDH in an NIH-sponsored prospective trial. Although in utero repair appeared to improve pulmonary function, as evidenced by fewer days of mechanical ventilation

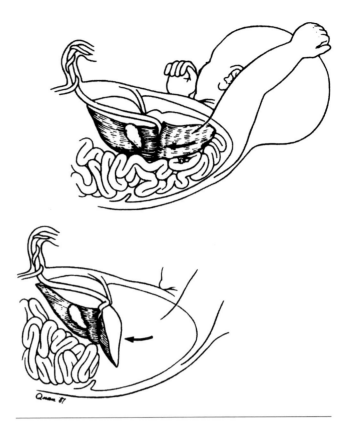

FIGURE 56-5 Attempts to reduce the herniated fetal liver (arrows) cause fetal deterioration and demise; autopsy and angiogram studies have documented kinking of the umbilical vein with compromise of venous return. (From Harrison MR, Langer JC, Adzick NS, et al. Correction of congenital diaphragmatic hernia in utero V. Initial clinical experience. *J Pediatr Surg.* 1990;25:50; with permission.)

and less need for ECMO, fetal surgery did not improve survival in these infants. Overall mortality was extremely low in both the fetal surgery group (25%) and the comparison group (12%), suggesting that liver down CDH may have a more benign postnatal course regardless of treatment.[31]

Diaphragmatic hernias in which a major portion of the liver is incarcerated in the chest ("liver up" CDH) are impossible to repair in utero because reducing the liver back into the abdomen results in acute obstruction of umbilical venous return and fetal death (Fig. 56-5).[23,32] Diagnostic techniques using color flow Doppler imaging of the umbilical and portal vessels now allow accurate detection of liver herniation.[33] Fetuses with liver herniation have never been successfully repaired completely in utero despite extensive efforts using a variety of techniques.[23]

PLUG: *PLUG THE LUNG UNTIL IT GROWS*

In utero treatment of these "liver up" CDH fetuses has required a fundamentally different approach. In the course of exploring the pathophysiology of CDH, experimental work has shown that fetal tracheal obstruction can correct the pulmonary hypoplasia associated with CDH.[34-39] Throughout gestation, the fetal lung produces lung fluid that exits through the trachea into the amniotic fluid. External drainage

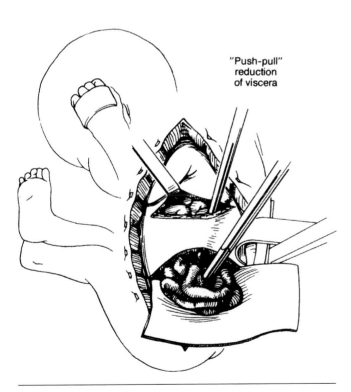

FIGURE 56-4 The CDH "two-step." The viscera (stomach, bowel, spleen) are reduced through the defect and out onto the abdominal patch by gently pushing from the thoracic incision and pulling from the abdominal incision. (From Harrison MR, Adzick NS, Flake AW, et al. The CDH Two-Step: A Dance of Necessity. *J Pediatr Surg.* 1993;28(6):814; with permission.)

"Push-pull" reduction of viscera

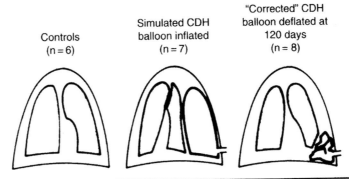

Viability	6/6 Lived	6/6 Died	5/5 Lived (with respiratory distress)
Lungweight	123.2 ± 25.4	49.6 ± 6.6	79.1 ± 6.0
Lungweight Bodyweight	3.42 ± 0.30	1.71 ± 0.03	2.26 ± 0.14
Aircapacity	222.5 ± 47.9	58.8 ± 7.6	151 ± 10.0
Aircapacity Bodyweight	6.24 ± 0.84	2.37 ± 0.12	4.55 ± 0.32

FIGURE 56-6 Tracheal occlusion can be used to treat diaphragmatic hernia. Diaphragmatic hernias were created in fetal lambs that then either underwent tracheal ligation or a sham operation. In the lambs with ligated tracheas, the viscera were reduced and the lungs were much bigger. (From Hedrick MH, Estes JM, Sullivan KM, et al. Plug the Lung Until it Grows (PLUG): A new method to treat congenital diaphragmatic hernia in utero. *J Pediatr Surg.* 1994;29(5):613; with permission.)

of fetal lung fluid in experimental animals retards lung growth resulting in pulmonary hypoplasia,[40,41] whereas tracheal obstruction markedly accelerates lung growth, resulting in pulmonary hyperplasia.[34–44] In fetal lambs with surgically created diaphragmatic hernias, tracheal obstruction expands the fetal lung, pushing the viscera back into the abdomen and producing lungs that are larger and functionally better at birth than untreated controls (Fig. 56-6).[34–39] In order to apply this strategy of tracheal obstruction to human fetuses with CDH, we developed techniques to achieve temporary tracheal occlusion that did not damage the fetal trachea and could be easily reversed at birth. The PLUG (*P*lug the *L*ung *U*ntil it *G*rows) procedure takes advantage of this phenomenon. Using the fetal lamb model, we developed and tested a variety of techniques including an internal occlusion device (plug) made of water-impermeable, expandable, polymeric foam that can be placed through the larynx, and external occlusion devices such as metal clips.[36]

We applied this strategy of temporary tracheal occlusion in 8 human fetuses with CDH and liver herniation at 25–28 weeks gestation. With ongoing experimental and clinical experience, the technique of tracheal occlusion evolved from an internal plug (2 patients) to an external clip (6 patients) and a technique was developed for unplugging the trachea at the time of birth EXIT (*E*x *U*tero *I*ntrapartum *T*reatment).[44] Translaryngeal placement of a foam plug appeared to be simple and easy to reverse at birth, but produced tracheomalacia in the first successful case and incomplete occlusion in the second case. External metal clips were used for the next 6 patients. Placement of 2 opposing large hemoclips with an

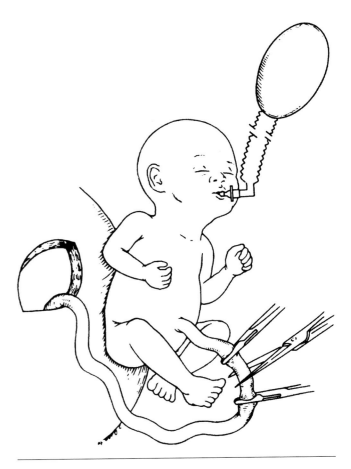

FIGURE 56-7 The crux of the EXIT procedure is securing the airway before the cord is divided.

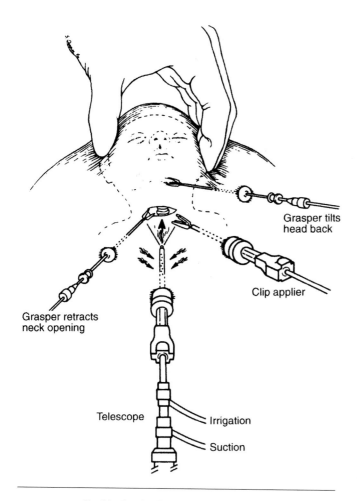

FIGURE 56-8 Positioning for fetoscopic tracheal occlusion with maternal laparotomy.

attached monofilament suture for removal at birth proved to be the most efficacious method of tracheal occlusion with minimal tracheal damage.

The time in gestation when the fetal tracheal obstruction is created also evolved. Because our experimental and clinical work showed that the fetal lung enlarged quite rapidly in response to tracheal occlusion, we have delayed the time of repair from 24 weeks to 26–28 weeks of gestation in order to have a more mature lung and fetus at delivery.

To optimize delivery of a fetus with a tracheal clip in place, we modified the anesthetic and surgical technique of cesarean delivery to maintain feto-placental circulation while the fetal airway is secured (Fig. 56-7). The mother is anesthetized using high doses of inhaled halogenated agents supplemented with single doses of nitroglycerin or terbutaline as necessary to insure complete uterine relaxation throughout the procedure. The fetal head and shoulders are delivered through the previous hysterotomy, but the lower torso and umbilical cord remain within the uterus. Because the umbilical circulation provides gas exchange, there is adequate time to expose the fetal neck, pass a bronchoscope, remove an internal plug or

external clip, secure the airway with an endotracheal or tracheostomy tube, suction lung fluid, administer surfactant, and begin ventilation—all before the umbilical cord is divided and the baby delivered.

Two fetuses had a foam plug placed inside the trachea: the first showed dramatic lung growth in utero and survived, and the second (who had a smaller plug to avoid tracheomalacia) showed no demonstrable lung growth and died at birth. Two fetuses had external spring loaded, aneurysm clips placed on the trachea: 1 was aborted due to tocolytic failure, and the other showed no lung growth (presumed leak) and died 3 months after birth. Four fetuses had metal clips placed on the trachea: all showed dramatic lung growth in utero with reversal of pulmonary hypoplasia documented after birth. However, all died of nonpulmonary causes.[46]

Temporary occlusion of the fetal trachea accelerates fetal lung growth and ameliorates the often fatal pulmonary hypoplasia associated with severe CDH. Although the strategy is physiologically sound and technically feasible, complications encountered during the evolution of these techniques have limited survival. In our prospective randomized trial fetuses who had a tracheal balloon showed lung growth but delivered early, so their survival was no different than fetuses who did not have fetal intervention but were delivered and cared for in the same tertiary center.[17] There is also concern about other effects of tracheal occlusion. Accumulating evidence suggests that tracheal obstruction may also delay or depress pulmonary maturation and surfactant production.[47,48] Although further evolution of this technique is required before it can be recommended as

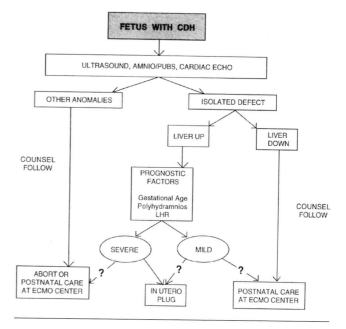

FIGURE 56-9 Algorithm for management of the fetus with CDH. (Adapted from Harrison MR, Langer JC, Adzick NS, et al. Correction of congenital diaphragmatic hernia in utero V. Initial clinical experience. *J Pediatr Surg.* 1990;25:54; with permission.)

therapy for fetal pulmonary hypoplasia, promising results have been reported using percutaneous fetal___ tracheal occlusion and subsequent deflation or removal of the balloon prior to vaginal delivery.[18,49]

FUTURE DIRECTIONS

Fetendo: Fetal Endoscopic Treatment

A major advance is the recent development of less invasive procedures that allow fetal repair without opening the uterus using video-assisted fetal endoscopy (Fetendo) (Fig. 56-8).[50–52] Fetendo may decrease preterm labor by decreasing uterine injury. Urinary tract obstruction has been corrected using this technique and work is ongoing to allow endoscopic tracheal occlusion. New miniaturized instruments and new techniques are making minimally invasive fetal surgery a reality.

Neonatal Lung Transplantation

Cadaveric, or living-related donation of a more mature reduced size lung (pulmonary lobe or segment) may work and help solve the critical donor shortage.[53] In utero transplantation of hematopoietic stem cells from the lung donor may induce tolerance and facilitate graft survival.[54]

CONCLUSION

We are continuing to refine surgical techniques and patient selection criteria to help fetuses with CDH. The pulmonary hypoplasia that limits survival is an underdevelopment of both the parenchyma and the pulmonary vascular bed, and appears to be reversible both experimentally and clinically. However, many weeks or even months are required. ECMO is limited to 1–2 weeks, and while useful for marginal babies, it clearly cannot salvage severely affected babies. Long-term support or replacement of lung function after birth will require either an artificial placenta or neonatal lung transplantation. Repair before birth with continued support on the "placental ECMO" while the fetal lung grows and recovers would be ideal. However repair in utero with continued gestation has proven to be a formidable challenge. Unraveling the pathophysiology of induced preterm labor and development of minimally invasive surgical techniques will promote the success of in utero treatment of CDH.

The family's dilemma in choosing management is particularly difficult because the natural history of fetal CDH is quite variable. Although some new sonographic parameters look promising, there are no prognostic criteria that adequately predict which fetus will survive and which will die. Optimal management of severely affected fetuses remains an unsolved problem (Fig. 56-7). For fetuses without liver herniation, repair before birth using a 2-step procedure that allows reduction of the viscera, reconstruction of the diaphragm, and enlargement of the abdomen to accept the returned viscera is physiologically sound and technically feasible but does not appear to improve survival. Fetuses with liver herniation into the chest have never been successfully repaired in utero, despite extensive efforts using a variety of techniques. For these fetuses, we are testing the concept that tracheal obstruction can ameliorate hypoplasia by accelerating the growth and development of the fetal lung before birth.

References

1. Harrison MR, Adzick NS, Estes JM, et al. A prospective study of the outcome for fetuses with diaphragmatic hernia. *JAMA*. 1994;271: 382.
2. Harrison MR, Jester JA, Ross NA. Correction of congenital diaphragmatic hernia in utero: the model: intrathoracic balloon produces fatal pulmonary hypoplasia (part I). *Surgery*. 1980;88:174.
3. Harrison MR, Bressack MA, Churg AM, et al. Correction of congenital diaphragmatic hernia in utero. Simulated correction permits fetal lung growth with survival at birth (part II). *Surgery*. 1980;88: 260.
4. Adzick NS, Outwater KM, Harrison MR, et al. Correction of congenital diaphragmatic hernia in utero: an early gestational fetal lamb model for pulmonary vascular morphometric analysis (part IV). *J Pediatr Surg*. 1985;20:673.
5. Harrison MR, Ross NA, de Lorimier AA. Correction of congenital diaphragmatic hernia in utero: development of a successful surgical technique using abdominoplasty to avoid compromise of umbilical blood flow (part III). *J Pediatr Surg*. 1981;16:934.
6. Soper RT, Pringle KC, Scofield JC. Creation and repair of diaphragmatic hernia in the fetal lamb: techniques and survival. *J Pediatr Surg*. 1984;19:33.
7. Chinn DH, Filly RA, Callen PW. Congenital diaphragmatic hernia diagnosed prenatally by ultrasound. *Radiology*. 1083;148:119.
8. Adzick NS, Harrison MR, Glick PL, et al. Diaphragmatic hernia in the fetus: prenatal diagnosis and outcome in 94 cases. *J Pediatr Surg*. 1985;20:357.
9. Adzick NS, Vacanti JP, Lillehei CW, et al. Fetal diaphragmatic hernia: ultrasound diagnosis and clinical outcome in 38 cases. *J Pediatr Surg*. 1989;24:654.
10. Stringer MD, Goldstein RB, Filly RA, et al. Fetal diaphragmatic hernia without visceral herniation. *J Pediatr Surg*. 1995;30:1264.
11. Bohn D, Tanura M, Perrin D. Ventilatory predictors of pulmonary hypoplasia in congenital diaphragmatic hernia, confirmed by morphologic assessment. *J Pediatr*. 1987;111:423.
12. Burge DM, Atwell JD. Could the stomach site help predict outcome in babies with left sided congenital diaphragmatic hernia diagnosed internally? *J Pediatr Surg*. 1989;24:567.
13. Geggel RL, Murphy JD, Langleben D. Congenital diaphragmatic hernia: arterial structural changes and persistent pulmonary hypertension after surgical repair. *J Pediatr*. 1985;107:457.
14. Goodfellow T, Hyde I, Burge DM. Congenital diaphragmatic hernia: the prognostic significance of the site of the stomach. *Br J Radiol*. 1987;60:993.
15. Adzick NS, Harrison MR, Glick PL. Maternal outcome after fetal surgery. *J Pediatr Surg*. 1986;21:477.
16. Crawford DC, Wright VM, Drake DP, et al. Fetal diaphragmatic hernia: the value of fetal echocardiography in the prediction of postnatal outcome. *Br J Obstet Gynaecol*. 1989;96:705.
17. Metkus AP, Filly RA, Stringer MD, et al. Sonographic predictors of survival in fetal diaphragmatic hernia. *J Pediatr Surg*. 1996;31: 148.

18. Harrison MR, Keller RL, Hawgood SB, et al. A randomized trial of fetal endoscopic tracheal occlusion for severe fetal congenital diaphragmatic hernia. *N Engl J Med.* 2003;349(20):1916–1924.

19. Fletcher JC, Jonsen AR. Ethical considerations in fetal treatment. In: Harrison MR, Golbus MS, Filly RA, eds. *The Unborn Patient: Prenatal Diagnosis and Treatment.* Philadelphia: Saunders; 1991; 14.

20. Longaker MT, Golbus MS, Filly RA. Maternal outcome after open fetal surgery: a review of the first 17 human cases. *JAMA.* 1991;265: 737.

21. Nakamaya KD, Harrison MR, Seron-Ferre M. Fetal surgery in the primate: uterine electromyographic response to operative procedure and pharmacologic agents (part III). *J Pediatr Surg.* 1984;19:333.

22. Sharland GK, Lockhart SM, Heward AJ. Prognosis in congenital diaphragmatic hernia. *Am J Obstet Gynecol.* 1992;166:9.

23. Harrison MR, Adzick NS, Flake AW, et al. Correction of congenital diaphragmatic hernia in utero: hard-earned lessons (part VI). *J Pediatr Surg.* 1993;28:1411.

24. Tibboel D, Bos AP, Pattenier JW. Preoperative stabilization with delayed repair in congenital diaphragmatic hernia. *Zeitschrift fuer Kinderchirurgie.* 1989;44:139.

25. Harrison MR, Adzick NS. Fetal surgical techniques. *Semin Pediatr Surg.* 1993;2:136.

26. Bond J, Harrison M, Slotnick R, et al. Cesarean delivery and hysterotomy using an absorbable stapling device. *Obstet Gynecol.* 1989;74:25.

27. Jennings RW, Adzick NS, Longaker MT, et al. Radiotelemetric fetal monitoring during and after open fetal operation. *Surg Gynecol Obstet.* 1993;176:59.

28. Jennings RW, MacGillivray TE, Harrison MR. Nitric oxide inhibits preterm labor in the rhesus monkey. *J Matern Fetal Med.* 1993;2:170.

29. Harrison MR, Adzick NS, Longaker MT. Successful repair in utero of a fetal diaphragmatic hernia after removal of viscera from the left thorax. *N Engl J Med.* 1990;322:1522.

30. Harrison MR, Adzick NS, Flake AW, et al. The CDH two-step: a dance of necessity. *J Pediatr Surg.* 1993;28:813.

31. Harrison M, Adzick N, Bullard K, et al. In utero repair of congenital diaphragmatic hernia: a prospective trial. Unpublished data.

32. MacGillivray TE, Jennings RW, Rudolph AM, et al. Vascular changes with in utero correction of diaphragmatic hernia. *J Pediatr Surg.* 1994;29:992.

33. Bootstaylor BS, Filly RA, Harrison MR, et al. Prenatal sonographic predictors of liver herniation in congenital diaphragmatic hernia. *J Ultrasound Med.* 1995;14:515.

34. Wilson JM, DiFiore JW, Peters CA. Experimental fetal tracheal ligation prevents the pulmonary hypoplasia associated with fetal nephrectomy: possible application for congenital diaphragmatic hernia. *J Pediatr Surg.* 1993;28:1433.

35. Hedrick M, Estes J, Sullivan K, et al. Plug the lung until it grows (PLUG): a new method to treat congenital diaphragmatic hernia in the fetus. *J Pediatr Surg.* 1994;29:612.

36. DiFiore JW, Fauza DO, Slavin R, et al. Experimental fetal tracheal ligation reverses the structural and physiological effects of pulmonary hypoplasia in congenital diaphragmatic hernia. *J Pediatr Surg.* 1994;29:248.

37. Bealer JF, Skarsgard ED, Hedrick MH, et al. The 'PLUG' odyssey: adventures in experimental fetal tracheal occlusion. *J Pediatr Surg.* 1995;30:361.

38. Beierle EA, Langham MR, Cassin S. In utero lung growth in fetal sheep with diaphragmatic hernia and tracheal stenosis. *J Pediatr Surg.* 1996 Jan;31(1):141–6.

39. Luks FI, Gilchrist BF, Jackson BT, et al. Endoscopic tracheal obstruction with an expanding device in the fetal lamb model: preliminary considerations. *Fetal Diagn Ther.* 1996 Jan–Feb;11(1):67–71.

40. Carmel J, Friedman F, Adams F. Fetal tracheal ligation and tracheal development. *Am J Dis Child.* 1965;109:452.

41. Alcorn D, Adamson T, Lambert T. Morphologic effects of chronic tracheal ligation and drainage in the fetal lamb lung. *J Anat.* 1976;22:649.

42. Moessinger AC, Harding R, Adamson TM, et al. Role of lung fluid in growth and maturation of the fetal sheep lung. *J Clin Invest.* 1990;86:1270.

43. Hooper SB, Man VKM, Harding K. Changes in lung expansion after pulmonary DNA synthesis and IGFII gene expression in fetal sheep. *Am J Physiol.* 1993;265 suppl:L403.

44. Hooper SB, Harding R. A major determinant of the growth and functional development of the fetal lung. *Clin Exp Pharmacol Physiol.* 1995;22:235.

45. Mychaliska GB, Bealer JF, Graf JL, et al. Operating on placental support: the ex utero intrapartum treatment procedure. *J Pediatr Surg* 1997;32(2):227–30.

46. Harrison M, Adzick N, Flake AW, et al. Correction of congenital diaphragmatic hernia in utero VIII: Response of the hypoplastic lung to tracheal occlusion. *J Pediatr Surg.* 1996;31(10):1339–48.

47. O'Toole SJ, Sharma A, Karamanoukian HL, et al. Tracheal ligation does not correct the surfactant deficiency associated with congenital diaphragmatic hernia. *J Pediatr Surg.* 1996;31:546.

48. Bullard KM, Sonne J, Hawgood S, et al. Tracheal ligation increases cell proliferation but decreases surfactant protein in fetal murine lungs in vitro. *J Pediatr Surg.* 1997;32(2):207–11.

49. Deprest J, Jani J, Gratacos E, et al. FETO Task Group. Fetal intervention for congenital diaphragmatic hernia: the European experience. Semin Perinatol. 2005 Apr;29(2):94–103.

50. Estes JM, MacGillivray TE, Hedrick MH, et al. Fetoscopic surgery for treatment of congenital anomalies. *J Pediatr Surg.* 1992;27: 950.

51. Skarsgard ED, Meuli M, VanderWall KJ, et al. Fetal endoscopic tracheal occlusion ('Fetendo-PLUG') for congenital diaphragmatic hernia. *J Pediatr Surg.* 1996;31(10):1335–8.

52. VanderWall KJ, Bruch SW, Meuli M, et al. Fetal endoscopic ('Fetendo') tracheal clip. *J Pediatr Surg.* 1996 Aug;31(8):1101–3.

53. Crombleholme TM, Adzick NS, Hardy K, et al. Pulmonary lobar transplantation in neonatal swine: a model for treatment of congenital diaphragmatic hernia. *J Pediatr Surg.* 1990;25:11.

54. Mychaliska GB, Rice HE, Tarantal AF, et al. In utero hematopoietic stem cell transplants induce tolerance for postnatal kidney transplantation in monkeys. *Surgical Forum.* 1996;47:443–445.

FETAL SURGERY—OPEN: CONGENITAL CYSTIC ADENOMATOID MALFORMATION

Darrell L. Cass / N. Scott Adzick

INTRODUCTION

Prenatal ultrasound and improved fetal diagnosis has provided new insight into the pathophysiology and natural history of congenital cystic adenomatoid malformation (CCAM). Using this technology, we have developed new management strategies aimed at improving the outcome of fetuses with this potentially fatal disease.

Congenital cystic adenomatoid malformation is a rare, congenital lung tumor for which the actual incidence remains unknown. The lesion was first described as a distinct pathologic entity by Ch'in and Tang[1] in 1949. Prior to that time CCAM was grouped under the general diagnosis of congenital cystic lung disease, along with bronchopulmonary sequestration, congenital lobar emphysema, bronchogenic cyst, and congenital cystic bronchiectasis.

A careful morphological description of CCAM was published by Stocker[2] in 1977. Grossly cystic adenomatoid malformation is a discrete, intrapulmonary mass that contains cysts ranging in diameter from less than 1 mm to over 10 cm. Microscopically, these malformations are characterized by an "adenomatoid" increase in terminal respiratory structures that form various sizes, intercommunicating cysts. Histologically, CCAM is distinguished from other lesions and normal lung by: (1) polypoid projections of the mucosa, (2) an increase in smooth muscle and elastic tissue within cyst walls, (3) an absence of cartilage (except that found in "entrapped," normal bronchi), (4) the presence of mucous secreting cells, and (5) the absence of inflammation. Although the tissue within these malformations does not function in normal gas exchange, there usually are connections with the tracheobronchial tree as evidenced by air trapping that frequently develops during postnatal resuscitative efforts.

Congenital cystic adenomatoid malformation occurs slightly more often in the left lung.[4,5] The lesion usually involves an entire pulmonary lobe, although as many as 17% are multilobar.[4] Rarely these lesions are bilateral, in which case they are uniformly fatal.[2–6]

There have been several attempts to classify CCAM based on histologic and clinicopathologic criteria. Stocker classified CCAM into 3 types based primarily on cyst size.[2] Type I CCAM consist of single or multiple large, thick-walled cysts, generally greater than 2 cm in diameter. Microscopically, these cysts have a noticeable increase in elastic tissue and smooth muscle, and are lined by mature ciliated, pseudostratified columnar epithelium. Type II lesions consist of numerous, smaller, evenly spaced cysts, usually less than 1 cm in diameter. These cysts are thinner-walled and lined by cuboidal to tall, columnar ciliated epithelium. In Stocker's classic description, Type II CCAM had a high association with other congenital defects. Type III lesions are bulky, firm, homogeneous masses that contain only microscopic cystic spaces (generally, less than 5 mm in diameter). Histologically, these lesions consist of abundant bronchiolar-like airspaces lined by ciliated cuboidal epithelium. Type III CCAM are the only truly "adenomatoid" malformations.

Adzick and colleagues have classified prenatally diagnosed CCAM into 2 categories based on gross anatomy and ultrasound findings.[7] Macrocystic CCAM contain single or multiple cysts that are 5 mm in diameter or larger and appear cystic on prenatal sonogram. Microcystic lesions are more solid, containing cysts smaller than 5 mm in diameter, and appear echogenic on prenatal ultrasound.

Since Stocker's initial series, other authors have reported an 11–21% incidence of associated congenital lesions in patients with CCAM.[4,5] The most common anomalies are renal, cardiac, gastrointestinal and craniofacial, and include: renal agenesis and Potter syndrome, tetralogy of Fallot, truncus arteriosus, VSD, congenital diaphragmatic hernia, intestinal atresias, and macrocephaly.

EMBRYOLOGY

The embryologic origin of CCAM remains speculative. Because of the segmental location of these lesions, the lack of cartilage, and the spectrum of associated congenital malformations, it is thought that these tumors arise between the 24th and 49th day of development.[2] These hypotheses remain unproven, however, as CCAM has never been diagnosed prior to the 16th week gestation by either autopsy or prenatal sonography.

Most pathologists consider CCAM a hamartoma, a developmental abnormality with excess of 1 or several tissue components. It is speculated that these lesions result from a localized arrest of the developing tracheobronchial bud.[2,8,9] Despite the resulting abnormal bronchial development, mesenchymal tissues proliferate leading to an overgrowth of bronchiolar-like air spaces and a paucity of normal alveoli.

Unlike bronchopulmonary sequestration (BPS), which is thought to arise as an aberrant outpouching from the developing foregut with systemic vascular supply, CCAM derives blood supply from the pulmonary circulation.[10] Because the natural history of sequestration appears to be different from that of CCAM,[6] it is important to use color flow Doppler when evaluating fetal lung masses in an effort to demonstrate systemic arterial blood supply to these lesions. Demonstration of a pulmonary tumor with a feeding vessel from the aorta is pathognomonic of bronchopulmonary sequestration.

NATURAL HISTORY

The natural history and clinical spectrum of fetuses with CCAM is quite variable and appears to depend on the size and secondary physiologic derangements caused by these tumors. As with all congenital, intrathoracic, space-occupying lesions,

CCAM produces a mass effect that can lead to both ipsilateral and contralateral pulmonary hypoplasia. Large malformations can produce mediastinal deviation or "shift," polyhydramnios and hydrops fetalis. Fetal hydrops is nearly always a predictor of fetal death.[11,12]

Polyhydramnios, seen with 50–70% of fetuses with CCAM, likely results from esophageal compression by the thoracic mass and decreased fetal swallowing of amniotic fluid.[5,7] This concept is supported by the frequent absence of fluid in the stomach of fetuses with large thoracic tumors and marked mediastinal shift, and the reappearance of stomach fluid and the resolution of polyhydramnios after effective fetal treatment.[12] Polyhydramnios is a marker for large thoracic tumors and often leads to prenatal ultrasound in the evaluation of maternal size to dates discordance.

Hydrops fetalis, seen in nearly 50% of fetuses with CCAM, refers to a pathologic increase of fluid in serous cavities or soft tissues of the fetus.[5,6] It is characterized sonographically by the presence of diffuse skin and scalp edema, or by the collection of fluid in more than 1 serous cavity (pleural, pericardial, or abdominal). Although CCAM is only a rare cause of nonimmune fetal hydrops (2% in 1 series), it is the most common intrathoracic lesion that can cause this derangement.[13] As we have demonstrated experimentally in a sheep model, fetal hydrops likely results from the mass lesion causing extreme mediastinal shift with vena cava and cardiac compression.[14] In some cases, hydrops may be exacerbated by loss of protein from the CCAM into the amniotic fluid leading to hypoproteinemia and decreased fetal oncotic pressure.[15] The presence of fetal hydrops may be the most important influence on fetal outcome.

CCAM can present as a fatal lesion in a fetus or neonate or as a relatively mild lesion that causes recurrent infections or minimal respiratory difficulty in an infant or child. Approximately 60–70% of patients with congenital cystic adenomatoid malformation will present at birth with respiratory distress that can result from air trapping, mediastinal compression, and pulmonary hypoplasia.[2,4,6] These patients usually require ventilatory support. In severe cases with large tumors and significant pulmonary hypoplasia, extracorporeal membrane oxygenation may be required. Once stabilized, these patients require resection of the tumor and relief of the mass effect.

Ten to 24% of patients with cystic adenomatoid malformation will be asymptomatic at birth.[2,4,6] These patients will present months to years later with repeated pneumonia or spontaneous pneumothorax that leads to further evaluation of the thorax. Rarely, CCAM is diagnosed as late as the teenage or adult years.[4,16,17] CCAM and other congenital lung lesions can rarely degenerate to malignancy. Embryonal rhabdomyosarcoma,[18] bronchioalveolar carcinoma,[19] myxosarcoma[20] and squamous cell carcinoma[21] have all been described to arise in association with congenital cystic lung lesions and CCAM. Although primary lung tumors are rare in the first 2 decades of life, 4% of these are associated with CCAM and other congenital cystic lung lesions.[19]

In early observations, 14–24% of CCAM were noted at stillbirth.[2,4] This observation suggested that there may be a different natural history for this disease when diagnosed antenatally.

ANTENATAL DIAGNOSIS OF CCAM

Most patients with CCAM are now diagnosed by obstetrical sonogram, either serendipitously or during the investigation of suspected maternal polyhydramnios or preterm labor. The diagnosis has been made sonographically as early as 16 weeks gestation;[22] however, most fetuses are diagnosed between 21 and 24 menstrual weeks.[5,11] Since the first report of prenatal diagnosis of CCAM by Garrett[22] in 1975, there have been over 210 cases reported in the world's literature.[5,23–35]

The classification and sonographic appearance of CCAM influences the differential diagnosis.[6] Macrocystic lesions can be difficult to distinguish from congenital diaphragmatic hernia (CDH). Demonstration of an intact diaphragm and the absence of intrathoracic peristalsis in herniated intestine or stomach help to exclude this diagnosis. Amniography with intrapartum single-section CT scan has occasionally been used to differentiate between CDH and CCAM. Prenatal sonography has been used to successfully diagnose CCAM in the presence of CDH.[23] New imaging modalities such as echoplanar magnetic resonance imaging and half Fourier single-shot turbo spin echo, or HASTE, may be useful prenatal imaging modalities in the future.[36] Microcystic CCAM are highly echogenic, which helps to distinguish these lesions from other solid tumors such as neuroblastoma. Bronchogenic or unilocular cysts are usually found next to major bronchi. Bronchopulmonary sequestration, particularly intralobar BPS, can be difficult to distinguish from CCAM. Demonstration of vascular supply from the thoracic or abdominal aorta by color flow Doppler is diagnostic for sequestration. Newer color Doppler modalities, such as enhanced or power Doppler, may be useful in distinguishing BPS from CCAM, and we have also found ultra-fast fetal MRI to be helpful.

Thorpe-Beeston and Nicolaides have recently reviewed 132 cases of prenatally diagnosed, pathologically proven or suspected CCAM.[5] Review of this series demonstrates the clinical features and natural history of fetuses with this malformation. The mean gestational age at diagnosis was 24.5 weeks (range 17–39 weeks). Fifty-nine percent of the lesions were macrocystic, 41% were microcystic. Eighty-six percent of the lesions were unilateral with a slight left-sided predominance (left—51% vs. right—35%), while 14% of the cases had bilateral involvement. Overall, 11% of the patients had associated malformations; however, the incidence was higher if the lesions were bilateral (28% vs. 10%), or microcystic (18% vs. 8%). Polyhydramnios was seen in 46% of the cases, and fetal hydrops was seen in 43%. In this cohort of 132 patients, 44 families elected to undergo pregnancy termination and 61 patients survived (representing 69% of those cases not undergoing termination, 46% of all cases). Thorpe-Beeston found that the likelihood of survival was slightly higher for macrocystic than for microcystic lesions (74% vs. 58%).

We have recently reviewed our own experience with 132 fetuses with CCAM, of which 55 (44%) had large lesions with associated hydrops. In this hydropic group, 12 fetuses were aborted, 24 died perinatally, and 19 underwent fetal therapy since hydrops is a predictor of perinatal demise. Of the 77 CCAM cases without hydrops, 70 have been successfully resected after birth. Many of these patients required ventilatory support, and 5 required ECMO. Seven patients with "shrinking" lesions have been followed without surgery.

ACCURACY OF PRENATAL DIAGNOSIS

Accurate intrauterine diagnosis of CCAM is based on a variety of factors including: (1) sonographic appearance of the mass (density, consistency, shadowing, vascularity), (2) mass location (left vs. right, anterior vs. posterior, unilateral vs. bilateral), and (3) associated findings (displacement of other viscera, other anomalies, fetal hydrops, polyhydramnios, systemic arterial supply). Although sonographic prenatal diagnosis is becoming increasingly sophisticated, diagnostic errors are still possible.

There have been few studies that have tried to evaluate the accuracy of prenatal sonography for diagnosing CCAM and other echogenic chest masses. McCullagh and colleagues at the Children's Hospital of Lewisham, London compared the postnatal diagnosis in 13 consecutive patients with a prenatal ultrasound diagnosis of CCAM (mean age at diagnosis = 22 weeks).[31] In this cohort the prenatal diagnosis has been confirmed pathologically in only 5 patients (38%). In 2 patients postnatal studies suggest CCAM, however the patients have yet to undergo resection. In 4 cases pathologic examination found bronchopulmonary sequestration ($n = 2$), bronchial atresia ($n = 1$), and lobar hyperplasia ($n = 1$). In 2 of 13 cases (15%), the abnormality was seen to regress spontaneously in utero. Postnatally, these patients remain asymptomatic without radiologic abnormalities.

King and colleagues at the Liverpool Maternity Hospital in the United Kingdom reviewed 17 consecutive patients that had echogenic chest masses on prenatal sonogram.[37] They compared prenatal diagnosis to postnatal or pathologic diagnosis. In this series, congenital diaphragmatic hernia was correctly diagnosed in 8 of 10 (80%) fetuses, bronchopulmonary sequestration in 4 of 5 (80%) fetuses, and tracheal atresia in 1 of 2 (50%) fetuses. In 1 fetus with hydrops and bilateral echogenic lungs, a diagnosis of CCAM was incorrectly made. Following termination the pathologic diagnosis of tracheal atresia was made. Additionally, there were 3 fetuses in which the diagnosis was inconclusive between CCAM and CDH. Two of 3 of these patients had CDH. One of these 3 patients had a suspected diagnosis of BPS by postnatal CT scan. Of the 5 patients with suspected BPS, 3 (60%) showed spontaneous regression on serial sonogram.

These studies suggest that it is important for fetuses with suspected CCAM and other anatomic malformations to be evaluated by experienced sonographers at centers that specialize in prenatal diagnosis and therapy. The accuracy of prenatal diagnosis will likely be greater in those centers that evaluate the largest number of patients. Clinicians who counsel families with these fetuses must be familiar with inaccuracies in prenatal diagnosis, as well as all possible treatment options.

DISAPPEARING LUNG LESIONS

Although the antenatal diagnosis of a large CCAM is overall an ominous finding, the natural history of these lesions is variable. A small percentage of these tumors can decrease in size and even disappear before birth. There have been 8 cases of pathologically proven, spontaneously regressing cystic adenomatoid malformation.[38,39] Interestingly, in 6 of 8 of these patients the lesion was located on the right side. There have been at least 23 more patients reported that have had prenatal sonographic findings suggestive of regressing CCAM, but the diagnosis has not been confirmed by pathology.[32,34,40–44] The percentage of cases that undergo spontaneous regression is not known for certain. Based on our experience at the University of California San Francisco and the Children's Hospital of Philadelphia as many as 15% of cases may decrease in size on serial ultrasound exam. Other authors have reported regression in from 13–17% of suspected cases of prenatally diagnosed CCAM.[5,45]

The reason for regression of congenital cystic adenomatoid malformation is not clear. Decompression of cystic lung fluid into the tracheobronchial tree or involution from outgrowing the blood supply are possible explanations. It is also possible that fetuses with disappearing cystic lung lesions have an erroneous diagnosis of CCAM. These patients may have bronchopulmonary sequestration, or another lung lesion that has a higher likelihood of decompression or involution. Sequestrations appear to undergo antenatal regression in as many as 66% of fetuses.[37,38,45] Recently, an echogenic lung mass was seen to resolve after relief of an obstructing mucous plug by postnatal bronchoscopy.[46] Thus far, we have no biochemical or sonographic marker that allows us to predict which CCAM will regress and which fetuses will develop hydrops and subsequent in utero demise. As a result, fetuses with CCAM must be followed closely with serial sonograms and families must be counseled appropriately. Fetal hydrops, however remains an accurate predictor of perinatal demise and is an indication for prenatal therapy in selected patients.

FETAL THERAPY

From insight into the antenatal natural history of CCAM we now know that as many as 50% of fetuses will develop hydrops and die perinatally.[6,7,11] Recent technological advances in obstetrical ultrasound has enabled the development of fetal therapy and new management strategies that are directed at altering this poor prognosis. Macrocystic CCAM may theoretically benefit from cyst decompression in order to decrease tumor size and to reverse or prevent mediastinal shift, polyhydramnios, and hydrops. There have been many reports in which thoracentesis was used in an effort to decompress large, macrocystic CCAM.[24,47–49] From these reports and from our own experience, it appears that cyst aspiration usually offers only short term decompression of dominant cysts. Fetal thoracentesis is limited by the rapid reaccumulation of cyst fluid and does not appear to alter the long-term outcome of these fetuses.

Thoracoamniotic shunts offer a theoretical advantage by providing continued drainage of the accumulating fluid in these lesions. The first successful thoracoamniotic shunts for CCAM were reported in 1987.[50,51] Nicolaides reported the placement of a "Rocket" double pigtail catheter into a large cystic lesion at 24 weeks gestation.[50] The shunt decompressed the lesion until spontaneous delivery occurred at 38 weeks. Clark reported successful percutaneous thoracoamniotic shunt placement and decompression of a macrocystic CCAM in a hydropic 20-week fetus.[51] Decompression of the lesion lead to resolution of mediastinal shift and hydrops, and the delivery of a 37-week infant who underwent uneventful resection of the CCAM. Despite these reports of early successes, the overall experience with thoracoamniotic shunts has been less favorable.

There have been another 22 cases of CCAM in the literature for which prenatal thoracoamniotic shunt placement was attempted.[5,25,52] Many of these shunts dislodged or clogged after relatively short periods of time. Moreover, catheters do not provide adequate drainage of multilobed cysts. Although the placement of catheters is less invasive than open fetal surgery, thoracoamniotic shunts appear to have limited usefulness for long-term therapy. In fetuses in whom nonimmune hydrops fetalis develops early, fetal surgery may provide the best option for ultimate survival. Additionally, when catheters do not adequately drain multicystic masses or when the sonographic appearance of the cyst is microcystic, surgery may be the only remaining option for fetal salvage.

FETAL SURGERY

The most worrisome prenatal presentation of CCAM is a large microcystic or multicystic tumor with hydrops that is not amenable to catheter decompression. In this subset of patients, fetal surgical resection may provide the only opportunity for survival. We have now performed fetal surgery on 13 such infants between 21 and 29 weeks' gestation with CCAM and hydrops.[11,53,54] Our results have been encouraging. In the 8 fetal patients who survived, CCAM resection led to resolution of hydrops, impressive in utero lung growth, and normal postnatal development. Following resection fetal hydrops resolved over a period of 1–2 weeks, and the mediastinum returned to the midline within 3 weeks.

We have learned valuable lessons from the 5 fetal patients who died. In the first case, resection was too late as preoperative labor and maternal preeclampsia persisted postoperatively, leading to premature delivery of a nonviable infant. From this experience we learned that the maternal hyperdynamic state referred to as the "mirror syndrome" cannot be reversed solely by treatment of the underlying fetal condition. This preeclamptic state is also seen with molar pregnancies and other fetal conditions that are associated with placentomegaly, and may be caused by a factor released by poorly perfused placental tissue that leads to endothelial cell injury.[55,56] Until the pathophysiology of the maternal mirror syndrome is understood, earlier intervention before the onset of placentomegaly and the re-

lated maternal preeclamptic state may be the only approach to salvage these doomed fetuses.

In another case, fetal resection of the right middle and lower lobes was a technical success at 21 weeks' gestation, but the fetus died in utero 8 hours postoperatively. Autopsy failed to reveal the cause of death. This case demonstrates the need for better postoperative fetal monitoring and treatment. In a third case, uncontrolled intraoperative uterine contractions led to fetal death, highlighting the need for better management of preterm labor. The remaining 2 unsuccessful cases were grossly hydropic fetuses at 21 weeks gestation who died after induction of maternal anesthesia or immediately after fetal thoracotomy.

This series demonstrates that in highly selected cases fetal CCAM resection is reasonably safe, technically feasible, reverses hydrops, and allows sufficient lung growth to permit survival. The clinical focus must now shift from the technical details of the fetal surgical procedure to the crucial need for better postoperative maternal-fetal monitoring and effective detection and treatment of preterm labor.

PRENATAL MANAGEMENT STRATEGY

The initial evaluation begins with an ultrasound to confirm the diagnosis, amniocentesis or percutaneous blood sampling to exclude chromosomal anomalies, and a fetal echocardiogram to rule out congenital heart disease. If an associated life-threatening anomaly is present or if the mother is sick with the mirror syndrome, then the family is counseled. For isolated fetal thoracic masses, the fetus undergoes a prognostic evaluation. If the fetus is not hydropic, then the mother is followed closely by serial ultrasonography. Fetuses with CCAM who do not have hydrops have a good chance for survival in the setting of maternal transport, planned delivery, and immediate resuscitation and surgery at a tertiary center with ECMO capability. Occasionally some of these lesions will shrink in size. At birth, babies that are asymptomatic and have evidence of a regressing CCAM should still be considered for surgical resection due to the long-term risks of infection, pneumothorax, and malignant degeneration.

If the fetus is hydropic at presentation or if hydrops develops during serial follow-up, then management depends on the gestational age and the degree of lung maturity. For those fetuses older than 32–34 weeks' gestation, betamethasone administration and early delivery should be considered so that the lesion can be resected ex utero. For those fetuses younger than 32 weeks' gestation, fetal surgical intervention should be entertained.

POSTNATAL MANAGEMENT

The fetus with CCAM should be referred to an institution that has appropriate staff and intensive care facilities to manage a critically ill neonate. At birth the newborn should be evaluated to confirm the diagnosis and to exclude associated anomalies. The pulmonary status should be monitored closely because of the risk of acute deterioration from air trapping, as well as pulmonary hypoplasia. Complete resection of the CCAM, usually by lobectomy, is the treatment of choice because of the risks of infection or malignant degeneration.[3,16,57,58] Incomplete resection of the tumor often leads to air leak at the surgical margin and usually requires reoperation.[16,57,58]

CONCLUSIONS

Overall, our experience with CCAM has been encouraging. Using recent advancements in prenatal ultrasound and fetal diagnosis we have gained new appreciation for the natural history of these lesions and new understanding for predictors of perinatal demise. This insight together with technologic advancements has allowed the development of fetal therapies that appear to improve the outcome of patients with this malformation. The evolution in the treatment of CCAM clearly demonstrates the integral role that ultrasound plays in providing accurate and timely prenatal diagnosis and therapy.

References

1. Ch'in KY, Tang MY. Congenital adenomatoid malformation of one lobe of a lung with general anasarca. *Arch Pathol.* 1949;48:221–229.

2. Stocker JT, Madewell JE, Drake RM. Congenital cystic adenomatoid malformation of the lung: classification and morphologic spectrum. *Hum Pathol.* 1977;8:155–171.

3. Halloran LG, Silverberg SG, Salzberg AM. Congenital cystic adenomatoid malformation of the lung. *Arch Surg.* 1974;104:715–719.

4. Miller RK, Sieber WK, Yunis EJ. Congenital cystic adenomatoid malformation of the lung: a report of 17 cases and review of the literature. *Pathol Ann.* 1980;1:387–407.

5. Thorpe-Veeston JG, Nicolaides KH. Cystic adenomatoid malformation of the lung: prenatal diagnosis and outcome. *Prenatal Diagn.* 1994;14:677–688.

6. Morin L, Crombleholme TM, D'Alton ME. Prenatal diagnosis and management of fetal thoracic lesions. *Sem Perinatol.* 1994;18:228–253.

7. Adzick NS, Harrison MR, Glick PL, et al. Fetal cystic adenomatoid malformation: prenatal diagnosis and natural history. *J Pediatr Surg,* 1985;20:483–488.

8. Moerman P, Fryns JP, Vandenberghe K, et al. Pathogenesis of congenital cystic adenomatoid malformation of the lung. *Histopathology.* 1992;21:315–321.

9. Cachia R, Soboonya RE. Congenital cystic adenomatoid malformation of the lung with bronchial atresia. *Hum Pathol.* 1981;12:947–950.

10. Skandalakis JE, Gray SW, Symbas P. Pulmonary circulation. In: Skandalakis JE, Gray SW, eds. *Embryology for Surgeons: The Embryological Basis for the Treatment of Congenital Anomalies.* 2nd ed. Baltimore, MD: Williams and Wilkins; 1994:451–490.

11. Adzick NS. Fetal cystic adenomatoid malformation of the lung: diagnosis, perinatal management, and outcome. *Semin Thorac Cardiovasc Surg.* 1994;6:247–252.

12. Neilson IR, Russo P, Laberge JM, et al. Congenital adenomatoid malformation of the lung: current management and prognosis. *J Pediatr Surg.* 1991;26:975–981.

13. Holzgreve W. The fetus with nonimmune hydrops. In: Harrison MR, Golbus MS, Filly RA, eds. *The Unborn Patient: Prenatal Diagnosis and Treatment.* 2nd ed. Philadelphia, PA: W.B. Saunders Co; 1991: 228–245.

14. Rice HE, Estes JM, Hedrick MH, et al. Congenital cystic adenomatoid malformation: a sheep model of fetal hydrops. *J Pediatr Surg.* 1994;29:692–696.

15. Adzick NS. The fetus with a cystic adenomatoid malformation. In: Harrison MR, Golbus MS, Filly RA, eds. *The Unborn Patient: Prenatal Diagnosis and Treatment.* 2nd ed. Philadelphia, PA: W.B. Saunders Co; 1991:320–327.

16. Coran AG, Drongowski R. Congenital cystic disease of the tracheobronchial tree in infants and children: experience with 44 consecutive cases. *Arch Surg.* 1994;129:521–527.

17. Patz EF Jr, Muller NL, Swensen SJ, et al. Congenital cystic adenomatoid malformation in adults: CT findings. *J Comput Assist Tomogr.* 1995;19:361–364.

18. Murphy JJ, Blair GK, Fraser GC, et al. Rhabdomyosarcoma arising within congenital pulmonary cysts: Report of three cases. *J Pediatr Surg.* 1992;27:1364–1367.

19. Benjamin DR, Cahill JL. Bronchoalveolar carcinoma of the lung and congenital cystic adenomatoid malformation. *Am J Clin Pathol.* 1991;95:889–892.

20. Stephanopoulos C, Catsaros MR. Myxosarcoma complicating a cystic hematoma of the lung. *Thorax.* 1963;18:144–145.

21. Usui Y, Takabe K, Takayama S, et al. Minute squamous cell carcinoma arising in the wall of a congenital lung cyst. *Chest.* 1991;99:235–236.

22. Garrett WJ, Kossoff G, Lawrence R. Gray-scale echography in the diagnosis of hydrops due to fetal lung tumor. *J Clin Ultrasound.* 1975;3:45–50.

23. Ryan CA, Finer NN, Etches PC, et al. Congenital diaphragmatic hernia: associated malformations-cystic adenomatoid malformation, extralobar sequestration, and laryngotracheoesophageal cleft: two case reports. *J Pediatr Surg.* 1995;30:883–885.

24. Obwegeser R, Deutinger J, Bernaschek G. Fetal pulmonary cyst treated by repeated thoracocentesis. *Am J Obstet Gynecol.* 1993;169:1622–1624.

25. Bernaschek G, Deutinger J, Hansmann M, et al. Feto-amniotic shunting-report of the experience of four European centres. *Prenatal Diagn.* 1994;14:821–833.

26. Sherer DM, Abramowicz JS, Metlay LA, et al. Nonimmune fetal hydrops caused by bilateral Type m congenital cystic adenomatoid malformation of the lung at 17 weeks' gestation. *Am J Obstet Gynecol.* 1992;167:503–505.

27. Murotsuki J, Uehara S, Okamura K, et al. Prenatal diagnosis of congenital cystic adenomatoid malformation of the lung by fetal lung biopsy. *Prenatal Diagn.* 1994;14:637–639.

28. Lagrew DC Jr, Morgan MA, Branigan T, et al. Type I fetal cystic adenomatoid malformation of the lung with hydrops at 18 weeks' gestation: a case report. *J Perinatol.* 1994;14:316–318.

29. Sweeney WJ, Kuller JA, Chescheir NC, et al. Prenatal ultrasound findings of linear nevus sebaceous and its association with cystic adenomatoid malformation of the lung. *Ob. Gyn.,* 1994;83(suppl 5 pt 2):860–862.

30. Taguchi M, Shimizu K, Oxaki Y, et al. Prenatal diagnosis of congenital cystic adenomatoid malformation of the lung. *Fetal Diagn Ther.* 1993;8:114–118.

31. McCullagh M, MacConnachie I, Garvie D, et al. Accuracy of prenatal diagnosis of congenital cystic adenomatoid malformation. *AJDC.* 1994;71(suppl):F111–F113.

32. Revillon Y, Jan D, Plattner V, et al. Congenital cystic adenomatoid malformation of the lung: prenatal management and prognosis. *J Pediatr Surg.* 1993;28:1009–1011.

33. dell'Agnola CA, Tadini B, Mosca F, et al. Prenatal ultrasonography and early surgery for congenital cystic disease of the lung. *J Pediatr Surg.* 1992;27:1414–1417.

34. Dumez Y, Mandelbrot L, Radunovic N, et al. Prenatal management of congenital cystic adenomatoid malformation of the lung. *J Pediatr Surg.* 1993;28:36–41.

35. Etches PC, Tierney AJ, Demianczuk NN. Successful outcome in a case of cystic adenomatoid malformation of the lung complicated

by fetal hydrops, using extracorporeal membrane oxygenation. *Fetal Diagn Ther*. 1884;9:88–91.

36. Baker PN, Johnson IR, Gowland PA, et al. Estimation of fetal lung volume using echo-planar magnetic resonance imaging. *Obstet Gynecol*. 1994;83:951–954.

37. King SJ, Pilling DW, Walkinshaw S. Fetal echogenic lung lesions: prenatal ultrasound diagnosis and outcome. *Pediatr Radiol*. 1995;25:208–210.

38. MacGillivray TE, Harrison MR, Goldstein RB, et al. Disappearing fetal lung lesions. *J Pediatr Surg*. 1993;28:1321–1325.

39. Budorick NE, Pretorius DH, Leopold GR, et al. Spontaneous improvement of intrathoracic masses diagnosed in utero. *J Ultrasound Med*. 1992;11:653–662.

40. Hatjis CG, Wall P. Type II congenital cystic adenomatoid malformation of the lung with a mediastinal shift: a case report. *J Reprod Med*. 1992;37:753–756.

41. Mashiach R, Hod M, Friedman S, et al. Antenatal ultrasound diagnosis of congenital cystic adenomatoid malformation of the lung: spontaneous resolution in utero. *J Clin Ultrasound*. 1993;21:453–457.

42. Sonek JD, Foley MR, Iams JD. Spontaneous regression of a large intrathoracic fetal lesion before birth. *Am J Perinatol*. 1991;8:41–43.

43. Sakala EP, Furness ME, Perrott WS, et al. Spontaneous in utero regression of antenatally diagnosed solid fetal chest masses: a report of two cases. *J Reprod Med*. 1994;39:531–536.

44. Glaves J, Baker JL. Spontaneous resolution of maternal hydramnios in congenital cystic adenomatoid malformation of the lung: antenatal ultrasound features: a case report. *Br J Obstet Gynecol*. 1983;90;1065–1068.

45. Sakala EP, Perrott WS, Grube GL. Sonographic characteristics of antenatally diagnosed extralobar pulmonary sequestration and congenital cystic adenomatoid malformation. *Obstet Gynecol Surv*. 1994;49:647–655.

46. Meizner I, Rosenak D. The vanishing fetal intrathoracic mass: consider an obstructing mucous plug. *Ultrasound Obstet Gynecol*. 1995;5:275–277.

47. Chao A, Monoson RF. Neonatal death despite fetal therapy for cystic adenomatoid malformation: a case report. *J Reprod Med*. 1990;35:655–657.

48. Nugent CE, Hayashi RH, Rubin J. Prenatal treatment of Type I congenital cystic adenomatoid malformation by intrauterine fetal thoracentesis. *J Clin Ultrasound*. 1989;17:675–677.

49. Kyle PM, Lange IR, Menticoglou SM, et al. Intrauterine thoracentesis of fetal cystic lung malformations. *Fetal Diagn Ther*. 1994;9:84–87.

50. Nicolaides KH, Blott M, Geenough A. Chronic drainage of fetal pulmonary cyst. *Lancet*. 1987;i:618.

51. Clark SL, Vitale DJ, Minton SD, et al. Successful fetal therapy for cystic adenomatoid malformation associated with second trimester hydrops. *Am J Obstet Gynecol*. 1987;157:294–295.

52. Nicolaides KH, Azar GB. Thoraco-amniotic shunting. *Fetal Diagn Ther*. 1990;5:153–164.

53. Kuller JA, Yankowitz J, Goldberg JD, et al. Outcome of antenatally diagnosed cystic adenomatoid malformations. *Am J Obstet Gynecol*. 1992;167:1038–1041.

54. Harrison MR, Adzick NS, Jennings RW, et al. Antenatal intervention for congenital cystic adenomatoid malformation. *Lancet*. 1990;336:965–967.

55. Goodlin RC. Mirror syndromes. In: Goodlin RC, ed. *Care of the Fetus*. New York, NY: Masson; 1979:48–50.

56. Dekker GA, van Geijn HP. Hypertensive disease in pregnancy. *Curr Opin Obstet Gynecol*. 1992;4:10–27.

57. Buntain WL, Isaacs H, Payne VC, et al. Lobar emphysema, congenital cystic adenomatoid malformation, pulmonary sequestration, and bronchogenic cyst in infancy and children: a clinical group. *J Pediatr Surg*. 1974;9:85–93.

58. Nishibayashi SW, Andrassy RJ, Wooley MM. Congenital cystic adenomatoid malformation: a 30-year experience. *J Ped Surg*. 1981;16:704–706.

CHAPTER 58

FETAL PHARMACOLOGIC THERAPY FOR MENDELIAN DISORDERS

Roderick F. Hume, Jr.

INTRODUCTION

Fetal therapy is now possible for several classical Mendelian disorders of metabolism. The history of metabolic disease began in 1908 when Garrod presented the concept that certain diseases of lifelong duration arise because an enzyme governing a single metabolic step is reduced in activity, or missing altogether.[1] LaDu verified this hypothesis through biochemical studies reported on the nature of the defect of tyrosine metabolism in alkaptonuria in 1958.[2] McKusick's catalog of inherited diseases is now staggering both in the number of disorders, and the rapidity with which the molecular basis of these disorders are being characterized.[3] The molecular and biochemical understanding of these inborn errors of metabolism now allows better care for patients with these individually rare diseases.[4] The improved quality of life finds more affected families choosing to face the risks of reproduction, challenging us in the field of prenatal diagnosis and fetal therapy.[5,6]

Fetal pharmacologic therapy of metabolic disorders occurs in several distinct clinical scenarios. The fetus may be considered the passive victim of a maternal metabolic derrangement such as maternal phenylketonuria (PKU).[7] The primary goal of maternal therapy is to optimize the fetal environment to minimize the risk for fetal damage of an otherwise unaffected fetus. Rarely the maternal adaptation to pregnancy may precipitate a clinical disease state in a previously asymptomatic individual; such as the manifesting ornithine transcarbamolase deficiency (OTC) heterozygote,[8,9] or Acute Intermittent Porphyria (AIP).[10] The fetus may even share the inherited defect with its mother, as described for PKU.[7] Optimal maternal care is then required for the well-being of both the mother and her fetus. Finally, the fetus may have the primary metabolic disorder, such as congenital adrenal hyperplasia (CAH), in which case the in utero therapy may have maternal risks as a secondary problem.[11]

Whether the metabolic defect is primarily maternal or fetal, there are only two basic modes of fetal therapy: indirect (transplacental or maternal), and direct (invasive or fetal). Fetal therapy may include nutritional management, pharmacological agents (drugs, vitamins, or hormones), transfusion of blood products, or transplantation of human stem cells. The latter represents the first real attempts at curative, genetic therapy.[12,13] However, the most common form of fetal therapy remains maternal transplacental therapy and will be the focus of this chapter. The goals of such fetal therapy include (1) to normalize the fetal compartment (PKU), (2) to optimize embryonic development (MMA or Wilson), or (3) to achieve drug levels within the fetus to treat a specific disorder (fetal arrythmia), or accelerate fetal lung maturation. Direct, invasive, fetal therapy is the only known mode of fetal therapy for certain conditions such as fetal transfusion for severe anemias, isoimmunization, or par-

vovirus infection. Intra-amniotic instillation of medications for hormonal replacement in hypothyroidism, antibiosis for some TORCH agents, and fetal arrythmia have been reported. Intramuscular fetal injections of perioperative medications such as curare have been useful in fetal therapeusis. Intravascular access for direct drug infusion, transfusion, or HSCT offer the most promising method to assure the control of fetal doses delivery. This may allow a better fetal therapeutic response with a decreased maternal risk. Classical mendelian disorders, or inherited errors of metabolism, in which fetal pharmacology therapy has been reported will be the primary focus of this review.

FETAL METABOLIC DISORDERS

The in utero fetal therapies currently employed for inborn errors of metabolism evolved from successful ex utero therapies for which some irreversible sequelae or fetal maldevelopment remained after the institution of neonatal therapy. The success of the neonatal screening programs for PKU and congenital hypothyroidism have been monumental. The prevention of mental retardation through early recognition and the application of rather simple nutritional therapy or hormonal replacement has proven that inherited errors of metabolism could be corrected. However, irreversible fetal damage could not be addressed by neonatal therapy for some individuals.[14]

FETAL GOITER/CONGENITAL HYPOTHYROIDISM

Neonatal goiter has been recognized since antiquity. Advanced sonographic evaluation and biochemical analysis of the amniotic fluid allows in utero diagnosis and therapy of fetal goiter.[15-18] The thyrotoxic effects of maternal therapy upon the fetal thyroid have also been recognized and optimal maternal therapeutic schemas reported.[19] Approximately 20% of congenital hypothyroidism is due to inborn errors of metabolism, or single gene defects.[20] These disorders include autosomal recessive familial congenital nongoitrous hypothyroidism,[21] autosomal dominant peripheral insensitivity to T4,[22] and X-linked pseudohypoparathyroidism la.[23] Fetal therapy may be required in these conditions to avoid irreversible damage already present at birth.

CONGENITAL ADRENAL HYPERPLASIA

Congenital Adrenal Hyperplasia offers the first example of an inborn error of metabolism inherited by the fetus to be treated in utero with prevention of fetal malformation as the primary goal. The history of CAH is quite unique. Line 32 of the Clay Tablet K2007 in the Nineveh Royal Library from circa 2,000 British Columbian states, "when a woman gives birth to an infant that has no penis, the master of the house will be enriched by the harvest of his field."[24] This is probably the earliest written reference to CAH virilization of the female fetus. Males may also inherit the AR disorder of steroid metabolism, most commonly 21-hydroxylase deficiency. The clinical spectrum of disease associated with CAH ranges from a critically ill salt-wasting variety, to mild virilization precociously in males, or ambiguously in females. Prominent clitiromegaly with labial fusion can resemble the male genitalia so much as to lead to the misclassification of newborn sex identity. This disorder can be life threatening if the salt-wasting variety of adrenal insufficiency is present. When recognized at birth steroid replacement therapy is initiated which decreases the androgen excess. Since CAH is inherited as an AR, and only the females will be affected by the anomaly, the birth defect risk is 1 in 8. However virilization of the female fetus may already have occurred during weeks 10–16 of gestation. Therefore, prenatal in utero therapy aimed at the prevention of virilization may begin prior to the determination of gender or disease status.[11,25–27] The fetal adrenal gland can be pharmacologically suppressed by maternal replacement doses of dexamethasone.[11] The 21-hydroxylase enzyme defect impairs the metabolism of cholesterol to cortisol, creating excessive 17-hydroxy progesterone, which can be used for prenatal diagnosis. Alternate pathway metabolism shifts this precursor to androstenedione and other androgens. Consequently, genetic females are exposed to high levels of androgens and can become masculinized. The abnormal differentiation can vary from mild clitoral hypertrophy to complete formation of a phallus and apparent scrotum. In the first attempt to prevent this birth defect, Evans and colleagues administered dexamethasone, a fluorinated steroid, to an at-risk mother beginning in the tenth week of gestation. Maternal estriol and cortisol values indicated rapid and sustained fetal and maternal adrenal gland suppression.[11] Forest and David using the same protocol of 0.25 mg of dexamethasone qid, but beginning at 9 weeks reported the successful prevention of external genitalia masculinization in several pregnancies at risk for the severe form of 21 hydroxylase deficiency CAH.[25,27]

This disorder was linked to chromosome 6 using HLA haplotypes as the informative marker. Subsequent gene mapping identified the 21 hydroxylase gene locus to be within the HLA gene cluster. Molecular heterogeneity is the rule with most CAH individuals being compound heterozygotes at the molecular level. The clinical phenotype does show a correlation with the molecular genotypic abnormality.[28] Utilization of CVS and molecular markers for the diagnosis of CAH can now assign disease status and gender sooner allowing maternal steroid therapy to be avoided in males or unaffected females. Due to a few reported cases of masculinization following the 9 weeks initiation protocol, we now begin steroid suppressive therapy at 7 weeks, and continue therapy until delivery, or confirmation of an unaffected fetus, due to the recognised risks associated with maternal dexamethasone therapy. The fundamental principles addressed by these treatment efforts can be extended to other medical fetal therapies. The concepts of a thorough informed consent procedure, thorough documentation of progress, and high-risk obstetric management have generally been followed by investigators in these fields.

METHYLMALONIC ACIDEMIA, MMA

Methylmalonic acidemia is related to a functional vitamin B12 deficiency. Coenzymatically active B12 is required for the conversion of methylmalonyl-coenzyme A to succinyl-coenzyme A. Genetically determined etiologies for methylmalonic acidemia include defects in methylmalonyl-coenzyme A mutase or in the metabolism of vitamin B12 to the coenzymatically active form, adenosylcobalamin, by the converting enzyme. Some patients respond to large dose B12 therapy which can enhance the amount of the active holoenzyme (mutase apoenzyme plus adenosylcobalamin). Ampola and colleagues were the first to attempt prenatal diagnosis and treatment of a B12-responsive variant of methylmalonic acidemia.[29] The diagnosis of MMA was made posthumously by chemical analysis of blood and urine of the proband who died of severe acidosis and dehydration at 3 months of age. At 19 weeks gestation an amniocentesis was performed to make the prenatal diagnosis in the subsequent pregnancy. Elevation of methylmalonic acid content was documented in the cell-free amniotic fluid. Cultured amniocytes had defective propionate oxidation, undetectable levels of adenosylcobalamin, and normal succinate oxidation and methylmalonyl-coenzyme A mutase activity in the presence of added adenosylcobalamin. These studies established the diagnosis of MMA due to deficient synthesis of adenosylcobalamin. Maternal methylmalonyl aciduria was confirmed at 23 weeks gestation, which confirmed this diagnosis. The maternal methylmalonic aciduria is known to be associated with fetal MMA, and not to be present in maternal heterozygotes carrying a normal fetus. The maternal urine values offer an excellent monitoring tool for fetal therapy.

Cyanocobalamin (10 mg/day) was administered orally to the mother in divided doses. A slight reduction in maternal urinary methylmalonic acid excretion was achieved, and only a marginal increase in maternal serum B12 levels. Therefore, at 34 weeks gestation, 5 mg of cyanocobalamin per day as an intramuscular injection was initiated. The maternal serum B12 level rose sixfold above normal, and the maternal urinary excretion of methylmalonic acid progressively decreased to slightly above normal by delivery. Amniotic fluid MMA levels were 3–4 times the normal mean level despite prenatal treatment. Postnatally the diagnosis of MMA was confirmed. The neonate suffered no acute neonatal complications, and had an extremely high serum level of B12. In this case the prenatal therapy certainly improved the fetal and secondarily the maternal biochemistry. Whether there was any significant clinical benefit to this fetus cannot be sufficiently addressed. Nyhan has suggested that an increased frequency of minor anomalies may be associated with untreated fetal MMA.[30] Thus, very early or perhaps even prophylactic treatment with vitamin B12 prior to prenatal diagnosis for the at-risk fetus may be indicated for the optimal therapy of B12-responsive MMA. It seems likely that reduction of the fetal burden of MMA should have developmental benefit, and could reduce the neonatal risk. However, this remains speculative.

The report of Ampola and colleagues was the first example of the treatment of a vitamin-responsive inborn error of metabolism in utero. Further studies are needed to establish the risk-to-benefit ratio of this therapeutic approach.

MULTIPLE CARBOXYLASE DEFICIENCY

Biotin-responsive multiple carboxylase deficiency is an inborn error of metabolism in which the mitochondrial biotin-dependent enzymes, pyruvate carboxylase, propionyl-coenzyme A carboxylase, and beta-methylcrotonyl-coenzyme A carboxylase have diminished activity. Metabolism in patients and in vitro cultured cells can be restored toward normal levels by biotin supplementation. Such therapy has been utilized for fetuses affected with this severe disorder of metabolism. Roth and colleagues treated a fetus without the benefit of prenatal diagnosis in a case in which two siblings had died of MCA.[31] The first sibling died at 3 days of age, and in the second sibling the diagnosis was made posthumously in the neonatal period. Because of the severe neonatal manifestations and the relative harmlessness of biotin, oral administration of this compound was given to the mother at a dose of 10 mg/day. No untoward effects were noted, and the maternal urinary biotin excretion increased by a 100-fold as measured in the urine. Dizygotic twins were subsequently delivered at term. Cord blood and urinary organic acid profiles were normal. Cord blood biotin concentrations were 4- and 7-fold greater than normal. Both neonatal courses were unremarkable. Cultured fibroblasts of twin B had virtually complete deficiency of all three carboxylase activities, while twin A was normal.

Packman and colleagues have also reported the successful prenatal therapy for a fetus at risk for MCD.[32] These reports provide compelling evidence that biotin administration effectively prevents neonatal complications in certain patients with biotin-responsive multiple carboxylase deficiency. No toxicity has been observed. Further experience with vitamin responsive disorders will be useful in the determination of the optimal mode and dose interval for fetal therapy.

MENKES

Hurley and colleagues have investigated possible deleterious effects of prenatal copper administration on mice with the recessive mutant "crinkled" gene.[33] This is speculated to be the mouse homologue of Menkes disease in the human. Dietary supplementation of copper sulfate partially ameliorated the effects of the crinkled gene in the offspring. Copper nitrilotracetate appeared to be superior to copper sulfate in increasing postnatal survival and body copper content of the mutant offspring of heterozygotes. Postnatal supplementation was not effective.

These studies may lead to insights relevant to prenatal treatment of Menkes syndrome, a sex-linked disorder characterized by progressive degeneration of neurologic function in infants. Howell believes that Menkes can be reliably diagnosed in utero by demonstrating abnormally increased copper uptake in cultured amniocytes incubated in a high copper medium. Menkes, like the mouse homologue, has proven refractory to postnatal copper therapy; it is conceivable that prenatal therapy may be of benefit.

MATERNAL METABOLIC DISORDERS

PKU

Classic phenylketonuria (PKU) is a molecularly heterogeneous metabolic disorder caused by deficient activity of the enzyme phenylalanine hydroxylase (PAH). The phenylalanine hydroxylase gene has been localized to chromosome 12q22–q24. Detailed molecular analysis suggests that genotype can predict phenotype.[34,35] PAH is a hepatic enzyme that catalyzes hydroxylation of phenylalanine (phe) to tyrosine (tyr).[36,37] This block in phe metabolism results in the accumulation of phe and its metabolites which then lead to progressive, severe, irreversible mental retardation. Pregnancies in untreated females with high levels of phe may spontaneously abort or show intrauterine growth retardation.[38] Elevated phe levels found in untreated maternal PKU are teratogenic. Children of PKU women may have mental retardation, dysmorphic facies, microcephaly and congenital heart disease. There appears to be a dose-response relationship between the severity of these manifestations and the mother's plasma level of phenylalanine during pregnancy.[39–42]

There are >1600 known women with PKU in the United States and Canada who are of childbearing age. In the preliminary report of an ongoing prospective, longitudinal study involving 213 pregnant women with PKU the outcomes of 134 pregnancies found optimal fetal outcomes with phenylalanine levels <600 umol/L (<10 mg/dl) during the first trimester. Not surprisingly, treatment initiated in the third trimester showed little benefit. Infants with congenital heart disease were born to mothers with phenylalanine levels greater than 10 mg/dl.[43,44]

A case report of 2 children, one with PKU and one without PKU were born from untreated pregnancies in a mother with PKU. Both were microcephalic at birth, and both had congenital anomalies. Both children are mentally retarded (IQ < 50), have hypoplasia of the corpus callosum and enlarged cerebral ventricles. However, only the PKU infant showed intrauterine growth retardation.[7] This case highlights the need for maternal biochemical control. Despite screening programs for almost 3 decades, undiagnosed maternal PKU represents an ongoing public health challenge.[45,46]

GALACTOSEMIA

Galactosemia is a disorder of galactose metabolism generally diagnosed during the neonatal period, with an incidence of approximately one in 50,000. Classic galactosemia is inherited as an autosomal recessive trait. Deficiency of the enzyme galactose-1-phosphate uridyltransferase (GALT) results in the inability to metabolize galactose, and leads to accumulation of galactose-1-phosphate.[47] The GALT locus associated with classic galactosemia has been localized to chromosome 9p13.

Pregnant women who are asymptomatic carriers can be detected by testing the activity of galactose-1-phosphate uridyltransferase in their red blood cells. Galactosemia can be diagnosed in infants at birth by determination of the enzyme activity level in red blood cells. Prenatal diagnosis has been reported using enzymatic assays in amniotic fluid cells and in chorionic villi tissue. An assay has been reported measuring the level of galactitol in amniotic fluid.

Pregnancies in women with galactosemia have been reported.[48,49] These cases demonstrate that dietary control does slightly lower the amount of galactitol in the amniotic fluid, but the amount of galactitol remaining is still high enough that fetal diagnosis can be made. Dietary restriction did not adversely affect the outcome of these neonates. Presently, the only treatment is dietary restriction after birth to maximize chances of normal growth and mental development. The assertion that the institution of a maternal galactose restricted diet for the fetus with this disorder may alter the severity of the neonatal symptoms remains speculative at this time.

GAUCHER DISEASE

Gaucher disease is a lysosomal storage disorder characterized by glucocerebroside accumulation principally in the reticuloendothelial system. It is the most common lysosomal storage disorder. The disease is inherited in an autosomal recessive manner, as a variable defect in the enzyme acid beta-glucosidase. The incidence in Ashkenazi Jews is 1 in 2500, with carrier frequency based upon molecular studies about 1 in 10 to 1 in 8 in this population. Three types of the disorder have been described.[50]

The type of disease is consistent within a sibship, although the extent of morbidity may vary between siblings; modifier genes or other epigenetic factors may be present. The correlation between any specific mutation and outcome is variable, making counseling difficult.[51-54] The basis for phenotype/genotype correlations in Gaucher Disease Type I have been proposed within the Ashkenazi population in whom 4 mutant alleles account for >90% of the mutations: N370S, 84GG, L444P, and IVS 2[+1].[55] The N370S/N370S individual has the milder disease with median onset at 31 years. In contrast the L444P homozygous genotype is associated with the neuronopathic type 2 or 3. Compound heterozygotes have phenotypes which fall between these extremes. The prediction of severity of phenotype may allow presymptomatic, or early symptomatic therapy, which is currently reserved for the severely affected individual. Enzyme therapy and bone marrow transplantation have been successful in the treatment of this disorder. Clinical trials of enzyme replacement therapy in type 1 disease using Ceredase®, a modified form of acid beta-glucosidase derived from human placenta, have been conducted in nonpregnant individuals and found to be effective.[56,57] Gaucher disease (type 1) in pregnancy has been described for a series of 47 pregnancies in 17 women.[58] Gene therapy may hold great promise for selected Gaucher families.

CYSTINOSIS

Cystinosis, a disorder of lysosomal cystine transport, is characterized by the intralysosomal accumulation of cystine.[59] Cystine is the dimer of the amino acid cysteine. Cystinosis is inherited in an autosomal recessive manner; the incidence is ~1 in 200,000. There are three forms of the disease. Prior to the era of renal transplantation, many patients did not survive past adolescence, secondary to renal failure. Recent reports have described successful pregnancy in patients with cystinosis and renal allografts. The placenta in one pregnancy showed cystine crystals on the maternal side but not on the fetal side.[60] With early diagnosis and the use of cysteamine to bind cystine crystals, renal function may be preserved and renal transplantation may be avoided. However, the fetal effects of cysteamine are unknown. The need for fetal therapy has not been established.

ORNITHINE TRANSCARBAMYLASE DEFICIENCY

Ornithine transcarbamylase (OTC) deficiency is an X-linked disorder caused by a defect an enzyme required for urea synthesis from ammonia. This enzyme defect results in elevation of ammonia levels throughout the body tissues. The gene for this urea cycle enzyme, which is 1 of 6 enzymes involved in urea synthesis, maps to chromosome Xp21. Approximately one third of cases result from a new mutation.

Some women who are carriers may not experience hyperammonemia until pregnancy or delivery, in which postpartum coma may be the presenting symptom.[8,9] Intravenous sodium benzoate, sodium phenylacetate and arginine hydrochloride have been used to treat hyperammonemia by forming compounds with ammonia that are readily excreted in the urine. The orphan drug benzoate/phenyacetate (Ucephan®) has been approved for patients with urea cycle disorders.[61]

ACUTE INTERMITTENT PORPHYRIA

Acute intermittent porphyria is an acute-onset hepatic porphyria, inherited as an autosomal dominant trait. The enzymatic defect results in a 50% reduction in the activity of PBG deaminase. The gene has been localized to chromosome 11q24. However, only 10% of patients with the enzyme defect are clinically affected. Because of this urine must be examined for PBG and d-ALA during an acute attack. Normal results virtually exclude AIP. Erythrocytes can also be examined for activity of PBG deaminase.[62]

In pregnancy, older surveys reported exacerbation of AIP in 95% of patients, with maternal death rates of 30–40%. More recent surveys suggest a lower attack rate (25%) and mortality (0–2%). The periods of disease exacerbation appear to be during early pregnancy or the puerperium. Not surprisingly, diagnosis before pregnancy improves outcome.[10,63,64]

WILSON DISEASE

Wilson disease is an autosomal recessive, multisystem disorder characterized by abnormal accumulations of tissue copper. The putative gene for Wilson disease has been mapped to 13q14. Prior to the introduction of chelation therapy in 1956 by Walshe, Wilson disease was a progressively debilitating and fatal disease. Since the introduction of D-penicillamine, a cupriuretic chelating agent, several pregnancies have been described.[65–69] Recurrent abortion is not uncommon in untreated Wilson disease, perhaps on the basis of direct embryotoxicity from elevated tissue copper; successful zinc therapy has been reported.[70]

However, chelating agents may be teratogenic.[71,72] Lysyl oxidase is copper-dependent and is involved in cross-linking collagen and elastin. Penicillamine dose-related teratogenesis has been described in rats. Several infants exposed to this drug, including 1 with Wilson disease, were found to have transient cutis laxa. One had inguinal hernias, low-set ears, and joint mobility. However, discontinuing therapy may be catastrophic for the mother or have significant neonatal sequelae. In 1 case, a gravida with 2 prior successful pregnancies and known Wilson disease deliberately stopped penicillamine therapy, developed CNS findings, fulminant hepatic failure, hemolytic crisis, and died post-partum.[73] In a second case, copper deposition was found on the maternal side of the placenta, but not on the fetal side. Copper levels in umbilical serum and amniotic fluid were remarkably elevated. The neonate showed hepatomegaly.[74] Thus, both fetal and maternal risks must be weighed before modifications in therapy are attempted.

SUMMARY

Over the course of the past decades, there have been tremendous advances in our ability to diagnose and treat fetal disorders. In addition to the disorders presented there have been a growing number of reports of pregnancy in cases of maternal metabolic disease.[75–87] The diagnosis of Mendelian defects have become considerably more sophisticated, and more common. Such prenatal diagnoses have led to the possibility for fetal therapy which has clearly been shown to be of benefit in congenital adrenal hyperplasia, the prevention of neural tube defects, and can alter metabolism in several other disorders for which there is still considerable question as to clinical efficacy. Nevertheless, these disorders serve as a paradigm for continued and enhanced treatment of the fetus as a patient, and one for which therapies can be devised that are effective in producing better outcomes.

References

1. Garrod A. Inborn errors of metabolism (Croonian lectures), *Lancet.* 1908;2:1–7, 73–79, 142–148, 214–220.
2. LaDu BN. The nature of the defect of tyrosine metabolism in alcaptonuria, *J Biol Chem.* 1958;230:251–260.
3. McKusick VA, Francomano CA, Antonarakis SE. *Mendelian Inheritance in Man.* 12th edition. Baltimore: Johns Hopkins University Press, 1996.
4. Scriver CR, Beaudet AL, Sly WS, et al. eds. *The Metabolic and Molecular Basis of Inherited Disease.* 7th edition. New York: McGraw-Hill, 1997.
5. Schulman JD, Simpson JL. *Genetic Diseases in Pregnancy: Maternal Effects and Fetal Outcome.* New York: Academic Press, 1981.
6. Evans MI. *Reproductive Risks and Prenatal Diagnosis.* Norwalk: Appleton & Lange, 1992.
7. Levy HL, Lobbregt D, Sansaricq C, Snyderman SE. Comparison of phenylketonuric and nonphenylketonuric sibs from untreated pregnancies in a mother with phenylketonuria. *Am J Med Genet.* 1992; 44:439–442.
8. Am PH, Hauser ER, Thomas GH, et al. Hyperammonemia in women with a mutation at the ornithine carbamoyltransferase locus: a cause of postpartum coma. *N Engl J Med.* 1990;322:1652–1655.
9. Horwich AL, Fenton WA. Precarious balance of nitrogen metabolism in women with a urea-cycle defect. *N Engl J Med.* 1990;322:1668–1670.
10. Kanaan C, Veille JC, Lakin M. Pregnancy and acute intermittent porphyria. *Obstet Gynecol Surv.* 1989;44:244–249.
11. Evans MI, Chrousos GP, Mann DL. Pharmacologic suppression of the fetal adrenal gland in utero: attempted prevention of abnormal external genital masculinization in suspected congenital adrenal hyperplasia. *JAMA.* 1985;253:1015.
12. Johnson MP, Drugan A, Miller OJ, et al. Genetic correction of hereditary disease. *Fetal Therapy.* 1989;4(1):28–39.
13. Schulman JD. Treatment of the embryo and the fetus in the first trimester: current status and future possibilities. *Am J Med Gen.* 1990;35(2):197–200.
14. Fisher DA, Klein AH. Thyroid development and disorders of thyroid function in the newborn. *N Engl J Med.* 1981;304:702–712.
15. Carswell F, Kerr MM, Hutchison JH. Congenital goitre and hypothyroidism produced by maternal ingestion of iodides. *Lancet.* 1970;1:1242–1243.
16. Davidson KM, Richards DS, Schatz DA, et al. Successful in utero treatment of fetal goiter and hypothyroidism. *N Engl J Med.* 1991;324(8):543–546.
17. Sagot P, David A, Yvinec M, et al. Intrauterine treatment of thyroid goiters. *Fetal Diagn Ther.* 1991; 6:28–33.
18. Hatjis CG. Diagnosis and successful treatment of fetal goitrous hyperthyroidism caused by maternal Grave's disease. *Obstet Gynecol.* 1993;81:837–839.
19. Momotani N, Noh J, Oyanagi H. Antithyroid drug therapy for Grave's disease during pregnancy. Optimal regimen for fetal thyroid status. *N Engl J Med.* 1986;315:24–28.
20. New England Congenital Hypothyroidism Collaborative. Characteristics of infantile hypothyroidism discovered on neonatal screening. *J Pediatr.* 1984;104:539–544.
21. White CW, Wiedermann BL, Kirkland RT. Hereditary congenital nongoitrous hypothyroidism. *Am J Dis Child.* 1981;135:568–569.
22. Hamon P, Bovier-La PM, Robert M. Hyperthyroidism due to selective pituitary resistance in thyroid hormone in a 15-month old boy: efficacy of 0-thyroxine therapy. *J Clin Endocrinol Metabol.* 1988;67:1089–1093.

23. Levine MA, Jap TS, Hung W. Infantile hypothyroidism in two sibs: an unusual presentation of pseudohypoparathyroidism type Ia. *J Pediatr*. 1985;107:919–922.

24. Stevenson RE. Causes of human anomalies: an overview and historical perspective. In: *Human Malformations and Related Anomalies*. New York: Oxford University Press: 1993:8–9.

25. David M, Forrest M. Prenatal treatment of congenital adrenal hyperplasia resulting from 21-hydroxylase deficiency. *J Pediatr*. 1984;105:799–803.

26. Pang S, Pollack MS, Marshall RN, et al. Prenatal treatment of congenital adrenal hyperplasia due to 21-hydroxylae deficiency. *N Engl J Med*. 1990;322(2):111–115.

27. Forest MG, David M. Prevention of sexual ambiguity in children with 21-hydroxylase deficiency by treatment in utero. *Pediatrie*. 1992;47(5):351–357.

28. Miller WL. Genetics, diagnosis, and management of 21-hydroxylase deficiency. *J Clin Endocrinol Metabol*. 1994;78(2):241–246.

29. Ampola MG, Mahoney MJ, Nakamura E. Prenatal therapy of a patient with vitamin B responsive methylmalonic acidemia. *N Engl J Med*. 1975;293:313.

30. Nyhan WL. Prenatal treatment of methylmalonic aciduria. *N Engl J Med*. 1975;293:353.

31. Roth KS, Yang W, Allen L. Prenatal administration of biotin: biotin responsive multiple carboxylase deficiency. *Pediatr Res*. 1982;16:126.

32. Packman S, Cowan MJ, Golbus MS. Prenatal treatment of biotin responsive multiple carboxylase deficiency. *Lancet*. 1982;1:1425.

33. Hurley LS, Bell LT. Genetic influence on response to dietary manganese deficiency in mice. *J Nur*. 1974;104:133.

34. Okano Y, Eisensmith RC, Guttler F, et al. Molecular basis of phenotypic heterogeneity in phenylketonuria. *N Engl J Med*. 1991;324:1232–1238.

35. Scriver CR. Phenylketonuria—genotypes and phenotypes [editorial]. *N Engl J Med*. 1991;324:1280–1282.

36. Scriver CR, Clow CL. Phenylketonuria:epitome of human biochemical genetics. Part I. *N Engl J Med*. 1980;303:1336–1342.

37. Scriver CR, Clow CL. Phenylketonuria: epitome of human biochemical genetics. Part II. *N Engl J Med*. 1980;303:1394–1400.

38. Shaw D, Macleod PM, Applegarth DA. Recurrent abortion and amnioacid abnormalities. *J Inher Metab Dis*. 1991;14:851–852.

39. Lenke RR, Levy HL. Maternal phenylketonuria and hyperphenylalaninemia: an international survey of the outcome of untreated and treated pregnancies. *N Engl J Med*. 1980;303:1202–1208.

40. American Academy Pediatric Committee on Genetics: Maternal phenylketonuria. *Pediatrics*. 1991;88:1284–1285.

41. Matalon R, Michals K, Azen C, et al. Maternal PKU Collaborative Study: the effect of nutrient intake on pregnancy outcome. *J Inher Metab Dis*. 1991;14:371–374.

42. Rouse B, Lockhart L, Matalon R, et al. Maternal phenylketonuria pregnancy outcome: a preliminary report of facial dysmorphology and major malformations. *J Inher Metab Dis*. 1990;13:289–291.

43. Koch R, Hanley W, Levy H, et al. A preliminary report of the collaborative study of maternal phenylketonuria in the United States and Canada. *J Inher Metab Dis*. 1990;13:641–650.

44. Platt LD, Koch R, Azen C, et al. Maternal phenylketonuria collaborative study, obstetric aspects and outcome: the first 6 years. *Am J Obstet Gynecol*. 1992;166:1150–1162.

45. Dorland L, Poll-The BT, Duran M, et al. Phenylpyruvate, fetal damage, and maternal phenylketonuria syndrome. *Lancet*. 1993;341:1351–1352.

46. Hanley WB, Clarke JTR, Schoonheyt WE. Undiagnosed phenylketonuria in adult women: a hidden public health problem. *Can Med Assoc J*. 1990;143:513–516.

47. Waggoner DD, Donnell GN, Buist NRM. Long-term prognosis in galactosemia: results of a survey of 350 cases. In: Donnell GN, ed. *Galactosemia: new frontiers in research*. NICHD/NIH publication 1993;93–3438.

48. Jakobs C, Kleijer WJ, Bakker HD, et al. Dietary restriction of maternal lactose intake does not prevent accumulation of galactitol in the amniotic fluid of fetuses affected with galactosaemia. *Prenatal Diagnosis*. 1988;8:641–645.

49. Tedesco TA, Morrow G, Meilman WJ. Normal pregnancy and childbirth in a galactosemic woman. *J Pediatr*. 1972;81:1159–1162.

50. Grabowski GA. Gaucher disease: enzymology, genetics and treatment. In: Harris H, Hirschhorn K, ed. *Advances in Human Genetics*. Vol 21, New York: Plenum Press, 1993.

51. Beaudet AL. Gaucher's disease [editorial]. *N Engl J Med*. 1987;316:619–621.

52. Zimran A, Gross E, West C, et al. Prediction of severity of Gaucher's disease by identification of mutations at DNA level. *Lancet*. 1989;2:349–352.

53. Sidransky E, Sherer DM, Ginns EI. Gaucher disease in the neonate: a distinct Gaucher phenotype is analogous to a mouse model created by targeted disruption of the glucocerebrosidase gene. *Pediatr Res*. 1992;32:494–498.

54. Zlotgora J, Zaizov R, Klibansky C, et al. Genetic heterogeneity in Gaucher disease. *J Med Genet*. 1986;23:319–322.

55. Sibille A, Eng CM, Kim S-J, et al. Phenotype/genotype correlations in Gaucher disease type I: clinical and therapeutic implications. *Am J Hum Gen*. 1993;52:1094–1101.

56. Barton NW, Brady RO, Dambrosia JM, et al. Replacement therapy for inherited enzyme deficiency-macrophage-targeted glucocerebrosidase for Gaucher disease. *N Engl J Med*. 1991;324:1464–1470.

57. Fallet S, Grace ME, Sibille A, et al. Enzyme augmentation in moderate to life-threatening Gaucher disease. *Pediatr Res*. 1992;31:496–502.

58. Zlotogora J, Sagi M, Zeigler M, et al. Gaucher disease type I and pregnancy. *Am J Med Genet*. 1989;32:475–477.

59. Gahl WA. Cystinosis: progress in a prototypic disease. *Ann Intern Med*. 1988;109:557–569.

60. Reiss RE, Kuwabara T, Smith ML, et al. Successful pregnancy despite placental cystine crystals in a woman with nephropathic cystinosis. *N Engl J Med*. 1988;319:223–226.

61. Hauser ER, Finkelstein JE, Valle D, et al. Allopurinol-induced orotidinuria: a test for mutations at the ornithine carbamoyltransferase locus in women. *N Engl J Med*. 1990;322:1641–1645.

62. Sassa S, Kappas A. Lack of effect of pregnancy or hematin on erythrocyte porphobilinogen deaminase activity in acute intermittent porphyria. *N Engl J Med*. 1993;321:192–193.

63. Milo R, Neuman M, Klein C, et al. Acute intermittent porphyria in pregnancy. *Obstet Gynecol*. 1989;73:450–452.

64. Kantor G, Rolbin SH. Acute intermittent porphyria and caesarean delivery. *Can J Anaesth*. 1992;39:282–285.

65. Marecek Z, Graf M. Pregnancy in penicillamine-treated patients with Wilson's disease. *N Engl J Med*. 1975;293:1300–1302.

66. Walshe JM. Pregnancy in Wilson's disease. *Quart J Med*. 1977;46:73–83.

67. Walshe JM. The management of pregnancy in Wilson's disease treated with trientine. *Quart J Med*. 1986;58:81–87.

68. Dupont P, Irion O, Beguin F. Pregnancy in a patient with treated Wilson's disease: a case report. *Am J Obstet Gynecol*. 1990;163:1527–1528.

69. Chin RKH. Pregnancy and Wilson's disease. *Am J Obstet Gynecol*. 1991;165:488–489.

70. Schagen van Leeuwen JH, Christiaens GCML, Hoogenraad TU. Recurrent abortion and the diagnosis of Wilson disease. *Obstet Gynecol*. 1991;78:547–549.

71. Linares A, Zarranz J, Rodriguez-AlarcOn J, et al. Reversible cutis laxa due to maternal D-penicillamine treatment. *Lancet*. 1979;2:43.

72. Rosa FW. Teratogen update: penicillamine. *Teratology*. 1986;33:127–131.

73. Oga M, Matsui N, Takanobu A, et al. Copper disposition of the fetus and placenta in a patient with untreated Wilson disease. *Am J Obstet Gynecol*. 1993;169:196–198.

74. Shimono N, Ishibashi H, Ikematsu H, et al. Fulminant hepatic failure during perinatal period in a pregnant woman with Wilson disease. Gastroenterologica Japonica. 1991;26:69–73.

75. Marks F, Ordorica S, Hoskins I, et al. Congenital hereditary fructose intolerance and pregnancy. *Am J Obstet Gynecol*. 1989;160:362–363.

76. Kamoun PP, Chadefaux B. Eleventh week amniocentesis for prenatal diagnosis of some metabolic diseases. *Prenatal Diagnosis*. 1991;11(9):691–696.

77. Farber M, Knappel RA, Binkiewicz A, et al. Pregnancy and vonGierke disease. *Obstet Gynecol*. 1976;47:226–228.

78. Johnson MP, Compton A, Drugan A, et al. Metabolic control of Von Gierke disease (Glycogen storage disease type IA) in pregnancy: maintenance of euglycemia with cornstarch. *Obstet Gynecol*. 1990;75:507–510.

79. Van Calcar SC, Harding CO, Davidson SR, et al. Case reports of successful pregnancy in women with maple syrup urine disease and propionic acidemia. *Am J Med Genet*. 1992;44:641–646.

80. Baxi LV, Rubeo TJ, Katz B, et al. Porphyria cutanea tarda and pregnancy. *Am J Obstet Gynecol*. 1983;146:333–334.

81. Lamon JM, Frykholm BC. Pregnancy and porphyria cutanea tarda. *Johns Hopkins Medical J*. 1979;145:235–237.

82. Malina L, Lim CK. Manifestation of familial porphyria cutanea tarda after childbirth. *Brit J Dermatol*. 1988;188:243–245.

83. Wendel U, Baumgartner R, van der Meer SB, et al. Accumulation of odd-numbered long-chain fatty acids in fetuses and neonates with inherited disorders of propionate metabolism. *Pediatric Res*. 1991;29(4):403–405.

84. Popli S, Leehey DJ, Molnar ZV, et al. Demonstration of Fabry's disease deposits in placenta. *Am J Obstet Gynecol*. 1990;163(2):464–465.

85. Dumontel C, Girod C, Dijoud F, et al. Fetal Niemann-Pick disease type C: ultrastructural and lipid findings in liver and spleen, Virchows Archiv -A. *Pathological Anatomy & Histopathol*. 1993;422(3):253–259.

86. Chung SR, Katayama S, Lebo R, et al. Restriction enzyme analysis of Norrie disease pedigrees. Asia-Oceania *J Obstet Gynecol*. 1992;18(3):255–261.

87. Bonduell M, Lissens W, Goossens A, et al. Lysosomal storage diseases presenting as transient or persistent hydrops fetalis. *Genetic Counseling*. 1991;2(4):227–232.

FOLIC ACID AND PREVENTION OF NEURAL TUBE DEFECTS

Elisa Llurba / Ellen J. Lansberger / Mark I. Evans

INTRODUCTION

Neural tube defects (NTDs) used to be the second most prevalent prenatal anomaly in the United States, only less frequent than cardiac malformations. Worldwide, there are 400,000 such defects.[1] NTDs can be separated into 2 main categories, abnormalities of the skull and brain, including anencephaly, acrania, or encephalocele; and malformations of the spine, including meningocele, meningomyelocele, or spina bifida.

Anencephaly is defined as a congenital absence of a major portion of the brain, skull, and scalp. The cerebral hemispheres develop without a cranial cover, and the exposure to amniotic fluid damages the brain. Encephalocele refers to the herniation of cranial contents through a defect in the skull. These conditions are usually lethal within the first days of life. Meningocele is a defect in the vertebrae through which the meningeal sac protrudes. In 90% of cases, neural tissue also protrudes into the meningeal sac, known as meningomyelocele. Spina bifida refers to both meningocele and meningomyelocele. Approximately 90% of these defects are not covered by skin (open neural tube defect) and are associated with spinal nerve damage below the level of the lesion. Disorders in motor, bowel, and bladder function are of various severities depending on the level of the lesion. Intelligence may be normal, but over 50% of affected individuals have a learning disability. It has been estimated that as many as 25% of patients may have an IQ below 50.[2] Hydrocephalus and the Arnold-Chiari malformation (elongation and downward displacement of the hindbrain) are often associated.[3] "Closed" spina bifida is a subtle malformation of the caudal neural tube; these defects are difficult to diagnose. They may not be recognized until adult life, basically in form of cutaneous defects or lipomas in lumbosacral region.[4]

Neural tube defects result from failure of the neural tube to fuse during early embryogenesis, between the third and fifth week of gestation.[5] At 18 days after fertilization, the primitive neural plate forms 2 lateral neural folds with a central neural groove. The lateral edges of these folds fuse in the mid-portion of the embryo, forming the neural tube. The fusion of the neural tube goes from the cranial to the caudal portion finishing by 26 days of development.

The etiology of NTD is not always clear. Mostly the disorder emerges as a multifactorial trait. Both genetic background and nutritional status influence the incidence. In more than 97% of cases, there is no prior family history of NTD.[6] It has been reported that 12% of cases have an identifiable cause.[7] These include chromosomal abnormalities (trisomy 18, triploidy), single gene mutations (Meckel-Gruber syndrome), maternal disease (diabetes mellitus, hyperthermia), or maternal exposure to teratogens (alcohol, valproic acid) (Table 59-1).

The most common risk factor is a previous affected family member. The risk of recurrence varies depending on the underlying population risk. Prospective studies have shown a recurrence risk of 1.5–3% in the general United States population.[8–10] The risk in Britain is about 4.4%.[11] In the United States when there are 2 affected siblings, the risk of recurrence of neural tube defects rises to 5.7%[8,12] with an increase as high as 12% in 1 British study.[13]

INCIDENCE

The incidence of NTD varies among different communities around the world. These variations are functions of genetic background, location, and nutritional status. Historically, before screening was implemented, the most affected population in the world was in Northern Ireland where the incidence was reported to be as high as 1 in 130 births.[14,15] Americans of Irish ancestry have a rate lower than in Ireland per se, but still considerably higher than the incidence in whites in the United States in general. The Japanese in Japan have among the lowest incidence,[16] about 0.23 per 1,000 live births, yet Japanese in Hawaii have an incidence double that of Japan.

There has been a gradual decline overall of NTDs in the United States ever since the depression in the 1930s when there was a virtual epidemic. The general conclusion has been that NTDs are partially precipitated by functional folic acid deficiencies, which are particularly common in poor diets, especially those lacking in fruits and green vegetables.[17] In 1973, the Food and Drug Administration allowed an increase in the amount in folic acid in multivitamin formulations.[18] The rate of NTD dropped from 2 per 1,000 live births reported for the years 1968 through 1972 to 1.3 per 1,000 from 1974 through 1978. After prenatal diagnosis and screening with maternal serum alpha-fetoprotein (MSAFP) was implemented across the United States in the mid-1980s, the rate of live births affected with NTDs decreased in the 1990s to less than 1 per 1,000.[19] Several changes in the epidemiological characteristics of neural tube defects have been observed since the introduction of screening programs. The detection is higher for anencephaly; therefore the proportion of spina bifida and combined fetal anomalies with NTD has increased. The incidence of NTDs in the white population has decreased relative to that in other races due to higher utilization of screening in white population. However, recently a great impact lowering the rate of NTDs has been achieved as a result of mandatory fortification of grain and flour with folic acid since 1998. There has been a reported decrease of 19% in the incidence of NTD in live births from 1996 to 2001 of livebirths (Fig. 59-1).[20]

The decline in NTD also has been observed in other countries, particularly those with historically high rates. In the

TABLE 59-1	DISORDERS ASSOCIATED WITH NTD
Folate deficiency	
Maternal hyperthermia	
Trisomy 13	
Trisomy 18	
Turner syndrome	
Triploidy	
Amniotic band syndrome	
Limb defects	
Body wall defects	
Meckel-Gruber syndrome	
Walker-Warburg syndrome	

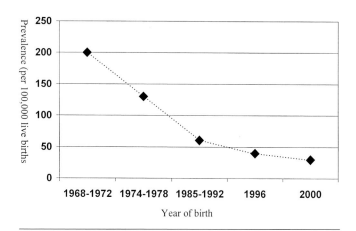

FIGURE 59-1 Prevalence of NTD among U.S. population (19,20).

United Kingdom, the decrease began in the early 1970s and continued after the introduction of folic acid fortification of breakfast cereals in 1985 and bread in 1991. As dietary folic acid consumption increased, the reported rate of decline of NTDs in this population was from 10.4% to 5.2% per year.[15] In Canada, greater than a 50% decrease in NTD has been reported since fortification with folic acid in 1998.[21] Mild decreases also have been reported in Mediterranean countries without fortification, basically due to screening programs. In France, between 1979 and 1994 the prevalence of NTD remained stable, but the incidence at birth dropped by almost 100% for anencephaly and 60% for spina bifida due to ultrasound diagnosis and termination of pregnancies.[22] In many European countries without fortification, there is a recommendation for women to supplement with folic acid in the periconceptional period, but few women actually take folate supplements prior to their pregnancies.[23,24] In China, a larger public health campaign was conducted advocating supplementation with 400 μg/day in the periconceptional period. The incidence of NTD decreased 79% in that population.[25] In South America, where abortion is illegal, a trend toward an increase of NTD has been noted.[26,27] As a result, Chile initiated a fortification program in 2000.[27] In view of the successful fortification programs in United States and Canada, other countries are planning fortification measures.

SCREENING OF NTD WITH MATERNAL SERUM ALPHA-FETOPROTEIN

Screening for NTD has 2 main steps: maternal serum alpha-fetoprotein in the second trimester of pregnancy and early diagnosis by ultrasound examination. The relationship between AFP and the presence of NTD has been known for over 3 decades. Brock and Sutcliffe first described the measurement of amniotic fluid AFP to diagnose NTDs.[28] AFP in maternal serum was subsequently utilized for the prenatal diagnosis of neural tube defects.[29] In the mid-1970s in the United

Kingdom, and in the mid-1980s in the United States, routine prenatal screening became widely accepted.

AFP is a glycoprotein that is synthesized sequentially by the yolk sac and the fetal gastrointestinal tract and liver. AFP levels in fetal plasma are maximal at 12–13 weeks gestation. After maturation of the fetal liver, plasma AFP levels decline and albumin gradually becomes the principal plasma protein of the fetus. Fetal AFP enters the fetal urine and consequently the amniotic fluid. Peak concentrations of amniotic fluid AFP are reached at 12–14 weeks gestation and steadily decline parallel to the fetal serum concentration. Amniotic fluid AFP passes into maternal circulation, probably by diffusion through the membranes or the placenta. AFP appears in low concentrations in maternal serum; its concentration peaks at 28–32 weeks gestation. Maternal serum levels of AFP can be measured as early as the first trimester. For screening purposes, maternal serum AFP (MSAFP) is measured between 15–20 weeks gestation, when the increase is linear. Because the distribution of MSAFP values do not follow a normal curve, parametric statistics are not appropriate, therefore, the results are expressed as multiples of the median (MoM) for gestational age.

In most labs, an MSAFP result $\geq$2.5 MoM or $\geq$4.5 MoM in twins is considered abnormally elevated and indicates the need for further testing.[30] Approximately, 2–3% of women screen positive. About 5–10% of the patients with an elevated MSAFP will have a fetus with an NTD or with some other significant congenital anomaly. The likelihood of a defect increases with the level of serum AFP. The positive predictive value of an MSAFP between 2.5–2.9 MoM for NTD is about 1.45%, with the predictive value as high as 13.4% if the MSAFP is above 7 MoM; overall, the risk of having an affected fetus is about 4.5% for an MSAFP value above 2.5 MoM.[31,32] MSAFP levels above 8.00 MoM are associated with large structural anomalies or with fetal death before 20 weeks of gestation.[32] In a low-risk population, MSAFP screening for NTD can detect 71–75% of all neural tube defects.[33] The sensitivity for anencephaly has been reported as high as 91%. The detection rate reaches nearly 100% for fetuses affected with abdominal wall defects.[34]

A large number of variables affect the concentration of MSAFP. Fetal maternal hemorrhage within 2 weeks before the sample can increase MSAFP due to an elevation of fetal red cells in maternal circulation.[35] The principal cause of false positive MSAFP screening is an error in gestational age dating. If gestational age is underestimated, the MSAFP may be higher than expected. Conversely, if gestational age is overestimated, the MSAFP may be falsely decreased. Moreover, correction for maternal weight, smoking status, number of fetus, and maternal race increases the sensitivity of the test.[36] Recently, the correction for diabetic status has been shown to be obsolete. Differences in MSAFP values are more related to obesity in the diabetic patient than glucose levels per se, leading to an overcorrection.[37] Weight corrections with truncations at both extremes have also been reevaluated recently and found to still be valid.[38]

Unexplained elevations of MSAFP levels have long been associated with adverse pregnancy outcomes.[39–41] In the absence of fetal malformations, MSAFP elevations probably are the result of transplacental leakage of AFP from the fetal to the maternal circulation.[42] The increased leakage of AFP may be caused by functional or structural abnormalities of the placenta. Yaron et al.[43] reported a 10-fold increase for miscarriage, 5-fold increase of risk for intrauterine fetal death, 2- to 3-fold increased risk for intrauterine growth restriction, oligohydramnios and abruptio placentae. Preterm delivery and gestational hypertension were also associated with elevation of MSAFP. On the other hand, a low MSAFP value was associated with an 11-fold increased risk for chromosomal defects and 3-fold increase for fetal intrauterine death.[40]

ULTRASOUND EXAMINATION

Only 5–10% of women with elevated MSAFP have been found to be carrying a fetus affected with a neural tube defect. The MSAFP is a screening test which only identifies those who need further testing. As with any rare event, the positive predictive values of the tests for NTD are low. The next diagnostic step should be easy to perform, inexpensive, and noninvasive. It should, however, give a definitive answer. When MSAFP screening was implemented in mid-1970s, prenatal ultrasound technology was vestigial. Therefore, amniocentesis for amniotic fluid AFP testing used to be performed as the next step for screen-positive cases.[7] This test had a high sensitivity and specificity for detection of NTD. However, even half of cases with high AFP in amniotic fluid were normal fetuses, mainly due to amniotic fluid sample contamination with fetal blood.[8,9] Another problem with the test was the cost and risk of this invasive procedure.[44] With increased experience and improved resolution of the equipment, the sensitivity of ultrasound for diagnosis of NTD has increased dramatically. Therefore, amniocentesis for AFP levels in amniotic fluid has progressively diminished, and targeted sonographic evaluation is currently offered as the main test for the detection of NTD.

In high-risk pregnancies, as determined by MSAFP, targeted sonographic evaluation of the fetus for NTD is remarkably accurate when performed by experienced sonographers. In a recent study by Lenon and Gray,[45] the sensitivity was reported to be 97%, the specificity was 100%, and the positive and negative predictive values also approached 100%. These results are similar to those found in other reported studies. In an Australian study the sensitivity for anencephaly achieved 100% even in low risk population, and for spina bifida was 89%.[46] For screening purposes, however, the detection rate for NTD in the general population was 79.4% for all defects,[34] and only 60% for spina bifida.[46] These results in a general population are similar to that of MSAFP. A higher level of sensitivity was achieved combining MSAFP and second trimester ultrasound.[34,46]

The ultrasonographic findings in a fetus affected by a neural tube defect have been well characterized. The diagnosis of anencephaly is usually easy, even in the late first trimester of pregnancy, when the ossification of the normal skull should be completed.[47]

Encephalocele usually occurs in the occipital region in Caucasians, whereas in fetuses of Southeast Asian ethnicity, the frontal location is more common.[48] Encephalocele is associated with other congenital anomalies in 40% of cases, with a high association with renal cystic disease.[49] Other brain anomalies could be associated, like ventriculomegaly, agenesis of corpus callosum, and microcephaly. The sonographic appearance of the cystic mass is diverse in both size and content; it can appear as a purely cystic mass, solid mass, or combined. The cystic mass is always associated with a bony defect.

The ultrasound diagnosis of meningomyelocele is more difficult. The diagnosis is based on a cystic mass protruding from the vertebrae without skin covering the defect. The morphology of the spine is also abnormal. Since the association with anomalies in the posterior fossa was described, the rate of diagnosis of spina bifida has increased.[50] An indirect finding in almost all cases of spina bifida is the abnormality in the anatomy of the posterior fossa, called Dandy-Walker malformation type 2. Herniation of the cerebellar vermis through the foramen magnum with displacement of the forth ventricle downward causes obliteration of the cisterna magna and forms the "banana sign." This is due to the posterior convexity of the cerebellum within the posterior cranial fossa in more than 95% of the cases (Fig. 59-2). The other common finding is the "lemon" sign due to the scalloping of frontal bones (Fig. 59-3).[50,51] Posterior fossa should be examined in all anomaly scans performed in the second trimester as recommended by the American Institute of Ultrasound in Medicine and American College of Obstetrics and Gynecology.

The risk for chromosomal anomalies in women with elevated MSAFP is about 0.5%, the same as the general population.[45] Amniocentesis for AF-AFP levels or detection of chromosomal abnormalities are offered when patients present with ultrasound findings suspicious of a chromosomal abnormality, very high levels of AFP despite a normal scan, or inability to adequately visualize fetal anatomy.

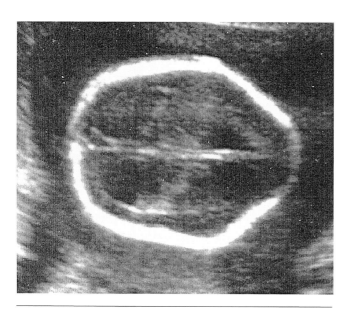

FIGURE 59-2 Transverse view of a fetal head demonstrating the "lemon sign" in a fetus with meningomylocele.

PREVENTION OF NTD

The association between folic acid deficiency and the incidence of neural tube defects has long been appreciated. Epidemiological observations have explored differences in socioeconomic status, seasonal variation, prevalence in different countries, and the association between poor diets and the incidence of NTDs.[17] These variations are a function of both genetic background and nutritional status. The general consensus has been that NTDs are partially precipitated by functional folic acid deficiencies, which are particularly common in poor diets lacking in fruits and green vegetables.[17] In 1976, Smithells et al.[52] first reported the relationship between vitamin deficiencies and NTDs. It seemed that periconceptional vitamins supplements containing folic acid decreased the incidence of NTDs compared with controls, but the treatments were not randomized.[52,53] Laurence et al. performed a randomized trial of supplementation with 400 μg/day with similar results, but statistical significance was not reached.[54] At the same time, an animal study found a relationship between folic acid deficiency at a certain time of gestation and the development of NTD.[55] A randomized trial of folic acid supplementation in of high-risk women with a prior affected child was conducted in 1991.[56] This resulted in a 72% reduction in the recurrence risk among women receiving 4 mg/day of folic acid. Supplementation was proven to be effective when serum concentrations were raised throughout the period of conception and up to the 30 days after conception, at which time the neural tube closes. It became commonplace to recommend folic acid supplementation at 4 mg/day for women who previously had an affected child.

Unfortunately, the vast majority of NTDs occur to women with no previous history. Observational studies, nonrandomized intervention studies and randomized controlled trials have been carried out in the past 2 decades to demonstrate whether or not folic acid taken in the periconceptional period could also effectively reduce the primary incidence of NTDs.[57–59] Pilot studies on the primary incidence have been much more difficult to control and required much larger numbers. The data were always confounded by biases, such as the overall health status and likelihood of taking vitamin supplementation. There has always been the concern of bias between patients who would pay attention to their health care and who would be willing to actually take prenatal vitamins versus those who would not. A recent review of the Cochrane database[60] of 4 trials involving 6,425 women showed that periconceptional folate supplementation reduced the incidence of NTD by 72%. There was no increase in miscarriage, ectopic pregnancy or stillbirth, although there was a possible increase in multiple gestations.

At the same time, organizations such as the American Public Health Association,[61] were suggesting that doctors taking care of pregnant patients had an "obligation" to ensure that anyone who might be pregnant be put on folic acid before they became pregnant. However, less than 30% of women were using supplements with 400 μg per day in the gestational period as recommended,[62] although 70% of them were aware of the preventive role of folic acid.[24,62] This low compliance is partially explained by the fact that more that 50% of pregnancies in United States are unplanned. A study conducted in Germany in 1995 concluded that important factors affecting awareness and use of folic acid were socioeconomic status and level of education.[63]

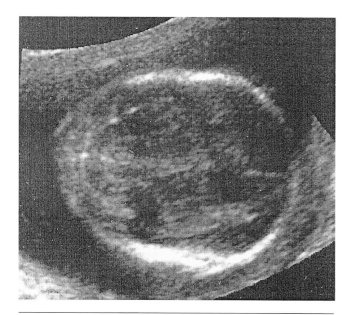

FIGURE 59-3 Fetal head in suboccipital bregmatic view demonstrating the "banana sign" which derives from anterior curving of the cerebellar hemispheres together with obliteration of the cisterna magna.

All these efforts in prevention and in prenatal diagnosis resulted in a decrease of NTD at birth in the 1990s to less than 1 per 1,000.[64] However, during this period of time, more than primary prevention, the main causal factor that accounted for the decline in NTDs at birth was the impact of prenatal diagnosis.[64] In addition, the decrease in the incidence was greater among women with better socioeconomic and educational status. This group of the population was more likely to receive both prenatal care and information about supplementation.[65]

In view of the suggested evidence that folic acid supplementation could reduce the incidence of both recurrences and primary incidences, in 1996 the United States Food and Drug Administration mandated that by January 1998, all breads and grains sold in the United States be fortified with folic acid.[66] The FDA estimated that fortification with folic acid would have increased the average consumption of folic acid by about 70–130 μgr/d.[67] Although this is only about one fourth of the total intake recommended in the periconceptional period, it was thought that amount would provide additional folic acid in the normal diet to rise to the optimal levels in the normal pregnant population.

U.S. birth certificate data have shown a 19% decline in NTDs in 2001 births compared with the incidence of NTDs in 1996, before mandatory fortification was instituted.[68] Although these results are positive and statistically significant, the decrease in NTDs was less than the decline predicted on the basis of observational studies.[69,70] It was estimated that if fortification added 100 μg of folic acid to the average daily diet of reproductive-aged women, this would result in a 23% decrease in NTD. However, recent data[71] suggested that fortification of cereal-grain food products in the United States has increased typical folic acid consumption by more than 200 μg, approximately twice the increment predicted by the FDA.[67,72] The prediction for these levels should lead to 41% reduction.[69] Another prediction study showed an 18% and 35% reduction in NTDs for 100 μg and 200 μg, respectively.[70]

One of the possible explanations for the discrepancy in findings is that some of these studies collected data from birth certificates. An evaluation of the accuracy of birth certificate data on birth defects showed that such data had a 67–86% sensitivity to report anencephaly and 40% for spina bifida.[73,74] Moreover, about 71% of women carrying a fetus with this defect decide to terminate their pregnancy,[75] and therefore these cases would be lost in birth certificates studies. Another limitation is that national birth certificates do not include fetal deaths or stillbirths, which are common occurrences in fetuses with NTDs.[76] Therefore, complete data regarding number of fetuses affected with NTDs are difficult to obtain and probably underestimate the overall incidence. This would decrease the apparent impact of folic acid fortification. If all these limitations are considered, it is possible that the decrease would be near that initially predicted. A recent study conducted in Canada after the fortification of grain products in 1998, showed a more than 50% reduction in NTD, when data from live births, stillbirths,

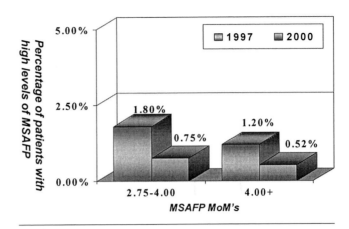

FIGURE 59-4 Decreasing percentage of high MSAFP's with folic acid fortification.

and terminations of pregnancies have been studied.[77] Another study[78] in the US population supported the fact that there has been an impact in the incidence on NTDs after fortification. MSAFP levels were used as a surrogate for the likelihood of NTDs. Comparative data from 1997 and 2000, after fortification was instituted, showed a 32% decrease in the number of high MSAFPs (Fig. 59-4). This significant decrease in MSAFP likely reflects primary prevention of NTDs through folic acid fortification.

GENETIC SUSCEPTIBILITY FOR NTD AND FOLIC ACID INTAKE

Despite the known evidence relating folic acid intake to prevention of NTDs, the underlying pathophysiologic mechanism is unknown. Folate plays an important role serving as a methyl donor in DNA synthesis, purine-pyrimidine metabolism and protein synthesis. The reduced folate coenzyme 5, 10-methylene tetrahydrofolate catalyses the main rate-limiting step during the DNA synthesis. Reduced folate is also a cofactor in the synthesis of homocysteine to methionine, an important factor for protein synthesis. These activities help cell proliferation and gene expression.[79] Cells are highly susceptible to folate deficiency during states of increased folate turnover. All these activities are increased during pregnancy; therefore pregnant women are particularly prone to develop relative deficiencies. Other possible influences include insufficient diet, the hemodilution of pregnancy, increased plasma clearance and genetic disorders that might affect production, transport, and metabolism.[80]

Genetic background, either of the mother or the fetus, may play an important role in the development of NTDs. In dichorionic pregnancies, 1 of the fetuses could be affected by the defect, while the other could be completely normal, despite the fact that each fetus is exposed to the same folate status from their mother. There is an increased acknowledgment regarding folate biochemistry and genetic polymorphisms in relation to folate-dependent metabolic pathways. The most studied polymorphism is in the gene for the production of the enzyme methylenetetrahydrofolate reductase (MTHFR). A tyrosine is substituted for cysteine at base pair 667 in the gene producing this enzyme, resulting in the C677T MTHFR polymorphism. MTHFR plays a significant role in the synthesis of methionine from homocysteine. When folate intake is deficient, individuals who are homozygous (T/T) for the abnormal gene have lower levels of the MTHFR enzyme and elevated blood homocysteine concentrations.[59,81] TT homozygosity in the fetus may be a risk factor for development of NTDs.[82] Other variants for folate-related genes include methionine reductase (MTRR) and methionine synthase (MTR), both of which have been associated with an increased risk of NTD, especially when folate status is low.[83] Moreover, infants with both the MTRR and MTR mutant genotype had a 5-fold increased risk of NTD.[84] The association between the MTHFR polymorphisms and NTDs has been described only in some populations, however, suggesting that these genetic polymorphisms are not the main contributing factor in the etiology of NTDs.[85]

FURTHER EFFECTS OF FOLIC ACID FORTIFICATION DURING PREGNANCY

Numerous epidemiological and clinical studies have demonstrated that folic acid intake has health implications in addition to NTD prevention. Folic acid interventions may also decrease the incidence of other birth defects, epithelial cancers, neurological problems, and cardiovascular disease. There is concern, however, about the risks associated with increasing folate levels within populations.

Observational studies have also shown a reduction in the incidence in other birth defects, in addition to NTDs.[86–88] There seems to be a lower rate of cleft palate and cardiac defects among pregnant women who have taken folic acid supplementation in the preconceptional months and during the first trimester of pregnancy. Data from a randomized controlled trial held in Hungary in 1994,[89] showed an increase in multiple births in women who were treated by folic acid. In a recent review of the Cochrane database, the pooled relative risk of multiple gestations was 1.4 for women with folic acid supplementation, but there was no significant increase in spontaneous abortion.[60] There was also some evidence that folic acid increases the number of miscarriages; there was a 16% relative risk of spontaneous abortion in patients with supplementation.[60] It has been suggested that a possible cause for the observed increase in both multiple gestations and spontaneous abortion is that folic acid may facilitate early fetal survival. In multiple gestations, where the nutrition requirements are high, a spontaneous abortion of 1 of the fetuses is frequent in early pregnancy.[90] The Hungarian study[60] also showed that there was an increase in fertility of women on folic acid sup-

plements and more live births in these women. It is known that MTHFR polymorphisms are associated with decreased fetal viability and recurrent miscarriage in early pregnancy. Therefore, women with this polymorphism could be able to get pregnant with folic acid supplementation and fortification.[91] Increased multiple gestations, a trend towards increased early miscarriage and fertility, has been explained with 2 concepts: "pseudoabortifacient"[92] and "terathanasia".[94] Most pregnancy losses occur early in pregnancy, before the recognition of a miscarriage. "Pseudoabortifacient" means that high levels of maternal folic acid may prolong pregnancies that otherwise would result in miscarriage.[92] "Terathanasia" is the mechanism by folic acid would reduce NTD and other birth defects by selective spontaneous abortion.[92,94] Selective spontaneous abortion together with the real antiteratogenic effect of folic acid may contribute to the reduction in NTD and other birth defects.[94] All these collateral effects on fertility and reproduction have been described after supplementation and fortification programs were implemented. There should be concern about the trend toward spontaneous abortion, and further epidemiological studies are required to appropriately ascertain the effect of folic acid in this and other aspects of human reproduction. Currently, the evidence is that folic acid supplementation and fortification results in more livebirth infants with fewer congenital malformations. This represents the biggest, single step in the reduction of birth defects.

There is also an association of folic acid with hypertension in pregnancy. A high level of homocysteine is a risk factor for gestational hypertension and preeclampsia.[95] MTHFR polymorphisms are associated with an increased risk of preeclampsia.[96,97] Folic acid supplementation has been proven to decrease plasma levels of homocysteine.[95,98] High plasma levels of homocysteine are also associated with an increase risk of cardiovascular disease.[99] Preeclampsia and cardiovascular diseases have in common endothelial damage and high rates of abnormal lipid profiles.[100] Women with a history of preeclampsia in their pregnancies are more likely to develop cardiovascular problems later in life.[101] Nevertheless, the effects on the incidence of preeclampsia have not been consistent. In Canada, the rate of preeclampsia has not changed after fortification.[102] However, another North American study showed a significant decrease in gestational hypertension and preeclampsia after supplementation.[103]

FOLIC ACID FORTIFICATION AND EFFECTS ON GENERAL POPULATION

It has been estimated that diet and nutrition, related mostly to low intakes of fruits, vegetables, and grains, contribute to about one third of preventable cancers. Population studies have described the association between folic acid intake and the incidence of cancer, especially, colon cancer.[104,105] A large prospective study from the Netherlands showed a 34%

decrease in the occurrence of colon cancer, but this protective effect was found only in men.[106] Individuals who are homozygous for the MTHFR polymorphism (T/T), in the presence of adequate folate intake, have a 40% decreased incidence of colon cancer, compared with those who are heterozygous (C/T) or have normal genotypes (C/C).[107] However, another common polymorphism of the MTHFR gene (1p36) is associated with an increased risk of cancer especially in older men and those with high alcohol intake.[108] Gastric cancer was found to be less prevalent in patients with atrophic gastritis who were taking folic acid supplementation.[109]

The incidence of other epithelial cancers is also influenced by folic acid intake. In the prospective study conducted in the Netherlands,[110] folic acid intake was inversely associated with lung cancer, even in people who smoked. Breast cancer has also been associated with folic acid intake. 32,826 women in the Nurses' Health Study were followed for the development of breast cancer.[111] The risk for women with the highest folate intake was 27% less than women with the lowest folate intake. This protective effect was even more significant for women who consumed alcohol. An interesting case-control study investigated the risk factors for acute lymphoblastic leukemia in childhood. They found that maternal folic acid supplementation during pregnancy reduced the risk of this leukemia in the offspring by 60%. The protective effect was independent of the time of initiation of the supplements and the duration of the intake during pregnancy.[112]

The pathophysiologic mechanisms underlying the protective effect of folic acid on the occurrence of cancer is not well established. Folate is essential for the synthesis, methylation, and repair of DNA. Folate metabolism promotes genome stability by avoiding uracil incorporation into DNA and by methylation of DNA. Folate depletion may play a role in disruption of DNA integrity and repair. Those 2 reactions influence the mutation rates, 1 of the basic mechanisms for the initiation of certain cancers.[113,114] However, since folic acid acts as a rate-limiting nutrient, cell proliferation is promoted in already established cancers in the presence of high levels of folic acid.[115] Future interventional studies are needed to provide evidence for the protective effect of folic acid, to determine the optimal dose and duration, and to target subpopulations in which additional efforts in prevention would be beneficial.

On the other hand, research is being carried out to determine the potential beneficial impact of folic acid fortification to decrease the rate of cardiovascular disease. Blood homocysteine levels decrease as folic acid levels increase. High blood homocysteine levels seem to be an independent risk factor for cardiovascular disease.[99] The relative risk of cardiovascular disease among individuals homozygous for MTHFR C677T variant is increased 16%.[116] This association was stronger among populations with classically low intake of folic acid, such as British and Chinese populations.[117] There is evidence that folic acid together with vitamins B6 and B12 could prevent atherosclerotic disease. It has been shown that these supplements could prevent reanastomosis and vascular events after coronary angioplasty.[118]

Folate deficiency is also associated with neurological problems. The importance of folic acid in the nervous system has been recognized for all ages, but especially in the elderly. Folic acid deficiency in the older population contributes to aging of brain processes, which increase the risk of vascular dementia and Alzheimer's disease.[119]

Prior to mandating folic acid fortification, there had been a concern about the effects of high doses of folic acid in subpopulations. The daily upper limit of intake set by the FDA was 1 mg.[67] However, it has been suggested that between 0.5–5% of adults consume more than 1 mg folic acid per day.[120] With high doses of folate there is a risk of masking the diagnosis of pernicious anemia, by delaying the diagnosis of an underlying vitamin B12 or cobalamin deficiency, even beyond the point of irreversible neurological damage has yet occurred.[121] Recent studies have also suggested that folic acid decreases the anti-inflammatory efficacy of methotrexate therapy in rheumatoid arthritis[122] and some anticonvulsive drugs.[123] There is a paucity of information about the effects of the fortification on children. It was estimated that 15–25% of children under 8 years could have intakes of folic acid above 300 μg per day.[124]

CONCLUSIONS

Overall, the introduction of folic acid fortification of breads and grains in the United States has proven to be a profoundly successful public health experiment achieving both a diminution of the rate of NTDs, congenital heart defects, and cleft palate. This represents the biggest, single step in the reduction of birth defects to date.

Numerous epidemiological and clinical studies have demonstrated the potential benefits associated with improving folic acid levels. This intervention has reduced not only the incidence in NTDs, the primary objective of this program, but also has decreased the occurrence of other birth defects, epithelial cancers, and cardiovascular disease in some studies. It is still too early to know the long-term impact of this intervention in the general population. Folate metabolism and its regulations are still not completely understood. Individual genetic backgrounds related to the metabolism of folate play an important role in the pathophysiology of some diseases. Thus, certain genetic groups will benefit from increased folic acid intake more than others. There is concern about the increased risk of multiple gestations and miscarriage reported for some groups. However, the general consideration is that folic acid supplementation and fortification results in more livebirth infants with fewer congenital malformations. At the present time, known benefits far outweigh known risks both in pregnancy and in the general population. Future interventional studies may provide supportive evidence for the protective effect of folic acid and determine the optimal dose and duration. Targeted subpopulations should be identified in which the efforts in prevention are cost-effective.

Finally, the actual scenario in prenatal diagnosis is changing with the trend toward performing screening for fetal chromosomal abnormalities during the first trimester of pregnancy. As first trimester screening with nuchal translucency and serum biochemical markers becomes more common, the incidence of anomalies diagnosed in the second trimester will further decrease. The move towards first trimester screening will accelerate the phenomenon of diminishing incidence of elevated MSAFPs. Therefore, as the incidence decreases, the cost-effectiveness of screening will decrease, and the positive predictive value of second trimester MSAFP will decrease as well. We should then consider higher cut-off values of abnormal MSAFP to decrease the false positive rate. This will improve cost effectiveness and additionally, alleviate maternal anxiety due to false positive results and the subsequent evaluation with possible unnecessary procedures.

Further efforts are needed to optimize folic acid intake among women from disadvantaged groups with poor nutritional status. There is concern that there may be lower consumption of fortified breakfast cereals and enriched grain products in women of low socioeconomic status.[65] Nevertheless, even with suboptimal consumption, the important contribution of the mandatory fortification is that it makes prevention possible in a nonsocial-class dependent fashion by ensuring availability to all women of childbearing age. The benefits of fortification include the primary prevention of major anomalies, fetal demise, and the potential decrease incidence of termination of these pregnancies. Overall, the introduction of folic acid supplementation of breads and grains in the United States has proven to be a profoundly successful public health experiment.

References

1. Reider MJ. Prevention of neural tube defects with periconceptional folic acid. *Clin Perinatol*. 1994;21:483–503.
2. Budorick NE, Pretorius DH, Nelson TR. Sonography of the fetal spine: technique, imaging, findings, and clinical implications. *Am J Roentgenol*. 1995;164:421–428.
3. Watson WJ, Chescheir NC, Katz VL, et al. The role of ultrasound in the evaluation of patients with elevated maternal serum alpha-fetoprotein: a review. *Obstet Gynecol*. 1991;78:123.
4. Schut L, Pizzi EJ, Bruce DA. Occult spinal dysraphism, myelomeningocele. In: McLaurin RL, ed. *Title*. New York, NY: Grune and Stratton, Inc; 1997.
5. Arley LB. *Developmental Anatomy: A Textbook and Laboratory Manual of Embryology*. 7th ed. Philadelphia, PA: WB Saunders; 1965.
6. Holmes LB, Driscoll SG, Atkins L. Etiologic heterogeneity of neural tube defects. *N Engl J Med*. 1976;294:365.
7. Main DM, Menutti MT. Neural tube defects: issues in prenatal diagnosis and counselling. *Obstet Gynecol*. 1986;67:1–6.
8. Milunsky A. Prenatal detection of neural tube defects: experience with 20,000 pregnancies (part VI). *JAMA*. 1980;244:2731.
9. Crandall BF, Matsumoto M. Routine amniotic fluid alpha-fetoprotein measurement in 34,000 pregnancies. *Am J Obstet Gynecol*. 1984;149:744.
10. Cowchock S, Ainbender E, Prescott G, et al. The recurrence risk of neural tube defects in United States: a collaborative study. *Am J Med Genet*. 1980;5:390.
11. Laurence KM, Beresford A. Continence, friends, marriage and children in 51 adults with spina bifida. *Dev Med Child Neurol Suppl*. 1975;35:123.
12. Evans MI, O'Brien JE, Dvorin E, et al. Biochemical screening. In: Gleicher N, ed. *Principles and Practice of Medical Therapy in Pregnancy*. 3rd ed. Appleton and Lange, 1998.
13. Carter CO. Recurrence risks for common malformations. *Practitioner*. 1974;213:667.
14. Little J, Elwood JM. Geographical variation. In: Elwood JM, Little J, Elwood JH, eds. *Epidemiology and Control of Neural Tube Defects*. Oxford, England: Oxford University Press; 1992:96–145.
15. Murphy M, Whiteman D, Stone D, et al. Dietary folate and the prevalence of neural tube defects in British Isles: the past two decades. *Br J Obstet Gynaecol*. 2000;107:885–889.
16. Ehara H, Ohno K, Ohtani K, et al. Epidemiology of spina bifida in Tottori Prefecture, Japan, 1976–1995. *Pediatr Neurol*. 1998;19:109–203.
17. Elwood JM, Elwood JH. *Epidemiology of Anencephaly and Spina Bifida*. New York, NY: Oxford University Press; 1980.
18. Walker E. FDA issues regulations for vitamins. *Mod Nurs Home*. 1973;31(5):4.
19. Olney RS, Mulinare J. Trends in neural tube defect prevalence, folic acid fortification and vitamin supplement use. *Sem Perinatol*. 2002;26:277–285.
20. Honein MA, Paulozzi LJ, Mathews TJ, et al. Impact of folic acid fortification of the US food supply on the occurrence of neural tube defects. *JAMA*. 2001;285:2981–2986.
21. Persad VL, Van den Holf MC, Dubé JM, et al. Incidence of open neural tube defects in Nova Scotia after folic acid fortification. *CAMJ*. 2002;6:167:241–245.
22. Alembik Y, Dott B, Roth MP, et al. Prevalence in neural tube defects in northeastern France, 1979–1994: impact of prenatal diagnosis. *Ann Genet*. 1997;40(2):69–71.
23. Vollset SE, Lande B. Knowledge and attitudes of folate, and use of dietary supplements among women of reproductive age in Norway 1998. *Acta Obstet Gynecol Scand*. 2000;79:513–519.
24. de Walle HE, Cornel MC, de Jong-van den Berg LT. Three years after the dutch folic acid campaign: growing socio-economic differences. *Prev Med*. 2002;35:65–69.
25. Berry RJ, Li Z, Erickson JD, et al. for the China-US Collaborative Project for Neural Tube Defect Prevention. Prevention of neural tube defects with folic acid in China. *N Engl J Med*. 1999;341:1485–1490.
26. International Clearinghouse for Birth Defects Monitoring Systems. Annual report 1997. Rome, Italy: International Centre for Birth Defects; 1997.
27. Nazer J, Lopez-Camelo J, Castilla EE. ECLAMC: 30-year study of epidemiological surveillance of neural tube defects in Chile and Latin America. *Rev Med Chil*. 2001;129:531–539.
28. Brock DJ, Sutcliffe RG. Alpha-fetoprotein in the antenatal diagnosis of anencephaly and spina bifida. *Lancet*. 1972;ii:197.
29. Schell DI, Drugan A, Brindley BA, et al. Combining ultrasonography and amniocentesis for pregnant women with elevated maternal serum alpha-fetoprotein: revising the risk estimate. *J Reprod Med*. 1990;35:543–546.
30. Drugan A, Dvorin E, O'Brien JE, et al. Alpha-fetoprotein. *Curr Opin Obstet Gynecol*. 1991;3:230–234.
31. Reichler A, Hume R, Drugan A, et al. Risk of anomalies as a function of level of elevated maternal serum alpha-fetoprotein. *Am J Obstet Gynecol*. 1994;171:1052–1055.
32. Killam WP, Miller RC, Seeds JW. Extremely high maternal serum alpha-fetoprotein levels at the second trimester screening. *Obstet Gynecol*. 1991;71:257–261.

33. Richards DS, Seeds JW, Katz VL. Maternal serum alpha-fetoprotein with normal ultrasound: is amniocentesis always appropriate? a review of 26069 screened patients. *Obstet Gynecol.* 1988;1:203.

34. Jorgensen FS, Valentin L, Salvesen KA, et al. MULTISCAN—a Scandinavian multicenter second trimester obstetric ultrasound and serum screening study. *Acta Obstet Gynecol Scand.* 1999;78:501–510.

35. Brock DJH, Bolton AE, Monaghan JM. Prenatal diagnosis of anencephaly through maternal serum alpha-fetoprotein measurements. *Lancet.* 1973;ii:923–924.

36. Evans MI, O'Brien JE, Dvorin E, et al. Similarity of insulin-dependent diabetics' and non-insulin-dependent diabetics' levels of beta-hCG and unconjugated estriol with controls: no need to adjust as with alpha-fetoprotein. *J Soc Gynecol Investig.* 1996;3:20–22.

37. Evans MI, Harrison H, O'Brien JE, et al. Maternal weight correction for alpha-fetoprotein: mathematical truncations revisited. *Genet Test.* 2002;6:221–223.

38. Los FJ, Dewolf BT, Huisjes HJ. Raised maternal serum alpha-fetoprotein levels and spontaneous feto-maternal transfusion. *Lancet.* 1979;ii:1210.

39. Macri JN, Weiss RR, Tillitt R, et al. Prenatal diagnosis of neural tube defects. *JAMA.* 1976;236:1251–1254.

40. Milunsky A, Alpert E, Neff R, et al. Prenatal diagnosis of neural tube defects: maternal serum alpha-fetoprotein screening. *Obstet Gynecol.* 1980;55:60–66.

41. Brock DJ, Barron L, Jelen P, et al. Maternal serum alpha-fetoprotein measurements as an early indicator of low birth-weight. *Lancet.* 1977;2:267–268.

42. Katz VL, Chescheir NC, Cefalo RC. Unexplained elevations of maternal serum alpha-fetoprotein. *Obstet Gynecol Surv.* 1990;45:719–726.

43. Yaron Y, Cherry M, Kramer RL, et al. Second trimester maternal serum marker screening: MSAFP, β-hCG, estriol, and their various combinations as predictors of pregnancy outcome. *Am J Obstet Gynecol.* 1999;181:968–974.

44. Vintzileos AM, Ananth CV, Fisher AJ, et al. Cost-benefit analysis of targeted ultrasonography for prenatal detection of spina bifida in patients with an elevated concentration of second trimester maternal-serum alpha-fetoprotein. *Am J Obstet Gynecol.* 1999;180:1227–1233.

45. Lennon CA, Gray DL. Sensitivity and specificity of ultrasound for the detection of neural tube and ventral wall defects in a high-risk population. *Obstet Gynecol.* 1999;94:562–566.

46. Chan A, Robertson E, Haan EA, et al. The sensitivity of ultrasound and serum alpha-fetoprotein in population-based antenatal screening for neural tube defects, South Australia 1986–1991. *Br J Obstet Gynaecol.* 1995;102:370–376.

47. Chatzipapas IK, Whitlow BJ, Economides DL. The "Mickey Mouse" sign and the diagnosis of anencephaly in early pregnancy. *Ultrasound Obstet Gynecol.* 1999;13:196–199.

48. Richards CG. Frontoethmoidal meningoencephalocele: a common and severe congenital abnormality in South East Asia. *Arch Dis Child.* 1992;67:717–719.

49. Kalien B, Robert E, Harris J. Associated malformations in infants and fetuses with upper or low neural tube defects. *Teratology.* 1998;57:56–63.

50. Nicolaides KH, Campbell S, Gabbe SG, et al. Ultrasound screening for spina bifida: cranial and cerebral signs. *Lancet.* 1986;2:72–74.

51. van den Hof MC, Nicolaides KH, Campbell J, et al. Evaluation of the lemon and banana signs in one hundred thirty fetuses with open spina bifida. *Am J Obstet Gynecol.* 1990;162:322–327.

52. Smithells RW, Sheppard S, Schorah CJ. Vitamin deficiencies and neural tube defects. *Arch Dis Child.* 1976;51:944.

53. Schorah CJ, Smithells RW, Scott J. Vitamin B12 and anencephaly. *Lancet.* 1980;19:880.

54. Laurence KM, James N, Miller MH. Double blind randomised controlled trial of folate treatment before conception to prevent recurrence of neural tube defects. *BMJ.* 1981;282:1509.

55. Wald NJ, Polani PE. Neural tube defects and vitamins: the need for a randomised clinical trial. *Br J Obstet Gynecol.* 1984;91:516.

56. Medical Research Council Vitamin study research group. Prevention of neural tube defects: results of the MRC Vitamin Study. *Lancet.* 1991;338:131–137.

57. Czeizel AE, Dudas I. Prevention of the first occurrence of neural tube defects by periconceptional vitamin supplementation. *N Engl J Med.* 1992;327:1832–1835.

58. Werler MM, Shapiro S, Mitchell AA. Periconceptional folic acid exposure and risk of occurrent neural tube defects. *JAMA.* 1993;269:1257–1261.

59. Berry RJ, Li Z, Erickson JD, et al. for the China-US Collaborative Project for Neural Tube Defect Prevention. Prevention of neural tube defects with folic acid in China. *N Engl J Med.* 1999;341:1485–1490.

60. Lumley J, Watson L, Watson M, et al. Periconceptional supplementation with folate and/or multivitamins for preventing neural tube defects. (Cochrane Review) In: The Cochrane Library, Issue 3, 2001. Oxford, England: Update Software.

61. CDC. Recommendations for the use of folic acid to reduce the number of cases of spina bifida and other neural tube defects. *MMWR Morb Mortal Wkly Rep.* 1992;41(no RR-14).

62. CDC. Knowledge and use of folic acid by women of childbearing age. *MMWR Morb Mortal Wkly Rep.* 1999;48:325–327.

63. Morin P, De Walls P, St-Cyr-Tribble D, et al. Pregnancy planning: a determinant of folic acid supplements use for the primary prevention of neural tube defects. *Can J Public Health.* 2002;93:259–263.

64. Erickson JD. Folic acid and prevention of spina bifida and anencephaly: 10 years after the U.S. Public Health Service recommendation. *MMWR Morb Mortal Wkly Rep.* 2002;51:1–3.

65. Meyer RE, Siega-Ritz AM. Socioeconomic patterns in spina bifida birth prevalence trends-North Carolina, 1995–1999. *MMWR Morb Mortal Wkly Rep* 2002;51:12–19.

66. Food and Drug Administration. Food Standards. *Federal Register.* 1996;61:8781–8797.

67. Food and Drug Administration. Food labelling: health claims and label statements; folate and neural tube defects. *Federal Register.* 1993;58:53254–53295.

68. Honein MA, Paulozzi LJ, Mathews TJ, et al. Impact of folic acid fortification of the US food supply on the occurrence of neural tube defects. *JAMA.* 2001;285:2981–2986.

69. Wald NJ, Law M, Jordan R. Folic acid food fortification to prevent neural tube defects. *Lancet.* 1998;351:834.

70. Daly S, Mills JL, Molloy AM, et al. Minimum effective dose of folic acid for food fortification to prevent neural tube defects. *Lancet.* 1997;350:1666–1669.

71. Quinlivan EP, Gregory JF. Effect of food fortification on folic acid intake in the United States. *Am J Clin Nutr.* 2003;77:221–225.

72. Choumenkovitch SF, Selhub J, Wilson PWF, et al. Folic acid intake from fortification in United States exceeds prediction. *J Nutr.* 2002;132:2792–2798.

73. Watkins ML, Edmonds L, McClearn A, et al. The surveillance of birth defects. *Am J Public Health.* 1996;86:731–734.

74. Piper JM, Mitchel EF, Snowden M, et al. Validation of the 1989 Tennessee birth certificates using maternal and newborn hospital records. *Am J Epidemiol.* 1993;737:758–768.

75. Cunningham G, Tompkinson DG. Cost and effectiveness of the California triple marker, prenatal screening program. *Genet Med.* 1999;1:199–206.

76. Little J, Elwood M. Fetal loss. In: Elwood JM, Little J, Elwood JH, eds. *Epidemiology and Control of Neural Tube Defects.* New York, NY: Oxford University Press; 1992:324–334.

77. Persad VL, van den Holf MC, Dubé JM, et al. Incidence of open neural tube defects in Nova Scotia after folic acid fortification. *CMAJ.* 2002;6:241–245.

78. Evans MI, Llurba E, Landsberger EJ, et al. Impact of folic acid fortification in the United States: markedly diminished high maternal serum alpha-fetoprotein values. *Obstet Gynecol.* 2004;103:474–479.

79. Shoiania AM. Folic acid and vitamin B12 deficiency in pregnancy and the neonatal period. *Clin Perinatol.* 1984;11:433.

80. Botto LD, Yang Q. Methylenetetrahydrofolate reductase gene variants and congenital anomalies: a HuGE review. *Am J Epidemiol.* 2000;151:862–877.

81. Bailey LB, Gregory JF. Polymorphisms of methylenetetrahydrofolate reductase and other enzymes: metabolic significance, risks and impact on folate requirement. *J Nutr.* 1999;129:919–922.

82. Wilson A, Platt R, Wu Q. A common variant in methionine synthetase reductase combined with low cobalamin (vitamin B12) increases risk for spina bifida. *Mol Gen Metab.* 1999;67:317–323.

83. Zhu H, Wicker NJ, Shaw GM, et al. Homocysteine remethylation enzyme polymorphisms and increased risk for neural tube defects. *Mol Genet Metab.* 2003;78:216–221.

84. Finnell RH, Shaw GM, Lammer EJ, et al. Does prenatal screening for 5,10-methylenetetrahydrofolate reductase (MTHFR) mutations in high-risk neural tube defects pregnancies make sense? *Genet Test.* 2002;6:47–52.

85. Czeizel AE, Toth M, Rockenbauer M. Population-based case control study of folic acid supplementation during pregnancy. *Teratology.* 1996;53:345–351.

86. Shaw GM, O'Malley CD, Wasserman CR. Maternal periconceptional use of multivitamins and reduced risk of conotruncal heart defects and limb deficiencies among offspring. *Am J Med Genet.* 1995; 59:536–545.

87. Werler MM, Hayes C, Louik C. Multivitamin supplementation and risk of birth defects. *Am J Epidemiol.* 1999;150:675–682.

88. Czeizel AE, Metneki J, Dudas I. The higher rate of multiple births after periconceptional multivitamin supplementation: an analysis of causes. *Acta Genet Med Gemmellol (Roma).* 1994;43:175–184.

89. Lumley J, Watson L, Watson M, et al. Modelling the potential impact of population-wide periconceptional folate/vitamin supplementation on multiple births. *Br J Obstet Gynaecol.* 2001;108:937–942.

90. Nelen WL, Blom HJ, Thomas CM, et al. Methylenetetrahydrofolate reductase polymorphism affects the change in homocysteine and folate concentrations resulting from low dose folic acid supplementation in women with unexplained recurrent miscarriages. *J Nutr.* 1998;128:1336–1341.

91. Hook EB. Folic acid: abortifacient or pseudoabortifacient? *Am J Med Genet.* 2000;301–302.

92. Windham GC, Shaw GM, Todoroff K, et al. Miscarriage and use of multivitamins and folic acid. *Am J Med Genet.* 2000;90:261–262.

93. Hook EB, Czeizel AE. Can terathanasia explain the protective effect of folic acid supplementation on birth defects? *Lancet.* 1997; 350:513–12.

94. Vollset SE, Refsum H, Irgens LM, et al. Plasma total homocysteine, pregnancy complications, and severe pregnancy outcome: the Hordaland Homocysteine Study. *Am J Clin Nutr.* 2000;71:962–968.

95. Wang J, Trudinger BJ, Duarte N. Elevated circulating homocysteine levels in placental vascular disease and associated pre-eclampsia. *Br J Obstet Gynaecol.* 2000;107:935–938.

96. Grandone E, Margaglione M, Colaizzo D. MTHFR polymorphisms and genetic susceptibility to preeclampsia. *Thromb Haemost.* 1997;77:1052–1054.

97. Kupferminc MJ, Eldor A, Steinman N, et al. Increased frequency of genetic thrombophilia in women with complications of pregnancy. *N Engl J Med.* 1999;340:9–13.

98. Homocysteine Lowering Trialists' Collaboration. Lowering blood homocysteine with folic acid based supplements: meta-analysis of randomised trials. *BMJ.* 1998;316:894–898.

99. Hankey GJ, Eikelboom JW. Homocysteine and vascular disease. *Lancet.* 1999;354:407–413.

100. Gratacos E. Lipid-mediated endothelial dysfunction: a common factor to preeclampsia and chronic vascular disease. *Eur J Obstet Gynecol Reprod Biol.* 2000;92:63–66.

101. Smith GC, Pell JP, Walsh D. Pregnancy complications and maternal risk of ischemic heart disease: a retrospective cohort study of 129,290 births. *Lancet.* 2001;357:2002–2006.

102. Ray JG, Mandani MM. Association between folic acid food fortification and hypertension or preeclampsia in pregnancy. *Arch Intern Med.* 2002;162:1776–1779.

103. Hernandez-Diaz S, Werler MM, Louik C, et al. Risk of gestational hypertension in relation to folic acid supplementation during pregnancy. *Am J Epidemiol.* 2002;156:806–812.

104. Eichholzer M, Luthy J, Moser U, et al. Folate and the risk of colorectal, breast and cervix cancer: the epidemiological evidence. *Swiss Med Wkly.* 2001;131:539–549.

105. Flood A, Caprario L, Chaterjee N, et al. Folate, methionine, alcohol, and colorectal cancer in a prospective study of women in the United States. *Cancer Causes Control.* 2002;13:551–561.

106. Konings EJ, Goldbohm RA, Brants HA, et al. Intake of dietary folate vitamers and risk of colorectal carcinoma: results from the Netherlands Cohort Study. *Cancer.* 2002;95:1421–1433.

107. Ma J, Stampfer MJ, Giovannucci E, et al. Methylenetetrahydrofolate reductase polymorphism, dietary interactions, and risk of colorectal cancer. *Cancer Res.* 1997;57:1098–1102.

108. Heijmans BT, Boer JM, Suchiman HE, et al. A common variant of methylenetetrahydrofolate reductase gene (1p36) is associated with an increased risk of cancer. *Cancer Res.* 2003;63:1249–1253.

109. Zhu S, Mason J, Shi Y, et al. The effect of folic acid on the development of stomach and other gastrointestinal cancers. *Chin Med J (Engl).* 2003;116:15–19.

110. Voorrips LE, Goldbohm RA, Brants HA, et al. A prospective cohort study on antioxidant and folate intake and male lung cancer risk. *Cancer Epidemiol Biomarkers Prev.* 2000;9:357–365.

111. Zhang SM, Willet WC, Selhub J, et al. Plasma folate, vitamin B6, vitamin B12, homocysteine, and risk of breast cancer. *J Natl Cancer Inst.* 2003;95:373–380.

112. Thompson JR, Gerald PF, Willoughby ML, et al. Maternal folate supplementation in pregnancy and protection against acute lymphoblastic leukaemia in childhood: a case-control study. *Lancet.* 2001;358:1935–1940.

113. DePinho RA. The age of cancer. *Nature.* 2000;408:248–254.

114. Choi SW, Mason JB. Folate and carcinogenesis: an integrated scheme. *J Nutr.* 2000;130:129–132.

115. McNulty, McPartlin JM, Weir DG, et al. Folate catabolism is increased during pregnancy in rats. *J Nutr.* 1993;123:1089–1093.

116. Klerk M, Verhoef P, Clarke R, et al. for the MTHFR Studies Collaboration group. MTHFR 667C→T polymorphism and risk of coronary heart disease: a meta-analysis. *JAMA.* 2002;288:2042–2043.

117. Wilson PWF. Homocysteine and coronary heart disease: how great is the hazard? *JAMA.* 2002;288:2042–2043.

118. Schnyder G, Roffi M, Flammer Y, et al. Effect of homocysteine-lowering therapy with folic acid, vitamin 12, and vitamin B6 on clinical outcome after percutaneous coronary intervention: the Swiss Heart Study: a randomized controlled trial. *JAMA.* 2002;288:973–979.

119. Reynolds EH. Folic acid, ageing, depression, and dementia. *BMJ.* 2002;324:1512–1515.

120. Lewis CJ, Crane NT, Wilson DB, et al. Estimated folate intakes: data updated to reflect food fortification, increased bioavailability, and dietary supplement use. *Am J Clin Nutr*. 1999;70:198–207.

121. Sauberlilich HE, Dowdy RP, Skala JH. *Laboratory Tests for the Assessment of Nutritional Status*. Cleveland, OH: CRC Press; 1974.

122. van Ede AE, Laan RF, Rood MJ, et al. Effect of folic or folinic acid supplementation on the toxicity and efficacy of methotrexate in rheumatoid arthritis: a forty-eight-week, multicenter, randomized, double-blind, placebo-controlled study. *Arthritis Rheum*. 2001;44:1515–1524.

123. Lewis DP, van Dyke DC, Willhite LA, et al. Phenytoin-folic acid interaction. *Ann Pharmacother*. 1995;29:726–735.

124. Bailey LB, Gregory JF. Folate metabolism and requirements. *J Nutr*. 1999;129:779–782.

EVALUATION OF THE FETAL CARDIOVASCULAR SYSTEM

Jack Rychik

INTRODUCTION

Congenital heart disease is the most common form of congenital anomaly found in the human species. It occurs in approximately 8 per 1000 live births and in approximately 10–12 per 1000 pregnancies. Congenital abnormalities of cardiac structure usually exist without manifestation of symptoms until separation from placental circulation at birth; hence, it can be easily missed during fetal life, unless carefully searched for. Recent advancements in ultrasound technology, improved operator skill, and greater popular interest in fetal imaging, in general, have led to an increased frequency, and improved accuracy of diagnosis of congenital heart disease prior to birth.

The ability to peer into the womb and observe the growing fetus has furthered our understanding of human development as well as significantly impacted our management strategies for treatment of congenital heart disease. While conventional diagnosis of congenital heart disease typically takes place in infancy and childhood, this arbitrary point in time is now changed as more and more patients are identified in the third and second trimesters of gestation (Fig. 60-1). This change has resulted in a substantial expansion of the field of fetal cardiology—from both a diagnostic and a potential interventional perspective—with a multidisciplinary interest abided by maternal-fetal medicine specialists, ultrasonographers, radiologists, pediatric cardiologists and surgeons.

In this chapter, we review the physiology of the developing fetal cardiovascular system and the basic tenets of the fetal echocardiographic evaluation and discuss a variety of disease processes that affect the fetal cardiovascular system.

UNIQUENESS OF THE FETAL CARDIOVASCULAR SYSTEM

The fetal cardiovascular system differs from the mature adult system in many ways. First, the structural elements of the fetal myocardium are unique. Early fetal myocytes can undergo replication with development of "hyperplasia" or an increase in cell number, while mature adult myocytes undergo "hypertrophy" or increase in cell size. In fact, the myocardium is limited in its ability to increase cell number much beyond the early postnatal period. Second, the fetal heart is much stiffer than the adult heart, with impaired relaxation relative to the adult. Fetal myocardium is composed of approximately 60% noncontractile elements, versus 30% in the adult heart.[1] The uptake of calcium via the sarcoplasmic reticulum differs in the fetus from the adult, impairing relaxation properties during diastole.[2]

Cardiac stroke volume in the fetus is limited in comparison with that after birth because of extrinsic compression of the heart. Cardiac output and blood flow are a factor of stroke volume and heart rate; it may explain why the fetus is limited in its ability to increase cardiac output to meet demands in various disease states unless there is a substantial increase in heart rate. In the fetus, the ventricles exist under a constraint exerted by the chest wall, fluid-filled lungs, and pericardium, resulting in a limited ability for the ventricle to expand and a reduced ventricular preload.[3] With the first few breaths of life, the lungs expand and lung fluid is expelled or resorbed, thereby freeing the ventricle from this constraint. In conjunction with increased pulmonary venous return, left ventricular preload is increased with resultant increase in stroke volume.

The fetal circulation is quite unique. Unlike those in the postnatal circulation, in which the pulmonary and systemic circulations are in series (deoxygenated blood is pumped by the right side into the lungs, returns as oxygenated blood to the left side, and is pumped out to the body), the fetal right and left flows are in parallel, with oxygenation taking place at a site external to the fetus, the placenta. Structures, such as the *ductus venosus, patent foramen ovale*, and the *ductus arteriosus*, provide unique blood flow pathways specific to the fetus (Fig. 60-2).

The circulation prior to birth is designed in such a manner that it appears to be quite adaptive to the fetal needs. The placenta is a richly vascularized organ and of extremely low vascular resistance. Two fetal iliac arteries originating from the descending aorta give rise to 2 umbilical arteries that exit the fetus and course toward the placenta. The umbilical arteries carry an admixture of deoxygenated arterial blood toward the oxygenating organ, the placenta. A single venous structure, the umbilical vein, carries richly oxygenated blood back to the fetus through the umbilical cord. The umbilical vein inserts into the ductus venosus, a structure that traverses the liver and connects into the inferior vena cava just as it enters the right atrium. The angle at which the ductus venosus inserts into the inferior vena cava–right atrial junction, is such that the stream of flow is directed toward the foramen ovale, into the left atrium and left ventricle. In this manner, the most richly oxygenated blood returning from the placenta is directed toward the developing organs most in need of oxygen delivery—the myocardial and cerebral circulations—both of which are perfused by the left ventricle. Similarly, the most deoxygenated blood in the fetus drains from the superior vena cava and is directed toward the tricuspid valve. This column of blood is then ejected by the right ventricle into the main pulmonary artery. The pulmonary vasculature is of very high resistance during prenatal life; hence, little flow enters the pulmonary circulation, and the majority of flow is directed toward the ductus arteriosus, descending aorta, and the umbilical arteries. The fetal cardiovascular architecture is designed to maximize delivery of oxygenated blood to the organs in the greatest need,

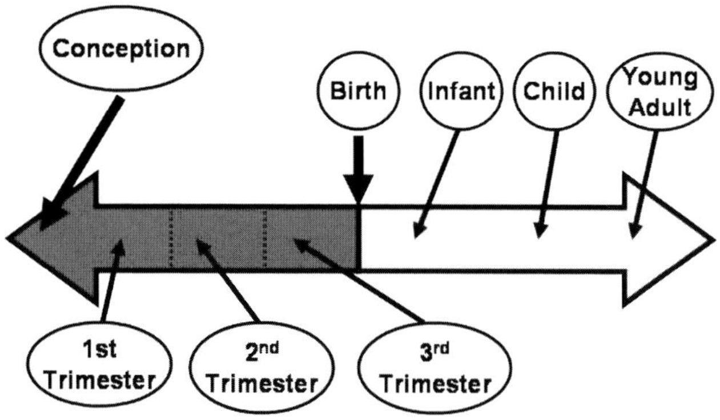

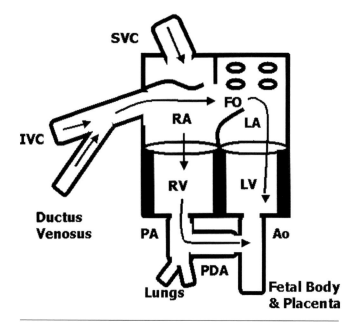

FIGURE 60-1 The timeline for detection and diagnosis of congenital heart disease. Conventional timing is upon the manifestation of symptomatology, at either birth, infancy, or childhood. Current trends are leading toward greater detection of congenital heart disease prior to birth either in the second or in the third trimester of gestation. Current techniques for suspicion of heart disease are evolving for use during the first trimester with the ultimate goal of determining who is at risk at the time of conception.

FIGURE 60-2 Schematic drawing of the fetal circulation. Ductus venosus flow (highly oxygenated) is channeled right to left across the foramen ovale and into the left atrium and left ventricle. This blood is then delivered to the upper portion of the body. Superior vena caval flow (highly deoxygenated) is directed toward the tricuspid valve and right ventricle and ejected across the ductus arteriosus to the lower part of the body.

and to deliver the most deoxygenated blood in the most direct manner possible to the placenta.

FETAL ECHOCARDIOGRAPHY: WHY PERFORM?

Fetal echocardiography utilizes the science of biological ultrasound to examine the developing fetal cardiovascular system. The first ultrasonic images of the human fetal heart were generated more than 25 years ago.[4] Since then, the modalities of 2-dimensional and Doppler imaging have added much to our understanding of the fetal heart; however, skepticism existed early on as to the role of fetal echocardiography in clinical care.

Is ultrasound scanning of the fetus helpful in diagnosing congenital heart disease? The answer depends on the way in which the fetal echocardiographic evaluation is performed. In a landmark study by Ewigman et al., more than 15,000 pregnant women underwent routine prenatal ultrasound evaluation.[5] The investigators found very little impact on perinatal outcome and concluded that routine ultrasound scanning was not helpful. Of note, the cardiac examination consisted of only a "4-chamber view." In other words, if the operator could count the presence of 4 chambers of the heart, the fetus was considered to have a normal cardiovascular system. Buskens et al. reported on the ultrasonic evaluation of nearly 7000 pregnant women performing the "4-chamber view" alone and compared the fetal examination findings with those from the postnatal echocardiogram.[6] They reported only 4.5% sensitivity for detection of congen-

ital heart disease. Utilizing a different approach to imaging, Stumpflen et al. reported on data from a single center in which more than 3000 women were scanned.[7] Operators were trained to perform a detailed fetal examination consisting of the "4-chamber view," identification of the right and left outflow tracts, and application of pulse-wave Doppler and color Doppler flow imaging. In their series, sensitivity and specificity for the detection of congenital heart disease were 86% and 100%, respectively, a marked improvement over the previous reports. These studies highlight the fact that methodology and technique used in performing fetal echocardiography are essential in defining its utility. Proper technique, training, equipment, and fund of knowledge all contribute to the very effective diagnostic yield of fetal echocardiography as it currently exists today.

Let us assume that a skilled examination provides for a complete and accurate prenatal diagnosis—does a correct fetal diagnosis of congenital heart disease impact patient outcome? Intuitively, one would predict that identification of congenital heart disease prior to birth would provide some benefit to the newborn. In the current era of rapid neonatal diagnosis, efficient interhospital transport, and excellent surgical results, differences in early operative outcome between prenatally and postnatally diagnosed infants have not been uniformly seen.[8] Some centers have begun to report differences in outcome, in particular for complex lesions. Tworetzky et al., at the University of California in San Francisco, found improved

TABLE 60-1	POTENTIAL BENEFITS OF PRENATAL DIAGNOSIS OF CONGENITAL HEART DISEASE

- Information/parental education
- Parental counseling/choice of termination
- Psychological/social preparation
- Choice of site for care
- Stable transition from pre- to postnatal life
- Reduction in acidosis
- Improved surgical survival
- Improved neurological outcome
- Long-term benefits
- Cost-effective

survival for first-stage palliation of hypoplastic left heart syndrome in prenatally diagnosed infants when compared with infants diagnosed after birth.[9] An important contributing factor to overall improvement may be the better physiological state of prenatally diagnosed infants. Verheijen et al. reported on a multicenter study in which comparison was made of the metabolic state of infants with and without prenatal diagnosis of congenital heart disease.[10] They found that prenatal diagnosis improved infant blood pH and lactate levels to a significant degree.

There are many potential benefits to the prenatal diagnosis of congenital heart disease (Table 60-1). We live in an era in which information is a critical commodity. Parents are strongly desirous of any and all information concerning their unborn child, as witnessed by the current interest in "fetal photography" and the 3-dimensional rendering of facial images of the fetus that are now commercially available. Knowledge of the presence of a fetus with congenital heart disease allows the family to prepare for the rigors of care necessary for an infant with a birth defect. Parents have the opportunity to spend time learning about the anomaly, the management, and lifelong ramifications. They can meet with physicians and nurses to discuss and develop a treatment strategy and can tour facilities such as the delivery suites and the intensive care unit. Prior knowledge of a congenital heart defect allows a family to investigate and choose a site for delivery and care, one that is experienced in the management of the lesion. Alternatively, some families may choose to terminate a pregnancy after the identification of serious congenital heart disease. Knowledgeable, compassionate, and nondirected counseling must accompany the revelation of the diagnosis. Emotional support should be available to families as they move through this decision process. Physicians and nurses offering such counseling must be fully aware of the latest strategies and outcomes for congenital heart disease so that families can make educated and informed decisions.

Of great promise is the possibility that prenatally diagnosed infants with congenital heart disease will do better in the long term than those diagnosed after birth. Much investigational focus is currently aimed at neurological outcome after repair of congenital heart disease. Studies have demonstrated impaired neurocognitive outcome and deficits in school performance in some children after surgical repair of congenital heart disease.[11] Prenatal diagnosis may have a positive impact on these long-term neurocognitive parameters, since the occurrence of hypotension, hemodynamic instability, and acidosis in the early neonatal period should be minimized. In addition, prenatal diagnosis may prove to be cost-effective in both the short and long terms if hospital outcome is improved and late complications are minimized.[12]

As a consequence of the increasing number of fetal echocardiograms performed, standards of practice are shifting. In a recent review of newborns with complex congenital heart disease admitted to the Cardiac Intensive Care Unit at The Children's Hospital of Philadelphia, more than half were diagnosed prenatally. The impact of this changing trend on overall outcome is of great interest and will be the subject of much study in the years to come.

FETAL ECHOCARDIOGRAPHY: IN WHOM, WHEN, AND HOW?

Fetal echocardiography can provide detailed information about the cardiovascular system, and precise and reliable diagnosis of complex congenital heart disease can be made prior to birth. In addition, fetal echocardiography provides insight into the pathophysiology of complex disease processes that can affect the developing cardiovascular system. High-quality fetal cardiovascular imaging is being performed with increasing frequency. From 1998 to 2004, fetal echocardiograms performed at The Children's Hospital of Philadelphia have more than tripled in number, with more than 1500 studies currently performed annually. While many pediatric cardiologists have become interested in developing the skills necessary to

TABLE 60-2	INDICATIONS FOR PERFORMANCE OF THE FETAL ECHOCARDIOGRAM

Maternal indications
- Family history of coronary heart disease
- Heritable disorders (Marfan syndrome, etc.)
- Metabolic disorders (diabetes, phenylketonuria, etc.)
- Teratogen exposure (lithium, etc.)
- Rubella infection
- Maternal autoimmune disease (Lupus, Sjogren syndrome, etc.)
- In vitro fertilization
- Advanced maternal age >40 yrs

Fetal indications
- Aneuploidy
- Extracardiac abnormality
- Fetal heart beat irregularity
- Fetal hydrops
- Increased nuchal translucency (first trimester)
- Abnormal obstetrical ultrasound screen

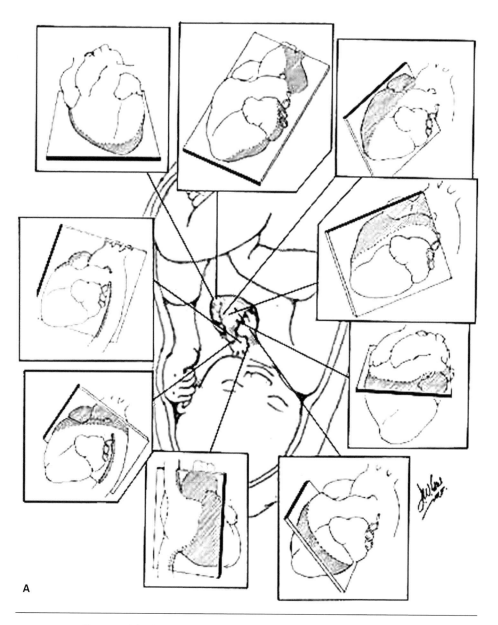

FIGURE 60-3 Tomographic views used for imaging of the fetal heart. Nine standardized views have been established. (Reprinted with permission from American Society of Echocardiography, 2004.)

perform fetal echocardiography, maternal-fetal medicine specialists, perinatologists, and ultrasound radiologists have also mastered these skills and may perform high-quality scanning. Guidelines for performance of fetal echocardiography were recently established by the American Society of Echocardiography.[13]

Indications for performing a fetal echocardiogram can be divided into those that are *maternal* or *fetal* (Table 60-2). A family history of congenital heart disease is a common indication for referral for fetal echocardiography. Maternal diabetes mellitus is a risk factor for congenital heart disease and should prompt examination. Maternal diabetes can also cause an increase in fetal ventricular wall thickness, resulting in a hypertrophic cardiomyopathy that can deleteriously affect ventricular function after birth. Maternal exposure to a teratogen or maternal infection with rubella may increase the likelihood of fetal heart disease. Maternal autoimmune disease such as lupus erythematosus or Sjogren disease can lead to diseases of the fetal conduction system or development of fetal cardiomyopathy.[14] Oftentimes, identification of fetal heart block may be the heralding sign of maternal autoimmune disease in an otherwise healthy, asymptomatic mother. Serological assessment of the mother will reveal her to be positive for SS-A or SS-B antibodies. Recent data confirm an increased incidence of congenital anomalies in fetuses conceived via in vitro fertilization techniques, in particular, through intracytoplasmic injection;[15,16] hence, all such women should have careful fetal echocardiography performed.

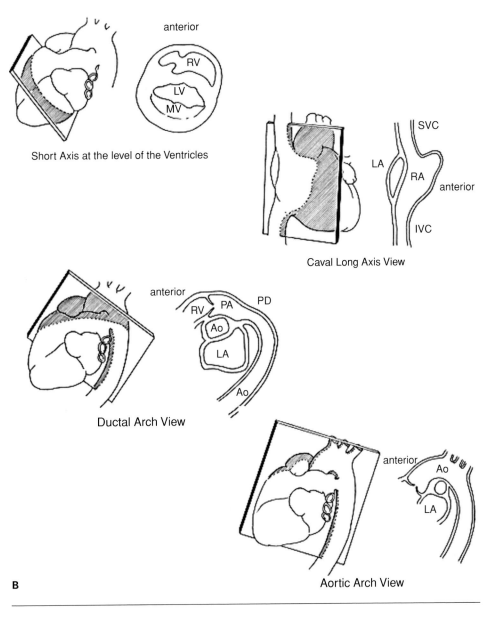

FIGURE 60-3 *Continued.*

Fetal indications include the presence of aneuploidy (e.g., trisomies 13, 18, or 21) or extracardiac anomalies (e.g., diaphragmatic hernia, teratoma). The presence of fetal hydrops should precipitate an investigation of possible cardiac causes via fetal echocardiography. Fetal heart beat irregularity or suspicion of a structural abnormality on routine obstetrical screening should lead to a more detailed and comprehensive fetal echocardiogram. Recently, great interest has been generated in the use of first-trimester (10–13 weeks' gestation) imaging of the posterior aspect of the fetal neck, looking at "nuchal translucency." Data suggest that fetuses with increased nuchal translucency have a significantly increased incidence of congenital heart disease, even in the absence of aneuploidy.[17,18] Some investigators have predicted that increased nuchal translucency

may become the most reliable predictor of the presence of congenital heart disease, although the mechanism as to why this occurs is poorly understood.

The optimal timing for performance of the fetal echocardiogram is at approximately 18–20 weeks' gestation. The earliest 4-chamber view can be obtained from the abdominal approach at approximately 14 weeks, although visualizing the outflow tracts at this age can be difficult. Oftentimes, image resolution and acoustic windows diminish after 34 weeks when the amniotic fluid-to-infant mass ratio decreases. Transvaginal fetal echocardiography, using specially designed ultrasound transducers, can be performed at 10–12 weeks, with good visualization of cardiac chambers, but views are limited because of restrictions in mobility of the transducer and an inability to

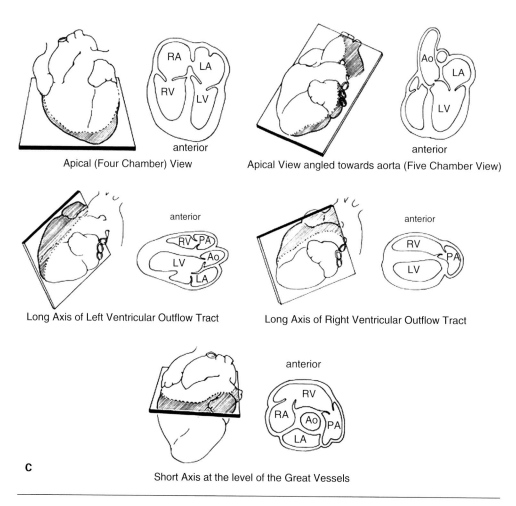

Apical (Four Chamber) View   Apical View angled towards aorta (Five Chamber View)

Long Axis of Left Ventricular Outflow Tract   Long Axis of Right Ventricular Outflow Tract

C

Short Axis at the level of the Great Vessels

FIGURE 60-3 *Continued.*

optimize scanning angles.[19] Nevertheless, transvaginal echocardiography can be a useful modality as a screening tool for congenital heart disease in high-risk patients and is being offered with increasing frequency.

As lesions and disease processes are dynamic in the growing fetus, identification of congenital heart disease or other disorders of the cardiovascular system requires repeat, serial fetal echocardiographic evaluation. It is our current practice to monitor fetuses with congenital heart disease with echocardiographic scans every 4–6 weeks to observe for developmental progression or physiological changes that may occur. Progressive structural changes may include development of worsening outflow tract or valvar stenosis,[20] or impairment of ventricular growth with worsening of ventricular hypoplasia.[21,22] Physiologic changes may include development of atrioventricular valve regurgitation or ventricular dysfunction.[23] Identification of these changes during gestation may radically alter the postnatal management strategies. Many fetuses with arrhythmia, hydrops, progressive disease processes, or those undergoing treatment require more frequent surveillance, as necessary.

Specific instrumentation is necessary to perform fetal echocardiography. Fetal imaging is carried out using ultra-sound frequencies of 3–7 MHz. Echocardiographic modalities of 2-dimensional, pulsed Doppler, continuous wave Doppler, and color Doppler flow imaging should all be available. In contrast to general obstetrical ultrasound, still frame storage of images is inadequate for analysis of the fetal cardiovascular system. Since the heart is a dynamic structure undergoing continuous change in a spacial-temporal manner, images must be analyzed, stored, and reviewed in motion. Videotape storage or digital media are currently available and provide excellent quality for review and analysis.

The fetal echocardiogram should be performed in a standardized and systematic way. Imaging views have been suggested by the American Society of Echocardiography[13] and are illustrated in Fig. 60-3. These views provide for a comprehensive assessment of the fetal cardiovascular system. A complete fetal echocardiogram should include a series of 2-dimensional tomographic sweeps through the fetal heart, color Doppler evaluation and pulse Doppler interrogation of cardiac inflow, outflow, venous returns, and arterial structures. The technical views and structures imaged are listed in Table 60-3.

TABLE 60-3 | ESSENTIAL COMPONENTS OF THE FETAL ECHOCARDIOGRAPHIC EXAMINATION

Feature	Essential Component
Anatomic overview	Fetal number and position in the uterus
	Establish stomach position and abdominal situs
	Establish cardiac position
Biometric examination	Cardiothoracic ratio
	Biparietal diameter
	Femur length
Cardiac imaging views/sweeps	Four-chamber view
	Four-chamber view angled toward great arteries ("5-chamber" view)
	Long-axis view (left ventricular outflow)
	Long-axis view (right ventricular outflow)
	Short-axis sweep (cephalad angling includes "3-vessel" view)
	Caval long-axis view
	Ductal arch view
	Aortic arch view
Doppler examination	Inferior and superior vena cava
	Pulmonary veins
	Hepatic veins
	Ductus venosus
	Foramen ovale
	Atrioventricular valves
	Semilunar valves
	Ductus arteriosus
	Transverse aortic arch
	Umbilical artery
	Umbilical vein
Measurement data	Atrioventricular valve diameter
	Semilunar valve diameter
	Main pulmonary artery
	Ascending aorta
	Branch pulmonary arteries
	Transverse aortic arch
	Ventricular length
	Ventricular short-axis dimensions
Examination of rhythm and rate	M-mode of atrial and ventricular wall motion
	Doppler examination of atrial and ventricular flow patterns

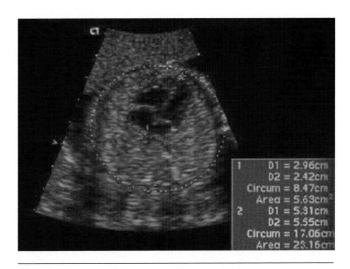

FIGURE 60-4 Cardiac area and thoracic area ratio measurement. This ratio should normally be less than 0.33.

FETAL ECHOCARDIOGRAPHY: EVALUATING THE FETAL CARDIOVASCULAR SYSTEM

CARDIAC STRUCTURE

A variety of parameters are used in the fetal echocardiogram to distinguish the abnormal from the normal. A simple measure of cardiac status is determining the heart size. Fetal cardiomegaly is assessed by comparing the measured cross-sectional area of the heart relative to the cross-sectional area of the chest wall (Fig. 60-4). The "cardiothoracic area ratio" should normally be less than 0.33, or upon visual inspection, one should be able to normally fit 3 hearts in the chest.[24]

Structural abnormalities of the heart can be readily discerned using 2-dimensional fetal echocardiography. An understanding of the full spectrum of congenital heart disease is necessary to confidently distinguish the normal from the abnormal. An in-depth discussion of such is beyond the scope of this chapter. Nonetheless, a simple checklist can be helpful in identifying and screening for the majority of cases of congenital heart disease.

A normal heart is present on fetal echocardiography if one can

1. *Identify the presence of 4 cardiac chambers*: Two atria of relative equal size and 2 ventricles of relative equal size;
2. *Identify the presence of 2 great vessels arising from the heart*: The (a) *pulmonary artery*, which arises from the right ventricle and bifurcates (splits) close to its ventricular origin into the branch pulmonary arteries and the ductus arteriosus, and the (b) *aorta*, which arises from the left ventricle and does not bifurcate but gives rise to the head vessels;
3. *Identify the crossing trajectory of the 2 great vessels*: As the great vessels arise just above their origin from the heart,

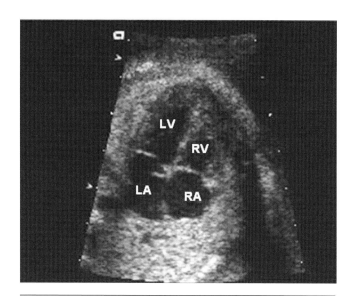

FIGURE 60-5 Normal 4-chamber view of the fetal heart. LA = left atrium; LV = left ventricle; RA = right atrium; RV = right ventricle.

they should cross each other at an angle of approximately 30–45 degrees, and not travel in parallel; and

4. *Confirm that the pulmonary artery is larger than the aorta.*

Confirmation of each of the above parameters, in the order listed, adds incremental confidence to the diagnosis of a structurally normal heart. Identifying 4 good-size cardiac chambers will rule out the presence of ventricular hypoplasia, but not conotruncal abnormalities of the great vessels such as trans-

position of the great vessels. The presence of 2 great vessels rules out pulmonary or aortic hypoplasia type syndromes. Absence of the normal crossing trajectory of the 2 great vessels and visualization of the vessels arising from the heart in parallel suggest a conotruncal anomaly such as transposition of the great vessels or double-outlet right ventricle. A pulmonary artery that is smaller than the aorta suggests tetralogy of Fallot or a form of anomaly manifesting pulmonary stenosis.[25] Some examples of simple and complex lesions are shown in Figs. 60-5 to 60-12. Images of a normal heart obtained via transvaginal fetal echocardiography are displayed in Fig. 60-13.

Structural abnormalities of the heart rarely result in any disturbance of fetal well-being; hence, nearly all will make it to term without hydrops or heart failure. Marked hypoplasia of the right or left ventricle or even severe outflow tract obstructions are of little hemodynamic consequence since (1) the placenta, not the fetal lungs, provide for oxygenation and (2) fetal structures such as the ductus arteriosus and foramen ovale allow for bypass of abnormally developed structures and maintenance of flow. In cases of right-sided heart structural disease, flow across the foramen ovale is right-to-left and the left ventricle can provide for fetal perfusion. Similarly, if the left ventricle is poorly developed, flow across the foramen ovale is left-to-right, and the right ventricle can then perfuse the fetal body via the patent ductus arteriosus. In contrast, the following conditions can adversely affect the fetus via manifesting as fetal instability: (1) genetic or chromosomal abnormalities; (2) hemodynamically significant atrioventricular valve regurgitation; or (3) ventricular dysfunction, or myocardial (pump) failure.

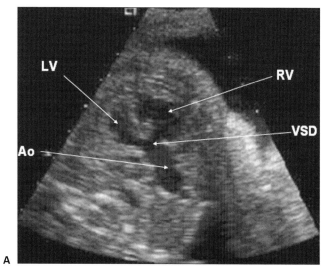

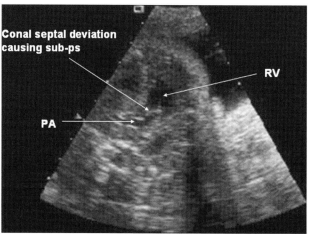

FIGURE 60-6 A fetal heart with tetralogy of Fallot. Panel (**A**) demonstrates the presence of a large ventricular septal defect and large overriding aorta (Ao). The pulmonary artery (PA) is not seen in this panel; however, with anterior angulation the small PA can be seen. The portion of the ventricular septum just beneath the great vessels called the "conal septum" can be seen deviated into the right ventricular outflow tract causing subpulmonic obstruction. This is one of the hallmark findings in tetralogy of Fallot.

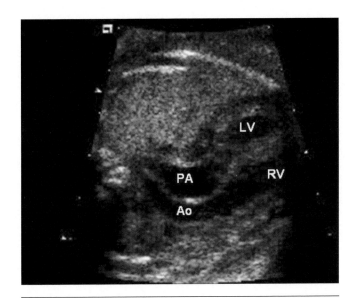

FIGURE 60-7 An example of transposition of the great arteries in the fetus. Both great vessels arise from the heart in parallel, suggesting a conotruncal anomaly. The aorta (Ao) is seen arising from the right ventricle (RV), and the pulmonary artery (PA) is seen arising from the left ventricle (LV).

Congenital heart disease can progress in the fetus. For example, pulmonary stenosis with a patent pulmonary valve identified at 18 weeks' gestation can progress to pulmonary atresia with subsequent right ventricular hypoplasia in some cases.[26] Dramatic changes with progression in left-sided heart anomalies have been reported. For example, aortic stenosis with a dilated poorly functional left ventricle at 16 weeks may

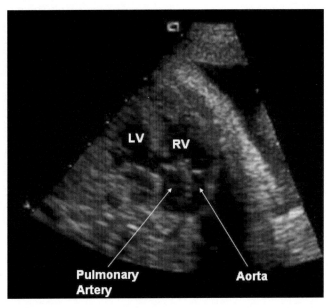

FIGURE 60-9 An example of double-outlet right ventricle. Note the large ventricular septal defect beneath the great vessels, both of which arise from the right ventricle.

undergo "arrest of left ventricular development" with manifestation of hypoplastic left heart at birth.[21,27] Identification of precisely who will progress from a simple lesion to a more complex lesion cannot yet reliably be determined.

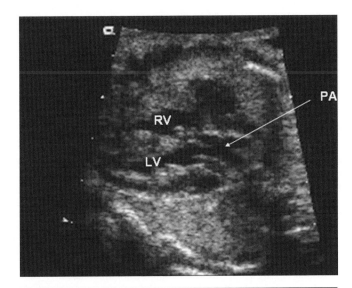

FIGURE 60-8 An example of transposition of the great arteries. The great vessel arising from the left ventricle bifurcates early and is the pulmonary artery.

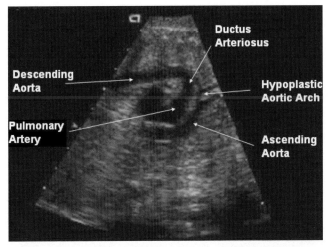

FIGURE 60-10 An example of a case of severe aortic arch hypoplasia. Both vascular arches of the fetal circulation are seen—the hypoplastic aortic arch and the ductal arch arising from the pulmonary artery and connecting to the descending aorta. This fetus will likely require patency of the ductus arteriosus at birth to maintain the fetal circulatory pathways and provide for systemic perfusion. Prostaglandin infusion should be offered to the neonate after delivery.

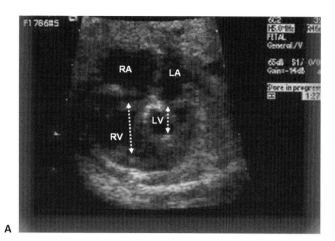 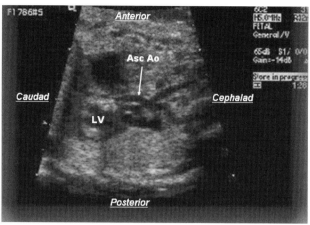

FIGURE 60-11 An example of hypoplastic left heart syndrome. This is one of the most commonly diagnosed forms of heart disease in the fetus due to its ease in recognition. Note the size discrepancy in ventricular length between the right ventricle and the left ventricle, with the left ventricle not reaching the cardiac apex, and approximately ½ the length of the RV (right ventricle). LA = left atrium; RA = right atrium.

DOPPLER ECHOCARDIOGRAPHY

Application of Doppler techniques to various anatomical sites within the cardiovascular system allows for an understanding of hemodynamic processes. Normal patterns of blood flow at these various sites have been established—deviations from these normal patterns of flow suggest pathology. Derangements of the fetal cardiovascular system commonly result in alteration of ventricular compliance and "stiffness" of the ventricles with elevation in atrial filling pressures, reflected as impediment to forward flow or reversal of direction of flow in the venous system.[28,29]

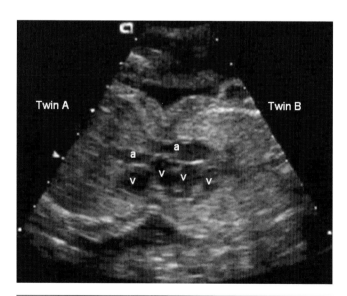

FIGURE 60-12 An example of fetal thoracopagus (conjoined twins, joined at the chest). The twins share a single heart with 2 atria (a) and 4 identifiable ventricles (v) all combined into 1 amalgam of cardiac mass.

The following are sites commonly interrogated and analyzed via Doppler echocardiography in the fetus:

- *Atrioventricular valves*: There are normally 2 peaks of flow across the tricuspid or mitral valve, representing (1) early "passive" diastolic filling with opening of the valve and (2) active diastolic filling in relation to atrial contraction. In the fetus, the second wave (atrial contraction) is normally of higher velocity[30] (Fig. 60-14). When ventricular compliance is altered, fusion of the 2 waveforms can occur. The fusion is also seen in early gestation (<16 weeks) and during periods of rapid heart rate (tachycardia).
- *Inferior vena cava*: Flow is normally phasic, with a small amount of reversal[31] (Fig. 60-15). An increased wave of reversal is seen under conditions of altered right ventricular compliance, anatomical restriction to flow such as a restrictive foramen ovale in the face of right-sided obstructive disease, or in situations of ventricular dysfunction.
- *Ductus venosus*: Flow is normally phasic, and all forward with no reversal (Fig. 60-16). The presence of any degree of reversal in a fetus (>17 weeks' gestation) is pathological and suggests elevated right atrial pressure.[28,32]
- *Umbilical artery*: Pulsatile flow with a systolic and diastolic phase is noted in each of the 2 umbilical arteries. Assessment of umbilical arterial flow provides important information on the health of the placenta.[29] The placenta is an organ of very low vascular resistance; hence, there should normally be a large amount of diastolic flow present in the umbilical artery. Diminished diastolic flow reflects elevated placental resistance and is seen in a variety of diseases including infection, fetal intrauterine growth retardation, maternal preeclampsia, or the twin-twin transfusion syndrome (TTTS). Placental vascular resistance can be measured by analyzing umbilical arterial flow and calculating the pulsatility index, which is equal to (systolic velocity − diastolic velocity)/

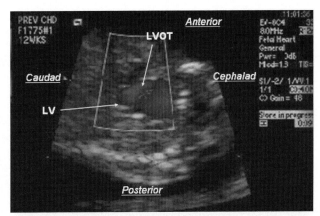

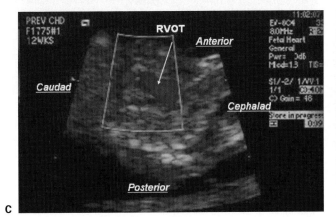

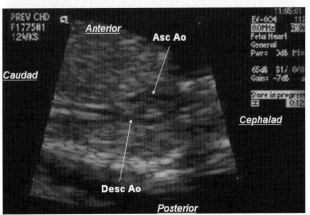

FIGURE 60-13 Transvaginal echocardiography. (**A**) Full view of fetal length, with heart noted centrally. (**B**) Zoom resolution view of the left ventricular outflow tract (LVOT) and then in (**C**), the right ventricular outflow tract (RVOT) with each crossing the other at an appropriate angle, suggesting the presence of normally related great arteries. (**D**) An image of the aortic arch including the ascending aorta (Asc Ao) and descending aorta (Desc Ao).

time-velocity integral, or area under the Doppler spectral curve (Fig. 60-17).

- *Umbilical vein*: Continuous low-velocity, nonpulsatile flow is normally expected in the umbilical vein[33] (Fig. 60-17).

BLOOD FLOW DISTRIBUTION WITHIN FETAL VASCULAR SYSTEMS

Early work performed before the era of Doppler echocardiography by Rudolph and colleagues established the patterns of flow in the mammalian fetal heart, using sheep models and microspheres.[34] Doppler echocardiography techniques have confirmed many of Rudolph's findings in the human. Recently, investigators have started to look at select regional blood flow patterns in the fetus in both the normal and diseased states. For example, it was initially believed that pulmonary blood flow remained fixed in utero throughout gestation with less than 20% of the combined right and left ventricular cardiac outputs delivered to the lungs. Elegant studies performed by Rasanen et al. have demonstrated that the amount of blood

flow to the pulmonary circulation increases with gestational age, with up to one third of the combined cardiac output delivered to the lungs near term.[35] In addition, the pulmonary circulation exhibits dynamic lability with an increase in flow in the presence of maternal exposure to supplemental oxygen, but only at a point in gestation well into the third trimester and not before. These studies provide insight into the development of the pulmonary vasculature with implications toward a better understanding of fetal factors that may contribute toward persistence in elevated pulmonary vascular resistance after birth.[36] For example, there may be a way to diagnose infants at risk for persistent pulmonary hypertension by assaying for the health of the pulmonary vascular resistance while still in utero.

With tools now available to quantify fetal pulmonary blood flow and fetal pulmonary vascular resistance, a multitude of questions can be raised and answered. For example, what are the effects of various structural heart anomalies on these patterns of pulmonary blood flow and hence pulmonary vascular development in the fetus? In many cardiac lesions, pulmonary vascular development is believed to be secondarily

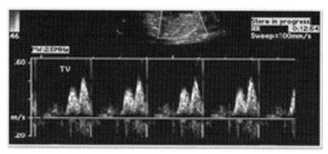

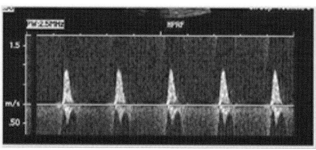

FIGURE 60-14 Doppler spectral display of the tricuspid inflow pattern. Top panel is the normal flow pattern expected with a "double-peak." The bottom panel is from a fetus with an abnormally hypertrophied heart and displays a Doppler tricuspid inflow pattern with a single peak.

affected by the structural rerouting of blood flow; conversely, the status of the resultant pulmonary vasculature after birth can seriously impact outcome at surgical repair. Information gleamed about the pulmonary circulation in the fetus may have

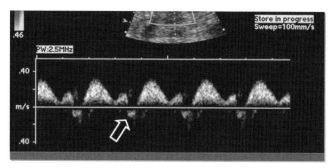

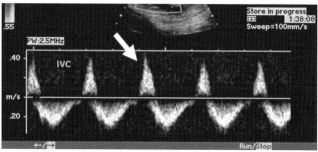

FIGURE 60-15 Inferior vena cava flow. Top panel is a Doppler spectral display from a normal fetus with a small amount of flow reversal (open arrow). Bottom panel is from a fetus with poor right ventricle compliance and demonstrates an increased degree of flow reversal (closed arrow).

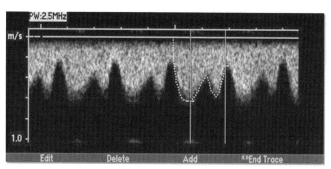

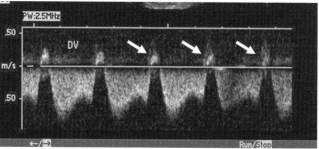

FIGURE 60-16 Ductus venosus flow. Top panel is the normal flow pattern with continuous forward flow. The bottom panel demonstrates some reversal of flow (arrows), suggesting a stiff abnormal heart.

important implications for improving postnatal management and survival in some patients.

Another vascular region of tremendous interest in the fetus is the cerebrovascular system. Numerous investigators have clearly demonstrated the presence of neurocognitive deficits in children who have undergone repair of complex congenital heart disease.[37,38] The cause of these findings may be multifactorial including factors such as conduct of the surgery, type of cardiopulmonary bypass used, genetic influences, or subtle structural neuroanatomical abnormalities. Another variable may be an alteration in fetal blood flow patterns to the cerebral circulation based on the structural heart disease present in utero. The widely accepted premise that cardiac output is maintained in most forms of congenital heart disease in the

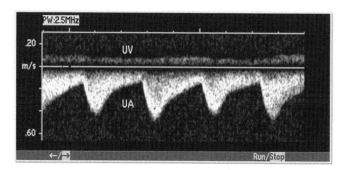

FIGURE 60-17 Doppler sample obtained from the umbilical cord. Both the umbilical artery (UA) and the umbilical vein (UV) flow patterns are displayed. Note the pulsatile systolic and diastolic components to the UA flow, while UV flow is continuous, nonpulsatile, and of low velocity.

fetus, simply because the fetus survives to term, may be a gross misconception. Subtle differences in regional blood flow, previously unrecognized, may occur with developmental consequences.

Investigational work initially performed by Donofrio[39] and further developed by Kaltman et al. in our laboratory[40] suggested a marked variability in Doppler-derived cerebrovascular blood flow resistance based on the type of congenital heart disease present. Kaltman et al. found a higher cerebrovascular resistance in the fetus with tetralogy of Fallot in comparison with the normal gestationally matched control and a lower cerebrovascular resistance in the fetus with hypoplastic left heart syndrome in comparison with the normal control. These findings suggest a marked variability in blood flow to the brain, which is influenced by the cardiac anomaly at hand. In addition, it demonstrates an adaptive attempt at fetal regional cerebrovascular flow autoregulation, on the basis of the heart defect present. This can be explained in the following manner. In tetralogy of Fallot, the presence of pulmonary stenosis and a large ventricular septal defect force the normal complement of right ventricular blood flow into the left ventricle. Hence, aortic flow is markedly increased in comparison to normal as it contains both the normal quantity of left ventricular inflow consisting of flow across the foramen (right to left) and pulmonary venous return, as well as the additional right ventricular blood flow. As the ascending aorta and the carotid vessels witness an increased volume of blood flow, the cerebrovascular circulation attempts to compensate and regulate by increasing resistance in order to maintain a controlled steady quantity of flow, in essence limiting cerebral overcirculation. However, in hypoplastic left heart syndrome, the aorta witnesses a decreased volume of blood flow in comparison to normal, since in the absence of a functional left ventricle, nearly all of the flow in the transverse aorta is via retrograde perfusion from the ductus arteriosus. Hence, in an attempt to increase cerebral blood flow volume, cerebrovascular resistance drops to encourage a shift in flow distribution to the brain. Cerebrovascular resistance is therefore affected by the architecture of the heart and the unique patterns of cardiac blood flow generated.

Whether these findings correlate with the neuroanatomical abnormalities seen after birth in infants with hypoplastic left heart syndrome[41] or with the abnormalities seen on subsequent cognitive testing is yet to be determined. As surgical outcomes for even the most complex forms of congenital heart disease continue to improve, the opportunity arises for further research in the quality of life of these survivors, with neurocognitive outcome a paramount focus. This data suggests that factors present prior to birth will likely play a role.

RHYTHM DISTURBANCES IN THE FETUS

Fetal heart rates normally range between 120 and 180 beats per minute with synchronous atrial and ventricular contraction. Transient increase in heart rate can be seen during fetal activity while transient fetal bradycardia can be noted during maternal abdominal compression, with temporary cord compression. Electrocardiography (ECG) is difficult, but not impossible to perform in the fetus. Fetal ECG signals are weak because of the distance to the maternal abdominal surface as well as interference from maternal ECG signal. Computer processing algorithms can provide impressions of fetal electrical activity, but reliable fetal ECG monitoring is still not clinically available. Conventionally, fetal arrhythmia is diagnosed by observation of the mechanical sequelae of electrical activity—namely, motion of the cardiac structures and blood flow patterns via fetal echocardiography.

Premature atrial contractions (PACs) are the most common arrhythmia seen in the fetus.[42] These are typically associated with a floppy atrial septum touching the back of the atrium during the various phases of the cardiac cycle. Maternal nicotine or excessive caffeine intake and placental insufficiency may contribute. PACs are benign and typically resolve after birth.

Maternal autoimmune disease resulting in SS-A or SS-B antibodies can result in fetal conduction system abnormalities and development of compete heart block.[43] Early signs of heart block such as first or second degree can be discerned on fetal echocardiography by measuring the time intervals between onset of flow across the mitral valve in conjunction with atrial contraction (a wave) and onset of flow across the aortic valve. This interval is called the "mechanical" PR interval and can provide information about the delay in conduction at the atrioventricular node (Fig. 60-18).[44] This time interval for the fetus should be less than 130 milliseconds. Although controversial, recent data support the notion that steroids can improve outcome of the fetus with maternal autoimmune-derived complete heart block.[43] Although once damaged, the atrioventricular node cannot be revived, and inhibition of the ongoing destruction by use of immunosuppressives such as steroids may result in a higher intrinsic ventricular rate, thereby maintaining cardiac output and preventing the onset of fetal hydrops. In addition, the ongoing immune process may lead to direct myocardial damage and development of cardiomyopathy. Steroid use may limit the development of myocardial damage that can occur independent of the damage caused to the atrioventricular node. It has been our practice to use 4–8 mg per day of dexamethasone at the earliest sign of heart block in at-risk patients. In addition, we have had success with the use of beta agonists, in particular albuterol. Allen et al. reported success, using intravenous albuterol (Salbutamol, product name in the United Kingdom) in increasing intrinsic ventricular rate and eliminating fetal hydrops.[45] Although intravenous albuterol is not currently available in the United States, we have had success defined by increasing fetal heart rate from 45 to 50 beats per minute with resolution of large pericardial effusion using oral albuterol at maximum dose of 4 mg 4 times daily.[46]

In the fetus, rapid heart rates seem to be well-tolerated for relatively long periods of time, even days. These rapid heart rhythms may include supraventricular tachycardia (SVT) (rates of 220–280 beats per minute) or atrial flutter, with rapid

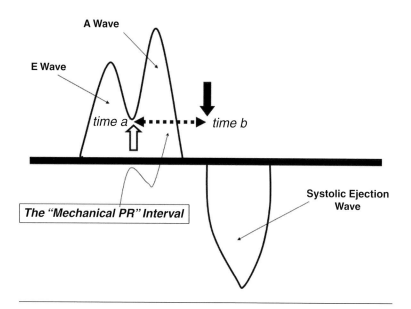

A Wave

E Wave

time a ◄┄┄┄► *time b*

The "Mechanical PR" Interval

Systolic Ejection
Wave

FIGURE 60-18 Diagram of the "Mechanical PR" interval. Time is measured from the onset of flow of the second peak of atrioventricular valve inflow, the "A wave," until the onset of systolic flow during ejection. The time corresponds to that between onset of atrial contraction (time a) and systolic flow (time b) and reflects the time between the "P wave" and the QRS complex on the electrocardiogram. This measure allows for assessment of the onset of heart block. Normal mechanical PR interval should be less than 130 milliseconds.

conduction (may be more than 300 beats per minute). SVT is distinguished from atrial flutter in the fetus by identifying a 1:1 ratio of motion of the atria and ventricles on fetal echocardiography. Ultimately, elevated heart rates may impair ventricular filling resulting in diminished cardiac output. Myocardial dysfunction can occur following prolonged periods of tachyarrhythmia resulting in impaired perfusion and hydrops. Treatment with transplacental therapy such as maternal administration of digoxin, amiodarone, or sotalol is effective in most cases.[47] Oftentimes, direct administration of drug to the fetus via umbilical vein puncture or intramuscular injection is necessary. Failure of therapeutic measures in treating either brady or tachyarrhythmias in the viable fetus should prompt consideration of delivery and direct administration of treatment to the premature infant, if impending fetal demise seems imminent and the potential for extrauterine survival is present.

FETAL CARDIOVASCULAR DISEASE: NONCONGENITAL HEART DISEASE

A variety of anomalies and disorders other than primary congenital heart disease may affect the fetal cardiovascular system.

1. Congenital diaphragmatic hernia is associated with congenital heart disease in approximately 10% of cases.[48] Abdominal contents in the thoracic cavity may limit pulmonary vascular development that can impact neonatal physiology. A number of findings are seen on fetal

echocardiography in these patients. Branch pulmonary artery measurements may reveal smallness on the side of the hernia, commensurate with the degree of pulmonary hypoplasia present.[49] In addition, mild left ventricular hypoplasia can be seen in accordance with limited right-to-left flow across the foramen and decreased fetal pulmonary venous return as a consequence of pulmonary hypoplasia.

2. Chest masses such as congenital cystic adenomatoid malformation (CCAM) can grow to giant size, resulting in compression of the thoracic contents and a cardiac tamponade-type physiology.[50] Hydrops can be seen when cardiac compression is significant, with a high likelihood of fetal demise. Changes in the echocardiography-derived Doppler filling patterns across the tricuspid and mitral valves may herald the findings of impending tamponade and fetal hydrops.

3. Arteriovenous malformations such as sacrococcygeal teratoma (SCT) or vein of Galen malformations can result in massive degrees of increased venous return and volume overload on the fetal heart.[51] Since the fetal heart tolerates volume loads poorly, fetal hydrops and demise are possible if these vascular lesions are large with high-volume loads. One measure of the consequence of these lesions is the fetal combined cardiac output. This can be calculated via echocardiography and is the sum of ejection volumes across both the pulmonary (right ventricle) and aortic (left ventricle) tracts. Normal fetal combined cardiac outputs range from 400 to 500 ml/min per kg, while the fetus with SCT may manifest values as high as more than 1000 ml/min per kg.[52] At these elevated levels, one can commonly see cardiomegaly, ventricular dilation, and atrioventricular valve regurgitation.

4. Maternal diabetes can increase the risk of development of congenital heart disease. In addition, elevated levels of maternal glucose can trigger hyperinsulinism in the fetus that promotes cardiac hypertrophy. Asymmetric septal hypertrophy of the fetal heart may occur, with development of left ventricular outflow tract obstruction as well as ventricular stiffness and diastolic dysfunction.

5. TTTS is a poorly understood phenomenon that occurs in diamniotic, monochorionic twins. It is the leading cause of morbidity and mortality in twin patients. The condition results in the development of hypovolemia in 1 twin (donor) and hypervolemia in the other twin (recipient), caused by a shift of volume from donor to recipient through placental vascular connections. In addition to volume shifts, there is also a transfer of mediators between the twins. In response to hypovolemia, there is activation of the renin-angiotensin system and release of vasoactive mediators such as endothelin-1 and other agents that cross the placental circulation into the recipient twin. These mediators, in conjunction with the volume load, can lead to

development of cardiomyopathy in the recipient twin. The process can be identified in the recipient twin by changes in the cardiovascular system consisting of ventricular dilation, atrioventricular valve regurgitation, and ventricular wall thickening. Various degrees of myocardial dysfunction can occur, first in the right ventricle and then in the left ventricle. As the disease progresses to its most serious form, reversal of flow in the ductus venosus can be seen as well as pulsations in the umbilical vein, findings suggestive of marked abnormality of ventricular compliance. As the disease progresses, there is a high incidence of fetal demise if the process is not abated.[53]

Curiously, some fetuses adapt to the volume load by developing progressive right ventricular hypertrophy with pulmonary stenosis or pulmonary atresia.[54] When these fetuses are born, their heart can have an identical appearance to that of pulmonary atresia with intact ventricular septum, a form of congenital heart disease. This phenomenon of TTTS emphasizes the notion of fetal flow and volume parameters influencing structural development of the heart, even late into the second trimester of gestation. The pathophysiology of TTTS may offer clues as to the development of other forms of congenital heart disease earlier in gestation.

DAWN OF A NEW ERA: THE FRONTIER OF FETAL SURGERY

As it currently stands, the practice of fetal cardiology is predominantly limited to diagnostics. Pharmacological intervention is available for fetal arrhythmias, but structural heart disease is currently not easily amenable to in utero repair. However, a number of centers are developing exciting new techniques that are altering the approach to cardiac lesions currently at high risk for infant repair.

Pioneers in the field of fetal surgery have established surgical techniques for safely accessing the human fetus during midgestation.[55,56] In principle, these techniques are reserved for anomalies in which the fetus is at risk for demise or in which postnatal outcome is extremely poor without intervention. Fetal surgery has been successfully performed with life-saving result in cases of giant CCAM and early hydrops, giant SCT with high output cardiac failure, and in some cases of congenital diaphragmatic hernia. Currently, a National Institutes of Health–sponsored randomized trial is under way to compare the outcome for fetal surgery for myelomeningocele with conventional postnatal surgery.[57] Of note, myelomeningocele is not a life-threatening anomaly, and postnatal management is highly successful; however, the objective of fetal intervention in this case is to alter and modify development in utero, in the

hopes of resulting in an improved outcome at birth and possible avoidance of a lifetime of morbidity.

This model of fetal myelomeningocele repair is very similar to that seen in congenital heart disease, in which the cardiac anomaly may not manifest itself clinically in utero, but only after birth, and the treatment after birth may have a relatively good survival outcome. As previously described, some cardiac lesions start out as much simpler anomalies at 18–20 weeks' gestation and progress into more severe forms over time.[21]

An example of such is the concept of potentially relieving outflow tract obstruction in fetal aortic stenosis via balloon valvuloplasty. The objective is to promote forward flow through the left ventricle and theoretically prevent the development of hypoplastic left heart syndrome. Using a percutaneous or maternal laparotomy approach, technical success with this procedure has been achieved by the group in Boston;[58] however, it is unclear whether the natural history of the lesion was impacted. Clearly identifying candidates who will benefit the most from fetal balloon valvuloplasty is difficult, as the factors that definitively predict development of left ventricular hypoplasia in the fetus have yet to be reliably established. Efforts are under way to more closely study this issue and map the natural history and progression of congenital heart disease in the fetus, in order to better identify specific factors that will predict for the progression of simple lesions into more complex ones.

Although fetal intervention and surgery for congenital heart disease loom on the horizon, many obstacles must still be overcome. Fetal cardiopulmonary bypass is difficult to achieve with the potential for devastating effects on placental function.[59] In addition, we have observed a number of deleterious effects of noncardiac fetal surgery on the fetal

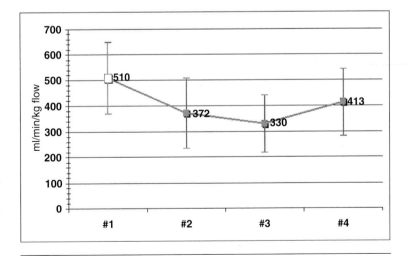

FIGURE 60-19 Graph of serial measures of combined cardiac output in ml/min per kg for fetuses undergoing surgery for repair of myelomeningocele. *X*-axis numbers reflect various time intervals: #1, prior to surgery; #2, after maternal anesthetic and maternal incision, but prior to fetal incision; #3, at fetal incision; and #4, after fetal surgery. Note the decrease in cardiac output at the time of fetal incision, which may be related to a number of factors.

cardiovascular system.[52] We performed continuous echocardiographic monitoring of 83 fetuses undergoing fetal surgery, 51 of whom had surgery for fetal myelomeningocele, an anomaly with no cardiovascular consequences. A number of findings were observed including a decrease in combined cardiac output (Fig. 60-19), constriction of the ductus arteriosus, and development of new atrioventricular valve regurgitation and diminished ventricular shortening during the surgery. In the majority, these findings were short-lived and limited to the surgical period, but in some they persisted up to 48 hours thereafter. Maternal anesthetic agents or other factors may be the cause; however, these findings illustrate the need for cautious study of these procedures as new and innovative interventions continue to develop.

SUMMARY

Through advances in imaging, we are currently able to visualize and understand many aspects of the developing fetal cardiovascular system, previously unknown. Fetal echocardiography provides a "window to the womb," which is changing the way congenital heart anomalies are detected. Fetal echocardiography will provide a way for prenatal interventional treatment to safely, effectively, and reliably take place, which will dramatically alter the way we treat many forms of congenital heart disease.

References

1. Friedman WF. The intrinsic physiologic properties of the developing heart. *Prog Cardiovasc Dis.* 1972;15:87–111.
2. Mahoney L. Calcium homeostasis and control of contractility in the developing heart. *Sem Perinatol.* 1996;20:510–519.
3. Grant DA. Ventricular constraint in the fetus and newborn. *Can J Cardiol.* 1999;15:95–104.
4. Kleinman CS, Hobbins JC, Jaffe CC, et al. Echocardiographic studies of the human fetus: Prenatal diagnosis of congenital heart disease and cardiac dysrhythmias. *Pediatrics.* 1980;65:1059–1067.
5. Ewigman BG, Crane JP, Frigoletto FD, et al. Effect of prenatal ultrasound screening on perinatal outcome. RADIUS Study Group. *N Engl J Med.* 1993;329:821–827.
6. Buskens E, Grobbee DE, Frohn-Mulder IM, et al. Efficacy of routine fetal ultrasound screening for congenital heart disease in normal pregnancy. *Circulation.* 1996;94:67–72.
7. Stumpflen I, Stumpflen A, Wimmer M, et al. Effect of detailed fetal echocardiography as part of routine prenatal ultrasonographic screening on detection of congenital heart disease. *Lancet.* 1996;348:854–857.
8. Mahle WT, Clancy RR, McGaurn SP, et al. Impact of prenatal diagnosis on survival and early neurologic morbidity in neonates with the hypoplastic left heart syndrome. *Pediatrics.* 2001;107:1277–1282.
9. Tworetzky W, McElhinney DB, Reddy VM, et al. Improved surgical outcome after fetal diagnosis of hypoplastic left heart syndrome. *Circulation.* 2001;103:1269–1273.
10. Verheijen PM, Lisowski LA, Stoutenbeek P, et al. Lactacidosis in the neonate is minimized by prenatal detection of congenital heart disease. *Ultrasound Obstet Gynecol.* 2002;19:552–555.
11. Mahle WT. Neurologic and cognitive outcomes in children with congenital heart disease. *Curr Opin Pediatr.* 2001;13:482–486.
12. DeVore GR. Influence of prenatal diagnosis on congenital heart defects. *Ann N Y Acad Sci.* 1998;847:46–52.
13. Rychik J, Ayres N, Cuneo B, et al. American Society of Echocardiography guidelines and standards for performance of the fetal echocardiogram. *J Am Soc Echocardiogr.* 2004;17:803–810.
14. Jaeggi ET, Fouron JC, Silverman ED, et al. Transplacental fetal treatment improves the outcome of prenatally diagnosed complete atrioventricular block without structural heart disease. *Circulation.* 2004;110:1542–1548.
15. Koivurova S, Hartikainen AL, Gissler M, et al. Neonatal outcome and congenital malformations in children born after in-vitro fertilization. *Hum Reprod.* 2002;17:1391–1398.
16. Hansen M, Kurinczuk JJ, Bower C, et al. The risk of major birth defects after intracytoplasmic sperm injection and in vitro fertilization. *N Engl J Med.* 2002;346:725–730.
17. Ghi T, Huggon IC, Zosmer N, et al. Incidence of major structural cardiac defects associated with increased nuchal translucency but normal karyotype. *Ultrasound Obstet Gynecol.* 2001;18:610–614.
18. McAuliffe FM, Hornberger LK, Winsor S, et al. Fetal cardiac defects and increased nuchal translucency thickness: A prospective study. *Am J Obstet Gynecol.* 2004;191:1486–1490.
19. Gembruch U, Knopfle G, Bald R, et al. Early diagnosis of fetal congenital heart disease by transvaginal echocardiography. *Ultrasound Obstet Gynecol.* 1993;3:310–317.
20. Hornberger LK, Sanders SP, Sahn DJ, et al. In utero pulmonary artery and aortic growth and potential for progression of pulmonary outflow tract obstruction in tetralogy of Fallot. *J Am Coll Cardiol.* 1995;25:739–745.
21. Hornberger LK, Sanders SP, Rein AJ, et al. Left heart obstructive lesions and left ventricular growth in the midtrimester fetus. A longitudinal study. *Circulation.* 1995;92:1531–1538.
22. Trines J, Hornberger LK. Evolution of heart disease in utero. *Pediatr Cardiol.* 2004;25:287–298.
23. Levin MD, Gaynor JW, Tian Z, et al. Prevalence of perinatal atrioventricular valve regurgitation in the single ventricle: From the fetus, through birth, and initial palliative surgery. *J Am Soc Echocardiogr.* 2004 (abstract).
24. Paladini D, Chita SK, Allan LD. Prenatal measurement of cardiothoracic ratio in evaluation of heart disease. *Arch Dis Child.* 1990;65:20–23.
25. DeVore GR, Siassi B, Platt LD. Fetal echocardiography. VIII. Aortic root dilatation—A marker for tetralogy of Fallot. *Am J Obstet Gynecol.* 1988;159:129–136.
26. Tulzer G, Arzt W, Franklin RC, et al. Fetal pulmonary valvuloplasty for critical pulmonary stenosis or atresia with intact septum. *Lancet.* 2002;360:1567–1568.
27. Danford DA, Cronican P. Hypoplastic left heart syndrome: Progression of left ventricular dilation and dysfunction to left ventricular hypoplasia in utero. *Am Heart J.* 1992;123:1712–1713.
28. Reed KL, Chaffin DG, Anderson CF, et al. Umbilical venous velocity pulsations are related to atrial contraction pressure waveforms in fetal lambs. *Obstet Gynecol.* 1997;89:953–956.
29. Makikallio K, Vuolteenaho O, Jouppila P, et al. Ultrasonographic and biochemical markers of human fetal cardiac dysfunction in placental insufficiency. *Circulation.* 2002;105:2058–2063.
30. Harada K, Rice MJ, Shiota T, et al. Gestational age- and growth-related alterations in fetal right and left ventricular diastolic filling patterns. *Am J Cardiol.* 1997;79:173–177.
31. Huisman TW, van den Eijnde SM, Stewart PA, et al. Changes in inferior vena cava blood flow velocity and diameter during breathing

movements in the human fetus. *Ultrasound Obstet Gynecol.* 1993;3:26–30.

32. Sherer DM, Fromberg RA, Divon MY. Prenatal ultrasonographic assessment of the ductus venosus: A review. *Obstet Gynecol.* 1996;88:626–632.

33. Reed KL, Anderson CF. Changes in umbilical venous velocities with physiologic perturbations. *Am J Obstet Gynecol.* 2000;182:835–838.

34. Edelstone DI, Rudolph AM. Preferential streaming of ductus venosus blood to the brain and heart in fetal lambs. *Am J Physiol.* 1979;237:H724–H729.

35. Rasanen J, Wood DC, Debbs RH, et al. Reactivity of the human fetal pulmonary circulation to maternal hyperoxygenation increases during the second half of pregnancy: A randomized study. *Circulation.* 1998;97:257–262.

36. Broth RE, Wood DC, Rasanen J, et al. Prenatal prediction of lethal pulmonary hypoplasia: The hyperoxygenation test for pulmonary artery reactivity. *Am J Obstet Gynecol.* 2002;187:940–945.

37. Bellinger DC, Wypij D, duDuplessis AJ, et al. Neurodevelopmental status at eight years in children with dextro-transposition of the great arteries: The Boston Circulatory Arrest Trial. *J Thorac Cardiovasc Surg.* 2003;126:1385–1396.

38. Mahle WT, Wernovsky G. Neurodevelopmental outcomes in hypoplastic left heart syndrome. *Semin Thorac Cardiovasc Surg Pediatr Card Surg Annu.* 2004;7:39–47.

39. Donofrio MT, Bremer YA, Schieken RM, et al. Autoregulation of cerebral blood flow in fetuses with congenital heart disease: The brain sparing effect. *Pediatr Cardiol.* 2003;24:436–443.

40. Kaltman J, Di H, Tian Z, et al. Impact of congenital heart disease on cerebrovascular blood flow dynamics in the fetus. *Ultrasound Obstet Gynecol.* 2004;25:32–36.

41. Galli KK, Zimmerman RA, Jarvik GP, et al. Periventricular leukomalacia is common after neonatal cardiac surgery. *J Thorac Cardiovasc Surg.* 2004;127:692–704.

42. Reed KL, Sahn DJ, Marx GR, et al. Cardiac Doppler flows during fetal arrhythmias: Physiologic consequences. *Obstet Gynecol.* 1987; 70:1–6.

43. Jaeggi ET, Fouron JC, Silverman ED, et al. Transplacental fetal treatment improves the outcome of prenatally diagnosed complete atrioventricular block without structural heart disease. *Circulation.* 2004;110:1542–1548.

44. Van Bergen AH, Cuneo BF, Davis N. Prospective echocardiographic evaluation of atrioventricular conduction in fetuses with maternal Sjogren's antibodies. *Am J Obstet Gynecol.* 2004;191:1014–1018.

45. Groves AM, Allan LD, Rosenthal E. Therapeutic trial of sympathomimetics in three cases of complete heart block in the fetus. *Circulation.* 1995;92:3394–3396.

46. Sivarajah J, Huggon IC, Rosenthal E. Successful management of fetal hydrops due to congenitally complete atrioventricular block. *Cardiol Young.* 2003;13:380–383.

47. Oudijk MA, Michon MM, Kleinman CS, et al. Sotalol in the treatment of fetal dysrhythmias. *Circulation.* 2000;101:2721–2726.

48. Cohen MS, Rychik J, Bush DM, et al. Influence of congenital heart disease on survival in children with congenital diaphragmatic hernia. *J Pediatr.* 2002;141:25–30.

49. Sokol J, Bohn D, Lacro RV, et al. Fetal pulmonary artery diameters and their association with lung hypoplasia and postnatal outcome in congenital diaphragmatic hernia. *Am J Obstet Gynecol.* 2002;186:1085–1090.

50. Mahle WT, Rychik J, Tian ZY, et al. Echocardiographic evaluation of the fetus with congenital cystic adenomatoid malformation. *Ultrasound Obstet Gynecol.* 2000;16:620–624.

51. Silverman NH, Schmidt KG. Ventricular volume overload in the human fetus: Observations from fetal echocardiography. *J Am Soc Echocardiogr.* 1990;3:20–29.

52. Rychik J, Tian Z, Cohen MS, et al. Acute cardiovascular effects of fetal surgery in the human. *Circulation.* 2004;110:1549–1556.

53. Rychik J. Fetal cardiovascular physiology. *Pediatr Cardiol.* 2004;25:201–209.

54. Lougheed J, Sinclair BG, Fung Kee Fung K, et al. Acquired right ventricular outflow tract obstruction in the recipient twin in twin-twin transfusion syndrome. *J Am Coll Cardiol.* 2001;38:1533–1538.

55. Harrison MR. Surgically correctable fetal disease. *Am J Surg.* 2000;180:335–342.

56. Harrison MR. Fetal surgery: Trials, tribulations, and turf. *J Pediatr Surg.* 2003;38:275–282.

57. Johnson MP, Sutton LN, Rintoul N, et al. Fetal myelomeningocele repair: Short-term clinical outcomes. *Am J Obstet Gynecol.* 2003;189:482–487.

58. Tworetzky W, Wilkins-Haug L, Jennings RW, et al. Balloon dilation of severe aortic stenosis in the fetus. Potential for prevention of hypoplastic left heart syndrome: Candidate selection, technique, and results of successful intervention. *Circulation.* 2004;110:2125–2131.

59. Khandelwal M, Rasanen J, Ludormirski A, et al. Evaluation of fetal and uterine hemodynamics during maternal cardiopulmonary bypass. *Obstet Gynecol.* 1996;88:667–671.

PRENATAL CARDIAC THERAPY

Charles S. Kleinman

In his classic text, *Congenital Diseases of the Heart,* Dr. Abraham M. Rudolph introduced the concept that the pathophysiology of congenital heart disease afflicting neonates can best be understood if one considers that neonatal physiology reflects many months of fetal adaptation to structural anomalies that originate during embryogenesis.[1] Once the tubular embryonic heart has undergone looping (initiated at 4 weeks postfertilization), with subsequent migration of the atrioventricular canal and truncus arteriosus, and intracardiac septation (completed by 8–10 weeks of gestation), flow volume subsequently determines the relative sizes of cardiac chambers and blood vessels leading toward and from the heart. Ventricular wall thickness directly reflects ventricular systolic blood pressure.

Dr. Rudolph's concepts, based on extensive physiologic observations in chronically instrumented fetal lambs provide the foundation upon which much of the clinical teaching of trainees in the field of neonatal cardiology is based.

The initial observations of human fetal cardiac structure and function that were made in our laboratory at Yale in 1977 provided some of the first evidence that the experimental observations in the lamb fetal heart, in large part, held for the developing human, as well.

It was not until we were well underway with our physiologic observations that we recognized the potential for the use of fetal echocardiography to provide diagnostic information that could be put to clinical use. Although the literature in 1977 already contained isolated case reports of prenatally diagnosed congenital heart malformations, our studies were the first to attempt to define clinical indications for prenatal screening for congenital heart disease, and the first to describe a clinical screening program for congenital heart disease.[2]

A review of the bibliographies of the other reports in this volume demonstrates the fact that reports of prenatal cardiac diagnosis and treatment did not appear in the literature until more than a decade after reports of fetal ultrasound diagnoses of complex anomalies of many other organ systems. In addition, the literature was replete with descriptions of fetal treatment for anomalies of other organ systems many years before our first reports of fetal cardiac therapy.[3]

The relatively "late start" of the field of fetal cardiology provided those of us who became involved with this field a distinct advantage over those who preceded us in devising fetal treatment protocols. For example, the great expectations that accompanied the introduction of shunting techniques to decompress fetal hydrocephalus were soon dashed when it was realized that the technique decreased mortality, but resulted in the survival of infants with terrible neurodevelopmental disabilities.[4] Similar early disappointments that accompanied procedures to palliate obstructive uropathy underscored the importance of defining the degree of renal damage in candidates for fetal therapy before undertaking invasive therapy.[5]

A desire to learn from the experience of our predecessors, rather than risk repeating their disappointments, made us circumspect in considering whether the ability to diagnose fetal heart disease justifies moving directly to efforts at fetal treatment, despite the potential glamour of such endeavors.

Having demonstrated the usefulness of fetal echocardiography for the observation of fetal cardiac structural development and cardiovascular physiology, we attempted to assemble a fund of knowledge that provides an understanding of the pathophysiology of heart disease in the human fetus, in addition to a detailed understanding of the normal and abnormal transitional circulation. Such information has allowed the development of aggressive treatment protocols for the management of the transitional circulation of infants born with complex forms of congenital heart disease, and has facilitated the provision of such treatments for these infants. Recently, reports have appeared documenting that such information and treatments may allow these fetuses to avoid lactic acidosis in the neonatal period, and demonstrating enhanced survival prospects for infants born with certain specific forms of congenital heart disease (e.g., transposition of the great arteries, hypoplastic left heart syndrome, coarctation of the aorta).[6–10]

It has been suggested by Harrison that the frustration of encountering a neonate with a surgical condition who has already deteriorated into an unsalvageable state by the time of birth should not lead directly to fetal surgery. In fact, such frustration could be channeled to fuel efforts to understand the pathophysiology of the condition, to define the natural history of the condition, and to define the expected frequency with which the particular diagnosis will be encountered (usually serendipitously). Once such information is in hand a rational risk/benefit analysis, considering the feasibility of fetal treatments, the potential risks of proposed surgical or medical interventions versus the potential benefits to be derived, the pharmacology and pharmacokinetics of potential drug therapies, and consideration that such therapies are affecting both the mother and fetus, must take place.[11]

Any discussion of in utero cardiac therapy for the human fetus must, therefore, be predicated on a complete understanding of normal and abnormal fetal cardiovascular physiology, including the physiology of the transitional circulation, both in health and disease.

FETAL CARDIOVASCULAR PHYSIOLOGY

Although similar in appearance to the postnatal heart and cardiovascular system, the circulatory system of the fetus has unique properties that allow the developing heart to adapt gradually to anatomic and blood flow perturbations with little, if any, detectable impact on overall fetal well-being.

The existence of fetal shunt pathways at the level of the foramen ovale, ductus arteriosus, and ductus venosus allows the 2 fetal ventricles to function in parallel with 1 another, rather than in series, with the only "connection" between the 2 ventricles across the systemic or pulmonary vascular beds. This parallel circuitry of the fetal circulatory system, with unrestricted interconnection of the 2 circulations at the level of ventricular inflow (the foramen ovale) and outflow (the ductus arteriosus) imparts a unique "redundancy" to the fetal cardiovascular system. In the event that flow through 1 portion of the heart or cardiovascular system is blocked owing to an anatomic (e.g., stenosis or atresia) or physiologic (e.g., poor muscular compliance or fibrosis) impedance, alternative pathways, or detours, are available to allow blood to bypass obstructions and reach their target organs. This vascular detour, or "deviation road," phenomenon provides the otherwise fragile fetus with a remarkable ability to survive in the face of seemingly lethal structural deficiencies. The most dramatic example is the remarkable survival of so many fetuses in whom the left heart structures are underdeveloped or completely undeveloped. It became apparent quite early in our experience with fetal echocardiography that the hypoplastic left heart syndrome could be diagnosed reliably, not only on the basis of identification of small, or absent, left heart (it is difficult to claim positive identification of an undeveloped structure) structures, but also on the basis of identification of a reciprocal enlargement of right heart structures (such as the right ventricle, pulmonary artery, and ductus arteriosus). It is the parallel circuitry that provides the basis for the observation that in the fetal heart "form follows function" (low flow through a region of the circulatory system results in small structures, whereas the reciprocal volume overload of the structures through which flow is detoured results in enlargement of those structures). In other words, the finding of disproportion of structures that are, in the normal fetus, relatively equal in size (e.g., right versus left ventricle; right versus left atrium), actually represents a proportionate response that preserves blood flow distribution to the fetal body. Alternatively, in situations in which there is an abnormal volume overload on given structures (e.g., the right ventricle and right atrium in the presence of tricuspid regurgitation; the right ventricle and pulmonary artery in the presence of pulmonary regurgitation; the left atrium and left ventricle in the presence of mitral regurgitation) disproportionate enlargement of structures represents evidence of a pathologic flow abnormality on the ipsilateral side of the circulation, rather than a compensatory redistribution of flow from the opposite side of the circulation. Such alternative explanations for a given appearance of the 4-chamber anatomy of the fetal heart are discussed, not to intimidate the reader, but to emphasize the importance of complete evaluation and understanding of anatomy and physiology before jumping to conclusions regarding diagnosis, solely on the basis of rote memory, or pattern recognition. Disproportionate right ventricular enlargement during the late second or early third trimester, for example, may be consistent with, but is certainly not diagnostic of, coarctation of the aorta.

It is essential, therefore, that the fetal cardiologist not only be adept at imaging the fetal heart, recognizing abnormal cardiac anatomy, and pigeonholing these findings into accurate anatomic diagnoses, but that he or she is also adept at interpreting these findings as reflections of details of cardiovascular physiology, including flow patterns within the great arteries, great veins, and the unique fetal shunt pathways.

It is widely known that the fetal right ventricle is normally "dominant" when comparing its workload to that of the fetal left ventricle. In the third trimester fetal lamb the ratio of right ventricular to left ventricular output is 2:1. Doppler flow studies in the human suggest that the right ventricle, although dominant, contributes approximately 55% of the combined output of the 2 fetal ventricles, whereas the left ventricle contributes approximately 45%. This is in keeping with speculation offered many years ago by Dr. Rudolph, who considered the relative blood flow needed to satisfy the oxygen transport requirements of the relatively larger human brain versus that of the lamb brain. Doppler flow studies in the human fetus have suggested that although pulmonary blood flow is quite low, because of high pulmonary vascular resistance, the human fetal lung receives a higher proportion of combined ventricular output than the lamb fetus. As pregnancy progresses, and differential growth of individual organs takes place, there is a gradual redistribution of regional fetal blood flow, reflective of metabolic demands, growth in organ mass, and altered vascularity of the individual organs.[1,12]

FETAL MYOCARDIAL PERFORMANCE

The ability of the fetus to withstand acute and chronic alterations in preload and afterload is determined, in large part, by intrinsic properties of fetal myocardium, which differ substantially from those of neonatal and mature myocardium. Over 30 years ago Friedman, working with isolated muscle strips as well as with whole heart preparations from fetal lambs, demonstrated that fetal ventricular myocardium is less compliant than mature myocardium. This results in a higher end-diastolic pressure at any given end-diastolic volume in the fetal heart. In addition, the same studies demonstrated a lower contractility of fetal ventricular myocardium. Fetal ventricular myocardium develops less active tension when contracting from any given end-diastolic length or volume. Such myocardial properties predict limited preload and afterload reserve for the intact fetal heart.[13]

Friedman attempted to explain the differences between fetal and mature myocardial function on the basis of light microscopic differences between the two. Adult myocardium contains larger myocytes, with an orderly, longitudinal, orientation, with very little space between the contractile elements. On the other hand, fetal myocardium contains smaller myocytes, with a more disorderly, random, orientation of contractile elements, with significant fluid-filled and fibroblast-containing interstitial space between the contractile elements. Subsequent electron micrographic studies have confirmed the consistent difference between myocyte size, relative myofibrillar disarray, and lower myofibrillar density of fetal compared with mature myocardium. In addition, the latter studies also demonstrated a relative paucity of mitochondria and sarcoplasmic reticula in fetal versus mature ventricular myocardium. The latter implies a relative disadvantage in energy metabolism and calcium flux in the fetal heart. Subsequent studies have demonstrated that as the heart matures that there is a progressive organization of myofibrils. As the myofibrils organize there is a proliferation of mitochondria. These mitochondria undergo ultrastructural maturation, with an increase in the density of cristae, at the same time that the mitochondria distribute in a more orderly fashion, along the myofilaments.[14]

Ascuitto and Ross-Ascuitto[15] demonstrated fundamental differences in substrate metabolism between the mature and the developing myocardium. Fetal and neonatal myocardium predominantly depends on glucose metabolism; a switch over to fatty acid metabolism occurs at some time during infancy. Such fundamental differences in myocardial metabolism may explain differences in the efficiency of the heart, and may have important implications regarding the time of onset and recognition of the manifestations of metabolic myopathies in the fetus and neonate.[15]

The relative paucity of sarcoplasmic reticulum and T-tubules in fetal myocardium results in a limitation of intracellular stores of Ca^{++} ion. This relative unavailability of intracellular ion renders the fetal myocardium particularly dependent on transsarcolemmal calcium transport, both for muscle contraction and, presumably, for muscle relaxation.[16]

CLINICAL IMPLICATIONS

CALCIUM FLUX

This dependence on the calcium exchange channels within the sarcolemma renders the immature myocardium particularly susceptible to the actions of calcium channel blocking agents. When these agents were originally introduced, one of their frequent uses related to their profound effect on the atrioventricular node, and their efficacy in the treatment of supraventricular tachycardia in the infant. Subsequent experience, however, demonstrated a potentially devastating negative impact on myocardial contractility in the immature heart, which led to the abandonment of these agents in children under 1–2 years of age.[17]

PRELOAD AND AFTERLOAD RESERVE

The intact fetal heart, therefore, has intrinsic properties that render it more susceptible to hemodynamic stress than the mature heart. The fetal left ventricle demonstrates significantly more functional reserve than the right ventricle, which functions in utero at a higher relative end-diastolic volume (preload) and higher afterload than postnatally. The fetal left ventricle has a greater potential to increase stroke volume in response to enhanced preload than does the right ventricle.

In addition, the fetal right ventricle is much more sensitive to acutely increased afterload stress than the left ventricle. The latter becomes clinically relevant because of the unique role of the fetal ductus arteriosus in determining afterload on the fetal right ventricle. The large right ventricular stroke volume bypasses the vasoconstricted pulmonary vascular bed, owing to the large ductus arteriosus, which allows 80–90% of the right ventricular stroke volume to pass into the descending aorta, and, eventually largely enter the low-resistance umbilical circulation.

In practical terms, it is difficult to postulate a clinical scenario in which an isolated normal fetal left ventricle is suddenly exposed to increased afterload. On the other hand, the fetal right ventricle is in a significantly more vulnerable position. Any situation resulting in prenatal constriction of the ductus arteriosus results in increased impedance to right ventricular ejection. Ultrasound studies in the human fetus suggest a physiologic partial narrowing the ductus arteriosus in late gestation. This may be associated with a relative exaggeration of the physiologic ventricular disproportion that renders the right ventricle to appear dilated and somewhat less contractile than the fetal left ventricle near term. This relative dilation may be ameliorated in some fetuses if there is a relative relaxation of the degree of vasoconstriction in the pulmonary vascular bed, allowing an increase in pulmonary blood flow in the near-term human fetus.

Pathologic constriction of the fetal ductus arteriosus was implicated years ago as 1 of the underlying mechanisms to explain the etiology of persistent pulmonary hypertension of the neonate. It was noted that the mothers of some neonates who presented with this syndrome had been ingesting large doses of aspirin, or other nonsteroidal anti-inflammatory drugs (NSAIDs).[18] Such medications, through their inhibition of the action of cyclooxygenase, inhibit the production of prostaglandins. As our understanding of the mechanism for controlling the patency of the ductus arteriosus evolved, it was recognized that intrinsic fetal production of prostaglandin E$_2$ was necessary to prevent constriction of vascular smooth muscle within the wall of this blood vessel that results in the obliteration of the vessel lumen. This became clinically relevant in the care of premature infants with persistence of the ductus arteriosus, resulting in pulmonary edema that complicated management of neonatal respiratory distress syndrome, in whom administration of cyclooxygenase inhibitors such as indomethacin facilitated ductal closure. Prenatal ductal closure, resulting from maternal ingestion of NSAIDs, could result in increased pulmonary arteriolar smooth muscle thickening and constriction owing to trapping of right ventricular output in the main pulmonary artery, at high pressure, and forcing this blood through the vasoconstricted pulmonary arterioles. In the rare cases of spontaneous prenatal ductal closure that have been encountered, the usual clinical scenario is the finding of right ventricular dilation, poor right ventricular contraction, and tricuspid regurgitation.[19]

These same findings have been recognized as the hallmark of acute ductal closure, resulting from the use of NSAIDs for tocolysis, especially in association with the uterine irritability that follows invasive fetal therapy.

Acutely increased right ventricular afterload may result from altered placental function. Acute placental insufficiency, resulting from such conditions as preeclampsia or abruptio placenta, may be associated with acute right ventricular failure, resulting from acute afterload mismatch and disordered myocardial oxygen supply and demand.

The increased interest in potential prenatal therapies for conditions that, on their surface, might appear somewhat far afield from fetal heart disease, require detailed knowledge of fetal flow physiology.[20] Careful surveillance of fetal cardiovascular function may provide early indications for intervention in monochorionic twins with twin-to-twin transfusion syndrome. Such surveillance may also provide insights into the relative impact of potential therapies, such as fetoscopic laser or radiofrequency ablation of bridging placental vessels versus amnioreduction of polyhydramnios around the recipient twin.[21–27]

NONIMMUNE HYDROPS FETALIS

We became aware of the proclivity of fetuses to develop anasarca as the manifestation of cardiovascular failure very early in our clinical investigations.[28,29] Rudolph, in the most recent revision of his text, *Congenital Diseases of the Heart*, attempts to explain this phenomenon.[30]

Consider that edema formation is determined by the reciprocal relationship between hydrostatic pressure, and its tendency to drive fluid from the vascular space into the interstitial space, and plasma oncotic pressure, and its tendency to suck interstitial fluid back into the vascular space. This fundamental relationship is influenced, as well, by the intrinsic leakiness of the capillary wall (filtration coefficient) to fluid, as well as the permeability of the capillary wall to protein (which determines the oncotic gradient between the intravascular and interstitial spaces). In addition, the steady state of fluid flux between the vascular and interstitial spaces is determined, in part, by the compliance of the interstitial space, with regard to its ability to accommodate the added volume of edema fluid. Finally, the ability of the lymphatic system to scavenge fluid from the interstitial space, and return it to the venous end of the intravascular space, is the final determinant of whether there is a net accumulation of fetal edema. Studies of fetal lymphatic flow suggest that the characteristics of the fetal vascular system have a significant baseline balance toward interstitial fluid accumulation that is swept dry by avid lymphatic drainage. On the other hand, even a modest increase in systemic venous pressure only increases hydrostatic pressure, increasing the tendency for fluid extravasation, but also moves venous pressure closer to the critical outflow pressure, at which lymphatic drainage abruptly drops.[30]

In other words, the fetus, because of the fine balance between hydrostatic and oncotic pressure, the intrinsic properties of the capillary wall and the interstitial space, and the susceptibility of lymphatic drainage to acute obstruction in the face of increased systemic venous pressure, functions on a razor's edge of fluid balance, between normality and hydrops fetalis. The limitation in preload and afterload reserve of fetal right, more than left, ventricle increases the susceptibility toward increased systemic venous pressure in the face of acute changes in vascular dynamics.

It is little wonder that acutely increased right ventricular afterload, in face of acute ductal constriction or placental insufficiency, or acute right ventricular preloading, in the face of acute-onset tricuspid regurgitation or acute trapping of systemic venous return in the right heart, secondary to impaired right-to-left shunting across the foramen ovale, may result in hydrops fetalis. Similarly, it has become increasingly apparent that fetuses who deteriorate into a hydropic state in the face of sustained tachy- or bradyarrhythmias are usually manifesting diastolic, rather than systolic, dysfunction. This should come as no small surprise; our understanding of the clinical manifestations of congestive heart failure in the mature cardiovascular system has turned attention toward the diastolic dysfunction that underlies most of the symptomatology of these patients.

The baseline limitation in diastolic relaxation and compliance of the fetal ventricles renders the fetal heart particularly susceptible to sustained tachycardia or bradycardia. Severe fetal tachycardia results in marked foreshortening of the diastolic filling period of the fetal ventricles. This shortening in diastolic filling is particularly disadvantageous to a heart in which active myocardial relaxation is not facilitated by rapid reuptake of Ca^{++} by sarcoplasmic reticulum, and in which diastolic compliance is impaired. Inadequate diastolic emptying results in increased end diastolic volume and pressure within the right atrium and systemic veins, and results in augmented atrial backflow in the systemic veins. The retrograde flow pattern in the systemic veins is quite similar to the characteristic flow pattern in the hepatic and pulmonary veins of mature patients with restrictive cardiomyopathy. In the presence of fetal atrial flutter, the ventricular response rate is rapid, but usually less than, the atrial rate. The venous flow pattern is further perturbed by atrial contractions that occur against a closed atrioventricular valve, resulting in more prominent retrograde flow in the fetal inferior vena cava. These retrograde atrial pulsations result in increased atrial and venous mean diastolic pressure, increased hydrostatic pressure, increased extravasation of plasma protein into the interstitial space, and, ultimately, may result in passive hepatic congestion and impaired serum albumin production.[31] These factors all predispose the fetus with sustained tachycardia to the development of hydrops fetalis, independent of the impact of tachycardia on ventricular systolic performance. The latter may ultimately deteriorate, but is not usually the immediate precursor of hydrops fetalis in the tachycardic fetus.

Some disagreement remains regarding the inherent danger of intermittent tachycardia to the human fetus, and predicting, in advance, the development of hydrops fetalis in a particular fetus with tachycardia.[32,33] A realistic risk/benefit analysis, which provides a necessary foundation for the formulation of a rational treatment algorithm, requires that one identify the fetus at greatest risk of hemodynamic deterioration (eg, death or the development of hydrops fetalis) in advance of such deterioration to provide timely treatment. It is not universally accepted, for example, that every fetus with intermittent, or even sustained, tachycardia is in imminent danger of sudden death or the development of hydrops fetalis. It is, however, generally accepted that the hydropic fetus is unlikely (but even this is not certain) to improve spontaneously. It is also well established that in the presence of hydrops fetalis maternal absorption and transplacental transfer of medications such as digoxin is impaired.[34]

In an effort to identify clinical findings predictive of early deterioration into hydrops fetalis in the tachycardic fetus, we identified the importance of determining the atrial contraction sequence. In the presence of tachycardia originating in the left, rather than right, atrium (e.g., reentry tachycardia with a left-sided bypass tract or atrial flutter arising within the left atrium) the onset of left atrial contraction, a fraction of a second prior to right atrial contraction, results in a transient increase of left atrial pressure. If left atrial pressure surpasses that in the right atrium the atrial septum primum, which represents the flap valve that ultimately apposes to the atrial septum and closes the foramen ovale postnatally, closes transiently in utero. Prenatal partial closure of the foramen ovale in the fetal patient with atrial tachycardia arising in the left atrium may trap systemic venous return in the right atrium and inferior vena cava, resulting in a disproportionate increase in mean systemic venous pressure. This, we believe, in turn, renders this subgroup of tachycardic fetuses at highest risk for early deterioration into a hydropic state.[35,36]

Alternatively, fetuses with severe bradycardia, are susceptible, as well, to the development of hydrops fetalis. The most frequently encountered sustained fetal bradycardia is congenital complete atrioventricular block. Previous studies have demonstrated that these fetuses fall into 2 major categories: (1) those with congenital complete block and associated congenital heart disease. These fetuses usually have abnormalities of cardiac anatomy at the atrioventricular junction (e.g., atrioventricular discordance [atrioventricular inversion, or congenitally corrected transposition of the great arteries], or visceral heterotaxia and left atrial isomerism); or (2) those with normal intracardiac anatomy in whom maternal serum contains high concentrations of autoantibodies (anti–SS-A or anti–SS-B) that may cross the placenta to cause autoimmune damage to the fetal atrioventricular conduction tissue. Such fetuses may also sustain autoimmune damage to cardiac contractile elements, resulting in an autoimmune myocarditis.[37]

In such fetuses, bradycardia results in prolonged atrial and ventricular diastolic filling times, resulting in increased filling volumes. Harkening back to the initial studies of myocardial performance of fetal myocardium, the limited compliance of fetal ventricular myocardium results in a higher diastolic pressure at any given diastolic volume. The atrioventricular dissociation between atrial and ventricular electrical activation and mechanical responses results in *cannon waves,* which are the product of atrial contraction against a closed atrioventric-

ular valve. These cannon waves result in a further increase in mean right atrial and systemic venous pressure, all of which predispose to the development of fetal anasarca.

THE EVOLUTION OF FETAL CONGENITAL HEART DISEASE

The characteristics of the circulation that impart a remarkable ability of the fetus to adapt, in a relatively undisturbed fashion, to the presence of major structural cardiac malformations also present the aspiring fetal cardiologist with the challenge of predicting the end result of flow perturbations that may be detected early in gestation. It has become apparent that these protective properties may result in a gradual progression of fetal cardiac structural abnormalities that reflect relative flow volumes and pressures within cardiac chambers and blood vessels.[38–45]

Postnatal experience has demonstrated that patients with severe tricuspid regurgitation, such as those with Ebstein malformation of the tricuspid valve, may, in the presence of a widely patent ductus arteriosus, be unable to generate an adequate pressure head to open the pulmonary valve. In such cases it may be difficult, if not impossible, to distinguish pulmonary valvular atresia from pseudo-atresia, in which the valve, although perforate, cannot be opened.[46,47] It has been demonstrated over the course of gestation that pseudo-atresia of such valves may progress to acquired, true atresia, thus representing the ultimate manifestation of the form follows function characteristics of the fetal circulation.

Conversely, low flow volume through the foramen ovale toward the left atrium and ventricle may result in progressive growth lag of left heart structures.[43] Low flow through a uni- or bicommissural aortic valve may beget further growth failure of the left heart, with compensatory enlargement and increased flow through the right heart. This disproportionate growth may provide the first diagnostic clue to the presence of congenital heart disease. The foramen ovale allows redistribution of venous return. The widely patent ductus arteriosus allows redistribution of arterial output, to provide adequate systemic flow to developing fetal vital organs, and equalizes systolic and diastolic pressure in the main pulmonary trunk and the ascending aorta. Low flow through the aortic valve may be, in some cases, inadequate to open the valve at all. In such situations the aortic valve may become imperforate, resulting in acquired aortic atresia.

IN UTERO CARDIAC THERAPY

The ability to diagnose structural or functional heart disease prenatally has, predictably, led to a growth of interest in the potential for prenatal therapy. It is, of course, necessary to identify fetal conditions that, if left untreated, result in fetal death, or compromised condition that render the neonate into a condition resulting in a lower likelihood of cure or functional survival than would be the case if the fetus were to undergo the proposed therapy. It is essential, of course, to consider the potential risks to both the mother and fetus, whose states of well-being are inextricably interwoven.

The rapidity with which the ability to diagnose heart disease in the fetus was followed by proposals for prenatal therapy was remarkable, especially when one considers the initial response to our initial publication on the subject.[2] In the 1981 edition of the *Yearbook of Cardiology*, Dr. Alexander Nadas, the revered Chairman of the Department of Cardiology at the Boston Children's Hospital, and 1 of the pioneers of pediatric cardiology, reviewed our publication. He pointed to the potential that these observations could have regarding research into fetal cardiac function, but expressed doubts that the information could have clinical importance. This was based on the assumption that prenatal cardiac diagnosis would be limited by the resolution of ultrasound to late gestation, at a time when termination of pregnancy was no longer legally feasible. Termination of pregnancy was, at the time, viewed as the only active intervention available.[48]

Our own experience convinced us that fetuses with sustained tachycardia and cardiovascular compromise could constitute a subgroup of patients who, under specific circumstances, including extreme prematurity and accurate arrhythmia diagnosis, could be candidates for prenatal drug therapy. Initial treatment efforts involved oral administration of antiarrhythmic agents to the pregnant woman. Even fetal antiarrhythmic therapy has evolved in a more invasive direction over the past decades, including injection of medication directly into the amniotic fluid, intramuscular administration of medication directly to the fetus, and direct, repetitive, administration of intravenous medication through the fetal umbilical vein.[34,49-52]

Direct instrumentation of the fetal heart was initially attempted in an effort to institute transcatheter pacing of a moribund fetus with congenital complete heart block and hydrops fetalis.[53] Subsequently there have been several reports of attempted catheter treatment of congenital cardiac malformations, with varied success.

Several centers have investigated techniques for the institution of surface cooling and rewarming, and for the provision of cardiopulmonary bypass in fetal animal models.[54,55]

FETAL ANTIARRHYTHMIC THERAPY

THE FETUS WITH TACHYCARDIA

The administration of antiarrhythmic therapy to the pregnant mothers of fetuses with sustained supraventricular tachycardia represent the first examples of successful prenatal cardiac therapy that reported in the medical literature. We attempted to bring some order and reason to the evaluation and treatment of these fetuses, without a clear understanding of how

frequently this condition occurs during pregnancy. We were, however, reassured by the existence of a body of literature that described the use of the, at the time, available antiarrhythmic agents for the treatment of pregnant women with cardiac arrhythmias of their own. This literature was replete with information concerning the pharmacology and pharmacokinetics of these medications in the pregnant woman and fetus.[56-62]

We concentrated our attention on the use of fetal ultrasound, in the absence of sensitive and accurate fetal electrocardiography, to develop algorithms for the analysis of the electrophysiologic mechanisms underlying clinical fetal arrhythmias.[49,50,63] m-Mode echocardiography, by providing information concerning cardiac motion against time, allows evaluation of the temporal sequence of mechanical responses of cardiac structures to electrical stimulation of atrial or ventricular structures. Using pulsed- or color Doppler recordings of flow against time allows a similar temporal sequencing of the underlying mechanical, and immediately preceding electrical events.

Using these techniques we concluded that the most commonly encountered sustained fetal tachycardia, supraventricular tachycardia, is most frequently (90–95%) a result of electrical reentry at the atrioventricular junction, usually by way of an accessory connection between atrial and ventricular myocardium, and less frequently via the atrioventricular node itself.[49,50,64,65] Supraventricular tachycardia resulting from electrical macroreentry circuits typically presents with a monotonous fetal heart rate of 240–260 beats/min, and is usually exquisitely sensitive to treatment with antiarrhythmic agents that alter conduction velocity and/or refractoriness of the atrioventricular node or accessory pathways. Such agents include digoxin, propranolol, flecainide, and sotalol, among others. Multiple publications have described treatment protocols for this arrhythmia. Our group has approached these patients conservatively, reserving treatment for fetuses who appear to have no reasonable alternative. The characteristics that identify such patients are the development of hydrops fetalis in the face of sustained arrhythmia at a gestational age that is early enough to preclude safe delivery and postnatal treatment. In such cases we begin therapy with medications that have a relatively broad therapeutic margin, with a low risk of proarrhythmia (unwanted precipitation or exacerbation of arrhythmia) in the fetus or pregnant woman.[59,66]

Atrial flutter, with electrical reentry confined completely within the atrial muscle, is more frequently associated with structural heart disease than is supraventricular tachycardia. This rhythm disturbance is more recalcitrant to medical therapy than supraventricular tachycardia, both in the neonate and the fetus.

Although an overview of the literature may leave the reader with the impression that the goal of clinical investigation has been to identify the single medication that can safely and effectively treat all fetal tachyarrhythmias, regardless of underlying electrophysiology, such an agent does not exist. A review of the literature provides the reader with a more complete review of the use of ultrasound to ascertain arrhythmia mechanism, and the application of this information to develop an algorithm for rational management of fetal tachycardia.[49,50]

The recent introductions of Doppler tissue imaging for evaluation of the temporal activation sequence of the fetal heart,[67] and magnetocardiography,[68] for the evaluation of the morphology of electrical events versus time in the fetal heart, offer powerful tools for the diagnosis of fetal arrhythmias that may supplant the currently employed echocardiographic techniques for arrhythmia diagnosis. The magnetocardiogram also offers the potential for more accurate and safer monitoring of the effect of potent antiarrhythmic medications on the fetal heart.

THE FETUS WITH BRADYCARDIA

As noted, the most important sustained bradyarrhythmia is congenital complete heart block. Such fetuses may develop hydrops fetalis, which may occur in the subgroup of fetuses with associated congenital heart disease. The association of clinical heart failure with congenital heart block, with or without congenital heart disease, represents an absolute indication for electrical pacemaker therapy in the neonate.[69] Hydrops fetalis in the presence of complete heart block in utero is a dire finding. The association of hydrops fetalis, complete heart block, and complex congenital heart disease is almost invariably fatal, with or without fetal therapy.[70]

The initial report of the application of electrical pacemaker therapy for fetal congenital heart block involved a fetus presenting with congenital heart block in the absence of congenital heart disease.[71] This fetus, with heart block presumably arising on the basis of immune complex-mediated damage to fetal conduction tissue and myocardium, presented with severe bradycardia and hydrops fetalis. In desperation, the treating physicians placed a pacing catheter within the fetal heart via percutaneous puncture of the maternal abdomen, uterus, and fetal thorax and ventricular wall. Fetal ventricular capture was demonstrated, without clinical improvement in the fetus. Subsequent attempts to utilize similar techniques had similarly discouraging outcomes.

Laboratory models of complete heart block have been created in fetal lambs, with subsequent resolution of hydrops fetalis following fetal exteriorization and surgical implantation of permanent pacemakers connected to epicardial pacing leads. An attempt to implant a pacemaker in this fashion in a human fetus was unsuccessful. Although it may well be that some human fetuses with heart block and hydrops fetalis have deteriorated solely because of bradycardia, we are concerned that some neonates do not respond to pacing alone, whether that pacing is ventricular demand pacing or the more physiologic, dual-chamber technique. We have postulated that this subgroup of patients has sustained immune-mediated damage to the contractile elements of the heart by the same mechanism that has damaged the conduction system.[72–75]

Although it has been demonstrated that the administration of β-mimetic agents to the pregnant woman can increase the intrinsic fetal heart rate by as much as 50%, we have not been impressed that such treatment ameliorates hydrops fetalis in affected fetuses.[37,76]

We reported a preliminary experience with the administration of absorbable corticosteroid to pregnant women whose fetuses have developed high-grade second- or recent-onset third-degree heart block in the presence of high maternal titers of anti–SS-A and/or anti–SS-B. In this small subgroup of patients, there was demonstrable improvement in atrioventricular conduction that we attributed to amelioration of the immune-mediated inflammatory response of the fetal atrioventricular conduction tissue. This report has spawned a multicenter study designed to evaluate the impact of maternally administered corticosteroid on echocardiographically estimated fetal atrioventricular conduction intervals in a population of fetuses whose mothers have high anti–SS-A or –SS-B antibodies.[77,78]

MEDICAL TREATMENT OF CONGESTIVE HEART FAILURE IN THE FETUS

The medical literature is replete with anecdotal reports of the administration of digoxin to pregnant women whose fetuses have evidence of impaired cardiac pump function. These have included cases in which structural heart disease (eg, aortic stenosis) is associated with ventricular dysfunction and hydrops fetalis and in whom the initiation of digoxin therapy is temporally associated with improved ventricular shortening and resolution of hydrops fetalis, with subsequent postnatal salvage of the child.[79,80] We have had similar personal experiences with 2 fetuses with similar presentation with hydrops fetalis and aortic stenosis. In addition, we witnessed a close temporal association between the initiation of maternally administered digoxin and improved ventricular shortening and resolution of hydrops fetalis in several fetal patients who were presumed to have viral myocarditis, with viruses such as adenovirus, parvovirus, and Coxsackievirus. In these cases, fetomaternal infection with the virus has been confirmed by maternal and fetal blood and amniotic fluid PCR. In 2 fetuses who had initial improvement, with eventual neonatal demise, adenoviral genome was detected by PCR on the infant's myocardial tissue. We also recently demonstrated improved myocardial shortening, and improved right ventricular dP/dT (calculated from the tricuspid regurgitant flow waveform) in 2 fetuses with progressively dilating right ventricles,[81] with progressive tricuspid regurgitation and abnormal inferior vena caval flow waveforms, in the face of large hemangiomas with significant arteriovenous shunting. The findings of cardiomegaly, tricuspid regurgitation, and abnormal venous Doppler in the vena cavae were quite similar to those described by Tulzer et al.[82] in justification of the invasive pulmonary balloon valvuloplasties of 2 fetuses with pulmonary stenosis/atresia.

We recently used digoxin to empirically treat a fetus with severe dilated cardiomyopathy and marked cardiomegaly, bilateral atrioventricular valve regurgitation, and abnormal venous pulsatility, and demonstrated a remarkable improvement in biventricular shortening, partial amelioration of atrioventricular valve regurgitation, and improved biventricular dP/dT. This fetus survived pregnancy and delivery, and ultimately underwent successful cardiac transplantation, only to be diagnosed to have an electron transport defect that was not identifiable in the studies performed on skeletal muscle biopsy prior to transplant. The same enthusiasm that we have criticized in others has led us to prescribe empirical treatment, without having done our homework with regard to ascertaining the mechanism of action of digoxin in the fetus.

On the other hand, this medication has been in use for over 200 years, and is still being administered largely on an empiric basis. Although the popularity of this agent for the treatment of congestive heart failure waxes and wanes every few years, recent studies have suggested some rationale for its inclusion in the therapeutic arsenal. It is, however, unclear whether the salutary effects are related to Na^+/K^+-ATPase inhibition, and enhanced calcium availability to the myofilaments, or whether alterations of catecholamine concentration/effect alters the neuroendocrine manifestations of congestive heart failure. The underlying rationale for its use remains, "it works." Although it is possible that some of the fetuses we and others have observed to improve in the days following digoxin administration spontaneously recovered from the underlying pathology that caused circulatory failure, and digoxin administration was simply serendipitous, in the last case we cited (with an electron transfer deficiency), at least, the underlying nature of the cardiomyopathy would not logically have spontaneous improvement after having demonstrated severe biventricular dilated myopathy. In any event, the centuries of use of this medication, in gravid and nongravid women, convinced us that if one monitors the mother and fetus carefully for evidence of contraindications to the administration of digoxin (ventricular preexcitation; severe maternal hypokalemia), or for indications calling for modulation of digoxin dose (e.g., maternal renal failure or concomitant treatment with medications that alter digoxin clearance [e.g., quinidine, amiodarone]) that, at the very least, you are unlikely to harm either the mother or fetus.

INTERVENTIONAL CARDIAC CATHETERIZATION OF THE HUMAN FETUS

AORTIC BALLOON VALVULOPLASTY

Motivated by a dismal postnatal outcome for fetuses diagnosed to have critical aortic stenosis prenatally, the group from Guy's Hospital in London embarked on an innovative program for percutaneous cardiac catheterization and aortic balloon valvuloplasty of fetuses with this condition. The initial experience was unsuccessful, although the feasibility of percutaneous entry of the maternal abdomen, uterus, and fetal chest and left ventricle, with subsequent wire entry of the ascending aorta,

passage of an angioplasty balloon catheter, and subsequent retrieval of the system,[83] was established. Ultimately, this group performed a total of 4 such procedures, and reported the first survivor.[84] These initial reports suggested that balloon valvuloplasty was feasible but that the prognosis for the fetus depended on the ability to relieve aortic stenosis and to prevent or reverse damage to the left ventricular myocardium. Despite the survival of a single patient, this group declared a moratorium on such procedures until a clearer appreciation of hemodynamics and improvement in catheter technology was in place.[85]

Follow-up studies from that same center, only a few years later, documented improved survival in neonates who had not undergone fetal intervention, undermining the rationale for the introduction of fetal intervention as an alternative approach to an otherwise hopeless condition.[86]

Almost a decade later Kohl et al. summarized the world experience with such techniques.[87] This report included 12 fetuses, including the 4 cases from Guy's Hospital. At the time of this review, the child from the Guy's experience represented the sole survivor. The conclusion was that the high failure rate was related to the selection of severe cases for treatment, technical problems during the procedure, and high postnatal operative mortality among patients who survived pregnancy. The conclusion of this paper was that: "Improved patient selection and technical modifications in interventional methods may hold promise to improve outcome in future cases." This, I believe, is problematic. If one reviews this report at arm's length we are presented with a "world experience" that added 8 attempts, at multiple centers, without a single success. In any other situation, the inability to duplicate the single success of the initial investigators would have cast a cloud of doubt over the technique, at least until a fundamental review of the technique and its indications had taken place! In this situation, the honest eagerness of the investigators to provide help for an unfortunate patient population, and their personal conviction that this technique should work, may have influenced their level of enthusiasm for a "therapy in search of an indication."

It was not until the group from Boston Children's Hospital issued a press release resulting in a front-page article in the *New York Times* that the next page was written in this story.[88] This article summarized the case of a surviving infant who had undergone a similar (the exact details of the modifications in the Guy's Hospital technique have not yet been published) valvuloplasty, not to necessarily prevent fetal or neonatal death from aortic stenosis, but to prevent evolution of the fetal condition into "hypoplastic left heart syndrome." This changed indication for invasive treatment was based on serial observations of left ventricular development among fetuses initially presenting with severe aortic outlet obstruction and poor left ventricular performance. It is well documented that some of these fetuses, especially in the presence of left ventricular fibroelastosis and reversed, left-to-right, shunting at the level of the foramen ovale go on to develop left ventricular hypoplasia.[89] By relieving left ventricular outlet obstruction, this group maintains that this child was spared a lifetime of cardiac disability related to living with palliated single ventricular physiology. It is clear that some fetal patients with severe left ventricular outlet obstruction will develop left ventricular failure, and ultimately manifest growth failure of left heart structures. The subgroup of patients alluded to by the Guy's Hospital group and the subsequent multicenter report did not appear to evolve toward left ventricular hypoplasia, although several of those patients could be candidates for single ventricular management, because of the presence of an irretrievably damaged left ventricle. Once again, the challenge is not to identify the irretrievably damaged left ventricle, but to identify the left ventricle that is certainly going to become irretrievably damaged in the absence of intervention. At this point, one can only look forward to the publication of a series of such patients from Boston to evaluate critically the selection criteria for this procedure and the details of the procedure itself.

PULMONARY BALLOON VALVULOPLASTY

A recent report in *The Lancet* documents the performance of pulmonary balloon valvuloplasty in 2 fetuses with severe right ventricular outlet obstruction ("complete or 'almost complete' pulmonary atresia"), right ventricular compromise, and "imminent" hydrops fetalis. Both fetuses survived and have biventricular circulatory systems. It remains to be seen whether such therapy is justified, and whether these fetuses survived because of, rather than in spite of, what was done for (to) them.[82]

FUTURE DIRECTIONS

We have recently been involved in conversations with our colleagues at Boston Children's Hospital, who have informed us of a preliminary experience in balloon atrial septoplasty of fetuses with hypoplastic left heart syndrome and restrictive foramen ovale. Such fetuses can be identified to have obstruction to pulmonary venous return on the basis of visualization of a small foramen ovale, the identification of a high-velocity jet of left-to-right atrial shunting, or on the basis of marked retrograde atrial flow in the pulmonary venous flow waveform.[90–94] These fetuses represent the sickest of neonates with congenital heart disease, typically presenting with critical cyanosis, secondary to pulmonary edema that results from severe pulmonary venous obstruction. In the absence of a mitral valve for left atrial outflow these infants depend on the foramen ovale for outlet of pulmonary venous blood from the left atrium. The first breath in the neonate results in a dramatic drop in pulmonary resistance, which allows an immediate flood of blood flow through the pulmonary vascular bed. This translates into an immediate torrential increase in pulmonary venous return. If there is a severe obstruction to pulmonary venous return, these neonates become severely distressed and cyanotic, to the point where survival past the immediate postdelivery period may be problematic. Such neonates have an extremely poor prognosis for survival, even when diagnosed prenatally. Typically, such neonates require emergent cardiac catheterization with static

dilation or stent placement within the atrial septum to allow decompression of the pulmonary veins.[95] Even those neonates who survive these procedures are at extremely high risk for subsequent Norwood palliation or cardiac transplantation.[96] Some of these neonates may, alternatively, be managed with immediate institution of extracorporeal membrane oxygenation, followed by cardiac surgical management of the hypoplastic left heart and atrial flow restriction. The potential for decompressing the left atrium of these fetuses, well before delivery, would be extremely attractive, if it could be accomplished at minimal maternal risk. Even a low-to-moderate risk to the fetus would be justifiable. Such patients represent the most ideal potential candidates for fetal therapy, because the natural history of their native condition is well known to be virtually hopeless, even with the timely provision of aggressive neonatal therapy.

HOW DO WE GET "ON BOARD?"

It is important to consider not only the role of such techniques for the management of these patients, but also to consider whether there is a rational justification to replicate programs of this sort. This decision should be based not solely on the natural desire to keep one's own center at the cutting edge, but should also be based on an estimation of just how many of these patients are likely to be encountered in a given region or "super-region" during any single year. There is a minimum "critical mass" of patients that necessary to hone a team to perform these procedures and to maintain clinical skills. It may well be that certain therapies should be reserved for superspecialized centers that receive referrals from collaborating diagnostic centers.

CONCLUSION

In conclusion, the widespread availability of high-resolution fetal echocardiographic imaging has resulted in a proliferation of prenatal screening programs for congenital heart disease. In addition, the close collaborations that have developed between pediatric/fetal cardiologists and perinatologists have resulted in an increased appreciation of the potential that echocardiography has to explain the hemodynamic impact of extracardiac structural and medical abnormalities on the fetal circulatory system. In addition, these studies may also be used to evaluate the impact of medical and invasive therapies that may be offered to the pregnant woman and her fetus.

The increased understanding of fetal cardiovascular development and physiology has, predictably, led to a surge of interest in the development of fetal treatment protocols for structural and functional heart disease. To a large extent, this interest stems from a sense that prenatal diagnosis will provide only a marginal improvement in outcome for fetuses with major cardiac abnormalities, if the information is solely employed to facilitate postnatal care, because the management of some cardiac lesions remains problematic from a surgical viewpoint. In recent years, an appreciation of the natural evolution of structural heart disease over the course of gestation, during fetal circulatory adaptation to an abnormal structural template that was established during organogenesis, has led to the belief that fetal intervention, at a critical period during development, may alter the remodeling process. In particular, the potential for preserving the potential for a 2-ventricular anatomic repair, thus avoiding multiple palliations into a single-ventricular "Fontan" circulation, has fueled a recent resurgence of interest in the potential for fetal cardiac surgery or interventional catheterization.

To be sure, these initial reports are encouraging. We must, however, be circumspect in our approach to such treatments, remembering the sad lessons learned by our forbearers in the field of fetal treatment, when they learned that some fetal treatments could improve survival of fetuses who became hopelessly impaired neonates and toddlers.

It is essential that we evaluate prospective treatments in a careful and rational fashion, remembering that the pregnant woman who is offered a glimmer of hope for her fetus is not always in a position to be totally analytical when considering whether to assent to well-intentioned, but unproved, therapies.

Determining whether to attempt such therapy, or whether to refer one's patients to another practitioner for such therapy, should be based on a complete understanding of the pathophysiology of the underlying abnormality and the rationale underlying the proposed therapy. In addition, it is essential that there be an open discussion of these treatments, with a sharing of positive and negative results.

One should consider, as well, whether press releases, resulting in dissemination of spectacular results by the media, should be made in advance of preparation, peer review, and impending publication of the information in a reputable medical journal. The downside risks inherent in presenting unproven therapies to a susceptible public and potential patient population certainly outweigh the gains to be derived from the notoriety associated with communication by sound bite.

References

1. Rudolph AM. *Congenital Diseases of the Heart.* Chicago: Yearbook; 1974.
2. Kleinman CS, Hobbins JC, Jaffe CC, et al. Echocardiographic studies of the human fetus: Prenatal diagnosis of congenital heart disease and cardiac dysrhythmias. *Pediatrics.* 1980;65:1059–1067.
3. Adamsons K Jr. Fetal surgery. *N Engl J Med.* 1966;275:204–206.
4. Clewell WH. Congenital hydrocephalus: treatment in utero. *Fetal Ther.* 1988;3:89–97.
5. McLorie G, Farhat W, Khoury A, et al. Outcome analysis of vesicoamniotic shunting in a comprehensive population. *J Urol.* 2001;3:1036–1041.
6. Verheijen PM, Lisowski LA, Stoutenbeek PH, et al. Prenatal diagnosis of congenital heart disease affects preoperative acidosis in the newborn patient. *J Thorac Cardiovasc Surg.* 2001;121:798–803.
7. Verheijen PM, Lisowski LA, Stoutenbeek, et al. Lactic acidosis in the neonate is minimized by prenatal detection of congenital heart disease. *Ultrasound Obstet Gynecol.* 2001;19:552–555.
8. Bonnet D, Coltri A, Butera G, et al. Detection of transposition of the great arteries in fetuses reduces neonatal morbidity and mortality. *Circulation.* 1999;99:916–918.
9. Tworetzky W, McElhinney DB, Reddy VM, et al. Improved surgical outcome after fetal diagnosis of hypoplastic left heart syndrome. *Circulation.* 2001;103:1269–1273.
10. Franklin O, Burch M, Manning N, et al. Prenatal diagnosis of coarctation of the aorta improves survival and reduces morbidity. *Heart.* 2002;87:67–69.
11. Harrison MR, Golbus MS, Filley RA, eds. *The Unborn Patient.* 2nd ed. Philadelphia: WB Saunders; 1991.
12. Rudolph AM, Heymann MA: Circulatory changes during growth in the fetal lamb. *Circ Res.* 1970;57:289–297.
13. Friedman WF: The intrinsic physiologic properties of the developing heart. In Friedman WF, Lesch M, Sonnenblick EH, eds: *Neonatal Heart Disease.* New York: Grune & Stratton; 1973:87–111.
14. Anderson PAW. The heart and development. *Semin Perinatol.* 1996;20:482–509.
15. Ascuitto RJ, Ross-Ascuitto NT. Substrate metabolism in the developing heart. *Semin Perinatol.* 1996;20:542–563.
16. Mahony L. Calcium homeostasis and control of contractility in the developing heart. *Semin Perinatol.* 20:510–519.
17. Garson A Jr. Medicolegal problems in the management of cardiac arrhythmias in children. *Pediatrics.* 1987;79:84–88.
18. Levin DL, Mills LJ, Weinberg AG. Hemodynamic, pulmonary vascular, and myocardial abnormalities secondary to pharmacologic constriction of the fetal ductus arteriosus. A possible mechanism for persistent pulmonary hypertension and transient tricuspid insufficiency in the newborn infant. *Circulation.* 1979;60:360–364.
19. Huhta JC, Moise KJ, Fisher DJ, et al. Detection and quantitation of constriction of the fetal ductus arteriosus by Doppler echocardiography. *Circulation.* 1987;75:406–412.
20. Reed KL, Appleton CP, Anderson CF, et al. Doppler studies of vena cava flows in human fetuses. Insights into normal and abnormal cardiac physiology. *Circulation.* 1990;81:498–505.
21. Hecher K, Diehl W, Zikulnig L, et al. Endoscopic laser coagulation of placental anastomoses in 200 pregnancies with severe mid-trimester twin-to-twin transfusion syndrome. *Eur J Obstet Gynecol Reprod Biol.* 2000;92:135–139.
22. Quintero RA, Morales WJ, Allen MH, et al. Staging of twin-to-twin transfusion syndrome. *J Perinatol.* 1999;19:550–555.
23. Simpson LL, Marx GR, Elkadry EA, et al. Cardiac dysfunction in twin-to-twin transfusion syndrome: a prospective, longitudinal study. *Obstet Gynecol.* 1998;92:557–562.
24. Simpson PC, Trudinger BJ, Walker A, et al. The intrauterine treatment of fetal cardiac failure in a twin pregnancy with an acardiac, acephalic monster. *Am J Obstet Gynecol.* 1983;147:842–844.
25. Umur A, van Gemert MJ, Ross MG. Fetal urine and amniotic fluid in monochorionic twins with twin-twin transfusion syndrome: simulations of therapy. *Am J Obstet Gynecol.* 2002;185:996–1003.
26. Wee LY, Fisk NM. The twin-twin transfusion syndrome. *Semin Neonatol.* 2002;7:187–202.
27. Zosmer N, Bajoria R, Weiner E, et al. Clinical and echographic features of in utero cardiac dysfunction in the recipient twin in twin-twin transfusion syndrome. *Br Heart J.* 1994;72:74–79.
28. Kleinman CS, Donnerstein RL, DeVore GR, et al. Fetal echocardiography for evaluation of in utero congestive heart failure: a technique for study of nonimmune fetal hydrops. *N Engl J Med.* 1982;306:568–575.
29. Silverman NH, Kleinman CS, Rudolph AM, et al. Fetal atrioventricular valve insufficiency associated with nonimmune hydrops. A

two-dimensional echocardiography and pulsed Doppler ultrasound study. *Circulation.* 1985;72:825–831.

30. Rudolph AM. *Congenital Diseases of the Heart.* 2nd ed. Armonk, NY: Futura; 2001.

31. Nimrod C, Davies D, Harder J, et al. Ultrasound evaluation of tachycardia-induced hydrops in the fetal lamb. *Am J Obstet Gynecol.* 1987;57:655–661.

32. Simpson LL, Marx GR, D'Alton ME. Supraventricular tachycardia in the fetus: conservative management in the absence of hemodynamic compromise. *J Ultrasound Med.* 1997;16:459–464.

33. Simpson JM, Milburn A, Yates RW, et al. Outcome of intermittent tachyarrhythmias in the fetus. *Pediatr Cardiol.* 1997;18:78–82.

34. Weiner CP, Thompson MIB. Direct treatment of fetal supraventricular tachycardia after failed transplacental therapy. *Am J Obstet Gynecol.* 1988;158:570–573.

35. Kleinman CS, Dubin AM, Nehgme RA, et al. Left atrial tachycardia in the human fetus: Identifying the fetus at greatest risk for developing nonimmune hydrops fetalis. In: *Proceedings of the Second World Congress of Pediatric Cardiology and Cardiac Surgery.* Armonk, NY: Futura; 1999.

36. Rudolph AM, Heymann MA. Cardiac output in the fetal lamb: the effect of spontaneous and induced changes of heart rate on the right and left ventricular output. *Am J Obstet Gynecol.* 1976;124:183–189.

37. Schmidt KG, Ulmer HE, Silverman NH, et al. Perinatal outcome of fetal congenital complete atrioventricular block: a multicenter experience. *J Am Coll Cardiol.* 1991;17:1360–1366.

38. Allan LD, Crawford DC, Tynan MJ. Evolution of coarctation of the aorta in intrauterine life. *Br Heart J.* 1984;52:471–473.

39. Feit L, Copel JA, Kleinman CS. Foramen ovale size in the normal and abnormal fetal heart. An indicator of transatrial flow physiology. *Ultrasound Obstet Gynecol.* 1991;1:313–319.

40. Fesslova V, Papa M, DeCaro E, et al. Evolution of left ventricular disease in the fetus. Case report. *Fetal Diagn Ther.* 1999;14:60–62.

41. Hornberger LK, Benacerraf BR, Bromley BS, et al. Prenatal detection of severe right ventricular outflow tract obstruction: pulmonary stenosis and pulmonary atresia. *J Ultrasound Med.* 1994;13:743–750.

42. Hornberger LK, Bromley B, Lichter E, et al. Development of severe aortic stenosis and left ventricular dysfunction with endocardial fibroelastosis in a second trimester fetus. *J Ultrasound Med.* 1996;15:651–654.

43. Hornberger LK, Sanders SP, Rein AJ, et al. Left heart obstructive lesions and left ventricular growth in the midtrimester fetus. A longitudinal study. *Circulation.* 1995;92:1531–1538.

44. Mielke GT, Mayer R, Hassberg D, et al. Sequential development of fetal aortic valve stenosis and endocardial fibroelastosis during the second trimester of pregnancy. *Am Heart J.* 1997;133:607–610.

45. Sharland GK, Chita SK, Fagg NL, et al. Left ventricular dysfunction in the fetus: Relation to aortic valve anomalies and endocardial fibroelastosis. *Br Heart J.* 1991;66:419–424.

46. Freedom R, Culham G, Moes F, et al. Differentiation of functional and structural pulmonary atresia: Role of aortography. *Am J Cardiol.* 1978;41:914–920.

47. Smallhorn JF, Izukawa T, Benson L, et al. Non-invasive recognition of functional pulmonary atresia by echocardiography. *Am J Cardiol.* 1984;54:925–926.

48. Nadas AS. *Yearbook of Cardiology—1981.* Chicago: Yearbook; 1981:86–88.

49. Kleinman CS, Nehgme RA, Copel JA. Fetal cardiac arrhythmias: diagnosis and therapy. In: RK Creasy, R Resnik, eds. *Maternal Fetal Medicine.* 4th ed. Philadelphia: WB Saunders;1995:301–318.

50. Kleinman CS, Copel JA, Nehgme RA. The fetus with cardiac arrhythmia. In MR Harrison, MI Evans, NS Adzick, W Holzgreve, eds. *The Unborn Patient: The Art and Science of Fetal Therapy.* Philadelphia: WB Saunders; 2001:417–441.

51. Hansmann M, Gembruch U, Bald RK, et al. Fetal tachyarrhythmias: transplacental and direct treatment of the fetus. A report of 60 cases. *Ultrasound Obstet Gynecol.* 1991;1:162–167.

52. Younis JS, Granat M. Insufficient transplacental digoxin transfer in severe hydrops fetalis. *Am J Obstet Gynecol.* 1987;157:1268–1269.

53. Strasburger JF, Kugler JD, Cheatham JP, et al. Nonimmunologic hydrops fetalis associated with congenital aortic valvular stenosis. *Am Heart J.* 1984;108:1380–1382.

54. Slate RK, Stevens MB, Verrier ED, et al. Intrauterine repair of pulmonary stenosis in fetal sheep. *Surg Forum.* 1985;36:246–247.

55. Turley K, Vlahakes GI, Harrison MR, et al. Intrauterine cardiothoracic surgery: The fetal lamb model. *Ann Thorac Surg.* 1982;34:422–426.

56. DeWolff D, deSchepper J, Verhaaren H, et al. Congenital hypothyroid goiter and amiodarone. *Acta Paediatr Scand.* 1988;77:616–618.

57. Evans MI, Pryde PG, Reichler A, et al. Fetal drug therapy. *West J Med.* 1993;159:325–332.

58. Gladstone GR, Hordof A, Gersony WM. Propranolol administration during pregnancy: effects on the fetus. *J Pediatr.* 1975;86:962–964.

59. Morganroth J. Risk factors for the development of proarrhythmic events. *Am J Cardiol.* 1987;59:32E–37E.

60. Roden DM. Risks and benefits of antiarrhythmic therapy. *N Engl J Med.* 1994;305:785–791.

61. Rogers MC, Willerson JT, Goldblatt A, et al. Serum digoxin concentrations in the human fetus, neonate and infant. *N Engl J Med.* 1972;287:1010–1014.

62. Ward RM. Pharmacological treatment of the fetus: clinical pharmacokinetic considerations. *Clin Pharmacokinet.* 1995;28:343–350.

63. Kleinman CS, Donnerstein RL, Jaffe CC, et al. Fetal echocardiography. A tool for evaluation of in utero cardiac arrhythmias and monitoring of in utero therapy: analysis of 71 patients. *Am J Cardiol.* 1983;51:237–243.

64. Gillette PC: The mechanisms of supraventricular tachycardia in children. *Circulation.* 1980;54:133–139.

65. Naheed ZJ, Strasburger JF, Deal BJ, et al. Fetal tachycardia: Mechanisms and predictors of hydrops fetalis. *J Am Coll Cardiol.* 1996;27:1736–1740.

66. Wellens JHH, Durrer D. Effect of digitalis on atrioventricular conduction and circus movement tachycardia in patients with the Wolff-Parkinson-White syndrome. *Circulation.* 1973;47:1229–1236.

67. Rein AJ, Levine JC, Nir A. Use of high-frame rate imaging and doppler tissue echocardiography in the diagnosis of fetal ventricular tachycardia. *J Am Soc Echocardiogr.* 2001;14:149–151.

68. Van Leeuwen P, Schussler, et al. Magnetocardiography for assessment of fetal heart actions. *Geburtshilfe Frauenheilkd.* 1995;55:642–646.

69. Michaelsson M, Engle MA. Congenital complete heart block: an international study of the natural history. *Cardiovascular Clin.* 1972;4:85–101.

70. Anandakumar C, Biswas A, Chew SS, et al. Direct fetal therapy for hydrops secondary to congenital atrioventricular heart block. *Obstet Gynecol.* 1996;87:835–837.

71. Carpenter RJ, Strasburger JF, Garson A Jr., et al. Fetal ventricular pacing for hydrops secondary to complete atrioventricular block. *J Am Coll Cardiol.* 1986;8:1434–1436.

72. Assad RS, Jatene MB, Moreira LF, et al. Fetal heart block: A new experimental model to assess fetal pacing. *Pacing Clin Electrophysiol.* 1994;17:1256–1263.

73. Kikuchi Y, Shiraisi H, Igarashi H, et al. Cardiac pacing in fetal lambs: intrauterine transvenous cardiac pacing for fetal complete heart block. *Pacing Clin Electrophysiol.* 1995;18:417–423.

74. Mrotsuki J, Okamura K, Watanabe T, et al. Production of complete heart block and in utero cardiac pacing in fetal lambs. *J Obstet Gynaecol.* 1995;21:223–239.

75. Walkinshaw SA, Welch CR, McCormack J, et al. *In utero* pacing for congenital heart block. *Fetal Diagn Ther.* 1994;9:183–185.

76. Koike T, Minakami H, Shiraishi H, et al: Fetal ventricular rate in case of congenital complete heart block is increased by ritodrine. Case report. *J Perinat Med.* 1997;25:216–218.

77. Copel JA, Buyon JP, Kleinman CS. Successful *in utero* therapy of fetal heart block. *Am J Obstet Gynecol.* 1995;173:1384–1390.

78. Harris JP, Alexson CG, Manning JA, et al: Medical therapy for the hydropic fetus with congenital complete atrioventricular block. *Am J Perinatol.* 1993;10:217–219.

79. Bitar FF, Byrum CJ, Kveselis DA, et al. In utero management of hydrops fetalis caused by critical aortic stenosis. *Am J Perinatol.* 1997;14:389–391.

80. Schmider A, Henrich W, Dahnert I, et al. Prenatal therapy of non-immunologic hydrops fetalis caused by severe aortic stenosis. *Ultrasound Obstet Gynecol.* 2000;16:275–278.

81. Kleinman CS, Donnerstein RL. Ultrasonic assessment of cardiac function in the intact human fetus. *J Am Coll Cardiol.* 1985;5(Suppl 1):84S–94S.

82. Tulzer G, Arzt W, Franklin RC, et al. Fetal pulmonary valvuloplasty for critical pulmonary stenosis or atresia with intact septum. *Lancet.* 2002;360:1567–1568.

83. Maxwell D, Allan L, Tynan MJ. Balloon dilatation of the aortic valve in the fetus. A report of two cases. *Br Heart J.* 1991;65:256–261.

84. Allan LD, Maxwell DJ, Carminati, et al. Survival after fetal aortic balloon valvoplasty. *Ultrasound Obstet Gynecol.* 1995;5: 90–91.

85. Kohl T, Szabo X, Suda K, et al. Fetoscopic and open transumbilical fetal cardiac catheterization in sheep. Potential approaches for human fetal cardiac intervention. *Circulation.* 1997;95:1048–1053.

86. Simpson JM, Sharland GK. Natural history and outcome of aortic stenosis diagnosed prenatally. *Heart.* 1997;77:205–210.

87. Kohl T, Sharland G, Chaoui R, et al. World experience of percutaneous ultrasound-guided-guided balloon valvuloplasty in human fetuses with severe aortic valve obstruction. *J Am Coll Cardiol.* 2000;15:1230–1233.

88. Grady D. Operation on fetus's heart valve called a 'science fiction' success. *New York Times.* February 25, 2002:1.

89. Berning R, Silverman NH, Villegas M, et al. Reverse shunting across the ductus arteriosus or atrial septum in utero heralds severe congenital heart disease. *J Am Coll Cardiol.* 1993;27:481–486.

90. Better DJ, Apfel HD, Zidere V, et al. Pattern of pulmonary venous blood flow in the hypoplastic left heart syndrome in the fetus. *Heart.* 1999;81:646–649.

91. Better DJ, Kaufman S, Allan LD. The normal pattern of pulmonary venous flow on pulsed Doppler examination of the human fetus. *J Am Soc Echocarfdiogr.* 1996;9:281–285.

92. Crowe DA, Allan LD. Patterns of pulmonary venous flow in the fetus with disease of the left heart. *Cardiol Young.* 2001;11:369–374.

93. Lenz F, Machlitt A, Hartung J, et al. Fetal pulmonary venous flow pattern is determined by left atrial pressure: report of two cases of left heart hypoplasia, one with patent and the other with closed interatrial communication. *Ultrasound Obstet Gynecol.* 2002;19:392–395.

94. Rychik J, Rome JJ, Collins MH, et al. The hypoplastic left heart syndrome with intact atrial septum: atrial morphology, pulmonary vascular histopathology and outcome. *J Am Coll Cardiol.* 1999;34: 554–560.

95. Cheatham JP. Intervention in the critically ill neonate and infant with hypoplastic left heart syndrome and intact atrial septum. *J Interv Cardiol.* 2001;14:357–366.

96. Graziano JN, Heidelberger KP, Ensing GJ, et al. The influence of a restrictive atrial septal defect on pulmonary vascular morphology in patients with hypoplastic left heart syndrome. *Pediatr Cardiol.* 2002;23:146–151.

Abramowicz J, Jaffe R. Diagnosis and intrauterine management of enlargement of the cerebral ventricles. *J Perinat Med.* 1988;16: 165–173.

Horsfall AC, Li JM, Maini RN. Placental and fetal cardiac laminin are targets for cross-reacting autoantibodies from mothers of children with congenital heart block. J Autoimmun 1996;9:561–568.

Yagel S, Weissman A, Rotstein Z, et al. Congenital heart defects: Natural course and in utero development. *Circulation.* 1997;96: 550–555.

CHAPTER 62

FETAL GENETIC THERAPY—SOMATIC

Yuval Yaron / Avi Orr-Urtreger

INTRODUCTION

Gene therapy refers to the correction of a disease state by introduction of foreign nucleic acid sequences designed to target the affected tissue. During the 1990s we have witnessed an explosion of experimental studies and clinical trials applying gene therapy to almost every discipline of medicine. Now, at the dawn of the new millennium and with the completion of the Human Genome Project, gene discoveries will lend themselves to the development of gene therapy for many disorders. However, postnatal gene therapy may come too late in those genetic disorders, which are already manifest in newborns with irreversible organ damage.

Prenatal diagnosis of genetic conditions became available almost 50 years ago with the introduction of amniocentesis and chorionic villous sampling (CVS). Until recently however, there was little hope for prenatal therapy, and most families whose fetus was diagnosed with a severe genetic condition could opt only for the termination of pregnancy. For such disorders, in utero gene therapy (IUGT) may offer a reasonable solution.

The development of high resolution sonography and the improvement of relatively safe procedures such as fetoscopy have made minimally invasive administration of therapeutic genes to the fetus *in utero* a real possibility. In addition to the prevention of prenatal irreversible damage, IUGT also allows targeting and expanding the stem cell population, which may be inaccessible later in life, and may avoid the immune response against the foreign therapeutic protein product.

However, there are considerable technical and ethical issues regarding IUGT. Before this mode of therapy can be applied in clinical practice, it is mandatory that extensive research be applied in appropriate animal models to test for efficiency and safety of the therapies for both the fetus and the mother.[1,2] Until these requirements are satisfied, human IUGT should be considered a premature technique, despite the great promise it holds for the future.[3] This chapter will review the state of the technology of IUGT and describe the studies that still need to be performed before it would be appropriate to consider human IUGT.[4,5]

THERAPEUTIC GENE DESIGN

Gene therapy may be applied to diseases that have a clear genetic cause, such as inborn errors of metabolism. It may also prove beneficial to conditions in which Genetics play an important role in multifactorial disorders such as cancer, diabetes, and cardiovascular disease. Finally, gene therapy may be a logical approach in combating viral disease, in which the viral genome is a potential target for intervention. Various approaches to gene therapy have been developed and therapeutic genes are designed accordingly.

GENE REPLACEMENT THERAPY

Loss-of-function mutations are responsible for a wide range of human diseases. These mutations result in the absence, reduction, or faulty production of essential proteins such as enzyme, structural, or a membrane receptor proteins. Theoretically, restoring the lost function can be achieved by introducing the normal or wild-type gene in a manner that would facilitate production of the missing gene product in the affected tissues at the appropriate time and quantity. This approach appears to be the most likely to be used in IUGT.

GENE INDUCTION

In many biological systems there is a certain degree of redundancy because certain functions can be achieved by more than one protein. This may be taken advantage of in gene design for IUGT. Certain genes that are expressed in early stages of fetal development are normally suppressed at a later stage. They are replaced by other genes that, under normal circumstances, are sequentially "turned-on." If, however, the latter genes are mutated or defective, a disease state results. To overcome this, the primordial genes may be induced to express their function once again. An example may be found in the globin system: fetal γ-globin is replaced by β-globin at a latter stage in development. In cases of β-thalassemia, in which the β-globin genes are mutated, γ-globin production may overcome some of the serious prenatal complications associated with the disease.

VIRALLY DIRECTED ENZYME PRODRUG THERAPY

Suicide Genes

Suicide genes encode nonmammalian enzymes that have the ability to convert a relatively nontoxic prodrug into a highly cytotoxic agent. Cells genetically transduced to express such genes essentially commit metabolic suicide in the presence of the appropriate prodrug. Such metabolic suicide genes may include viral enzymes like the varicella zoster or herpes simplex-derived thymidine kinase (HSV-Tk1). Introduction of the HSV-Tk1 gene confers sensitivity to the antiherpes drug ganciclovir. Only cells transfected with these enzymes metabolize the prodrug thereby causing cell death.[6,7] The enzyme phosphorylates the nontoxic ganciclovir to a potent DNA synthesis inhibitor.[8] The selective effect of such suicide genes can further be perfected by employment of a triggering mechanism. Such an approach takes advantage of the unique production of embryonic and fetal molecules by some tumors. For example, the alphafetoprotein (AFP) gene which is normally expressed in fetal liver is transcriptionally inactive in the adult, but is reactivated in hepatocellular carcinoma. Thus it can be utilized in creating a hepatocarcinoma-specific gene-targeting mechanism. A hybrid gene can be constructed consisting of HSV-Tk1 gene under the control of the human AFP gene promoter. This hybrid gene can then be introduced into AFP-producing hepatoma cells. Although the gene construct can transfect many cell types, only AFP producing cells will express the HSV-Tk1 gene, thus rendering them increasingly sensitive to ganciclovir treatment.[9] This approach may be applied to the therapy of various forms of cancers and to viral infections.

Gene Suppression Therapy

Foreign genes may be employed to oppose the expression of, what are usually, dominant genes that cause disease ranging from cancer to viral infections. This approach may also be utilized to oppose the expression of genes that are responsible for genetic diseases caused by a mutated protein, which assumes an altered function which is responsible for the disease manifestations, such as the sickling of red blood cells (RBCs) induced by hemoglobin S (HbS) in sickle-cell anemia.

Ribozymes and Antisense RNA

It is believed that RNA molecules were evolutionary the first class of molecules that possessed enzymatic activity. Ribozymes are a class of RNA molecules that can perform catalytic activity in the absence of proteins. Specifically, they hybridize to and cleave target mRNA molecules, thereby preventing their translation into specific proteins. This approach may have therapeutic application by targeting ribozymes to specific mRNA of key proteins implicated in disease states where a negative dominant effect predominates.[10] In addition, oligonucleotide sequences may be designed to target promoter regions of certain genes, thus blocking the binding of regulatory molecules that activate the gene and rendering it inactive.[11]

GENE-DELIVERY TECHNIQUES

With the completion of the Human Genome Project an ever-increasing number of disease-associated genes are now revealed. This knowledge, coupled with advances in recombinant DNA technology, have resulted in the fact that construction of therapeutic-gene sequences is a relatively straightforward task. In contrast, the rate-limiting step toward successful gene therapy, and in particular IUGT, has remained in the development of safe and efficient gene-delivery techniques. Such techniques should bring the therapeutic gene into the target tissue where it is to be expressed at the appropriate time and quantity, in a manner that does not endanger the fetus or the mother. Most gene-delivery techniques are based on various viral vectors, however, nonviral vectors are also investigated as they may be less risky.

VIRAL VECTORS

By far, the most widely employed techniques for gene delivery make use of viral vectors. Many protocols use an *ex vivo* approach: cells are removed from the patient, genetically modified, and then re-implanted. This approach, however, is both cumbersome and costly, requires high-tech facilities, and, most importantly, is limited to cell types that can be obtained and cultured readily such as blood cells. This approach cannot be applied to solid tissues and nondividing cells such as muscle cells or neurons. The *in vivo* approach for gene delivery by viral vectors can greatly facilitate gene therapy protocols of the future by enabling transfection into nondividing cells. However, before in vivo gene therapy may safely be employed for IUGT, some significant problems must be overcome. Ideally, therapeutic genes should be expressed exclusively in the relevant cell type and be free of any untoward effects on healthy cells. Several different types of viral vectors have been employed for gene delivery.

Retroviruses

Retroviruses have 2 identical single-stranded RNA genomes packaged into a viral particle, composed of a viral-encoded envelope, or *env* protein, which is embedded in a lipid bilayer derived from the host plasma membrane. The viral core consists of virally encoded enzymes, such as reverse transcriptase (RT) and integrase, that are essential for viral replication and integration of the viral DNA into the host genome. Because the retroviral genome is integrated into the host genome, the transgenic cells retain the new genetic information through subsequent cell divisions, the integration results in a relatively stable transgene. However, vector titers however are low, require dividing cells for effective transfection to occur, and, thus, are unsuitable for nondividing cells like neurons or muscle cells.

Adenoviruses

Adenoviral (AV) vectors usually do not incorporate their DNA into the genome of the host cell and generally remain within the host cell as episomes. This is of concern because it may limit the longevity of the expressed transgene. However, unlike retroviruses, they do not require actively dividing cell lines and high titers can be generated. Such vectors, therefore, would be more suitable for targeting nondividing cells. This is especially true for the treatment of muscle cells, in particular myoblasts because myoblasts have an abundance of beta 3/beta 5-integrin, which is the main component of the internalization receptor for AV. This could contribute, among other things, to the relatively high susceptibility of myoblasts to AV infection and AV-mediated gene transduction.[12]

Adeno-Associated Virus

The adeno-associated virus (AAV) is a nonpathogenic integration of DNA vectors in which all viral genes have been removed and helper virus cotransfection is virtually eliminated. These vectors tend to persist in infected cells for prolonged periods of time, with no significant untoward effect on the host.

Like AV vectors, AAV vectors may also persist in an episomal state. Although AAV vectors may exhibit a relative preference for actively dividing cells, they do not require host cell proliferation. AAV is unique among eukaryotic DNA viruses in its ability to integrate at a specific site within the human chromosome (19q13.3–qter) and for this reason, as well as being it is nonpathogenic, has become an increasingly attractive vector for gene delivery.

NONVIRAL VECTORS

Unlike the risks associated with viral transfection, nonviral gene delivery techniques appear to be as safe as conventional pharmaceutical products. In contrast with the stable transfection of cells by some viral vectors, nonviral gene delivery techniques induce only a transient gene expression, a concept known as "gene therapeutics." Currently, various nonviral vectors are being assessed in a variety of experimental studies and clinical trials of gene therapy for a number of disorders, including cystic fibrosis, cancer, and peripheral vascular disease.[13] One such technique is lipofection, in which DNA plasmids carrying the therapeutic genes are entrapped in lipid vesicles (liposomes). These liposomes act as vehicles that deliver the gene to the target cells where they are only transiently expressed. This is due to the fact that they do not incorporate into the host genome.[14] This approach is particularly promising in treatment of diseases that are manifested in epithelial lining of various organs, making them accessible to surface delivery methods. The treatments are usually well tolerated and no adverse respiratory, cardiac, immunologic, or other organ toxicity were detected.[15]

The physiological process of receptor-mediated endocytosis (RME) can also be exploited to deliver genetic material to specific cell types. This approach uses antibodies or ligands with an affinity to a specific cell-membrane receptor (e.g., transferrin), and are known to undergo endocytosis. These are complexed with the therapeutic gene through a covalently bound polycationic linker molecule (e.g., polylysine).[16] The complexes in turn, bind to the cell surface receptor and are endocytized into the endosomal compartment of the cell. Certain steps must be taken to avoid degradation of the DNA and to assist endosomal escape of the DNA into the cytosol where it is to be expressed.[16]

GENE TARGETING

Once introduced into the target cells, the therapeutic gene may be integrated into the host cell genome or remain as cytoplasmic episomes. Integration of novel DNA into the genome carries the potential of durable gene expression and propagation of the therapeutic gene into daughter cells. However, nonsite-specific viral vectors integrate randomly into the host genome. This has the potential risk of disrupting functional genes, and is known as insertional mutagenesis. This could result in a loss of gene function, defective regulation and gene expression, or an altered gene product. To overcome this problem, therapeutic genes may be designed in a manner that would ensure their integration into predetermined loci within the genome. This may be achieved by homologous recombination where the therapeutic gene is flanked by DNA sequences homologous to the genomic target locus. This approach takes advantage of the endogenous recombinational machinery of the cell which favors crossing-over between homologous sequences. This results in insertion of the therapeutic gene (if 1 crossover occurs) or replacement of the genomic sequence with the therapeutic gene (if 2 occur).[17]

SAFETY OF IN UTERO GENE THERAPY

The issue of safety is crucial one. Although gene therapy is considered experimental in children and adults and detrimental effects of viral vectors has been well documented, the fetal response to gene transfer and the potential risk it carries are far from understood. Several studies have approached this issue.

SAFETY OF THE MOTHER

The issue of safety should take into consideration both the treated fetus and the mother. Given the fact that standard obstetrical invasive procedures pose little risk to the mother, there should be minimal risk by actual technique of gene transfer to the fetus. However, one must take into consideration the effects of the viral vector itself, e.g., the accidental transfer of the viral vector into the maternal blood stream.

Studies in sheep have shown that the actual risk for this is low.[18] There is also some concern that once transfected, fetal blood-borne viral vectors may infect the placental tissue and thereby gain access to maternal circulation.[19] Additional animal studies are required to fully address this issue, especially in cases where multiple injections of high-titer vector are performed.[4] Further harm to the mother could occur if only partial amelioration of a lethal fetal condition is partially treated. In such a case, a fetus, which that would be aborted otherwise, would succumb to the disease at a later stage in pregnancy, and require second or even third trimester termination.

SAFETY OF THE FETUS

The fetus may obviously gain from IUGT, but may be at risk from some of the complications associated with the procedure. Technical advances in ultrasonographically directed needle procedures are considered to be relatively safe, and have an approximate risk for the fetus of 1–3%. One of the most obvious risks in IUGT is that the viral vector itself may induce damage, either directly by its inherent pathogenic effects or indirectly to an immune response mounted by the fetus causing tissue damage. Some recent experiments addressed this issue. Prenatal exposure to an E1, E3-deleted AV vector in fetal sheep was associated with a high degree of pathology and mortality not likely to be related to complications of the surgical or anesthetic procedures. Particularly, inflammatory and fibrotic responses were observed in the lungs.[20] However, in early gestation, AV delivery to sheep does not seem to elicit an immune response.[21] With IUGT there is also the risk of insertional mutagenesis associated with random insertion of the therapeutic gene possibly interrupting key genetic loci that may lead to developmental disruption and even tumorigenesis. Finally, there is the theoretical risk of germ-line alteration, yet this has not been the case in several animal studies of mice and sheep,[22] but this issue needs further investigation to establish the overall incidence of germ line transmission and whether the degree of risk may be acceptable.[4]

ESTABLISHING THE APPROPRIATE TIMING OF IUGT

It is obvious that if IUGT is to prevent prenatal irreversible damage, early intervention is necessary. However, it is important to establish the optimal window of opportunity for therapy to be both beneficial and safe. It appears that administration of IUGT at various gestational ages results in different patterns of therapeutic gene expression in different tissues. For example, following in utero intravascular administration of replication-deficient AV in a murine model, the patterns of gene expression were distinct for each stage of virus administration. Moreover, individual organ gene expression varied with the timing of injection, with the largest number of organs expressing the transgene when embryos were injected at 15 days post conception.[23] Furthermore, it appears that early IUGT may be advantageous because of a lack of immune response and persistence of transgene expression. This suggests that fetal exposure to the foreign transgene protein and to the viral-vector antigens may induce tolerance when introduced early in gestation.[24] The optimal window of opportunity for IUGT in humans is still to be established.

ANIMAL STUDIES AND CLINICAL TRIALS

CYSTIC FIBROSIS

Cystic fibrosis (CF) is an autosomal recessive disease caused by a mutation of the cystic fibrosis transmembrane conductance regulator (CFTR) gene. The CFTR protein is a chloride-ion transporter that regulates transmembrane voltage. Reduced or absent cyclic adenosine monophosphate (cAMP)-mediated chloride transport in epithelial-lined organs is responsible for the clinical manifestations. The disease is characterized mainly by accumulation of mucus in the lung that predisposes to inflammation. Other affected organs include the gastrointestinal tract and the reproductive system. Studies with experimental animals demonstrate that the human CFTR cDNA could be transferred to the airway epithelium using an adenoviral vector (Ad-CFTR), with expression of the human CFTR gene lasting for at least 6 weeks.[25] The first human trial of gene therapy for CF was initiated in 1993 and included 4 patients with CF who received the Ad-CFTR by instillation to their nasal or bronchial epithelium.[26] Both the CFTR protein and mRNA, undetectable prior to treatment, were observed in about 14% of one patient's epithelium cells, and mRNA alone in another patient for 1 week. However after 10 days, no expression was found.[26] Liposome-mediated treatment has also been attempted in CF patients. The restoration rate of CFTR activity was only 20%, peaking 3 days post-treatment, and reverting to pretreatment levels after a week.[27] Present gene-delivery methods do not appear to induce permanent CFTR gene expression in the respiratory system.

For gene therapy to be effective in CF repeated administrations need to be performed. This would obviously limit the use of AV vectors because of their potential to induce an immune response. To overcome this problem it may be advantageous to perform IUGT. To assess whether the IUGT could attain a high level of organ-specific gene transfer to the fetal lung late in gestation without the immunogenic response a recombinant AV-mediated transfer of the beta-galactosidase marker gene to the lung of late gestation fetal sheep was performed using a fetoscopic technique.[28] The study demonstrated that transgene expression was greatest in the distal pulmonary parenchyma, particularly in type II pneumocytes, and extended out to the pleura. There was no evidence of acute toxicity or immune response. This suggests that IUGT for CF may be feasible. Additional modifications in the therapeutic gene design, e.g., the development of transgenes with tissue-specificity, may improve efficiency. In the case of CF, tissue specific expression cassettes have been developed for airway epithelia and may prove useful in IUGT.[29]

INBORN ERRORS OF METABOLISM

Numerous experimental studies have addressed the feasibility of gene therapy for a wide variety of metabolic disorders characterized by lack or complete deficiency of essential enzymes. Most of these studies are still in the early stages of animal model and in vitro human cell-cultures studies.

Gaucher Disease

This common inherited metabolic disorder, is an excellent candidate for targeted gene therapy using hematopoietic stem cells (HSC). The feasibility of introducing the human glucocerebrosidase (GC) gene into hematopoietic progenitors with long-term expression using a variety of retroviral vectors has been demonstrated in several animal models.[30] Subsequently, it was shown that GC enzyme expression can be detected in peripheral blood lymphocytes more than 12 months after transplantation, and has a transduction efficiency of up to 95% in hematopoietic stem-cells (CD34+).[31] This provides encouraging data for the future use of gene therapy for this disease. IUGT may be reserved in the future for the most severe form, acute neuronopathic type II Gaucher.

Maple Syrup Urine Disease (MSUD)

Maple syrup urine disease (MSUD) is an autosomal recessive disease caused by a deficiency of branched-chain keto acid dehydrogenase, a mitochondrial multienzyme complex responsible for the decarboxylation of leucine, isoleucine, and valine. The complex consists of 3 subunits (E1, E2, and E3), and mutations in any subunit result in MSUD. No satisfactory treatment for MSUD is currently available.[32] To assess the feasibility of gene therapy for this disease, a retroviral vector containing the human E2 cDNA was used to restore leucine decarboxylation activity in fibroblasts derived from a MSUD patient with a mutation in the E2 subunit. Decarboxylation activity in transduced cells was restored to 93% of the wild-type level. Correct targeting of the expressed wild-type E2 protein to mitochondria was demonstrated by comparing the immunofluorescent pattern of E2 and a mitochondrial marker protein. Stable expression of enzyme activity has been achieved for at least 7 weeks. These results demonstrate the capacity for phenotypic correction of a gene defect whose product is a part of a multienzyme complex.[32] Given the severity of some forms of the disease, it may be a candidate for IUGT.

IMMUNOLOGICAL DISORDERS

Adenosine Deaminase Deficiency

Historically, the adenosine deaminase (ADA) gene was the first to be used in a postnatal gene-therapy clinical trial aimed at achieving an actual medical cure.[33] Adenosine deaminase deficiency is a severe and fatal immunodeficiency syndrome with profound T-lymphocytopenia. Affected individuals have variable defects of both T- and B-lymphocyte function and greatly increased morbidity and mortality caused by frequent viral and bacterial infection, which leads to death in early childhood. Classical treatments include administration of the missing enzyme linked to PolyEthylen Glycol (PEG-ADA), as well as bone marrow transplantation. Despite its severity, the disease is not complex from the genetic point of view. Theoretically, restoration of a functional ADA gene into the patient's lymphocytes should result in clinical improvement.

In 1990, a clinical trial was initiated using retroviral-mediated transfer of the ADA gene into the T-cells of 2 ADA-deficient children who did not respond to conventional PEG-ADA administrations.[33] Peripheral blood lymphocytes were collected, cultured ex vivo, infected with a retroviral vector expressing the ADA cDNA, and re-infused into the patients. This procedure was repeated monthly for 2 years. Subsequently, both children have been reported to have ADA-positive circulating lymphocytes. Gene treatment ended after 2 years, but integrated vector and ADA gene expression in T-cells persisted.[34,35] Several other teams have tried similar approaches for treating ADA deficiency by gene therapy with varying success.[36–38] While IUGT for this disorder would probably be successful, there is no indication that prenatal IUGT would be superior to postnatal gene therapy.

Hematological Disorders

These disorders, which include hemoglobin synthesis and coagulation defects, are, at least theoretically, more readily amenable to gene therapy since circulating blood cells can easily be reached for both ex vivo and in vivo gene therapy. Several studies have addressed hematological disorders as candidates for gene therapy.

The Thalassemias

Mutations at the α-globin locus are a common class of mutations in humans that result in various forms of α-thalassemia. Deletion of all 4 adult α-globin genes results in the perinatal lethal condition manifested by hydrops fetalis. It has been demonstrated that introduction of a human α-globin transgene can ameliorate the severity of the disorder in a mouse thalassemia-model, providing hope for human gene therapy of this disorder.[39] To be relevant to the human disease, however, effective therapy requires IUGT to avoid the severe prenatal complications.

The main pathophysiologic feature of β-thalassemia is the accumulation of unpaired α-globin chains in erythrocytes that alter membrane stability and result in early cell destruction. One option for correcting the imbalance is through the induction of fetal hemoglobin (HbF) synthesis. It has been shown that, in vitro, erythropoietin increases erythroid precursors cells programmed to produce HbF in humans and β-minor globin in mice. By introducing AAV-mediated erythropoietin gene transfer into mouse muscle, it was possible to attain robust and sustained secretion of erythropoietin in β-thalassemic mice. This resulted in a stable correction of anemia associated with improved RBC morphology, increased β-minor globin synthesis, and decreased amounts of α-globin chains bound to erythrocyte membranes. If this were shown to be effective in humans, then correction of the prenatal defect by IUGT may bring the fetus to viability without the prenatal sequellae.[40]

Another option for treatment of β-thalassemia is increasing γ-globin gene expression and reverting to an early fetal condition where HbF predominates. The possibility of activating the γ-globin gene expression by triplex-forming-oligonucleotide (TFO) directed at targeted mutagenesis was recently evaluated.[41] Using a psoralen-conjugated TFO designed to bind to a site overlapping with an Oct-1 binding site at the -280 region of the γ-globin gene, targeted mutagenesis of the Oct-1 binding site has been achieved by transfecting the in vitro formed plasmid-oligo complex into human normal fibroblast (NF) cells. These results suggest that targeted mutagenesis at the Oct-1 binding site can lead to a condition similar to hereditary persistence of fetal hemoglobin (HPFH). This may provide a novel approach for gene therapy of β-thalassemia and sickle cell disease by IUGT.[41]

Coagulation Disorders

Coagulation disorders are also potential candidates for gene therapy and IUGT. Hemophilia B, a model of coagulation disorders, is characterized by an X-linked deficiency of factor IX.

It has previously been suggested that keratinocytes in the skin might provide a suitable target cell for delivery of factor IX to the systemic circulation in patients with hemophilia B. Experiments in transgenic mice demonstrated that human factor IX can be efficiently synthesized in the skin by keratinocytes and secreted across the epidermal basement membrane to reach the systemic circulation where significant levels can be attained.[42] To evaluate the applicability of such an approach to IUGT, an E1/E3-deleted AV vector carrying the human coagulation factor IX gene was administered into the amniotic cavities of mid- to late-gestation mouse fetuses. The transgenic protein was found to be produced in the fetal skin, mucosae, and amniotic membranes and was shown to be present for several days after birth of healthy pups. This approach for IUGT of hemophilia B may prevent hemorrhagic complications during delivery such as intracranial bleeding.[43]

NEUROMUSCULAR DISORDERS

Duchenne Muscular Dystrophy

Transfer of myoblasts, the stem-cell precursors of muscle fibers, is yet another potential use of stem-cell therapy. Duchenne muscular dystrophy (DMD) is a paradigm for such disorders. It is a lethal X-linked disorder, caused by mutations in the dystrophin gene which is an exceptionally large gene (2.3 megabase, 79 exons) mapped to chromosome region Xp21. A lack of dystrophin results in muscle degeneration leading to progressive weakness and death by the second decade of life. Theoretically, donor myoblasts injected into muscles of affected patients may fuse with host muscle fibers, thus contributing nuclei, which are capable potentially of replacing the deficient dystrophin. Myoblast implantation has had some success in animal models but little, if any, effect on DMD patients.[44] There have been several attempts at postnatal myoblast transfer therapy for DMD. Morandi et al. performed myoblast transplantation in 3 DMD patients from HLA-matched donors. However, 3 months later, biopsies from the injected muscles failed to demonstrate dystrophin expression by immunocytochemistry and RT-PCR.[45] Mendell et al. injected donor myoblasts once a month for 6 months into the biceps brachii muscles of 12 boys with DMD. Six months after the final myoblast transfer, the presence of dystrophin was assessed with the use of specific antibodies. No significant improvement in muscle strength was noted although in 1 patient, 10% of muscle fibers expressed donor-derived dystrophin, 3 others had less than 1% donor dystrophin, and the remaining 8 had none.[46] Miller et al. evaluated myoblast implantation in 10 boys (5–10 years old) with DMD. Using RT-PCR, evidence of myoblast survival and dystrophin mRNA expression was obtained in 3 patients after 1 month and in 1 patient after 6 months.[47] The lack of success in treatment of DMD by postnatal myoblast therapy underscore the value of in utero myoblast cell therapy.

Duchenne muscular dystrophy demonstrates the problems associated with somatic gene therapy due to the enormous size of the gene and the large number of target cells that need to be treated. Gene therapy, based on the introduction of dystrophin gene constructs by retroviral or AV vectors, has also been successful in animal models.[48] Adenoviral vectors may be a potentially effective delivery system for muscle disease, provided immature muscle cells are abundant in the muscle. This is because myoblasts have an abundance of beta 3/beta 5-integrin, which is the main component of the internalization receptor for adenoviruses.[12] Unfortunately, the level of beta 3/beta 5-integrin is about 3 times lower in mature myotubes than in myoblast precursors. Another drawback of adenoviruses is that the maximal size of a gene insert is only about 7.5 kb. This is obviously not sufficient to accommodate the whole dystrophin gene, but may be enough to accommodate a dystrophin minigene (6.3 kb) that may confer partial dystrophin activity.[49] Although the minigene encodes a truncated protein, its expression has been shown in a mouse model to protect muscle fibers against the degeneration process that affects the dystrophin-deficient myofibers.[6]

Neurological Disorders

Treatment of central nervous system (CNS) diseases poses a significant challenge because of complex functions of the nervous system and the permanent damage caused by numerous genetic disorders in utero. One of the modes of therapy that is being investigated is the potential use of CNS-derived neural progenitor cells. These cells would be good candidates for multiple cell-based therapies for neural diseases. Further identification of the molecules that direct the differentiation of adult neural progenitors may allow their activation in vivo to induce self-repair.[50] Experiments have shown that clones of neural stem cells (NSCs) isolated from human fetal telencephalon have a self-renewing capacity and give rise to all fundamental neural lineages in vitro. Following transplantation into germinal zones of the newborn mouse brain they were found to participate in all aspects of normal development, including normal migration patterns, and dissemination into various regions of the CNS, where they differentiate into developmentally and regionally appropriate cell types. Indeed, these cells were shown to correct a genetic metabolic defect in neurons and glia cells in vitro. It may be envisioned that cells genetically engineered to express therapeutic genes may facilitate IUGT for neurodegenerative disorders.[51]

ETHICAL IMPLICATIONS

At the present time, IUGT is still considered experimental and ethical issues need to be considered before this technique becomes clinically available. It is clear that before IUGT is considered for human clinical trials, thorough evaluation of safety and efficacy is to be developed in appropriate animal models. Although preliminary animal studies show great promise, many more problems remain. There are still the potential risks for the mother, such as infection or preterm labor, by the invasive procedure, and adverse effects of the viral vectors and the immune response. Obviously, the fetus who stands to gain from IUGT is also at risk for these complications. Such issues are the concern of most scientists who are studying the potential uses of IUGT. Those who oppose IUGT commonly focus on a different set of moral concerns. Concern has been expressed about the possibility that IUGT may lead to the uptake and expression of genetic material in cells not intended as the targets of gene therapy. The greatest concern is the possibility that genetic material may be incorporated into the germ-line of subjects, and lead to permanent changes that will be passed on to future generations.[52] The possibility of germ-line transmission of the transgene may, in theory occur inadvertently or as a deliberate action in a process termed germ-line gene therapy (GLGT).

There has been a great deal of controversy concerning both the technical feasibility and the ethical acceptability of human germ-line modification for the prevention of serious disease. It is argued by some that this technique constitutes a slippery slope towards the Orwellian concept of "human genetic engineering," and that GLGT has a potential for misuse in trait enhancement and "neo-eugenics."[53] Some proponents of IUGT claim that its use in the form of GLGT for the purpose of trait-enhancement is certainly deplorable, yet maintain that potential future misuse should not be allowed to prevent the legitimate development of a technology that can save lives and relieve suffering. Furthermore, they suggest that the theoretical specter of germ-line transfer should not deter attempts at IUGT, as most proposed protocols involve second-trimester fetuses, by which time all organ systems have formed. Moreover, all published data to date indicate that germ-line gene transfer is highly unlikely, or may not even be possible, using present techniques.[54] A practical view is that most likely candidates for IUGT are not likely to live to reproductive age, and even if they do, inadvertent germ-line transmission would produce an individual incapable of reproducing.[52] Others do not even eschew GLGT and view it as another form of IUGT that is merely a step further.[55] Some suggest that there is merit in continuing the discussion about human germ-line intervention in order to carefully compare with alternative strategies for preventing genetic disease.[56]

Opponents of IUGT maintain that there are very few examples in which existing alternatives (gamete donation and preimplantation genetic diagnosis [PGD]) would not allow families affected by genetic disease to have genetically related children.[57] It has been claimed that the whole issue of IUGT is becoming a hypothetical one because of the advent of PGD.[58] Given the current state of postnatal gene therapy, some would claim that it is premature to embark on a project that is more complicated and poses a risk to both the fetus and mother. There is currently a prohibition on human GLGT, and laws against it have been established in many countries. The United Kingdom's Gene Therapy Advisory Committee prohibited direct injection of viral vectors into fetuses for the purpose of IUGT on safety and ethical grounds. The United States National Institutes of Health Recombinant DNA Advisory Committee is establishing working groups that will discuss various aspects of IUGT and review proposed clinical trials.[59] As recently stated by Caplan and Wilson:

The real moral challenge facing in utero gene therapy is to find ways to insure that the review of protocols is adequate, that those undertaking trials are competent to do so; that adequate financing exists to permit fair access to clinical trials; and that careful procedures are worked out for insuring informed consent, equity in subject selection and adequate oversight and review for the earliest clinical studies, in which the prospect of direct benefit to the fetus is tiny or non-existent. In our view, that is where the efforts of researchers, policy makers, regulators and ethicists ought to be directed.[52]

References

1. Senut MC, Gage FH. Prenatal gene therapy: can the technical hurdles be overcome? *Mol Med Today*. 1999;5:152–156.
2. Douar AM, Themis M, Coutelle C. Fetal somatic gene therapy. *Mol Hum Reprod*. 1996;2:633–641.
3. Moulton G. Panel finds in utero gene therapy proposal is premature. *J Natl Cancer Inst*. 1999;91:407–408.
4. Zanjani ED, Anderson WF. Prospects for in utero human gene therapy. *Science*. 1999;285:2084–2088.
5. Yang EY, Flake AW, Adzick NS. Prospects for fetal gene therapy. *Semin Perinatol*. 1999;23:524–534.
6. Trinh QT, Austin EA, Murray DM, et al. Enzyme/prodrug gene therapy: comparison of cytosine deaminase/5-fluorocytosine versus thymidine kinase/ganciclovir enzyme/prodrug systems in a human colorectal carcinoma cell line. *Cancer Res*. 1995;55:4808–4812.
7. Mullen CA. Metabolic suicide genes in gene therapy. *Pharmacol Ther*. 1994;63:199–207.
8. Kun LE, Gajjar A, Muhlbauer M, et al. Stereotactic injection of herpes simplex thymidine kinase vector producer cells (PA317-G1Tk1SvNa.7) and intravenous ganciclovir for the treatment of progressive or recurrent primary supratentorial pediatric malignant brain tumors. *Hum Gene Ther*. 1995;6:1231–1255.
9. Ido A, Nakata K, Kato Y, et al. Gene therapy for hepatoma cells using a retrovirus vector carrying herpes simplex virus thymidine kinase gene under the control of human alpha-fetoprotein gene promoter. *Cancer Res*. 1995;55:3105–3109.
10. Sullivan SM. Development of ribozymes for gene therapy. *J Invest Dermatol*. 1994;103(5 Suppl):S85–S89.
11. Janicek MF, Sevin BU, Nguyen HN, et al. Combination anti-gene therapy targeting c-myc and p53 in ovarian cancer cell lines. *Gynecol Oncol*. 1995;59:87–92.
12. Acsadi G, Jani A, Huard J, et al. Cultured human myoblasts and myotubes show markedly different transducibility by replication-defective adenovirus recombinants. *Gene Ther*. 1994;1:338–340.
13. Ledley FD. Non-viral gene therapy. *Curr Opin Biotechnol*. 1994;5:626–636.
14. Alton EW, Middleton PG, Caplen NJ, et al. Non-invasive liposome-mediated gene delivery can correct the ion transport defect in cystic fibrosis mutant mice. *Nat Genet*. 1993;5:135–142.
15. Nabel EG, Yang Z, Muller D, et al. Safety and toxicity of catheter gene delivery to the pulmonary vasculature in a patient with metastatic melanoma. *Hum Gene Ther*. 1994;5:1089–1094.
16. Phillips SC. Receptor-mediated DNA delivery approaches to human gene therapy. *Biologicals*. 1995;23:13–16.

17. Morrow B, Kucherlapati R. Gene targeting in mammalian cells by homologous recombination. *Curr Opin Biotechnol*. 1993;4:577–582.

18. Porada CD, Tran N, Eglitis M, et al. In utero gene therapy: transfer and long-term expression of the bacterial neo(r) gene in sheep after direct injection of retroviral vectors into pre-immune fetuses. *Hum Gene Ther*. 1998;9:1571–1585.

19. Tsukamoto M, Ochiya T, Yoshida S, et al. Gene transfer and expression in progeny after intravenous DNA injection into pregnant mice. *Nat Genet*. 1995;9:243–248.

20. Iwamoto HS, Trapnell BC, McConnell CJ, et al. Pulmonary inflammation associated with repeated, prenatal exposure to an E1, E3-deleted adenoviral vector in sheep. *Gene Ther*. 1999;6:98–106.

21. Yang EY, Cass DL, Sylvester KG, et al. Fetal gene therapy: efficacy, toxicity, and immunologic effects of early gestation recombinant adenovirus. *J Pediatr Surg*. 1999;34:235–241.

22. Ye X, Gao GP, Pabin C, et al. Evaluating the potential of germ line transmission after intravenous administration of recombinant adenovirus in the C3H mouse. *Hum Gene Ther*. 1998;9:2135–2142.

23. Schachtner S, Buck C, Bergelson J, et al. Temporally regulated expression patterns following in utero adenovirus-mediated gene transfer. *Gene Ther*. 1999;6:1249–1257.

24. Yang EY, Kim HB, Shaaban AF, et al. Persistent postnatal transgene expression in both muscle and liver after fetal injection of recombinant adenovirus. *J Pediatr Surg*. 1999;34:766–772.

25. Korst RJ, McElvaney NG, Chu CS, et al. Gene therapy for the respiratory manifestations of cystic fibrosis. *Am J Respir Crit Care Med*. 1995;151(3 pt 2):S75–S87.

26. Crystal R, McElvaney M, Rosenfeld M, et al. Administration of an adenovirus containing the human CFTR cDNA to the respiratory tract of individuals with cystic fibrosis. *Nat Genet*. 1994;8:42–50.

27. Caplen NJ, Alton EW, Middleton PG, et al. Liposome-mediated CFTR gene transfer to the nasal epithelium of patients with cystic fibrosis. *Nat Med*. 1995;1:39–46.

28. Sylvester KG, Yang EY, Cass DL, et al. Fetoscopic gene therapy for congenital lung disease. *J Pediatr Surg*. 1997;32:964–969.

29. Chow YH, O'Brodovich H, Plumb J, et al. Development of an epithelium-specific expression cassette with human DNA regulatory elements for transgene expression in lung airways. *Proc Natl Acad Sci U S A*. 1997;94:14695–14700.

30. Wei JF, Wei FS, Samulski RJ, et al. Expression of the human glucocerebrosidase and arylsulfatase A genes in murine and patient primary fibroblasts transduced by an adeno-associated virus vector. *Gene Ther*. 1994;1:261–268.

31. Nimgaonkar M, Bahnson A, Kemp A, et al. Long-term expression of the glucocerebrosidase gene in mouse and human hematopoietic progenitors. *Leukemia*. 1995;(9 suppl 1):S38–S42.

32. Mueller GM, McKenzie LR, Homanics GE, et al. Complementation of defective leucine decarboxylation in fibroblasts from a maple syrup urine disease patient by retrovirus-mediated gene transfer. *Gene Ther*. 1995;2:461–468.

33. Culver K, Anderson F, Blaese R. Lymphocyte gene therapy. *Hum Gene Ther*. 1991;2:107–109.

34. Blaese RM, Culver KW, Miller AD, et al. T lymphocyte-directed gene therapy for ADA-SCID: initial trial results after 4 years. *Science*. 1995;270:475–480.

35. Kohn D, Weinberg KI, Parkman P, et al. Gene therapy for neonates with ADA-deficient SCID by retroviral-mediated transfer of the human ADA cDNA into umbilical cord CD34+ cells [abstract]. *Blood*. 1993;82 (suppl 1):315a.

36. Bordignon C, Notarangelo LD, Nobili N, et al. Gene therapy in peripheral blood lymphocytes and bone marrow for ADA-immunodeficient patients. *Science*. 1995;270:470–475.

37. Kohn DB, Weinberg KI, Nolta JA, et al. Engraftment of gene-modified umbilical cord blood cells in neonates with adenosine deaminase deficiency. *Nat Med*. 1995;1:1017–1023.

38. Parkman R, Weinberg K, Crooks G, et al. Gene therapy for adenosine deaminase deficiency. *Ann Rev Med*. 2000;51:33–47.

39. Paszty C, Mohandas N, Stevens ME, et al. Lethal alpha-thalassemia created by gene targeting in mice and its genetic rescue. *Nat Genet*. 1995;11:33–39.

40. Bohl D, Bosch A, Cardona A, et al. Improvement of erythropoiesis in beta-thalassemic mice by continuous erythropoietin delivery from muscle. *Blood*. 2000;95:2793–2798.

41. Xu XS, Glazer PM, Wang G. Activation of human gamma-globin gene expression via triplex-forming oligonucleotide (TFO)-directed mutations in the gamma-globin gene 5′ flanking region. *Gene*. 2000;242:219–228.

42. Alexander MY, Bidichandani SI, Cousins FM, et al. Circulating human factor IX produced in keratin-promoter transgenic mice: a feasibility study for gene therapy of hemophilia B. *Hum Mol Genet*. 1995;4:993–999.

43. Schneider H, Adebakin S, Themis M, et al. Therapeutic plasma concentrations of human factor IX in mice after gene delivery into the amniotic cavity: a model for the prenatal treatment of haemophilia B. *J Gene Med*. 1999;1:424–432.

44. Pagel CN, Morgan JE. Myoblast transfer and gene therapy in muscular dystrophies. *Microsc Res Tech*. 1995;30:469–479.

45. Morandi L, Bernasconi P, Gebbia M, et al. Lack of mRNA and dystrophin expression in DMD patients three months after myoblast transfer. *Neuromuscul Disord*. 1995;5:291–295.

46. Mendell JR, Kissel JT, Amato AA, et al. Myoblast transfer in the treatment of Duchenne's muscular dystrophy. *N Engl J Med*. 1995;333:832–838.

47. Miller RG, Sharma KR, Pavlath GK, et al. Myoblast implantation in Duchenne muscular dystrophy: the San Francisco study. *Muscle Nerve*. 1997;20:469–478.

48. Morgan JE. Cell and gene therapy in Duchenne muscular dystrophy. *Hum Gene Ther*. 1994;5:165–173.

49. Karpati G, Acsadi G. The principles of gene therapy in Duchenne muscular dystrophy. *Clin Invest Med*. 1994;17:499–509.

50. Shihabuddin LS, Palmer TD, Gage FH. The search for neural progenitor cells: prospects for the therapy of neurodegenerative disease. *Mol Med Today*. 1999;5:474–480.

51. Flax JD, Aurora S, Yang C, et al. Engraftable human neural stem cells respond to developmental cues, replace neurons, and express foreign genes. *Nat Biotechnol*. 1998;16:1033–1039.

52. Caplan AL, Wilson JM. The ethical challenges of in utero gene therapy. *Nat Genet*. 2000;24:107.

53. Penticuff J. Ethical issues in genetic therapy. *J Obstet Gynecol Neonatal Nurs*. 1994;23:498–501.

54. Anderson WF. Risks inherent in fetal gene therapy. *Nature*. 1999;397:383.

55. Resnik D. Debunking the slippery slope argument against human germ-line gene therapy. *J Med Philos*. 1994;19:23–40.

56. Wivel NA, Walters L. Germ-line gene modification and disease prevention: some medical and ethical perspectives. *Science*. 1993;262:533–538.

57. King D, Shakespeare T, Nicholson R, et al. Risks inherent in fetal gene therapy. *Nature*. 1999;397:383.

58. Pergament E, Bonnicksen A. Preimplantation genetics: a case for prospective action. *Am J Med Genet*. 1994;52:151–157.

59. Wadman M. NIH launches discussion of in utero gene therapy. *Nature*. 1998;395:420.

CHAPTER 63

FETAL GENETIC THERAPY—STEM CELLS

Heung Bae Kim / Aimen F. Shaaban / Alan W. Flake

INTRODUCTION

Cellular transplantation offers the opportunity to treat a variety of genetic disorders by replacing absent or defective cells with functionally normal cells. Bone marrow transplantation (BMT), as a form of cellular transplantation, is at present the only curative therapy for a number of congenital hematologic diseases. The rationale behind BMT is that the successful engraftment and proliferation of even a single normal hematopoietic stem cell (HSC) can repopulate a patient's marrow and provide normal hematopoiesis for life. Although BMT is an established therapy in the treatment of many diseases,[1–3] broad application is limited by the requirement for an immunologically matched donor and need for ablation of the recipient's bone marrow with toxic chemotherapy or radiation. The more mismatched the donor marrow the greater the chance of graft rejection, graft-versus-host disease (GVHD), and a poor patient outcome.[4]

Recent advances in ultrasound technology and molecular biology have made possible the prenatal diagnosis of an increasing number of congenital diseases. As a result, prenatal therapy can now be realistically entertained as a therapeutic option in many of these disorders. The rationale for prenatal intervention is most compelling in those cases where irreversible damage has been done by the time of birth. Numerous cases of successful prenatal therapy have already been reported in the treatment of some lethal fetal diseases such as transfusion for erythroblastosis fetalis[5] as well as fetal surgical intervention for anatomic malformations.[6] Another compelling reason for fetal intervention is there may be some biological advantages relative to postnatal therapy. The unique fetal environment might allow the treatment of some diseases with decreased morbidity and mortality, improved cost effectiveness, and improved outcomes in comparison to those of postnatal therapy. In this chapter, we will review the rationale and experimental support for in utero cellular transplantation, particularly focusing on HSC transplantation. The potential applications and limited clinical experience with in utero HSC transplantation will also be discussed.

BACKGROUND

The first observation that the in utero transfer of hematopoietic cells could result in long-term hematopoietic chimerism was made by Owen in 1945.[7] Owen noted that dizygotic cattle twins, which share a common placental circulation in utero, were red blood cell chimeras after birth. Subsequent experiments demonstrated tolerance to donor specific skin grafts in some of these natural hematopoietic chimeras.[8] Naturally occurring hematopoietic chimerism has also been demonstrated in primates[9–11] and humans.[12] The New World primate, Saguinus oedipus, has a high incidence of dizygotic twinning with stable bone marrow and peripheral blood chimerism with as high as 80% donor cells in some animals.[13] In humans, chimerism has also been noted in some cases of monochorionic, dizygotic twinning.[14] These naturally occurring examples of hematopoietic chimerism prove that the early fetal transfer of allogeneic cells can engraft and provide stable hematopoiesis in an otherwise normal host.

The classic studies in 1953 by Billingham, Brent, and Medawar gave the first experimental support for the concept of "actively acquired tolerance."[15] They demonstrated that prenatal or neonatal exposure to a foreign antigen in mice can result in specific transplantation tolerance to that antigen later in life. Although these early studies did not evaluate the presence of hematopoietic chimerism, they remain a cornerstone in our understanding of prenatal cellular transplantation.

Fleishman and Mintz provided the first evidence that in utero transplantation of hematopoietic stem cells could correct a genetic defect.[16] They showed that normal allogeneic hematopoietic cells could successfully engraft in an anemic mouse model following in utero transplantation. Furthermore, engraftment of transplanted HSCs resulted in a progressive expansion of the donor-cell pool and the rescue of mice that otherwise would have died in the neonatal period. More recently, Blazar et al. successfully engrafted severe combined immunodeficiency (SCID) mice with normal HSCs after in utero transplantation. These chimeric animals demonstrated normal donor T and B cell function as adults.[17]

Successful engraftment of allogeneic HSCs has also been achieved in hematopoietically normal fetal mice,[18,19] sheep,[20] goats,[21] and monkeys.[22] The best characterized of these systems is the allogeneic sheep model. Intraperitoneal transplantation of allogeneic fetal liver derived from HSCs into early-gestation fetal lambs results in long-term multilineage hematopoietic chimerism without the need for myeloablation, immunosuppression, or evidence of GVHD. Levels of donor cell engraftment in this model are in the range of 10–20% following a single intraperitoneal injection. Follow-up of these animals has demonstrated stable engraftment in the bone marrow and peripheral blood for over 5 years. This model has provided some basic observations on the biology of in utero cellular transplantation. The gestational age at the time of transplantation affected the ability to successfully engraft a normal recipient; thus, confirming the concept of an immunologic "window of opportunity." Late-gestational transplantation resulted in a failure of engraftment; the loss of ability to engraft roughly corresponds to the gestational age at which fetal lambs reject allogeneic skin grafts.[23,24]

In other experiments, the effects of cell dose were examined. Increasing doses of donor cells initially increased engraftment, but engraftment rapidly reached a plateau suggesting a saturation of available receptive sites, or "niches." If this hypothesis were true, then the transplantation of cells in divided doses should allow the development of new niches between the administration of doses and improve engraftment. This was shown to be the case because the serial transplantation of the same total number of cells in 3 divided doses produced higher levels of engraftment.[25] Finally, the allogeneic sheep model confirmed the extreme susceptibility of the fetus to GVHD. Transplantation of adult bone marrow uniformly resulted in lethal GVHD, whereas T-cell depleted adult bone marrow did not. Unfortunately, T-cell depleted marrow also had a greatly diminished ability to engraft. Reconstitution of the donor cell inoculum with even small numbers of T-cells restored the ability to engraft.[26] Although the allogeneic sheep model has been quite informative, allogeneic models in other species have demonstrated great variability in engraftment. This variability remains unexplained.

Remarkably, fetal cellular transplantation can even extend across widely disparate species barriers. Xenogeneic hematopoietic chimerism has been achieved after in utero HSC transplantation in several combinations including transplants between rat-mouse,[27] human-mouse,[28] human-sheep,[29] and human-baboon species.[30] Comparison of the human-sheep model to the allogeneic sheep model has shown that the major difference between allogeneic and xenogenic transplantation is the requirement for higher doses of xenogenic cells to achieve engraftment and relatively low levels of peripheral donor-cell expression. This latter requirement is probably secondary to a lack of species-specific hematopoietic growth factors.[31]

In summary, there is a large body of experimental evidence to support the feasibility of in utero HSC transplantation. In the presence of a selective advantage for normal donor cells, in utero transplantation can correct hematopoietic disorders. Even in a normal host, stable hematopoietic chimerism can be achieved, although usually at low levels. The primary limitation to the successful clinical application of in utero HSC transplantation will most likely be the low levels of engraftment and peripheral expression because these low levels are inadequate to treat the majority of potential target diseases. The future of in utero HSC transplantation will depend on the development of strategies to successfully provide a competitive advantage for donor cell engraftment and peripheral expression.

THE FETUS AS A STEM CELL RECIPIENT

The fetus offers a unique receptive environment which may favor engraftment and survival of donor HSCs relative to the postnatal environment. Postnatal BMT generally requires myeloablative radiation or chemotherapy regimens in order to achieve engraftment. The final goal of postnatal BMT is the complete replacement of all hematopoietic elements with donor cells. In contrast, engraftment following in utero transplantation is based on competition for available hematopoietic niches, and its goal is to achieve an adequate level of mixed hematopoietic chimerism to ameliorate disease. The availability of receptive niches relates to the ontogeny of fetal hematopoiesis. Human fetal hematopoiesis progresses in

an orderly fashion beginning in the yolk sac at around the third week of gestation.[32] During the sixth week, hematopoietic cells migrate from the yolk sac and populate the liver. The liver remains the predominant hematopoietic organ until the end of the second trimester, at which time bone marrow hematopoiesis predominates. Although the bone marrow begins to form during the twelfth week of gestation, the first hematopoietic elements are not present until around 15 weeks. Migration of HSCs from the fetal liver to the bone marrow is not complete until 34 weeks of gestation. This process is presumably controlled by a sequential expression of homing receptors and their corresponding ligands in the various organs and HSCs, respectively. This orderly progression of HSC migration and the dramatic expansion of the fetal hematopoietic compartment results in the availability of microenvironmental niches during the second and third trimesters for occupation by donor cells. Hematopoietic stem cells transplanted during this window of opportunity can effectively compete with migrating host cells for available niches. In the end, engraftment and proliferation of stem cells will depend on their ability to compete effectively against other cells. Studies of HSC homing after in utero transplantation suggest that the pattern of engraftment recapitulates ontogeny.[33]

In addition to the availability of space in the bone marrow for HSCs to engraft, the fetus also offers an immunologic advantage to the transplantation of foreign cells. Normal immunologic development includes a period of fetal immunologic unresponsiveness. Antigens present during this period are processed as "self" by the developing immune system and, therefore, are not rejected. There is strong evidence that the fetal thymus plays a major role in the determination of self-recognition. Pre-T-cells migrate from the fetal liver or bone marrow to the developing thymus where the cells undergo a series of maturational steps to form mature peripheral T-cells. These steps include positive selection of clones capable of recognizing self-MHC followed by negative selection of T-cell clones which recognize self antigen in association with self-MHC.[34] This process eliminates the majority of T-cells entering the thymus and results in the mature T-cell repertoire capable of reacting against foreign antigens. While the first hematopoietic cells appear in the thymus by 9 weeks, mature T-cells are not found in the circulation until 14–16 weeks of gestation.

Thus, the developing fetus has several potential advantages as a recipient of foreign cells. There is a "window of opportunity" early in the second trimester, prior to population of the bone marrow and prior to immunologic maturity, during which the fetus should be receptive to transplantation of foreign hematopoietic stem cells. Transplantation during this period can theoretically be performed without both HLA matching and the need for myeloablation. In the human fetus, the window would appear to be prior to 14 weeks of gestation, although for immunodeficiency states, it may extend much later. Another benefit of prenatal transplantation is that the uterus is the ideal sterile environment eliminating the risk of infection during the 2–4 month period of bone marrow reconstitution seen after postnatal BMT. Finally, fetal therapy may prevent early clinical manifestations of the disease and avoid the complications of postnatal therapy including recurrent infections, multiple transfusions, and growth retardation.

RISKS OF IN UTERO STEM CELL TRANSPLANTATION

The risks of in utero stem cell transplantation are low but not negligible. The risk of procedure-related fetal loss has been estimated to be approximately 1%, which is based on experience with intraperitoneal transfusions for fetal anemia.[5] Although uncommon, infection is another potential complication of in utero injections. In one report, prenatal transplantation of fetal liver was followed by a septic abortion within 24 hours.[35] Another potential risk of in utero stem cell transplantation is GVHD. The fetus is particularly susceptible to GVHD, and the risk is proportional to the number of mature T-cells transplanted. The use of first trimester fetal liver as a source of stem cells minimizes this risk because the number of mature T-cells in fetal liver prior to 14 weeks gestation is negligible. Despite this advantage, the fetal liver yields a limited number of cells and is not a renewable source of stem cells should donor-specific postnatal HSC transplantation be necessary. In addition, fetal tissue, which is obtained by the usual methods, has a high degree of microbial contamination.[36]

In contrast, the use of adult bone marrow provides a renewable, relatively infection-free, and ethically acceptable alternative to fetal liver. The major disadvantage with the use of adult bone marrow is the risk of GVHD. It has been shown in experimental sheep models that unprocessed adult bone marrow engrafts well, but results in the occurrence of uniformly lethal GVHD.[37] Fortunately, current methods of bone marrow enrichment allow nearly a complete depletion of T-cells while producing a rich population of primitive HSCs. Until fetal tissue can be expanded in culture and stored for future use, T-cell depleted adult bone marrow is probably the safest and most practical source of donor hematopoietic cells.

DISEASES AMENABLE TO PRENATAL TREATMENT

Recent advances in prenatal diagnosis such as chorionic villus sampling (CVS) and detection of fetal cells in the maternal circulation[38] have made it possible to diagnose an increasing number of genetic disorders during the first trimester.[39,40] In utero stem cell transplantation could potentially be used to treat any disorder that can be diagnosed early in gestation and treated by postnatal BMT. These include diseases in 3 categories: immunodeficiency states, hemoglobinopathies, and inborn errors of metabolism.

It is important, however, to recognize that each candidate disease, which potentially could be treated using in utero stem cell transplantation, is biologically unique and needs to be considered individually in the context of prenatal transplantation. For example, although experimental evidence suggests that in utero transplantation into normal hosts usually results in low levels of hematopoietic chimerism, some disease states might

provide the transplanted cells a survival advantage over the host cells. This survival advantage could result in peripheral amplification of engraftment and possibly adequate levels of mixed chimerism to cure the disease. In other diseases, relatively minimal levels of chimerism may be all that is required to successfully treat the disease. Finally, the induction of immunologic tolerance may allow postnatal BMT from the same donor to "boost" the level of engraftment. It has been shown in experimental work that microchimerism is sufficient to induce tolerance to subsequent donor-specific cellular or organ transplantation.[19]

Immunodeficiency States

Congenital immunodeficiency syndromes are a diverse group of diseases that may offer some advantages for in utero cellular therapy. In circumstances of defective T-cell function, HSC transplantation potentially can be performed at a later gestational age than in a recipient with a normal immune system. This defect prolongs the window of opportunity for prenatal therapy. In some of these disorders, a competitive advantage exists for normal cells that leads to improved engraftment levels after cellular transplantation.

The best example of a disease in which normal cells have a competitive advantage is SCID syndrome. A variety of genetic mutations have been identified that result in SCID, but the most common is the X-linked recessive form, which has recently been found to result from the mutation of the gene encoding the common gamma-chain component of the cytokine receptor superfamily, including receptors for IL-2, IL-4, IL-7, IL-9, IL-15, and possibly IL-13.[41] Patients affected by X-linked SCID have a severely dysfunctional immune system caused by both B- and T-cell defects.

Mature T-cells are usually absent due to a block in T-cell development caused by the simultaneous inactivation of multiple cytokine receptors. In this environment, cells, which have a normal cytokine response, should have a competitive survival advantage, and allow a small number of engrafted HSCs to produce a clinically significant number of mature circulating T-cells. Support for this concept comes from clinical success with HLA-matched sibling BMT that can be performed without myeloablation.[42] Other immunodeficiency diseases, such as chronic granulomatous disease[43] or hyper IgM syndrome,[44] would not be expected to provide a competitive advantage for normal cells. However, these diseases could still be amenable to prenatal therapy because even low levels of chimerism might ameliorate clinical disease.

Hemoglobinopathies

Sickle cell anemia and thalassemia syndromes are the most prevalent diseases potentially treatable by prenatal stem cell transplantation. These diseases are characterized by abnormal hemoglobin production resulting in defective red blood cells (RBCs). Both diseases can be diagnosed during the first trimester[45] and both have been cured by postnatal BMT, although this is not routinely recommended because of the associated morbidity and mortality. In both diseases, clinical cure can be achieved by attaining a threshold level of normal peripheral RBCs. From experience with postnatal BMT, we know that stable mixed chimerism with donor cell levels between 10 and 20% are sufficient to ameliorate disease in sickle cell disease as well as α-thalassemia.[46,47] As in some of the immunodeficiency states, a survival advantage exists for normal RBCs. For sickle cell disease, the average life span of affected red blood cells in the periphery is 10–20 days (normal life span = 120 days) while in thalassemia, most cells (80%) never leave the bone marrow, whereas those that do have a shortened life span. Therefore, even low levels of bone marrow HSC engraftment might be sufficient to produce clinically significant normal hemoglobin levels.

Inborn Errors of Metabolism

This is a heterogeneous group of diseases that results from a deficiency of specific lysosomal enzymes and leads to the accumulation of substrates such as mucopolysaccharides or glycogen. The particular pattern of substrate accumulation in various organs determines the degree of organ injury and the clinical manifestations of the disease. Affected organs include the brain, liver, heart, and bones. The goal in the treatment of these diseases is to replace the missing enzyme by engraftment of normal cells in the affected organs. BMT has been shown to be effective in producing mononuclear cells which can differentiate into a variety of cell types in different organs, including Kupffer cells in the liver, Langerhans cells in the skin, alveolar macrophages in the lung, and glial cells in the central nervous system. In some cases, postnatal BMT has been shown to arrest the progression of disease, but has not been shown to correct existing injury.[48] In many of these diseases, injury begins prior to birth; so, prenatal therapy would be optimal. In addition, the development of the blood-brain barrier in postnatal animals might prevent transplanted cells from entering the central nervous system. Although prenatal therapy for inborn errors of metabolism has great theoretical appeal, inborn errors of metabolism are currently thought to be the least likely group of diseases to be successfully treated using in utero HSC transplantation.

CLINICAL EXPERIENCE WITH IN UTERO HEMATOPOIETIC STEM CELL TRANSPLANTATION

To date, there have been 23 clinical reports of in utero stem cell transplantation, but only a few have demonstrated engraftment (see Table 63-1). Several attempts have been made to treat, by in utero stem cell transplantation, the hemoglobinopathies and some inborn errors of metabolism, but none of the studies have shown any benefit despite the presence of low level chimerism in some cases. In contrast, the immunodeficiency diseases have shown promise, probably to the weakened immune status of the recipients and the selective competitive advantage of normal donor cells.

Touraine reported the first successful treatment of bare lymphocyte syndrome (BLS) and SCID using in utero fetal liver transplantation. In both cases, fetal liver donor cells were transplanted via umbilical vein injection at 28 weeks (BLS) and 26 weeks (SCID) of gestation. The child with BLS was reported to have 10% donor lymphocytes by HLA analysis at birth and 26% at 1 year of age. Although the child was reported to be clinically free of infection, he required isolation for 16 months and received 7 postnatal fetal liver transplants. He has continued to require immunoglobulin replacement. The results from the patient transplanted for SCID are equally difficult to assess. Published data confirmed the presence of Y-chromosomes by polymerase chain reaction analysis, but this was also complicated by multiple postnatal fetal liver and thymus transplants. There has been no report of immunologic function, but the patient has achieved delayed T-cell reconstitution.

Recently, Flake et al. reported the first unequivocally successful case of a genetic disease cured by prenatal stem cell transplantation.[49] In this case, a fetus was diagnosed with X-linked SCID at 12 weeks of gestation by CVS. Paternal bone marrow was collected, enriched for stem cells, and simultaneously depleted of T-cells. The fetus received 3 in utero stem cell transplants at 16, 17.5, and 18.5 weeks of gestation via ultrasound-guided intraperitoneal injection. The child was delivered at 36 weeks and cord blood analysis revealed that all of his T-cells were of paternal origin, whereas all of his B-cells, monocytes, and natural killer (NK) cells were of host origin. Similar results were found on blood analysis at 3 and 6 months of age. The child has shown in vitro evidence of normal immune function as well as donor-specific tolerance in a mixed lymphocyte reaction. He has received 4 doses of IV immunoglobulins during his life for low IgG titers, but is currently producing lower-normal-levels of IgG and has specific humoral response to vaccinations. He has had 2 upper respiratory infections and 1 episode of otitis media which all resolved normally. Otherwise, his growth and development have been normal and he is currently a healthy 2-year-old boy.

A second successful case has recently been reported by Wengler in which a similar protocol was used to treat a fetus with X-linked SCID.[50] This fetus received 2 injections of enriched paternal bone marrow via ultrasound-guided intraperitoneal injection at 21 and 22 weeks of gestation. At birth, analysis of cord blood indicated that this child was also a split chimera with T-cells of paternal origin and B-cells, monocytes, and NK cells of recipient origin.

SUMMARY

In utero stem cell transplantation has tremendous potential as a therapy for selected congenital disorders. This is supported by extensive experimental work and limited clinical success. The advantages of in utero transplantation include an immunologically naïve recipient with receptive hematopoietic niches

TABLE 63-1 | CLINICAL IN UTERO STEM CELL TRANSPLANTATIONS REPORTED TO DATE

Diagnosis	Gestation	Donor Source	Route	Postnatal BMT?	Outcome	Engraftment	Reference
IMMUNODEFICIENCY STATES							
BLS	28	FL and thymus	UV	Yes (7)	Alive—requires immunoglobulin	Yes	51
SCID	20	Maternal BM	IP/UV	N/A	TAB 26 weeks	No	52
SCID	26	FL	UV	Yes (Multiple)	Alive-requires Immunoglobulin	Yes	51
X-linked SCID	16, 17.5, 18.5	Paternal BM	IP	No	Alive and well	Yes-100% donor T-cells	49
X-linked SCID	21, 22	Paternal BM	IP	No	Alive and well	Yes-100% donor T-cells	50
Chediak-Higashi	19	Maternal BM	IP	Yes	Born with disease	No	52
CGD	18	FL		N/A	In utero death	?	53
HEMOGLOBINOPATHIES							
α-Thalassemia	15, 31	FL	IP/UV	No	Alive-transfusion dependent	No	54
α-Thalassemia	18	Maternal BM	IP	N/A	TAB 24 weeks	Yes	52
α-Thalassemia	13	Paternal BM			Born with disease	No	55
α-Thalassemia	12	FL	IP	No	Alive—one transfusion	Yes-0.9% HgbA	51
α-Thalassemia	17	FL	UV	N/A	Died in utero	N/A	51
α-Thalassemia	25	Sibling BM	IP	Unknown	Born with disease	No	56
α-Thalassemia	18	FL	UV	No	Alive	No	54
α-Thalassemia	14	FL		N/A	Septic abortion	N/A	35
Sickle cell	13	FL	IP	No	Alive	No	54
INBORN ERRORS OF METABOLISM							
Globoid cell leukodystrophy	13	Paternal BM (5% T-cells)	IP	N/A	Died in utero at 20 weeks	Yes	57
Metachromatic leukodystrophy	34	Paternal BM	IP	Unknown	Born with disease	No	56
Metachromatic leukodystrophy	23	Paternal BM	IP	Unknown	Born with disease	No	56
Hurler Syndrome	14	FL		Unknown	Born with disease	?	35
Neimann-Pick disease	14	FL			Alive and well	?	53
HEMOLYTIC DISEASE							
Rh disease	17	Maternal BM	UV	No	Healthy	No	58
Rh disease	12	Maternal BM	IP	No	Healthy	No	59

Abbreviations: BLS—Bare Lymphocyte Syndrome; SCID—Severe Combined Immunodeficiency; CGD—Chronic Granulomatous Disease; FL—Fetal Liver; BM—Bone Marrow; UV—Umbilical Vein; IP—Intraperitoneal

that allow engraftment of HLA mismatched donor cells without fear of rejection or need for myeloablation. In addition, the uterus offers the ideal sterile environment during hematopoietic reconstitution, which make this a cost effective alternative to postnatal BMT. Although there have been a few successful cases, broad application of in utero stem cell transplantation awaits improved understanding of the mechanisms underlying stem cell homing, engraftment, and proliferation. Improved methods of donor cell collection and processing, as well as ex vivo expansion and storage, will increase the safety of this technique. The limited clinical success thus far supports caution against rapid, widespread application pending an improved understanding of stem cell biology and the proper clinical indications for in utero intervention.

References

1. Parkman R. Overview: bone marrow transplantation in the 1990s. *American Journal of Pediatric Hematology-Oncology.* 1994;16: 3–5.
2. Vermylen C, Cornu G. Bone marrow transplantation for sickle cell disease. The European experience. *American Journal of Pediatric Hematology-Oncology.* 1994;16:18–21.
3. Giardini C, Galimberti M, Lucarelli G. Bone marrow transplantation in thalassemia. *Annual Review of Medicine.* 1995;46:319–330.
4. Rowe JM, Ciobanu N, Ascensao J, et al. Recommended guidelines for the management of autologous and allogeneic bone marrow transplantation. A report from the Eastern Cooperative Oncology Group (ECOG) [see comments]. *Annuals of Internal Medicine.* 1994;120:143–158.
5. Moise KJ, Jr. Intrauterine transfusion with red cells and platelets. *Western Journal of Medicine.* 1993;159:318–324.
6. Flake AW, Harrison MR. Fetal surgery. *Annual Review of Medicine.* 1995;46:67–78.
7. Owen RD. Immunogenetic consequences of vascular anastomoses between bovine twins. *Science.* 1945;102:400–401.
8. Anderson D, Billingham RE, Lampkin GH, et al. The use of skin grafting to distinguish between monozygotic and dizygotic twins in cattle. *Heredity.* 1951;5:379–397.
9. Wislocki GB. Observations on twinning in marmosets. *American Journal of Anatomy.* 1939;64:445–483.
10. Benirschke K, Brownhill LE. Further observations on marrow chimerism in marmosets. *Cytogenetics.* 1962;1:245–257.
11. Benirschke K, Anderson JM, Brownhill LE. Marrow chimerism in marmosets. *Science.* 1962;138:513–515.
12. van Dijk BA, Boomsma DI, de Man AJ. Blood group chimerism in human multiple births is not rare. *American Journal of Medical Genetics.* 1996;61:264–268.
13. Picus J, Aldrich WR, Letvin NL. A naturally occurring bone-marrow-chimeric primate. I. Integrity of its immune system. *Transplantation.* 1985;39:297–303.
14. Gill TJ. Chimerism in humans. *Transplantation Proceedings.* 1977; 9:1423–1431.
15. Billingham RE, Brent L, Medawar PB. 'Actively acquired tolerance' of foreign cells. *Nature.* 1953;172:603–606.
16. Fleischman RA, Mintz B. Prevention of genetic anemias in mice by microinjection of normal hematopoietic stem cells into the fetal placenta. Proceedings of the National Academy of Sciences of the United States of America. 1979;76:5736–5740.
17. Blazar BR, Taylor PA, Vallera DA. In utero transfer of adult bone marrow cells into recipients with severe combined immunodeficiency disorder yields lymphoid progeny with T- and B-cell functional capabilities. *Blood.* 1995;86:4353–4366.
18. Howson-Jan K, Matloub YH, Vallera DA, et al. In utero engraftment of fully H-2-incompatible versus congenic adult bone marrow transferred into nonanemic or anemic murine fetal recipients. *Transplantation.* 1993;56:709–716.
19. Carrier E, Lee TH, Busch MP, et al. Induction of tolerance in nondefective mice after in utero transplantation of major histocompatibility complex-mismatched fetal hematopoietic stem cells. *Blood.* 1995;86:4681–4690.
20. Flake AW, Harrison MR, Adzick NS, et al. Transplantation of fetal hematopoietic stem cells in utero: the creation of hematopoietic chimeras. *Science.* 1986;233:776–778.
21. Pearce RD, Kiehm D, Armstrong DT, et al. Induction of hemopoietic chimerism in the caprine fetus by intraperitoneal injection of fetal liver cells. *Experientia.* 1989;45:307–308.
22. Harrison MR, Slotnick RN, Crombleholme TM, et al. In-utero transplantation of fetal liver haemopoietic stem cells in monkeys. *Lancet.* 1989;2:1425–1427.

23. Zanjani ED, Ascensao JL, Flake AW, et al. The fetus as an optimal donor and recipient of hemopoietic stem cells. *Bone Marrow Transplantation.* 1992;10:107–114.
24. Silverstein AM, Prendergast RA. Fetal response to antigenic stimulus. IV. Rejection of skin homografts by the fetal lamb. *Journal of Experimental Medicine.* 1964;119:955–964.
25. Flake AW, Zanjani ED. Cellular therapy. *Obstetrics & Gynecology Clinics of North America.* 1997;24:159–177.
26. Crombleholme TM, Harrison MR, Zanjani ED. In utero transplantation of hematopoietic stem cells in sheep: the role of T cells in engraftment and graft-versus-host disease. *Journal of Pediatric Surgery.* 1990;25:885–892.
27. Rice HE, Hedrick MH, Flake AW. In utero transplantation of rat hematopoietic stem cells induces xenogeneic chimerism in mice. *Transplantation Proceedings.* 1994;26:126–128.
28. Pallavicini MG, Flake AW, Madden D, et al. Hemopoietic chimerism in rodents transplanted in utero with fetal human hemopoietic cells. *Transplantation Proceedings.* 1992;24:542–543.
29. Zanjani ED, Pallavicini MG, Ascensao JL, et al. Engraftment and long-term expression of human fetal hemopoietic stem cells in sheep following transplantation in utero. *Journal of Clinical Investigation.* 1992;89:1178–1188.
30. Shields LE, Bryant EM, Easterling TR, et al. Fetal liver cell transplantation for the creation of lymphohematopoietic chimerism in fetal baboons. *American Journal of Obstetrics & Gynecology.* 1995;173:1157–1160.
31. Flake AW, Hendrick MH, Rice HE, et al. Enhancement of human hematopoiesis by mast cell growth factor in human-sheep chimeras created by the in utero transplantation of human fetal hematopoietic cells. *Experimental Hematology.* 1995;23:252–257.
32. Metcalf D, Moore MAS. Embryonic aspects of haemopoiesis. In: Haemopoietic cells. Amsterdam, London: North-Holland Pub. Co. Frontiers in Biology; Vol. 24. 1971:Chapter 4. p. 172–271.
33. Zanjani ED, Ascensao JL, Tavassoli M. Homing of liver-derived hemopoietic stem cells to fetal bone marrow. *Transactions of the Association of American Physicians.* 1992;105:7–14.
34. Weissman IL. Developmental switches in the immune system. *Cell.* 1994;76:207–218.
35. Cowan MJ, Golbus M. In utero hematopoietic stem cell transplants for inherited diseases. *American Journal of Pediatric Hematology-Oncology.* 1994;16:35–42.
36. Rice HE, Hedrick MH, Flake AW, et al. Bacterial and fungal contamination of human fetal liver collected transvaginally for hematopoietic stem cell transplantation. *Fetal Diagnosis & Therapy.* 1993;8: 74–78.
37. Zanjani ED, Lim G, McGlave PB, et al. Adult haematopoietic cells transplanted to sheep fetuses continue to produce adult globins. *Nature.* 1982;295:244–246.
38. Cheung MC, Goldberg JD, Kan YW. Prenatal diagnosis of sickle cell anaemia and thalassaemia by analysis of fetal cells in maternal blood [see comments]. *Nature Genetics.* 1996;14:264–268.
39. Puck JM. IL2RGbase: a database of gamma c-chain defects causing human X-SCID. *Immunology Today.* 1996;17:507–511.
40. Embury SH. Advances in the prenatal and molecular diagnosis of the hemoglobinopathies and thalassemias. *Hemoglobin.* 1995;19:237–261.
41. Noguchi M, Yi H, Rosenblatt HM, et al. Interleukin-2 receptor gamma chain mutation results in X-linked severe combined immunodeficiency in humans. *Cell.* 1993;73:147–157.
42. Buckley RH, Schiff SE, Schiff RI, et al. Haploidentical bone marrow stem cell transplantation in human severe combined immunodeficiency. Seminars in Hematology. 1993;30:92–101; discussion 102–104.
43. Bjorgvinsdottir H, Ding C, Pech N, et al. Retroviral-mediated gene transfer of gp91phox into bone marrow cells rescues defect in host defense against Aspergillus fumigatus in murine X-linked chronic granulomatous disease. *Blood.* 1997;89:41–48.

44. Hollenbaugh D, Wu LH, Ochs HD, et al. The random inactivation of the X chromosome carrying the defective gene responsible for X-linked hyper IgM syndrome (X-HIM) in female carriers of HIGM1 [see comments]. *Journal of Clinical Investigation.* 1994;94:616–622.

45. Tuzmen S, Tadmouri GO, Ozer A, et al. Prenatal diagnosis of beta-thalassaemia and sickle cell anaemia in Turkey. *Prenatal Diagnosis.* 1996;16:252–258.

46. Andreani M, Manna M, Lucarelli G, et al. Persistence of mixed chimerism in patients transplanted for the treatment of thalassemia. *Blood.* 1996;87:3494–499.

47. Walters MC, Patience M, Leisenring W, et al. Bone marrow transplantation for sickle cell disease [see comments]. *New England Journal of Medicine.* 1996;335:369–376.

48. Navarro C, Fernandez JM, Dominguez C, et al. Late juvenile metachromatic leukodystrophy treated with bone marrow transplantation; a 4-year follow-up study. *Neurology.* 1996;46:254–256.

49. Flake AW, Roncarolo MG, Puck JM, et al. Treatment of X-linked severe combined immunodeficiency by in utero transplantation of paternal bone marrow [see comments]. *New England Journal of Medicine.* 1996;335:1806–1810.

50. Wengler GS, Lanfranchi A, Frusca T, et al. In-utero transplantation of parental CD34 haematopoietic progenitor cells in a patient with X-linked severe combined immunodeficiency (SCIDXI). *Lancet.* 1996;348:1484–1487.

51. Touraine JL, Raudrant D, Rebaud A, et al. In utero transplantation of stem cells in humans: immunological aspects and clinical follow-up of patients. *Bone Marrow Transplantation.* 1992;9:121–126.

52. Diukman R, Golbus MS. In utero stem cell therapy. *Journal of Reproductive Medicine.* 1992;37:515–520.

53. Touraine JL. In utero transplantation of fetal liver stem cells into human fetuses. *Journal of Hematotherapy.* 1996;5:195–199.

54. Westgren M, Ringden O, Eik-Nes S, et al. Lack of evidence of permanent engraftment after in utero fetal stem cell transplantation in congenital hemoglobinopathies. *Transplantation.* 1996;61:1176–1179.

55. Jones DR, Bui TH, Anderson EM, et al. In utero haematopoietic stem cell transplantation: current perspectives and future potential. *Bone Marrow Transplantation.* 1996;18:831–837.

56. Slavin S, Naparstek E, Ziegler M, et al. Clinical application of intrauterine bone marrow transplantation for treatment of genetic diseases–feasibility studies. *Bone Marrow Transplantation.* 1992;9:189–190.

57. Blakemore K, Bambach B, Moser H, et al. Engraftment following in utero bone marrow transplantation for globoid cell leukodystrophy. *American Journal of Obstetrics & Gynecology.* 1996;174:312.

58. Linch DC, Rodeck CH, Nicolaides K, et al. Attempted bone-marrow transplantation in a 17-week fetus [letter]. *Lancet.* 1986;2:1453.

59. Thilaganthan B, Nicolaides KH, Morgan G. Intrauterine bone-marrow transplantation at 12 weeks' gestation [letter]. *Lancet.* 1993; 342:243.

Ethical, Legal, and Social Issues

PSYCHOSOCIAL ISSUES IN PRENATAL DIAGNOSIS

David W. Britt

There are several large-scale trends that are affecting the nature of psychosocial phenomena in prenatal diagnosis throughout the world. In the developed world, there is a growing awareness of "shifting the focus away from short-term technocentric medical advances to concentrate on the broader public health issues…[to a] focus on the effectiveness of prenatal care interventions on longer-term benefits for women and children's health."[1] These are encouraging reactions to technological change because they are based, on at least implicitly, an awareness of the fact that there are no purely technological fixes to the quality of prenatal care is associated with prenatal diagnosis.

There are other trends, however, about which we should be less sanguine. In the developed world there is a progressive concentration of wealth and income among a small minority of (usually Caucasian, in the United States) individuals. This inequality-of-wealth trend is coupled with trends that have led Feagin, for example, to estimate that by the midpoint of the 21st century Caucasians will be a minority in the United States, and there will be greater segregation among Caucasians and minorities than at present.[2] Because of rapid technological change in the United States, such shifts in wealth *may* be somewhat more rapid than in other countries, but inequality of wealth (and related trends) are phenomena that hardly are limited to the United States. In short, in the U.S. at least, wealth appears to becoming more and more concentrated in the hands of a small number of Caucasians, whereas the country is becoming more multicultural and, thus, at risk of becoming more segregated.

Against the historical backdrop, consider that we also live in period of astonishing growth in genetic knowledge, which has powerful implications for the future of prenatal diagnosis as well as many other aspects of healthcare.[3,4] Addressing questions is a continuing concern, e.g., technology raises such questions as who should have access to such knowledge about individuals and for what purpose, and what are the tradeoffs between fostering universal health care and underwriting high-tech breakthroughs.[4,5,6] Such questions become more pressing to ask, but more difficult to answer as access to resources becomes more concentrated by class. When only the wealthy or well insured can gain access to effective prenatal diagnosis, the bias may work in both blatant and subtle ways.

Nsiah-Jefferson has reviewed how class bias and racism has promoted a fundamental shift in the birth-control movement in the United States.[7] What started out as a *right* for the privileged became a *duty* for the poor. This same shift is suggested in Lippman's discussion of biomedical prevention:

Given that prevention is increasingly the goal of biomedicine, with what speed will the disabilities and variations that *can* be prevented because prenatal tests for them exist become those that *should* be prevented, with testing thereby reshaping eugenics into a private process of 'selection by prevention.'[8]

As other prevention theorists have suggested, there is a difference between prevention and control over one's options.[9] With regard to prenatal diagnosis, there is a difference between preventing illness and promoting informed consent with respect to options. One cannot understand the implications of the tensions between prevention and control without appreciating the power and cultural differences that exist between counselor/physician and patient in developed countries.[7] Nor can one ignore the fact that such issues are writ large in developing countries, where some have estimated that 95% of the world's future children will be born.[10]

One may examine such issues as a community or nation-wide on at least 3 levels: access, control and equity. Given "what is so antiseptically called a 'positive' diagnosis," these issues, through the lens of the diagnostic counseling session and the context surrounding the individual woman, may have a variety of meanings depending on context.[7,11] Nonetheless, she and her family will decide, what tests to take serially, counseling to seek, actions to take. In this chapter, rather than seeking to exhaustively review the many studies of these 3 levels, a context-sensitive perspective is presented to help integrate discussions across the 3 levels. Tunis has called for a focus on "individual-difference variables."[12] Although I agree that understanding the woman as a person extends us beyond a simple, presumptively rational understanding of "what is going on," I believe the real leverage is at the cultural and contextual levels. The same individual-difference variables may have a variety of outcomes and meanings in different combinations of context.

DESCRIBING CONTEXT

Contexts have usually been presented in the social sciences, initiated by Bronfenbrenner in developmental psychology and Strauss in grounded theory, as a tree-ring-like set of contexts that implicate one another.[13,14] Closer to the individual are microcontexts and furthest away are macrocontexts. This approach has stimulated much thought amongst a generation of scholars concerned with health issues, but it makes analysis less realistic in at least 2 respects. First, it does not capture the multiple ways that contexts may intersect with one another to create combinations of contexts. And, second, it does not suggest a useful tool for helping scholars and practitioners study the applied implications of combinations of contexts, which are more clearly present in the work of Becker, Britt, and Ragin.[15−17]

Contexts are composed of cultural, situational and biographical factors that intersect with one another in multiple ways and form different configurations or combinations of contexts. At its core there are elements of current and past pregnancies, Britt et al. have called *proximate decision context*.[18] The major sources of contextual variation that intersect with the proximate decision are familial, cultural, technological, and institutional contexts. Other authors have discussed, in detail, several of these contexts. Hence, I'll discuss only 1 at length: institutional context.

In seeking to understand the institutional context relevant in a given situation, one must move beyond an understanding of the role of organized groups such as HMOs and financial/insurance barriers that are a substantial part of the environment within which patients and providers interact.[7] One must move beyond the structure of laws and regulations that characterize a particular society, though these often permit a relatively subtle understanding of the possible interactions between providers and patients.[5,19,20] It is necessary to understand that in the particular environment under consideration—where environment serves as a short-hand way of referring to the combination of contexts wherein such transactions occur and women also make decisions—medical professionals construct an active or passive collaboration with their patients and colleagues. One aspect of the institutional context is understanding how receptive the clinic is. Another aspect is understanding the general structure of the medical setting in terms of what it presents as routine tests—as opposed to more nonroutine tests that require the patient to make decisions.[21,22,23] One should also understand the discipline and training of the medical professional because genetic counselors tend to differ from physicians. Integral to such a discussion would be the assessment of the gender of these individuals *in combination with* where they practice. Women physicians outside the United States, for example, have been shown to be more pessimistic about disabilities and more willing to abort fetuses with genetic disorders than their male counterparts.[24] Furthermore, one should understand the level of collaboration or conflict among the generalists and professionals who do or do not interact in a particular case.[25,26] Three things should stand out from these examples. First, other than personality characteristics of individual patients, many factors are important in understanding the phenomena associated with prenatal diagnosis. Second, combinations of these factors are critical for understanding the nature of context as it affects action. Third, there is no substitute for careful, detailed, qualitative, and comparative analysis of such situations.

These contexts, as well as their change over time, may be studied on a single or multiple levels. So, for example, one might examine the impact of various factors on the level and/or rate of aggregate uptake in prenatal diagnostic services across countries. Some aspects of uptake will be a straightforward function of the extent of resource commitment at a national level.[27] In part, the impact of resource commitment will be mediated by the level of professionalization of prenatal diagnostic services and the extent to which networks of physicians and counselors have been built;[28] and, finally, part of the effect of national commitments will be mediated by how cost-effective funds are utilized.[29] Such factors speak to a relatively rational process of implementation and development of prenatal

diagnostic services. Other aspects of cross-country or cross-cultural analysis, however, introduce the possibility of more complicated aspects of the development process. For example, cultures vary in the extent to which they can integrate scientific and nonscientific thinking.[30,31] Although work on such matters has been done, there is much dialog that needs to take place regarding the diffusion of prenatal diagnostic technologies and the conditions under which they may be successfully integrated into a society.[19] All of this leaves us with the conclusion that we can say little about collective uptake and that there will be much disagreement about what factors are important and how much progress has been made.

Successful implementation, however, is problematic in and of itself. If one were to examine the inequality of access within and across countries, or the extent of coerciveness in a particular system, the nature of the analysis would be quite different.[7,11,32] For most practitioners, however, such analyses become more relevant as they embrace a level of analysis that touches on how context shapes an individual's series of decisions regarding her involvement in prenatal diagnostic services or how a patient and her counselors/physicians construct counseling sessions.

To appreciate the role of context we must jointly consider prediagnostic services at 2 levels of analysis: first, in terms of contradictions and tensions for the society as a whole and, second, counseling session. Several scholars have examined problematic aspects of the counseling interview.[22–24,31,33,34] Two critical factors in such discussions are the level of trust of medical authorities and education of the patients. By considering the implications of these 2 complex elements in the form of a simple typology, the critical nature of their combination.[35]

Trust in medical professionals is an especially complicated dimension. At its heart, however, is a question regarding how tensions resulting from genetic reasoning are dealt with in particular cultures. The existence of tension is an unavoidable consequence of advancements in the technical knowledge of genetics. There will be uneven development both within and across countries.[19] Where development is more pronounced, however, there will be accompanying modes of dissemination, training, and credentialing as the medical professions, whose knowledge base is fundamentally altered by this growing knowledge, struggle to adapt to the sea change of information.

At the societal level there may be considerable tension between those who want to explain health/disease and normality/abnormality in terms genetics, and those who see this approach as at best reductionist and at worst controlling and hostile. Lippman, for example, uses the term *geneticization* to refer to a medical model couched in the language of genetics that gives priority to differences among individuals on the basis of their DNA codes.[8] As the human genome project and its aftermath proceed, such a "scientific" position and its potential for eugenic implications may become more dominant in a given society.[3] Nelkin and Lindee suggest the implications go much farther than scientists and medical professionals talking to one another:

Eugenics is not simply gross coercion of individuals by the state. Rather, it can be productively understood as a constellation of beliefs about the importance of genetics in shaping human health and behavior, the nature of worthwhile lives, the interests of society, and, especially, reproductive responsibility.[36]

One characteristic of the dominant rhetoric is that beliefs about genetics may become taken-for-granted, routine aspects of culture. This has immediate implications for prenatal diagnosis. Santalahti et al., for example, ascribe the high participation rate in prenatal screening tests in Finland to the "great *trust* [my emphasis] placed in Finnish maternity care, and from the general tendency to assume that whatever care is offered has been carefully considered and is the best available."[23] Such trust is a double-edged sword. On the one hand, it leads to high participation in maternal care centers: "Practically all pregnant Finnish women (99.9%) attend maternity care centers, which have a very positive image . . . [resulting in] an exceptionally low perinatal mortality rate (6% in 1994)."[23] On the other hand, offering serum screening as part of maternity care implies general approval for the screening process.[33] Hence, it may decrease the chances of *active* decision making on the part of women living in such circumstances. Santalahti et al. estimated that only a minority of their sample made an active decision whether or not to participate in serum screening.[24] The rest accepted it as a routine part of medical care.

At the same time, there may be strong cultural forces at work that minimally emphasize the gulf between "science-speaking genetics counselors and their multicultural patient populations."[30] Taken further, such a gulf might lead to what Fletcher, following Capron, has called *genicity*:[4,37]

A public reaction to advances in human genetics, that is, fear, images of mad scientists and Nazi eugenics, and a sense that there were no longer any mystery about human beings . . . focused especially on reproduction and manipulation of genes for *eugenic* [my emphasis] purposes.

Genicity and geneticization are too complicated to be thought of as polar opposites of a single dimension. Not only are the concepts inherently multidimensional, they also reflect a constantly changing tug of war for the dominant and legitimate position regarding genetic knowledge. Yet they do serve as convenient short-hand ways of referring to the different clusters of phenomena that should be considered as part of the assessment of trust. On one extreme, geneticization rules. Genetics is considered both legitimate and relevant for explaining disease, and the medical establishment is trusted to apply this knowledge in a carefully considered manner that puts the interests of the patient first. On the other extreme, genicity rules. Genetics is considered a fundamental threat to humanity, yet the medical establishment is not trusted to apply this knowledge for the common good.

The second critical factor that must be considered is the extent of education and general knowledge of women who will undergo prenatal testing. The variations in general levels of literacy and specific genetic knowledge are enormous both within and across nations and cultures. Literacy is also an indicator for how relatively powerful women are in their families, work places, and communities. Therefore, variation on this dimension is at least as multidimensional and complicated as variation in issues of trust. Hence, any discussion here risks oversimplification. Yet again, considering the extremes is a useful exercise. On one pole are situations in which the majority of women are educated and genetic knowledge (at least with respect to the role of genetics in their pregnancies) is relatively high. On the other pole are women with less education and less well-developed understanding of the potential implications of genetics in their pregnancies.

This leaves us with a typology that crosses patient education and trust in medical authorities. Where patients are relatively well-educated and informed, and where there is reasonable trust in medical authorities, the chances of a *shared collective definition* of the counseling interview are good. Genetic counselors and primary-care/OBGYN physicians will be well informed, but importantly, the gulf in knowledge between the counselor and his or her patient will be less pronounced than between an expert and women, who are less-well educated and informed. Consequently, the negative consequences of such a gulf, reinforced by differences in social class and race, which have been eloquently spoken to by Nsiah-Jefferson, Rapp, and others, should be blunted.[7,11,31] In turn, an informed discussion of information and options may be negotiated within a climate of trust and mutual respect.

The downside, however, lies in how fragile *shared mutual definition* is. Its continuance rests on increasing professionalization of those medical professionals who interact with patients around medical issues not only in terms of their knowledge of genetics but also in terms of their capacities for developing rapport with their patients. Frankel's work on doctor-patient interactions has shown us, as medical issues become more complicated and have more serious consequences for patients, that much effort and training is required to assure medical personnel are able to listen, empathize and develop rapport with their patients.[38]

Where women are less well-informed or educated, it is more realistic to think in terms of a *collective fiction* than a shared collective definition.[39] Under such conditions, the legitimacy and power of the medical authorities in the situation allows them to simply impose (intentionally or unintentionally) their own definition of what is happening and what is important. Press and Browner have spoken powerfully of the nature of such situations in the United States, but such dynamics are not peculiar to developed countries.[39]

Also, consider how this becomes more complicated as cultural differences provide another element of the combinatorial context. Rapp, for example, has spoken of how many elements come together as women make decisions regarding testing and other matters:

Class, racial and ethnic markers, experiences with, and attitudes toward, a range of disabilities all strongly influence a woman's responses to the [amniocentesis] test. We need to insist simultaneously on the collective and individual nature of these orienting *features each woman brings to her encounter* [my emphasis] with prenatal testing. It matters whether one is African-American, Polish or Irish-Catholic, middle-class or working class or poor. But it also matters whether this is a first or fourth pregnancy, whether you have experienced difficulties in getting or staying pregnant, whether you had a cousin with Down syndrome or a neighbor who was hemophiliac."[11]

Such analyses become even more complicated when features of the larger culture and *features individual physicians/counselors bring to the encounter* are considered. Otano, for example, describes the painful situation confronting physicians and patients in Argentina.[40] After prenatal diagnosis, physicians are put in the position of telling their patients that abortion is illegal. Over 400,000 illegal abortions are performed each year, and of the high maternal mortality rate a third are attributable to the lack of safety in such procedures. Here trust becomes a much more complicated achievement and burden, with institutional conflict between the Church and the medical establishment being played out in the counseling interview.

Training in listening skills and empathy can only go so far—even in those situations where there exists a fundamental trust of medical authorities to act in the interest of their patients. More dramatic and longer-term solutions are required to shift what are essentially collective fictions to negotiated collective definitions. The basic concepts of access and support are not mysterious, but there needs to be innovative experimentation in different contexts to find ways of conveying the meaning of genetic information and supporting the legitimacy of choice. In some cases this may mean using the knowledge that counselors provide may shape how women understand the meaning and purpose of screening and also reinforce the legitimacy of women's choice.[41] But the search for effective ways of clarifying meaning and supporting women's choices (and their right to choose) must go beyond careful randomized control studies.[42] Such carefully controlled studies, ironically, are much more likely where they may be least needed—in those situations where medical personnel are already well trained in developing informed consent and women feel empowered to make choices.

Finally, there are those situations in which trust is not vested in the medical establishment, either because of a past history of untrustworthy actions (as with the Tuskegee experiments), conflicts within the culture regarding scientific and nonscientific reasoning, or locally as a result of past experiences of a woman and her friends and family. Under such conditions, regardless of whether or not the patient is educated or not the chances of hostility and distrust are high.

Short-term fixes cannot be effective in such situations. A general strategy that might be effective in some contexts is working through community institutions where there is a lot of contact and the patient's experience with these high-contact institutions has been benign. Under such conditions medical clinics might be able to "borrow the credibility" of their more trusted counterparts.

THE ROLE OF CONTEXT IN INDIVIDUAL DECISIONS

Britt et al. have developed the idea of *proximate decision context* as a way of representing the intersection of various features of a woman's pregnancy history as she is making a decision regarding whether to keep or terminate a pregnancy where Down syndrome has been diagnosed.[44] As with Rapp, the central concern aims at the differential meaning of combinations of elements that make up one's individual experience and social context.[11]

One strategy for balancing and integrating the various contextual elements that may be relevant to understanding decision making and reactions to engagement in the testing and confronting the possibility of termination is to focus on distinctly different combinations of contextual elements. Such "framing" permits the researcher to explore in depth, using a variety of methods and perspectives, the implications of particular combinations of contextual elements. So, for example, Rapp has concentrated on multi-cultural populations with less privileged educational and scientific backgrounds in New York City.[31]

Such diverse studies allow us to begin to understand the limits of contextual constraints on prenatal diagnostic phenomena. For example, Porter and Macintyre reported that women are prone to assume that the care that they are provided has been well thought out and may even be the best for them.[44] The power of the medical gaze in this respect may be shown by noting that a similar phenomenon has been found in 2 very different populations and contexts. Santalahti et al. report this in their Finnish sample.[23] Press and Browner report a similar finding in their California study of AFP screening for neural tube defects.[39] Where women are well informed, such trust may be warranted, and a collective definition of screening situation may be gained. Where women are less well informed, a collective fiction is more likely wherein women become unthinking conspirators in a collective fiction.

Context is not all contemporaneous.[46] On a more specific level, however, the ongoing stream reflects the nature of the decision processes: it is not a single decision but a series of decisions to which researchers must be sensitive and about which practitioners must be informed.[47] Women and their families have a series of decisions to make. Each time they passively or actively make decisions regarding testing, they alter the situational context in which they and others construct encounters with one another and make decisions. At several points they may drop out of the process. Yet there may be some meaningful continuity to their choices. Santilahti et al., for example, report that Finnish women who had an acquaintance with someone who was disabled were less likely to participate in a screening program.[23] Further, if they did participate, they were less likely to decide to abort given a positive indication. Such findings speak to the powerful, continuing influence of our social and psychological contexts. Yet it is also the case that as women move from one stage to another they are wittingly or unwittingly creating additional contexts within which decisions must be made—even if in a passive and deferential manner they let the "authoritative" counselors and physicians dictate what should be done.[39]

The context in which various tests take place is important in understanding the impact of events. As Rapp and others have shown, the *meaning* of events may change dramatically as the context changes.[31] Experience and meaning are conditioned by the situation in which events take place. Britt et al., for example, have shown that the experience of anxiety by itself does not undermine the effectiveness of a bonding intervention in multifetal reduction procedures.[48] It is only when this anxiety involves an unresolved moral dilemma that it interferes with the facilitation of a shift from grieving over reduced embryos to a focus on the life-affirming aspects of getting a complicated pregnancy back on course.

TOWARD A CROSS-CONTEXT, CLINICALLY RELEVANT RESEARCH AGENDA

As prenatal diagnosis changes with the development of new technologies and areas of professional development, it is crucial that the boundaries of clinically relevant research be as broad as possible. To focus too narrowly on individual or even contextual factors in the diagnostic process runs the risk of research becoming nothing more than an academic exercise. Yet to focus too narrowly on what appear to be clinical options runs the risk of research serving to support a "collective fiction" that is every bit as real as that discussed by Press and Browner for patient-doctor interactions.[39]

McCormick and Siegel capture part of this argument in their discussion of Agency for Health Care Policy and Research (AHCPR):[1]

AHCPR holds the main responsibility at the federal level for examining the relationship between how health care is organized, financed and delivered and the care outcomes and health of those it is intended to serve. Since its inception, ACHPR has struggled to balance the need for rigorous research that addresses questions of what works with the impatience of stakeholders in the health care system for solutions rather than ever more refined questions.[1]

Balancing rigor and practicality is not enough, however. The nature of rigor needs to be examined as emphasis on context and meaning move to the foreground. Rigor should take on a dual meaning of plausibly eliminating alternative hypotheses and being clinically relevant.[16] Finally, the nature of what is practical must be examined not only for contextual limits but

also for the role of powerful vested interests in shaping the nature of prenatal diagnosis.[11,39]

References

1. McCormick MC, Siegel J. *Prenatal Care: Effectiveness and Implementation.* New York: Cambridge University Press; 1999.
2. Feagin J. Invited Plenary Address, Midwest Sociological Association Meetings, Chicago, IL, April 2000.
3. Alta Charo R. Effect of the human genome initiative on women's rights and reproductive decisions. *Fetal Diagn Ther.* 1993;8:148–159.
4. Fletcher J. The long view: How genetic discoveries will aid health care reform. *J Women's Health.* 1998;7:817–823.
5. Rothenberg KH. The law's response to reproductive genetic testing: Questioning assumptions about choice, causation and control. *Fetal Diagn Ther.* 1993;8:160–163.
6. Britt D, Butler B, Hulen A, et al. Low Birth Weight Patterns: Assessing Telemedical Access Inequality in Arkansas. Society of Maternal Fetal Medicine 24th Annual Meeting, New Orleans, February 2–7, 2004. American Journal of Obstetrics and Gynecology (In press).
7. Nsiah-Jefferson L. Access to reproductive genetic services for low-income women and women of color. *Fetal Diagn Ther.* 1993;8:107–127.
8. Lippman A. Prenatal genetic testing and geneticization: Mother matters for all. *Fetal Diagn Ther.* 1993;8:175–188.
9. Rappoport J. Terms of empowerment/exemplars of prevention: Toward a theory for community psychology. *Am J Comm Psychol.* 1987;15:121–148.
10. Galjaard H. Gene technology and social acceptance. *Pathologie Biologie.* 1997;45:250–255.
11. Rapp R. Sociocultural differences in the impact of amniocentesis: An anthropological research report. *Fetal Diagn Ther.* 1993;8:90–96.
12. Tunis SL. Prenatal diagnosis of fetal abnormalities: Psychological impact. In: Singson JL, Elias S, eds. *Essentials of Prenatal Diagnosis.* New York: Churchill Livingstone; 1994.
13. Bronfenbrenner U: Contexts of child rearing: Problems and prospects. *Am Psychologist.* 1979;34:844–850.
14. Strauss AL and Corbin J. Basics of Qualitative Research: Grounded Theory Procedures and Techniques (1990) (book).
15. Becker HS. *Tricks of the Trade.* Chicago: University of Chicago Press; 1998.
16. Britt DW. *A Conceptual Introduction to Modeling: Qualitative and Quantitative Perspectives.* Mahwah, NJ: Lawrence Erlbaum; 1997.
17. Ragin C. *The Comparative Method: Moving Beyond Qualitative and Quantitative Strategies.* Berkeley: University of California Press; 1987.
18. Britt DW, Risinger ST, Mans M, et al. Devastation and Relief: Conflicting meanings in discovering fetal anomalies. *Ultrasound in Obstetrics and Gynecology.* 2002;20:1–5.
19. Novaes HMD. Social impacts of technological diffusion: Prenatal diagnosis and induced abortion in Brazil. *Social Science and Medicine.* 2000;50:41–51.
20. Rothenberg KH. Genetic discrimination and health insurance: A call for legislative action. *J Am Med Women's Assoc.* 1997;52:43–44.
21. Evans WJ. A comparative analysis of prenatal-clinic receptivity (unpublished doctoral dissertation, Wayne State University), 2000.
22. Press N, Browner CH. Characteristics of women who refuse an offer of prenatal diagnosis. *Am J Med Genet.* 1998;78:433–445.
23. Santalahti P, Hemminki E, Aro AR, et al. Participation in prenatal screening tests and intentions concerning selective termination in Finnish medical care. *Fetal Diagn Ther.* 2000;14:71–79.

24. Wertz DC. Is there a "Women's Ethic" in genetics: A 37-nation survey of providers. *J Am Med Women's Assoc.* 1997;52:33–38.

25. Spickard A Jr, Gabbe SG, and Christianson JF. Mid-career burnout in generalist and specialist physicians. *Journal of the American Medical Association.* 2000;288(12):1447–1450.

26. Berman DR, Johnson TRB, Apgar BS, et al. Model of family medicine and obstetrics-gynecology collaboration in obstetric care at the University of Michigan. *Obstetrics and Gynecology.* 2000;96(2):3087–3313.

27. Chakravarty A, Purandare H, Gogate S, et al: Development and delivery of prenatal diagnostic services on the Indian subcontinent. Presentation at the 10th International Conference on Prenatal Diagnosis and Therapy, Barcelona, Spain. June 21, 2000.

28. Papp Z: Prenatal genetic counselling services in Hungary, 1976–2000. Presentation at the 10th International Conference on Prenatal Diagnosis and Therapy, Barcelona, Spain. June 19, 2000.

29. Alonzo A, Valiente A, Moreno F, et al: Fluorescence in situ hybridization (FISH) on supernatant medium. An alternative for failed conventional amniotic fluid culture. Poster presented at the 10th International Conference on Prenatal Diagnosis and Therapy, Barcelona, Spain. June 21, 2000.

30. Chadwick R, ten Have H, Husted J, et al. Genetic screening and ethics: European perspectives. *J Med Philosophy.* 1998;23:255–273.

31. Rapp R. Communicating about chromosomes: Patients, providers and cultural assumptions. *J Am Med Women's Assoc.* 1997;52:28–32.

32. Newell C. The social nature of disability, disease and genetics: A Response to Gilliam Persson, Holtug, Draper and Chadwick. *J of Med Ethics.* 1999;25:172–175.

33. Santalahti P, Aro AR, Hemminki E, et al. On what grounds do women participate in prenatal screening? *Prenat Diagn.* 1998;18:153–165.

34. Santalahti P, Hemminki E, Latikka AM, et al. Women's decision-making in prenatal screening. *Social Science and Medicine.* 1998;46:1067–1076.

35. Becker HS. *Tricks of the Trade.* Chicago: University of Chicago Press;1998.

36. Nelkin D, Lindee M. The revival of eugenics in American popular culture. *J Am Med Women's Assoc.* 1997;52:45–46.

37. Capron AM. Unsplicing the gordian knot. Legal and ethical issues in the "new genetics." In: Milinsky A, Annas GJ, eds. *Genetics and The Law, III.* New York: Plenum Press; 1985.

38. Frankel RM and Stein TS. *The Four Habits of Highly Effective Clinicians: A Practical Guide.* CA: Kaiser Permanente.

39. Press NA, Browner CH. 'Collective fictions.' Similarities in reasons for accepting maternal serum alpha-fetoprotein screening among women of diverse ethnic and social class backgrounds. *Fetal Diagn Therap.* 1993;8:97–106.

40. Otono L: First trimester diagnosis without legal abortion? Presentation at the 10th International Conference on Prenatal Diagnosis and Therapy, Barcelona, Spain. June 21, 2000.

41. Press N, Browner CH. Why women say yes to prenatal diagnosis. *Social Science and Medicine.* 1997;45:979–989.

42. Thornton JG, Hewison J, Lilford RJ, et al. A randomized trial of three methods of giving information about prenatal testing. *Br Med Journal.* 1995;28:1127–1130.

43. Britt DW, Risinger ST, Miller V, et al. Determinants of parental decisions after the prenatal diagnosis of Down Syndrome: Bringing in context. *Am J Med Genet.* 2000;93:410–416.

44. Porter M, Macintyre S: What is, must be best: A research note on conservative or deferential responses to antenatal care provision. *Social Science and Medicine.* 1984;11:1197–1200.

46. Maines D. The social construction of meaning. *Contemp Soc.* 2000;29:577–584.

47. Roelofsen EEC, Kamerbeek LI, Tymstra TJ: Chances and choices: Psychosocial consequences of maternal serum screening. A report from the Netherlands. *J Repro Infant Psych.* 1993;11:41–47.

48. Britt DW, Mans M, Risinger S, et al. The impact of career interests, unresolved moral dilemmas and procedural anxiety on the effectiveness of an MFRP coping and bonding intervention. *Journal for the Society of Gynecologic Investigation.* 2002;9;105A.

CHAPTER 65

ETHICS AND PRENATAL DIAGNOSIS: CROSS-CULTURAL CONSIDERATIONS

John C. Fletcher

INTRODUCTION

This chapter concerns ethical issues in prenatal diagnosis with attention to cross-cultural considerations. Two main sources of international research and discussion inform its content. The first source is the results of 2 international surveys of medical geneticists' views on ethical problems in practice. These surveys* were conducted in 1985 (19 nations) and in 1994 (37 nations) by Dorothy C. Wertz.[1,2,3] The second source is a consensus development process of the World Health Organization (WHO) since 1992 to develop proposed guidelines for medical genetics and genetic services.[4,5] The material in the tables below stems from WHO deliberations. These guidelines are proposed for policy makers and members of professional societies in different nations to use as points of departure for debate and shape their own guidelines for ethical issues in genetic services.

RESOURCES IN MEDICAL ETHICS FOR PROVIDERS OF PRENATAL DIAGNOSIS

In at least 4 ways, ethical concerns in medical genetics are different than those of Western medical ethics that focus largely on duties of the physician-patient relationship. First, genetic information may affect an entire family, rather than only the individual. Secondly, genetic discoveries may be predictive of future adverse events in an individual or family member's health. Third, genetic information and the choices of the present may affect future generations. Fourth, medical genetics has a tradition of nondirectiveness in counseling. Indeed, the term "patient" is not fitting for the role of many who seek genetic services, including prenatal diagnosis. They are not sick or physically suffering. The terms "counselee" or "pregnant woman" will be used frequently below instead of "patient," in recognition of this important difference.

What are resources for ethical problems in providing prenatal diagnosis? Such providers may be specialists in medical genetics as well as in other medical fields, e.g., obstetrics and gynecology, maternal-fetal medicine, pediatrics, internal medicine, etc. They are socially and morally located within the traditions and practice of medicine. For this reason, ethical principles which provide a major ethical framework for medicine are also relevant to ethical issues in prenatal diagnosis. Table 65-1 depicts 4 principles that are resources for ethical guidance in medicine. The primary ethical concerns of Western medical ethics are for the wellbeing of individual patients, although 3 principles (beneficence, nonmaleficence, and justice) are also relevant to the health and wellbeing of populations.[6] The bearing of these principles on ethical issues in providing prenatal diagnosis will be noted in subsequent tables. Other resources for ethics include the character traits of committed health professionals, knowledge of the most ethically significant cases in the field, and knowledge of the moral perspectives of those who criticize or oppose the one or more uses of prenatal diagnosis in society.

The principle of respect for autonomy includes: a) respecting the self-determination and choices of autonomous persons, and b) protecting persons with diminished autonomy, e.g., young children, mentally retarded persons, and those with other mental impairments.

The principle of beneficence (L. "bene" = good) is the source of Western physicians' obligation to give highest loyalty to the welfare of individual patients. Beneficence also bears upon concern for and improving the health of a whole population.

Nonmaleficence (L. "male" = evil, harm) is the source of the traditional medical norm of "do no harm," prevent harm altogether, or, if harm cannot be avoided to minimize harm to patients.

Justice is the source of several moral norms. On the individual level, the norm of fairness requires giving each person what is due to him or her. The norm of distributive justice underlies society's obligation to allocate resources according to need. The norm of equity guides the quest for equal consideration and treatment of all peoples around the world.

Justice and Genetic Services

Worldwide, at least 5,000 specialists practice medical genetics.[7] At present, the majority of them (about 3,330) work in developed Western nations, which have an overall approximate ratio of geneticist to population of 1:222,000, as compared to 1 of 1:700,000 for Eastern European nations and 1:3,700,000 for developing nations. As deaths from other causes (e.g., infant infections and malnutrition) decline in developing nations, genetics will assume a larger role. Prevention and care of genetic diseases and birth defects concern persons in every nation. Genetic disabilities occur with similar frequencies in developed and developing nations and irrespective of the socioeconomic status of individuals. At all levels of society children born with genetic disadvantages have higher risks to get sick and to die of environmental causes such as infections and malnutrition. For these reasons, if a right to health care is to be meaningful, such a right must include access to services for the diagnosis, treatment, and prevention of genetic disorders.

Correction of dramatic variation between levels of genetic services in developed and developing nations is an overriding ethical concern, considering claims of justice and equity. In ethics, "ought" implies "can." However, it is unfair to impose an "ought" where the agent or group lacks the means

---

*At several places it will be noted that "most medical geneticists" support a particular moral position. The data to support the statement were gathered in the 1994 survey and discussed in an overview article by Dr. Wertz cited at reference 3.

TABLE 65-1	ETHICAL PRINCIPLES IN MEDICINE

Respect for the autonomy of persons: respecting self-determination of patients and protecting persons with diminished autonomy;

Beneficence: highest priority to the welfare of patients and maximizing benefits to their health; also applies to concern for the health of populations;

Nonmaleficence: avoiding harm to patients or, at least, minimizing harm;

Justice: to give persons their due and distribute benefits of medicine fairly in society, according to need.

or power to act upon it. Thus, the imperatives of the 4 principles have little moral weight or force in respect to human genetics in nations where few or no genetic services exist at all.

ETHICAL ISSUES IN PRENATAL DIAGNOSIS

Prenatal diagnosis, a key feature of genetic services, includes all methods of ascertaining the health of the developing fetus; biochemical screening (maternal serum alpha-fetoprotein (MSAFP), triplemarker screening), ultrasound, amniocentesis, and chorionic villus biopsy. Newer methods, such as fluorescent in situ hybridization (FISH) technologies[8] and experimental isolation of fetal cells from maternal blood.[9,10] In

the first trimester of pregnancy raise no new ethical problems and require no lengthy discussion here. A national advisory group on ethical issues in human reproduction called for careful ethical reflection on the potential for mass screening by fetal cell isolation.[11] However, if this technique is eventually proved and used in early prenatal care, the same ethical requirements would apply as in maternal serum testing for levels of alpha-fetoprotein: voluntariness, pretest counseling, informed consent, and if findings were suggestive of aneuploidy, a recommendation would follow for prenatal diagnosis by a more definitive method to confirm the early finding.[12] The technique itself presents no new ethical problems, but widespread use in practice would require much effort and ingenuity to satisfy ethical requirements.

Although utilization of prenatal diagnosis may be envisioned on a larger scale, its primary purpose must continue to give particular couples information about the health status of the fetus so that they can make plans for the future. It may also help the physician to prepare for a difficult birth.

Proposed ethical guidelines for the provision of prenatal diagnosis appear in Table 65-2. Guidelines 1–5 will be discussed in this section, followed by a section on counseling prior to prenatal diagnosis, which includes discussion of guidelines 6–8.

Equitable Access to Services and the Woman's Role

The prenatal diagnostic services that exist in a nation should be available equitably to all who need them, regardless of ability to pay, if there is a medical indication for the service.

Respondents to the 1985 survey stated that the most serious ethical problem facing medical genetics globally was to meet the need for services with equity. This is still the leading ethical issue in prenatal diagnosis in terms of magnitude and number of lives affected. When prenatal diagnosis is a scarce resource, medical geneticists and other providers should be able to prioritize allocation in terms of (1) seriousness of the genetic condition, and (2) level of risk. In setting such priorities, providers should assume that most couples requesting prenatal diagnosis may change their minds after learning that the fetus is affected, regardless of the couple's stated intentions.

To insure equitable access, counselors should not make willingness to abort affected fetuses a precondition to receive prenatal diagnosis. Social justice also requires societal support for the costs of medically indicated treatment after birth for children with disabilities

TABLE 65-2	PROPOSED ETHICAL GUIDELINES FOR PRENATAL DIAGNOSIS

1. Equitable distribution of genetics services, including prenatal diagnosis, is owed first to those with the greatest medical need, regardless of ability to pay, or any other considerations (justice).

2. If prenatal diagnosis is medically indicated, it should be available regardless of a couple's stated views on abortion. Prenatal diagnosis may, in some cases, be used to prepare for the birth of a child with a disorder (autonomy).

3. Prenatal diagnosis is done only to give parents and physicians information about the health of the fetus. The use of prenatal diagnosis for paternity testing, except in cases of rape or incest or for gender selection, apart from sex-linked disorders, is not acceptable (nonmaleficence).

4. Prenatal diagnosis should be voluntary in nature. The prospective parents should decide whether a particular genetic disorder warrants prenatal diagnosis or termination of a pregnancy with an affected fetus, rather than the doctor or the government (autonomy).

5. Prenatal diagnosis solely for relief of maternal anxiety, in the absence of medical indications, should have lower priority in allocation of resources than prenatal diagnosis with medical indications (justice).

6. Counseling should precede prenatal diagnosis (nonmaleficence).

7. Physicians should disclose all clinically relevant findings to the pregnant woman or couple (autonomy).

8. The woman and/or couple's choices in an affected pregnancy should be respected and protected, within the framework of the law and culture of the nation. The couple, not the professional or the government, should make the choice (autonomy).

due to genetic causes. Such support will vary between nations, depending on their resources for health care.

The status of women in particular societies strongly influences the place of prenatal diagnosis in the health care system, as well as the centrality of the role of the pregnant woman in decision making. The woman's role will vary widely in different cultural settings. In any case, the pregnant woman should have an important role in making decisions about prenatal diagnosis because she is the one who will give birth and be responsible for caring for the child. Most geneticists around the world believe that the woman or the couple, not the doctor or the government, should be the primary decision makers.

Effects of Differential Use by Different Social Groups

Inequitable access is unjust and can produce further social inequality as those in different social groups avail themselves of the services unequally. In many countries, women who have prenatal diagnosis tend to be better educated and to have higher incomes than those who do not have prenatal diagnosis. The better off and better educated are using prenatal diagnosis at disproportionate rates to other classes.[13] For example, if this trend continues in the United Kingdom, "the two-income family that has postponed child-raising until their mid-thirties would become the primary customers for chromosome analysis. This prospect challenges the British sense of fairness and the belief that health care is a right rather than a privilege."[14]

Women who receive prenatal diagnosis today are not always the women whose pregnancies have the highest genetic risk. The age distribution in childbearing suggests that poor women who lack access to contraception account for a disproportionate share of the births to women over 40. People from lower socio-economic groups are also at greater risk for exposures to environmental hazards, both at home and at work, that may cause fetal disorders. Although substance abuse and male battering of pregnant women occur in all social classes, these problems are less likely to receive consistent treatment among poor women.

In the future, differential uses of prenatal diagnosis and selective abortion by different social groups could lead to an unbalanced distribution of genetic disorders among social classes.

It will be the educated, articulate, vocal, and economically privileged who will use the system most effectively and for whom there will be the most marked fall in births of affected children. Further, the burden of caring for handicapped children might increasingly fall on those who can least afford it and are least able to press for better services.[15]

Equitable access to genetic services is also a strong response to criticism that prenatal diagnosis is, in its consequences, the moral equivalent of social eugenics.[16] The integrity of the parents' freedom to choose prenatal diagnosis and to act upon its results is the most authentic refutation of this charge. Equitable access preserves freedom of choice among the majority of couples, regardless of income, to seek prenatal diagnosis as well as deciding to continue or terminate a pregnancy with an affected fetus. Kitcher's[17] important work on social ethics and prenatal diagnosis counts the costs

to freedom of choice by the trends of domination of access by the economically advantaged and of scarce economic and social support for children with disabilities. Kitcher shows how, if these trends continue, many couples will choose abortion, mainly influenced by stark economic realities of a noncaring society, rather than within the freedom of a wider context of a reasonable level of assurance of economic and social support, in which to assess the degree of pain, suffering, and disability of an affected child-to-be.

Equity and Parents' View of Abortion

Instead of choosing to terminate a pregnancy with an affected fetus, some couples use prenatal diagnosis to prepare for the birth of a child with a disability. The majority of medical geneticists regard this aim as a medically indicated use of prenatal diagnosis. If treatments for genetic disorders do continue to improve, there will be less likelihood of abortion and prenatal diagnosis could be used more frequently to prepare for the births of children needing treatment. Prenatal diagnosis should be *offered* to all pregnant women at elevated risk, regardless of their views on abortion. It is unfair not to offer prenatal diagnosis on the basis of an individual or couple's views. Offering does not mean urging or coercing. It means simply presenting information about prenatal diagnosis.

It is likely that women who request prenatal diagnosis with the stated intention of preparing for the birth of a child with a disorder do so hoping for favorable results and to continue their pregnancies with less anxiety. Indeed, reducing anxiety among pregnant women at higher genetic risk is a justified use of prenatal diagnosis. If risk to the fetus is minimal, helping couples to prepare themselves for the birth of an affected child, provided that they understand and accept the risks to the fetus, is an ethically acceptable use of the procedure.[18] Some couples use the knowledge that the fetus is affected to make early plans for treatment, housing, and education. Some unfortunate couples use test results of a lethal abnormality to prepare for the short life and certain death of an infant after delivery.[19] Other couples change their minds about abortion after learning that the fetus is affected. To refuse prenatal diagnosis is to prejudge a couple's behavior when, in fact, it is difficult to predict a couple's final response to knowledge that the fetus is affected.

Indications for Prenatal Diagnosis

The term "indications" means a medical, psychological, or social rationale justifying the procedure. The discussion below applies mainly to invasive and relatively costly procedures (e.g., amniocentesis and chorionic villus biopsy) that provide a definitive diagnosis.

Medical Indications: Pregnancies at Elevated Risk

Medical indications include all factors leading to elevated risk, e.g., advanced maternal age, family history of a genetic disorder, knowledge of an abnormal gene in the family, a previous child with a disorder, or suspect findings (i.e., by ultrasonography in an ongoing pregnancy). In several nations, many government commissions and professional bodies have agreed upon medical indications for prenatal diagnosis, beginning in the United States in 1979.[20] There is less agreement worldwide, however, about the status of nonmedical indications based on psychological or social arguments or on what disorders are sufficiently serious to warrant prenatal diagnosis. These controversial questions are discussed below.

Nonmedical Requests for Prenatal Diagnosis

These requests include (1) sex selection, in the absence of an X-linked disorder; (2) prenatal paternity testing; and (3) tissue typing for possible organ donation after birth.

Prenatal Diagnosis and Parental Preference of Sex

Respondents stated that sex selection was the hardest ethical issue for them on the 1985 survey. This issue requires considerable discussion.

In 1994, 47% of 2,903 medical geneticists and counselors in 37 nations reported at least 1 parental request for sex selection by prenatal diagnosis.[21] These cases involve 3 ethical issues. First, there is an issue of professional ethics: whether providers of prenatal diagnosis ought to cooperate with parents who openly make this request or covertly seek such knowledge to act upon it. Whether abortion is justified as a means to this end is a second and more general issue. A third is whether couples ought to choose the sex of their children, and if so, under what conditions.

Sex selection is a major problem in some nations. China,[22] India,[23] and Turkey[24] now legally prohibit prenatal diagnosis for this purpose. The laws were enacted due to serious population loss of females, imbalance of the sex ratio, inequity to those in greater medical need of prenatal diagnosis, and flagrant contradiction to the social ideal of gender equality.

Despite these laws, the use of prenatal diagnosis for sex selection continues in these and other developing nations with a strong preference for sons. A large number of procedures are performed for sex selection rather than detection of fetal abnormalities. Ultrasound, although not always accurate, is affordable even to villagers and poses no known risk to the mother.

In some Asian nations, sex selection adds to an already unbalanced sex ratio due to neglect of female children. An estimated 60 to 100 million women are missing from the world's population.[25,26] These figures include 29 million in China and 23 million in India. In the United States there are 105 women to every 100 men. In Africa and Latin America the proportions of women and men are roughly equal. In much of Asia, including Pakistan, Afghanistan, Turkey, Bangladesh, India, and China, there are fewer than 95 women for every 100 men.[27] Families in these nations desire sons for economic reasons. Where most people have no social security or retirement pensions, sons are responsible to care for parents in their old age. Daughters usually leave the parental family to live with their husbands and to help care for their parents-in-law. Even if a daughter stays in the parental home, she seldom has the earning power to support her parents. In some nations, a daughter represents a considerable economic burden because her family must pay a dowry to her husband's family in order to arrange a marriage. A son's religious duties at the parents' funerals, although often cited as a reason for son preference, are of lesser importance than economic factors. These religious duties can be performed by other male relatives.

Direct requests for prenatal diagnosis for sex selection are likely to remain few in Western nations because (1) the absence of a strong cultural preference for children of a particular gender and (2) personal and cultural objections to use of abortion for this purpose. Although the majority of North Americans believe that abortion should be available to others in a wide variety of situations, including sex selection, few would use it themselves.[28] Information about fetal sex is almost always communicated to parents who wish to know by providers of prenatal diagnosis. Some clinics in the United Kingdom withhold the information unless specifically requested.[29,30]

Geneticists and counselees in the United States rely heavily on the principle of autonomy in facing the issue of sex selection. In the 1985 and 1994 surveys, geneticists were given a case of a couple with 4 healthy girls who want prenatal diagnosis to identify the gender of the fetus. The couple stated that they would abort a female fetus. In 1985, 34% would perform prenatal diagnosis for this couple and 28% would offer a referral. In the 1994 survey, despite much discussion in the bioethics literature and strong public opposition by 2 national bodies to sex selection,[33,34] 34% would still perform it and 38% would refer. The 1994 survey included 473 genetics counselees. Almost as many counselees as geneticists thought that doctors ought to respect a couple's request for sex selection, although their responses to questions about abortion show that almost none of them would ask for sex selection themselves. What respondents say they would do or what they prefer on a questionnaire is almost certainly unreliable in estimating the actual incidence of sex selection procedures in the United States, a figure that remains unknown. However, one must assume from these findings that respect for autonomy is a prevailing value among geneticists and counselees, and in specific cases this respect would extend to sex selection.

McCullough and Chervenak[35] perceive a "strong consensus" against gender identification by prenatal diagnosis and challenge the reasoning of those who support it as speculative and incomplete. Their arguments aside for the moment, the results of the 1994 survey point to anything but a "strong consensus."[36] In a 37 nation study of 2903 geneticists and counselors, 29% would perform prenatal diagnosis in the case above and 20% would offer referral. The percentage who would perform prenatal diagnosis in the United States (34%) was exceeded by Mexico (38%), Cuba (62%), and Israel (68%). These data point to a trend toward honoring such requests, rather than a consensus against it. The reasoning of respondents who would cooperate appeals almost exclusively, as do McCullough and Chervenak, to autonomy-based arguments. These authors and most respondents had almost no discussion of harmful societal consequences or of principles other than autonomy, such as justice. McCullough and Chervenak also argue, but without any evidence, that gender identification could be beneficial in giving the pregnant woman's spouse time to adjust to the information and reducing a potential for coercion. This is an important ethical question that deserves empirical research.

Robertson,[37] after discussing some reasons to oppose the use of prenatal diagnosis and abortion for sex choice, vigorously defends autonomy-based gender choice in a future context of effective preconceptual methods of sex determination. His arguments will probably prevail in the future, barring a biological disaster or social revolution followed by rigid controls on methods of reproduction. If preconceptual sex selection were limited to balancing gender in 2- or 3-child families in open societies where equality for women was protected, this use would likely be socially benign.

Neither Robertson nor McCullough and Chervenak consider 2 additional reasons to oppose sex selection by prenatal diagnosis: (1) the further harm done to equitable access by use of a resource by recipients in no medical need compared with those at higher genetic risk, and (2) the precedent that sex selection sets for eugenic uses of genetic information. Narrowing the purpose of prenatal diagnosis to information about the health status of the fetus helps to prevent future genetic "tinkering" with traits that may be culturally desirable but have little to do with disease. On the premise that gender is not a disease, it follows that cooperating with sex selection negates the medical uses of prenatal diagnosis to detect serious disorders in the fetus and undermines the major moral reason that justifies prenatal diagnosis and abortion of a pregnancy with an affected fetus—the prevention of untreatable genetic disease. The use of prenatal diagnosis for sex selection is a precedent that places society on a "slippery slope" toward selection on cosmetic grounds, such as height, weight, or eye, hair or skin color. Some parents may select for particular purposes, eg, weight.[38] For these reasons, the Council of Europe forbade sex selection, except to avoid sex-linked hereditary disease, in the use of any technique of medically assisted reproduction.[39]

Ethical arguments in favor of sex selection in general, including preconceptual selection, are that (1) sex choice would enhance the quality of life for a child of the "wanted" sex; (2) sex choice would provide a better quality of life for the family that has the sex balance it desires; (3) sex choice would provide a better quality of life for the mother, because she would undergo fewer births and her status in the family would be enhanced; (4) sex choice would help to limit the population.[40] According to these arguments, families that have the gender "balance" they desire would be happier. Further, children of the "unwanted" gender, usually female, would be spared the abuse, neglect, and early death in childhood that is their documented fate,[41] which may occur to a lesser extent elsewhere. It is also argued that women would not be abused by their husbands for not bearing children of the desired sex. In this view, women would not suffer repeated pregnancies and births in order to produce at least 1 child of the desired sex, usually a son. The population dimension of the argument is that couples would not have more children than they could afford in order to have a child of the desired sex. Many couples in developing nations would prefer to have at most 2 children. These couples could limit their family size and still have a son to support them in their old age, instead of continuing to have children until they have a son. The threat of world overpopulation might recede.

Each of the arguments above can be effectively countered. Arguments that sex selection will lead to a better quality of life for families, children, or women are comprehensible only in the context of a sexist society that gives preferential treatment to one sex, usually the male. Instead of selecting sex, societies should work to improve quality of life by making society less sexist. Efforts need to be directed towards equality of the sexes and against gender stereotyping, including the stereotyping of fetuses.[42,43] Although sex selection could prevent some abuse of unwanted female children and their mothers in the short run, it does not correct the underlying abuses, namely the social devaluation of women in many parts of the world and the gender stereotyping of children of both sexes in the rest of the world.

There is no good evidence that sex selection will reduce population growth in developing nations. Effective contraceptives and education of women in developing nations, as well as increased opportunities for their employment outside the home are more effective means of reducing population growth than sex selection. In developed nations, sex selection will likely have no effect on population size, because most couples will not have more children than they wish in order to have a child of a particular sex.[44]

Warren recently argued that even though some uses of sex preselection could be socially harmful and harm women, it is impossible at this stage of history to know sufficiently what all of the consequences of the practice would be. She also acknowledges that there are nonsexist reasons for wanting children of both genders in a family, e.g., to increase knowledge and experience of the other gender. She opposes a categorical rejection based on either negative social consequences or loyalty to equality between the genders.[45] She is right that arguments based on moral absolutes are likely to yield little sound guidance in practice because of the complexities of living. To some it is an absolute that all sex selection, including selection for the "balanced family" desired in some Western nations, perpetuates gender stereotyping and sexism.[46] In an ideal nonsexist society, there would be no reason to select one sex over the other. However, such societies probably will never exist yet some will continue to make progress in overcoming sexism. Even where sexism is evident, every act of gender selection that does not involve abortion or embryo selection is not morally wrong such as the desire to balance gender. One can oppose sexist social practices and still morally balance gender in one's family, if a safe method of preconceptual sex determination were available.

There is no need in the United States for state laws prohibiting sex selection by prenatal diagnosis because it is probably not occurring with sufficient magnitude to warrant such actions. Also, such laws would be a pretext for more intrusion into reproductive freedom. Providers of prenatal diagnosis do not have to accede to counselee requests or even to offer referrals. In cases where providers suspect that sex selection is likely to occur, they may consider withholding information about fetal sex until after the legal time limit for abortion has passed. The information is not related to the health of the fetus. In this event, the provider should inform the couple of the reason for withholding the information.

Prenatal Paternity Testing

In cases where paternity is uncertain, the woman or her partner(s) may request prenatal diagnosis solely for paternity testing. It is not clear whether withholding prenatal paternity testing would reduce or increase the number of abortions in situations where paternity is dubious. Withholding prenatal testing could increase interpersonal dishonesty. Openness is often the most beneficial alternative, especially in view of the child's future relationships with others. Each situation must be evaluated individually in the light of social, cultural, and family norms. Medical geneticists must acknowledge procedural risks to the fetus and should inform the woman as well as the man of these risks.

Prenatal paternity testing can also be used for forensic purposes, if pregnancy occurs after rape or incest. In cases where the pregnancy may have resulted from criminal assault, it is especially important to know the truth about paternity so that the woman can make a decision about abortion. Probably few would question the use of prenatal diagnosis if rape or incest has occurred.

Tissue-Typing for Organ or Marrow Donation

Sometimes a couple with a seriously ill child wish to know whether their fetus, once born, will be able to serve as a donor of bone marrow or other organ transplants for the living child.[47] Information about the fetus would enable them to make plans for the living child's future. This information, however, would also enable them to "save time" by aborting a fetus with an incompatible tissue type and conceiving another fetus that might have tissue suitable for a transplant. Professionals sometimes suspect that the latter motive underlies requests for prenatal diagnosis. Parents are understandably concerned over the health of their living child and deserve sympathy in these situations. They fear that time will run out before they can find a suitable donor. Nevertheless, if they are considering the fetus primarily as an organ donor, they are using that fetus as a means to an end rather than as an end in itself. A fetus should not be regarded as a tissue preparation for someone else, even if the transplant procedure may be harmless to the donor. Restraint would be strongly advisable in matters relating to tissue-typing because the temptation that it provides a couple to think of a fetus in terms of benefit to someone else. In order to prevent possible harm to the fetus, it is advisable to wait until birth for tissue-typing.

Voluntary Use and "Less Serious" Conditions

There is no consensus among providers of prenatal diagnosis or in society on a definition of a "serious" genetic condition. Conditions and their consequences once frequently fatal in childhood, e.g., cystic fibrosis, are now medically treatable and more socially acceptable, and many affected individuals reach adulthood. Some individuals with Down syndrome hold jobs, albeit in protected work places. Many who would once have been bedridden can now propel themselves in wheelchairs. People with hearing, visual, or motor disabilities can now enter many public buildings, apartments, and businesses as the result of laws requiring accessibility. In other words, many disabilities are less "serious" than they were formerly because of medical, legal, and social advances.

On the other hand, in many cases, medicine has extended life without being able to treat the basic mental or neurological problems. Parents can grow old while still caring for an adult child with a mental disability.

Prenatal diagnosis reveals disorders that some medical professionals might not consider "serious," such as sex chromosome abnormalities, but which society continues to stigmatize. Some parents who want small families of 1 or 2 children may decide that a boy with XXY (Klinefelter syndrome) for example, is not the son they want. Although the boy will reach puberty with proper treatment, he will be infertile (a condition that many fathers associate, falsely, with impotence), may look different from his peers, and may have learning or behavioral problems. A couple may decide that they do not wish to invest their resources in a child if they could choose otherwise. Another example: a couple belonging to a social group that places a high value on a woman's ability to bear children may decide that a girl with 45,X (Turner syndrome) would be an economic burden. On account of her infertility, no one in that cultural group may marry her. Parents vary greatly in their perceptions of seriousness. What one couple finds acceptable, another may find extremely serious in terms of their personal expectations for the child, their culture's expectations, their economic situation, or their goals for their own lives.[48] Although use of abortion may follow a range of perceived seriousness that starts with severe mental retardation (total inability to communicate), early death, or extreme physical disability as the most serious,[49] a small percentage of couples might consider, for example, development of Alzheimer disease at age 60 a condition that warranted termination before birth, especially if they themselves had cared for a parent with Alzheimer disease. Even though they might not be living to care for the child when the child reaches 60, they might consider the future suffering for the child as a serious defect.

Following the principle of autonomy, physicians should respect the wishes of fully informed and counseled parents and let them exercise the freedom to decide what they consider serious, even if the majority would not agree with that decision. There are cultural as well as individual differences in how people define health and disease.[50] Unless society is willing to raise the child, the decision is best left to the parents who will actually raise the child.[51,52,53,54]

It would be dangerous to create medical, legal, or social definitions of "serious," because these could infringe on couples' lives in several ways. First of all, a disorder now considered "serious," such as Down syndrome, could become less "serious" in its effects because of improved education and training. If Down syndrome were to be redefined as no longer "serious," prolife activists could promote legislation to prevent abortion after prenatal diagnosis for this and other disorders.

At the other extreme, a cultural majority could define a condition as "serious" when it is in fact treatable. This majority could enforce its views on people who hold minority views by refusing social supports for children with this condition. In order to accommodate minority as well as majority views in pluralistic societies, it is wise public policy to leave all such decisions to parents, even if some decisions appear to be made on "frivolous" grounds. The alternatives to a parent-centered policy are: (1) to forbid any abortions after prenatal diagnosis, or (2) to allow abortions only for disorders where there is evidence that death or total neurological devastation shortly after birth would be expected. In the second alternative, society (or the government) would specify a list of abortable disorders. The first alternative would force some parents to accept burdens that they are unable to bear. The second alternative is based on the view that the previable fetus and the newborn are equal. Most people around the world do not share this view. This alternative would impose one moral view of the equality of the previable fetus and newborn upon all. Forbidding abortion could also encourage pediatric euthanasia.

Accommodating all views, however, could leave the door open to some "cosmetic" decisions, for example, with regard to height and weight. Extreme variants in both weight and height are "medical" conditions and doctors are ethically obligated to disclose major variations from the norm.

The best approach to prenatal diagnosis for so-called "less serious" conditions is to provide the most complete, unbiased education possible. This is especially important if parents have no experience with the disorder in question. What parents do after learning that the fetus is affected depends to a great extent on what the provider, counselor, or genetic support group tells them. For example, fewer parents decide to abort for sex chromosome disorders if provided with thorough, unbiased counseling.[55]

Maternal Anxiety

Maternal anxiety, in the absence of a known factor for elevated risk, is at the borderline of medical indications. In some nations with a large laboratory capacity it is considered a medical indication. In nations with limited laboratory capacity, it may be considered a waste of scarce resources. In deciding whether to perform prenatal diagnosis solely on the basis of maternal anxiety and the mother or couple's request, justice should be the primary concern. Unless public health resources are virtually unlimited, it is unfair to provide this service because it means depriving others of a needed service. It also poses an unnecessary risk to the fetus. Morbid anxiety in either parent, clinically confirmed by a psychiatrist or psychologist, warrants the service on humanitarian grounds. Sometimes this occurs in women who have cared for people with severe disabili-

ties. A woman experiencing the usual anxieties of pregnancy, however, should not receive prenatal diagnosis solely on this ground.

PRETEST AND POSTTEST COUNSELING

Prenatal diagnosis should be provided in a supportive, noncoercive atmosphere that allows couples to make choices that are best for them in view of their values and parenting goals.[56] This includes pre- and posttest counseling and full disclosure of test results. Within the legal provisions of each nation, safe and affordable abortion services should be available. Proposed guidelines for pretest counseling appear in Table 65-3.

Counseling Prior to Prenatal Diagnosis

The principles of respect for persons and nonmaleficence require that women know the purpose of the tests that are being offered. This applies to all forms of prenatal diagnosis. A woman should know, before a blood test for MSAFP, that this test may be the first step on the road to a decision about abortion. She should have the right and the power to refuse such testing if she does not wish to face such a decision. If possible, decisions about testing should be made by the couple together. If a couple cannot agree among themselves, the woman should make the final decision because it is her body that is involved.

Content of Counseling

Prior counseling need not always be elaborate. Too strict demands for counseling could be a misuse of scarce resources. Such counseling should be provided for both high-risk families (advanced maternal age, family history of genetic disorder, previous child with a genetic disorder, suspect clinical or laboratory findings in pregnant women) and low-risk families (routine biochemical screening or MSAFP testing). Ideally, both groups should receive counseling covering the topics in Table 65-3 above. In practice, it may be necessary to abbreviate counseling for those at low risk.

Prior counseling has practical advantages in the provision of genetics services. It makes postprocedure counseling (for those with results showing that the fetus is affected) much less difficult because counselees are somewhat prepared, helps to facilitate communication, and prevent unexpected emotional crises. Prior counseling may not be possible for primary care physicians who have many patients and limited time. Basic counseling need not be done by physicians themselves. Trained healthcare workers, written material, and audio-visual materials could be sufficient. Women receiving ultrasound should also receive counseling before the procedure, but the counselor should also explain that ultrasound may identify conditions that can be corrected or ameliorated before birth.

Timing of Counseling Prior to Prenatal Diagnosis

Scheduling prenatal diagnosis immediately after counseling reduces the likelihood that a woman will abstain from the procedure. In order to avoid the appearance of pressure or

TABLE 65-3	**PROPOSED GUIDELINES FOR COUNSELING PRIOR TO PRENATAL DIAGNOSIS**

Counseling should, at a minimum, include these points:

1. Name(s) and general characteristics of the major disorder(s) that the test may identify. The list of disorders need not be exhaustive. The characteristics of the disorder(s) should be described also in terms of their effects on the future child, on the parents, and on family life.
2. Possibilities for treatment of the disorder(s) and availability of supportive care.
3. Description of the likelihood (risk) that the fetus may have the disorder(s). Risks should be expressed in several ways (as a percent, proportion, and verbally).
4. The possibility of findings that the fetus is affected as well as any fortuitous or unexpected findings.
5. Alternatives available if the fetus is affected, for example, carrying the fetus to term and caring for the child at home; placing the child in an institutional setting, if available; placing the child for adoption; termination of pregnancy; prenatal treatment for the fetus or early treatment after birth.
6. The possibility of ambiguous results for the material examined in amniocentesis or chorionic villus biopsy, or for ultrasound.
7. Information that the test may not help the baby.
8. Information that the test does not guarantee a healthy baby because there are many disorders that cannot be identified before birth.
9. The medical risks to fetus and mother posed by the testing procedure. Pretest counseling makes posttest counseling (if the fetus is affected) much less difficult because prospective parents are somewhat prepared.
10. Noninvasive screens used early in pregnancy, such as MSAFP, may be the first step on the road to prenatal diagnosis and a possible decision about abortion.
11. Costs of the test and sources of reimbursement for the mother or couple, if applicable.
12. Names and addresses of genetic support groups or organizations for persons with genetic disorders.

coercion, it may be preferable to have a waiting period of 1 to 7 days between counseling and prenatal diagnosis. This can pose a hardship for women who must travel long distances, however. To avoid this hardship, women who have traveled to a clinic for counseling should have a choice to proceed with the procedure on the same day. An alternative would be for a community-based counselor to travel to the family's home or neighborhood health center to provide the pretest counseling. The woman could then decide whether or not to travel to the clinic for prenatal diagnosis.

Full Disclosure of Test Results

All test results relevant to genetic disorders or fetal malformations should be disclosed. These include sex chromosome abnormalities and disorders that may not be considered serious.

Ambiguous or Conflicting Results

Ambiguous or conflicting test results should be disclosed. Although uncertainty may cause anxiety, it is better to disclose an ambiguous result before birth than to have the patient face an unexpected surprise after birth. New or controversial interpretations of test results should be disclosed.

Normal Test Results

All normal test results, including those from MSAFP measurements and 2- or 3-marker testing, should be disclosed promptly because testing arouses anxiety in many people.

Disclosure to Husband or Partner

Although both parents should ultimately know the test results, priority should be given to the woman. She should have control over information about both her body and her fetus. If she has difficulty telling her partner, the physician or counselor should work with her toward a solution that will provide least harm to all concerned.

In some cases, a woman may ask that her spouse or partner be told the results first. This request should be honored, but the medical geneticist has the responsibility to make sure that the woman is acting voluntarily and receives the information in a timely fashion.

Disclosure to a Couple's Other Children

Many parents wonder whether to disclose prenatal test results (or even the fact that they have been tested) to their affected or unaffected children. The benefits and harms of disclosure will vary in individual cases. This is a decision best left to the parents. The physician should not tell a couple's minor children, but should be prepared to discuss with the couple the potential benefits and harms of disclosure to children.

Timing and Method of Disclosure to Parents

In order to maximize a couple's options speed is of the essence. All disclosure that the fetus is affected should be in person to allow maximum support and counseling. In practice, this may, on rare occasions, be impossible. The benefits of in-person counseling may be outweighed by the anxiety of waiting. If there is a strong need, basic information can be transmitted sensitively by telephone, and then followed by a clinic appointment. This information should be conveyed only to the woman, however. In rural areas where counselees may have to travel long distances to a clinic, more of the counseling may have to be by telephone. Thus, the counselor should take care to insure privacy. If a telephone is not available, it may, very exceptionally, be necessary to use other means for prompt communication, for instance adequately trained rural community health workers could visit the woman's home to deliver the basic information.

Post-Test Counseling After Findings of an Affected Fetus

Full Information About the Disorder

One of the most troubling issues in genetics is counseling, after diagnosing an affected fetus, when abortion is an option. The opportunities are ripe for counselor bias and presentation of information intended to influence the decision making process. Geneticists in the 1995 survey stated that one of the most difficult questions concerned how to counsel nondirectively after prenatal diagnosis.[57] The survey presented them with personal choices about abortion in a list of 24 conditions. A majority of M.D. geneticists would abort for 15 of the 24 conditions. In the United States, 85% would abort for Down syndrome, 92% for severe, open spina bifida, 73% for cystic fibrosis, 72% for Huntington disease, and 56% for achondroplasia. A substantial minority (31%) would abort for severe obesity in the absence of a genetic syndrome. They stated that they would be as "unbiased as possible" for all conditions except anencephaly, trisomy 13, and cases involving parental selection of sex. If one appreciates the influences of metacommunication in counseling, the values and beliefs of the counselor will make their presence felt.

Outside the United States, the majority of M.D. geneticists would present purposely slanted information in all 24 conditions. A variety of motivations lay behind optimistic or pessimistic counseling: to influence decisions to terminate, to reflect religious opposition to abortion, or to protect children with particular disorders. Outside of the United States and some English-speaking nations, "nondirective" counseling does not exist.

Although these findings are sobering, it is necessary to outline the ethical requirements of posttest counseling. It should include a description of the full range of severity of the disorder, from least to most affected, and a description of the most usual symptoms characterizing people with the disorder. These symptoms should be described in terms of their functional effects rather than in medical terms. Counseling should describe how a person with the disorder develops over the entire life course—from birth to death. The counselor should make it clear, if affected persons experience physical pain or suffering. The counselor should describe the possible range of effects of the disorder on family life (including the marriage) as well as financial and emotional costs, possibilities for treatment, education, and supportive living in special settings or in the community. If the counselor offers referral to families who have children or siblings with the disorder, care must be taken to offer a sufficient number to represent different parental views and different degrees of severity of the disorder, if relevant. The counselor may also present the option of carrying the child to term and placing it for adoption as an option, but only if adoption is a realistic possibility.

Counseling Both Parents

Ideally, a couple should be seen together. However, the mother may be seen alone if she desires. At the outset of counseling, the counselor should explain to both parents that they should not feel guilty. Their actions did not cause the disorder, nor did it result from the woman's or the man's behavior before or during pregnancy. It is especially important that this information reach the husband, in order to prevent blame falling upon the wife. Counseling should be accompanied by some form of ongoing evaluation that enables the counselor to see whether the couple actually understands the information provided. There should be evidence of full understanding before the woman or couple is encouraged to make a decision.

Counseling When Parental Behavior Leads to Birth Defects

When parental behavior (e.g., maternal smoking, drug or alcohol abuse, failure to stay on the phenylketonuria diet, or physical abuse by a woman's partner) has led to abnormalities in the fetus or child, it may be counterproductive to make the parents feel guilty. Although the fetus or child is damaged, this is not the same as child abuse and should not be referred to legal authorities. Usually the mother had diminished control over her body, especially if she was addicted. The goal of counseling should be to prevent further damage to the fetus or child. This may mean educating the parents; offering the possibility of abortion, offering a supportive environment; on a voluntary basis (preferably a residential institution); where the mother can continue her pregnancy without drugs or alcohol and on the proper diet, or providing support services for the family and the child.

Abortion Counseling

For women considering abortion, the counselor should describe the various methods available and the attendant risks and discomforts of each. Methods should be offered by health care systems on the basis of minimum discomfort and complications for the woman rather than convenience for the doctor.

If a woman chooses abortion, she should be made aware that, while most women recover emotionally and return to their usual activities within a month, some feel lingering grief and a few undergo clinically significant depression.[58,59] She should be told of the availability of counseling or support groups.

Timing of Abortion Relative to Counseling

A waiting period of at least a day between counseling and abortion is desirable, for several reasons. It allows the woman and partner some time for deliberation after the initial shock of receiving test results. Also, it reduces the possibility of regretting an over hasty decision.

On the other hand, some women must travel long distances to clinics and cannot afford to spend an extra day near the clinic. In view of these potential hardships, which affect many people, a flexible policy seems best. A mandatory waiting period could impose undue hardship. The counselor should suggest that a couple take some time to come to a decision. Support should be available, in the form of inexpensive, subsidized lodging near the clinic, for those who need time to reach a decision. However, prompt abortion services should also be available if a woman needs or wishes them. No woman should have to wait more than a day after she has decided to have an abortion.

ABORTION OF A PREGNANCY WITH AN AFFECTED FETUS

Respecting Different Cultural Perspectives

There are many different cultural perspectives about when human life begins. Given the diversity of views, it is unlikely that there will ever be universal agreement on this issue. Therefore, it is best to proceed on the basis of acknowledgement of, and respect for, the views of others. This means that abortion procedures should be available even if only acceptable to, or used, by a minority of a nation's people. Such procedures should be supported by public health funds and provided free of charge. No woman should be coerced into having any procedure or coerced into carrying a child to term.

The following discussion centers on abortion of a pregnancy where the fetus is affected. It is difficult to completely separate the issue of abortion for genetic conditions from abortion on social grounds or abortion on request because, in most nations, there are no medical standards for hereditary disorders or fetal malformations that may warrant abortion. Instituting such standards in pluralistic societies could be oppressive because different cultural groups may hold different views about the relative seriousness of different conditions. Setting medical standards for "seriousness" of hereditary disorders in the context of prenatal diagnosis and abortion would also place the balance of power in the hands of politicians and administrators, instead of women and couples. The most ethical approach, therefore, is to leave such abortion choices within the wider context of elective abortion, and to let women and couples decide upon the seriousness of a condition, in view of their personal and social situations.

Nations with laws forbidding genetically indicated abortions have an obligation to examine the conditions under which prenatal diagnosis is offered. It burdens women significantly to offer prenatal diagnosis without the possibility of safe, affordable abortion. Professionals who perform prenatal diagnosis in a country where abortion is illegal need not abandon women who learn that the fetus is affected. If necessary, the professional can refer her outside the country.

In degree of controversy, abortion following prenatal diagnosis outranks any other ethical problem in this area. However, far fewer persons are adversely affected, compared to those harmed by no access to services. Also, the incidence of selective abortions for genetic reasons is no more than 1% of all abortions,[60] vastly fewer than elective abortions because of social causes, failed contraception, or personal reasons. Some women do not choose abortion after learning of genetic abnormalities (e.g., in disorders such as cystic fibrosis).[61] Abortion choices are, however, a special source of emotional suffering for the reasons shown in Table 65-4.

TABLE 65-4	WHY ARE ABORTION CHOICES AFTER PRENATAL DIAGNOSIS SO DIFFICULT?
1.	The choice usually involves a wanted pregnancy.
2.	Many people attribute a higher moral status to the fetus at midtrimester and at viability.
3.	Many parents, who have already viewed the fetus on ultrasound, will have endowed it with the qualities of a living child.
4.	There is a wide spectrum of severity in some chromosomal and Mendelian disorders.
5.	Improved treatments for some disorders have led to longer life spans for some affected persons.
6.	Knowledge of selective abortion could harm the mental health of living children (siblings of the fetus), who have the same genetic condition.

Difficulties of Abortion Choices

Most pregnancies that proceed as far as prenatal care and prenatal diagnosis are "wanted" pregnancies, even if they were not wanted or intended at the time of conception. There are different degrees of wantedness, but usually by the time a woman receives a second trimester prenatal test result she has started to think of herself as a mother. This may be why many women who, would not hesitate to abort an unwanted pregnancy for personal reasons, feel emotional pain and guilt about aborting when there is something wrong with the fetus. The mother who learns that her fetus is affected must make her decision on the basis of the fetus's characteristics. She must also live with her decision. If she aborts, she may feel grief similar to the loss of a child. If she carries to term, she and her family will be responsible for the child's care.

Many people believe that a second-trimester fetus has greater moral status and deserves greater respect than a first-trimester fetus. Christianity, Islam, and Judaism have historically placed greater value on second-trimester fetuses. Women's experience of pregnancy makes second-trimester abortions emotionally difficult because the fetus has begun to move. A woman having prenatal diagnosis may have seen the fetus on ultrasound and may have begun the process of maternal-infant bonding.[62]

Some of the more common genetic disorders diagnosed prenatally, including Down syndrome and sex chromosome abnormalities such as XXY, vary widely among individuals in terms of effects on daily living. Some children with Down syndrome, given maximum educational opportunities and support, may be able to hold unskilled jobs in protected environments or read at an elementary level. Other children with Down syndrome, given the same level of support, may have IQs of less than 30 and require lifetime institutional or parental care. In many nations, optimum education and support are not currently available, and children with genetic disorders are unlikely to reach their full potential, especially if a family has few resources of its own. Children with Down syndrome do not ordinarily suffer and are often happy individuals. The "suffering," if any, is that of the family. Women making abortion decisions, if fully informed, have to weigh the possibility that the aborted fetus might have had a happy life after birth against the possibility that the child would have low potential and would require care that the parents might be unable or unwilling to provide.

Improved treatment for some disorders and improved medical care in general have compounded the problem of abortion choices. Not too long ago, the life expectancy of a child with Down syndrome was markedly lower than average: few reached middle age. Now, at least in developed nations, many people with Down syndrome can expect to reach middle age or beyond. The increase in life expectancy has important implications for care. It is not uncommon for parents in their 80s to have total responsibility for the care of children with Down syndrome in their 50s (an age where many persons with Down syndrome will have developed Alzheimer's disease). When the parents die, the care usually falls on the siblings of the affected individual. Women making abortion decisions now have to consider that, if they carry the fetus to term, they and their partners may be required to care for the child for the rest of their natural lives rather than for a short term.

Couples who are already the parents of a child with a genetic disorder not causing mental retardation, e.g., cystic fibrosis, are frequently concerned that by aborting a fetus with the same disorder they are rejecting their already living child. They may be concerned that if the child were to know about the abortion, the child will have lower self-esteem or feel worthless. Careful counseling about if and how to inform the child can overcome this potential problem.

Some groups, especially some of those representing persons with disabilities, have expressed concern that abortion of genetically affected fetuses will direct societal attention and resources away from caring for living persons with genetic conditions, or will obscure environmental causes of birth defects. These concerns will be addressed under section 5.

In view of the psychological distress that choices about abortion choices present for women, followup is in order for all women who learn that the fetus is affected, whatever their decision. Bereavement therapy or support groups should be available, if women request it.

Twin and Other Multifetal Pregnancies

Ethical problems arise after prenatal diagnosis of 1 abnormal twin[63] or in multifetal pregnancies in which the number of fetuses threatens the mother's ability to carry them all to viability. In the former cases, parents may desperately want to have a normal child, but are unable to care for a child with a disability. The latter cases, also marked by desperation, usually follow infertility treatments, including in vitro fertilization (IVF).[64] Families using IVF for genetic reasons should be told, before initiating an IVF program, that the procedure may result in a multifetal pregnancy that may require a decision about fetal reduction. Both situations call for a position to do the least harm

in a "lifeboat" type of ethical emergency. The principle of proportionality is clearly relevant here. Selective termination of 1 twin with a disorder or malformation is ethically more complex than selective abortion of a single fetus. Risk of dangers to the wellbeing of the presumed normal twin and the mother (i.e., the risks of clotting, hemorrhage, and shock). The act of termination is not morally different, in kind, from selective abortion, although the considerations are more complex.

Third Trimester Abortions

Anomalies are now more frequently discovered in the third trimester because of high resolution ultrasound examinations. Decisions about third-trimester abortion pose particular ethical difficulties because the fetus is often viable, albeit requiring extraordinary medical intervention and reduced likelihood of normal life. There are no crosscultural acceptable lines of demarcation indicating the severity of the fetal defects for which third-trimester abortion could be ethically allowable. Sometimes the result of denying abortion is a "born fetus" that spends agonizing days or weeks in a neonatal intensive care unit before dying.[65]

McCullough and Chervenak reported clinical research[66] in their careful ethical analysis of this complex issue. They develop[67] a 3-part schema classifying fetal anomalies by degree of probability of antenatal diagnosis and degree of probability of outcome. Based on this assessment, McCullough and Chervenak make recommendations to the pregnant woman for: 1) either nonaggressive management (allowing the fetus to die after delivery) or termination of pregnancy, 2) either aggressive (all available management alternatives) or nonaggressive management, and 3) aggressive management (for fetuses that can survive with minimal deficits) and recommend against the other 2 options. They are appropriately silent about any resort to legal alternatives in cases of maternal refusal of the third option.

Legal third-trimester abortions should be limited to situations for which second-trimester abortion was not possible because the fetal condition was not diagnosable in the second trimester. Decisions that can be made in the second trimester must not be postponed until the third trimester. If abortion is legal in the third trimester, it should be performed in a manner that provides adequate analgesia to the woman, does not cause the fetus to undergo prolonged suffering, and does not provoke the woman to change her mind (futilely) during the 4 to 5 days that may be required for dilating the cervix and for vaginal delivery.[68] Procedures that deliver a living fetus that subsequently takes hours, days, or weeks to die are ethically unacceptable; they do not save meaningful life and only lengthen suffering for both fetus and family.

In most cases, fetal therapy will not be a feasible alternative. However, in cases where therapy is available but involves an intervention in the mother's body, the situation is analogous to Cesarean section, though with potentially greater risks and less likelihood of successful outcome. The mother should have final decision over whether or not fetal therapy is performed.

EFFECTS OF PRENATAL DIAGNOSIS ON ATTITUDES TOWARDS PERSONS WITH DISABILITIES

Some advocates for the disabled and feminist critics of prenatal diagnosis fear that increased use will shift social resources away from people with disabilities.[69–72] Others argue that no evidence has appeared during the period in which prenatal diagnosis has been available.[73,74]

In reviewing this topic, it is important to remember that many birth defects are not purely genetic in origin. Common causes of birth-associated disability are prematurity, low birth weight and environmental exposure.[75] Altogether, chromosomal disorders (e.g., Down syndrome), single-gene disorders (e.g., Tay-Sachs and fragile-X syndrome), and developmental malformation syndromes account for about 43% of individuals with IQs under 50.[76,77] Accidents at birth, prematurity, environmental or substance exposures, and unknown factors (possibly including some multifactorial genetic factors) account for the remaining 57%. It is important not to let the availability of genetic tests lead to the illusion that most disabilities are avoidable through prenatal diagnosis. Some fetal malformations cannot yet be diagnosed prenatally. Even disorders that can be diagnosed prenatally, such as Tay-Sachs, will not be tested for in low-risk groups and will continue to appear. Other disorders, such as neurofibromatosis, have a high new mutation rate. This means that disabilities will always occur, regardless of prenatal diagnosis. Society needs to be prepared to offer support to persons with disabilities. Even if every pregnancy underwent chromosomal prenatal diagnosis and testing for neuraltube defects (an unlikely event, given the negative risk-benefit ratio for younger women) and every woman chose abortion of affected fetuses (also an unlikely event), children would still be born with genetic conditions or congenital malformations (unsuspected inborn errors of metabolism, new mutations, etc.).

Social and economic programs to prevent prematurity and low birthweight should go hand-in-hand with public education about genetics and use of prenatal diagnosis. Prevention of disabilities—through adequate maternal nutrition, prenatal care, prevention of substance abuse or physical abuse, and prenatal diagnosis—is not at crosspurposes to increased support for living people with disabilities. It is illogical to argue that supports for people with disabilities will be reduced if there are fewer such persons. Much of the concern expressed by people with disabilities stems from the potential symbolic impact of widespread use of prenatal diagnosis on people's perception of disabilities in general. Public education about disability is one way of addressing these concerns.

The world is unlikely to have fewer persons with disabilities in the future. As societies age, we can expect more, rather than fewer, persons with disabilities of all types, including mental disabilities. It is therefore important to increase, rather than to contemplate decreasing, supports for persons with disabilities. It is also important to prevent mandatory use of either prenatal diagnosis or its results.

Coercion should be avoided. There should be protection for the views of minorities who believe in the protection of all life. This does not mean that society should bear the costs of all aggressive life support when treatment is ultimately futile; withholding such support is ethically permissible and is allowed by many world religions, although the degree of ethical stringency differs among them on this issue. The main point is that the availability of genetic tests must not be allowed to create an illusion that most disabilities are preventable and therefore unacceptable to society.

References

1. Wertz DC, Fletcher JC. *Ethics and Human Genetics: A Cross-Cultural Perspective.* Heidelberg: Springer-Verlag; 1989.
2. Wertz DC, Fletcher JC. Geneticists approach ethics: an international survey. *Clin Genet.* 1993;43:104–110.
3. Wertz DC. Society and the not-so-new genetics: what are we afraid of? Some future predictions from a social scientist. *J Contemp Health Law & Policy.* 1997;13:299–345.
4. Hereditary Diseases Programme. *Guidelines on ethical issues in medical genetics and provision of genetics services.* Geneva: World Health Organization, 1995.
5. Hereditary Diseases Programme. *Proposed international guidelines on ethical issues in medical genetics and genetic services.* Geneva: World Health Organization, 1997.
6. Beauchamp TL. Childress JF. *Principles of Biomedical Ethics.* 4th ed. New York: Oxford University Press; 1995.
7. See note 4, preface.
8. D'Alton ME, Malone FD, Chelmow D, et al. Defining the role of fluorescence in situ hybridization on uncultured amniocytes for prenatal diagnosis of aneupolidies. *Am J Ob & Gyne.* 1997;176:769–774.
9. Lamvu G, Kuller JA. Prenatal diagnosis using fetal cells from the maternal circulation. *Obstet & Gynecol Surv.* 1997;52:433–437.
10. Lo YM, Corbetta N, Chamberlain PF, et al. Presence of fetal DNA in maternal plasma and serum. *Lancet* 1997;350:485–487.
11. National Advisory Board on Ethics in Reproduction. Isolating fetal cells in maternal blood—the importance of ethical reflection. *Naber Report.* 1996;2:12,5.
12. Elias S, Annas GJ. *Reproductive Genetics and the Law.* Chicago: Year Book Medical Publishers; 1987:68–76.
13. Halliday J, Lumley J, Watson L. Comparison of women who do and do not have amniocentesis or chorionic villus sampling. *Lancet.* 1995;345:704–709.
14. Harris R, Wertz DC. Ethics and Medical Genetics in the United Kingdom. In: Wertz DC, Fletcher JC, eds. *Ethics and Human Genetics: A Cross-cultural Perspective.* Heidelberg: Springer-Verlag; 1989:388–418.
15. See note 9 at p. 405.
16. Duster T. *Backdoor to Eugenics.* New York: Routledge; 1990.
17. Kitcher P. *The Lives to Come.* New York: Simon & Schuster; 1996:199.
18. Clark SL, DeVore GR. Prenatal diagnosis for couples who would not consider abortion. *Obstet & Gynecol.* 1989;73:1035–1037.
19. Chitty LS, Barnes CA, Berry C. Continuing with pregnancy after a diagnosis of lethal abnormality; experience of five couples and recommendations for management. *Brit Med J.* 1996;313:478–480.
20. National Institutes of Health. *Antenatal diagnosis.* Bethesda, MD: NIH Publ. No. 80–1973, 1979;I 39–42.

21. Wertz DC, Fletcher JC. Ethical and social issues in prenatal sex selection: a survey of geneticists in 37 nations. *Soc Sci Med.* 1998 Jan; 46(2):255–273.

22. *New York Times.* New Chinese law prohibits sex-screening of fetuses. 1994;A5.

23. Jayaraman KS. India bans the use of sex screening tests. *Nature.* 1994;370:320.

24. Calaca C, Akin A. The issue of sex selection in Turkey. *Hum Reprod.* 1995;10:1631–1632.

25. Sen A. More than 100 million women are missing. *NY Rev Books.* 1990;20:61–66.

26. Coale AJ, Banister J. Five decades of missing females in China. *Demog.* 1994;31:459–479.

27. United Nations. *The world's women, 1970–1990: trends and statistics.* New York: United Nations; 1991.

28. Wertz DC, Rosenfield JM, Janes SR, et al. Attitudes toward abortion among parents of children with cystic fibrosis. *Am J Publ Healt.* 1991;81:992–996.

29. Hulten M, Needham P. Preventing infanticide. *Nature.* 1987;325:190.

30. Wertz DC, Fletcher JC. Fatal knowledge? Prenatal diagnosis and sex selection. *Hastings Cent Rep.* 1989;19:21–27.

31. United States. President's Commission for the Study of Ethical Problems in Medicine and Biomedical and Behavioral Research. *Screening and counseling for genetic conditions.* Washington, DC: US Government Printing Office; 1983:58.

32. Institute of Medicine. Committee on Assessing Genetic Risks. *Assessing genetic risks.* Washington, DC: National Academy Press; 1994:105.

33. McCullough LB, Chervenak FA. Ethics in Obstetrics and Gynecology. New York: Oxford University Press; 1994:210–211.

34. See note 21.

35. Robertson JA. Genetic selection of offspring characteristics. *Boston U Law Rev.* 1996;76:454–463.

36. See note 19.

37. Council of Europe. Convention on human rights and biomedicine. Article 14. Strasbourg, 1966.

38. Warren MA. *Gendercide: The Implications of Sex Selection.* Totowa, NJ: Rowman & Allenheld; 1985.

39. Verma IC, Singh B. Ethics and medical genetics in India. In: Wertz DC, Fletcher JC, eds. *Ethics and Human Genetics: A Cross-cultural Perspective.* Heidelberg: Springer-Verlag; 1989:250–270.

40. Rothman BK. *The Tentative Pregnancy.* New York: Norton; 1986.

41. Sjögren, B. Parental attitudes to prenatal information about the sex of the fetus. *Acta Obstet Gyn Scand.* 1988;67:43–46.

42. Dixon RD, Levy DE. Sex of children: a community analysis of preferences and predetermination attitudes. *Sociol Quart.* 1985;26:251–271.

43. Warren MA. The ethics of sex preselection. In: Alpern KD, ed. *The Ethics of Reproductive Technology.* New York: Oxford University Press; 1992:232–246.

44. Overall C. *Ethics and Human Reproduction: A Feminist Analysis.* Boston: Allen & Unwin; 1987.

45. Clark RD, Fletcher JC, Peterson G. Conceiving a fetus for bone marrow donation: an ethical problem in prenatal diagnosis. *Prenat Diag.* 1989;9:329–334 (retraction in *Prenat Diag.* 1990;10:549).

46. Ekwo EE, Kim JO, Gosselink C. Parental perceptions of the burden of disease. *Am J Med Genet.* 198;955–963.

47. See note 28.

48. Payer L. *Medicine and Culture: Varieties of Treatment in the USA, England, West Germany, and France.* New York: Penguin Books; 1988.

49. Powledge TM, Fletcher JC. Guidelines for the ethical, legal, and social issues in prenatal diagnosis. *N Engl J Med.* 1979;300:168.

50. Juengst ET. Prenatal diagnosis and the ethics of uncertainty. In: Monagle JF, Thomasma DC, eds. *Medical Ethics: A Guide For Health Professionals.* Rockville, MD: Aspen; 1988.

51. Danish Council of Ethics. *Fetal diagnosis and ethics: a report.* Ravnsborggade 2-4, DK-2200 Copenhagen N; 1991:58.

52. Cowan RS. Genetic technology and reproductive choice: an ethics for autonomy. In: Kevles DJ, Hood L, eds. *Code of Codes: Scientific and Social Issues in the Human Genome Project.* Cambridge, MA: Harvard University Press; 1992:244–263.

53. Holmes-Siedle M, Ryyanen M, Lindenbaum RH. Parental decisions regarding termination of pregnancy following prenatal detection of sex chromosome abnormalities. *Prenat Diag.* 1987;7:239–244.

54. Council of Europe. Recommendation R(90)13 of the Committee of Ministers to member states on prenatal genetic screening, prenatal genetic diagnosis, and associated genetic counseling. In: Texts of the Council of Europe on Biomedical Matters. Strasbourg;1993:53–55, CDBI/INF (93)2.

55. See note 3, pp. 336–7.

56. Black RB. Psychosocial issues in genetic testing and pregnancy loss. *Fetal Diagn Ther.* 1993;8(suppl 1).

57. Black RB: A 1 and 6 month follow-up of prenatal diagnosis patients who lost pregnancies. *Prenat Diagn.* 1989;9:795–799.

58. See note 1, p. 322.

59. See note 28.

60. Fletcher JC, Evans MI. Maternal bonding in early fetal ultrasound examinations. *N Engl J Med.* 1983;308:392–393.

61. Stewart KS, Johnson MP, Quintero RA, et al. Congenital abnormalities in twins: selective termination. *Curr Opinion in Ob & Gyn.* 1997;9:136–139.

62. Evans MI, Fletcher JC, Zador IE, et al. Selective first-trimester termination in octuplet and quadruplet pregnancy: clinical and ethical issues. *Obstet Gynecol.* 1988;71:289–296.

63. Fletcher JC, Isada NB, Pryde PG, et al. Fetal intracardiac potassium chloride injection to avoid the hopeless resuscitation of an abnormal abortus: II. Ethical issue. *Ob & Gyn.* 1992;80:130–133.

64. Chervenak FA, McCullough LB. An ethically justified, clinically comprehensive management strategy for third-trimester pregnancies complicated by fetal anomalies. *Obstet Gynecol.* 1990;75:311–316.

65. See note 33, pp. 211–223.

66. Hearn WO. *Abortion Practice.* Boulder, CO: Alpenglo Graphics; 1990.

67. Schroeder-Kurth TM, Huebner J. Ethics and medical genetics in the Federal Republic of Germany. In: *Ethics and Human Genetics. A Cross-cultural Perspective.* Heidelberg: Springer-Verlag; 1989:156–175.

68. Asch A. Disability: I. Attitudes and social perspectives. In: Reich WT, ed. *Encyclopedia of Bioethics.* 2nd ed. New York: Simon & Schuster Macmillan; 1995:602–608.

69. See note 40.

70. Asch A, Geller G. Feminism, bioethics, and genetics. In: Wolf SM, ed. *Feminism and Bioethics. Beyond Reproduction.* New York: Oxford University Press; 1996:318–350.

71. Motulsky A, Murray J. Will prenatal diagnosis with selective abortion affect society's attitude toward the handicapped? In: Berg K, Tranoy KE, eds. *Research Ethics.* New York: Alan R. Liss; 1983.

72. Wertz DC, Fletcher JC. A critique of some feminist challenges to prenatal diagnosis. *J Women's Health.* 1993;2:173–188.

73. Yankauer A. What infant mortality tells us. *Am J Publ Health.* 1990;80:653–659.

74. See note 20, p. I–29.

75. See note 32, p. 72.

AN ETHICAL FRAMEWORK FOR FETAL THERAPY

Frank A. Chervenak / Laurence B. McCullough

INTRODUCTION

Research into new forms of fetal therapy raise a number of scientific, clinical, and ethical challenges for physicians. At this time, the most significant area, clinically and ethically, in which fetal therapy is now being developed is fetal surgery. Therefore, we make fetal therapy the major focus of this chapter.

Research in fetal surgery involves repair of a fetal anomaly either through a hysterotomy or endoscopy. Such invasive procedures create risks of harm yet potential benefit to both the pregnant woman and the fetal patient. The risks for pregnant women include morbidity and (rarely) mortality associated with major surgery and anesthesia, psychosocial risks of losing a pregnancy or living with the burden of iatrogenic injury to a future child, and risks to future pregnancies from uterine rupture. Risks for the fetal patient include iatrogenic prematurity and injury, and (rarely) death from anesthesia and surgical procedures. Potential benefits of fetal surgery are reduction of mortality and/or improvement in functional status for the fetal patient and future child; and, consequently, psychosocial benefit to the pregnant woman and her family. Although fetal surgery has been attempted to correct a variety of fetal anomalies, including meningomyelocele, diaphragmatic hernia, cystic adenomatoid malformation of the lung, and sacrocogygeal terratoma, at this time fetal surgery should not be considered or offered to pregnant women as standard fetal therapy. Indeed, investigation in this area is being conducted under research protocols at a small number of centers of excellence.[1–6]

Medical innovation, especially regarding surgical interventions, has frequently been unmanaged: interventions have gone from innovation to standard of care without adequate scientific and ethical evaluation.[7] Mammary artery ligation for the management of angina is a classic example of this phenomenon. Poorly managed and evaluated surgical innovation can impair scientific progress and put the health and lives of patients at unnecessary risk. Fetal surgery, until recently, has had a history of unmanaged innovation, but has impacted far fewer patients. Recent innovations in fetal surgery for spina bifida, a relatively common anomaly that is usually diagnosed in the second trimester, raise the possibility of fetal surgery for a greater number of patients.[1–5] These developments challenge physicians to conduct ongoing innovations in fetal surgery in an ethically responsible fashion,[8] for which there is widespread support in the professional community.[9] This chapter provides a comprehensive ethical framework for the responsible management of fetal therapy research from innovation to standard of care, and applies this framework to an analysis of research on fetal surgery for spina bifida because it is an important, controversial area of such research.

We base our 5-part framework on a central concept of obstetric ethics—the concept of the fetus as a patient.[10] We, first, identify ethical criteria for preliminary investigation for new fetal therapies; second, identify ethical criteria for initiation of clinical trials and for assessment of the results of such trials, ie, whether they establish a standard of care; third, describe the informed consent process that should be followed for research; fourth, consider whether selection criteria should include abortion preferences of the woman; and, fifth, consider whether practicing physicians have an obligation to offer referral to clinical trials of investigation of new fetal therapies. We, then, apply this 5-part ethical framework to investigational fetal surgery for spina bifida.

THE FETUS AS A PATIENT

To say that something has moral status means that we have obligations to protect and promote its interests. The authors have argued elsewhere that the concept of the fetus as a patient should not be understood in terms of the independent moral status of the fetus, ie, some feature(s) of the fetus that are independent of other entities—including the pregnant woman, physician, and the state—generates obligations to it.[10,11] We believe that all such attempts to establish independent moral status to the fetus end in failure because there are irreconcilable differences among the theological methods that have been deployed over the centuries of debate about the independent moral status of the fetus.[10]

Another, more clinically useful, line of argument is that the moral status of the fetus depends on whether it is reliably expected to achieve the relatively unambiguous moral status of becoming a child and, still later, the unambiguous moral status of becoming a person. When reliable links exist between a fetus and its later achieving the moral status of a child and then person, the fetus is a patient. There are 2 such links that pertain: one to the viable and the other to the previable fetus.

The first link between a fetus and its later achieving moral status as a child, and then person, is viability: the ability of the fetus to exist ex utero. Viability requires levels of technological intervention necessary to support immature or impaired anatomy and physiology through delivery when childhood begins, and into the second year of life, a time at which, it has been argued, personhood exists.[10] Viability is therefore *not* an intrinsic characteristic of the fetus, but a function of *both* biology and technology. In developed countries, fetal viability occurs at approximately the 24th week of gestational age, as determined by competent and reliable ultrasound dating.[12] When the viable fetus and the pregnant woman are presented to the physician, the viable fetus is a patient.

The second link between a fetus and its later achieving moral status as a child, and then person, is the autonomous decision of the pregnant woman to continue a previable pregnancy to viability and thus to term. This is because the only link between a previable fetus and its later achieving moral status as a child, and later person, is the pregnant woman's autonomy, which is exercised in the decision not to terminate her pregnancy, because technological factors do not exist that can sustain the previable fetus ex utero. When the pregnant woman decides not to terminate her pregnancy and when the previable fetus and pregnant woman are presented to the physician, the previable fetus becomes a patient.[10]

In summary, the viable fetus, when the pregnant woman presents for medical care, is a patient. The previable fetus is a patient as a function of the pregnant woman's decision to confer this status on the fetus and present herself for care. We cannot overemphasize that the existence of a fetal research project does not establish that the fetus is a patient, because, by definition, research interventions have not been established as clinically beneficial to the fetus. A pregnant woman's decision to enroll in scientific investigation of a new fetal therapy does not mean that the previable fetus irrevocably has the status of being a patient because before viability the pregnant woman can withdraw the status of being a patient from her fetus even after having earlier conferred that status.

Beneficence is an ethical principle that obligates the physician to seek a greater balance of clinical goods over clinical harms in patient care.[10] When the fetus is a patient, the physician has beneficence-based obligations to protect its life and health. These obligations must in all cases be considered along with beneficence-based and autonomy-based obligations to the pregnant woman.[10,11] Therefore, ethical criteria to guide innovation in fetal therapy must take account of beneficence-based obligations to the fetal patient and beneficence-based and autonomy-based obligations to the pregnant woman.[6] Failure to consider *all* of these obligations results in an inadequate ethical framework to guide innovations in fetal therapy.

ETHICAL CRITERIA FOR A INITIATION AND ASSESSMENT OF CLINICAL TRIALS OF NEW FETAL THERAPIES

Innovation in fetal therapy should begin with animal models that are carefully designed, sufficiently powered, and rigorously evaluated. The next step is the design of an intervention and its implementation in the form of a single case or limited case series. In our view, this approach is necessary to determine the feasibility, safety, and efficacy of new fetal therapies. Potential subjects should be protected from potentially harmful innovation.

We now identify 3 criteria, all of which must be satisfied, in order to conduct preliminary investigations in an ethically responsible fashion, ie, one that takes into account beneficence-based obligations to the fetal patient and beneficence-based and autonomy-based obligations to the pregnant woman. The previable fetus is a patient in these cases because by virtue of the woman's decision to continue her pregnancy, in order to have the opportunity to gain the potential benefits of the innovation. She remains free to withdraw that status before

viability. The viable fetus is a patient in these cases by virtue of viability.

1. The proposed fetal therapy is reliably expected, on the basis of previous animal studies, either to be lifesaving or to prevent serious and irreversible disease, injury, or handicap for the fetus;
2. Among possible alternative designs, the proposed fetal therapy is designed in such a way as to involve the least risk of mortality and morbidity to the fetal patient (which is required by beneficence and will satisfy the U.S. research requirement of minimized risk to the fetus);[13] and
3. On the basis of animal studies and analysis of theoretical risks both for the current and future pregnancies of the woman, the mortality risk to the pregnant woman is reliably expected to be low and the risk of disease, injury, or handicap to the pregnant woman is reliably expected to be low or manageable.[6]

The first 2 criteria implement beneficence-based obligations to the fetal patient. Research on animal models should reliably suggest that there would be therapeutic benefit without disproportionate disease-related or iatrogenic fetal morbidity or mortality. If animal studies result in high rates of mortality or morbidity for the fetal subject, then therapeutic innovation should not be introduced to human subjects until these rates improve in subsequent animal studies.

The third criterion, although it does not directly involve the fetus, is important because fetal therapy, especially fetal surgery, is also invasive to the pregnant woman. This criterion reminds investigators that the willingness of a subject, in this case the pregnant woman, to consent to risk does not by itself establish whether the risk to benefit ratio is favorable. Instead, investigators have an independent beneficence-based obligation to protect human subjects from unreasonably risky research and should use beneficence-based, risk-benefit analyses. The phrase "maternal-fetal surgery" is useful if it reminds investigators of the need for such comprehensive clinical ethical analysis. If this phrase is used to systematically subordinate fetal interests to maternal interest and rights, thus undermining the concept of the fetus as a patient in favor of the concept that the fetus is merely a part of the pregnant woman, we reject this phrase.

Randomized clinical trials commence when clinical equipoise emerges from the innovation. Clinical equipoise means that there is "a remaining disagreement in the expert clinical community, despite the available evidence, about the merits of the intervention to be tested."[14] Brody notes that one challenge here is identifying how much disagreement can remain for there still to be equipoise.[14] Lilford has suggested that if, reliably measured, two thirds of the expert community, measured reliably, then no longer disagrees, equipoise is not satisfied.[15] When the experimental intervention is more harmful than nonintervention, equipoise cannot be achieved.

We propose that the satisfaction of the previous 3 criteria with slight modifications should count as equipoise in the expert community.

1. The initial case series indicates that the proposed fetal therapy is reliably expected either to be lifesaving or to prevent serious and irreversible disease, injury, or handicap;
2. Among possible alternative designs, the proposed fetal therapy continues to involve the least risk of morbidity and mortality to the fetus; and
3. The case series indicates that the mortality risk to the pregnant woman is reliably expected to be low and the risk of disease, injury, or handicap to the pregnant woman, including for future pregnancies, is reliably expected to be low or manageable.[6]

One good test for the satisfaction of the first and third criteria is significant trends in the data from the case series. When equipoise has been achieved on the basis of these 3 criteria, randomized clinical trials should commence. They should have relevant and clearly defined primary and secondary endpoints and a design adequately powered to measure these endpoints.

The above 3 criteria can be used in a straightforward manner to define rules for terminating such a clinical trial. When the data support a rigorous clinical judgement that the first or third criterion is not satisfied, the trial should be stopped. When the clinical trial is completed, its outcome can be assessed to determine whether the innovative fetal therapy should be regarded as standard of care. The trial results should meet the following 3 criteria in order to establish the innovation as standard of care:

1. The proposed fetal therapy has a significant probability of being lifesaving or preventing serious or irreversible disease, injury, or handicap for the fetus;
2. The proposed fetal therapy involves low mortality and low or manageable risk of serious and irreversible disease, injury, or handicap to the fetus; and
3. The mortality risk to the pregnant woman is low and the risk of disease, injury or handicap is low or manageable, including for future pregnancies.[6]

Brody has underscored the value of data safety and monitoring boards to prevent investigator bias and to protect subjects.[14] Such boards should be used in research on fetal therapies, especially to ensure adherence of the abovementioned ethical criteria as a basis for monitoring such research.

INFORMED CONSENT

The informed consent process should always be led by physicians competent to explain the surgical and anesthetic interventions, alternatives, benefits, and risks. Having a physician lead the consent process who is not involved in the research project is an acceptable alternative only if that physician possesses the requisite competence.

Like all consent processes for human subject research,[16] counseling the pregnant woman about initial innovation or clinical trials should be rigorously nondirective, in that the physician should not recommend for or against participation. Investigators should emphasize the distinction between research and treatment to prevent therapeutic misconception. This is the be-

lief of patients that research, like treatment, will be beneficial and not involve disadvantages that do not occur in the therapeutic setting, e.g., the beliefs that the purpose of a randomized trial is to treat his or her condition or that his or her physician will select the best treatment for his or her condition.[17] The words "treatment" or "therapy," therefore, should *not* be used by investigators to describe the intervention. The investigators should be explicit about the fact that the surgical and anesthetic techniques are research or experimentation. Potential subjects in a case series should be told about the results of animal studies and potential subjects in clinical trials should be told about the results of the case series. The nature of the surgical and anesthetic procedures should be described to the pregnant woman in detail, including the risks to both her and the fetus. The alternatives of termination of pregnancy and of postpartum management must be presented, along with their benefits and risks.

In the consent process, words such as "mother," "father," and "baby" should *not* be used by investigators, because these suggest moral relationships and moral statuses that do not apply.[18] Words such as "pregnant woman," "potential father," "fetus," and "fetal patient" should be used instead. The pregnant woman should be clearly informed that she is under no obligation to the fetal patient to enroll it in a clinical research project.

Clinical experience teaches that in fetal research there can be considerable internal and external pressure on women to enroll. Therefore the consent process should be altered to mitigate these effects. The woman should have time to reflect on her decision, ask questions, and have her questions answered to her satisfaction. To protect a woman from being coerced, her husband or partner and other family members should be reminded that while they may have strong views for or against her participation, their role should be to support and respect her decision-making process and its outcome. Their relationship to her is primarily an obligation to respect and support her decision. Family members do not have the right to make decisions for her. Family members may be involved in the informed consent process according to the woman's preferences in this matter.

Principal investigators should insure that everyone involved in the consent process takes a strictly nondirective approach. While not currently required in federal consent regulations, prospective monitoring of the consent process, e.g., in random sampling, should be used to enforce a nondirective approach.

Publicity about either a case series investigation or a clinical trial should be nondirective because it is the first step in the informed consent process. Press releases, media interviews, patient education materials, Web sites, and other forms of publicity should be strictly nondirective. The above restrictions on word choice should be followed strictly. "Science by press conference" should be avoided. The data and safety monitoring board should assume oversight responsibilities in these areas.

Investigators may face an ethical challenge when a pregnant woman refuses to enter a randomized trial and insists on access to a proposal fetal therapy. Depending on the results of the trial, the investigator should explain that the assumption that the proposed intervention would benefit the fetal patient has no scientific basis and that, on balance, the experimental intervention could turn out to be harmful. Acquiescing to such requests only encourages and potentially exploits false hopes. The ethically justified response is to refuse all such requests, no matter how insistent. Institutional review boards should refuse requests for compassionate exceptions.

SELECTION CRITERIA BASED ON ABORTION PREFERENCE

In general, it is an accepted feature of study design in general that clinical trials should be conducted in such a way as to control for the idiosyncratic effects of patients' preferences on results. This, for example, justifies such strategies as randomization and blinding.

For research on fetal therapies this general rule of study design raises 2 significant ethical problems. First, from the perspective of investigators, to get the cleanest results about outcomes for fetuses and future children one would not want any pregnancies in which fetal research occurred to result in elective abortions. Second, from the perspective of pregnant women who would accept elective termination, it might be desirable to prevent, through abortion before viability, adverse outcomes of fetal research.

To address the first problem, study design would exclude women who indicated any willingness to consider elective abortion. To address the second problem, study design would exclude women who were opposed to abortion. These solutions share a disabling ethical problem: such a study design decides for the pregnant woman whether the previable fetus is or is not a patient, an unjustifiable violation of her autonomy in favor of research considerations.

To avoid this unacceptable ethical problem, there should be no exclusion criteria in research on fetal therapies based on willingness to countenance elective abortion. Study designs would therefore have to include elective abortion and birth of adversely affected infants as endpoints. In addition, investigators should understand that the decision of a pregnant woman to enroll herself and her previable fetus in research does not mean that she has irrevocably conferred the status of being a patient on the previable fetus-subject. In the informed consent process principal investigators should emphasize this point.

COOPERATION OF PRACTICING PHYSICIANS WITH CLINICAL INVESTIGATION

It is widely accepted that physicians are justified in informing their patients about relevant clinical investigations, and with the patients' consent, referring them to the investigators. In our view, there is also an ethical obligation to do so. The justification for this ethical obligation cannot appeal to benefit the pregnant woman or fetal patient because, by definition, the existence of clinical investigation does not establish clinical benefit. However, there is an obligation to future patients,

pregnant women and fetuses alike, to establish whether investigative fetal intervention improves the current standard of care or not. Physicians should take seriously their obligation to future patients to assure that innovation has the opportunity to be validated scientifically and ethically, rather than introduced in an unmanaged fashion or simply ignored.

APPLICATION OF ETHICAL FRAMEWORK TO INVESTIGATIONAL SURGERY FOR SPINA BIFIDA

Research on the surgical management of spina bifida in fetuses has been controversial and is currently being applied to this common fetal anomaly. Animal investigation of fetal surgery for spina bifida suggested that there would be therapeutic benefit without disproportionate morbidity or mortality.[2] The 3 criteria for investigation with human subjects of feasibility, safety, and efficacy were therefore satisfied.

The results of the case series reported in the literature and clinical experience meet the 3 criteria for equipoise. There has been reduction in the Arnold-Chiari malformation and subsequent reduction in the necessity for shunt placement with the prevention of mortality and morbidity associated with this malformation. Improvement in spinal cord function and overall functional status and quality of life have not been clearly demonstrated. The intervention continues to have very low rates of fetal mortality and maternal morbidity.[3,4]

Equipoise having been established, it is both ethically justified and warranted to undertake a well designed, randomized clinical trial in the few centers qualified to perform the procedure. Such a trial should have well defined endpoints. There are 2 main clinical concerns about spina bifida. First, it results in loss of motor and sensory function of the lower extremities, as well as bowel and bladder impairment. Second, the associated Arnold-Chiari malformation results in hydrocephalus with its resultant shunt dependency and complications. The primary endpoints of the clinical trial should address these outcomes as well as rates of fetal and maternal surgical complications and iatrogenic prematurity.

Equipoise means that there is no established benefit for the procedure and that it should be investigated according to scientific standards. This means that the procedure should not be offered outside the context of a clinical trial, even in response to the most urgent requests of pregnant women or referral by colleagues for the procedure. This restriction is a powerful antidote to the problem of the technological imperative, i.e., the idea that if something can be done it should be done.

Rules for termination of the study should be established at the beginning of the trial and their application should be based on statistical evidence of clear net benefit or net harm. The data and safety monitoring board should approve the study design and endpoints, define the stopping rules, and set up a procedure to closely monitor the trial, including recruitment of patients and the informed consent process.

The informed consent process should be rigorously nondirective, which will be challenging for physicians who have participated in the innovation phase and have championed the procedure. Expressions of clinical judgment about the benefits of the procedure or other forms of enthusiasm have no place in the informed consent process for a randomized clinical trial. Consent forms, as well as websites and other marketing materials, should take great care with word choice, as described above. In particular, there should be no use of words such as "treatment" or "therapy." Instead, "research," "experimental intervention," and the like should be used. The use of such language in both oral and written communication is a powerful antidote to the problem of therapeutic misconception.[17] It should also be made abundantly clear to the pregnant woman and her partner that she is under no obligation to place herself or her fetus in the clinical trial because no benefit from the procedure has been established and it might prove, on balance, to be harmful.

Selection criteria should make no reference to the woman's willingness to terminate or continue pregnancy before or during the trial. The consent process should make clear to her that her preferences for the disposition of her pregnancy will be respected, just as they would in a nonexperimental, clinical setting.

Participating centers should report the results of the research at professional meetings and in the scientific literature. Only after reports have appeared in the scientific literature should inquiries by the lay press be accommodated and addressed.

Referring physicians should be clear that the procedure remains experimental and is available in a clinical trial. They should emphasize that this means that the benefits and risks of the procedure have not been established and, therefore, there is no obligation on the part of the pregnant woman or her fetus to enroll in the trial. Her judgment about the importance of her obligation to future pregnancies and fetal patients should be explored nondirectively.

CONCLUSION

It has long been recognized that the development of new fetal therapies raises significant ethical issues.[19,20] In this chapter we provided an ethical framework for responsibly managing the transition from initial innovation of fetal therapies to clinical trials, and then to offering the therapies to pregnant women as a standard of care for the management of fetal anomalies. We have shown that the informed consent process for innovation and research should be strictly nondirective, and emphasized that the pregnant woman has no ethical obligation to enroll the fetal patient and herself in such investigations. We have also shown that selection criteria based on abortion preference, pro or con, have no place in the ethical design of fetal research. We also argued that the practice community has an obligation to offer referral to clinical investigation of new fetal therapies.

In our view, the ethical integrity of all forms of fetal research is just as important as their scientific integrity. The current controversy concerning clinical investigation of fetal surgery for spina bifida, as well as still-to-be-developed fetal therapies, can be reliably addressed using this ethical framework.

References

1. Harrison MR, Golbus MS, Filly RA, eds. *UnbornPatient.* 2nd ed. Orlando: Grune & Stratton; 1991.
2. Meuli M, Meuli-Simmen C, Hutchins GM, et al. In utero surgery rescues neurological function at birth in sheep with spina bifida. *Nat Med.* 1995;1:342–347.
3. Bruner JP, Tulipan N, Paschall RL, et al. Fetal surgery for myelomeningocele and the incidence of shunt-dependent hydrocephalus. *JAMA.* 1999;282:1819–1825.
4. Sutton LN, Adzick NS, Bilaniuc LT, et al. Improvement in hindbrain herniation demonstrated by serial fetal magnetic resonance imaging following fetal surgery for myelomeningocele. *JAMA.* 1999; 282:1826–1831.
5. Simpson JL. Fetal Surgery for Myelomeningocele. Promise, progress and problems. *JAMA.* 1999;282:1873–1874.
6. Chervenak FA, McCullough LB. A comprehensive ethical framework for fetal research and its application to fetal surgery for spina bifida. *Am J Obstet Gynecol.* 2002;187:10–14.
7. Frader JE, Caniano DA. Research and innovation in surgery. In: McCullough LB, Jones JW, Brody BA, eds. *Surgical Ethics.* New York: Oxford University Press; 1998:216–241.
8. Lyerly AD, Gates EA, Cefalo RC, et al. Toward the ethical evaluation and use of maternal-fetal surgery. *Obstet Gynecol.* 2001;98:689–697.
9. Lyerly AD, Cefalo RC, Socol M, et al. Attitudes of maternal-fetal specialists concerning maternal-fetal surgery. *Am J Obstet Gynecol.* 2001;185:1052–1058.
10. McCullough LB, Chervenak FA. *Ethics in Obstetrics and Gynecology.* New York: Oxford University Press; 1994.
11. Chervenak FA, McCullough LB, Birnbach D: Ethics: an essential dimension of obstetric anesthesia. *Anes Analg.* In press.
12. Chervenak FA, McCullough LB. The limits of viability. *J Perinat Med.* 1997;25:418–420.
13. Department of Health and Human Services. *Regulations for the protection of human subjects.* 45 CFR 46.
14. Brody BA. *The Ethics of Biomedical Research: An International Perspective.* New York: Oxford University Press; 1998.
15. Lilford RJ. The substantive ethics of clinical trials. *Clin Obstet Gynecol.* 1992;35:837–845.
16. Faden RR, Beauchamp TL. *A History of Theory of Informed Consent.* New York: Oxford University Press; 1986.
17. Appelbaum PS, Roth LH, Lidz CW, et al. False hopes and best data: consent to research and the therapeutic misconception. *Hastings Cont Rep.* 1987;17:20–24.
18. DeCrespigny L, Chervenak F, McCullough L. Mothers and babies, pregnant women and fetuses. *Br J Obstet Gynaecol.* December 1999; 106(12):1235–1237.
19. Barclay WR, McCormick RA, Sidbury JB, et al. The ethics of in utero surgery. *JAMA.* October 2, 1981;246(14):1551–1552, 1554–1555.
20. Fletcher JC, Jonsen AR. Ethical considerations of fetal therapy. In: Harrison MR, Golbus MS, Filly RA, eds. *Unborn Patient.* 2nd ed. Orlando: Grune & Stratton; 1990:159–170.

LEGAL ISSUES IN GENETIC DIAGNOSIS AND COUNSELING

Charles W. Fisher / Carol Tarnowsky / Pamela A. Boland

Scientific advances now make it possible to control conception, to discover fetal injury, to detect genetically transmitted anomalies or defects prior to and after conception, and, in some cases, to treat and cure certain in utero abnormalities. A woman may choose to terminate a pregnancy by abortion when there is fear that the fetus will be born with significant, incorrectible defects or injuries.[1] As a consequence of the United States Supreme Court's decision in *Roe v. Wade*, these extraordinary advances in medical science are unfortunately accompanied by new risk factors for medical legal liability. In today's litigious society, virtually every aspect of patient care is scrutinized for potential liability with the ultimate goal of monetary recovery. Heightened awareness of the potential for lawsuits arising out of genetic counseling, diagnosis, and treatment will arm the health care provider with greater protection in those particular situations most likely to result in a potential lawsuit.

Some prenatal diagnostic issues present medical dilemmas that will not, and cannot, be easily solved by legal rulings or advice. For instance, liability for prenatal diagnostic ultrasound is one of the most common litigation scenarios in the area of genetics, both in terms of the failure to perform an ultrasound and the failure to identify anomalies. While first trimester ultrasound for gestational dating would *limit* potential legal exposure for failing to diagnose an in utero abnormality, late second trimester ultrasound provides more medical diagnostic information but, especially in cases of office ultrasound, exposes the physician to *greater liability* for abnormalities that might remain undiagnosed (or allegedly be missed) while performing ultrasounds at 16–22 weeks gestation.

This is merely one situation in which the question will eternally be asked whether or not one should perform a test or diagnostic procedure that may not be absolutely required since it may extend one's potential liability for failing to diagnose an abnormality. Legally, although you may not have a duty to perform a particular test or procedure,[2] *once you undertake the duty you are required to perform it within the standard of care.*[3]

It would be impossible to thoroughly discuss each and every potential fact scenario, diagnostic procedure, and so on, in the space provided for this chapter. Additionally, each state may have its own particular legal application for liability, damages, remedies, and criteria for such things as the age at which elective terminations can be performed. The object, therefore, of this chapter, is to address legal liability from the standpoint of those cases that are either commonly encountered, or that could subject the health care provider to significant monetary exposure.

We have therefore selected three areas for discussion:

1. Common legal claims in genetic testing and diagnosis;
2. Consent and informed consent for medical diagnosis and treatment of minors;
3. The pros, cons, and the current state of knowledge of chorionic villus sampling (CVS).

The health care provider should be mindful that there are certain professional witnesses or "experts" who are willing to say nearly anything for a price. These witnesses are often dishonest and outright fraudulent in their testimony. Although their medical positions as to the standard of care should be looked on with askance, they should not be ignored, as they are the very persons who may create your legal liability. Knowledge of their activities, as well as the lawsuit claims that they are willing to support, may provide insight for the health care provider as to procedural protections to safeguard his practice of the standard of care (consent forms, documentation, instructions, etc).

COMMON LEGAL CLAIMS IN GENETIC TESTING & DIAGNOSIS

The causes of actions that arise in the area of genetics generally target failure to perform appropriate testing or a failure to appropriately interpret the results of such tests. The legal claims made by a plaintiff, however, fall into category(ies) of wrongful death, wrongful life, wrongful birth, and negligent infliction of emotional distress, which are defined below. Most of the cases in this field have arisen subsequent to the United States Supreme Court's partial legitimization of abortion in *Roe v. Wade* (410 U.S. 113, 35 L.Ed. 2d 147, 93 S. Ct. 705 (1973)).[4]

Understanding specific legal claims that can be made, and the types of damages that can be recovered, is quite helpful to understanding what the lawsuit is about, how the physician should document in order to make the best attempts, and what the physician can expect if a lawsuit is filed.

WRONGFUL DEATH

In a wrongful death claim, plaintiff's estate contends that a death occurred that would have or could have been prevented by appropriate medical treatment. In the area of genetics, a wrongful death plaintiff alleges that appropriate testing or appropriate interpretation of test results would have revealed an abnormality that could have been treated in-utero or at delivery and that, had the same been done, death could have been avoided. Damages for wrongful death generally include the loss of companionship and mental anguish.

WRONGFUL BIRTH[5]

A *parent's* claim for wrongful birth rests upon the injury to the mother by virtue of the physician's negligence resulting in the deprivation of the right to make an informed choice to prevent the child's conception or to terminate the pregnancy via an abortion. Courts considering wrongful birth claims have been almost unanimous in recognizing a cause of action against a physician where it is alleged that, but for the defendant's negligence, the parent would have terminated the congenitally or genetically defective fetus by abortion.[6]

In courts recognizing this cause of action,[7] the parents must establish that a breach of duty by the physician deprived them of the opportunity to accept or reject the continuance of the pregnancy. The clear majority of courts considering these types of medical malpractice claims have concluded that there is a legally cognizable injury proximately caused by a breach of duty.[8]

The damages generally allowable are those that flow from this breach of duty; that is, the parents are generally entitled to the extraordinary expenses attendant in the care and treatment of the afflicted child but are generally offset by the cost of raising a normal child. That is, there are always costs associated with raising any child, and the parents should not be entitled to recover costs such as food, clothing, etc.

In cases of severe genetic defects but with an extended life expectancy, medical costs could certainly range in the millions of dollars. Because the legal liability of the parents to support their child terminates, depending upon the state, between the ages of 18–21, some courts also permit parents to recover the extraordinary costs associated with the child's affliction after the child has reached the age of majority. These courts reason that, under common law, where a child is incapable of supporting himself because of physical or emotional disabilities, the parents' obligation to support continues beyond the child's age of majority.[9]

In contrast to damages permissible in a wrongful death case, courts generally do not allow damages for loss of companionship or parental pain and suffering in a wrongful birth claim.[10] Such damages for wrongful birth have always been a difficult issue for the courts, for courts have found it philosophically impossible to determine the benefit/loss ratio between the joy the child brings to the lives of his/her parents and the disappointment in having a child afflicted with some genetic defect.

WRONGFUL LIFE

The wrongful life claim is one brought by the *child*, with a defect or anomaly, whose life would have been terminated via abortion but for the negligence of the defendant in failing to so inform the parent of the potentially anomalous child.[11] This is the other side of the wrongful birth claim; here, the child contends to have suffered harm or damage as a result of medical malpractice thus entitling the child to recover the extraordinary expenses associated with his/her disability.

Courts have systematically rejected wrongful life claims on two related grounds.[12] Initially, the courts have proven unwilling to hold that a child can recover damages for achieving life. The threshold problem has been the assertion by the infant plaintiff not that she should have been born without defect but that she should not have been born at all.

The essence of this claim is that the negligent conduct deprived the child's mother from obtaining an abortion, which would have terminated the fetus' existence. Resting on the belief that all human life, no matter how burdened by disability,

is, as a matter of law, always preferable to nonlife, the courts have declined to find that an infant afflicted by a genetic or congenital impairment has suffered a legally cognizable injury. Again, the courts have overwhelmingly determined that life hindered by disability is preferable to no life at all.[13]

The second basis relied upon by those courts in declining to recognize the wrongful life claim is the difficulty, if not impossibility, of measuring appropriate damages. The traditional tort remedy is compensatory in nature. The basic rule of tort compensation is to place the plaintiff in the position that s/he would have occupied absent the defendant's negligence.[14]

Applying this general rule, the damages recoverable on behalf of a child for wrongful life are thus limited to those necessary to restore the child to the position he would have occupied were it not for the alleged malpractice of the physician or other health-care provider. In a wrongful life case, there is no allegation that but for the defendant's negligence the child would have had a healthy, unimpaired life. Rather, the claim is that without the defendant's negligence, the child would never have been born. Thus, the cause of action involves of a calculation of damages dependent upon the relative benefits of an impaired life as opposed to no life at all, a comparison that courts have deemed the law not equipped to make.[15]

LACK OF INFORMED CONSENT

Where diagnostic tests are not offered to maternal patients, the parents may subsequently file a cause of action alleging the physician's failure to obtain informed consent. Specifically, plaintiffs maintain that a physician's failure to inform a patient about the benefits and risks of various types of treatments and tests, such as the MSAFP or amniocentesis, render the patient's "decision" to forego them uninformed.

There is a division among the jurisdictions regarding what constitutes informed consent in the area of prenatal testing. In a recent Maryland case, *Reed v. Campagnolo*,[16] the court found that a patient's informed consent must be to some treatment, and where a physician never proposes prenatal testing, plaintiff cannot establish this element. Whether the physician has a duty to offer or recommend the tests is analyzed in relation to the professional standard of care, and application of that standard may or may not produce a result identical with the informed consent criterion of what reasonable persons would want to know.[17]

The leading Maryland case on the issue of informed consent, *Sard v. Hardy*,[18] discussed the doctrine only in the context of treatment actually proposed by the physician. The Maryland court noted that the doctrine "follows logically from the universally recognized rule that a physician, treating a mentally competent adult under nonemergency circumstances, cannot properly undertake to perform surgery or administer other therapy without the prior consent of his or her patient. In order for the patient's consent to be effective, it must have been an "informed" consent, one that is given after the patient has received a fair and reasonable explanation of the contemplated treatment or procedure."[19] The doctrine of informed consent thus imposes upon a physician, before subjecting a patient to medical treatment, the duty to explain the procedure to the patient and to warn the patient of any material risks or dangers inherent in the treatment to thereby enable the patient to make an intelligent and informed choice about whether to undergo treatment.[20]

The duty to make full disclosure to patients requires a physician to reveal to the patient the nature of the patient's ailment, the nature of the proposed treatment, the probability of the success of the contemplated treatment and its alternatives, and the risks of unfortunate consequences associated with the proposed treatment.[21]

The *Reed* court noted that New York courts have held that a cause of action sounding in informed consent requires an affirmative act by the physician. In *Karlsons v. Guerinot*,[22] the plaintiffs contended that the defendant physician's failure to inform the plaintiffs of the risks involved with the mother's pregnancy, including the risk that she would give birth to a deformed child, gave rise to a cause of action for failing to obtain an informed consent to continuation of the pregnancy and to the delivery of the infant.[23]

In denying the cause of action, the court noted that actions based upon the doctrine of informed consent exist only where the injury suffered arises from an affirmative violation of the patient's physical integrity and, where nondisclosure is concerned, these risks are directly related to such affirmative treatment. Where the resultant harm arises not out of any affirmative violation of the woman's physical integrity and where the alleged undiagnosed risks do not relate to any affirmative treatment but to the condition of pregnancy itself, plaintiff has alleged the basis of an action of medical malpractice but not one of informed consent.[24]

The *Reed* court denied plaintiffs' recovery on this theory, noting that plaintiffs sought a rule that the appropriate tests for predictive genetic counseling would be determined by what reasonable persons similarly situated would want to know. The court determined, however, that the rule cannot focus exclusively on the plaintiff; rather, a fair rule would have to look at all of the possible tests that might be given and evaluate the reasons for excluding some and perhaps recommending one or more other tests. This requires expert testimony.[25]

Reaching a contradictory result was the State of Michigan in *Blair v. Hutzel Hospital*,[26] wherein the court determined that a physician's failure to advise an obstetrical patient about the availability of an MSAFP test subjected the physician to liability by depriving her of a substantial opportunity to achieve a better result.

As the Michigan Court of Appeals noted, a patient treats with a physician in order to improve opportunities to avoid, ameliorate, or reduce physical harm. An obstetrical patient treats with a physician to obtain the best possible care during pregnancy and to achieve the best possible outcome.[27] Thus, the court reasoned, the physician has a duty to ensure that a woman makes informed decisions regarding her procreative options, including the option of abortion. The failure to so inform a pregnant patient of testing that would afford her in-

formation upon which to base such a decision, is a breach of that duty.[28]

The court concluded that the element of causation is satisfied if a plaintiff can establish that the defendant's negligence in providing that information deprived her of a substantial opportunity to learn of the risks of bearing a child with birth defects and that, had she been provided with such information, she would have obtained an abortion.[29]

Again, whether a physician is required to offer to perform a diagnostic procedure will be the subject of debate in a negligence area. Where plaintiffs establish through expert testimony that a physician was negligent in failing to advise a patient of available testing and to offer the same to her, plaintiff may, in some jurisdictions, successfully bring a lack of informed consent claim in addition to the others discussed herein. Should the physician undertake the duty to discuss prenatal diagnostic testing, he or she undertakes the duty to thoroughly explain the same to afford the patient with a sufficient knowledge base upon which to base her informed consent.

NEGLIGENT INFLICTION OF EMOTIONAL DISTRESS

In addition to seeking compensation for the extraordinary expenses inherent in managing and treatment of a child with a disability, parents often seek damages for their emotional distress, which they contend to be a natural and foreseeable consequence of the injury sustained and thus should be compensable as well. There are various analyses applied throughout the United States with some jurisdictions specifically prohibiting recovery of emotional damages for prenatal or labor events, some allowing recovery due to the close nexus between a mother and her unborn child, and some allowing recovery only where the emotional distress has manifest itself in physical injury. The following is a brief overview of this negligence tort along with an example of the varied approaches taken within different jurisdictions.

Initially, the tort of negligent infliction of emotional distress was almost exclusively confined to cases in which the plaintiff sustained psychic injury as a direct result of witnessing the traumatic infliction of injury on a close relative by defendant's negligent act. In order to recover under this cause of action, a plaintiff was required to establish that he or she likewise sustained "physical impact." The evolutionary development of this tort later allowed for recovery without physical impact for a plaintiff who had witnessed harm come about to a close relative so long as the plaintiff was within the "zone of danger" of the negligent force of harm.

Under the "zone of danger rule," a bystander who is in a zone of physical danger and who, because of the defendant's negligence, has reasonable fear for his own safety is given a right of action for physical injury or illness[30] resulting from emotional distress.

Parents of an unborn child are not ipso facto in the zone of danger for negligence involving that child.[31] Thus, some jurisdictions have deemed parents to be outside of the zone of danger and precluded from recovering damages when negligent genetic counselling results in the birth of a hemophiliac child,[32] when hospital personnel allow a newborn to fall off a delivery table,[33] and when negligence is a factor in the delivery of a stillborn child.[34]

Interestingly, at least one jurisdiction that permits no bystander recovery for emotional distress damages nevertheless makes an exception for a mother during the birth of her child.[35] Specifically, the State of Connecticut has held that a mother is not a mere bystander at the birth of her own child,[36] reasoning that "to infer that a mother is a bystander at the birth of her infant manifests a basic misunderstanding of the duty owed a patient by a physician. In such circumstances, . . . the two are within the zone of danger, and the doctor owes a duty to each."[37] Connecticut courts thus determined that, contrary to being a witness or bystander to the inflicted injury, a plaintiff-mother is the very person to whom the obstetrician owes a duty and the very person directly injured by the physician's breach of that duty.[38] Under this analysis, when a child is injured due to negligent obstetrical care, the mother and child are joint victims of malpractice, not separate entities.[39] "To suggest that a mother engaging in the process of labor and delivery is a bystander to the event, or to try to sever out concerns for her own well-being versus concerns for the child within her, defies logic and reason. A mother's concerns during delivery for her own welfare and that of her child are so interwoven as to be legally inseparable. Where the child remains a part of the mother's physical being, concerns for the child's welfare during delivery procedures are concerns for the mother's well being."[40]

The seminal case in the area of bystander recovery is *Dillon v. Legg*, 68 Cal 2d 728, 69 Cal Rptr 72, 441 P2d 912 (1968), a decision that established a rule that a mother who was in close proximity and was an eyewitness to the striking of her child by an automobile could recover for physical injury resulting from emotional shock caused to her, even though the mother was not herself in the "zone of danger." *Dillon* extended liability to a bystander beyond the zone of danger and enunciated a test of reasonable foreseeability. To determine if the injury to the bystander was reasonably foreseeable, the court formulated 3 guidelines: (1) whether plaintiff was located near the scene of the accident as contrasted with one who was a distance away from it; (2) whether the shock resulted from a direct emotional impact upon plaintiff from the sensor and contemporaneous observance of the accident, as contrasted with learning of the accident from others after its occurrence; and (3) whether plaintiff and the victim were closely related, as contrasted with an absence of any relationship or the presence of only a distant relationship.[41]

The evolution of bystander recovery law in California after *Dillon* provides a background against which to view recovery by a parent for the negligent infliction of emotional distress as a result of injury to the parent's child. In *Jansen v. Children's Hosp Medical Center of East Bay*,[42] the court rejected a mother's claim for damages for emotional trauma caused by witnessing the progressive decline and ultimate death of her daughter in the hospital. The mother alleged that the child's

death resulted from malpractice by the hospital. The court found that *Dillon*'s requirement of sensory and contemporaneous observance of the accident, as contrasted with learning of the accident from others after its occurrence, contemplated a sudden and brief event causing the child's injury.

In *Justus v. Atchison*,[43] the court denied the claims of fathers who had witnessed the negligent delivery of their stillborn infants. The court found that the shock sustained by the father occurred when they were informed of the deaths of their infants later rather than at the time they observed the deaths contemporaneously with the event. Thus, although *Justus* implicitly approved *Jansen*'s sudden occurrence requirement, the case essentially involved a situation where the fathers were unaware of the connection between the defendants' conduct and the injury to their children.

Ochoa v. Superior Court of Santa Clara County,[44] found the "sudden occurrence" of *Jansen* and *Justus* to be an unwarranted restriction of the *Dillon* guidelines.[45] In *Ochoa*, a 13-year-old boy became seriously ill while confined to juvenile hall. His parents, to no avail, strenuously objected to the inadequate medical treatment their son was receiving. He died the day after he was admitted to the infirmary. *Ochoa* confirmed that parents were permitted to recover, even though the injury producing event was not sudden or accidental and even though its negligent cause was not immediately apparent. The court held that "when there is observation of the defendant's conduct and the child's injury and also contemporaneous awareness that the defendant's conduct or lack thereof is causing harm to the child, recovery is permitted."[46] In *Ochoa*, the mother's observation of her son's pain and suffering and his deteriorating condition, at the same time the defendants were failing to either properly care for him or to accede to her entreaties that she be allowed to obtain treatment for him, formed the basis of the emotional distress for which she sought recovery.

The view enunciated in *Ochoa* was reaffirmed in *Thing v. LaChusa* (48 Cal 3d 644, 257 Cal Rptr 865, 771 P2d 814 (1989)). The *Thing* court cautioned that the dictum in *Ochoa* suggesting that the factors noted in the *Dillon* guidelines were not essential in determining whether a plaintiff is a foreseeable victim of the defendant's negligence should not be relied upon.[47] In *Thing*, the court held that a mother who did not witness the accident in which an automobile struck and injured her son could not recover damages from the driver for emotional distress because "[s]he did not observe defendant's conduct and was not aware that her son was being injured."[48]

The *Thing* court repudiated foreseeability in emotional distress cases and formulated the test that a plaintiff may recover damages for emotional distress caused by observing the negligently inflicted injury of a third person only if the plaintiff (1) is closely related to the injury victim, (2) is present at the scene of the injury producing event at the time it occurs and is then aware that it is causing injury to the victim, and (3) as a result suffers serious emotional distress—a reaction beyond that which would be anticipated in a disinterested witness and which is not an abnormal response to the circumstances.[49]

Cases from other jurisdictions have followed *Dillon* and its progeny in requiring that the emotional impact to the immediate family member who is a bystander to medical malpractice must result from the sensory and contemporaneous observance of the tortuous conduct. For example, New Jersey disallowed recovery for parents of a 10-month old whose death was caused by medical misdiagnosis because there was no personal observation of a "shocking" event;[50] Connecticut declined to follow California cases and denied recovery for a daughter whose mother died as a result of medical malpractice that the daughter "may have observed;[51] Michigan recognized a cause of action for parents of a viable infant who was stillborn after medical providers failed to heed the parents' requests for evaluation and wherein the parents witnessed efforts to resuscitate the child;[52] Pennsylvania dismissed a complaint of the husband and daughter of decedent where neither alleged to have personally observed medical malpractice against the decedent;[53] New Jersey denied recovery by parents of a child who died 3 days after birth as a result of a condition that the physicians failed to diagnose and treat because the misdiagnosis was not an event observed by the parents.[54]

As the examples referenced illustrate, courts in the various jurisdictions approach actions for negligent infliction of emotional distress on a case-by-case basis. Further, although it is foreseeable that persons other than the injured party will suffer psychological trauma at witnessing an injury to a loved one, foreseeability of injury alone does not justify imposing liability for negligently caused emotional distress. Policy considerations dictate that courts establish restrictions on recovery for emotional distress, notwithstanding the sometimes arbitrary results.

TYPICAL MEDICAL/LEGAL SCENARIOS

Medical/legal claims in genetics arise generally as to issues of testing, interpretation, and follow-up. Subjects of dispute are usually the following:

(a) Failure to offer an alphafetoprotein (AFP) test;
(b) Failure to offer a double or a triple prenatal screen;
(c) Failure to offer an amniocentesis;
(d) Failure to act on abnormal results of either an AFP or an amniocentesis and the legal consequences thereof (proximate cause);
(e) Failure to perform an amniocentesis on a patient when the requesting patient will be younger than 35 years of age at delivery;
(f) Failure to diagnose an abnormality on ultrasound that is either treatable or could lead to early termination and potential damage recovery;
(g) Late diagnosis of chromosomal abnormality (after 24 weeks) and the failure to refer patient; and
(h) Damages for failure to terminate a normal baby and an abnormal baby.

These subjects are best illustrated by the case examples below. Both a legal theory for the action and the collectable damages are discussed.

CASE 1—FAILURE TO OFFER AFP

During prenatal care, the patient's obstetrician fails to offer her the option of an AFP test. Subsequently, the patient delivers an infant afflicted with Down syndrome. Karyotype testing reveals that the child indeed has a genetic abnormality. Thereafter, the mother sues the obstetrician for failing to offer an AFP test to diagnose the genetic abnormality.

Two separate causes of action will likely be contemplated: wrongful birth and wrongful life. Almost every court in the United States has allowed an action for wrongful birth in this circumstance, reasoning that the parent would have terminated the child, and the family would have avoided the delivery of a genetically defective infant. The courts have overwhelmingly disallowed wrongful life claims, reasoning that it is better to be born alive with a genetic defect rather than to have no life as a result of the pregnancy termination.

In contesting a cause of action based upon the failure to offer an AFP test, it should be remembered that the alphafetoprotein test is only about 25 percent accurate in screening for genetic defects. Therefore, *more likely than not*, an alphafetoprotein test will not raise the risk factor for genetic defect. Several states have addressed whether such a cause of action can be maintained in the absence of the usual "preponderance of the evidence" requirement. States are divided on this issue, some disallowing the cause of action because it is impossible to prove this element by a preponderance of evidence while others allow the action to proceed while limiting damages to the extent of the percentage of likelihood that the genetic defect would have been determined (24% times the dollar amount of damages). Those courts that have allowed such a cause of action to continue have actually changed the historical tort preponderance of the evidence requirement.

CASE 2—FAILURE TO OFFER DOUBLE OR TRIPLE SCREENING

A patient treating with her physician is not offered triple screening or double screening tests for genetic defects. Subsequently the child is born with an abnormal karyotype. The patient sues the physician contending that the patient would have terminated had she known a genetic defect existed. An alphafetoprotein test was performed but did not reveal an abnormality.

One of the significant questions in this particular case is whether or not the standard of care required double or triple screening. Currently, authors are divided on this issue, some recommending double screening while others recommend triple screening. However, it would appear that the current standard of care in 1997 requires at least double screening, which will enhance the ability to determine possible genetic defects by a significant factor well above alphafetoprotein tests alone.

The causes of action are essentially the same as those in Case 1; however, there is a distinction between the 2 factual situations, since with double screening and/or triple screening, the ability to determine possible genetic defects is probably above 50%. This, therefore, creates a real cause of action by way of the "preponderance of evidence" in every state.

CASE 3—FAILURE TO OFFER AMNIOCENTESIS

A 36 year old patient receiving prenatal care is not offered amniocentesis due to oversight. The patient receives double screening, the results of which are negative, but ultimately delivers a child afflicted with Trisomy 18. The patient, who would have terminated at or before 24 weeks, now brings a lawsuit against her physician for failure to offer an amniocentesis. The obstetrician responds by indicating that double screening was performed, which was negative.

Clearly, the standard of care requires that amniocentesis be offered to patients who will be 35 years or older at the time of delivery.

From a legal standpoint, double screening is not a defense because amniocentesis is nearly 100% accurate in determining abnormal karyotypes. Therefore, liability is fairly clear in this situation. The only real issue will be the amount of damages, which is dependent upon the particular jurisdiction and the needs of the particular child.

CASE 4—FAILURE TO TERMINATE A NORMAL CHILD

A husband and wife seek consultation and genetic karyotyping from their obstetrician to determine the gender of their child prior to 24 weeks. The family wishes to have a male child, having had several female children previously. Karyotyping is done through amniocentesis; however, there is a typographical error in the laboratory report, and the parents are advised that they are going to have a male child. At the time of birth, however, the mother and father discover that they have their sixth female child and are upset with the obstetrician and the hospital. The family sues both the obstetrician and the hospital alleging medical malpractice.

This is a cause of action *only* for wrongful birth. Since there is nothing abnormal about the child that was born, it cannot be a cause of action for wrongful life with damages due to a genetic abnormality.

Although there clearly was an error in diagnosis and management, the real question remains as to whether or not there is a cause of action. Courts have been reluctant to grant causes of action for wrongful birth under these circumstances where a normal, healthy child is born, regardless of gender. Many courts have determined that the happiness and joy brought to a family by a child as compared to whatever negative feelings the family has for that child due to the sex, or the birth itself,

it not actionable. Courts have determined that it is impossible for jurors to place values on the positive and negatives of such situations and render any type of verdict. Other courts have felt that it is against public policy for one to bring a lawsuit that essentially wishes that there child was dead.

A separate cause of action, similar to that of wrongful pregnancy, may be available to the mother seeking recovery for the discomfort and restrictions of pregnancy from 24–40 weeks where she establishes that she would have terminated the pregnancy prior to 24 weeks had gender been known. If married, the woman's spouse has a cause of action for loss of consortium for the disruption of his life occasioned by the continued pregnancy. However, as one can plainly see, this fact scenario would present very little damage potential.

Damages for the cost of raising a normal child have not yet been recognized by any courts in the United States. Therefore, these types of actions have very limited potential and limited exposure pending a change in the law.

CASE 5—FAILURE TO INFORM PATIENT OF ABNORMAL KARYOTYPE UNTIL AFTER 24 WEEKS

A patient visits her physician prenatally and informs the doctor that she had a child previously affected by Krabbe disease, a genetic syndrome. The physician orders a battery of laboratory tests, and it is determined by comparing her enzyme activity levels to controls that she likely is carrying another Krabbe affected baby in her current pregnancy. However, the physician fails to review the laboratory report when it arrives and does not discover this fact until the patient is 27 weeks. In the state where the physician practices, it is illegal to terminate the child at 24 weeks or greater. Upon discovering the error, the physician does not advise the patient of any of this, as he feels it is too late to terminate the pregnancy. Subsequently, the child is born and appears normal. Within a year, however, the child deteriorates neurologically secondary to Krabbe's disease and dies. The mother, having already gone through this previously now witnesses her second child dying from Krabbe's disease over the one year of life, suffering a slow neurological deterioration. As a result of this, the mother has a nervous breakdown, must quit her job, and becomes physically disabled to the point that she can no longer function in her normal household environment and take care of the family. The family brings a lawsuit against the obstetrician.

Causes of action in this scenario include wrongful birth and wrongful life as well as a potential claim for negligent infliction of emotional distress. Again, negligent infliction of emotional distress refers to those situations where a parent witnesses injury to a close relative immediately within the zone of danger, such as where a child is struck by a car in the presence of a parent, and where such parent frequently suffers some type of physical ailment arising from the emotional distress suffered at the time of the stressful incident. Although various legal defenses could be brought as to the "immediacy" of injury since this particular case extended over one year, this may become a fact question for the jury.

Wrongful birth damages would be limited to those expenses actually incurred up to the time of the child's death. Notably, the damages recoverable on the basis of the negligent infliction of emotional distress claim could certainly be a long term, future type of damages if the mother in this case were to continue to be plagued by some type of physical disability due to the psychological impact of losing a second child from Krabbe disease.

CASE 6—FAILURE TO PERFORM AMNIOCENTESIS UPON PATIENT REQUEST

A 24-year-old pregnant woman comes to her physician at 12 weeks and requests an amniocentesis for karyotype. A friend of this woman recently delivered a baby with Down syndrome, and the pregnant woman is now concerned that she may have a baby similarly afflicted. Because of this concern and in spite of the fact that she is only 24 years old, she nevertheless desires an amniocentesis. The doctor advises her that she is only 24 years old and that amniocentesis is not recommended for her at this point. The doctor does not perform an amniocentesis, nor does he refer her to a geneticist or a maternal/fetal medicine specialist. Subsequently, the mother delivers, and although the child does not have Down syndrome, the child does have Trisomy 13. The mother brings a cause of action against the obstetrician for failure to perform an amniocentesis.

Clearly the standard of care requires that amniocentesis be offered to those patients who will be 35 years or greater at the time of delivery. However, it is not clear that the standard of care requires performing an amniocentesis upon request. The standard of care is generally defined as what the "average physician would do under like or similar circumstances."

While this is somewhat nebulous, there are certainly those plaintiff experts who will testify that if a patient requests an amniocentesis, the standard of care requires that it be performed. The alternative would be for the physician to refer the patient to a specialist in either genetics or maternal-fetal medicine for further consultation. Regardless of whether or not one considers this to be the standard of care, the performance of an amniocentesis, which is a low-risk procedure, could easily be performed and would avoid the risk of a lawsuit such as this.

The causes of action are again those of wrongful birth and wrongful life. A particular twist to this case is whether or not a cause of action exists for having the Trisomy 13 baby. Arguably there is no legal proximate cause since the patient wanted testing for Down syndrome and did not have a Down syndrome baby. However, it undoubtedly would be the plaintiff's argument that the patient would not know of every possible genetic defect and, simply by referring to Down syndrome, had indicated that she wanted testing for any genetic defect, using the Down syndrome generically, not specifically.

The resolution of this issue would rest primarily upon the testimony of the plaintiff, her understanding of the issues, and the expressions of what she wanted or expected the doctor to do. The judge would then determine whether a factual or legal issue existed, the former of which would be a question for the jury, while the latter would be resolved by the judge

him/herself. Obviously, if the patient testified that she only wanted screening for Down syndrome and nothing else, then a dismissal for failure to show proximate cause, a legal issue, might be sought. On the other hand, if the patient uses the term "Down syndrome" as simply a generic expression to convey a desire to screen for all genetic anomalies, the issue would be a fact question for the jury.

CASE 7—FAILURE TO DIAGNOSE ABNORMALITY ON ULTRASOUND

Two different pregnant women see two different obstetricians. The first obstetrician performs an ultrasound at 12 weeks and dates the pregnancy but does not perform an ultrasound thereafter. The second obstetrician performs an ultrasound at 12 weeks and then again at 22 weeks. Both babies have a diaphragmatic hernia, but neither physician makes that diagnosis. In fact, it is visible on the 22-week ultrasound.

Both physicians are sued by their patients. With respect to obstetrician #1, the claim is that there should have been an ultrasound performed at 22 weeks. In the case of obstetrician #2, the claim is that the obstetrician missed the diaphragmatic hernia at 22 weeks.

There are several important issues in this factual scenario. First, does the standard of care require any ultrasound on a low-risk patient? Current medical literature would seem to indicate that it does not. However, the law requires that where one assumes a duty unimposed by any standard, the duty must be performed in a non-negligent manner. That is, once a physician elects to perform an ultrasound it must be performed and interpreted within the requisite standard of care.

The second issue is whether the standard of care requires a repeat ultrasound at 22 weeks as a follow-up to the 12-week ultrasound. Clearly the standard of care does not require the second ultrasound where it does not require the first. Because the standard of care does not require the performance of the subsequent ultrasound, obstetrician #1 may very well escape liability.

Obstetrician #2 will not be so lucky, for he voluntarily assumed a duty of care by performing the second ultrasound at 22 weeks. Even though there was no standard of care requirement to perform the ultrasound, he is now bound to appropriately interpret that ultrasound. Because he misinterpreted the ultrasound for which he voluntarily assumed a duty of care, he will be deemed negligent and faces liability.

This scenario unfortunately points out the unfair dichotomy that exists with respect to those physicians who decide to "do more" for their patient than the standard of care requires. The law unfortunately is absurdly applied in these situations. Obstetrician #1 can escape total and complete liability because he did not perform an ultrasound at 22 weeks, whereas obstetrician #2 faces liability because he voluntarily, without requirement, undertook to perform an ultrasound at 22 weeks and misinterpreted the ultrasound.

The cause of action will vary depending upon the outcome of the child. If the child survives at delivery but is afflicted by a significant abnormality that will affect him over the course of his life, plaintiffs will have a cause of action sounding in wrongful birth and wrongful life. Plaintiff will again need to establish that she would have terminated the pregnancy rather than to undergo a repair attempt.

If the diaphragmatic hernia is not repaired and the child dies shortly thereafter, the family has an action for wrongful death. In such a cause of action, plaintiffs allege that, had the abnormality been identified, the child could have been treated either in utero or at delivery, the diaphragmatic hernia immediately addressed and corrected, and the child's life saved. Damages for wrongful death generally include the loss of companionship and mental anguish. (Since the child is not a contributor of money to the family, lost wages would not be included).

CONSENT/INFORMED CONSENT FOR MINORS

In general, a minor, which in most states is a person under 18 years old, is considered incapable of consenting to medical care and treatment, and a parent or guardian must consent on the minor's behalf. A healthcare provider who provides medical treatment to a minor without obtaining the consent of the parent or legal guardian may be liable for battery for the unconsented to touching of a minor. This, at times, prevents a minor from seeking necessary medical care and inhibits a physician from providing such care.

Noting that many minors were foregoing necessary medical care, especially in the areas of contraception and pregnancy related care, most states either by case law or legislation have modified the above rule to permit minors, in certain circumstances, to consent to and obtain medical services without requiring that a parent or guardian render consent as well. While most states have laws similar to those discussed herein, a provider should consult with his/her legal counsel or health system risk manager to obtain the specific requirements of the state in which he/she practices.

COMMON LAW EXCEPTIONS

Consent in an Emergency Situation

When a minor requires emergent medical care and her parent or legal guardian is not readily available, a healthcare provider, under the legal doctrine of "implied consent," may treat the minor without consent in order to "protect the life or health of the child."[55] Documentation of both the medical emergency and attempts to locate a parent or guardian prior to treatment will be important for risk management purposes.

A provider should not "create" an emergency in order to render treatment for which consent has not been obtained. Further, where an emergency exists and a parent or legal guardian expressly communicates a refusal of treatment, the county probate court should be petitioned, if time permits, to secure an emergency order authorizing treatment. In a few cases, courts have held a physician liable to the parents of a minor for assault

and battery where treatment was rendered where the parents had repeatedly indicated a refusal to permit treatment.[56]

Mature Minors

When a minor is close to the age of majority and has the mental capacity to consent on her own behalf, courts on an occasional basis have found no liability against a physician or a hospital for failure to obtain parental consent.[57] Further, at least 1 state has taken a very broad interpretation of what constitutes a "mature minor" and allows a minor to consent if he/she is of "sufficient intelligence to understand and appreciate the consequences of the proposed surgical procedure."[58]

In the case of a "mature minor," the parents would not be responsible for payment for services rendered, but the mature minor would be. Thus, collection may be a problem. This situation commonly occurs when a minor requests contraception and does not want her parents to know. Providers will have to balance confidentiality concerns against the right to collect payment.

Emancipated Minors

The "emancipated minor" rule is another established exception which allows a minor to consent to her own medical treatment. "Emancipation" is the relinquishment of parental control and authority over the minor.[59] She is, in essence, acting as an adult and may consent to medical treatment. Although the laws vary slightly from state to state, in general minors are considered emancipated by marriage, active military service, economic independence, parental consent, and by conduct of the parent inconsistent with the subjection of control by his parent.[60] From a liability standpoint, the burden of proving emancipation will be placed on the healthcare provider who provides treatment to a minor. It will also be the provider's burden to prove that the minor is of sufficient maturity to consent. Thus, it is important to place evidence of emancipation in the minor's medical record. This evidence may include court documents, a marriage certificate, military service documents, or proof that the minor lives independently and is employed.

STATUTORY EXCEPTIONS

In recent years, most state legislatures have enacted statutes authorizing certain classes of minors to consent to various medical procedures. From a public policy standpoint, it is believed that a minor, if requesting treatment, should be allowed the highest level of care possible in order to improve the overall health of the community.

Nearly all states have established exceptions allowing a minor to consent to the treatment of pregnancy and pregnancy-related healthcare and the treatment of sexually transmitted diseases, including HIV and AIDS.[61] Increasingly common are statutes which allow a minor to consent to birth control.[62] Some states provide, however, that if a health professional believes that the minor is immature and thus incapable of consenting to such treatment, a parent/guardian may be notified or the requested treatment may be refused. Further, some statutes allow a healthcare provider, for medical reasons, to notify a parent or legal guardian (or putative father, if the minor is pregnant) regarding healthcare decisions. However, the provider may have to inform the minor that such notification may be given prior to providing treatment. Since laws vary from state to state, it is best to consult legal counsel or a health system risk management department regarding the requirements of a particular state.

In rendering pregnancy care to minors, issues that frequently arise and raise a potential "red flag" for a healthcare provider include what treatment constitutes "pregnancy-related treatment," whether the contemplated procedure is surgical in nature, and whether parental notification should be considered. For example, should a parent be informed if a pregnant minor requires an amniocentesis, which most physicians believe involves at least some risk to both the mother and fetus? A similar concern arises if a cesarean section is required. It is best not to establish too rigid a policy in handling these types of situations as experience has shown that individual factual situations play a large part in determining whether parental notification is appropriate. It is generally accepted, however, that in situations where a minor's life may be in danger, parental notification would likely take priority over the minor's confidentiality concerns.

Finally, in most states, even though the minor may give consent, a minor's parent or legal guardian remain responsible for payment. However, other considerations, such as the confidentiality concerns noted above, may prevent a provider from seeking payment from the minor's parent or legal guardian.

Sterilization

While there is legal authority in nearly all states allowing a minor to consent to many reproductive treatments and procedures, most states either specifically disallow a minor to consent to sterilization or are silent on the issue. The majority of the states consider sterilization an "extraordinary procedure" that can only be performed with the informed consent of an adult or pursuant to a court order.

Further, in the absence of a statute, some state courts have held that the courts lack the power to order sterilization of minors or other incompetent patients. A very recent trend, however, has been for some courts to decide that they have the authority to order a sterilization on a minor. In these cases, courts have held hearings to determine whether it is in the best interest of the minor to be sterilized. Courts typically examine the following factors in making their determination:

(1) The possibility that the minor could become pregnant, including whether the minor is in an environment where intercourse is possible.

(2) The possibility the minor will experience trauma or physiological or psychological damage if she becomes pregnant.

(3) Current levels of sexual activity.

(4) The inability of the minor to understand about reproduction or contraception.

(5) The feasibility and medical advisability of less drastic means of contraception.

(6) The ability of the minor to care for a child.

(7) Consent and permission from relevant family members.

(8) A demonstration that the party seeking sterilization are doing so in good faith and that their primary concern is for the best interest of the minor rather than his/her own convenience.

Finally, if it is determined that a minor is to undergo sterilization, either on an elective basis or for medical reasons, her insurance status must be considered. Many insurance companies and, in particular, Medicaid, outline stringent requirements, including waiting periods, informed consent, and less invasive alternatives discussions prior to authorizing the procedure.

Abortion

A minor's right to consent to abortion was established by the United States Supreme Court in 1976.[63] However, the Supreme Court has upheld the power of states to require parental consent under certain conditions.[64] Based upon the decisions of the Supreme Court, most states have enacted comprehensive statutory requirements with which a minor must comply in order to obtain an abortion in the absence of parental consent. Typically, these statutes include a hearing before a probate judge to ensure sufficient maturity, a detailed informed consent discussion, and a waiting period of 24–48 hours after the procedure has been explained to allow the minor to change her mind if she desires.[65] While some of the above requirements have undergone constitutional challenges, they have largely been upheld.

Courts have also held that noncompliance with statutory informed consent requirements are acceptable in emergency situations where a physician concludes that an abortion is a medical necessity. Factors to consider include whether allowing the pregnancy to continue would pose a threat to the minor's life or health or whether the pregnancy could cause severe and permanent psychological harm to her.

If an abortion is to be performed on a minor, it is suggested that there be a reasonable effort on the part of all persons involved to accurately determine the age of the minor requesting the procedure. One possible mechanism would be to consider whether the individual making the determination (based on information supplied by the minor) would be prepared to testify under oath that he had no substantial doubt as to the truth of the information given by the minor requesting the abortion.

A physician asked to perform an abortion an any girl under the age of 18 should also determine that the minor has the appropriate mental and emotional maturity to understand the nature, risk, and possible consequences of the procedure and should document such evidence in the medical record. It is essential that the potential risks and benefits of the procedure be fully explained to the minor by the physician. She should also be given an opportunity to discuss with the physician any questions she may have with regard to the proposed course of treatment.

It is further advisable for the medical staff to establish a minimum age (i.e., between 15 and 18 years) and to require a physician who has agreed to perform an abortion on a minor below that age to consult with other staff physicians as to the capacity of the minor to give informed consent. Although it may not be possible to set all-inclusive guidelines, it would seem reasonable to assume that as the age of the minor falls below the minimum age established as a guideline, the importance of such consultation and the depth of the inquiry required should correspondingly increase.

In the case of any such minor, the guidelines should recognize an affirmative obligation on the part of the attending physician and consultants to evaluate on a professional medical basis the possible risks and benefits of urging the minor to consult with her parent or legal guardian before undergoing the procedure. If the attending physician believes that it is in the minor's best interest for her parent to be informed and he is unable to obtain the minor's agreement to such procedure, it is believed that the physician would then be justified in withdrawing from the case.

A physician should not perform an abortion on a minor who objects but whose parent consents unless a court authorizes the performance of the abortion or it is necessary to prevent the minor's death or severe disability.

CHORIONIC VILLUS SAMPLING—INFORMED CONSENT AND LEGAL RISKS

CVS procedures have become an important part of the diagnostic regimen available for early prenatal testing. Currently, there are a number of lawsuits around the United States claiming that a particular CVS procedure caused transverse limb anomalies (or other defects) as a result of a vascular disruption during the pregnancy. Depending upon the article to which one refers, there either is or is not a correlation between CVS and transverse limb anomalies. For example, compare the report generated by the Centers for Disease Control and Prevention, which describes such a correlation, with the reports of the World Health Organization, which make no such finding. Regardless of the reports one believes to be accurate, the present state of knowledge, from a legal standpoint, probably requires that the patient be informed of the fact that some physicians feel that there is a risk of CVS and transverse limb anomalies at specific gestational ages. The specifics of that informed consent discussion will be elucidated below; however, an historical perspective that has led to the most recent set of lawsuits is worth understanding.

Prior to the Firth letter in *Lancet* on March 30, 1991, there was no information that chorionic villus sampling had the potential to cause limb abnormalities. In an anecdotal letter to *Lancet* on March 30, 1991, Dr. Firth described 5 babies in a cluster and requested that the rest of the world review their statistics to determine if this was a "real" finding.

Preceding this article, there had been research concluding that significant vascular disruption may cause limb abnormali-

ties if it occurred between 6 and 8 weeks of gestation. However, no research scientist had found data to suggest that CVS would cause enough of a vascular abruption to create a limb abnormality. There are several "so-called" experts who are currently testifying that prior reports of amniotic band syndromes after CVS put physicians on notice that CVS could cause limb anomalies from vascular disruption. Obviously, this did not and does not hold water, since the very articles on amniotic band syndrome following CVS pointed out that this same occurrence could happen with amniocentesis and was believed to result from a completely different mechanism unrelated to vascular disruption. Nevertheless, these experts do exist.

In August 1990, the FDA approved the CVS Trophican catheter. It is important to understand that this approval came after studying the potential effects of the CVS procedure *including fetal loss and fetal abnormality*. On August 9, 1990, the FDA reported that the procedure was "safe and effective" with reasonable assurance when used for its intended use. The most that was reported was a small increase of fetal loss above and beyond that of amniocentesis. Perhaps as important as the FDA approval is its reference to certain articles lending support to its decision. One of those articles came from the *Journal of the American Medical Association* (258(24)). In that article, at page 3562, the following statement is made:

Because CVS is performed early in pregnancy, it could conceivably interfere with placental function. This could be reflected in growth retardation, prematurity, and increased birth defects. *None of these complications have occurred in frequencies greater than those observed in the general pregnant population.* There is also the possible complication of spontaneous rupture of membranes with potential loss of the fetus following the procedure.

Thus, the United State government not only approved the catheter but discussed the risks and supported its discussion with the *Journal of the American Medical Association* (JAMA).

The JAMA article was not the only article that reviewed potential limb anomalies following CVS. In 1990, the *American Journal of Medical Genetics* (37:366–370), carried an article by Kaplan et al. addressing this specific issue. The statement from this particular group was as follows:

We conclude that exposure to CVS is not associated with an increased frequency of malformations or minor anomalies in infants compared with amniocentesis, . . .

This article also pointed out the following:

The possibility of litigation blaming CVS for congenital malformation exists.

The purpose of the article was to investigate concerns regarding disturbance of the chorion early in pregnancy, the possibility of congenital malformations, and the comparison of limb anomalies in CVS groups to the background rate.

Prior to Dr. Firth's 1991 letter to *Lancet*, the state of knowledge regarding CVS procedures clearly contradicted a conclusion that there was an increased risk of limb anomalies above and beyond the background rate when CVS was performed. *Prior to March 30, 1991, certainly no one should ever be blamed for not informing a patient of a potential or possible risk of transverse limb anomalies associated with CVS.*

The major question, however, is when the standard of care changed to require informed consent to include a discussion of the potential risk for transverse limb anomalies. Obviously, one letter, such as that of Dr. Firth, would not have an immediate impact and would not alter the standard of care even if a physician were to have read the *Lancet* article. Just as important as Dr. Firth's findings in his own grouping is the portion of his article that discusses the prior American and Canadian studies that found no such increased risk of abnormalities *in CVSs performed primarily at 10 weeks or greater rather than 6 to 8 weeks.* (As a matter of fact, it is very difficult to find reliable data showing that there is a true risk of statistical significance after 10–11 weeks.) Virtually every study that claims to have made such a finding has arguable accuracy.

It is plausible that the standard of care did not change until the publication of Dr. Barbara Burton's article in May of 1992. Her study was the first American investigation to specifically explore the CVS performed after 10 weeks gestation; Dr. Burton concluded that an increased risk of limb anomalies following CVS procedures indeed existed.

Although Dr. Burton's article has been criticized by some (especially since her fetal loss rate was higher than that of other institutions), the following statement published for the first time in an American study, probably changed the actual standard of care:

Further data are needed to confirm this association and to quantify the risks. Until such data are available, patients should be counselled that there appears to be an increased risk of limb malformations associated with CVS (See page 730).

Most institutions had probably already changed their counselling procedures, but until this article surfaced, one cannot say with certainty that the standard of care had actually changed. The publication of Dr. Burton's study and conclusions in an American medical journal thus became the most identifiable point at which one could view the standard of care as having changed, regardless of the accuracy of Dr. Burton's analysis. In fact, in close proximity to the publication of Dr. Burton's findings, newspapers began publishing articles supported by statements of prominent U.S. physicians indicating that this issue certainly raised the possibility of transverse limb anomalies and that the patient should be advised of the same.

From an historical perspective, one can come to the following conclusions:

1. Up until March of 1991, no one should be held responsible for a failure of informed consent regarding CVS and its potential association with transverse limb anomalies.
2. Between March of 1991 (Firth) and May of 1992 (Burton), probably one should not be held responsible for an alleged failure of informed consent since there clearly was a differ-

ence between the gestational ages studied by Dr. Firth and the gestational ages in the American and Canadian CVS groups.
3. After May of 1992, there appears to have been a duty to inform patients of a potential association between transverse limb anomalies and CVS procedures. Furthermore, it probably was better to perform the procedure after 10 weeks than before depending upon the patient's request.

Today, it is difficult to determine exactly what a patient should be told during a genetic counselling session, since the data is not clear. There are those experts who will testify regardless of what was said to the patient, that had the patient really "known" of the potential "real" risk, the patient would have refused the procedure. In fact, one of the current experts commonly used by plaintiffs in these cases has made the statement that certain institutions are generically violating the standard of care as too many of the patients at those institutions undergo CVS procedures. Therefore, an expert can determine, by the number of patients alone who consent to such a procedure, that an institution is per se violating the standard of care.

At a minimum, the following information needs to be conveyed to a patient:

1. CVS carries an increased risk of miscarriage above and beyond amniocentesis.
2. CVS has been reported by some authors to carry an increased risk of transverse limb anomalies above and beyond the background rate at specific gestational ages.
3. The patient should be given statistics from the local institution regarding CVS and reported transverse limb anomalies.
4. Upon request, the patient can be given references with some statistics on both sides of the issue.
5. When one views the actual, small risk factors quoted per 10,000, one can understand why item #4 above is an important feature to have available for discussion with the patient.

The World Health Organization now has upwards of 150,000 to 200,000 reported cases and yet has not shown any risk of transverse limb anomaly above and beyond the background rate, whereas the published CDC study looked at essentially a very small number of patients to arrive at the conclusions that an increased risk existed at specific gestational ages. Even in studies revealing an increased rate, however, transverse limb anomalies are reported in the range of 1.5–2.3 per 10,000 for the background rate, whereas CVS exposed rates are reported in the range of 1.4–7.4 per 10,000 (See the CDC study).

When a patient begins to understand that the risk may only be going from 2 per 10,000 to 7 per 10,000, the statistical chances are so diminished, that the risk factor may not dissuade a patient who is interested in first trimester diagnosis for psychological reasons. Quoting the actual rate per 10,000 is probably a better way to present it to a patient than simply saying that there may be a double, triple, or even 5- or 6-fold increase in the rate of transverse limb anomalies.

The so-called increased risk found by certain investigators has an apparently more dramatic impact on the investigators and their papers than does the information so obtained have on patients who are being counselled. Investigators who are finding a doubling or a tripling of the risk of CVS and its relationship to limb anomalies seem to lose focus on the fact that they are nevertheless dealing with very tiny numbers out of groupings of 10,000. An often overlooked portion of the CDC findings concludes that those patients who were provided with statistical data to assist them in the decision making process chose to undergo CVS despite the increased risk:

. . . One study demonstrated that perspective patients who were provided with formal genetic counselling including information about limb deficiencies and other risks and benefits, chose CVS at a rate similar to a group of perspective patients who were counselled before published reports of CVS-associated limb deficiencies (Cutillo DM et al. from *Prenatal Diagnosis* 1994;14:327–332).

Whatever increased risk that might exist is apparently not as substantial a factor to those patients who, for psychological and/or physical reasons, desire to have a CVS early on rather than wait until the second trimester for their diagnostic procedures. To these patients, the maternal concerns and social pressures apparently are of a greater impact than the small increased statistical risk described in some academic research papers.

In conclusion, it can be stated that there are no doubt going to be those "soapbox" experts who will testify rather regularly regarding informed consent, the standard of care, and cause and effect relationship between CVS and transverse limb anomalies at any gestational age. It is highly likely that the cause and effect relationship at specific gestational ages will eventually be attacked with a *Daubert* motion as to scientific reliability, especially in those cases when the CVS was done at 10–11 weeks.

In the meantime, the best defense is to provide the patient some information regarding the possible risk factors with CVS and to *document the same with a written consent form*. Most patients remember very little from informed consent discussions, especially as time passes. There are even those patients who, 6 months subsequent to having undergone surgery, cannot accurately recall the type of surgery performed or the reasons therefor. It is highly unlikely that a patient will recall the specifics regarding an informed consent discussion relative to CVS and its potential for causing transverse limb anomalies many months or years after its occurrence; additionally, it is common practice for a patient, now a plaintiff, to deny that such a discussion ever took place during a deposition or at trial.

References

1. See *Roe v. Wade*, 410 U.S. 113, 93 S. Ct. 705, 35 L. Ed. 2d 147 (1973).
2. While one may not have a duty to perform a test or other diagnostic procedure, however, the standard of care may nevertheless require that the patient be advised of the availability of such tests. For example, in May of 1985, the American College of Obstetrics and Gynecology (ACOG) stated that it is "imperative that every prenatal patient be advised of the availability of [the AFP] test and that [the physician's] discussion about the test and the patient's decision with respect to the test be documented in the patient's chart." In June of 1988, ACOG stated that pregnant women should "be made aware of the availability of MSAFP screening" and that "the testing should proceed in accordance with [1986] guidelines," which required the test to be performed for "patients who desire it."
3. See, e.g., *Williams v. Robinson*, 512 So. 2d 58, 69 A.L.R. 4th 861 (Alabama 1987); *Underwood v Holy Name of Jesus Hosp*, 289 Ala 216, 266 So.2d 773 (1972); *LaRaia v Superior Ct of Arizona*, 150 Ariz 118, 722 p.2d 286 (1986); *Huggins v Longs Drug Stores California, Inc*, 6 Cal 4th 124, 862 P.2d 148, 24 Cal. Rptr. 587 (1993); *Burgess v Superior Court*, 2 Cal 4th 1064, 831 P2d 1197, 9 Cal. Rptr. 2d 615 (1992); *Greenberg v Perkins*, 845 P2d 530 (Colo. 1993); *Clayton v Kelly*, 193 Ga. App. 45, 357 S.E.2d 865 (1987); *Smith v Hull*, 659 N.E.2d 185 (Indiana, 1996); *Johnston v Elkins*, 241 Kan. 407, 736 P.2d 935 (1987); *Burgess v Perdue*, 239 Kan 473, 721 P.2d 239 (1986); *Profitt v Bartolo*, 162 Mich App 35, 412 N.W.2d 232 (1986); *West v Sanders Clinic for Women, P.A.*, 661 So.2d 714 (Miss. 1995); *Parkell v Fitzporter*, 301 Mo 217, 256 S.W. 239 (1923); *Maguire v State*, 254 Mont 178, 835 P.2d 755 (1992); *Smith v Cote*, 128 N.H. 231, 513 A.2d 341 (1986); *Tufo v. Township of Old Bridge*, 278 N.J. Super 312, 650 A.2d 1044 (1995); *Sawh v Schoen*, 215 A.D.2d 291, 627 N.Y.S. 2d 7 (1995); *McEachern v Miller*, 268 N.C. 591, 151 S.E. 2d 209 (1966); *Truscott v Peterson*, 78 N.D. 498, 50 NW2d 245 (1951); *Schmitz v Blanchard Valley OB-GYN, Inc*, 63 Ohio App 3d 756, 580 N.E.2d 55 (1989); *Shaw v Kirschbaum*, 439 Pa. Super 24, 653 A2d 12 (1994); *Pope v St John*, 862 S.W.2d 657 (Tex. App. 1993); *C. S. v Nielson*, 98 Utah Adv Rep 4, 767 P.2d 504 (1988); *Vann v Harden*, 187 Va. 555, 47 S.E. 2d 314 (1948).
4. A thorough analysis of these types of cases can be found in five law journal and law review articles published since 1980: Note, Wrongful Birth Actions: The Case Against Legislative Curtailment, 100 Harv. L. Rev. 2017 (1987); Bell Legislative Intrusions Into the Common Law of Medical Malpractice: Thoughts About the Deterrent Effect of Tort Liability, 35 Syracuse L. Rev. 939 (1984); Collins, An Overview and Analysis: Prenatal Torts, Preconception Torts, Wrongful Life, Wrongful Death, and Wrongful Birth: Time for a New Framework, 22 J. Fam. L. 677 (1983–1984); Rogers III, Wrongful Life and Wrongful Birth: Medical Malpractice in Genetic Counseling and Prenatal Testing, 33 S.C.L.Rev. 713 (1982); Trotzig, The Defective Child and the Actions for Wrongful Life and Wrongful Birth, 14 Fam.L.Q. 15 (1980).
5. Note that wrongful life and wrongful birth claims are distinct from claims of wrongfuls conception or pregnancy. Liability for the latter is based upon a physician's negligence in performing a sterilization procedure or an abortion or the pharmacist's or pharmaceutical manufacturer's negligence in preparing or dispensing a contraceptive prescription. See *Phillips v. United States*, 508 F. Supp. 544, 545, n. 1 (D.S.C. 1981); see generally, Holt, Wrongful Pregnancy, 33 S.C.L.Rev. 759 (1983). While some states previously permitted recovery for the costs of raising a perfectly normal child, the overwhelming majority currently limits recovery to the costs of the pregnancy and birth and the related damages for pain and suffering, mental distress, lost wages, and loss of consortium.
6. See *Phillips v United States*, 508 F. Supp. 544, 545, n. 1 (D.S.C. 1981); see generally Rogers, Wrongful Life and Wrongful Birth: Medical Malpractice in Genetic Counseling and Prenatal Testing, 33 S.C.L.Rev. 713 (1982).
7. Note, Wrongful Birth Actions: The Case Against Legislative Curtailment, 100 Harv. L. Rev. 2017, 2018 n. 5 (1987), lists the following jurisdictions recognizing a cause of action for wrongful birth: Alabama, see *Robak v United States*, 658 F. 2d 471 (7th Cir. 1981); California, see *Andalon v Superior Court*, 162 Cal App 3d 600, 208

Cal Rptr 899 (1984); Florida, see *Moores v Lucas*, 405 So.2d 1022 (Fla. Dist. Ct. App. 1981); Illinois, see *Goldberg v Ruskin*, 128 I11 App 3d 1029, 471 N.E.2d 530, 84 I11 Dec 1 (1984), aff'd, 113 I112d 482, 499 N.E.2d 406, 101 I11 Dec. 818 (1986); Maine, see Me.Rev.Stat. Ann.tit.24 §2931(2) (1985); Michigan, see *Eisbrenner v Stanley*, 106 Mich App 357, 308 N.W.2d 209 (1981); New Hampshire, see *Smith v Cote*, 128 N.H. 231, 513 A.2d 341 (1986); New Jersey, see *Berman v Allan*, 80 N.J. 421, 404 A.2d 8 (1979); New York, see *Becker v Schwartz*, 46 N.Y.2d 401, 386 N.E.2d 807, 413 N.Y.S.2d 895 (1978); North Carolina, see *Gallagher v Duke Univ*, 638 F. Supp 978 (M.D.N.C. 1986); Pennsylvania, see *Gildiner v Thomas Jefferson Univ Hosp*, 451 F. Supp. 692 (E.D. Pa 1978); South Carolina, see *Phillips v United States*, 508 F. Supp. 544 (D.S.C. 1981); Texas, see *Jacosh v Theimer*, 519 S.W.2d 846 (Tex. 1975); Virginia, see *Naccash v Burger*, 223 Va. 406, 290 S.E.2d 825 (1982); Washington, see *Harbeson v Parke-Davis, Inc*, 98 Wash 2d 460, 656 P.2d 483 (1983), aff'd, 746 F.2d 517 (9th Cir. 1984); West Virginia, see *Jennifer S. v Kirdnual*, 332 S.E.2d 872 (W.Va. 1985); and Wisconsin, see *Dumer v St. Michael's Hospital*, 69 Wis.2d 766, 233 N.W.2d 372 (1975).

8. See, Alabama, *Robak v United States*, 658 F.2d 471 (7th Cir. 1981); Colorado, *Lininger v Eisenbaum*, 764 P.ed 1202 (Colo. 1988); Delaware, *Garrison v Medical Center of Delaware, Inc.* 581 A.2d 288 (Del. 1990); Florida, *Kush v Lloyd*, 616 So.2d 415 (1942); Idaho, *Blake v Cruz*, 108 Idaho 253, 698 P.2d 315 (1984); Illinois, *Siemieniec v Lutheran Gen'l Hospital*, 117 I11.2d 230, 111 I11. Dec. 302, 512 N.E. 2d 691 (1987); Kansas, *Arche v United States*, 247 Kan. 276, 798 P.2d 477 (1990); Michigan, *Proffitt v Bartolo* 162 Mich App 35, 412 N.W.2d 232 (1987); New Hampshire, *Smith v Cote*, 128 N.H. 231, 513 A. 2d 341 (1986); New Jersey, *Berman v Alla*, 80 N.J. 421, 404 A. 2d 8 (1979); New York, *Becker v Schwartz*, 46 N.Y. 2d 401, 413 N.Y.S. 2d 895, 386 N.E. 2d 807 (1978); South Carolina, *Phillips v United States*, 508 F. Supp. 544 (D.S.C. 1981); Texas, *Jacobs v Theimer*, 519 S.W. 2d 846 (Tex. 1975); Virginia, *Naccash v Burger*, 223 Va. 406, 290 S.E. 2d 825 (1982); Washington, *Harbeson v Parke-Davis, Inc*, 98 Wash. 2d 460, 656 P. 2d 483 (1983); West Virginia, *James G. v Caserta*, 175 W. Va. 406, 332 S.E. 2d 872 (1985); Wisconsin, *Dumer v St. Michael's Hosp*, 69 Wis. 2d 766, 233 N.W. 2d 372 (1975).

9. The some seventeen states permitting recovery have justified their action on grounds such as (1) encouraging an attitude of reverence for human life; (2) holding parents responsible for the care of children they bring into society; (3) improving the quality of human existence; (4) protecting the procreative rights of individuals; (5) holding tortfeasors liable for damages proximately caused by their actions; and (6) encouraging competent medical care for all.

10. See, e.g., *Becker v Schwartz*, 46 N.Y. 2d 401, 413, 386 N.E. 2d 807, 813, 413 N.Y.S. 2d 895, 901 (1978); *Jacobs v Theimer*, 519 S.W. 2d 846, 849 (Tex. 1975).

11. Rogers, Wrongful Life and Wrongful Birth: Medical Malpractice in Genetic Counseling and Prenatal Testing, 33 S.C.L.Rev. 713 (1982); Trotzig, The Defective Child and Actions for Wrongful Life and Wrongful Birth, 14 Fam.L.Q. 15 (1980).

12. A thorough analysis and discusion of causation issues in the wrongful life claim is contained in the dissenting opinions of Judge Wachtler appearing in the early case of *Becker v. Schwartz*, 46 N.Y. 2d 401, 417, 422, 386 N.E. 2d 907, 816–819, 413 N.Y.S. 2d 895, 904–907 (1978).

13. *Id.*

14. *Id.*

15. During the 1980s, however, the supreme courts of California, New Jersey, and Washington permitted children to pursue wrongful life actions limited to the recovery of special damages attributable to the extraordinary medical expenses expected to be incurred during the child's lifetime in the management, treatment, and care of congenital or genetic ailments. See *Turpin v. Sortini*, 31 Cal. 2d 220, 643 P.2d, 954, 182 Cal. Rptr. 337 (1982) (hereditary deafness); *Procanik v. Cillo*, 97 N.J. 339, 478 A.2d 755 (1984) (congenital rubella syn-drome); *Harbeson v. Parke-Davis, Inc*, 98 Wash. 2d 460, 656 P.2d 483 (1983) (fetal hydanatoin syndrome).

16. 332 Md 226, 630 A2d 1145 (1993).

17. *Id.*

18. 281 Md 432, 379 A2d 1014 (1977).

19. *Id.*

20. *Id.*

21. *Id.*

22. 57 AD2d 73, 394 NYS2d 933 (NY App Div 1977).

23. *Karlsons, supra* at 81, 394 NYS2d at 938.

24. *Id.* at 82, 294 NYS2d at 939; see also *Keselman v. Kingsboro Medical Group*, 156 AD2d 334, 335, 548 NYS2d 287, 228–289 (1989).

25. *Reed, supra* at 244.

26. 217 Mich App 502 (1996).

27. *Id.* at 511.

28. *Id.*

29. *Id.* at 5121–5512.

30. Courts have traditionally been reluctant to allow recovery for purely mental or emotional distress because such injuries are not easily foreseeable [cites-RICKEY, GUSTAFSON, WARGELIN]. Thus, historically, plaintiffs with a cause of action for the negligent infliction of emotional distress had to plead some contemporaneous physical injury resulting from a direct impact or as a physical manifestation of the emotional distress.

31. *Siemieniec v. Lutheran General Hospital*, 117 I112d 230, 512 NE2d 691 (1987).

32. *Siemieniec, supra*, 117 I11 2d at 260–62.

33. *Villamil v. Elmhurst Memorial Hospital*, 175 I11 App 3d 668, 529 NE2d 1181 (1988).

34. *Robbins v. Kass*, 163 I11 App 3d 927, 516 NE2d 1023 (1987).

35. *Smith v Humes*, Superior Court, judicial district of *Stamford-Norwalk at Stamford*, 1997 Conn Super LEXIS 2018, Docket No 950143884S (July 22, 1997) (Ryan, J).

36. See, e.g., *Golymbieski v. Equia.* Superior Court, judicial district of *Waterbury*, 1997 Conn Super LEXIS 1387, Docket No 125140 (May 22, 1997) (Fasano, J) (3 conn Ops 704); *Scalise v. Bristol Hospital*, Superior Court, judicial district of *Hartford-New Britain at Hartford*, 1995 Conn Super LEXIS 1983, Docket No. 525217 (July 5, 1995) (Corradino, J) (14 Conn L Rptr 534, 537).

37. *Britton v Borelli*, 7 Conn Law Trib No 25, p 11 (super Ct, June 5, 1981) (Moraghan, J), citing *Howard v Lecher*, 42 NY2d 109, 116, 397 NYS2d 363, 366 NE2d 64 (Cooke J, dissenting).

38. *Id.*

39. *Golymbieski v Squia, supra*, 3 Conn Ops 704; *Stapleton v SHE Medical Associates*, Superior Court, judicial district of *Hartford-New Britain at Hartford*, 1995 Conn Super LEXIS 1503, Docket No. 536586 (May 18, 1995) (Sheldon J).

40. *Golymbieski, supra*, 1997 Conn Super LEXIS 1387, 3 Conn Ops 704.

41. *Dillon*, 441 P2d at 920.

42. 31 Cap App 3d 22, 106 Cal Rptr 883 (1973).

43. 19 Cal 3d 564, 139 Cal Rptr 97, 565 P2d 122 (1977).

44. 39 Cal 3d 159, 216 Cal Rptr 661, 703 P2d 1 (1985).

45. *Id.* 703 P2d at 7.

46. *Id.* 703 P2d at 8.

47. See *Id.* 771 P2d at 830.

48. *Id.*

49. *Id.* 771 P2d at 8229–8830.

50. *Frame v Kothari.*, 115 NJ 638, 560 A2d 675 (1989).

51. *Maloney v Conroy*, 208 Conn 392, 545 A2d 1059 (1988). Note by contrast, that Connecticut allows bystander derivative liability only in the context of a mother's emotional distress related to prenatal and antenatal negligence. See footnotes through—and—accompanying text.

52. *Wargelin v Sisters of Mercy Health Corp*, 149 Mich App 75, 385 NW2d 732 (1986).

53. *Halliday v Beltz*, 356 Pa Super 375, 514 A2d 906 (1986).

54. *Lindenmuth v Alperin*, 197 NJ Super 385, 484 A2d 1316 (1984).
55. See *Sullivan* v *Montgomery* 155 Misc 448, 449–50; 279 NYS 575, 576–578 (1935); *Luka v Lowri*, 171 Mich 122 (1912); NY Pub Health Law, §2504.4; Montana Code Annotated, §41–405.
56. *See Zoski v Gaines*, 271 Mich 1 (1935).
57. *Younts v St. Francis Hospital and School of Nursing*, 205 Kan. 292, 469 P. 2d 330 (1970); *Bishop v Shurley*, 237 Mich 76, 221 NW2d 75 (1926); *Lacey v Laird*, 166, Ohio St 12, 139 NE2d 25 (1956; Miss Code Annotated, §41:41–3(h).
58. Miss Code Annotated, §41:41–3.
59. *Swenson v Swenson*, 241 Mo App 21, 227 SW2d 103, 105 (1950); *Lawson v Brown*, 349 F Supp 203 (WD Va 1972); Cal Civ Code §6922; Texas Statutes Annotated, §32-003.
60. *Murphy v Murphy*, 206 Misc 228, 229; 133 NYS 2d 796, 797 (Sup Ct 1954); Michigan Compiled Laws, §722.4.
61. Michigan Compiled Laws §§333.5127, 333.9132; Texas Compiled Laws, §32.003; California Civil Code, §6922.
62. Delaware 59 Laws, §708; California Civil Code, §6925.
63. *Planned Parenthood v Dunforth*, 428 US 52 (1976).
64. *Planned Parenthood v Casey*, 112 S Ct 2791 (1992).
65. Michigan Compiled Laws, §722.903, *et seq.*; Miss Code Annotated, §41:41–55; North Carolina General Statutes, §90-21.7, *et seq.*

CHAPTER 68

POLITICS AND GENETIC REPRODUCTIVE RISKS

Ruth S. Hanft

Rapid advances in genetic research as well as the ability to identify potential life threatening and disabling illnesses in utero have raised numerous economic, social, and ethical issues. Politics has always been part of the scientific discussion of research resource allocation, particularly the allocation of federal dollars. The role of interest groups, such as academic institutions and disease-specific organizations, that influence resource policy, has been recognized for a long time.[1] In recent years, the clash of values between "right to life" and "choice" groups have affected research and health-service delivery policy.

Since the late 1970s, the rapid rise of healthcare costs, concerns about the safety, efficacy, and cost effectiveness of new technologies have become major political issues, particularly as they relate to health insurance coverage under public and private programs. For example, insurers' policies on the payment for genetic screening and counseling vary widely because most insurance does not cover preventive or screening procedures. However, some states that regulate private health insurance have mandated such coverage.

In many states, to assure access to care for treatable hereditary diseases, public health departments and/or hospitals screen newborns for various hereditary diseases, yet coverage for specific diseases varies widely. Tandem mass spectrometry is beginning to spread. However, to some extent, politics determines which diseases are screened on the basis of the number of proponents for that disorder within the state. Some states provide the screening without charge, others charge fees. The end result is that access to screening varies widely by state and disease.[2] Access to screening of parents and fetuses also varies widely depending on the availability of the services and the ability of the individuals to pay.

Politics has dominated the dialogue on human reproduction and reproductive genetics and has gone beyond resolving disputes over shares of the resources to interfering with scientific independence and patient-physician relationship. At the federal level, numerous efforts have been made to restrain scientific research in the fields of reproduction and reproductive genetics and limit the transfer of new technologies to the whole population or specific subgroups. In addition, attempts by the government have been made to constrain the private dialogue between patient and provider concerning personal healthcare issues.

For the last 20 years, there has been substantial federal legislative decisions related to scientific research and care largely based on the right of reproductive choice and the status of embryos and fetuses. Overlapping these issues are issues of the right to die. Regarding the issue of abortion, the limits of abortion and challenges to *Roe v. Wade*[3] are the issues mainly argued by the public. The issue of abortion has affected basic research advances, for instance, the U.S. production and distribution of RU 486, research of embryos and fetal tissue and the availability of diagnostic procedures that predict

death and disability as well as prevent and treat diseases such as Parkinsonism, cancer, diabetes, and HIV. Current issues include:

1. Limits on abortion. Some states have legislation that requires parental notification of adolescent decisions to abort. Also, the existence of waiting periods for abortions after counseling and offering of alternatives to abortion.
2. The distribution of RU 486. Although the Food and Drug Administration has granted approval of RU 486, there were threats to boycott products of potential manufacturers as well as delays in the distribution of the product. Recently, the Food and Drug Administration refused to change regulations to permit the sale of over the counter postcortal pregnancy prevention drugs to adolescents.
3. Withholding of research resources on political grounds. There is a congressionally mandated ban against federal funding of fetal tissue research.[4] Stem cell research is controversial; opponents call it "lethal human experimentation."[5]
4. Restriction of access to technologies. Medical payment programs, particularly Medicaid, attempt to restrict access to health care programs for certain federal beneficiaries such as the military and federal employees.

THE FEDERAL POLITICAL DYNAMIC

ELECTION TIME

During the last 8 years of the twentieth century, the executive branch of government had been in the hands of the Democratic Party, which supported reproductive choice and fetal tissue and stem cell research. Despite the pro-choice stance of the administration, Congress, in both the House and Senate, was dominated by pro-life Republicans, who dominated and still dominate key authorizing and appropriation committees. Continual attempts have been made by the majority in Congress to restrict abortion, through legislation and riders to unrelated legislation, which have been, by and large, vetoed by President Clinton. In the Bush administration, the climate has changed dramatically. Both houses of Congress are dominated by Republicans.

Although stances on reproductive-genetic policies do not correspond to particular political parties, the power and support of the pro-life and/or religious right interest groups are stronger within the Republican Party. Some Republicans are pro-choice, yet the views of the Republican majority range from pro-life under any circumstance to abortion under special conditions, e.g., rape, incest, danger to the mother's life, or, in some cases, the genetic diagnoses of diseases such as Tay Sachs. By contrast, the issue of fetal tissue and brainstem research divides normally pro-life Republicans.

There is also no unanimity among Democrats over abortion, although a majority of Democrat office holders support choice. In heavily conservative Catholic and Evangelical districts there are Democrat representatives who are pro-life.

The 2000 election pitted pro-choice Al Gore against pro-life George W. Bush. In addition, there was a major failed attempt to recapture the House of Representatives by the Democrats, which could have lifted the ban on research. Both before and after the 2000 election, Republicans held a narrow majority of 5 seats in the House.

Particularly important for reproductive genetic policy is the composition of the Supreme Court, which has moved in the direction of states rights and limitations on choice. It is anticipated that President Bush will be able to appoint 2 justices of the 9 (with the consent of the Senate) during his first term. He has recently appointed one new justice replacing justice Renquist.

To understand the political impact on the reproductive and genetic issues, it is important to understand federal health policy and the interaction among the executive, legislative, and judicial branches of the federal government, states, and interest groups.

THE POLITICAL PROCESS

The U.S. Constitution establishes 3 co-equal branches of the federal government that create a "separation of powers" among the legislative, executive, and judicial branches of government. Unlike parliamentary systems, the party affiliation of the legislative and executive branches can be, and frequently are, different. There are, therefore, 3 loci of policy making that affect all issues, including those of reproductive rights and genetics. Currently, the party affiliation of the executive and the majority in both houses of Congress are the same.

The judicial branch, or the Supreme Court, in which judges are appointed for life, perform the function of interpreting state and federal laws in relation to the Constitution, particularly the Bill of Rights (the first 10 amendments to the Constitution) and federal-state roles and responsibilities.

The president, as the leader of the executive branch, plays a large role in the development and proposal of legislation and regulations. The president also proposes appointments to nonelected offices and takes administrative action through resource allocation of the budget. Serving as head of his political party, he speaks for the party yet to a lesser degree than in parliamentary systems.

For example, the president's budget is not only a resource allocation but a policy document. If agreed on by Congress, the allocation of resources for research, for instance the human genome project, becomes national policy. Unless overridden by a two thirds vote of Congress, a presidential veto of legislation or the threat of veto sets policy. President Clinton used the veto power or its threat to reverse a number of Congressional efforts to limit abortion. President Bush infrequently uses the veto since there is close agreement between the President and the Republican majorities in Congress. The regulatory process, as in the case of the "gag rule" on abortion advice, can establish national policy.

The 2 houses of Congress can have an impact at several points, e.g., the authorization of specific legislation, the authorization for the NIH or Title X of the Public Health Service (Family Planning), and the appropriation of federal funds. In the case of reproductive issues, there is language that specifically prohibits Medicaid use of federal dollars for abortion.

Congress, in particular the Senate, must approve the appointment of key officials in the executive branch and nominees to the Supreme Court. In effect, Congress has the power to veto presidential choices of appointees. For example, during the Clinton administration, there was an objection by senators to the appointment of Dr. Henry Foster, a noted obstetrician-gynecologist, as Surgeon General because he had performed a few abortions. When there is a split in political party between the legislative and executive branches, or the 2 branches of Congress, "gridlock" can occur on legislation and the budget. Gridlock occurred at the end of the Reagan administration, during the subsequent Bush administration, and in the final term of the Clinton administration.

The courts are the final arbiter on the constitutionality of specific legislation, regulation and federal-state disputes over authority.[6] They have played a major role in reproductive genetic policy through *Roe v. Wade* and several interpretations of state statutes, for instance *Planned Parenthood of S.E. Pennsylvania et al. v. Casey, 1992*. Because the President nominates the justices whose nominations are confirmed or denied by the Senate, the views of the President on research and abortion are critical. The abortion issue has played a major role in the selection and confirmation process as evidenced by Congressional denial of Robert Bork during the Reagan administration, and the statements of George W. Bush during the 2000 election that he would nominate justices who would pass a "litmus test" on abortion. He has since said he won't impose a litmus test, but will nominate candidates with a conservative approach to constitutional issues like.

Interest groups play a critical role in health policy through lobbying and political contributions. In recent years, the influence of campaign funding particularly so called soft money, has played a major role in elections and, consequently, is powerful within the executive and legislative branches of government. Many groups are involved in lobbying—from representatives of business and labor, to academic health centers and scientific groups—the right-to-life groups have had a substantial impact on issues of reproduction and reproductive genetics as evidenced by delays in the production and distribution of RU 486, the debate on late term abortion, or partial-birth abortion, and the restrictions on research.[7]

The Constitution also divides power between the states and federal government. The Tenth Amendment to the Constitution states, "The powers not delegated to the United States by the Constitution, nor prohibited by it to the States, are reserved to the States respectively, or to the people." In recent years, the states have played an increasing role in health and welfare policy. For example, although Medicaid is a federal-state program and Congress has restricted the use of federal Medicaid funds to pay for abortion, some states cover abortion under all or limited circumstances using state funding. States also regulate private health insurance, except for plans covered by the Employee Retirement Income Security Act (ERISA) legislation, and some have mandated coverage of infertility services and certain prenatal and newborn testing. Where interest groups have failed to overturn *Roe v. Wade*, they have influenced states to restrict or discourage abortion services through the legislation of waiting periods, parental consent, and prohibition of late term abortions. Many of these laws have been successfully challenged in federal courts.

HEALTHCARE FINANCING

In healthcare, the majority of financing and insurance decision making that affects reproduction and reproductive genetics, such as prenatal diagnosis, occurs in the private sector through the purchase of health insurance, enrollment in Health Maintenance Organizations (HMOs) or self-funding of health benefits by private employers. States and the federal government play roles in the regulation of health insurance and HMOs, except for self-funded or union employer plans that are regulated under ERISA.

The federal government, as an employer, also plays a role under the Federal Employees Health Benefits program and the military direct service and insurance programs for the armed services, their dependents, and retired military personnel. Finally, the federal government sets certain basic standards and limitations on Medicaid and Child Health Insurance plans, which are administered by the states.

There is little detailed knowledge of actual coverage of specific services under private health insurance, self-funded plans, and HMO policies. Decisions on the coverage of specific benefits are made by employers through collective bargaining or by HMOs. Preexisting condition clauses, exclusions for "investigative" or "experimental" procedures, and requirements that services be "medically necessary" have particular relevance to reproductive genetics. In addition, services such as in vitro fertilization, genetic testing, and pregnancy usually occur in one's early years of work, that is before young people are fully settled in employment. They may move in and out of insurance coverage, and they frequently have limited financial access to these services.

While there is better information on federal-state programs, the level of detail is insufficient to determine the coverage of services such as prenatal diagnosis. Medicaid is the primary finance mechanism to provide health services to low income people. Medicaid is a federal-state program in which the states have considerable flexibility to determine the specific services covered for eligible women and their children. Many states do not provide more than prenatal, delivery, and post partum services, and exclude services such as in vitro fertilization. Welfare reform has had an impact on the number of people covered by Medicaid, because coverage is available for 2 years after securing a job. Former welfare recipients generally enter the labor market in low-skilled, low-wage jobs where the employer does not provide health insurance benefits. Thus, when Medicaid eligibility expires the worker is uninsured.

Family planning services may or may not be covered under private plans, although most HMOs make these services available. Family planning is covered under Medicaid and under grants from Title X of the Public Health Service law.

THE ELECTION OF 2000 AND 2004 AND DRAMATIC CHANGES

The election of 2000 posed many questions that have influenced major changes in reproductive genetic and reproductive health policy. George Bush was elected President, while the Senate initially remained under Democratic control. The House majority was and is Republican. The Senate also came under Republican control at the midpoint of President Bush's first term. There were a number of scenarios for the outcome of the 2000 election, each of which would have vastly different consequences for reproductive health policy. The combinations and permutations are as follows:

The growing sophistication of prenatal diagnosis and therapy raises a conflict between a mother and her fetus. An early diagnosis may divide pro-life advocates because some would support abortion under exceptional conditions.[8] In addition, ethical concerns have been raised about the widespread potential availability of prenatal diagnosis of "minor conditions or characteristics."[9,10]

The most dramatic impact has been on the issue of stem cell research. The President has restricted federal funding of stem cell research to a small number of stem cell lives. Although the Republican party is split on the issue, no new lives from fetal tissue can be created using Federal dollars. Several states, notably California and New Jersey, are using state money for stem cell research.

On abortion policy, efforts continue to further restrict abortion.

FUTURE ISSUES IN REPRODUCTIVE GENETIC RESEARCH AND TESTING

RESEARCH

As technology advances new issues emerge. These include whether the ownership of genetic material and treatment modalities derived from genetic research, should be public or commercial property. The blurred distinction between federally funded research and private-sector development of specific diagnostic and treatment technologies grows more complex over time. In the absence of universal health insurance, and policies as to which technologies should be available to all, the issue of ownership can have major impact on access to beneficial technologies by subgroups of the population, particularly low income and minority populations.

INTRODUCTION OF NEW TECHNOLOGIES

There are 2 issues here. First, when does a technology leave the experimental or investigational stage and become recognized for purposes of insurance reimbursement. For example, it took many years after RU 486 was proven effective in Europe be-fore the Food and Drug Administration (FDA) approved it as safe and effective. Then, there were long delays in finding a manufacturer who would provide it to the American market. Consequently, the drug is not yet available.

Gene replacement therapy is another example. Although the FDA makes recommendations on certain technologies, it does not have authority in other areas. Also, there can be widespread differences in decisions made by different public and private insurance plans. For example, in the late 1990s new technologies entered the market before definitive assessment had been completed.

The second issue concerns genetic testing and under what circumstances there should be guidelines for the use and pay-ment of genetic testing, especially when it can lead to abortion under circumstances where there is no evidence of "serious defects to the fetus."[9,10]

PAYMENTS FOR PRENATAL DIAGNOSIS AND THERAPY

Private and public health insurance coverage of prenatal and newborn testing, therapy, and abortion varies widely. The United States has a patchwork of insurance coverage and over 45–47 million people are not covered by any health insur-ance. As described earlier, benefit packages for employees are largely determined by the employer, collective bargaining and the particular HMO or, in the case of public insurance, by Congress or state legislatures. During the past decade, em-ployers have been tightening up coverage because of cost con-straints and imposing greater coinsurance and copayments on services. Also, during this time, many small employers have dropped insurance coverage. In addition, welfare reform has reduced the number of people eligible for Medicaid. As de-scribed earlier, maternity care is also subject to preexisting condition clauses for new employees.

Although ultrasound, fetal monitoring, and amniocentesis are accepted as routine and frequently covered, newer diag-nostic and fetal treatment techniques are slower to be included in coverage, particularly in times of cost constraints. Efficacy and cost effectiveness studies will be increasingly necessary for new diagnostic and treatment modalities.

UNIVERSAL HEALTH INSURANCE COVERAGE

With the growing number of uninsured individuals and the increasing dissatisfaction with managed health plans, there was a renewed interest in expanding health insurance cov-erage through federal and/or state legislation. However, the budget deficit and constraints on state funding have slowed, if not stopped, their efforts. During the Clinton administration there was consensus with the Republican congress to develop a federal state program for low-income children.

If a serious effort were to be made to provide universal cov-erage, the major issues from the prospective of reproductive healthcare would be what services will or will not be covered

under any plan: family planning, genetic testing, fetal treat-ment, or abortion. Will coverage be federal or vary by state? If vouchers are used, will there be minimum coverage require-ments or an open market?

PRIVACY, CONFIDENTIALITY AND PATIENTS RIGHTS

The current situation regarding the privacy of patient records is that insurers, employers and governments routinely have ac-cess to patients' records. The rationale is to determine whether the provided medical services are "medically necessary."[11] A number of states have regulations to protect privacy and con-fidentiality of medical records. These regulations do not apply to self funded plans. Because health insurance, in general, is experience rated the threat remains that insurers and employers will seek such information, in order to reduce their exposure to medical care costs for those with a predisposition to genetic illness.

It is hypothesized, although there is no hard evidence, that individuals do not apply for health insurance payments for ge-netic testing because of the fear that it will affect employability of family members and the ability to obtain health insurance coverage at reasonable rate.

The debate over patients' rights, the ability to choose a personal physician and obtain a referral to a specialist, and coverage of specific services under managed care plans di-rectly affects reproductive screening for genetic risks and fetal intervention, because most of these services are not provided by primary care physicians, but require referral to obstetric and gynecological specialists in reproductive genetics.

CONCLUSIONS

It is difficult to predict what will happen during the remainder of the Bush administration, because both the issues and the political environment remain complex. In the fields of repro-duction and reproductive genetics, new advances are ongoing and usually raise religious, ethical, political issues. These is-sues range from federal funding of specific types of research to the rights of the mother and fetus, ie, who has choice under what circumstances; from the effectiveness of different diag-nostic and treatment modalities to who pays for what under what circumstances. Based on past experience, it is clear that the election and the political process, including appointments to the Supreme Court, have profound implications for the res-olution of many of these issues.

References

1. Strickland SP. *Politics, Science and Dread Disease.* Cambridge, MA: Harvard University Press; 1972:134–157.

2. *New York Times*. February 26, 2000.

3. *Roe v. Wade,* 410 U.S. 113, 93 S. Ct. 705, 35 L.Ed. 2d 147 (1970).

4. Kirchhoff. Progress or bust: the push to double NIH's budget. *Congressional Quarterly Weekly*. May 8, 1999:1060.

5. Munro N. Frontier ethics. *National Journal*. June 5, 1999: 1518.

6. *Marbury v. Madison,* 5 U.S. 137 at 177–178, 2l ed. 60 (1803).

7. *ADA v. Guam Society of Obstetricians and Gynecologists et al,* U.S. Lexus 7350, 61 U.S. L.W. 3399 (1992).

8. Mattingly S. The maternal fetal dyad. *Hastings Center Report*. 1992;22(1):13–18.

9. Andrews LB, Fullarton JE, Holtzman NA, et al. *Assessing Genetic Risks: Implications For Social Policy.* Washington, DC: National Academy Press: 1994.

10. Botkin J. Fetal privacy and confidentiality. *The Hastings Center Report*. 1995;25(5): September–October 1995.

11. Silberner J. Keeping confidence: capitol report. *The Hastings Center Report*. 1997;27(6), November–December 1997.

INDEX

Note: Numbers in italics indicate figures; those followed by *t* indicate tables.

A

Abdomen (fetal)
abdominal tumors, 336
abdominal wall defects, 248–252, 333–335, 599–600
gastroschisis, 251–252
omphalocele, 249–250
astomia, 240
calcifications, *248*
congenital agastria, 243
congenital duplication of the stomach, 242
congenital esophageal duplication, 241
congenital isolated esophageal atresia, 240–241
embryology, 239
esophageal atresia associated with tracheoesophageal
fistula, 241
esophageal stenosis, 241
esophagus, 240
expectation of ultrasound examination, 239
gallbladder, 247–248
gastrointestinal abnormalities, 239–40
large intestine, 245–246
larnyx and pharnyx, 240
laryngeal atresia, 240
laryngeal palsy, 240
liver, 246–247, 249*t*
microgastria, 243
nonvisualization of fetal stomach, causes of, 242*t*
normal and abnormal findings, 44
normal ultrasound appearance of upper GI tract, *241*
overview, 239–240
pyloric atresia, 243
small intestine, *243,* 243–245
spleen, 247, 249*t*
stomach, 241–242
stomach pseudomass, *242*
teratoma, 240
Abdominal dystocia, 261
Abetalipoproteinemia, 12*t*
Abnormalities. *See also* specific abnormality
incidence of in multifetal gestation, 572*t*
percent incidence of in twins/singletons, 572*t*
Abnormal reconstitution, 46
Abortion, 537–546. *See also* First trimester termination;
Second trimester termination; Selective termination;
Spontaneous abortion
of anomalous fetus in multiple gestations (second trimester),
543–545
counseling, 715–716
difficulty of choices after prenatal diagnosis, 716*t*
ethical issues, 716–717
first trimester, 537–538

illegal, 704
laws, 284, 571, 741
minor's right to consent to, 735–736
percentage of reported legal abortions, 539*t*
political issues, 741
presented as option for fetal anomalies, 581
privacy rights, 284
psychological aspects of, 524, 545–546
respecting different cultural perspectives on, 716–717
second trimester, 538–543
third trimester, 717
Abruptio placenta, 674
Acatalasia, 12*t*
Accessory lobe of the liver, 247
Accutane, 119
ACE inhibitors, 84*t*
Acentric chromosomes, 47
Acetylcholinesterase, 455, 476
Achalasia, 241
Achondrogenesis, 263, 265, *266*
Achondroplasia, 10, 12*t,* 53, 263, 266–267
Acne medications, 119–120
Acrania, 641
Acrocallosal syndrome, 214
Acrocentric chromosomes, 46
Actinomyces israelli, 152
Acute intermittent porphyria, 636–637
Acute lymphoblastic leukemia, 647
Adenine phosphoribosyltransferase deficiency, 488
Adeno-associated virus, 684–685
Adenosine deaminase deficiency, 687
Adenoviruses, 684
Adult polycystic kidney disease (APDK), 501, 502
Advanced maternal age
genetic counseling and, 72
as indication for amniocentesis, 415
as indication for biochemical screening, 277, 283–285
African-descended population, single gene disorders
and, 12*t*
Age determination. *See* Fetal age determination
Agency for Health Care Policy and Research (AHCPR), 705
Agenesis, 211, 257
of the corpus callosum (ACC), 214–215, 377
of the liver, 247
Aging
Down syndrome and maternal age, 20–22, 21*t,* 315–316
Down syndrome and paternal age, 21
folic acid intake and, 647
as indication for CVS, 433
risk of abnormalities with, 571
somatic mtDNA mutations and, 33–34

Aicardi's syndrome, 215
Air embolization, 572–573
Alcohol abuse, during pregnancy, 123–128
    diagnosing, 127
    effects of alcohol, 125–126
        low birth weight, 125
        neural development, 126
        neurobehavioral and neural abnormality, 125–126
        spontaneous abortion/stillbirths, 125
    paternal drinking, 125
    prevention, 127
    research issues, 126–127
Alcohol-related birth defects (ARBDs), 123
Alcohol-related neurodevelopmental disorders (ARNDs), 123
Allele drop out (ADO), 508
Alleles, 10
Allele-specific oligonucleotide hybridization, 497
Alloimmune thrombocytopenia (ATP), 444, 454
Alloimmunization, 443, 453
Alobar holoprosencephaly, 192, 212–213, *213*
Alpha-fetoprotein, 279–280, 417, 419
    failure of offer AFP test, 731
α-iduronidase, 487
α-l-antitrypsin deficiency, 499
α-thalassemia, 12*t*, 687
Alzheimer's disease, 647
American Collaborative Report, 435
American College of Medical Genetics, 475, 481
American College of Obstetricians and Gynecologists Ethics Committee, 577
Amino acid disorders, 489–490
    alcohol abuse and, 125
Aminophyllines, 143*t*
Aminopterin, 83*t*, 84
Amniocentesis, 415–419, *417*, 423, 449, 475–476. *See also* Early amniocentesis
    chromosome aberrations found in, 5
    fetal CMV infection and, 156
    indications for prenatal diagnosis by, 415–416, 416*t*
    interpretation of results, 417–418
    legal issues, 732, 733
    multiple gestations and, 418
    safety and complications of, 419
    special conditions for, 418
    technical aspects of, 416–417
    tetraploidy diagnosis from, 6
Amniodrainage, 462, 463–464
Amnioinfusion, 608
Amniomax, 475
Amniotic band syndrome (ABSd), 468, 642*t*
Amniotic fluid
    embolism, 469
    leakage, 419
    physiology of, 410
    ultrasound evaluation of, 410–411
Amputation, 468, 597
Analgesics, 142*t*
Anal rectal atresia, 246
Analyte-specific reagents, 481
Anasarca, 674, 675
Androgens, 84, 84*t*
Anemia, 345, 445
Anencephaly, 15, 178, *188, 209–210, 210,* 331, *332,* 575, 641, 643
Anesthetics, 143*t*
Aneuploidies, 5, 6, 19–30, 44, 475. *See also* Cytogenetics; Molecular cytogenetics; Trisomy 21 (Down syndrome)
    diagnosis using fetal cells from maternal blood, 507

Edwards syndrome, 19, 29
    high-resistance umbilical artery Doppler study, 343
    Patau syndrome, 19, 29
    second semester sonographic markers for
        Down syndrome, 309–317
        Edward syndrome, *317,* 317–321, *318, 319*
        Patau syndrome, *321,* 321–322, *322*
        triploidy, 322–324, *323*
        Turner syndrome, *324,* 324–325, *325*
    sex chromosome aneuploidy, 29–30
    smaller-than-expected fetus and, 433
Aneurism of the vein of galen, 331, 380, *381*
Angelman syndrome, 35, 36, 48, 439, 480, 481*t*, 486
Angiotensin-converting enzyme (ACE) inhibitors, 84*t*
Anhydramnios, 261, 606
Anomalies
    obstetrical management of (*See* Obstetrical management of anomalies)
    ultrasound diagnosis of, 187–194
Antiacne medications, 144*t*
Antiarrhythmic therapy
    fetal, 676–677
    maternal, 676
Antibiotics, 84*t*, 141, 142*t*
Anticipation phenomenon, 14, 37
Anticoagulants, 120, 144*t*
Anticonvulsant drugs, 83, 143*t*
    Carbamazepine (Tegeretol), 115
    Phenytoin, 114–115
    Trimethadione, 118
    Valproic acid, 115, 118
Antidepressant drugs, 118–119, 143*t*
    Fluoxetine, 118–119
    Lithium, 119
Antiemetics, 142*t*, 143*t*
Antihistamines, 142*t*
Antihypertensives, 85*t*
Antimalarials, 144*t*
Antimetabolites, 538
Antiprogestins, 538, 538*t*
Antipyretic drugs, 141, 142*t*
Antithyroid medications, 143*t*
Anti-tuberculosis therapy, 85*t*, 90, 142*t*
Aortic arch hypoplasia, *661*
Aortic balloon valvuloplasty, 678–679
Aortic stenosis, 678
Arachnoid cysts, 219, *220,* 378, *379*
Arachnoid granulations, congenital absence of, 217
ARBDs. *See* Alcohol-related birth defects (ARBDs)
ARNDs. *See* Alcohol-related neurodevelopmental disorders (ARNDs)
Arnold-Chiari malformation, 189, 212, 217, 218, 601, 641
Arrhythmia (fetal), 193, 345, 585
Arterio-venous anastomosis, 461
Arteriovenous malformations, 666
Arthrogryposis, 193
Ascertainment bias, 113
Ascites, *193, 259*
Ashkenazi Jewish population
    autosomal recessive disorders and, 12*t*, 501
    disease carrier frequencies, 74*t*
    single gene disorders and, 12*t*, 485
Asians, autosomal recessive disorders in, 12*t*, 501
Aspartylglucoseaminuria, 12*t*
Aspirin intake, maternal, 85*t*, 673
Assisted reproductive technologies (ARTs), 433, 561, 566*t*
    Down syndrome risk, 23–24
Astomia, 240
Ataxia telangiectasia, 7

Atherosclerotic disease, 647
Atrial flutter, 665–666, 676
Atrial septal defect (ASD), 15*t*
Atrioventricular valves, 662
Autoimmune disorders, persisting fetal cells in maternal blood and, 510
Autopsy. *See* Fetal autopsy
Autosomal aneuploidies, 44–46
Autosomal dominant disorders, 10–11, 12*t*
Autosomal dominant pedigree, 11*f*
Autosomal recessive inheritance, 11–13
    autosomal recessive pedigree, *13*
    characteristics, 12
    X-linked pedigree, *13*
Autosomal trisomies, 6
Avery, Oswald, 71

B
Bacteremia, post CVS, 434
Bacterial infections, and pregnancy, 149–152
    Group A beta-hemolytic streptococcus, 150–153
    Group B beta-hemolytic streptococci (GBS), 149–150
Bacteroidaceae, 152
Balanced rearrangements, 46–47
Balanced translocations, 478
Balloon atrial septoplasty, 679
Balloon valvuloplasty, 667
Banana sign, 189, *192, 212*
Basal ganglia, 33–34
Bayesian analysis, 452
BDIS, 598
Beckwith-Wiedemann Syndrome (BWS), 35–36, 599
Behavioral development, alcohol abuse and, 125
Bell syndrome, 498
Beneficence, 707, 722
Benzoate/phenyacetate (Ucephan®), 636
Benzodiazepines, 85*t*, 90
ß-globin genotype, 509
Beta hCG levels, 438
Beta human chorionic gonadotrophin, 279
ß-thalassemia, 10, 12*t*, 499, 509, 687
Bilateral club feet, *358*
Bilateral renal agenesis (BRA), 257, 501
Biochemical genetics, 485–490
    assay conditions, 488–489
    controls and blanks, 489
    enzyme preparations, 488
    fetal samples, 487–488
    genetic heterogeneity, 486–487
    mode of inheritance/family studies, 485–486
    nonenzymatic defects, 490
    separation and detection methods, 489–490
    substrates and cofactors, 489
Biochemical screening, 277–285, 415
    "advanced maternal age" and, 283–285
    for chromosome abnormalities, 279–282
    fundamental principles, 277–278
    integrated testing
        algorithmic questions, 282–283
        first trimester, 282
        Trisomy 18, 282
    for neural tube defects, 279
    public policy and ethical issues, 283
    screening *vs.* diagnostic tests, 278*t*
    two-step approach to fetal cell analysis, *281*
Bioinformatics, 514–515

Biomed 2 Programme, 459
Biopsies, tissue. *See* Tissue biopsies
Bipolar coagulation, 467
Birth control movement, in U.S., 701
Birth defects, 3. *See also* Fetal anomalies and birth defects
    environmental/occupatational exposure and, 140–141
    psychological reaction to, 523
Birth weight, effect of alcohol abuse on, 125
Blacks, autosomal recessive disorders in, 12*t*
Bladder (fetal), 257. *See also* Genitourinary tract abnormalities
    bladder outlet obstruction, 477
    enlarged, demonstrating keyhole sign, *258*
Blair v. Hutzel Hospital, 729
Bleeding, after CVS, 437
Blighted ovum, 6
Blood transfusion, fetal, 459
Bloom's syndrome, 7, 12*t*
Body stalk anomaly, 300
Body wall defects, 642*t*
Bone marrow donors, 502
Bone marrow transplantation, 691
Boston Children's Hospital, 679
Brachycephaly, 44
Bradyarrhythmia (fetal), 585–586
Bradycardia (fetal), 445, 674, 675, 677
Brain imaging. *See also* Neurosonography
    corpus callosum and midbrain structures, 369
    multiplanar display of midline structures, *360*
    posterior fossa, 369–371, *370*
    transvaginal fetal neuroscan, 365–369
Brain tumors (fetal), 221–222
Breast cancer, 501, 502, 647
    chemotherapy during pregancy, 178–179
Bronchial cyst, 610, 612*t*
Bronchioalveolar carcinoma, 628
Bronchogenic cysts, 628
Bronchopulmonary sequestration, 346
Brushfield spots, 44
Bulky disease, 180
Burton, Barbara, 737
BWS. *See* Beckwith-Wiedemann Syndrome (BWS)

C
Caffeine, 86*t*, 90–91, 665
Calcium flux, 673
Calymmatobacterium granulomatis, 152
Campomelic dysplasia, 268–269
Canadian Collaborative CVS-Amniocentesis Clinical Trial, 433
Canavan, 12*t*
Cancer. *See also* Chemotherapy, in pregnancy; specific type of cancer
    chemotherapeutic drugs, 144*t*
    folic acid intake and, 646
    radiation exposure and, 171, 173–174
Cannon waves, 675
Cannulas, 459–460
Capillary hemangiomata, 45
Carbamazepine (Tegeretol), 86*t*, 91–92, 115
Carbamyl phosphate synthetase deficiency, 451
Cardiac abnormalities, obstetric management of, 584
    diaphragmatic hernia, 586–587
    extrasystole, 585
    fetal arrhythmia, 585
    structural cardiac anomalies, 584–585
    sustained bradyarrhythmia, 585–586
    sustained tachyarrhythmia, 585
    ventral wall defects, 587–588
Cardiac function, 229

Cardiac imaging techniques, 227–229
Cardiac malformations, isotretinoin ingestion and, 120
Cardiac tamponade, 573, *573*
Cardiac therapy, 671–680
    aortic balloon valvuloplasty, 678–679
    clinical implications, 673–775
        calcium flux, 673
        nonimmune hydrops fetalis, 674
        preload and afterload reserve, 673–674
    evolution of fetal congenital heart disease, 675
    fetal antiarrhythmic therapy
        bradycardia and, 677
        tachycardia and, 676–677
    fetal cardiovascular physiology, 671–672
    fetal congestive heart failure and, 677–678
    fetal myocardial performance, 672–673
    future directions in, 679
    interventional cardiac catheterization of fetus, 678–679
    pulmonary balloon valvuloplasty, 679
    in utero, 675–676
Cardiovascular diseases
    folic acid and, 646, 647
    future of surgery for, 667–668
Cardiovascular system, evaluation of, 653–668. *See also* Heart and vascular
        malformations
    blood flow distribution, 663–665
    cardiac area/thoracic area ratio measurement, *659*
    cardiac structure, 659–661
    Doppler echocardiography, 662–663
    echocardiography
        essential components of, 659*t*
        indications for, 655–659, 655*t*
        purpose of, 654–655
    fetal circulation, *654*
    noncongenital heart disease, 666–667
    normal view of heart, *660*
    rhythm disturbances in the fetus, 665–666
    tomographic views used for imaging of fetal heart, *656–658*
    transposition of the great arteries, *661*
    uniqueness of fetal system, 653–654
Carrier detection, 501–502
C-banding, 41
CDH. *See* Congenital diaphragmatic hernia (CDH)
Cebocephaly, 45
Cell differentiation, 63–66
Cell membrane dysfunction, 10
Cell memory, 66
Central nervous system
    diagnosed with 3-D ultrasound, 359
    fetal genetic therapy and, 688
    fetopsy of tissue, 553–554
    obstetric management of anomalies, 582
    tumors, 346
Centromeric probes, 482
Cephalic pole malformations, 331
Cephaloceles, 211
Cephalocentesis, 195
Cerebellar hypoplasia, *380*
Cerebral parenchyma, progressive degeneration of, 331
Ceredase®, 636
Chain termination mutations, 10
Chang, 475
CHARGE association, 61
Charge flow separation, 506
CHD7, 61
Chelation therapy, 637
Chemical cleavage of mismatch (CCM), 499

Chemical matrix, 513
Chemotherapy, in pregnancy, 141, 144*t,* 177–182
    breast cancer, 178–179
    chemotherapeutic agents, classification of, 177–182
    colon cancer, 182
    leukemia, 179
    lymphoma, 179–181
    melanoma, 181–182
    ovarian cancer, 181
Chickenpox (varicella), 160
Chinese
    alpha thalassemia and, 12*t*
    autosomal recessive disorders and, 12*t*
Chlamydia trachomatis, 150–151
Chondroectodermal dysplasia, 269
Chorangioma, 409
Chorioamnionitis, 419, 608
Chorionicity, 349, 350*t*, 409
Chorionic villus sampling (CVS), 7, 423, 433–440, 449, 476–477, 487
    accuracy of, 438
    complications, 437–439
    confined placental mosaicism and, 439
    fetal virus infections and, 156
    indications, 433
    informed consent/legal risks, 736–738
    lab methodology, 476–477
    long-term infant development after, 438
    multiple gestations and, 433
    posterior early, *436*
    procedure, 433–435
    risk of fetal abnormalities following, 436–437
    safety of, 433, 435–436
    transcervical, *434,* 476
    trisomy rescue and, 36
Chorionic villous sampling (CVS), 92
Choroid plexus, 205, 331
Choroid plexus cysts (CPC), *192,* 219, *220,* 319–321, *334, 378*
    and chromosomal aneuploidy, 378*t*
Choroid plexus papillomas, 221
Christmas disease, 487
Chromatin-DNA, 65
Chromosomal aberrations, 41, 43–48
    autosomal aneuploidies, 44–46
    balanced rearrangements, 46–47
    diagnosis of indirect signs of, 337–339
    DiGeorge syndrome, 48
    frequency of, 43
    inversions, 47
    microdeletion syndromes, 48
    Miller-Dieker syndrome, 48
    numerical, 43–44
    Prader-Willi and Angelman syndromes, 48
    structural abnormalities, 46
    subtelomeric rearrangements, 48
    unbalanced rearrangements, 47–48
    velocardiofacial (VCF) syndrome, 48
    Williams syndrome, 48
Chromosomal anomalies, 5–8
    detected in amniocentesis, 415
    frequency of, 5*t*
    numerical, 5–7
    obstetric management of, 591
    structural, 7–8
Chromosomal breakage, 46
Chromosomal mosaicism, 7
Chromosome analysis requirements/guidelines, 475–476
Chromosome 15, 439, 482

Chromosomes, 3–5, 41. *See also* Chromosomal anomalies
Cimetidine, 119
Class bias, 701
Cleft lip and/or palate, 14, 15*t*, 45, *358*
Cleidocranial dysplasia, 271
Clinical equipoise, 722
Cloaca, developmental abnormalities of, 607
Cloacal anomalies, *259*
Cloning, 36
"Closed" spina bifida, 641
Clostridia, 152
Clubfoot, 193, *194, 358*
CNS-derived neural progenitor cells, 688
Coagulation disorders, 687–688
Cocaine, 86*t*, 100–101
College of American Pathologists (CAP), 475, 481
Colobomata, 45
Colon atresia, 246
Colon cancer, 182, 646–647
Colon duplication, 246
Color blindness, 14*t*
Colorectal cancer. *See* Colon cancer
Complete congenital heart block, 585
Computer and ultrasound, 383–385
Conception, and intercourse frequency, 135, 136*t*
Confidentiality, 744
Confined placental mosaicism, 439
Congenital adrenal hyperplasia, 633–634
Congenital agastria, 243
Congenital amputation, 597
Congenital anomalies, assessment and management of, 595–602
    abdominal wall defects, 599–600
    congenital cystic adenomatoid malformation, 599
    congenital diaphragmatic hernia, 599
    congenital heart disease, 597*t*
    ethical considerations, 601
    hydrops fetalis, 598–599, 598*t*, 599*t*
    interpretation of diagnostic studies, 595
    myelomeningocele, 601
    physical assessment, 596
    postnatal diagnostic studies, 597–598
    renal anomalies, 600–601
    resuscitation, 595–596
Congenital bullous epidermolysis, 449
Congenital cystic adenomatoid malformation (CCAM), 599, 627–631, 666
    accuracy of prenatal diagnosis, 629
    antenatal diagnosis of, 628–629
    disappearing lung lesions, 629
    embryology, 627
    fetal surgery, 630
    fetal therapy, 629–630
    natural history, 627–628
    postnatal management, 630–631
    prenatal management strategy, 630
Congenital cystic adenomatoid malformation (CCAM) shunt therapy, 610–613
    differential diagnosis in CCAM, 612*t*
    MRIs, *611, 612*
    prenatal evaluation, 610–611
    sonographic images, *611–613*
    technique, 611–612
Congenital diaphragmatic hernia (CDH), *191,* 599, 617–624, 628, 666
    algorithm for management of affected fetus, *623*
    experimental correction of simulated, *618*
    "liver up" and "liver down," 621
    maternal and fetal considerations, 619–621

    mortality rate, 618, 619
    prenatal diagnosis and prognosis, 618–619
    rationale for in utero intervention, 617
    sonography, 618
    in utero surgical correction, 617–621
        complete CDH repair, 621
        EXIT procedure, *622, 622*–623
        fetoscopic tracheal ternal laparotomy, *623*
        future directions in, 624
        maternal perioperative care, 620–621
        PLUG, 621–624
        tracheal occlusion, *622*
        "two-step" technique, *621*
Congenital dislocation of hip (CDH), 15*t*
Congenital esophageal atresia, 240–241
Congenital esophageal duplication, 241
Congenital heart disease, 14, 15*t*, 584–585, 597, 653. *See also* Cardiac therapy
    conditions associated with, 597*t*
    heart block, 677
    omphaloceles and, 599
    timeline for detection/diagnosis of, *654*
Congenital hypophosphatasia (perinatal lethal type), 270–271
Congenital hypothyroidism, 501, 633
Congenital ichthyosiform ertheraderma, 449
Congenital infection, 444, 454
Congenital mesoblastic nephroma, 261
Congenital nephrosis, 12*t*
Conjoined twins, 351–353, *355*
Conotruncal malformations, 232
Consanguinity, 12, 74
Contiguous gene syndromes, 47
Contraceptives
    barrier, 135
    oral, 113, 135
Cord
    cord occlusion, 466–468
        bipolar coagulation, 467
        fetoscopic cord ligation, 467
        laser coagulation, 466–467
        monopolar coagulation, 467
    entanglement, 350
    fetoscopic ligation, 467, 575
    fetoscopic surgery on, 461
Cordocentesis, 7, 443–446, 449, 453–448, 607
    complications/risk factors for, 445–446, 445*t*
    indications and applications for, 444–445, 444*t*, 454–447
    methods, 443–444, 453–454
Coronal planes, *203,* 203–204
Corpus callosum, 190
    absence of, 126
    agenesis of, *214,* 214–215
    neuroscan of, 370, *375*
Cortical cysts, *606*
Coumadin derivatives, 92–93
Coumarin derivatives, 86*t*, 120
Counseling, 703. *See also* Genetic counseling
    for abnormalities, 529–535
        facilitation of waiting period, 530–532
        indication for prenatal diagnosis, 529
        prenatal diagnostic techniques and, 529–530
    abortion counseling, 715–716
    of both parents, 715
    content of, 713
    decision-making process
        continuing the pregnancy, 534
        termination of pregnancy, 532–533
    followup, 534–535

Counseling (*contd.*)
  full disclosure of test results, 714
  post-test, after findings of affected fetus, 715–716
  prior to prenatal diagnosis, 713
  psychological aspects of pregnancy termination, 545–546
  selective termination of anomalous fetus in multiple gestations, 543
  in subsequent pregnancies, 535
  support groups, 531, 533, 535
  timing of, prior to prenatal diagnosis, 713–714, 714*t*
  when parental behavior leads to birth defects, 715
COX deficiency, 34–35
Cranial dysraphia, 211–212
Craniofacial anomalies, 468
  isotretinoin ingestion and, 119
Creatine phosphokinase (CPK), 451
Crick, Francis, 71
Cri du chat syndrome (5p deletion syndrome), 48, 481*t*
Curtis-Fitz-Hughes syndrome, 151
CVS. *See* Chorionic villus sampling (CVS)
Cyanocobalamin, 634
Cyclophosphamide, 86*t*, 93
Cyclopia, 45
Cyro-precipitate plug (amniopatch), 469
Cystic adenomatous malformation, 610, 612*t*
Cystic fibrosis, 12, 12*t*, 497, 499, 501, 502, 686
  genetic counseling for, 74
Cystic hygroma, 45, 324, 325, 331, 477
Cystinosis, 490, 636
Cytochrome C oxidase (COX) deficiency, 34–35
Cytogenetics, 455. *See also* Molecular cytogenetics
  amniocentesis, 475–476
  chorionic villus sampling (CVS), 476–477
  cystic hygroma fluid, 477
  fetal blood sampling, 477
  fetal skin biopsy, 477–478
  fetal urine, 477
  G-banded karyotypes, *478–480*
  issues common to all prenatal sample types, 478–480
  standard cytogenetic techniques, 41
Cytomegalovirus (CMV), 157–159, 158*t*, 221

D

Daffos, Fernand, 443, 453, 477
Dandy-Walker malformation, 187, *188*, 215, *216*, 331, *380*, 643
Darwin, Charles, 71
Databases, 61, 383
D&C (dilation and curettage), 537, 542
Decidua, 407
D&E (dilation and extraction), 539, 541, 541*t*
Deformations, 58, 58*t*, 141. *See also* specific deformation
deLange's syndrome, 215
Deletions, 47
De Lia, Julian, 461
Denaturing gradient gel electrophoresis (DGGE), 499
Deoxyribonucleic acid (DNA). *See* DNA
Determination, 63
Developmental anomalies, 346
Developmental delay, 8
Dexamethasone, 665
Diabetes, 14
  maternal, 666
  maternally inherited diabetes mellitus, 35
  non-insulin-dependent diabetes mellitus (NIDDM), 35

Diagnostic *vs.* screening tests, 278*t*
Diaphragmatic hernia, 610, 612*t*
Diastrophic dysplasia, 269
Diazepam, 455
Dicentric chromosomes, 47
Dichorionic twins, 349, *351*
Dictyotene, 4
Dicumarol, 120
Diethylstilbestrol, 87*t*, 93
DiGeorge syndrome, 42, 48, 481*t*, 482, 597
Digoxin, 87*t*, 677–678
Dilation and curettage (D&C), 537, 541*t*, 542
Dilation and extraction (D&E), 539, 541
Dillon v. Legg, 730
Dimeric inhibin A, 281
Diode laser, 460
Diphenylhydantoin, 87*t*, 93–94, 114
Disclosure
  of full information about disorder, 715
  of test results, 714
Discordant trisomy 18, 575
Disruption, 58, 141. *See also* specific disruption
Disseminated intravascular coagulopathy (DIC), 574
Distension medium and instruments, 460
Diuretics, *143*
Diverticulum, 241
DNA, 3, 41, 493
  chief classes of, 9
  cytogenetic principles, 41
  fetal DNA in maternal plasma, 509
  fingerprinting, 508
  "frameshift" mutations, 10, *10*
  methylation of, 35, 36
  molecular cytogenetic techniques, 41–43
  mutation in normal sequence of, 9–10
  nucleotide base pairing, *8*
  polymorphisms, 499
  reverse dot blot, 497
  southern blot analysis, 497–499, *498, 499*
  transcriptional regulation and, 65
  trinucleotide repeats, 494
Doe v. Bolton, 284, 571
Dominant disorders, 10
Doppler imaging
  abdominal wall defects, 333–335
  color flow, 331–339, 408, 621
  in diagnosis of indirect signs of chromosomal defects, 337–339
  Doppler Flow Velocity Waveform Study, 343
  echocardiography, 662–663, *664*
  fetal abnormalities in second trimester, 343–346
    chorioangioma of the placenta, 346
    developmental anomalies, 346
    fetal anemia, 345
    fetal cardiac anomaly, arrhythmia, 345
    organ identification, 346
    umbilical placental flow velocity waveforms, 343–345
  fetal lung masses and, 627
  malformations of the cephalic pole, 331
  malformations of the genito-urinary tract, 335–336
  malformations of the thorax, 331–333
  pulsed- and color-flow, 227, 228
  tissue imaging, 677
  of vascular anatomy, 345–346
Doppler resistance index, 444, 445, 454
Down, Langdon, 289, 309
Down syndrome. *See* Trisomy 21 (Down syndrome)
Drinking, maternal. *See* Alcohol abuse, during pregnancy

Drugs, 113–120. *See also* specific drug
  acne treatments, 119–120
  anticonvulsant, 114–115, 118
  antidepressants, 118–119
  ascertainment bias, 113
  coumarin derivatives, 120
  FDA use in pregnancy ratings, 114*t*
  H2 blockers, 119
  oral contraceptives, 113
  teratogen
    probable risk of, ranking, 115*t*
    Wayne State University rating system, 116–117*t*
  teratogenicity of, 141–144
Duchenne muscular dystrophy, 10, 13, 14*t*, 688
  tissue biopsies for, 443–443, 449, 451–453
Ductal closure, 673
Ductus venosus, 662, *664*
Duodenal atresia/stenosis, *244*
Duodenal ulcer, 15*t*
Dysmorphic features, 8
Dysmorphology, 63
Dysplasia, 58–59. *See also* specific dysplasia
Dysraphia, 211–212
Dystrophin, 443, 452, 453, 688
Dystrophin gene structure, *496*

E
Early amniocentesis, 418–419, 423–430
  amniotic fluid sampling and results
    accuracy of results, 425–426
    technique, 425
  comparing benefits and risks of, 424–425
  complications
    fetal needle trauma, 429
    musculoskeletal, 428–429, 428*t*
    postprocedure amniotic fluid leakage, 428
    post-procedure loss rate, 424, 426–428, 426*t*
  defined, 423
  embryology, 423–424
  evidence of bacterial and viral organisms, 429
  studies on, 424*t*
Eastern Europeans, autosomal recessive disorders and, 12*t*
Ebstein anomaly, 119
Echocardiography, 193, 585–586, 610, 671, 676. *See also* Heart and vascular malformations
  Doppler technique, 662–663
  imaging techniques, 227–229
  impact of, on obstetric management, 232–234
  increased nuchal translucency as indicator for, 300
  transvaginal, *663*
Echogenic bowel, 245
Echogenic intracardiac focus, 312–313, *313*
Echoplanar magnetic resonance imaging, 628
Ectodermal dysplasia, 14*t*
Ectopic kidneys, 257
Ectopic pregnancy, 543
Edema, *338*
Edwards syndrome. *See* Trisomy 18 (Edwards syndrome)
Electronic medical record (EMR), 383–385, *384*
Electrospray ionization (ESI), 513
Ellis-van Creveld syndrome, 215, 269
Emancipated minors, 734
Embryofetoscopy, 156
Embryogenesis, 63, *64*
Embryonal rhabdomyosarcoma, 628
Embryonic germinal disc, 468
Embryoscopy, in first trimester, 460–461

Emergency situations, consent for minors, 734
Encephalocele, *190,* 217, 641
Encephalomyopathies, 54
Endocardial cushion defect, 44
Endoscopes, 459
Endoscopic laser coagulation, 575
Endothelin, 445
Enteroviruses, 162
Environmental and occupational exposure, 131–146
  animal reproductive/developmental endpoints, 132
  dependent factors, 135*t*
  developmental toxicity or birth defects, 140–141
  epidemiology of reproductive failure, 136–137
  epidemiology of spontaneous abortion, 137–139
  exposure assessment, 134
  hazard characterization, 134
  hazard identification, 131, 133–134
  human reproductive/developmental endpoints, 131–132, 132*t*
  industrial and environmental exposures, 145–146
  infertility, causes of, 137*t*
  maternal, and miscarriage, 139
  multifactorial disorders and, 14, 15
  reproductive status among currently married women, 137*t*
  risk assessment, 131
  risk characterization, 134
  successful reproduction/development, 134–136
  timing of, in reproductive/developmental toxicity, 132–133, 133*t*
Env protein, 684
Enzymatic defects, 3
Epidermolysis bullosa lethalis, 449, 477
Epidermolytic hyperkeratosis, 449
Epigenetic phenomena, 36
Epilepsy, 14, 114
Epostane, 538*t*
Epstein-Barr virus (EBV), 160
Equipoise, 722, 724
Escherichia coli, 151–152
Eskimos, single gene disorders and, 12*t*
Esophagus, 240
  esophageal atresia, 240–241
  esophageal compression, 610
  esophageal stenosis, 241
Ethical issues
  beneficence, 707, 722
  biochemical screening and, 283
  cooperation of practicing physicians with clinical investigation, 724
  cross-cultural considerations, 707–718
    abortion, 716–717
    attitudes towards persons with disabilities, 718
    equitable access to services, 708–709
    equity and parents' view of abortion, 709
    indications for prenatal diagnosis, 709–710
    maternal anxiety, 713
    parental preference of sex, 710–712
    prenatal paternity testing, 712
    pretest and posttest counseling, 713–716
    resources for prenatal diagnosis providers, 707–708
    tissue-typing for organ or marrow donation, 712
    voluntary use and "less serious" conditions, 712–713
  ethical criteria for clinical trials of new fetal therapies, 722–723
  ethical principles in medicine, 708*t*
  fetal genetic therapy and, 688–689
  fetus as patient, 721–722
  informed consent, 723–724
  proposed prenatal diagnosis guidelines, 708*t*
  selection criteria based on abortion preference, 724
  selective termination and, 576–577

Ethical issues (*contd.*)
  spina bifida surgery, 724–725
  treatment of congenital malformations, 601
  in utero surgery, 619
Ethnic populations, 501
  autosomal recessive disorders in, 12
  Down syndrome risk, 24, *25*
  ethnic-based carrier screening, 74
  neural tube defects and, 643
  single gene disorders in, 12*t*
Etretinate, 97–98
Eugenics, 71, 702–703
EUROFOETUS project, 459, 464–465, 469
European MRC Working Party on the Evaluation of CVS, 435
Exencephalocele, 331
Exencephaly, 331
Exomphalos, 249
Exons, 493
Exsanguination, 573
Extra-amniotic prostaglandins, 540–541
Extracorporeal membrane oxygenation (ECMO), 617
Extralobar pulmonary sequestration, 610, 612*t*
Extrasystole, 585
Extremities, evaluation by 3-D ultrasound, 361

F
Fabry disease, 486, 489
Facial dysmorphism, 14
FACS, 505, 506
Factor XI deficiency, 12*t*
FADS. *See* Fetal akinesia deformation sequence (FADS)
Familial dysautonomia, 12*t*, 501
Familial hypercholesterolemia, 490
Familial Mediterranean fever, 12*t*
Family history of disorder/defects, genetic counseling and, 73
Family involvement, in grief process, 525–526
Fanconi anemia, 7
FASD. *See* Fetal alcohol spectrum disorders (FASD)
FASTER trial, 282
Fetal age determination, 387–393
  age curve used in, *394*
  choosing appropriate age estimate, 391–393
  fetal age defined, 387
  fetal age functions, 387–388
  first trimester, 388–390, *390*
  regression equations for, 388*t*
  report forms, *392*
  second and third trimesters, 390–391
  variability associated with estimates, 389*t*
Fetal akinesia deformation sequence (FADS), 60
Fetal alcohol abuse syndrome, 123–124. *See also* Alcohol abuse, during pregnancy
Fetal alcohol spectrum disorders (FASD), 123
Fetal anomalies and birth defects, 57–62. *See also* specific anomaly or birth defect
  association, 61
  categories of structural defects, *59*
  causes of, 58*t*
  classification of fetal and birth defects, 57–59
    deformation, 58, 58*t*
    disruption, 58
    dysplasia, 58–59
    malformation, 57–58, 58*t*
  common multiple congenital anomaly or dysplasia syndrome, 60*t*
  diagnostic approach to dysmorphic fetus, 59
  genetic counseling when evidence of, 73
  sequence, 60–61

  single-system defect, 59–60
  syndrome, 60
Fetal autopsy, 549–558
  of anomalous fetus selectively terminated, 544–545
  clinical information, 550
  dilatation and evacuation specimens, 555
  performance of, 551–555
    gross external examination, 552–553
    internal examination, 553
    microscopic evaluation, 555
    organs, 553–555
    weights and measures, 552
  perinatal pathologist and, 550
  permission for, 550
  photography, 557–558
  placental examination, 555–557
  radiological examination, 550–551, *551*
  report, 558
  role of clinician/pathologist, 544
  special studies, 557
Fetal blood sampling, 477, 488
  viral infections and, 156
Fetal brain imaging. *See* Neurosonography
Fetal-cell-specific markers, 506
Fetal cystic hygromas, 191
Fetal erythroblasts, 505, *508. See also* Maternal blood, diagnosis using fetal cells from
Fetal growth assessment, 393–402
  common misconceptions, 393–395
  growth rates, 398–399
  individualized, 400, 401–402
  long-term processes reflected, 394–395
  mathematical functions used in, 399*t*
  neonatal growth profile, 396*t*
  Prenatal Growth Assessment Score (PGAS), 402
  selection of anatomic parameters, 395–397
    other anatomical measurements, 396–397
    parameter sets *vs.* single parameters, 396, 397*t*
    postnatal parameters, 396
    prenatal parameters, 395–396, 396*t*
  size assessment, 397–398
  size curve used in, *395*
  third trimester normal growth period, *397*
  use of size/growth assessments, 400–402
Fetal hemolytic anemia, 247
Fetal hydantoin syndrome (FHS), 115
Fetal hydrops, 665
Fetal hypoglycemia, 125
Fetal karyotyping, 606, 607
Fetal liver biopsy, 449–451, 488
Fetal mosaicism, 5
Fetal muscle biopsy, 443–443, 451–453
Fetal phenytoin syndrome, 141
Fetal skin biopsy, 449–451, 477–478
  background, 455
  fetoscopy, 449
  genodermatoses and, 455–457
  safety of, 456–457
  technique, 455–456
  ultrasound-guided, 449–451
Fetal urine, 259, 477
Fetal warfarin syndrome (FWS), 120
Fetal weight, ultrasonographic estimations of, 252
Fetendo (fetal endoscopic treatment), *623, 624*
Feto-fetal transfusion syndrome, 461–465
Feto-protein studies, 455
Fetoscopic cord ligation, 467, 575

Fetoscopic laser occlusion of the chorioangiopagus vessels (FLOC), 463
Fetoscopic laser therapy, 674
Fetoscopy, 449, 459
    assessment of fetal viral infections and, 156
    cystoscopy, 605
    defined, 459
    fetal genetic therapy, 683
    genodermatoses and, 455
    registry of procedures, 469
Fibrochondrogenesis, 271
Fibrocystic renal dysplasia, *606*
Finns, single gene disorders and, 12*t*
First trimester biochemical screening, 282
First trimester termination, 537–538
    antimetabolites, 538
    antiprogestins, 538, 538*t*
    complications, 537
    medical methods, 537
    prostaglandins, 537–538
    surgical techniques, 537
FISH. *See* Fluorescence in situ hybridization (FISH)
5′ untranslated region, 493
5p Deletion syndrome (Cri du chat syndrome), 48
Flow velocity waveform study, 343
Fluorescence in situ hybridization (FISH), 41–43, 48, 281–282, 475, 480–483, 597
    balanced rearrangements and, 479
    centromeric probes, 482
    cystic hygroma fluid and, 477
    and diagnosis using fetal cells from maternal blood, 505–507
    fetal urine, 477
    in fetopsy, 557
    marker chromosomes and, 479, 482
    microdeletion syndromes, 482
    painting probes, 482
    prenatal interphase FISH, 482–483
    replacement technique for, 483
    study guidelines, 481
    subtelomeric probes, 481–482
Fluorescent activated cell sorter (FACS), 281, 505, 506
Fluoxetine (Prozac), 118–119
Folic acid
    and anticonvulsant drug use, 114
    decreasing percentage of high MSAFPs with, 645*t*
    deficiency of, 641
    effects on general population, 646–647
    health implications other than NTD prevention, 646
    NTD prevention and, 644–645
    NTD susceptibility and, 645–646
    prevention of neural tube defects and, 209
Food and Drug Administration (FDA), 481
    drug rating system, 113, 114*t*
    folic acid and, 641, 645
48,XXXX (tetrasomy X), 46
48,XXXY, 46
48,XXYY, 46
45,X karyotype, 479–480
49,XXXXX (pentasomy X), 46
47,XXX (Trisomy X) syndrome, 43, 46
47,XXY (Klinefelter syndrome), 43, 45–46
47,XYY syndrome, 43, 46
4p Deletion syndrome (Wolf-Hirschhorn syndrome), 48
Fragile X syndrome, 14*t*, 37–38, 54, 434, 498
    CVS an unreliable test for, 476
Frameshift mutations, *10*, 493
Free radicals, 33
French Canadians, autosomal recessive disorders and, 501

Friedreich ataxia, 54
Frontal plane, *203*
Fryns syndrome, 359
Full mutations, 498
Furosemide washout scan, 600

G
Galactosemia, 490, 635–636
Galactose-1-phosphate uridyltransferase (GALT), 635–636
Galen malformations, 219
Gallbladder
    abnormal, 247–248
    agenesis, 247–248
    normal, 247
GALT (galactose-1-phosphate uridyltransferase), 635–636
Galton, Francis, 71
Gardnerella vaginallis, 152
Gardner's syndrome, 11
Garrod, Archibald, 51, 71
Gas distension, 460
Gastric cancer, 647
Gastric pseudomass, *242*
Gastrointestinal tract. *See also* Abdomen (fetal), normal and abnormal findings
    fetopsy of, 554
Gastroschisis, *191,* 251–252, 600
Gaucher, 501
Gaucher disease, 488, 636, 686
G-banding, 41
GBS (Group B beta-hemolytic streptococci), 149–150
Gene dosage effect, 14
Gene induction, 683
Gene markers, 3
Gene replacement therapy, 683, 744
Gene structure/function, 8–9
Gene suppression therapy, 684
Genetic anticipation, 37
Genetic counseling, 71–78, 455. *See also* Counseling
    case studies, 75–77
    indications for, 72–75
    psychosocial, 75
Genetic defects/disease. *See also* specific defect or disease
    causes of, 3
    ethnic groups and, 12
    Mendel's experiments and, 3
    single gene disorders, 9–10, 14
Genetic liability, 15
Genetics
    genes and development, 63–69
        cell differentiation, 63–66
        morphogenesis, 66–68
        from theory to practice, 68–69
    genetic imprinting, 54
    interface between environment and gene, 64
    Mendelian (*See* Mendelian inheritance)
    mitochondrial inheritance, 54
    non-Mendelian inheritance, 54–55
    principles of, 3–15
        autosomal dominant inheritance, 10–11
        autosomal recessive inheritance, 11–13
        chromosomal anomalies, 5–8
        chromosomes/cell division, 3–5
        multifactorial inheritance, 14–15
        sex-linked inheritance, 13–14
        single gene disorders, 9–10
        structure/function of human gene, 8–9
    triplet repeats, 54–55, 54*t*

Genetic screening. *See* Molecular screening
Genetic therapy (fetal), 683–689. *See also* Stem cell transfer (fetal genetic
          therapy)
    animal studies/clinical trials, 686–687
    cystic fibrosis, 686
    establishing appropriate timing of, 686
    ethical implications, 688–689
    gene-delivery techniques, 684–685
    gene induction, 683
    gene targeting, 685
    immunological disorders, 687–688
    inborn errors of metabolism, 686–687
    neuromuscular disorders, 688
    safety of fetus, 685–686
    safety of mother, 685
    therapeutic gene design, 683–684
        gene replacement therapy, 683
        virally directed enzyme prodrug therapy, 683–684
Genicity, 703
Genital herpes simplex, 434
Genitourinary defects
    Doppler imaging of, 335–336
    obstetric management of, 588–589
Genitourinary tract, fetopsy of, 554
Genitourinary tract abnormalities, 257–261
    agenesis, 257
    cloacal anomalies, *259*
    horseshoe and pelvic kidneys, 257–258
    posterior urethral valve, 258–259
    renal cystic disease, 260–261
    renal pelvis dilation, 259–260, *260*
    renal tumors, 261
    ureteral pelvic junction obstruction, 258
    ureterovesicojunction, 258
    urinary tract dilatation or obstruction, 258
Genodermatoses, 455–457
Genomic imprinting, 5, 35–36
    Beckwith-Wiedemann Syndrome (BWS), 35–36
    epigenetic phenomena and, 36
    in human disease, 35
Genotypic characterization, 501
Germ cell tumors, 181
Germ-line gene therapy (GLGT), 689
Germline mosaicism, 36–37
Gestational age assessment, 140
Gestational sac volume, 362
Giemsa dye, 41
Globin gene, *497*
Glucocorticoids, 87*t*
Glucose intolerance, 35
Glycogen storage diseases, 449
GM$_2$ gangliosidosis, 489
Goiter, fetal, 633
Goldenhar syndrome, 215
Gomori trichome staining, 34
Gonococcal perihepatitis, 151
Graft-*versus*-host disease (GVHD), 515, 691, 693
Graves disease (maternal), 444, 454
"Greek mask," 48
Grief counseling, 533, 534, 545–546
Grief process, 525–526
Group A beta-hemolytic streptococcus, 150–153
Group B beta-hemolytic streptococci (GBS), 149–150
Group B streptococcus infection, 434
Growth Potential Realization Index, 402*t*
Growth restriction (severe, early onset), 444, 454
G6PD deficiency, 12*t*

Guy's Hospital cardiac techniques, 678–679
GVHD. *See* Graft-*versus*-host disease (GVHD)
Gynecomastia, 45

H
Haemophilus influenza, 493
Haemophilus influenzae, 150
Hamartoma, 627
Hamartoses, 597
Haplotype analysis, 493
Happy puppet (Angelman) syndrome, 35, 48
Harlequin ichthyosis, 449, 451
Hartmann's solution, 460
Hartnup disorder, 487
H2 blockers, 119
hCG (human chorionic gonadotropin), 138
Healthcare financing, 741, 743, 744
Heart, fetopsy of, 554
Heart and vascular malformations, 227–235. *See also* Cardiovascular system,
          evaluation of
    fetal cardiac function, 229
    fetal echocardiographic imaging, 227–229
        atrioventricular septal defect, *228*
        4-chamber view, *228,* 230–231, *232*
        indications for, 229–230
    fetal tumors, 235
    heart disease and chromosome abnormalities, 231–232
    prenatal surgical therapy, 234–235
Hemangiomas, 346, 437
Hematological disorders, 687
Hematopoietic stem cell transplantation, 624. *See also* Stem cell transfer
          (fetal genetic therapy)
Hemoglobinopathies, 501, 693–694
Hemolytic disease, 444, 445, 454, 695*t*
Hemophilias (A and B), 14*t,* 47, 486, 487, 499, 687
Hemophilus ducreyi, 152
Hemophilus vaginallis, 152
Hemorrhage, fetal-to-maternal, 437
Hepatic hemangioma, 346
Hepatitis C virus, 161–162
Hereditary pancreatitis, 11
Hereditary persistence of fetal hemoglobin (HPFH),
          687
Herpe simplex virus, 159
Herpesvirus family, 157, 160–162
Heterodisomy, 36
Heteroplasmy, 33, 54
Heterozygote detection, X-linked disorders and, 486
Heterozygous, 10, 11
H4 histone transcription, 65
HGPRT deficiency, 14*t*
Histology, 455
Hodgkin disease, 179–181
Holoacrania, 210
Holoprosencephaly, 45, *188,* 212–215
Holt-Oram syndrome, 272
Homeobox, 66
Homologous chromosomes, 3
Homoplasmy, 33
Homozygous, 10, 11
Horseshoe kidney, 257
Hox genes, 67
Human chorionic gonadotropin (hCG), 138
Human Genome Project (HGP), 71, 277, 529, 684
Human immunodeficiency virus (HIV), 162–164
    perinatal HIV transmission, 163*t*
Huntington disease, 11, 12*t,* 38, 501

Hurler syndrome, 487, 574
Hydramnios, 411
Hydranencephaly, 331
Hydrocephalus, *189*, 211, 212, *217*, 217–219, 641
    isotretinoin ingestion and, 120
    long term outcome of, 218*t*
    resolution strategies for management of, *196*
Hydrocephaly, 221, 331
    neuroscan of, 374–375, *376*
Hydronephrosis, *190*, 258, 260, 312, *360*, 605, 608
    597
Hydrops, 444–445, 454–447, 596
Hydrops fetalis, 598–599, 628, 674–675, 677
    conditions associated with, 598*t*
    diagnostic workup for, 599*t*
Hydrops fetoplacentalis, 469
Hydroureters, 605
Hydroxyurea (HU), 501
Hyperactivity, in children with fetal alcohol abuse syndrome,
        126
Hyperammonemia, 636
Hypercalcemia, 48
Hypercholesterolemia, 12*t*
Hyperechoic bowel, *312*
Hyperglycosylated hCG tests, 281
Hyperimidodipeptiduria, 488
Hyperosmolar urea, 540
Hyperphenylalaninemia, 487
Hypertelorism, 192
Hypertension, maternal, 646
Hyperthyroidism (fetal), 444, 454
Hypertonic saline, 540, 542
Hypervolemia, 666
Hypoglycemics, 143*t*
Hypogonadism, 45, 48
Hypoplastic left heart syndrome, *662*, 672, 678
Hypotelorism, 192
Hypotonia, 48
Hypotonicity, 44
Hypovolemia, 461, 666
Hypoxia, 331
    endothelial adaptation to, 445
Hysterotomy, 571, 573

I
Iatrogenic PPROM (iPPROM), 469
Idiopathic pleural effusion shunt therapy, 613–615
    complications, 614–15
    potential etiologies of isolated pleural effusions, 613*t*
    prenatal evaluation, 614
    selection criteria, 614*t*
    sonograms, *614*, *615*
Ileal atresia, 245
Iminoglycinuria, 12*t*
Immune thrombocytopenia (ITP), 444, 454
Immunodeficiency states, 693
Immunohistochemistry, 455, 507
Immunological disorders, 687–688
Imprinting, 36
Inborn errors of metabolism, 686–687
"Inborn errors of metabolism," 11
Inbreeding, 12
Indanpaan MAOIs, 118
Indicator dilution technique, 410
Indomethacin, 87*t*
Industrial exposure, 145–146
Infantile polycystic kidney, 260–261

Infection
    after CVS, 437
    in-utero, and effect on fetal brain, 221–222
Inferior vena cava, 662, *664*
Infertility
    causes of, 137*t*
    genetic counseling and, 73–74
    Klinefelter syndrome and, 46
    male, 502
    percentage of married women and, 137*t*
Inflammatory processes, 217
Influenza, 162
Informed consent, 195, 581, 723–724, 728–729
    chorionic villus sampling and, 736–738
    for minors, 734–736
Inherited disorders, 501
Iniencephaly, 210–211, *211*
Intercourse frequency, and conception, 135, 136*t*
Internet databases, 383, 384*t*
Intracranial cystic formations, 331
Intracranial hemorrhage, *193*
Intracranial teratomas, 221, 346
Intracytoplasmic fetal hemoglobin staining, 506
Intrahepatic alcohol injection, 575
Intrapartum infections, 159
Intrathoracic lesion, 628
Intrauterine Fetal Death (IUFD), 461, 464
Intrauterine growth retardation (IUGR), 125, 439
Introns, 493
In utero gene therapy, 683
Inversions, 7, 47, 417, 478
Inverted duplicated 15 markers, 482
Iodine, 143*t*
Ionizing radiation, exposure to, 7, 97, 169–174
    effects of, in pregnancy, 171–173
    fetal dose estimate, 170, 172*t*
    hereditary effects of, 171
    magnetic resonance imaging (MRI), 173
    maternal dose estimate, 171*t*
    nomenclature used, 169–170
    pathophysiology, 170–171
    radiobiology, 169–170
    radionuclide examinations, 173
    radiotherapy, 173–174
    safety measures, 174
Isodisomy, 36
Isotretinoin, 97, 113, 119–120

J
Jansen v. Children's Hospital Medical Center of East Bay,
        730
Japanese, single gene disorders and, 12*t*
Jarcho-Levin syndrome, 271
Jejunal atresia/stenosis, 244–245
Jeune syndrome, 269–270
Joubert's syndrome, 214
Justus v. Atchison, 730

K
Kallman syndrome, 481*t*
Karlsons v. Guerinot, 729
Karl Storz Endoskope, 459
Karyotype, 5, 193, 444, 454
    chromosome arrangement in, 41
    mosaicism diagnosis and, 7
Katz-Rothman, Barbara, 524
KCl, 543, 572, *573*

Kearns-Sayre and chronic progressive external ophthalmoplegia (KSS/CPEO), 34
Kennedy disease (spinal and bulbar muscular atrophy), 38–39
Ketotic hyperglycinemia, 488
Keyhole sign, *258*
Kidney malformations, 45
Kidney(s)
    biopsies, 443, 453
    horseshoe and pelvic, 257–258
    infantile polycystic, 260–261
    multicystic dysplastic, 260
    nonfunctioning multicystic, 600
    polycystic, 192
    polycystic kidney disease, 600
    tumors, 261
    ultrasound examination of, 178, 192
Kleinefelter syndrome (47,XXY), 6, 45–46
Krabbe disease, 485
KSS/CPEO. *See* Kearns-Sayre and chronic progressive external ophthalmoplegia (KSS/CPEO)

L
"Lambda sign," 349, *351*
Langer mesomelic dysplasia, 271–272
Large intestine
    abnormalities, 246
    normal, 245–246, *246*
Larnyx, 240
Laryngeal atresia, 240
Laryngeal palsy, 240
Laser coagulation, 460, 461–465
    operative technique, 462–463
    pathophysiology, 461
    results, 463–465
Leber hereditary optic neuropathy (LHON), 34
Leber optic neuropathy, 54
Legal issues
    chorionic villus sampling, informed consent/legal risks, 736–738
    consent/informed consent for minors
        common law exceptions, 734
        statutory exceptions, 734–736
    failure to diagnose abnormality, 733–734
    failure to offer amniocentesis, 732
    failure to perform amniocentesis upon patient request, 733
    lack of informed consent, 728–729
    negligent infliction of emotional distress, 729–731
    typical medical/legal scenarios
        failure to inform patient of abnormal karyotype before 24 weeks, 732–733
        failure to offer AFP, 731
        failure to offer double or triple screening, 731–732
        failure to terminate a normal child, 732
    wrongful birth, 727–728
    wrongful death, 727
    wrongful life, 728
Leigh syndrome, 35
Lemon sign, 189, *191*, 212
Lesch Nyhan syndrome (HGPRT deficiency), 14*t*
Leucine, 9
Leukemia, 647
    chemotherapy during pregnancy, 179
Limb circumference, 3-D ultrasound measurement of, 361
Limb defects, 642*t*
Limb reduction defects, 436, 437
Linear Energy Transfer, 169
Linkage, 499

Linkage analysis, 499
Lissencephaly, 48, 217
Listeria monocytogenes, 150
Lithium, 119
Lithium carbonate, 87*t*, 94
Liver
    abnormalities, 247
    biopsy (fetal), 449, 451
    herniation, 621
    normal, 246–247
    normal range of fetal liver length, 249*t*
    tumors, 346
Lobar holoprosencephaly, 212, 213–214, *214*
Locus-specific probes, 481
London Dysmorphology Database, 61
Lowe Oculo-Cerebro-Renal syndrome, 14*t*
Lung cancer, 647
Lungs, fetopsy of, 554
Lung transplantation, 624
Lung volume measurements, 362
Luteinizing hormone (LH), 4
Lymphatic system, fetopsy of, 554–555
Lymphoblasts, 281
Lymphoma, chemotherapy during pregnancy, 179–181
Lyon Birth Defect Registry, 118
Lysyl oxidase, 637

M
Macrocephaly, 195
Macrocystic lesions, 628
Macrocysts, 610–613
MACs, 505
Magenis, RE, 35
Magnetic activated cell sorting (MACS), 281, 505
Magnetic resonance imaging (MRI), 173
    cranial, 597
Magnetocardiography, 677
MALDI, 513–514
Malformations, 57–58, 141. *See also* specific malformation
    etiology of, 79
Maple syrup urine disease (MSUD), 687
Marfan syndrome, 12*t*, 54
Marker chromosomes, 478, 482
Maroteaux-Lamy syndrome, 490
MASA syndrome, 214
Mass spectrometry, 513–514, *514*
Maternal age, advanced, 44, 45
    aneuploidy and, 5
    chromosome rearrangements in, 8
    Down syndrome and, 27–28, 289, 290*t*, 297*t*
    trisomy and, 6
Maternal blood, diagnosis using fetal cells from, 281, 505–510
    determining erythroblasts of fetal origin, 508–509
    diagnosis of fetal aneuploidies, 507
    efficacy in the cytogenetic analysis fetal cells, 507
    fetal cell identification, 506–507
    fetal cells and disease, 510
    fetal DNA in maternal plasma, 509
    historical/technical overview, 505
    NICHD NIFTY study, 505–506
    optimization of recovery, 506
    PCR and Mendelian disorders, 507–508
    simultaneous analysis of fetal sex and rhesus D, *509*
    in vitro culture of enriched fetal cells, 509–510
Maternal cell contamination (MCC), 438–439
Maternal hyperthermia, 642*t*
Maternally inherited diabetes mellitus, 35

Maternal meiotic nondisjunction, 44

Maternal septicemia, 419

Maternal serum alpha-fetoprotein (MSAFP), 5, 438, 446
    genetic counseling for positive screen, 72
    neural tube defect screening with, 284, 641, 642–643
    risk of chromosome abnormalities with low levels of, 279

Maternal serum pregnancy associated plasma protein A (PAPP-A), 433

Matrix-assisted laser desorption/ionization (MALDI), 513–514

Mature minors, 734

McKusick, Victor, 10

Meckel-Gruber syndrome, 211, 215, 642*t*

Meconium ileus, 245

Median cleft face syndrome, 192

Median ("mid-sagittal") plane, 204–205

Mediterranean population
    autosomal recessive disorders and, 12*t*, 501
    single gene disorders and, 12*t*

Mega-cisterna magna, 215

Megacystis/microcolon syndrome, 300, 605, 608

Meiosis, 3–4, *4, 4t*, 10

Meiotic nondisjunction, 44

Melanoma, chemotherapy and, 181–182

MELAS. *See* Mitochondrial myopathy, encephalopathy, lactic acidosis,
    and stroke-like episodes (MELAS)

Membrane rupture, 438

Membranes, fetoscopic surgery on, 461

Mendel, Gregor, 10, 71
    experiments, 3
    hereditary theory, 5

Mendelian inheritance, 51–54. *See also* Genetics
    basic principles, 51
    exceptions to, 33–39
    patterns of Mendelian transmission
        autosomal dominant, 52–53, *53*
        autosomal recessive, 51–52, *52*
        sex linkage, *53,* 53–54, *54*
    pedigree analysis, 51, *52*

Meningocele, 211, 641

Meningo-encephalocele, 211

Meningomyelocele, *190,* 641
    "banana sign," 643, *644*
    "lemon sign," 643, *644*
    ultrasound diagnosis of, 643

Menkes, 635

Mental retardation, 6, 8
    Fragile X syndrome, 14
    microdeletion syndromes and, 48
    subtelomeric rearrangements and, 48

Meroacrania, 210

MERRF syndrome. *See* Myoclonus Epilepsy and Ragged-Red Fibers
    (MERRF) syndrome

Messenger RNA, 493

Metabolic disorders
    fetal
        congenital adrenal hyperplasia, 633–634
        fetal goiter/congenital hypothyroidism, 633
        Menkes, 635
        methylmalonic acidemia, MMA, 634–635
        multiple carboxylase deficiency, 635
    maternal
        acute intermittent porphyria, 636–637
        cystinosis, 636
        galactosemia, 635–636
        Gaucher disease, 636
        ornithine transcarbamylase deficiency, 636
        PKU, 635
        Wilson disease, 637

Metachromatic leukodystrophy, 485, 487, 490

Methionine reductase (MTRR), 646

Methionine synthase (MTR), 646

Methotrexate, 83*t*, 84

Methylation, 35, 36

Methylene blue, 87*t*, 94

Methylenetetrahydrofolate reductase (MTHFR), 646

Methylmalonic acidemia, 487, 634–635

Michigan Alcoholism Screening Test (MAST), 124, 127

Microarrays (DNA chips) with genomic clones, 483

Microcephaly, 44, 45, 126, 192, 211, 212

Microdeletion syndromes, 48, 481*t,* 482
    FISH probe procedures, 42

Microgastria, 243

Micrognathia, 359

Micromagnetic conjugated antibodies to CD71, 505

Microphthalmia, 45
    with linear skin defects syndrome, 486

Microsatellites, 439

Mid-coronal plane, 203–204

Mifepristone (RU486), 538*t*

Miller-Dieker syndrome, 48, 214, 481*t*

Mini-laparotomy, 462

Minors, consent/informed consent for
    common law exceptions, 734
    statutory exceptions, 734–736

Mirror syndrome, 630

Miscarriage. *See* Spontaneous abortion

Misoprostol, 87*t*, 94–95, 540

Missense mutation, 493

Mitochondrial genome and nuclear genome compared, 33

Mitochondrial inheritance, 33–35, 54
    mitochondrial disease, 34–35
    mitochondrial genome, *34*
    mitochondrial genome and nuclear genome compared, 33
    somatic mtDNA mutations and aging, 33–34

Mitochondrial myopathy, encephalopathy, lactic acidosis, and stroke-like
    episodes (MELAS), 34

Mitosis, 3, *4,* 4*t*

Modified Neonatal Growth Assessment Score (mNGAS), 402

Molar pregnancy, 44

Molecular cytogenetics, 41–43, 480–483
    centromeric probes, 482
    chromosome 15-derived markers, 482
    FISH study guidelines, 481
    marker chromosomes, 482
    microdeletion syndromes, 481*t,* 482
    painting probes, 482
    prenatal interphase FISH, 482–483
    subtelomeric probes, 481–482
    X chromosome-derived markers, 482

Molecular diagnostics, 493–499
    allele-specific oligonucleotide hybridization, 497
    glossary, 494*t*
    linkage, 499
    molecular genetics, 493
    mutational scanning, 499
    polymerase chain reaction, 493–496
    restriction endonuclease allele recognition, 496–497
    reverse dot blot, 497
    sequence analysis, 499
    southern blot analysis, 497–499

Molecular screening, 501–502
    carrier detection, 501–502
    nonclassical applications, 502
    presymptomatic detection, 501

Monoamine oxidase inhibitors (MAOIs), 118

Monoamniotic twins, 571
Monochorionic-diamniotic twins, 350, *352*
Monochorionic (MC) twins, 461–465. *See also* Nd:YAG laser coagulation of chorionic plate vessels
    cardiovascular function of, 674
    cord occlusion in, 466–468
    discordant congenital or acquired anomalies in, 466
Monochorionic-monoamniotic twins, 350–351
    "Lambda sign," *351*
Monogenic disorders. *See* Biochemical genetics
Monopolar coagulation, 467
Monopolar thermocoagulation, 575
Monosomy, 44, 47
Monosomy X (Turner syndrome), 6, 44, 45
Monozygotic twins, 571
    mortality rates, according to chorionicity and amnionicity, 350*t*
    type of, according to time of splitting, 350*t*
Morphogenesis, 63, 66–68
Mosaic aneuploidy, 6
Mosaicism, 44
    autosomal dominant traits and risk of, 52–53
    confined placental, 439
    fetal skin biopsy and, 477
    germline mosaicism, 36–37
    indicated in amniocentesis, 417
    somatic mosaicism, 37
Mosaic tetraploidy, 6
Mosaic tetrasomy 12p, 7
Mosaic trisomic villus mesenchyme, 439
MSAFP. *See* Maternal serum alpha-fetoprotein (MSAFP)
mtDNA (mitochondrial DNA). *See* Mitochondrial inheritance
Mucopolysaccharidoses, 451, 490
Mucopolysaccharidosis I, 487
Multicystic dysplastic kidney, 260
Multi-disciplinary Dysmorphology Database, 384, *385*
Multifactorial disorders, 3
Multifactorial inheritance, 14–15
    risk of recurrence, 15*t*
Multifetal pregnancy reduction, 354, 571. *See also* Selective termination
    changes in etiology of multifetal pregnancies, 562*t*
    CVS for triplets, *567*
    losses and very prematures starting by number, 564*t*
    losses by years, 563*t*
    maternal age and ART, 566*t*
    monogygotic twin pair as part of multiple, *565*
    outcomes, 562–565
    patient issues, 565–566
    pleural effusion following KCl injection, *563*
    procedures, 561–562
    ratio of observed to expected multiples, 562*t*
    reduced *vs.* "unreduced" triplets comparison, 565*t*
    risk reduction, 564*t*
    risks starting with triplets, *566*
    societal issues, 566–568
Multifetal pregnancy reduction (MFPR), 561–568
Multiplanar orthogonal display, 371, *372*
Multiple births, in U.S., 562*t*
Multiple carboxylase deficiency, 635
Multiple defect syndrome, 68
Multiple developmental defects, 141
Multiple gestations
    amniocentesis and, 418
    CVS and, 433
    first trimester ultrasound with nuchal translucency, 294–295
    late diagnosis of twinning, 354*t*
    monochorionic-diamniotic twins, 350
    placenta evaluation, 409

quadruplets, 349
selective termination of anomalous fetus in, 543–545
ultrasound in, 349–356
    acardiac twins, *355–356*
    conjoined twins, 351–353
    cord entanglement, *354*
    dichorionic twins, 349, *351*
    higher-order multifetal pregnancies, 354
    monochorionic-diamniotic twins, 350 *352*
    monochorionic-monoamniotic twins, 350–351
    monochorionic twins, 349–350, *353*
    TRAP sequence, 353–354
Mumps, 162
Muscle biopsy (fetal), 443–443, 451–453
Muscular dystrophy, 38
Mutagenic agents, 7
Mutational scanning, 499
Myelomeningocele, 601, 667
Myocardial dysfunction, 444–445, 454–447, 666
Myocarditis, 445
Myoclonus Epilepsy and Ragged-Red Fibers (MERRF) syndrome, 34
Myotonia, 38
Myotonic dystrophy, 11, 12*t*, 38
Myxosarcoma, 628

N

Nadas, Alexander, 676
Narcotic analgesics, 142*t*
NARP. *See* Neuropathy, ataxia, and retinitis pigmentosa (NARP)
Nd:YAG laser coagulation of chorionic plate vessels, 460, 461–465
    operative technique, 462–463
    pathophysiology, 461
    results, 463–465
Needle guide, 443, 453
Neisseria gonorrhoeae, 151
Neonatal respiratory distress syndrome, 673
Neonatal sepsis, 151
Neural tube defects, 14, 15*t*, 209–212, 641–648. *See also* Folic acid
    anencephaly, 209–210
    anticonvulsant medications and, 115
    biochemical screening for, 279
    categories of, 641
    CVS evaluation of not possible, 476
    disorders associated with, 642*t*
    dysraphia, 211–212
    genetic susceptibility for, 645–646
    incidence of, 641–642
    iniencephaly, 210–211
    MSAFP levels and, 284
    obstetric management of, 582–583
    prevalence of, 641, 642*t*
    prevention of, 644
    screening of, with maternal serum alpha-fetoprotein, 642–643
    sonography of, 376–377
    ultrasound examination, 643
Neuroblastoma, 346
Neurofibromatosis, 11
Neurological disorders, 688
Neuromuscular disorders, 688
Neuropathy, ataxia, and retinitis pigmentosa (NARP), 34
Neurosonography
    agenesis of the corpus callosum, 377
    aneurysm of the vein of galen, 380, *381*
    anterior fontanelle, *366*
    arachnoid cysts, 378, *379*
    brain structures described, *367, 368,* 368–369
    cerebellar hypoplasia, *380*

cerebral circulation, 207–209, *208*
cerebral cortex, *207*
choroid plexus cysts, *378*
coronal planes, 203–204
corpus callosum, *206*
corpus callosum and midbrain structures, 369, *375*
cystic brain lesions, 219–221
diagnosing fetal brain malformation, 209–222
embryology, *201,* 201–202, *202*
equipment, 199
fetal brain pathology, 373
fetal brain tumors, 221–222
hydrocephaly and ventriculomegaly, 215–219
intracranial hemorrhage, 380
midline anomalies, 212–215
neural tube defects, 376–377
porencephalic cyst, 378, *379*
posterior fossa, *205,* 369–371, *370, 380*
subarachnoid space, *373*
three-dimensional fetal neuroscan, 371–373
transvaginal approach, 199–201, *200, 373*
    nomenclature, 204*t*
    scanning planes and anatomy, 202–209
transvaginal fetal neuroscan technique, 365–369, *366*
using 2D and 3D transvaginal transfontanelle scanning, 373–374
ventriculomegaly and hydrocephaly, 374–375, *376*
Neutrophil alkaline phosphatase, 281
Nicholls, RD, 35
Nodular sclerosis, 180
Nondisjunction, 36, 37, 44–45
Non-Hodgkin lymphoma, 179–181
Nonimmune edema, 336
Nonimmune hydrops fetalis, 610, 674
    obstetric management of, 590
Non-insulin-dependent diabetes mellitus (NIDDM), 35
Nonketotic hyperglycinemia, 487
Nonmaleficence, 707
Nonsense mutation, 493
Nonsteroidal anti-inflammatory drugs (NSAIDs), 673–674
NOR-banding, 41
Northern blot, 495–496, 557
Northern Europeans, autosomal recessive disorders and, 12*t,* 501
Nuchal cystic hygroma, *193*
Nuchal translucency
    increased, and fetal abnormalities, 299–300*t*
    increased, and major cardiac defects, 298*t,* 299*t*
    increased, in chromsomally normal fetus, 296–301, 298*t,* 301*t*
    relationship between thickness of and various complications, 297*t*
Nuchal translucency measurement, 290–291, 433, 482
    prospective screening studies for Trisomy 21, 292*t,* 293*t*
    results of observational studies, 293*t*
Nuchal translucency thickness, and risk for chromosomal abnormalities, 291–292, 291*t*
Nuclear genome and mitochondrial genome compared, 33
Nuclear matrix-DNA, 65
Nucleated red blood cells, 281, 505. *See also* Maternal blood, diagnosis using fetal cells from

O

Oblique-1 and oblique-2 planes, 204–207
Obstetrical endoscopy, 459
Obstetrical management of anomalies, 579–591
    abortion option, 581
    aggressive management approach, 581–582
    chromosome anomalies, 591
    common clinical situations
        cardiac abnormalities, 584–586

central nervous system anomalies, 582
    CNS anomalies, 584
        neural tube defects, 582–583
        ventriculomegally, 583–584
    diagnosis of anomalies, 579–581
    fetal anomalies evaluation and management algorithm, 580*t*
    fetal management strategies, 580*t*
    genitourinary defects, 588–589
    informed consent, 581
    multispecialty representation, 581
    nonaggressive management approach, 582
    nonimmune hydrops fetalis, 590
    postpartum, 591
    skeletal dysplasias, 589–590
Obstructive uropathies, 605–610
    fetal urine parameters, 607*t*
    Fetendo (fetal endoscopy), 624
    MRI, *607*
    prenatal evaluation, 606–608
    ultrasounds, *606, 607*
    vesicoamniotic shunt placement
        complications, 609–610, *610*
        follow-up, 610
        patient selection, 608
        technique, 608–609, *609*
Occipital plane, *203,* 203–204
Occupational exposure. *See* Environmental and occupational exposure
Ochoa v. Superior Court of Santa Clara County, 730
Oculocutaneous albinism, 449
Oguchi disease, 12*t*
Oligohydramnios, 60, 192, *217,* 257, 258, 260, 261, 411, 438, 445, 600, 606–608
    sequence, *61*
Omphalocele, 45, 189, *191,* 211, 249–250, 599
1-cell disease, 488, 490
Online Mendelian Inheritance in Man (OMIM), 61
Operative fetoscopy, 459–470
    amniotic band syndrome (ABSd), 468
    clinical applications, 460–469
    complications of, 468–469
    cord occlusion in MC twins, 466–468
    feto-fetal transfusion syndrome, 461
    fetoscopic cord obliteration, 465
    in first trimester, 460–461
    instrumentation and techniques, 459–460
    laser coagulation, 461–465
    on placenta, cord, and membranes, 461
    selective termination in MC twins, 465–466
Oral contraceptives, 113
Organic acid disorders, 489–490
Organ system classification, 57
Organ transplant donors, 502
Ornithine carbamoyltransferase deficiency, 486, 488
Ornithine transcarbamylase deficiency, 449, 451, 636
Oromandibular-limb hypogenesis syndrome, 436, 437
Osteocalcin transcription, 65
Osteogenesis imperfecta, *194,* 263, 267, *267*
Osteoprogenitor cells, 65
Ovarian cancer, 181
Ovulation induction agents, 561
Oxazolidine-2, 4-diones, 88*t,* 95

P

Pacemaker, neonatal, 677
Painting probes, 481, 482
Pallister Killian syndrome, 7
Pancreas, 248

Pancuronium, 445
Paracentric inversions, 47
Partial agenesis of the corpus callosum (PACC), 214
Partial trisomies, 6
Parvovirus infection, 161, 445
Patau syndrome. *See* Trisomy 13 (Patau syndrome)
Paternal age, risk of Down syndrome and, 21, 28
Paternal drinking, mutagenic effects of, 125
Paternal meiosis II, 46
Paternal meiotic nondisjunction, 44
Paternity testing (prenatal), 712
Patient rights, 744
Pattern formation, 66*t*, 67
Patterns of inheritance, 71
PAX2, 68–69
PCR-mediated site-directed mutagenesis (PSM), 496
Pelvic inflammatory disease, 151
Pelvic kidney, 257–258
Pencillamine, 88*t*, 95, 637
Pentalogy of Cantrell, 599
Percoll gradient, 506
Percutaneous umbilical blood sampling (PUBS), 6, 443, 453
Pericentric inversions, 47
Pernicious anemia, 647
Phakomatoses, 12*t*
Pharmacogenomics, 518–519
Pharmacologic therapy (fetal), 633–637
    fetal metabolic disorders, 633–635
    maternal metabolic disorders, 636–637
Pharynx, 240
Phenindione, 120
Phenotypic abnormalities, 486
Phenotypic expression, variability of, 33
Phenylketonuria (PKU), 12*t*, 501, 635
Phenytoin, 114–115
PKU, 635
Placenta, 407–411
    amniotic fluid
        physiology of, 410
        ultrasound evaluation of, 410–11
    chorioangioma of, 346
    chorionicity, 349
    embryology of, 407
    fetoscopic surgery on, 461
    location and attachment, 407–408
    multiple gestations, 409
    placental lesions, 409
    size/shape of, 408–409
Placenta accreta, 408
Placental thrombosis, 437
Placental vascular disruption, 437
Placenta previa, 408
Planar images, 357
Platelet transfusion, prophylactic, 446
Pleural effusion(s). *See* Idiopathic pleural effusion shunt therapy
PLUG (Plug the Lung Until it Grows), 617
Point mutation, 493
Polarity genes, 66
Political issues, 741–744
    elections of 2000 and 2004, 743
    federal political dynamic, 741–743
    healthcare financing, 744, 741–743
    payments for prenatal diagnosis/therapy, 744
    political process, 742–743
    privacy/confidentiality/patient rights, 744
    reproductive genetic research/testing, future issues in, 743–744
    universal health insurance coverage, 744

Polycystic kidney disease (adult type), 12*t*
Polydactyly, 12*t*, 45, 597
Poly-FISH, 507
Polyhydramnios, 210, 461, 469, 575, 610, 619, 628
    gastroschisis and, 252
    renal tumors, *261*
Polymerase chain reaction, 493–496, *495*
    chromosome 21 identification, *508*
    and Mendelian disorders, 507–508
    mutiplex PCR, *495*
    northern blot, 495–496
Polymorphic restriction enzyme sites, *496*
Polymorphisms, 646
Polyploidy, 5, 43–44
Pompe disease, 488
POPRAS (Problem Oriented Perinatal Risk Assessment System), 383
Porencephalic cyst, 191, 378, *379*
Porencephaly, 191, 220, *221*
Porphyrias, 486
POSSUM, 61, 598
Posterior fossa, 369–371
    lesions of, *380*
Posterior urethral valve, 258–259
Postnatal diagnostic studies, 597–598
Postpartum management, after delivery of infant with congenital anomalies, 591
Postterm delivery, 139
Potter facies, 600
Potter's sequence of deformities, 257
Prader-Willi syndrome (PWS), 35, 36, 42, 48, 439, 480, 481*t*, 486, 597
Preeclampsia, 510, 646, 674
Pregnancy
    alcohol abuse during, 123–128
    bacterial infections and, 149–152
    chemotherapy in (See Chemotherapy, in pregnancy)
    drug use during (See Drugs)
    exposure to ionizing radiation during, 169–174
    life table of reproductive success, 138*t*
    prior chromosomal disorder, 73
    recurrent loss/stillbirth, and genetic counseling, 73
Preimplantation genetic diagnosis, 689
Premature atrial contractions, 665
Premature birth, 349
    environmental/occupational exposure and, 139–140
    feto-fetal transfusion syndrome and, 461
Premutation characteristic, 14
Premutations, 498
Prenatal diagnosis
    accuracy of, 629
    amniocentesis and, 415–416, 416*t*
    CDH and, 618–619
    ethical issues, 709–710
    guidelines, 708*t*
    payments for (political issue), 741
    psychological reaction to, 523–527
    resources for, 707–708
Prenatal Growth Assessment Score (PGAS), 402
Prenatal interphase FISH, 482–483
Preterm delivery, 139
(Preterm) prelabor rupture of the membranes (PPROM), 470–471
Primary hyperoxaluria type 1, 451
Privacy, 744
Progestins, 88*t*, 95–96
Pronuclear transplantation, 35
Prostaglandins, 537–538, 540, 541*t*
Protein coding genes, 9, *9*
Proteomics, 513–520

applications, 515–520
  analysis of unknown serum samples, *516*
  real time monitoring of disease, 518–520, *519*
  serum disease diagnosis, 515–517
  serum management of therapy toxicity, 518–520
  serum surrogates for disease pathway profiling, 517–518
  signal transduction pathway profiling, *518*
  bioinformatics, 514–515
  creating a proteomic "fingerprint," *516*
  mass spectrometry, 513–514
Proteus group, 152
Prozac, 118
Prune-belly syndrome, 258, 554, 605, 606
Pseudocholiesterase deficiency, 12*t*
Pseudo-Hurler polydystrophy, 488, 490
Pseudomosaicism, 7
Pseuoabortifacient, 646
Psu dic (15;15) markers, 482
Psychological reaction, to prenatal diagnosis and loss, 523–527
Psychoses, postabortal, 545
Psychosocial issues, 701–705
  boundaries of clinically relevant research, 705
  describing context, 701–704
  role of context in individual decisions, 704–705
Public policy, biochemical screening and, 283
PUBS. *See* Percutaneous umbilical blood sampling (PUBS)
Pulmonary balloon valvuloplasty, 677–679
Pulmonary hyperplasia, 622
Pulmonary hypoplasia, 257, 610, 622, 630
Pulmonary parenchymal hypoplasia, 617
Pulmonary shunts. *See* Congenital cystic adenomatoid malformation
    (CCAM) shunt therapy
Pulmonary stenosis, 15*t*
Pyelocaliceal retention, 258
Pyloric atresia, 243
Pyloric stenosis, 14, 15*t, 244*

Q
Q-banding, 41
QF-PCR, 483
Quadruplets, 349

R
Rachischises, 211
Racism, 701
Radial aplasia-thrombocytopenia syndrome, 272
Radiation exposure. *See* Ionizing radiation, exposure to
Radioactive isotopes, 96–97
Radiobiology, 169–170
Radio-frequency ablation, 575, 674
Radionuclide examinations, 173–174
Radiotherapy, 173–174
Ragged red fibers, 34
Rare sex-chromosome aneuploidies, 46
Reanastomosis, 647
Recessive trait, 10
Reciprocal translocation, 7, 46–47
Recombinant DNA technology, 684
Reed v. Campagnolo, 728
Renal anomalies, 600–601
Renal cystic disease, 260–261
Renal dysplasia, 443, 453
  ability of selected biochemical values to predict absence of, 259*t*
Renal function analysis, 606, 607–608, 607*t*
Renal isotope scan, 600
Renal pelvis dilation, 259–260, *260*
Renal tumors, 261, 346

Repetitive sequence probes, 481
Reproductive failure, aneuploidy and, 6
Reproductive toxicity, 136
Research financing, 741
Reserpine and Rauwolfia alkaloids, 143*t*
Restriction endonuclease allele recognition, 496–497
Restriction fragment length polymorphisms (RFLPs), 3, 499
Resuscitation, 595–596
Retinoblastoma, 11
Retinoids systemic administration, 88*t,* 97–98
Retinoids (topical administration), 88*t,* 98
Retroviruses, 684
Rett syndrome, 486
Reverse dot blot hybridization procedure, 497
Reverse transcriptase-polymerase chain reaction, 495–496
RFLPs. *See* Restriction fragment length polymorphisms (RFLPs)
Rheumatoid arthritis, 647
Rh ISO-immunization, 542
Rh-negative, 542
Rh$_o$ (D) immune globulin (RhoGAM), 598
Rhombomeres, 67
Rh sensitization, 438
Ribozymes and antisense RNA, 684
Ring chromosome, 47
RNA molecules, 684
Robertsonian translocation, 8, 45, 46, 480
Roberts-SC phocomelia, 272
Roe v. Wade, 284, 571
Rossavik growth model, 399
RU 486, 741
Rubella virus, 155, 156–157, 221–222
  congenital rubella sequelae, 157*t*
Rubenstein-Taybi syndrome, 214
Rupture of membranes, 438

S
Sacrococcygeal teratoma, 666
Sagittal planes, *204,* 204–207
Saline instillation, 541*t*
Salmonella typhi, 153
Sandhoff disease, 489
Sard v. Hardy, 728
Scalp defects, 45
Scheie syndrome, 487
Schizencephaly, 220
SCID syndrome, 691, 693
Second trimester termination, 538–543
  anomalous fetus in multiple gestations, 543–545
  complications, 541*t*
    bleeding, 542
    hypertonic saline, 542
    infection, 541
    mortality, 542
    retained products of conception, 541–542
    Rh ISO-immunization, 542
    uterine perforation, 540
  dilation and extraction (D&E), 539
  extra-amniotic prostaglandins, 540–541, 541*t*
  hyperosmolar urea, 540
  hypertonic saline, 540
  instillation techniques, 539
  prostaglandins, 540, 540*t*
  subsequent pregnancies and
    ectopic pregnancy, 542
    preterm delivery/low birthweight, 542–543
    secondary infertility, 542
    spontaneous abortion, 542

Sedatives, 142*t*, 143*t*

Segmentation genes, 66

SELDI, 513–514

Seldinger technique, 460

Selective termination, 571–577. *See also* Multifetal pregnancy reduction
  abnormality risks, 571, 572*t*
  of anomalous fetus in multiple gestations, 543–545
  bipolar forceps used in, 575–576, *576*
  data analysis, 576
  determining monochorionic/dichorionic pregnancy, 543
  diagnostic evaluation of aborted fetus, 544–545
  ethics, 576–577, 717
  historical data, 574
  identification of affected fetus, 543
  intravascular consumptive coagulopathy, 544
  in monochorionic twin gestations, 575–576
  overall results, 544, 574–575
  premature labor, 543
  techniques for, 543, 571–572, 572*t*, 575*t*
    air embolization, 572–573
    cardiac tamponade, 573
    by coagulation of umbilical cord, *576*
    exsanguination, 573
    hysterotomy, 571, 573
    KCl, 543, 572, *573*
  terminology, 571

Semilobar holoprosencephaly, 212, 213

Septostomy, 461

Sequence analysis, 499

Serotonin reuptake inhibitors (SSRIs), 118

Sertraline (Zoloft), 118

Serum alpha fetoprotein (maternal), 437

Serum disease diagnosis, 515–517

Serum fingerprints, 514, *515*

Severe combined immunodeficiency (SCID), 691, 693

Sex chromosome aneuploidies, 29–30, 45

Sex-linked inheritance, 13–14

Sex selection, 710–712

Sheaths, 459–460

Sherman paradox, 38, 494, 498

Shingles (zoster), 160

Short rib polydactyly syndrome, 267–268

Shunt procedures, 605–615
  congenital cystic adenomatoid malformation (CCAM), 610–613
  idiopathic pleural effusion, 613–615
  intrauterine, 195
  lower urinary tract obstruction, 259, 605–610
  thoracoamniotic, 630
  ventriculoperitoneal, 601

Sickle cell disease, 9–10, 12*t*, 496, 497, 501, 693–694

Signal transduction pathway profiling, *518*

Single gene disorders, 9–10

Single-stranded conformation polymorphism analysis (SSCP), 499

Single-system defect, 59–60

Situs inversus, 52

Sjögren-Larsson syndrome, 449, 450

Skeletal abnormalities, 597

Skeletal development, 263

Skeletal dysplasia(s), 263–273
  achondroplasia, 266–267
  asphyxiating thoracic dystrophy, 269–270
  campomelic dysplasia, 268–269
  chondroectodermal dysplasia, 269
  classification of, 263–264
  cleidocranial dysplasia, 271
  congenital hypophosphatasia, 270–271

diastrophic dysplasia, 269
  fibrochondrogenesis, 271
  Holt-Oram syndrome, 272
  Langer mesomelic cysplasia, 271–272
  long bone measurements, 263
  obstetric management of, 589–590
  osteogenesis imperfecta, *267*
  radial aplasia-thrombocytopenia syndrome, 272
  Roberts-SC phocomelia, 272
  short rib polydactyly syndrome, 267–268
  sonographic approach to, 264
  spondylocostal dysplasia type I, 271
  spondyloepiphyseal dysplasia congenita, 270
  thanatophoric dysplasia, 264–266

Skeletal system, fetopsy of, 554

Skin abnormalities, 597. *See also* Genodermatoses

Skin biopsy (fetal), 449

Small intestine
  abnormalities, 243–245, *244*
    duodenal atresia/stenosis, *244*
    echogenic bowel, 245
    ileal atresia, 245
    jejunal atresia/stenosis, 244–245
    meconium ileus, 245
    vulvulous, 245
  double-bubble sign, *189,* 244, 245*t*
  normal, *243*

Smead-Jones combined layered suture, 573

Smith-Lemli-Opitz syndrome, 597

Smith-Magenis syndrome, 481*t*

Smoking, 665
  and maternal serum AFP levels, 280
  risk of Down syndrome and, 24–25

Somatic mosaicism, 37

Sonographic survey, 606

Southern blot analysis, 434, 497–499, 557

Spatio-temperol image correlation, 358

Spectral karyotyping (SKY), 43

Spectrometer, 513
  basic components, *514*
  low and high resolution, *515*

Sphyngolipidoses, 12*t*

Spina bifada, 15, 189, *191, 192,* 211, 641, 643
  anticonvulsant medications and, 115, 118
  ethical issues regarding fetal surgery for, 724–725

Spinal and bulbar muscular atrophy (Kennedy disease), 38–39

Spinal defects, diagnosed with 3-D ultrasound, 359

Spinal dysraphia, 211–212

Spinal malformations, 641

Spinal rachischisis, 210

Spinocerebellar ataxia Type I (SCA1), 38

Spleen, 247

Splenomegaly, 247

Splicing, 493

Splicing abnormalities, 493

Spondylocostal dysplasia Type I, 271

Spondyloepiphyseal dysplasia congenita, 270

Spontaneous abortion, 5, 6, 136, 137–138
  alcohol and, 125
  distribution of early pregnancy loss by gestational age, 138*t*
  distribution of pregnancy loss among married couples, 137*t*
  effect of cycle day on, 136*t*
  epidemiiology of, 137–139
  fetoscopy and, 459
  folic acid and, 646
  maternal occupational/environmental exposure and, 139

Robertsonian translocations and, 8
in subsequent pregnancy after D&C, 542
tetraploidy and, 5–6
triploidy and, 5
Squamous cell carcinoma, 628
SRY, 480
Staphylococcus aureus, 152
Staphylococcus epidermis, 152–153
Stem cell transfer (fetal genetic therapy), 624, 691–695
  background, 691–692
  clinical experience with, 694, 695*t*
  diseases amenable to, 693–694
    hemoglobinopathies, 693–694, 695*t*
    hemolytic disease, 695*t*
    immunodeficiency states, 693, 695*t*
    inborn errors of metabolism, 694, 695*t*
  fetus as stem cell recipient, 692–693
  receptive environment of fetus, 692–693
  risks, 693
Sterilization, of minor or incompetent patients, 735
Steroids, 144*t*, 665
Steroid sulfatase deficiency, 481*t*
Stillbirths, 349
Stomach. *See also* Gastrointestinal tract
  causes of nonvisualization of, 242*t*
  congenital duplication of, 242
Storaz 27071Z, 455–456
Storz, Karl, 459
Streptococcus pyogenes. *See* Group A beta-hemolytic
      streptococcus
Streptomycin, 98
Structure-regulation paradigm, 65–66
Subtelomeric probes, 481–482
Subtelomeric rearrangements, 48
Suction curettage, 537, 541*t*
Suicide genes, 683–684
Supravalvular aortic stenosis, 48
Supraventricular tachycardia, 585, 665
Surface-enhanced laser desorption/ionization (SELDI), 513–514
SURUSS trial, 282
Syphilis, 151

T

T-ACE questionnaire, 127
Tachyarrhythmia (fetal), 585
Tachycardia (fetal), 674–677
Talipes equinovarus, 434
Tamponade, 666
Target genes, 66
Tay Sachs disease, 12, 12*t*, 451, 489, 501, 577
  biochemical tests indicating, 485, 486
  political issues, 741
Technology, political issues and, 741
Tegeretol, 115
Terathanasia, 646
Teratology, 79–101
  alcohol as a teratogen, 124
  environmental risk parameters or modifiers, 80–82
    stage of exposure, 80
    threshold concept and exposure magnitude, 80–81
  genetic counseling and, 74–75
  mechanisms of teratogenesis, 82–83, 83*t*
  overall teratogenic risk, 79–80
  principles of, 81–82
  therapeutic agents and drugs, 83–101
Teratoma, 191, 610, 612*t*
  Doppler imaging of, 345

pharyngeal, 240
  sacrococcygeal, *194,* 235, 666
Term delivery, 139
Terminal differentiation, 63
Termination of pregnancy. *See* Abortion; Selective termination
Testicular feminization, 14*t*
Tetracycline, 98
Tetralogy of Fallot, 15*t,* 482, *660*
Tetraploidy, 5–6, 43–44
Thalassemias, 497, 501, 687, 693–694
Thalidomide, 89*t,* 98–99, 113
Thanatophoric dysplasia, 263, *264, 264–266, 265*
Thing v. LaChusa, 730
Thoracoamniotic shunts. *See* Idiopathic pleural effusion shunt therapy
Thoracocentesis, *614*
Thoracopagus, *662*
Thorax, malformations of, 211, 331–333
Three-dimensional ultrasonography, 411
Thrombocytopenia, 446
Throphoblasts, 281
Thyroid dysfunction (maternal), 444, 454
Thyroid stimulating antibody (TSiG) (maternal), 444, 454
Tissue biopsies, 449–454
  fetal liver biopsy, 449, 451
  fetal muscle biopsy, 451–453
  fetal skin biopsy, 449
  fetoscopy, 449
  ultrasound-guided biopsies, 449–451
Tissue typing (for organ or marrow donation), 712
Tocolysis, 573
Toxins. *See* Environmental and occupational exposure
Toxoplasmosis, 443, 444, 453, 454
Toxoplasmosis, fetal intracranial, 221
Tracheal obstruction, 622
Tracheal occlusion, *622*
Tracheoesophageal fistula, 241
Tracheomalacia, 622
Tranquilizers, 143*t*
Transabdominal CVS, 434. *See also* Chorionic villus
      sampling (CVS)
Transabdominal ultrasonography, 407
Transcervical CVS, 433, *434. See also* Chorionic villus
      sampling (CVS)
Transcription, 9
Transcriptional regulation, 65
Transient vesicoperitoneal fistulas, 609
Translocation(s), 7–8, 46–47, 417
  reciprocal, 7
  Robertsonian, 8
Transvaginal echocardiography, *663*
Transvaginal fetal neuroscan, 365–369
  brain structures described, 368–369
  scanning planes employed by 2D scanning, 365–368
Trans-vaginal sonography (TVS), 349
Transverse limb reduction defect, 436
TRAP. *See* Twin reversed arterial perfusion sequence (TRAP)
Treponema pallidu (syphilis), 151
Tricuspid regurgitation, 675
Tricyclic derivatives, 118
Trimethadione, 113, 118
Trinucleotide repeat expansion, 37–39
  Fragile-X syndrome, 37–38
  Huntington disease, 38
  Myotonic dystrophy, 38
  Spinal and bulbar muscular atrophy, 38–39
  Spinocerebellar ataxia Type I, 38
Trinucleotide repeats, 494

Triplets
  incidence of chromosomal abnormalities in, 572*t*
  selective termination and, 575, 576
Triplex-forming-oligonucleotide, 687
Triploid conception, 5
Triploidy, 43–44, 322–324, *323*, 642*t*
  sonographic findings, 310*t*
Trisomy, 6, 44, 45
Trisomy 13 (Patau syndrome), 19, 29, 45, *321, 322,* 597, 642*t*
  omphaloceles and, 599
  second trimester sonographic markers for, 321–32, 321–322
Trisomy15, 439
Trisomy 18 (Edwards syndrome), 19, 29, 45, 193, *194, 317–319,* 642*t*
  biochemical screening for, 282
  Doppler imaging of, 343
  omphaloceles and, 599
  second trimester sonographic markers for, 310*t*
    choroid plexus cysts, 319–321
    sonography, 317–319
Trisomy 21 (Down syndrome), 41, 44–45. *See also* Aneuploidies
  abnormal serum markers in mother, 316
  advanced maternal age and, 415
  age-specific risk, 315–316
  balanced Robertsonian translocation and, 46
  fetal loss, 21–22, *22*
  fetal pyelectasis detected, 259
  first trimester ultrasound with nuchal translucency, 289–301
    absent nasal bone, *295,* 295–296, 296*t*
    combined first trimester screening, 292–301
    detection rate, 294*t*
    multiple pregnancies, 294–295
  general risk factors
    ethnic origin, 24, *25*
    medical/personal/environmental factors, 25
    smoking, 24–25
    twins, 24
    vaginal bleeding, 25
  genetics, 19–20
  individual risk assessment, 316–317
  low levels of MSAFP and risk of, 279, 280*t*
  maternal age and, 20–21, 21*t*
  measuring fetal nuchal translucency thickness, 290–293*t*
  mosaicism and, 6–7
  multiple recurrence, 22–23, 289
  natural history of, 19
  paternal age and, 21, 28
  patient-specific risks for, 289–290, 290*t*
  polymorphisms, 23
  in previous births, 22
  recurrence of, *23*, 45
  reproductive risk factors
    assisted reproduction, 23–24
    parity, 23
  risk screening, 25–29
    ageing oocyte hypothesis, 27
    allowing for covariables, 26
    compromised microcirculation hypothesis, 28
    delayed fertilization/sperm aging hypothesis, 28
    etiological hypotheses, 26
    gestational age, 26
    mitochondrial DNA mutuation hypothesis, 28–29
    premature reproductive aging hypothesis, 27–28
    production line hypothesis, 26–27
    relaxed selection hypothesis, 27
    test interpretation, 25–26
  second semester sonographic markers for, 309–317, 310*t*
    echogenic intracardiac focus, 312–313, *313*
    extremities, 314
    fetal ear/frontal lobe/cerebellar diameter/heart rate, 314
    gender, 313
    humerus, 311–312
    hydronephrosis, 312
    hyperechoic bowel, *312*
    iliac length and angle measurements, 313–314
    likelihood ratios, 316*t*
    long bone biometry, 310–311
    major anomalies, 313
    nasal bone, 309–310, *311*
    nuchal fold, 309, *310*
    sonographic scoring index, 315*t*
  selective termination in twin pregnancy, 574, 577
Trisomy rescue, 36
Trocars, 459–460
Trophocan™ catheter, 433
Truncus arteriosus, 482
Trunk anomalies, 468
Trypsin G-band technique, 475
TT homozygosity, 646
Tuberous sclerosis, 11
Tumors, Doppler imaging of, 345–346
Tumor suppressor genes, 54
Turner syndrome (monosomy X), 6, 44, 45, 231, 310*t, 324,* 324–325, *325,* 331, 642*t*
"Twin peak" sign, 349, *351*
Twin pregnancies
  according to zygocity, chorionicity, and amnionicity, 350
  amniocentesis and, 418
  anencephalic and normal dichorionic, *573*
  conjoined twins, 351–353, *355*
  CVS and, 433, *434*
  dichorionic twins, 349, *351*
  Down syndrome risk in, 24
  first trimester ultrasound with nuchal translucency, 294–295
  monochorionic-diamniotic, 350
  monochorionic-monoamniotic, 350–351
  monochorionic twins, 349–350, *353*
  risks of abnormalities in, 571
  selective termination of (*See* Selective termination)
  twin-to-twin transfusion syndrome (TTTS), 353
Twin reversed arterial perfusion sequence (TRAP), 353–354, 465–466, 575, 576
Twin-to-twin transfusion syndrome, 349, *353,* 575
  cardiovascular function in, 674
2,8-dihydroxyadenine urolithiasis, 488

U
Ultrasonography, three-dimensional, 357–362, 411
  advantages of, 357–358
  bilateral club feet, *358*
  cleft lip and palate, *359*
  diagnosis of central nervous system abnormalities, 359
  fetal extremities, 361
  limitations of, 362
  micrognathia diagnosis, 358
  spinal defect diagnosis, 359
  urogential anomalies, *360,* 360–361
  volume measurements, 361
Ultrasound evaluation, 433
Ultrasound examination, comprehensive
  abnormal fetal biometry, 192–193
  abnormal location/contour of a normal structure, 189–190
  absence of structure normally present, 178–179
  absent or abnormal fetal motion, 193
  aggressive management of pregnancy, 195–196

cephlocentesis, 195
    diagnosis of fetal anomalies, 187–194
    dilatation behind an obstruction, 188–189
    herniation through structural defects, 189
    management of pregnancy complicated by an anomaly, 194–196
    nonaggressive management of pregnancy, 195
    presence of additional structure, 190–192
    and subsequent termination of pregnancy, 195
Ultrasound-guided biopsies, 449–451
Umbilical artery imaging, *338*, 662, *664*
Umbilical artery resistance index, 445
Umbilical cord
    Doppler imaging of, *338, 339*
    pseudocysts of, 338
Umbilical placental flow velocity waveforms, 343–345, 344*t*
Umbilical vein imaging, 663, *664*
Umbilical vein puncture, 445
Umbilical venous pressure (UVP), elevated, 444–445, 454–447
Unbalanced rearrangements, 47–48
Unbalanced translocations, 478
Unconjugated estriol (uE3), 279–280
Unilateral renal agenesis, 257
Unilocular cysts, 628
Uniparental disomy (UPD), 36, 475, 480
    confined placental mosaicism and, 439
Universal health insurance coverage, 744
Ureteral pelvic junction obstruction, 258
Ureterovesicojunction abnormalities, 258
Urinary tract
    dilatation or obstruction, 258
    infections (UTI), 151
    obstruction, *552 (See also* Obstructive uropathies)
Urine, fetal, 477
Uterine duplication or atresias, 259
Uterine vascular disruption, 437

V
VACTERL, 61
Vaginal duplication or atresias, 259
Valproic acid, 115, 118
Valvuloplasty, 667
"Vanishing twin," 433
Variable number of tandem repeats (VNTRs), 439
Variant chromosomes, 478
Varicella-zoster virus (VZV), 160–161
Vascular anastomoses, 574
Vascular dementia, 647
Vascular embolization, 575
Vascular malformations. *See* Heart and vascular malformations
Vascular systems, blood flow distribution of, 663–665
Vas defferens, congenital absence of, 501
Vasodilators, 143*t*
VATER, 61
VCFS syndrome. *See* Velocardiofacial syndrome (VCFS)
Velocardiofacial syndrome (VCFS), 42, 48, 481*t, 482*
Ventral wall defects, 587–588
Ventricular spetal defect (VSD), 15*t*

Ventriculomegaly, 215, 217–219
    neonatal outcome of, 219*t*
    neuroscan of, 374–375
    obstetric management of, 583–584
Vesicoamniotic shunt procedure, 607–610
    complications, 609–610
    fetal urine parameters, 607*t*
    follow-up, 610
    patient selection, 608
    prenatal evaluation, 606–608
    technique, 608–609
Vesicocentesis, 259, 607
Vesico-ureteric reflux, 260
"Viking helmet," 214
Viral agents, and reproductive risks, 155–164
    cytomegalovirus, 157–159
    diagnostic approach, 155–56
    enteroviruses, 162
    Epstein-Barr virus, 160
    fetal effects of intrauterine infections, 156*t*
    hepatitus C, 161
    herpes simplex virus, 159
    HIV, 162–164
    influenza, 162
    mumps, 162
    parvovirus, 161
    rubella, 156–157
    varicella-zoster virus, 160
Virally directed enzyme prodrug therapy, 683–684
Viral vectors, 684–685
Voiding cystourethrogram (VCUG), 597, 600, 601
Volume measurements, with 3-D ultrasound, 361
Von Gierke's disease, 451
Vulvulous, 245

W
Walker-Warburg syndrome, 215, 642*t*
Warfarin, 92–93, 120
Watson, James, 71
Wayne State University Teratogen Rating System, 113, 116–117*t*
Wertz, Dorothy C., 707
Wharton's jelly, 338
Williams syndrome, 48, 481*t*
Wilms's tumor, 36
Wilson disease, 637
Wolf-Hirschhorn syndrome (4p deletion syndrome), 48, 481*t*

X
X chromosome-derived markers, 482
X-linked dominant syndromes, 215
X-linked hydrocephalus, 214
X-linked inheritance, 13–14*t*, 53–54
X-linked spastic paraplegia, 214

Z
Zygocity, 349, 350*t*